ICD-10-PCS

The complete official code set

Codes valid from October 1, 2021, through September 30, 2022

2022

optum360coding.com

Notice

ICD-10-PCS: The Complete Official Code Set is designed to be an accurate and authoritative source regarding coding and every reasonable effort has been made to ensure accuracy and completeness of the content. However, Optum360 makes no guarantee, warranty, or representation that this publication is accurate, complete, or without errors. It is understood that Optum360 is not rendering any legal or other professional services or advice in this publication and that Optum360 bears no liability for any results or consequences that may arise from the use of this book. Please address all correspondence to:

Optum360
2525 Lake Park Blvd
Salt Lake City, UT 84120

Our Commitment to Accuracy

Optum360 is committed to producing accurate and reliable materials. To report corrections, please visit www.optum360coding.com/accuracy or email accuracy@optum.com. You can also reach customer service by calling 1.800.464.3649, option 1.

Copyright

Acknowledgments

Marianne Randall, CPC, *Product Manager*

Anita Schmidt, BS, RHIA, AHIMA-approved ICD-10-CM/PCS Trainer, *Subject Matter Expert*

Karen Krawzik, RHIT, CCS, AHIMA-approved ICD-10-CM/PCS Trainer, *Subject Matter Expert*

LaJuana Green, RHIA, CCS, *Subject Matter Expert*

Stacy Perry, *Manager, Desktop Publishing*

Tracy Betzler, *Senior Desktop Publishing Specialist*

Hope M. Dunn, *Senior Desktop Publishing Specialist*

Katie Russell, *Desktop Publishing Specialist*

Kate Holden, *Editor*

Anita Schmidt, BS, RHIA, AHIMA-approved ICD-10-CM/PCS Trainer

Ms. Schmidt has expertise in ICD-10-CM/PCS, DRG, and CPT with more than 15 years' experience in coding in multiple settings, including inpatient, observation, and same-day surgery. Her experience includes analysis of medical record documentation, assignment of ICD-10-CM and PCS codes, and DRG validation. She has conducted training for ICD-10-CM/PCS and electronic health record. She has also collaborated with clinical documentation specialists to identify documentation needs and potential areas for physician education. Most recently she has been developing content for resource and educational products related to ICD-10-CM, ICD-10-PCS, DRG, and CPT. Ms. Schmidt is an AHIMA-approved ICD-10-CM/PCS trainer and is an active member of the American Health Information Management Association (AHIMA) and the Minnesota Health Information Management Association (MHIMA).

Karen Krawzik, RHIT, CCS, AHIMA-approved ICD-10-CM/PCS Trainer

Ms. Krawzik has expertise in ICD-10-CM, ICD-9-CM, CPT/HCPCS, DRG, and data quality and analytics, with more than 30 years' experience coding in multiple settings, including inpatient, observation, ambulatory surgery, ancillary, and emergency room. She has served as a DRG analyst and auditor of commercial and government payer claims, as a contract administrator, and worked on a team providing enterprise-wide conversion of the ICD-9-CM code set to ICD-10. More recently, she has been developing print and electronic content related to ICD-10-CM and ICD-10-PCS coding systems, MS-DRGs, and HCCs. Ms. Krawzik is credentialed by the American Health Information Management Association (AHIMA) as a Registered Health Information Technician (RHIT) and a Certified Coding Specialist (CCS) and is an AHIMA-approved ICD-10-CM/PCS trainer. She is an active member of AHIMA and the Missouri Health Information Management Association.

Product Updates

Significant updates to this manual will also be provided on our product updates page at Optum360coding.com, which can be accessed at the following:

https://www.optum360coding.com/ProductUpdates/
Password: PCS22UPD

Contents

What's New for 2022

The Centers for Medicare and Medicaid Services is the agency charged with maintaining and updating ICD-10-PCS. CMS released the most current revisions, a summary of which may be found on the CMS website at https://www.cms.gov/medicare/icd-10/2022-icd-10-pcs.

Due to the unique structure of ICD-10-PCS, a change in a character value may affect individual codes and several code tables.

Change Summary Table

2021 Total	New Codes	Revised Titles	Deleted Codes	2022 Total
78,136	191	62	107	78,220

ICD-10-PCS Code FY 2022 Totals, By Section

Medical and Surgical	67,754
Obstetrics	304
Placement	861
Administration	1,253
Measurement and Monitoring	422
Extracorporeal or Systemic Assistance and Performance	52
Extracorporeal or Systemic Therapies	46
Osteopathic	100
Other Procedures	78
Chiropractic	90
Imaging	2,977
Nuclear Medicine	463
Radiation Therapy	2,087
Physical Rehabilitation and Diagnostic Audiology	1,380
Mental Health	30
Substance Abuse Treatment	59
New Technology	264
Total	78,220

ICD-10-PCS Table Changes Highlights

- New rows added to root operation table Extraction in the Central Nervous System and Cranial Nerves body system, capturing body part values Brain and Cerebral Hemisphere

- New qualifier Orbital Atherectomy Technique added to root operation table Extirpation in the Heart and Great Vessels body system, Percutaneous approach, for body parts Coronary Artery, One; Coronary Artery, Two; Coronary Artery, Three Arteries; and Coronary Artery, Four or More Arteries

- New row added to root operation table Fragmentation in the Heart and Great Vessels body system, capturing body parts Coronary Artery, One; Coronary Artery, Two; Coronary Artery, Three Arteries; and Coronary Artery, Four or More Arteries

- New rows added to root operation table Replacement in the Heart and Great Vessels body system, adding body part Heart, Open approach, with Devices Biologic with Synthetic Substitute, Autoregulated Electrohydraulic and Synthetic Substitute, Pneumatic, and new rows added to body part Pulmonary Valve, device Zooplastic Tissue, to capture new Device qualifiers In Existing Conduit and Native Site

- New body part value Ventricle, Left, added to root operation table Restriction in the Heart and Great Vessels body system

- Approach value Percutaneous added to body parts Brachial Artery, Left, and Brachial Artery, Right, in the root operation table Bypass in the Upper Arteries body system

- New body part value Intracranial Artery added to root operation table Fragmentation in the Upper Arteries body system

- New approach values Via Natural or Artificial Opening and Via Natural or Artificial Opening Endoscopic added to root operation table Occlusion in the Lower Veins body system, body part Lower Vein

- New body part value Bone Marrow added to root operation table Extraction in the Lymphatic and Hemic Systems body system

- New body part values Liver; Liver, Right Lobe; and Liver, Left Lobe, added to root operation table Division in the Hepatobiliary System and Pancreas body system

- New row added specific to body part Tongue, Palate, Pharynx Muscle, to root operation table Division in the Muscles body system with two new approach values, Via Natural and Artificial Opening and Via Natural and Artificial Opening Endoscopic

- New device value added to body part Skull in the root operation table Insertion in the Head and Facial Bones body system to capture Infusion Device

- New device value for Spinal Stabilization Device, Vertebral Body Tether, added to root operation table Reposition in the Upper Bones body system for body part Thoracic Vertebra and root operation table Reposition in the Lower Bones body system for body part Lumbar Vertebra

- New rows added to root operation table Excision in the Lower Bones body system, specific to body parts Metatarsal, Right, and Metatarsal, Left, adding new qualifier value Sesamoid Bone(s) 1st Toe

- New rows added specific to body parts Shoulder Joint, Right, and Shoulder Joint, Left, adding new qualifier values Humeral Surface and Glenoid Surface to root operation tables Removal and Revision in the Upper Joints body system

- New substance Pathogen Reduced Cryoprecipitated Fibrinogen Complex, with qualifier Nonautologous, added to root operation table Transfusion, Circulatory, in the Administration section

- New approach Percutaneous Endoscopic added to root operation table Irrigation, Physiological Systems and Anatomical Regions, in the Administration section, for body part Peritoneal Cavity

- New row added to root operation table Measurement, Physiological Devices, in the Measurement and Monitory section for body system Central Nervous with Function/Device value Cerebrospinal Fluid Shunt and qualifier Wireless Sensor

- New qualifier Automated added to root operation table Performance, Physiological Systems, for body system Cardiac, Duration Continuous, Function Output

- New rows added for body part Liver to root operation table Fluoroscopy, Hepatobiliary System and Pancreas, in the Imaging section

- New row added to New Technology root operation table Extirpation, Cardiovascular System New Technology Group 7, and deleted rows for New Technology Group 1

- New body part Thoracic Aorta, Arch, added to New Technology root operation table Replacement, Cardiovascular System, with device Branched Synthetic Substitute with Intraluminal Device, New Technology Group 7

- New row added to New Technology root operation table Replacement, Skin, Subcutaneous Tissue, Fascia and Breast, to capture Device/Substance/Technology Bioengineered Allogeneic Construct, New Technology Group 7

- New device value Posterior (Dynamic) Distraction Device added to New Technology root operation table Reposition, Bones, New Technology Group 7

- New device value Interbody Fusion Device, Customizable, added to New Technology root operation table Fusion, Joints, New Technology Group 7

- Multiple Device/Substance/Technology values added to New Technology root operation table Introduction, Anatomical Regions

- New Device/Substance/Technology values Hyperimmune Globulin and High-Dose Intravenous Immune Globulin added to New Technology root operation table Transfusion, Anatomical Regions

- New row added in New Technology root operation table Measurement, Physiological Systems, for body part Central Nervous, Device/Substance/Technology Computer-aided Triage and Notification, New Technology Group 7, and body part Arterial, Device/Substance/Technology Pulmonary Artery Flow, Computer-Aided Triage and Notification, and body part Nose, Device/Substance/Technology Infection, Nasopharyngeal Fluid SARS-CoV-2 Polymerase Chain Reaction

- New row added to New Technology root operation table Introduction, Extracorporeal, for body part Extracorporeal, Device/Substance/Technology Nafamostat Anticoagulant, New Technology Group 7

- Seven new tables in New Technology section:
  — X2J   Cardiovascular System, Inspection
  — X2K   Cardiovascular System, Bypass
  — X2V   Cardiovascular System, Restriction
  — XD2   Gastrointestinal System, Monitoring
  — XDP   Gastrointestinal System, Irrigation
  — XFJ   Hepatobiliary System and Pancreas, Inspection
  — XWH   Anatomical Regions, Insertion

- Two deleted tables in the New Technology Section:
  — XR2   Joints, Monitoring
  — XW2   Anatomical Regions, Transfusion

New Definitions Addenda

Section 0 — Medical and Surgical Body Part Definitions

ICD-10-PCS Value	Definition	
Cervical Spinal Cord	Add	Dorsal root ganglion
Lumbar Spinal Cord	Add	Dorsal root ganglion
Metatarsal, Left	Add	Fibular sesamoid
	Add	Tibial sesamoid
Metatarsal, Right	Add	Fibular sesamoid
	Add	Tibial sesamoid
Neck	Add	Parapharyngeal space
	Add	Retropharyngeal space
Spinal Cord	Add	Dorsal root ganglion
Thoracic Spinal Cord	Add	Dorsal root ganglion

Section 0 — Medical and Surgical Device Definitions

ICD-10-PCS Value		Definition	
Add	Biologic with Synthetic Substitute, Autoregulated Electrohydraulic for Replacement in Heart and Great Vessels	Add	Carmat total artificial heart (TAH)
Add	Other Device	Add	Alfapump® system
	Stimulator Generator, Multiple Array for Insertion in Subcutaneous Tissue and Fascia	Add	PERCEPT™ PC neurostimulator
	Stimulator Generator, Single Array for Insertion in Subcutaneous Tissue and Fascia	Delete	InterStim® Therapy neurostimulator
		Add	InterStim™ II Therapy neurostimulator
	Stimulator Generator, Single Array Rechargeable for Insertion in Subcutaneous Tissue and Fascia	Add	InterStim™ Micro Therapy neurostimulator
	Synthetic Substitute, Pneumatic for Replacement in Heart and Great Vessels	Add	SynCardia (temporary) total artificial heart (TAH)

Section 0 — Medical and Surgical Device Aggregation Table

Specific Device		for Operation		in Body System		General Device	
Add	Spinal Stabilization Device, Vertebral Body Tether	Add	Reposition	Add	Lower Bones	Add	4 Internal Fixation Device
				Add	Upper Bones		

Section 3 - Administration Substance Definitions

ICD-10-PCS Value	Definition
Add Globulin	Add Gammaglobulin Add Hyperimmune globulin Add Immunoglobulin Add Polyclonal hyperimmune globulin
Hematopoietic Stem/Progenitor Cells, Genetically Modified	Add OTL-101 Add OTL-103 Add OTL-200
Add Other Anti-infective	Add AVYCAZ® (ceftazidime-avibactam) Add Ceftazidime-avibactam Add CRESEMBA® (isavuconazonium sulfate) Add Isavuconazole (isavuconazonium sulfate)
Add Other Antineoplastic	Add Blinatumomab Add BLINCYTO® (blinatumomab)
Add Other Therapeutic Substance	Add Idarucizumab, Pradaxa®(dabigatran) reversal agent Add Praxbind® (idarucizumab), Pradaxa®(dabigatran) reversal agent
Add Pathogen Reduced Cryoprecipitated Fibrinogen Complex	Add INTERCEPT Blood System for Plasma Pathogen Reduced Cryoprecipitated Fibrinogen Complex Add INTERCEPT Fibrinogen Complex

Section X — New Technology Root Operation Definitions

ICD-10-PCS Value	Definition
Add Bypass	Add Definition: Altering the route of passage of the contents of a tubular body part.
Add Insertion	Add Definition: Putting in a nonbiological appliance that monitors, assists, performs, or prevents a physiological function but does not physically take the place of a body part.
Add Inspection	Add Definition: Visually and/or manually exploring a body part.
Add Irrigation	Add Definition: Putting in or on a cleansing substance
Add Restriction	Add Definition: Partially closing an orifice or the lumen of a tubular body part.

Section X — New Technology Device/Substance/Technology Definitions

ICD-10-PCS Value	Definition
Add Antibiotic-eluting Bone Void Filler	Add CERAMENT® G
Add Axicabtagene Ciloleucel Immunotherapy	Add Axicabtagene Ciloleucel Add Yescarta®

ICD-10-PCS Value	Definition
Add Bioengineered Allogeneic Construct	Add StrataGraft®
Add Branched Synthetic Substitute with Intraluminal Device in New Technology	Add Thoraflex™ Hybrid device
Brexucabtagene Autoleucel Immunotherapy	Add Tecartus™
Delete Engineered Autologous Chimeric Antigen Receptor T-cell Immunotherapy	Delete Axicabtagene Ciloleucel Delete KYMRIAH Delete Tisagenlecleucel
Add Bromelain-enriched Proteolytic Enzyme	Add NexoBrid™
Add Ciltacabtagene Autoleucel	Add cilta-cel
Add High-Dose Intravenous Immune Globulin	Add GAMUNEX-C, for COVID-19 treatment Add hdIVIG (high-dose intravenous immunoglobulin), for COVID-19 treatment Add High-dose intravenous immunoglobulin (hdIVIG), for COVID-19 treatment Add Octagam 10%, for COVID-19 treatment
Add Hyperimmune Globulin	Add Anti-SARS-CoV-2 hyperimmune globulin Add HIG (hyperimmune globulin), for COVID-19 treatment Add hIVIG (hyperimmune intravenous immunoglobulin), for COVID-19 treatment Add Hyperimmune intravenous immunoglobulin (hIVIG), for COVID-19 treatment Add IGIV-C, for COVID-19 treatment
Add Idecabtagene Vicleucel Immunotherapy	Add ABECMA® Add Ide-cel Add Idecabtagene Vicleucel
Add Interbody Fusion Device, Customizable in New Technology	Add aprevo™
Add Lifileucel Immunotherapy	Add Lifileucel
Add Lurbinectedin	Add ZEPZELCA™
Add Nafamostat Anticoagulant	Add LTX Regional Anticoagulant Add Niyad™
Add Posterior (Dynamic) Distraction Device in New Technology	Add ApiFix® Minimally Invasive Deformity Correction (MID-C) System
Add Reduction Device in New Technology	Add Neovasc Reducer™ Add Reducer™ System
Add REGN-COV2 Monoclonal Antibody	Add Casirivimab (REGN10933) and Imdevimab (REGN10987) Add Imdevimab (REGN10987) and Casirivimab (REGN10933)
Add Satralizumab-mwge	Add ENSPRYNG™
Add Terlipressin	Add TERLIVAZ®
Add Tisagenlecleucel Immunotherapy	Add KYMRIAH® Add Tisagenlecleucel
Add Trilaciclib	Add COSELA™

List of Updated Files

2022 Official ICD-10-PCS Coding Guidelines
- Guidelines B3.7, B4.1c, B4.8, E.1a, and E.1b revised in response to public comment and internal review
- Downloadable PDF

2022 ICD-10-PCS Code Tables and Index (Zip file)
- Code tables for use beginning October 1, 2021
- Downloadable PDF, file name is pcs_2022.pdf
- Downloadable xml files for developers, file names are icd10pcs_tables_2022.xml, icd10pcs_index_2022.xml, icd10pcs_definitions_2022.xml
- Accompanying schema for developers, file names are icd10pcs_tables.xsd, icd10pcs_index.xsd, icd10pcs_definitions.xsd

2022 ICD-10-PCS Codes File (Zip file)
- ICD-10-PCS codes file is a simple format for nontechnical uses, containing the valid FY 2022 ICD-10-PCS codes and their long titles
- File is in text file format: file name is icd10pcs_codes_2022.txt
- Accompanying documentation for codes file: file name is icd10pcsCodesFile.pdf
- Codes file addenda in text format: file name is codes_addenda_2022.txt

2022 ICD-10-PCS Order File (Long and Abbreviated Titles) (Zip file)
- ICD-10-PCS order file is for developers, provides a unique five-digit "order number" for each ICD-10-PCS table and code, as well as a long and abbreviated code title.
- ICD-10-PCS order file name is icd10pcs_order_2022.txt
- Accompanying documentation for tabular order file: file name is icd10pcsOrderFile.pdf
- Tabular order file addenda in text format: file name is order_addenda_2022.txt

2022 ICD-10-PCS Final Addenda (Zip file)
- Addenda files in downloadable PDF: file names are tables_addenda_2022.pdf, index_addenda_2022.pdf, definitions_addenda_2022.pdf
- Addenda files also in machine readable text format for developers: file names are tables_addenda_2022.txt, index_addenda_2022.txt, definitions_addenda_2022.txt

2022 ICD-10-PCS Conversion Table (Zip file)
- ICD-10-PCS code conversion table is provided to assist users in data retrieval, in downloadable Excel spreadsheet: file name is icd10pcs_conversion_table_2022.xlsx
- Conversion table also in machine readable text format for developers: file name is icd10pcs_conversion_table_2022.txt
- Accompanying documentation for code conversion table: file name is icd10pcsConversionTable.pdf

Introduction

ICD-10-PCS: The Complete Official Code Set is your definitive coding resource for procedure coding in acute inpatient hospitals. In addition to the official ICD-10-PCS Coding System Files, revised and distributed by the Centers for Medicare and Medicaid Services (CMS), Optum360's coding experts have incorporated Medicare-related coding edits and proprietary features, such as coding tools and appendixes, into a comprehensive and easy-to-use reference.

This manual provides the most current information that was available at the time of publication. For updates to official source documents that may have occurred after this manual was published, please refer to the following:

- **CMS International Classification of Disease, 10th Revision, Procedural Coding System (ICD-10-PCS):**

    https://www.cms.gov/medicare/icd-10/2022-icd-10-pcs

- **CMS Inpatient Prospective Payment System Proposed Rule, FY2022**

    https://www.cms.gov/medicare/acute-inpatient-pps/fy-2022-ipps-proposed-rule-home-page

- **CMS Inpatient Prospective Payment System Proposed Rule, FY 2022 - Proposed, version 39, MS-DRG Grouper software, Definitions Manual files and Medicare Code Editor (MCE) files**

    https://www.cms.gov/Medicare/Medicare-Fee-for-Service-Payment/AcuteInpatientPPS/MS-DRG-Classifications-and-Software

- **American Hospital Association (AHA) Coding Clinics**

    https://www.codingclinicadvisor.com/

ICD-10-PCS Code Structure

ICD-10-PCS has a seven-character alphanumeric code structure. Each character contains up to 34 possible values. Each value represents a specific option for the general character definition. The 10 digits 0–9 and the 24 letters A–H, J–N, and P–Z may be used in each character. The letters O and I are not used so as to avoid confusion with the digits 0 and 1. An ICD-10-PCS code is the result of a process rather than as a single fixed set of digits or alphabetic characters. The process consists of combining semi-independent values from among a selection of values, according to the rules governing the construction of codes.

	Section	Body System	Root Operation	Body Part	Approach	Device	Qualifier
Characters:	1	2	3	4	5	6	7

A code is derived by choosing a specific value for each of the seven characters. Based on details about the procedure performed, values for each character specifying the section, body system, root operation, body part, approach, device, and qualifier are assigned. Because the definition of each character is also a function of its physical position in the code, the same letter or number placed in a different position in the code has a different meaning.

The seven characters that make up a complete code have specific meanings that vary for each of the 17 sections of the manual.

Procedures are then divided into sections that identify the general type of procedure (e.g., Medical and Surgical, Obstetrics, Imaging). The first character of the procedure code always specifies the section. The second through seventh characters have the same meaning within each section, but may mean different things in other sections. In all sections, the third character specifies the general type of procedure performed (e.g., Resection, Transfusion, Fluoroscopy), while the other characters give additional information such as the body part and approach.

In ICD-10-PCS, the term *procedure* refers to the complete specification of the seven characters.

Number of Codes in ICD-10-PCS

The table structure of ICD-10-PCS permits the specification of a large number of codes on a single page. At the time of this publication, there are 78,220 codes in the 2022 ICD-10-PCS.

ICD-10-PCS Manual

Index

Codes may be found in the index based on the general type of procedure (e.g., resection, transfusion, fluoroscopy), or a more commonly used term (e.g., appendectomy). For example, the code for percutaneous intraluminal dilation of the coronary arteries with an intraluminal device can be found in the Index under *Dilation*, or a synonym of *Dilation* (e.g., angioplasty). The Index then specifies the first three or four values of the code or directs the user to see another term.

Example:

Dilation
    Artery
        Coronary
            One Artery 0270

Based on the first three values of the code provided in the Index, the corresponding table can be located. In the example above, the first three values indicate table 027 is to be referenced for code completion.

The tables and characters are arranged first by number and then by letter for each character (tables for 00-, 01-, 02-, etc., are followed by those for 0B-, 0C-, 0D-, etc., followed by 0B1, 0B2, etc., followed by 0BB, 0BC, 0BD, etc.).

Note: The Tables section must be used to construct a complete and valid code by specifying the last three or four values.

Tables

The tables in ICD-10-PCS provide the valid combination of character values needed to build a unique procedure code. Each table is preceded by the first three characters of the code, along with their descriptions. In the Medical and Surgical section, for example, the first three characters contain the name of the section (character 1), the body system (character 2), and the root operation performed (character 3).

Listed underneath the first three characters is a table comprising four columns and one or more rows. The four columns in the table specify the last four characters needed to complete the ICD-10-PCS code. Depending on the section, the labels for each column may be different. In the Medical and Surgical section, they are labeled body part (character 4), approach (character 5), device (character 6), and qualifier (character 7). Each row in the table specifies the valid combination of values for characters 4 through 7.

Table 1: Row from table Ø27

Ø   Medical and Surgical
2   Heart and Great Vessels
7   Dilation   Definition: Expanding an orifice or the lumen of a tubular body part

Explanation: The orifice can be a natural orifice or an artificially created orifice. Accomplished by stretching a tubular body part using intraluminal pressure or by cutting part of the orifice or wall of the tubular body part.

Body Part Character 4	Approach Character 5	Device Character 6	Qualifier Character 7
Ø Coronary Artery, One Artery 1 Coronary Artery, Two Arteries 2 Coronary Artery, Three Arteries 3 Coronary Artery, Four or More Arteries	Ø Open 3 Percutaneous 4 Percutaneous Endoscopic	4 Intraluminal Device, Drug-eluting 5 Intraluminal Device, Drug-eluting, Two 6 Intraluminal Device, Drug-eluting, Three 7 Intraluminal Device, Drug-eluting, Four or More D Intraluminal Device E Intraluminal Device, Two F Intraluminal Device, Three G Intraluminal Device, Four or More T Intraluminal Device, Radioactive Z No Device	6 Bifurcation Z No Qualifier

For instance, table 1 above shows the first row from table Ø27 in ICD-10-PCS. The values Ø27 specify the section *Medical and Surgical (Ø)*, the body system *Heart and Great Vessels (2)*, and the root operation *Dilation (7)*. As shown, the root operation (Dilation) is also accompanied by its corresponding definition and explanation. Note, a definition of the root operation is provided for every table in ICD-10-PCS; however, an explanation may not always be applicable.

In total, this single row can be used to construct 240 unique procedure codes. The valid codes shown in table 2 (below) are constructed using the body part (character 4) value of Ø, Coronary artery, one artery, combined with all valid approach (character 5) values, device (character 6) values, and a qualifier (character 7) value of Z, No Qualifier.

Table 2: Code titles for dilation of one coronary artery (Ø27Ø)

Code	Title
027004Z	Dilation of Coronary Artery, One Artery with Drug-eluting Intraluminal Device, Open Approach
027005Z	Dilation of Coronary Artery, One Artery with Two Drug-eluting Intraluminal Devices, Open Approach
027006Z	Dilation of Coronary Artery, One Artery with Three Drug-eluting Intraluminal Devices, Open Approach
027007Z	Dilation of Coronary Artery, One Artery with Four or More Drug-eluting Intraluminal Devices, Open Approach
02700DZ	Dilation of Coronary Artery, One Artery with Intraluminal Device, Open Approach
02700EZ	Dilation of Coronary Artery, One Artery with Two Intraluminal Devices, Open Approach
02700FZ	Dilation of Coronary Artery, One Artery with Three Intraluminal Devices, Open Approach
02700GZ	Dilation of Coronary Artery, One Artery with Four or More Intraluminal Devices, Open Approach
02700TZ	Dilation of Coronary Artery, One Artery with Radioactive Intraluminal Device, Open Approach
02700ZZ	Dilation of Coronary Artery, One Artery, Open Approach
027034Z	Dilation of Coronary Artery, One Artery with Drug-eluting Intraluminal Device, Percutaneous Approach
027035Z	Dilation of Coronary Artery, One Artery with Two Drug-eluting Intraluminal Devices, Percutaneous Approach
027036Z	Dilation of Coronary Artery, One Artery with Three Drug-eluting Intraluminal Devices, Percutaneous Approach
027037Z	Dilation of Coronary Artery, One Artery with Four or More Drug-eluting Intraluminal Devices, Percutaneous Approach
02703DZ	Dilation of Coronary Artery, One Artery with Intraluminal Device, Percutaneous Approach
02703EZ	Dilation of Coronary Artery, One Artery with Two Intraluminal Devices, Percutaneous Approach
02703FZ	Dilation of Coronary Artery, One Artery with Three Intraluminal Devices, Percutaneous Approach
02703GZ	Dilation of Coronary Artery, One Artery with Four or More Intraluminal Devices, Percutaneous Approach
02703TZ	Dilation of Coronary Artery, One Artery with Radioactive Intraluminal Device, Percutaneous Approach
02703ZZ	Dilation of Coronary Artery, One Artery, Percutaneous Approach
027044Z	Dilation of Coronary Artery, One Artery with Drug-eluting Intraluminal Device, Percutaneous Endoscopic Approach
027045Z	Dilation of Coronary Artery, One Artery with Two Drug-eluting Intraluminal Devices, Percutaneous Endoscopic Approach
027046Z	Dilation of Coronary Artery, One Artery with Three Drug-eluting Intraluminal Devices, Percutaneous Endoscopic Approach
027047Z	Dilation of Coronary Artery, One Artery with Four or More Drug-eluting Intraluminal Devices, Percutaneous Endoscopic Approach
02704DZ	Dilation of Coronary Artery, One Artery with Intraluminal Device, Percutaneous Endoscopic Approach
02704EZ	Dilation of Coronary Artery, One Artery with Two Intraluminal Devices, Percutaneous Endoscopic Approach
02704FZ	Dilation of Coronary Artery, One Artery with Three Intraluminal Devices, Percutaneous Endoscopic Approach
02704GZ	Dilation of Coronary Artery, One Artery with Four or More Intraluminal Devices, Percutaneous Endoscopic Approach
02704TZ	Dilation of Coronary Artery, One Artery with Radioactive Intraluminal Device, Percutaneous Endoscopic Approach
02704ZZ	Dilation of Coronary Artery, One Artery, Percutaneous Endoscopic Approach

Table 3: Rows from table ØØH

Ø **Medical and Surgical**
Ø **Central Nervous System and Cranial Nerves**
H **Insertion**   Definition: Putting in a nonbiological appliance that monitors, assists, performs, or prevents a physiological function but does not physically
                          take the place of a body part
                          Explanation: None

Body Part Character 4		Approach Character 5	Device Character 6	Qualifier Character 7
Ø Brain Cerebrum Corpus callosum Encephalon		Ø Open	1 Radioactive Element 2 Monitoring Device 3 Infusion Device 4 Radioactive Element, Cesium-131 Collagen Implant M Neurostimulator Lead Y Other Device	Z No Qualifier
Ø Brain Cerebrum Corpus callosum Encephalon		3 Percutaneous 4 Percutaneous Endoscopic	1 Radioactive Element 2 Monitoring Device 3 Infusion Device M Neurostimulator Lead Y Other Device	Z No Qualifier
6 Cerebral Ventricle Aqueduct of Sylvius Cerebral aqueduct (Sylvius) Choroid plexus Ependyma Foramen of Monro (intraventricular) Fourth ventricle Interventricular foramen (Monro) Left lateral ventricle Right lateral ventricle Third ventricle	E **Cranial Nerve** U **Spinal Canal** Epidural space, spinal Extradural space, spinal Subarachnoid space, spinal Subdural space, spinal Vertebral canal V **Spinal Cord** Dorsal root ganglion	Ø Open 3 Percutaneous 4 Percutaneous Endoscopic	1 Radioactive Element 2 Monitoring Device 3 Infusion Device M Neurostimulator Lead Y Other Device	Z No Qualifier

Table 3, is split into three rows; values of characters must all be selected from within the same row of the table. Rows 1 and 2 have the same body part (character 4) value of Ø Brain and the same qualifier value (character 7) of Z No Qualifier. However, the approach (character 5) values are not the same for these two rows, and there is one additional device (character 6) value in row 1 that is not included in row 2. As shown in row 1, body part value Brain (Ø) with device value Radioactive Element, Cesium-131 Collagen Implant (4) can only be used with approach value Open (Ø). In other words, code ØØHØ34Z would be invalid as the approach value 3 is only applicable to row 2 and the device value 4 is only applicable to row 1. It would be inappropriate to build a code for body part Ø if all of the values are not contained in its own row.

Note: In this manual, there are instances in which some tables due to length must be continued on the next page. Each section must be used separately and value selection must be made within the same row of the table.

Character Meanings

In each section, each character has a specific meaning, and this character meaning remains constant within that section. Character meaning tables have been provided at the beginning of each body system in the Medical and Surgical section (Ø) and the Obstetric section (1) to help the user identify the character members available within that section. These tables have purple headers, unlike the official code tables that have green headers and **SHOULD NOT** be used to build a PCS code. Following is an excerpt of a character meaning table.

Table 4: Rows from Central Nervous System and Cranial Nerves - Character Meanings Table

Operation–Character 3		Body Part–Character 4		Approach–Character 5		Device–Character 6		Qualifier–Character 7	
1	Bypass	Ø	Brain	Ø	Open	Ø	Drainage Device	Ø	Nasopharynx
2	Change	1	Cerebral Meninges	3	Percutaneous	1	Radioactive Element	1	Mastoid Sinus
5	Destruction	2	Dura Mater	4	Percutaneous Endoscopic	2	Monitoring Device	2	Atrium
7	Dilation	3	Epidural Space, Intracranial	X	External	3	Infusion Device	3	Blood Vessel
8	Division	4	Subdural Space, Intracranial			4	Radioactive Element, Cesium-131 Collagen Implant	4	Pleural Cavity
9	Drainage	5	Subarachnoid Space, Intracranial			7	Autologous Tissue Substitute	5	Intestine
B	Excision	6	Cerebral Ventricle			J	Synthetic Substitute	6	Peritoneal Cavity
C	Extirpation	7	Cerebral Hemisphere			K	Nonautologous Tissue Substitute	7	Urinary Tract
D	Extraction	8	Basal Ganglia			M	Neurostimulator Lead	8	Bone Marrow
F	Fragmentation	9	Thalamus			Y	Other Device	9	Fallopian Tube
H	Insertion	A	Hypothalamus			Z	No Device	A	Subgaleal space
J	Inspection	B	Pons					B	Cerebral Cisterns

Sections

Procedures are divided into sections that identify the general type of procedure (e.g., Medical and Surgical, Obstetrics, Imaging). The first character of the procedure code always specifies the section.

The sections are listed below:

Medical and Surgical section
Ø   Medical and Surgical

Medical and Surgical-related sections
1   Obstetrics
2   Placement
3   Administration
4   Measurement and Monitoring
5   Extracorporeal or Systemic Assistance and Performance
6   Extracorporeal or Systemic Therapies
7   Osteopathic
8   Other Procedures
9   Chiropractic

Ancillary Sections
B   Imaging
C   Nuclear Medicine
D   Radiation Therapy
F   Physical Rehabilitation and Diagnostic Audiology
G   Mental Health
H   Substance Abuse Treatment

New Technology Section
X   New Technology

Medical and Surgical Section (Ø)

Character Meaning

The seven characters for Medical and Surgical procedures have the following meaning:

Character	Meaning
1	Section
2	Body System
3	Root Operation
4	Body Part
5	Approach
6	Device
7	Qualifier

The Medical and Surgical section constitutes the vast majority of procedures reported in an inpatient setting. Medical and Surgical procedure codes all have a first character value of Ø. The second character indicates the general body system (e.g., Mouth and Throat, Gastrointestinal). The third character indicates the root operation, or specific objective, of the procedure (e.g., Excision). The fourth character indicates the specific body part on which the procedure was performed (e.g., Tonsils, Duodenum). The fifth character indicates the approach used to reach the procedure site (e.g., Open). The sixth character indicates whether a device was left in place during the procedure (e.g.,

Synthetic Substitute). The seventh character is qualifier, which has a specific meaning for each root operation. For example, the qualifier can be used to identify the destination site of a *Bypass*. The first through fifth characters are always assigned a specific value, but the device (sixth character) and the qualifier (seventh character) are not applicable to all procedures. The value *Z* is used for the sixth and seventh characters to indicate that a specific device or qualifier does not apply to the procedure.

Section (Character 1)

Medical and Surgical procedure codes all have a first character value of Ø.

Body Systems (Character 2)

Body systems for Medical and Surgical section codes are specified in the second character.

Body Systems
Ø   Central Nervous System and Cranial Nerves
1   Peripheral Nervous System
2   Heart and Great Vessels
3   Upper Arteries
4   Lower Arteries
5   Upper Veins
6   Lower Veins
7   Lymphatic and Hemic Systems
8   Eye
9   Ear, Nose, Sinus
B   Respiratory System
C   Mouth and Throat
D   Gastrointestinal System
F   Hepatobiliary System and Pancreas
G   Endocrine System
H   Skin and Breast
J   Subcutaneous Tissue and Fascia
K   Muscles
L   Tendons
M   Bursae and Ligaments
N   Head and Facial Bones
P   Upper Bones
Q   Lower Bones
R   Upper Joints
S   Lower Joints
T   Urinary System
U   Female Reproductive System
V   Male Reproductive System
W   Anatomical Regions, General
X   Anatomical Regions, Upper Extremities
Y   Anatomical Regions, Lower Extremities

Root Operations (Character 3)

The root operation is specified in the third character. In the Medical and Surgical section there are 31 different root operations. The root operation identifies the objective of the procedure. Each root operation has a precise definition.

- *Alteration:* Modifying the natural anatomic structure of a body part without affecting the function of the body part

- *Bypass:* Altering the route of passage of the contents of a tubular body part

- *Change:* Taking out or off a device from a body part and putting back an identical or similar device in or on the same body part without cutting or puncturing the skin or a mucous membrane

- *Control:* Stopping, or attempting to stop, postprocedural or other acute bleeding

- *Creation:* Putting in or on biological or synthetic material to form a new body part that to the extent possible replicates the anatomic structure or function of an absent body part

- *Destruction:* Physical eradication of all or a portion of a body part by the direct use of energy, force, or a destructive agent

- *Detachment:* Cutting off all or a portion of the upper or lower extremities

- *Dilation:* Expanding an orifice or the lumen of a tubular body part

- *Division:* Cutting into a body part without draining fluids and/or gases from the body part in order to separate or transect a body part

- *Drainage:* Taking or letting out fluids and/or gases from a body part

- *Excision:* Cutting out or off, without replacement, a portion of a body part

- *Extirpation:* Taking or cutting out solid matter from a body part

- *Extraction:* Pulling or stripping out or off all or a portion of a body part by the use of force

- *Fragmentation:* Breaking solid matter in a body part into pieces

- *Fusion:* Joining together portions of an articular body part rendering the articular body part immobile

- *Insertion:* Putting in a nonbiological appliance that monitors, assists, performs, or prevents a physiological function but does not physically take the place of a body part

- *Inspection:* Visually and/or manually exploring a body part

- *Map:* Locating the route of passage of electrical impulses and/or locating functional areas in a body part

- *Occlusion:* Completely closing an orifice or lumen of a tubular body part

- *Reattachment:* Putting back in or on all or a portion of a separated body part to its normal location or other suitable location

- *Release:* Freeing a body part from an abnormal physical constraint by cutting or by use of force

- *Removal:* Taking out or off a device from a body part

- *Repair:* Restoring, to the extent possible, a body part to its normal anatomic structure and function

- *Replacement:* Putting in or on biological or synthetic material that physically takes the place and/or function of all or a portion of a body part

- *Reposition:* Moving to its normal location or other suitable location all or a portion of a body part

- *Resection:* Cutting out or off, without replacement, all of a body part

- *Restriction:* Partially closing an orifice or lumen of a tubular body part

- *Revision:* Correcting, to the extent possible, a portion of a malfunctioning device or the position of a displaced device

- *Supplement:* Putting in or on biological or synthetic material that physically reinforces and/or augments the function of a portion of a body part

- *Transfer:* Moving, without taking out, all or a portion of a body part to another location to take over the function of all or a portion of a body part

- *Transplantation:* Putting in or on all or a portion of a living body part taken from another individual or animal to physically take the place and/or function of all or a portion of a similar body part

The above definitions of root operations illustrate the precision of code values defined in the system. There is a clear distinction between each root operation.

A root operation specifies the objective of the procedure. The term *anastomosis* is not a root operation, because it is a means of joining and is always an integral part of another procedure (e.g., Bypass, Resection) with a specific objective. Similarly, *incision* is not a root operation, since it is always part of the objective of another procedure (e.g., Division, Drainage). The root operation *Repair* in the Medical and Surgical section functions as a "not elsewhere classified" option. *Repair* is used when the procedure performed is not one of the other specific root operations.

Appendix B provides additional explanation and representative examples of the Medical and Surgical root operations. Appendix C groups all root operations in the Medical and Surgical section into subcategories and provides an example of each root operation.

Body Part (Character 4)
The body part is specified in the fourth character. The body part indicates the specific anatomical site of the body system on which the procedure was performed (e.g., Duodenum). Tubular body parts are defined in ICD-10-PCS as those hollow body parts that provide a route of passage for solids, liquids, or gases. They include the cardiovascular system and body parts such as those contained in the gastrointestinal tract, genitourinary tract, biliary tract, and respiratory tract.

Approach (Character 5)
The technique used to reach the site of the procedure is specified in the fifth character. There are seven different approaches:

- *Open*: Cutting through the skin or mucous membrane and any other body layers necessary to expose the site of the procedure

- *Percutaneous*: Entry, by puncture or minor incision, of instrumentation through the skin or mucous membrane and any other body layers necessary to reach the site of the procedure

- *Percutaneous Endoscopic*: Entry, by puncture or minor incision, of instrumentation through the skin or mucous membrane and any other body layers necessary to reach and visualize the site of the procedure

- *Via Natural or Artificial Opening*: Entry of instrumentation through a natural or artificial external opening to reach the site of the procedure

- *Via Natural or Artificial Opening Endoscopic*: Entry of instrumentation through a natural or artificial external opening to reach and visualize the site of the procedure

- *Via Natural or Artificial Opening with Percutaneous Endoscopic Assistance:* Entry of instrumentation through a natural or artificial external opening and entry, by puncture or minor incision, of instrumentation through the skin or mucous membrane and any other body layers necessary to aid in the performance of the procedure

- *External*: Procedures performed directly on the skin or mucous membrane and procedures performed indirectly by the application of external force through the skin or mucous membrane

The approach comprises three components: the access location, method, and type of instrumentation.

Access location: For procedures performed on an internal body part, the access location specifies the external site through which the site of the procedure is reached. There are two general types of access locations: skin or mucous membranes, and external orifices. Every approach value except external includes one of these two access locations. The skin or mucous membrane can be cut or punctured to reach the procedure site. All open and percutaneous approach values use this access location. The site of a procedure can also be reached through an external opening. External openings can be natural (e.g., mouth) or artificial (e.g., colostomy stoma).

Method: For procedures performed on an internal body part, the method specifies how the external access location is entered. An open method specifies cutting through the skin or mucous membrane and any other intervening body layers necessary to expose the site of the procedure. An instrumentation method specifies the entry of instrumentation through the access location to the internal procedure site. Instrumentation can be introduced by puncture or minor incision, or through an external opening. The puncture or minor incision does not constitute an open approach because it does not expose the site of the procedure. An approach can define multiple methods. For example, *Via Natural or Artificial Opening with Percutaneous Endoscopic Assistance* includes both the initial entry of instrumentation to reach the site of the procedure, and the placement of additional percutaneous instrumentation into the body part to visualize and assist in the performance of the procedure.

Type of instrumentation: For procedures performed on an internal body part, instrumentation means that specialized equipment is used to perform the procedure. Instrumentation is used in all internal approaches other than the basic open approach. Instrumentation may or may not include the capacity to visualize the procedure site. For example, the instrumentation used to perform a sigmoidoscopy permits the internal site of the procedure to be visualized, while the instrumentation used to perform a needle biopsy of the liver does not. The term "endoscopic" as used in approach values refers to instrumentation that permits a site to be visualized.

Procedures performed directly on the skin or mucous membrane are identified by the external approach (e.g., skin excision). Procedures performed indirectly by the application of external force are also identified by the external approach (e.g., closed reduction of fracture).

Appendix A compares the components (access location, method, and type of instrumentation) of each approach and provides an example and illustration of each approach.

Device (Character 6)

The device is specified in the sixth character. There are four general types of devices:

- Biological or synthetic material that takes the place of all or a portion of a body part (e.g, skin graft, joint prosthesis).

- Biological or synthetic material that assists or prevents a physiological function (e.g., IUD).

- Therapeutic material that is not absorbed by, eliminated by, or incorporated into a body part (e.g., radioactive implant).

- Mechanical or electronic appliances used to assist, monitor, take the place of or prevent a physiological function (e.g., cardiac pacemaker, orthopedic pin).

Appendix F compares the general device types and provides examples of each.

While all devices can be removed, some cannot be removed without putting in another nonbiological appliance or body-part substitute.

When a specific device value is used to identify the device for a root operation, such as *Insertion* and that same device value is not an option for a more broad range root operation such as *Removal*, select the general device value. For example, in the body system Heart and Great Vessels, the specific device character for Cardiac Lead, Pacemaker in root operation *Insertion* is J. For the root operation *Removal*, the general device character M Cardiac Lead would be selected for the pacemaker lead.

ICD-10-PCS contains a PCS Device Aggregation Table (see appendix G) that crosswalks the *specific* device character values that have been created for specific root operations and specific body part character values to the *general* device character value that would be used for root operations that represent a broad range of procedures and general body part character values, such as Removal and Revision.

Instruments used to visualize the procedure site are specified in the approach, not the device, value.

If the objective of the procedure is to put in the device, then the root operation is *Insertion*. If the device is put in to meet an objective other than *Insertion*, then the root operation defining the underlying objective of the procedure is used, with the device specified in the device character. For example, if a procedure to replace the hip joint is performed, the root operation *Replacement* is coded, and the prosthetic device is specified in the device character. Materials that are incidental to a procedure such as clips, ligatures, and sutures are not specified in the device character. Because new devices can be developed, the value *Other Device* is provided as a temporary option for use until a specific device value is added to the system.

Qualifier (Character 7)

The qualifier is specified in the seventh character. The qualifier contains unique values for individual procedures. For example, the qualifier can be used to identify the destination site in a *Bypass*.

Medical and Surgical Section Principles

In developing the Medical and Surgical procedure codes, several specific principles were followed.

Composite Terms Are Not Root Operations

Composite terms such as colonoscopy, sigmoidectomy, or appendectomy do not describe root operations, but they do specify multiple components of a specific root operation. In ICD-10-PCS, the components of a procedure are defined separately by the characters making up the complete code. The only component of a procedure specified in the root operation is the objective of the procedure. With each complete code the underlying objective of the procedure is specified by the root operation (third character), the precise part is specified by the body part (fourth character), and the method used to reach and visualize the procedure site is specified by the approach (fifth character). While colonoscopy, sigmoidectomy, and appendectomy are included in the Index, they do not constitute root operations in the Tables section. The objective of colonoscopy is the visualization of the colon and the root operation (character 3) is *Inspection*. Character 4 specifies the body part, which in this case is part of the colon. These composite terms, like colonoscopy or appendectomy, are included as cross-reference only. The index provides the correct root operation reference. Examples of other types of composite terms not representative of root operations are *partial* sigmoidectomy, *total* hysterectomy, and *partial* hip replacement. Always refer to the correct root operation in the Index and Tables section.

Root Operation Based on Objective of Procedure

The root operation is based on the objective of the procedure, such as *Resection* of transverse colon or *Dilation* of an artery. The assignment of the root operation is based on the procedure actually performed, which may or may not have been the intended procedure. If the intended procedure is modified or discontinued (e.g., excision instead of resection is performed), the root operation is determined by the procedure actually performed. If the desired result is not attained after completing the procedure (i.e., the artery does not remain expanded after the dilation procedure), the root operation is still determined by the procedure actually performed.

Examples:

- Dilating the urethra is coded as *Dilation* since the objective of the procedure is to dilate the urethra. If dilation of the urethra includes putting in an intraluminal stent, the root operation remains *Dilation* and not *Insertion* of the intraluminal device because the underlying objective of the procedure is dilation of the urethra. The stent is identified by the intraluminal device value in the sixth character of the dilation procedure code.

- If the objective is solely to put a radioactive element in the urethra, then the procedure is coded to the root operation *Insertion*, with the radioactive element identified in the sixth character of the code.

- If the objective of the procedure is to correct a malfunctioning or displaced device, then the procedure is coded to the root operation *Revision*. In the root operation *Revision*, the original device being revised is identified in the device character. *Revision* is typically performed on mechanical appliances (e.g., pacemaker) or materials used in replacement procedures (e.g., synthetic substitute). Typical revision procedures include adjustment of pacemaker position and correction of malfunctioning knee prosthesis.

Combination Procedures Are Coded Separately

If multiple procedures as defined by distinct objectives are performed during an operative episode, then multiple codes are used. For example, obtaining the vein graft used for coronary bypass surgery is coded as a separate procedure from the bypass itself.

Redo of Procedures

The complete or partial redo of the original procedure is coded to the root operation that identifies the procedure performed rather than *Revision*.

Example:

A complete redo of a hip replacement procedure that requires putting in a new prosthesis is coded to the root operation *Replacement* rather than *Revision*.

The correction of complications arising from the original procedure, other than device complications, is coded to the procedure performed. Correction of a malfunctioning or displaced device would be coded to the root operation *Revision*.

Example:

A procedure to control hemorrhage arising from the original procedure is coded to *Control* rather than *Revision*.

Examples of Procedures Coded in the Medical Surgical Section

The following are examples of procedures from the Medical and Surgical section, coded in ICD-10-PCS.

- Suture of skin laceration, left lower arm: 0HQEXZZ

  Medical and Surgical section (0), body system *Skin and Breast* (H), root operation *Repair* (Q), body part *Skin, Left Lower Arm* (E), *External* Approach (X) *No device* (Z), and *No qualifier* (Z).

- Laparoscopic appendectomy: 0DTJ4ZZ

  Medical and Surgical section (0), body system *Gastrointestinal* (D), root operation *Resection* (T), body part *Appendix* (J), *Percutaneous Endoscopic* approach (4), No Device (Z), and No qualifier (Z).

- Sigmoidoscopy with biopsy: 0DBN8ZX

  Medical and Surgical section (0), body system *Gastrointestinal* (D), root operation *Excision* (B), body part *Sigmoid Colon* (N), *Via Natural or Artificial Opening Endoscopic* approach (8), *No Device* (Z), and with qualifier *Diagnostic* (X).

- Tracheostomy with tracheostomy tube: 0B110F4

  Medical and Surgical section (0), body system *Respiratory* (B), root operation *Bypass* (1), body part *Trachea* (1), *Open* approach (0), with *Tracheostomy Device* (F), and qualifier *Cutaneous* (4).

Obstetrics Section (1)

Character Meanings

The seven characters in the Obstetrics section have the same meaning as in the Medical and Surgical section.

Character	Meaning
1	Section
2	Body System
3	Root Operation
4	Body Part
5	Approach
6	Device
7	Qualifier

The Obstetrics section includes procedures performed on the products of conception only. Procedures on the pregnant female are coded in the Medical and Surgical section (e.g., episiotomy). The term "products of conception" refers to all physical components of a pregnancy, including the fetus, amnion, umbilical cord, and placenta. There is no differentiation of the products of conception based on gestational age.

Thus, the specification of the products of conception as a zygote, embryo or fetus, or the trimester of the pregnancy is not part of the procedure code but can be found in the diagnosis code.

Section (Character 1)
Obstetrics procedure codes have a first character value of *1*.

Body System (Character 2)
The second character value for body system is *Pregnancy*.

Root Operation (Character 3)
The root operations *Change, Drainage, Extraction, Insertion, Inspection, Removal, Repair, Reposition, Resection,* and *Transplantation* are used in the obstetrics section and have the same meaning as in the Medical and Surgical section.

The Obstetrics section also includes two additional root operations, *Abortion* and *Delivery*, defined below:

- *Abortion*: Artificially terminating a pregnancy
- *Delivery*: Assisting the passage of the products of conception from the genital canal

A cesarean section is not a separate root operation because the underlying objective is *Extraction* (i.e., pulling out all or a portion of a body part).

Body Part (Character 4)
The body part values in the obstetrics section are:

- *Products of conception*
- *Products of conception, retained*
- *Products of conception, ectopic*

Approach (Character 5)
The fifth character specifies approaches as defined in the Medical and Surgical section.

Device (Character 6)
The sixth character is used for devices such as fetal monitoring electrodes.

Qualifier (Character 7)
Qualifier values are specific to the root operation and are used to capture details of the procedure, such as whether forceps or a vacuum were used during an Extraction, the type of fluid taken out during a Drainage procedure, or the products of conception body system that was repaired.

Placement Section (2)

Character Meanings
The seven characters in the Placement section have the following meaning:

Character	Meaning
1	Section
2	Body System
3	Root Operation
4	Body Region
5	Approach
6	Device
7	Qualifier

Placement section codes represent procedures for putting a device in or on a body region for the purpose of protection, immobilization, stretching, compression, or packing.

Section (Character 1)
Placement procedure codes have a first character value of *2*.

Body System (Character 2)
The second character contains two values specifying either *Anatomical Regions* or *Anatomical Orifices*.

Root Operation (Character 3)
The root operations in the Placement section include only those procedures that are performed without making an incision or a puncture. The root operations *Change* and *Removal* are in the Placement section and have the same meaning as in the Medical and Surgical section.

The Placement section also includes five additional root operations, defined as follows:

- *Compression*: Putting pressure on a body region
- *Dressing*: Putting material on a body region for protection
- *Immobilization*: Limiting or preventing motion of an external body region
- *Packing*: Putting material in a body region or orifice
- *Traction*: Exerting a pulling force on a body region in a distal direction

Body Region (Character 4)
The fourth character values are either body regions (e.g., *Upper Leg*) or natural orifices (e.g., *Ear*).

Approach (Character 5)
Since all placement procedures are performed directly on the skin or mucous membrane, or performed indirectly by applying external force through the skin or mucous membrane, the approach value is always *External*.

Device (Character 6)
The device character is always specified (except in the case of manual traction) and indicates the device placed during the procedure (e.g., cast, splint, bandage, etc.). Except for casts for fractures and dislocations, devices in the Placement section are off the shelf and do not require any extensive design, fabrication, or fitting. Placement of devices that require extensive design, fabrication, or fitting are coded in the Rehabilitation section.

Qualifier (Character 7)

The qualifier character is not specified in the Placement section; the qualifier value is always *No Qualifier*.

Administration Section (3)

Character Meanings

The seven characters in the Administration section have the following meaning:

Character	Meaning
1	Section
2	Body System
3	Root Operation
4	Body System/Region
5	Approach
6	Substance
7	Qualifier

Administration section codes represent procedures for putting in or on a therapeutic, prophylactic, protective, diagnostic, nutritional, or physiological substance. The section includes transfusions, infusions, and injections, along with other similar services such as irrigation and tattooing.

Section (Character 1)

Administration procedure codes have a first character value of *3*.

Body System (Character 2)

The body system character contains only three values: *Indwelling Device, Physiological Systems and Anatomical Regions,* or *Circulatory System*. The *Circulatory System* is used for transfusion procedures.

Root Operation (Character 3)

There are three root operations in the Administration section.

- *Introduction*: Putting in or on a therapeutic, diagnostic, nutritional, physiological, or prophylactic substance except blood or blood products

- *Irrigation*: Putting in or on a cleansing substance

- *Transfusion*: Putting in blood or blood products

Body/System Region (Character 4)

The fourth character specifies the body system/region. The fourth character identifies the site where the substance is administered, not the site where the substance administered takes effect. Sites include *Skin and Mucous Membranes, Subcutaneous Tissue,* and *Muscle*. These differentiate intradermal, subcutaneous, and intramuscular injections, respectively. Other sites include *Eye, Respiratory Tract, Peritoneal Cavity,* and *Epidural Space*.

The body systems/regions for arteries and veins are *Peripheral Artery, Central Artery, Peripheral Vein,* and *Central Vein*. The *Peripheral Artery* or *Vein* is typically used when a substance is introduced locally into an artery or vein. For example, chemotherapy is the introduction of an antineoplastic substance into a peripheral artery or vein by a percutaneous approach. In general, the substance introduced into a peripheral artery or vein has a systemic effect.

The *Central Artery* or *Vein* is typically used when the site where the substance is introduced is distant from the point of entry into the artery or vein. For example, the introduction of a substance directly at the site of a clot within an artery or vein using a catheter is coded as an introduction of a thrombolytic substance into a central artery or vein by a percutaneous approach. In general, the substance introduced into a central artery or vein has a local effect.

Approach (Character 5)

The fifth character specifies approaches as defined in the Medical and Surgical section. The approach for intradermal, subcutaneous, and intramuscular introductions (i.e., injections) is *Percutaneous*. If a catheter is placed to introduce a substance into an internal site within the circulatory system, then the approach is also *Percutaneous*. For example, if a catheter is used to introduce contrast directly into the heart for angiography, then the procedure would be coded as a percutaneous introduction of contrast into the heart.

Substance (Character 6)

The sixth character specifies the substance being introduced. Broad categories of substances are defined, such as anesthetic, contrast, dialysate, and blood products such as platelets.

Qualifier (Character 7)

The seventh character is a qualifier and is used to indicate whether the transfused substance is *Autologous, Nonautologous, or Allogeneic* (related, unrelated, unspecified), or to further specify the substance.

Measurement and Monitoring Section (4)

Character Meanings

The seven characters in the Measurement and Monitoring section have the following meaning:

Character	Meaning
1	Section
2	Body System
3	Root Operation
4	Body System
5	Approach
6	Function/Device
7	Qualifier

Measurement and Monitoring section codes represent procedures for determining the level of a physiological or physical function.

Section (Character 1)

Measurement and Monitoring procedure codes have a first character value of *4*.

Body System (Character 2)

The second character values for body system are A, *Physiological Systems* or B, *Physiological Devices*.

Root Operation (Character 3)

There are two root operations in the Measurement and Monitoring section, as defined below:

- *Measurement*: Determining the level of a physiological or physical function at a point in time

- *Monitoring*: Determining the level of a physiological or physical function repetitively over a period of time

Body System (Character 4)

The fourth character specifies the specific body system measured or monitored.

Approach (Character 5)

The fifth character specifies approaches as defined in the Medical and Surgical section.

Function/Device (Character 6)

The sixth character specifies the physiological or physical function being measured or monitored. Examples of physiological or physical functions are *Conductivity, Metabolism, Pulse, Temperature,* and *Volume.* If a device used to perform the measurement or monitoring is inserted and left in, then insertion of the device is coded as a separate Medical and Surgical procedure.

Qualifier (Character 7)

The seventh character qualifier contains specific values as needed to further specify the body part (e.g., central, portal, pulmonary) or a variation of the procedure performed (e.g., ambulatory, stress). Examples of typical procedures coded in this section are EKG, EEG, and cardiac catheterization. An EKG is the measurement of cardiac electrical activity, while an EEG is the measurement of electrical activity of the central nervous system. A cardiac catheterization performed to measure the pressure in the heart is coded as the measurement of cardiac pressure by percutaneous approach.

Extracorporeal or Systemic Assistance and Performance Section (5)

Character Meanings

The seven characters in the Extracorporeal or Systemic Assistance and Performance section have the following meaning:

Character	Meaning
1	Section
2	Body System
3	Root Operation
4	Body System
5	Duration
6	Function
7	Qualifier

In Extracorporeal or Systemic Assistance and Performance procedures, equipment outside the body is used to assist or perform a physiological function. The section includes procedures performed in a critical care setting, such as mechanical ventilation and cardioversion; it also includes other services such as hyperbaric oxygen treatment and hemodialysis.

Section (Character 1)

Extracorporeal or Systemic Assistance and Performance procedure codes have a first character value of *5.*

Body System (Character 2)

The second character value for body system is A, *Physiological Systems.*

Root Operation (Character 3)

There are three root operations in the Extracorporeal or Systemic Assistance and Performance section, as defined below.

- *Assistance:* Taking over a portion of a physiological function by extracorporeal means

- *Performance:* Completely taking over a physiological function by extracorporeal means

- *Restoration:* Returning, or attempting to return, a physiological function to its natural state by extracorporeal means

The root operation *Restoration* contains a single procedure code that identifies extracorporeal cardioversion.

Body System (Character 4)

The fourth character specifies the body system (e.g., cardiac, respiratory) to which extracorporeal or systemic assistance or performance is applied.

Duration (Character 5)

The fifth character specifies the duration of the procedure.

Function (Character 6)

The sixth character specifies the physiological function assisted or performed (e.g., oxygenation, ventilation) during the procedure.

Qualifier (Character 7)

The seventh character qualifier specifies the type of equipment used, if any.

Extracorporeal or Systemic Therapies Section (6)

Character Meanings

The seven characters in the Extracorporeal or Systemic Therapies section have the following meaning:

Character	Meaning
1	Section
2	Body System
3	Root Operation
4	Body System
5	Duration
6	Qualifier
7	Qualifier

In extracorporeal or systemic therapy, equipment outside the body is used for a therapeutic purpose that does not involve the assistance or performance of a physiological function.

Section (Character 1)

Extracorporeal or Systemic Therapy procedure codes have a first character value of 6.

Body System (Character 2)

The second character value for body system is *Physiological Systems.*

Root Operation (Character 3)

There are 11 root operations in the Extracorporeal or Systemic Therapy section, as defined below.

- *Atmospheric Control*: Extracorporeal control of atmospheric pressure and composition

- *Decompression*: Extracorporeal elimination of undissolved gas from body fluids

  Coding note: The root operation *Decompression* involves only one type of procedure: treatment for decompression sickness (the bends) in a hyperbaric chamber.

- *Electromagnetic Therapy*: Extracorporeal treatment by electromagnetic rays

- *Hyperthermia*: Extracorporeal raising of body temperature

  Coding note: The term hyperthermia is used to describe both a temperature imbalance treatment and also as an adjunct radiation treatment for cancer. When treating the temperature imbalance, it is coded to this section; for the cancer treatment, it is coded in section *D Radiation Therapy*.

- *Hypothermia*: Extracorporeal lowering of body temperature

- *Perfusion*: Extracorporeal treatment by diffusion of therapeutic fluid

- *Pheresis*: Extracorporeal separation of blood products

  Coding note: Pheresis may be used for two main purposes: to treat diseases when too much of a blood component is produced (e.g., leukemia) and to remove a blood product such as platelets from a donor, for transfusion into another patient.

- *Phototherapy*: Extracorporeal treatment by light rays

  Coding note: Phototherapy involves using a machine that exposes the blood to light rays outside the body, recirculates it, and then returns it to the body.

- *Shock Wave Therapy*: Extracorporeal treatment by shock waves

- *Ultrasound Therapy*: Extracorporeal treatment by ultrasound

- *Ultraviolet Light Therapy*: Extracorporeal treatment by ultraviolet light

Body System (Character 4)

The fourth character specifies the body system on which the extracorporeal or systemic therapy is performed (e.g., skin, circulatory).

Duration (Character 5)

The fifth character specifies whether the procedure was performed once (single) or multiple times.

Qualifier (Character 6)

The sixth character for Extracorporeal or Systemic Therapies is *No Qualifier*, except for root operation Perfusion which has a sixth character qualifier of *Donor Organ*.

Qualifier (Character 7)

The seventh character qualifier is used in the root operation *Pheresis* to specify the blood component on which pheresis is performed and in the root operation *Ultrasound Therapy* to specify site of treatment.

Osteopathic Section (7)

Character Meanings

The seven characters in the Osteopathic section have the following meaning:

Character	Meaning
1	Section
2	Body System
3	Root Operation
4	Body Region
5	Approach
6	Method
7	Qualifier

Section (Character 1)

Osteopathic procedure codes have a first character value of *7*.

Body System (Character 2)

The body system character contains the value *Anatomical Regions*.

Root Operation (Character 3)

There is only one root operation in the Osteopathic section.

- *Treatment*: Manual treatment to eliminate or alleviate somatic dysfunction and related disorders

Body Region (Character 4)

The fourth character specifies the body region on which the osteopathic treatment is performed.

Approach (Character 5)

The approach for osteopathic treatment is always *External*.

Method (Character 6)

The sixth character specifies the method by which the treatment is accomplished.

Qualifier (Character 7)

The seventh character is not specified in the Osteopathic section and always has the value *None*.

Other Procedures Section (8)

Character Meanings

The seven characters in the Other Procedures section have the following meaning:

Character	Meaning
1	Section
2	Body System
3	Root Operation
4	Body Region
5	Approach
6	Method
7	Qualifier

The Other Procedures section includes acupuncture, suture removal, and in vitro fertilization.

Section (Character 1)
Other Procedure section codes have a first character value of *8*.

Body System (Character 2)
The second character values for body systems are *Physiological Systems and Anatomical Regions* and *Indwelling Device*.

Root Operation (Character 3)
The Other Procedures section has only one root operation, defined as follows:

- *Other Procedures*: Methodologies that attempt to remediate or cure a disorder or disease.

Body Region (Character 4)
The fourth character contains specified body-region values, and also the body-region value *None*.

Approach (Character 5)
The fifth character specifies approaches as defined in the Medical and Surgical section.

Method (Character 6)
The sixth character specifies the method (e.g., *Acupuncture, Therapeutic Massage*).

Qualifier (Character 7)
The seventh character is a qualifier and contains specific values as needed.

Chiropractic Section (9)

Character Meanings
The seven characters in the Chiropractic section have the following meaning:

Character	Meaning
1	Section
2	Body System
3	Root Operation
4	Body Region
5	Approach
6	Method
7	Qualifier

Section (Character 1)
Chiropractic section procedure codes have a first character value of *9*.

Body System (Character 2)
The second character value for body system is *Anatomical Regions*.

Root Operation (Character 3)
There is only one root operation in the *Chiropractic* section.

- *Manipulation:* Manual procedure that involves a directed thrust to move a joint past the physiological range of motion, without exceeding the anatomical limit.

Body Region (Character 4)
The fourth character specifies the body region on which the chiropractic manipulation is performed.

Approach (Character 5)
The approach for chiropractic manipulation is always *External*.

Method (Character 6)
The sixth character is the method by which the manipulation is accomplished.

Qualifier (Character 7)
The seventh character is not specified in the Chiropractic section and always has the value *None*.

Imaging Section (B)

Character Meanings
The seven characters in Imaging procedures have the following meaning:

Character	Meaning
1	Section
2	Body System
3	Type
4	Body Part
5	Contrast
6	Qualifier
7	Qualifier

Imaging procedures include plain radiography, fluoroscopy, CT, MRI, and ultrasound. Nuclear medicine procedures, including PET, uptakes, and scans, are in the nuclear medicine section. Therapeutic radiation procedure codes are in a separate radiation therapy section.

Section (Character 1)
Imaging procedure codes have a first character value of *B*.

Body System (Character 2)
In the Imaging section, the second character defines the body system, such as *Heart* or *Gastrointestinal System*.

Type (Character 3)
The third character defines the type of imaging procedure (e.g., MRI, ultrasound). The following list includes all types in the *Imaging* section with a definition of each type:

- *Computerized Tomography (CT Scan)*: Computer reformatted digital display of multiplanar images developed from the capture of multiple exposures of external ionizing radiation

- *Fluoroscopy*: Single plane or bi-plane real time display of an image developed from the capture of external ionizing radiation on a fluorescent screen. The image may also be stored by either digital or analog means

- *Magnetic Resonance Imaging (MRI)*: Computer reformatted digital display of multiplanar images developed from the capture of radiofrequency signals emitted by nuclei in a body site excited within a magnetic field

- *Other Imaging*: Other specified modality for visualizing a body part

- *Plain Radiography*: Planar display of an image developed from the capture of external ionizing radiation on photographic or photoconductive plate
- *Ultrasonography*: Real time display of images of anatomy or flow information developed from the capture of reflected and attenuated high frequency sound waves

Body Part (Character 4)
The fourth character defines the body part with different values for each body system (character 2) value.

Contrast (Character 5)
The fifth character specifies whether the contrast material used in the imaging procedure is *High Osmolar, Low Osmolar*, or *Other Contrast* when applicable.

Qualifier (Character 6)
The sixth character qualifier provides further detail regarding the nature of the substance or technologies used, such as *Unenhanced and Enhanced (contrast), Laser, or Intravascular Optical Coherence.*

Qualifier (Character 7)
The seventh character is a qualifier that may be used to specify certain procedural circumstances, the method by which the procedure was performed, or technologies utilized, such as *Intraoperative, Intravascular, or Transesophageal.*

Nuclear Medicine Section (C)

Character Meanings
The seven characters in the Nuclear Medicine section have the following meaning:

Character	Meaning
1	Section
2	Body System
3	Type
4	Body Part
5	Radionuclide
6	Qualifier
7	Qualifier

Nuclear Medicine is the introduction of radioactive material into the body to create an image, to diagnose and treat pathologic conditions, or to assess metabolic functions. The Nuclear Medicine section does not include the introduction of encapsulated radioactive material for the treatment of cancer. These procedures are included in the Radiation Therapy section.

Section (Character 1)
Nuclear Medicine procedure codes have a first character value of *C*.

Body System (Character 2)
The second character specifies the body system on which the nuclear medicine procedure is performed.

Type (Character 3)
The third character indicates the type of nuclear medicine procedure (e.g., planar imaging or nonimaging uptake). The following list includes the types of nuclear medicine procedures with a definition of each type.

- *Nonimaging Nuclear Medicine Assay:* Introduction of radioactive materials into the body for the study of body fluids and blood elements, by the detection of radioactive emissions
- *Nonimaging Nuclear Medicine Probe:* Introduction of radioactive materials into the body for the study of distribution and fate of certain substances by the detection of radioactive emissions; or alternatively, measurement of absorption of radioactive emissions from an external source
- *Nonimaging Nuclear Medicine Uptake:* Introduction of radioactive materials into the body for measurements of organ function, from the detection of radioactive emissions
- *Planar Nuclear Medicine Imaging*: Introduction of radioactive materials into the body for single-plane display of images developed from the capture of radioactive emissions
- *Positron Emission Tomography (PET) Imaging:* Introduction of radioactive materials into the body for three dimensional display of images developed from the simultaneous capture, 180 degrees apart, of radioactive emissions
- *Systemic Nuclear Medicine Therapy:* Introduction of unsealed radioactive materials into the body for treatment
- *Tomographic (Tomo) Nuclear Medicine Imaging*: Introduction of radioactive materials into the body for three dimensional display of images developed from the capture of radioactive emissions

Body Part (Character 4)
The fourth character indicates the body part or body region studied; with regional (e.g., *lower extremity veins*) and combination (e.g., *liver and spleen*) body parts commonly used.

Radionuclide (Character 5)
The fifth character specifies the radionuclide, the radiation source. The option *Other Radionuclide* is provided in the nuclear medicine section for newly approved radionuclides until they can be added to the coding system. If more than one radiopharmaceutical is given to perform the procedure, then more than one code is used.

Qualifier (Character 6 and 7)
The sixth and seventh characters are qualifiers but are not specified in the *Nuclear Medicine* section; the value is always *None*.

Radiation Therapy Section (D)

Character Meanings
The seven characters in the Radiation Therapy section have the following meaning:

Character	Meaning
1	Section
2	Body System
3	Modality
4	Treatment Site
5	Modality Qualifier
6	Isotope
7	Qualifier

Section (Character 1)

Radiation therapy procedure codes have a first character value of *D*.

Body System (Character 2)

The second character specifies the body system (e.g., central nervous system, musculoskeletal) irradiated.

Modality (Character 3)

The third character specifies the general modality used (e.g., beam radiation).

Treatment Site (Character 4)

The fourth character specifies the body part that is the focus of the radiation therapy.

Modality Qualifier (Character 5)

The fifth character further specifies the radiation modality used (e.g., photons, electrons).

Isotope (Character 6)

The sixth character specifies the isotopes introduced into the body, if applicable.

Qualifier (Character 7)

The seventh character may specify whether the procedure was performed intraoperatively.

Physical Rehabilitation and Diagnostic Audiology Section (F)

Character Meanings

The seven characters in the Physical Rehabilitation and Diagnostic Audiology section have the following meaning:

Character	Meaning
1	Section
2	Section Qualifier
3	Type
4	Body System/Region
5	Type Qualifier
6	Equipment
7	Qualifier

Physical rehabilitation procedures include physical therapy, occupational therapy, and speech-language pathology. Osteopathic procedures and chiropractic procedures are in separate sections.

Section (Character 1)

Physical Rehabilitation and Diagnostic Audiology procedure codes have a first character value of *F*.

Section Qualifier (Character 2)

The section qualifier *Rehabilitation* or *Diagnostic Audiology* is specified in the second character.

Type (Character 3)

The third character specifies the type. There are 14 different values, which can be classified into four basic types of rehabilitation and diagnostic audiology procedures, defined as follows:

Assessment: Includes a determination of the patient's diagnosis when appropriate, need for treatment, planning for treatment, periodic assessment, and documentation related to these activities

Assessments are further classified into more than 100 different tests or methods. The majority of these focus on the faculties of hearing and speech, but others focus on various aspects of body function, and on the patient's quality of life, such as muscle performance, neuromotor development, and reintegration skills.

- *Speech Assessment*: Measurement of speech and related functions

- *Motor and/or Nerve Function Assessment*: Measurement of motor, nerve, and related functions

- *Activities of Daily Living Assessment*: Measurement of functional level for activities of daily living

- *Hearing Assessment*: Measurement of hearing and related functions

- *Hearing Aid Assessment*: Measurement of the appropriateness and/or effectiveness of a hearing device

- *Vestibular Assessment*: Measurement of the vestibular system and related functions

Caregiver Training: Educating caregiver with the skills and knowledge used to interact with and assist the patient

Caregiver Training is divided into 18 different broad subjects taught to help a caregiver provide proper patient care.

- *Caregiver Training*: Training in activities to support patient's optimal level of function

Fitting(s): Design, fabrication, modification, selection, and/or application of splint, orthosis, prosthesis, hearing aids, and/or other rehabilitation device

The fifth character used in *Device Fitting* procedures describes the device being fitted rather than the method used to fit the device. Definitions of devices, when provided, are located in the definitions portion of the ICD-10-PCS tables and index, under section F, character 5.

- *Device Fitting*: Fitting of a device designed to facilitate or support achievement of a higher level of function

Treatment: Use of specific activities or methods to develop, improve, and/or restore the performance of necessary functions, compensate for dysfunction and/or minimize debilitation

Treatment procedures include swallowing dysfunction exercises, bathing and showering techniques, wound management, gait training, and a host of activities typically associated with rehabilitation.

- *Speech Treatment*: Application of techniques to improve, augment, or compensate for speech and related functional impairment

- *Motor Treatment*: Exercise or activities to increase or facilitate motor function

- *Activities of Daily Living Treatment*: Exercise or activities to facilitate functional competence for activities of daily living

- *Hearing Treatment*: Application of techniques to improve, augment, or compensate for hearing and related functional impairment

- *Cochlear Implant Treatment*: Application of techniques to improve the communication abilities of individuals with cochlear implant
- *Vestibular Treatment*: Application of techniques to improve, augment, or compensate for vestibular and related functional impairment

The type of treatment includes training as well as activities that restore function.

Body System/Region (Character 4)
The fourth character specifies the body region and/or system on which the procedure is performed.

Type Qualifier (Character 5)
The fifth character is a type qualifier that further specifies the procedure performed. Examples include therapy to improve the range of motion and training for bathing techniques. Refer to appendix J for definitions of these types of procedures.

Equipment (Character 6)
The sixth character specifies the equipment used. Specific equipment is not defined in the equipment value. Instead, broad categories of equipment are specified (e.g., aerobic endurance and conditioning, assistive/adaptive/supportive, etc.)

Qualifier (Character 7)
The seventh character is not specified in the Physical Rehabilitation and Diagnostic Audiology section and always has the value *None*.

Mental Health Section (G)

Character Meanings
The seven characters in the Mental Health section have the following meaning:

Character	Meaning
1	Section
2	Body System
3	Type
4	Qualifier
5	Qualifier
6	Qualifier
7	Qualifier

Section (Character 1)
Mental health procedure codes have a first character value of *G*.

Body System (Character 2)
The second character is used to identify the body system elsewhere in ICD-10-PCS. In this section it always has the value *None*.

Type (Character 3)
The third character specifies the procedure type, such as crisis intervention or counseling. There are 12 types of mental health procedures.

- *Psychological Tests:* The administration and interpretation of standardized psychological tests and measurement instruments for the assessment of psychological function

- *Crisis Intervention:* Treatment of a traumatized, acutely disturbed, or distressed individual for the purpose of short-term stabilization
- *Medication Management:* Monitoring and adjusting the use of medications for the treatment of a mental health disorder
- *Individual Psychotherapy:* Treatment of an individual with a mental health disorder by behavioral, cognitive, psychoanalytic, psychodynamic, or psychophysiological means to improve functioning or well-being
- *Counseling:* The application of psychological methods to treat an individual with normal developmental issues and psychological problems in order to increase function, improve well-being, alleviate distress, maladjustment, or resolve crises
- *Family Psychotherapy:* Treatment that includes one or more family members of an individual with a mental health disorder by behavioral, cognitive, psychoanalytic, psychodynamic, or psychophysiological means to improve functioning or well-being
- *Electroconvulsive Therapy:* The application of controlled electrical voltages to treat a mental health disorder
- *Biofeedback:* Provision of information from the monitoring and regulating of physiological processes in conjunction with cognitive-behavioral techniques to improve patient functioning or well-being
- *Hypnosis:* Induction of a state of heightened suggestibility by auditory, visual, and tactile techniques to elicit an emotional or behavioral response
- *Narcosynthesis:* Administration of intravenous barbiturates in order to release suppressed or repressed thoughts
- *Group Psychotherapy:* Treatment of two or more individuals with a mental health disorder by behavioral, cognitive, psychoanalytic, psychodynamic, or psychophysiological means to improve functioning or well-being
- *Light Therapy:* Application of specialized light treatments to improve functioning or well-being

Qualifier (Character 4)
The fourth character is a qualifier to indicate that counseling was educational or vocational or to indicate type of test or method of therapy.

Qualifier (Character 5, 6 and 7)
The fifth, sixth, and seventh characters are not specified and always have the value *None*.

Substance Abuse Treatment Section (H)

Character Meanings
The seven characters in the Substance Abuse Treatment section have the following meaning:

Character	Meaning
1	Section
2	Body System
3	Type
4	Qualifier
5	Qualifier
6	Qualifier
7	Qualifier

Section (Character 1)

Substance Abuse Treatment codes have a first character value of *H*.

Body System (Character 2)

The second character is used to identify the body system elsewhere in ICD-10-PCS. In this section, it always has the value *None*.

Type (Character 3)

The third character specifies the type of procedure. There are seven values classified in this section, as listed below:

- *Detoxification Services:* Detoxification from alcohol and/or drugs

- *Individual Counseling:* The application of psychological methods to treat an individual with addictive behavior

- *Group Counseling:* The application of psychological methods to treat two or more individuals with addictive behavior

- *Individual Psychotherapy:* Treatment of an individual with addictive behavior by behavioral, cognitive, psychoanalytic, psychodynamic, or psychophysiological means

- *Family Counseling:* The application of psychological methods that includes one or more family members to treat an individual with addictive behavior

- *Medication Management:* Monitoring and adjusting the use of replacement medications for the treatment of addiction

- *Pharmacotherapy:* The use of replacement medications for the treatment of addiction

Qualifier (Character 4)

The fourth character further specifies the procedure type. These qualifier values vary dependent upon the Root Type procedure (Character 3). Root type 2, *Detoxification Services* contains only the value Z, *None* and Root type 6, *Family Counseling* contains only the value 3, *Other Family Counseling*, whereas the remainder Root Type procedures include multiple possible values.

Qualifier (Character 5, 6 and 7)

The fifth through seventh characters are designated as qualifiers but are never specified, so they always have the value *None*.

New Technology Section (X)

General Information

Section X New Technology is a section added to ICD-10-PCS beginning October 1, 2015. The new section provides a place for codes that uniquely identify procedures requested via the New Technology Application Process or that capture other new technologies not currently classified in ICD-10-PCS.

Section X does not introduce any new coding concepts or unusual guidelines for correct coding. In fact, Section X codes maintain continuity with the other sections in ICD-10-PCS by using the same root operation and body part values as their closest counterparts in other sections of ICD-10-PCS. For example, the codes for the infusion of ceftazidime-avibactam, use the same root operation (Introduction) and body part values (Central Vein and Peripheral Vein) in section X as the infusion codes in section 3 Administration, which are their closest counterparts in the other sections of ICD-10-PCS.

Character Meanings

The seven characters in the new technology section have the following meaning:

Character	Meaning
1	Section
2	Body System
3	Root Operation
4	Body Part
5	Approach
6	Device/Substance/Technology
7	Qualifier

Section (Character 1)

New technology procedure codes have a first character value of *X*.

Body System (Character 2)

The second character values for body system combine the uses of body system, body region, and physiological system as specified in other sections in ICD-10-PCS.

Root Operation (Character 3)

The third character utilizes the same root operation values as their counterparts in other sections of ICD-10-PCS.

Body Part (Character 4)

The fourth character specifies the same body part values as their closest counterparts in other sections of ICD-10-PCS.

Approach (Character 5)

The fifth character specifies approaches as defined in the Medical and Surgical section.

Device/Substance/Technology (Character 6)

The sixth character specifies the key feature of the new technology procedure. It may be specified as a new device, a new substance, or other new technology. Examples of sixth character values are *blinatumomab antineoplastic immunotherapy, orbital atherectomy technology,* and *intraoperative knee replacement sensor*.

Qualifier (Character 7)

The seventh character qualifier is used exclusively to specify the new technology group, a number or letter that changes each year that new technology codes are added to the system. For example, Section X codes added for the first year have the seventh character value 1, *New Technology Group 1*, and the next year that Section X codes are added have the seventh character value 2, *New Technology Group 2*, and so on. Changing the seventh character value to a unique letter or number every year that there are new codes in the new technology section allows the ICD-10-PCS to "recycle" the values in the third, fourth, and sixth characters as needed.

New Technology Coding Instruction

Section X codes are standalone codes. They are not supplemental codes. Section X codes fully represent the specific procedure described in the code title, and do not require any additional codes from other sections of ICD-10-PCS. When section X contains a code title which describes a specific new technology procedure, only that X code is reported for the procedure. There is no need to report a broader, non-specific code in another section of ICD-10-PCS.

For example, code XW033G5 Introduction of Sarilumab into Peripheral Vein, Percutaneous Approach, New Technology Group 5, would be reported to indicate that Sarilumab was administered via peripheral vein. A separate code from table 3EØ in the Administration section of ICD-10-PCS would not be reported in addition to this code. The X section code fully identifies the administration of the sarilumab, and no additional code is needed.

The New Technology section codes are easily found by looking in the ICD-10-PCS Index or the Tables. In the Index, the name of the new technology device, substance or technology for a section X code is included as a main term. In addition, all codes in section X are listed under the main term New Technology. The new technology code index entry for sarilumab is shown below.

Sarilumab XWØ

New Technology
     Sarilumab XWØ

ICD-10-PCS Index and Tabular Format

The *ICD-10-PCS: The Complete Official Code Set* is based on the official version of the International Classification of Diseases, 10th Revision, Procedure Classification System, issued by the U.S. Department of Health and Human Services, Centers for Medicare and Medicaid Services. This book is consistent with the content of the government's version of ICD-10-PCS and follows their official format.

Index

The Alphabetic Index can be used to locate the appropriate table containing all the information necessary to construct a procedure code, however, the PCS tables should always be consulted to find the most appropriate valid code. Users may choose a valid code directly from the tables—he or she need not consult the index before proceeding to the tables to complete the code.

Main Terms

The Alphabetic Index reflects the structure of the tables. Therefore, the index is organized as an alphabetic listing. The index:

- Is based on the value of the third character
- Contains common procedure terms
- Lists anatomic sites
- Uses device terms

The main terms in the Alphabetic Index are root operations, root procedure types, or common procedure names. In addition, anatomic sites from the Body Part Key and device terms from the Device Key have been added for ease of use.

Examples:

Resection (root operation)

Fluoroscopy (root type)

Prostatectomy (common procedure name)

Brachiocephalic artery (body part)

Bard® Dulex™ mesh (device)

The index provides at least the first three or four values of the code, and some entries may provide complete valid codes. However, the user should always consult the appropriate table to verify that the most appropriate valid code has been selected.

Root Operation and Procedure Type Main Terms

For the *Medical and Surgical* and related sections, the root operation values are used as main terms in the index. The subterms under the root operation main terms are body parts. For the Ancillary section of the tables, the main terms in the index are the general type of procedure performed.

Examples:

Biofeedback GZC9ZZZ
Destruction
    Acetabulum
        Left 0Q55
        Right 0Q54
    Adenoids 0C5Q
    Ampulla of Vater 0F5C
Planar Nuclear Medicine Imaging
    Abdomen CW10

See Reference

The second type of term in the index uses common procedure names, such as "appendectomy" or "fundoplication." These common terms are listed as main terms with a "see" reference noting the PCS root operations that are possible valid code tables based on the objective of the procedure.

Examples:

Tendonectomy
    see Excision, Tendons 0LB
    see Resection, Tendons 0LT

Use Reference

The index also lists anatomic sites from the Body Part Key and device terms from the Device Key. These terms are listed with a "use" reference. The purpose of these references is to act as an additional reference to the terms located in the Appendix Keys. The term provided is the Body Part value or Device value to be selected when constructing a procedure code using the code tables. This type of index reference is not intended to direct the user to another term in the index, but to provide guidance regarding character value selection. Therefore, "use" references generally do not refer to specific valid code tables.

Examples:

CoAxia NeuroFlo catheter
    use Intraluminal Device
Epitrochlear lymph node
    use Lymphatic, Left Upper Extremity
    use Lymphatic, Right Upper Extremity
SynCardia Total Artificial Heart
    use Synthetic Substitute

Code Tables

ICD-10-PCS contains 17 sections of Code Tables organized by general type of procedure. The first three characters of a procedure code define each table. The tables consist of columns providing the possible last four characters of codes and rows providing valid values for each character. Within a PCS table, valid codes include all combinations of choices in characters 4 through 7 contained in the same row of the table. All seven characters must be specified to form a valid code.

There are three main sections of tables:

- Medical and Surgical section:
  - *Medical and Surgical* (0)
- Medical and Surgical-related sections:
  - *Obstetrics* (1)
  - *Placement* (2)
  - *Administration* (3)
  - *Measurement and Monitoring* (4)
  - *Extracorporeal or Systemic Assistance and Performance* (5)
  - *Extracorporeal or Systemic Therapies* (6)
  - *Osteopathic* (7)
  - *Other Procedures* (8)
  - *Chiropractic* (9)

- Ancillary sections:
  — *Imaging* (B)
  — *Nuclear Medicine* (C)
  — *Radiation Therapy* (D)
  — *Physical Rehabilitation and Diagnostic Audiology* (F)
  — *Mental Health* (G)
  — *Substance Abuse Treatment* (H)
- New Technology section:
  — *New Technology* (X)

The first three character values define each table. The root operation or root type designated for each table is accompanied by its official definition.

Example:

Table ØØF provides codes for procedures on the central nervous system that involve breaking up of solid matter into pieces:

Character 1, Section	Ø: Medical and Surgical
Character 2, Body System	Ø: Central Nervous System and Cranial Nerves
Character 3, Root Operation	F: Fragmentation: Breaking solid matter in a body part into pieces

Tables are arranged numerically, then alphabetically.

When reviewing tables, the user should keep in mind that:

- Some tables may cover multiple pages in the code book—to ensure maximum clarity about character choices, valid entries do

not split rows between pages. For instance, the entire table of valid characters completing a code beginning with 4A1 is split between two pages, but the split is between, not within, rows. This means that all the valid sixth and seventh characters for, say, body system *Arterial* (3) and approach *External* (X) are contained on one page.

- Individual entries may be listed in several horizontal "selection" lines.
- When a table is continued onto another page, a note to this effect has been added in red.

Body Part Definitions:

An exclusive Optum360 feature in the tables is the incorporation of the body part definitions provided in appendix E into the Medical and Surgical section (Ø) tables under their appropriate body part characters in the first column (character 4). This provides the user a direct reference to all anatomical descriptions, terms, and sites that could be coded to that particular body part value.

Paired body parts typically have values for the right and left side and in some cases a value for bilateral. These paired body parts often have the same list of inclusive body part definitions. When there are paired body parts with the same body part definitions, the first listed body part (usually the right side) contains the list of body part definitions while the second listed body part (usually the left side) contains a **See** instruction. This **See** instruction references the body part value that contains the body part definitions. In the table below, body part value P – Upper Eyelid, Left is followed by a **See** instruction that states **See** *N Upper Eyelid, Right*. All body part descriptions under value N also apply to body part value P.

Example:

Ø	**Medical and Surgical**
8	**Eye**
M	**Reattachment**

Definition: Putting back in or on all or a portion of a separated body part to its normal location or other suitable location
Explanation: Vascular circulation and nervous pathways may or may not be reestablished

Body Part Character 4	Approach Character 5	Device Character 6	Qualifier Character 7
N Upper Eyelid, Right Lateral canthus Levator palpebrae superioris muscle Orbicularis oculi muscle Superior tarsal plate	**X** External	**Z** No Device	**Z** No Qualifier
P Upper Eyelid, Left *See N Upper Eyelid, Right*			
Q Lower Eyelid, Right Inferior tarsal plate Medial canthus			
R Lower Eyelid, Left *See Q Lower Eyelid, Right*			

ICD-10-PCS Additional Features

Use of Official Sources

Color-coding, symbol, and other annotations in this manual that identify coding and reimbursement issues are derived from various official federal government sources, including the *Federal Register*, volume 86, number 88, May 10, 2021 ("Hospital Inpatient Prospective Payment Systems for Acute Care Hospitals and the Long Term Care Hospital Prospective Payment System and Proposed Policy Changes and Fiscal Year 2022 Rates; Proposed Rule") and the proposed, version 39, MS-DRG Grouper software, Definitions Manual files and Medicare Code Editor (MCE) files published with the fiscal 2022 IPPS proposed rule. For the most current files related to IPPS, please refer to the following:

- FY2022 IPPS Final Rule
  https://www.cms.gov/Medicare/Medicare-Fee-for-Service-Payment/AcuteInpatientPPS/IPPS-Regulations-and-Notices

- FY2022 Final Version 39, MS-DRG Grouper software
  https://www.cms.gov/Medicare/Medicare-Fee-for-Service-Payment/AcuteInpatientPPS/MS-DRG-Classifications-and-Software

Table Notations

Many tables in ICD-10-PCS contain color or symbol annotations that may aid in code selection, provide clinical or coding information, or alert the coder to reimbursement issues affected by the PCS code assignment. These annotations may be displayed on or next to a character 4, character 6, or character 7 value. Please note that some values may have more than one annotation; this is true most often with the character 4 value.

Refer to the color/symbol legend at the bottom of each page in the tables section for an abridged description of each color and symbol.

Annotation Box

An annotation box has been appended to all tables that contain color-coding or symbol annotations. The color bar or symbol attached to a character value is provided in the box, as well as a list of the valid PCS code(s) to which that edit applies. The box may also list conditional criteria that must be met to satisfy the edit.

For example, see Table 00F. Four character 4 body part values have a gray color bar. In the annotation box below the table, the gray color bar is defined as "Non-OR," or a nonoperating room procedure edit. Following the Non-OR annotation are the PCS codes that are considered nonoperating room procedures from that row of Table 00F.

Bracketed Code Notation

The use of bracketed codes is an efficient convention to provide all valid character value alternatives for a specific set of circumstances. The character values in the brackets correspond to the valid values for the character in the position the bracket appears.

Examples:

In the annotation box for Table 00F the Noncovered Procedure edit (NC) applies to codes represented in the bracketed code 00F[3,4,5,6]XZZ.

> 00F[3,4,5,6]XZZ Fragmentation in (Central Nervous System and Cranial Nerves), External Approach

The valid fourth character values (body part) that may be selected for this specific circumstance are as follows:

3	Epidural Space, Intracranial
4	Subdural Space, Intracranial
5	Subarachnoid Space, Intracranial
6	Cerebral Ventricle

The fragmentation of matter in the spinal canal, Body Part value U, is not included in the noncovered procedure code edit.

Color-Coding/Symbols

New and Revised Text

To highlight changes to the PCS tables for the current year, the new and revised text is provided in green font.

Medicare Code Edits

Medicare administrative contractors (MACs) and many payers use Medicare code edits to check the coding accuracy on claims. The coding edits provided in this manual include only those directly related to ICD-10-PCS codes used for acute care hospital inpatient admissions. These edits are based on the proposed, version 39, Medicare Code Editor (MCE) files published with the fiscal 2022 IPPS proposed rule.

The PCS related Medicare code edits are listed below:

- Invalid procedure code
- *Sex conflict
- *Questionable obstetric admission
- *Noncovered procedure
- *Limited coverage procedure

Starred edits above that are related to PCS issues are identified in this manual by symbols as described below.

Sex Edit Symbols

The sex edit symbols below are used to detect inconsistencies between the patient's sex and the procedure. The symbols below most often appear to the right of the body part (character 4) value but may also be found to the right of the qualifier (character 7) value:

♂ Male procedure only

♀ Female procedure only

QA **Questionable Obstetric Admission**

An inpatient admission is considered questionable when a vaginal or cesarean delivery code is assigned without a corresponding secondary diagnosis code describing the outcome of delivery. Both a delivery (ICD-10-PCS) code and an outcome-of-delivery (ICD-10-CM) code must be present to avoid errors in MS-DRG assignment. This symbol is found only in the Obstetrics Section, appearing to the right of the body part (character 4) value.

NC **Noncovered Procedure**

Medicare does not cover all procedures. However, some noncovered procedures, due to the presence of certain diagnoses, are reimbursed.

Lc Limited Coverage

For certain procedures whose medical complexity and serious nature incur extraordinary associated costs, Medicare limits coverage to a portion of the cost. The limited coverage edit indicates the type of limited coverage.

ICD-10 MS-DRG Definitions Manual Edits

An MS-DRG is assigned based on specific patient attributes, such as principal diagnosis, secondary diagnoses, procedures, and discharge status. The attributes (edits) provided in this manual include only those directly related to ICD-10-PCS codes used for acute care hospital inpatient admissions. These edits are based on the proposed, version 39, MS-DRG Grouper software and Definitions Manual published with the fiscal 2022 IPPS proposed rule.

Non-Operating Room Procedures Not Affecting MS-DRG Assignment

In the Medical and Surgical section (ØØ1-ØYW) and the Obstetric section (1Ø2-1ØY) tables **only,** ICD-10-PCS procedures codes that DO NOT affect MS-DRG assignment are identified by a **gray color bar** over the body part (character 4) value and are considered non-operating room (non-OR) procedures.

NOTE: The majority of the ICD-10-PCS codes in the Medical and Surgical-Related, Ancillary and New Technology section tables are non-operating room procedures that do not typically affect MS-DRG assignment. Only the Valid Operating Room and DRG Non-Operating Room procedures are highlighted in these sections, *see* Non-Operating Room Procedures Affecting MS-DRG Assignment and Valid OR Procedure description below.

Non-Operating Room Procedures Affecting MS-DRG Assignment

Some ICD-10-PCS procedure codes, although considered non-operating room procedures, may still affect MS-DRG assignment. In all sections of the ICD-10-PCS book, these procedures are identified by a **purple color bar** over the body part (character 4) value.

Valid OR Procedure

In the Medical and Surgical-Related (2WØ-9WB), Ancillary (BØØ-HZ9) and New Technology (X2A-XYØ) section tables **only,** any codes that are considered a valid operating room procedure are identified with a **blue color bar** over the body part (character 4) value and will affect MS-DRG assignment. All codes without a color bar (blue or purple) are considered non-operating room procedures.

Hospital-Acquired Condition Related Procedures

Procedures associated with hospital-acquired conditions (HAC) are identified with the **yellow color bar** over the body part (character 4) value. Appendix K provides each specific HAC category and its associated ICD-10-CM and ICD-10-PCS codes.

Combination Only

Some ICD-10-PCS procedure codes that describe non-operating room procedures can group to a specific MS-DRG but only when used in combination with certain other ICD-10-PCS procedure codes. Such codes are designated by a **red color bar** over the body part (character 4) value.

⊞ Combination Member

A combination member, which can be either a valid operating room procedure or a non-operating room procedure, is an ICD-10-PCS procedure code that can influence MS-DRG assignment either on its own or in combination with other specific ICD-10-PCS procedure codes. Combination member codes are

designated by a plus sign (⊞) to the right of the body part (character 4) value.

Note: In the few instances when a code is both a combination member and a non-operating room procedure affecting the MS-DRG assignment, the body part (character 4) value will have a purple color bar and the combination member icon.

See Appendix L for Procedure Combinations

Under certain circumstances, more than one procedure code is needed in order to group to a specific MS-DRG. When codes within a table have been identified as a Combination Only (**red color bar**) or Combination Member (⊞) code, there is also a footnote instructing the coder to *see Appendix L*. Appendix L contains tables that identify the other procedure codes needed in the combination and the title and number of the MS-DRG to which the combination will group.

Other Table Notations

AHA Coding Clinic:

Official citations from AHA's *Coding Clinic for ICD-10-CM/PCS* have been provided at the beginning of each section, when applicable. Each specific citation is listed below a header identifying the table to which that particular *Coding Clinic* citation applies. The citations appear in purple type with the year, quarter, and page of the reference as well as the title of the question as it appears in that *Coding Clinic's* table of contents. *Coding Clinic* citations included in this edition have been updated through second quarter 2021.

NT New Technology Add-on Payment

This symbol identifies procedure codes that involve new technologies or medical services that have qualified for a new technology add-on payment (NTAP). CMS provides incremental payment, in addition to the DRG payment, for technologies that have received the NTAP designation. This symbol appears to the right of the sixth character value.

Note: Only specific brand or trade named devices, substances, or technologies receive NTAP approval. The sixth character value in the PCS table provides a generalized description that may be applicable to several brand or trade names. Unless otherwise specified in the annotation box, refer to appendix H or I to determine the specific brand or trade name of the device, substance, or technology that is applicable to the new technology add-on payment. New technology add-on payments are not exclusive to the New Technology (X) section.

Appendixes

The resources described below have been included as appendixes for *ICD-10-PCS The Complete Official Code Set*. These resources further instruct the coder on the appropriate application of the ICD-10-PCS code set.

Appendix A: Components of the Medical and Surgical Approach Definitions

This resource further defines the approach characters used in the Medical and Surgical (Ø) section. Complementing the detailed definition of the approach, additional information includes whether or not instrumentation is a part of the approach, the typical access location, the method used to initiate the approach, related procedural examples, and illustrations all of which will help the user determine the appropriate approach value.

Appendix B: Root Operation Definitions

This resource is a compilation of all root operations found in the Medical and Surgical-related sections (Ø-9) of this PCS manual. It provides a definition and in some cases a more detailed explanation of the root operation, to better reflect the purpose or objective. Examples of related procedure(s) may also be provided.

Appendix C: Comparison of Medical and Surgical Root Operations

The Medical and Surgical (Ø) section root operations are divided into groups that share similar attributes. These groups, and the root operations in each group, are listed in this resource along with information identifying the target of the root operation, the action used to perform the root operation, any clarification or further explanation on the objective of the root operation, and procedure examples.

Appendix D: Body Part Key

When an anatomical term or description is provided in the documentation but does not have a specific body part character within a table, the user can reference this resource to search for the anatomical description or site noted in the documentation to determine if there is a specific PCS body part character (character 4) to which the anatomical description or site could be coded.

Appendix E: Body Part Definitions

This resource is the reverse look-up of the Body Part Key. Each table in the Medical and Surgical section (Ø) of the PCS manual contains anatomical terms linked to a body part character or value, for example, in Table ØBB the Body Part (character 4) of 1 is Trachea. The body part Trachea may have anatomical structures or descriptions that may be used in procedure documentation instead of the term trachea. The Body Part Definitions list other anatomical structures or synonyms that are included in specific ICD-10-PCS body part values. According to the body part definitions, in the example above, cricoid cartilage is included in the Trachea (character 1) body part.

Appendix F: Device Classification

This resource provides an explanation of how a device is defined in the ICD-10-PCS classification along with two tables. The first table groups devices used in the ICD-10-PCS tables into general categories, including a definition of each device type and related examples. The second table provides definitions of transplant and grafting tissue types and associated terminology that may be found in the documentation.

Appendix G: Device Key and Aggregation Table

The Device Key helps users code the appropriate PCS sixth character for device. Devices are listed alphabetically by brand name or commonly used medical terminology and are translated to the appropriate PCS language or value. The key also reflects the body system where the device is located. For example, a SAPIEN valve used for transaortic valve replacement translates to Zooplastic Tissue in Heart and Great Vessels.

The following symbol **NT** has been placed next to those devices that have received an NTAP (new technology add-on payment) designation. When the code for this device is applied to an inpatient encounter, CMS provides incremental payment in addition to the DRG payment.

The Aggregation Table crosswalks specific device character value definitions for specific root operations in a specific body system to the more general device character value to be used when the root operation covers a wide range of body parts and the device character represents an entire family of devices.

Appendix H: Device Definitions

This resource is a reverse look-up to the Device Key. The user may reference this resource to see all the specific devices that may be grouped to a particular device character (character 6).

Example:
The operative report states, "An internal fixation device was used to repair a fractured femur. Kirschner wire, bone screws and neutralization plate all used and left in the bone at the end of the procedure. "

Although PCS requires all devices left in the body to be coded and the operative report lists three different devices, a check in the device definitions shows that all of these devices are included in the PCS value "Internal Fixation Device" and require only one code.

The following symbol **NT** has been placed next to those devices that have received an NTAP (new technology add-on payment) designation. When the code for this device is applied to an inpatient encounter, CMS provides incremental payment in addition to the DRG payment.

Appendix I: Substance Key/Substance Definitions

The Substance Key lists substances by trade name or synonym and relates them to a PCS character in the Administration (3) or New Technology (X) section in the Substance (sixth character) or Qualifier (seventh character) column.

The Substance Definitions table is the reverse look-up of the substance key, relating all substance categories, the sixth- or seventh character values, to all trade name or synonyms that may be classified to that particular character.

The following symbol **NT** has been placed next to those substances/ technologies that have received an NTAP (new technology add-on payment) designation. When the code for this substance/technology is applied to an inpatient encounter, CMS provides incremental payment in addition to the DRG payment.

Appendix J: Sections B-H Character Definitions

In each ancillary section (B-H) the characters in a particular column may have different meanings depending on which section the user is working from. This resource provides the values for the characters in these sections as well as a definition of the character value.

Appendix K: Hospital Acquired Conditions

Hospital acquired conditions (HACs) are conditions that are considered reasonably preventable when occurring during the hospital admission and may prevent a case from grouping to a higher-paying MS-DRG. In certain instances the HACs are conditional, requiring a specific ICD-10-CM diagnosis code in combination with a specific ICD-10-PCS procedure code. This resource identifies these conditional HACs, listing the diagnosis and procedure codes that, in combination, may trigger a HAC edit. All codes, ICD-10-CM and ICD-10-PCS, are listed with their full descriptions.

Appendix L: Procedure Combination Tables

The procedure combination tables provided in this resource illustrate certain procedure combinations that must occur in order to assign a specific MS-DRG.

Appendix M: Coding Exercises and Answers

This resource provides the coding exercises with answers, and in some cases a brief explanation as to the reason that particular code was used.

ICD-10-PCS Official Guidelines for Coding and Reporting 2022

Narrative changes appear in **bold** text.

The Centers for Medicare and Medicaid Services (CMS) and the National Center for Health Statistics (NCHS), two departments within the U.S. Federal Government's Department of Health and Human Services (DHHS) provide the following guidelines for coding and reporting using the International Classification of Diseases, 10th Revision, Procedure Coding System (ICD-10-PCS). These guidelines should be used as a companion document to the official version of the ICD-10-PCS as published on the CMS website. The ICD-10-PCS is a procedure classification published by the United States for classifying procedures performed in hospital inpatient health care settings.

These guidelines have been approved by the four organizations that make up the Cooperating Parties for the ICD-10-PCS: the American Hospital Association (AHA), the American Health Information Management Association (AHIMA), CMS, and NCHS.

These guidelines are a set of rules that have been developed to accompany and complement the official conventions and instructions provided within the ICD-10-PCS itself. They are intended to provide direction that is applicable in most circumstances. However, there may be unique circumstances where exceptions are applied. The instructions and conventions of the classification take precedence over guidelines. These guidelines are based on the coding and sequencing instructions in the Tables, Index and Definitions of ICD-10-PCS, but provide additional instruction. Adherence to these guidelines when assigning ICD-10-PCS procedure codes is required under the Health Insurance Portability and Accountability Act (HIPAA). The procedure codes have been adopted under HIPAA for hospital inpatient healthcare settings. A joint effort between the healthcare provider and the coder is essential to achieve complete and accurate documentation, code assignment, and reporting of diagnoses and procedures. These guidelines have been developed to assist both the healthcare provider and the coder in identifying those procedures that are to be reported. The importance of consistent, complete documentation in the medical record cannot be overemphasized. Without such documentation accurate coding cannot be achieved.

Conventions

A1. ICD-10-PCS codes are composed of seven characters. Each character is an axis of classification that specifies information about the procedure performed. Within a defined code range, a character specifies the same type of information in that axis of classification.

> *Example:*
> The fifth axis of classification specifies the approach in sections Ø through 4 and 7 through 9 of the system.

A2. One of 34 possible values can be assigned to each axis of classification in the seven-character code: they are the numbers Ø through 9 and the alphabet (except I and O because they are easily confused with the numbers 1 and Ø). The number of unique values used in an axis of classification differs as needed.

> *Example:*
> Where the fifth axis of classification specifies the approach, seven different approach values are currently used to specify the approach.

A3. The valid values for an axis of classification can be added to as needed.

> *Example:*
> If a significantly distinct type of device is used in a new procedure, a new device value can be added to the system.

A4. As with words in their context, the meaning of any single value is a combination of its axis of classification and any preceding values on which it may be dependent.

> *Example:*
> The meaning of a body part value in the Medical and Surgical section is always dependent on the body system value. The body part value Ø in the Central Nervous body system specifies Brain and the body part value Ø in the Peripheral Nervous body system specifies Cervical Plexus.

A5. As the system is expanded to become increasingly detailed, over time more values will depend on preceding values for their meaning.

> *Example:*
> In the Lower Joints body system, the device value 3 in the root operation Insertion specifies Infusion Device and the device value 3 in the root operation Replacement specifies Ceramic Synthetic Substitute.

A6. The purpose of the alphabetic index is to locate the appropriate table that contains all information necessary to construct a procedure code. The PCS Tables should always be consulted to find the most appropriate valid code.

A7. It is not required to consult the index first before proceeding to the tables to complete the code. A valid code may be chosen directly from the tables.

A8. All seven characters must be specified to be a valid code. If the documentation is incomplete for coding purposes, the physician should be queried for the necessary information.

A9. Within a PCS table, valid codes include all combinations of choices in characters 4 through 7 contained in the same row of the table. In the example below, ØJHT3VZ is a valid code, and ØJHW3VZ is *not* a valid code.

Section:	Ø	**Medical and Surgical**
Body System:	J	**Subcutaneous Tissue and Fascia**
Operation:	H	**Insertion** Putting in a nonbiological appliance that monitors, assists, performs, or prevents a physiological function but does not physically take the place of a body part

Body Part	Approach	Device	Qualifier
S Subcutaneous Tissue and Fascia, Head and Neck **V** Subcutaneous Tissue and Fascia, Upper Extremity **W** Subcutaneous Tissue and Fascia, Lower Extremity	**Ø** Open **3** Percutaneous	**1** Radioactive Element **3** Infusion Device **Y** Other Device	**Z** No Qualifier
T Subcutaneous Tissue and Fascia, Trunk	**Ø** Open **3** Percutaneous	**1** Radioactive Element **3** Infusion Device **V** Infusion Pump **Y** Other Device	**Z** No Qualifier

A10. "And," when used in a code description, means "and/or," except when used to describe a combination of multiple body parts for which separate values exist for each body part (e.g., Skin and Subcutaneous Tissue used as a qualifier, where there are separate body part values for "Skin" and "Subcutaneous Tissue").

Example:

Lower Arm and Wrist Muscle means lower arm and/or wrist muscle.

A11. Many of the terms used to construct PCS codes are defined within the system. It is the coder's responsibility to determine what the documentation in the medical record equates to in the PCS definitions. The physician is not expected to use the terms used in PCS code descriptions, nor is the coder required to query the physician when the correlation between the documentation and the defined PCS terms is clear.

Example:

When the physician documents "partial resection" the coder can independently correlate "partial resection" to the root operation Excision without querying the physician for clarification.

Medical and Surgical Section Guidelines (section Ø)

B2. Body System

General guidelines

B2.1a. The procedure codes in Anatomical Regions, General, Anatomical Regions, Upper Extremities and Anatomical Regions, Lower Extremities can be used when the procedure is performed on an anatomical region rather than a specific body part, or on the rare occasion when no information is available to support assignment of a code to a specific body part.

Examples:

Chest tube drainage of the pleural cavity is coded to the root operation Drainage found in the body system Anatomical Regions, General.

Suture repair of the abdominal wall is coded to the root operation Repair in the body system Anatomical Regions, General.

Amputation of the foot is coded to the root operation Detachment in the body system Anatomical Regions, Lower Extremities.

B2.1b. Where the general body part values "upper" and "lower" are provided as an option in the Upper Arteries, Lower Arteries, Upper Veins, Lower Veins, Muscles and Tendons body systems, "upper" or "lower" specifies body parts located above or below the diaphragm respectively.

Example:

Vein body parts above the diaphragm are found in the Upper Veins body system; vein body parts below the diaphragm are found in the Lower Veins body system.

B3. Root Operation

General guidelines

B3.1a. In order to determine the appropriate root operation, the full definition of the root operation as contained in the PCS Tables must be applied.

B3.1b. Components of a procedure specified in the root operation definition or explanation as integral to that root operation are not coded separately. Procedural steps necessary to reach the operative site and close the operative site, including anastomosis of a tubular body part, are also not coded separately.

Examples:

Resection of a joint as part of a joint replacement procedure is included in the root operation definition of Replacement and is not coded separately.

Laparotomy performed to reach the site of an open liver biopsy is not coded separately.

In a resection of sigmoid colon with anastomosis of descending colon to rectum, the anastomosis is not coded separately.

Multiple procedures

B3.2. During the same operative episode, multiple procedures are coded if:

a. The same root operation is performed on different body parts as defined by distinct values of the body part character.

   Examples:

   Diagnostic excision of liver and pancreas are coded separately.

   Excision of lesion in the ascending colon and excision of lesion in the transverse colon are coded separately.

b. The same root operation is repeated in multiple body parts, and those body parts are separate and distinct body parts classified to a single ICD-10-PCS body part value.

   Examples:

   Excision of the sartorius muscle and excision of the gracilis muscle are both included in the upper leg muscle body part value, and multiple procedures are coded.

   Extraction of multiple toenails are coded separately.

c. Multiple root operations with distinct objectives are performed on the same body part.

   Example:

   Destruction of sigmoid lesion and bypass of sigmoid colon are coded separately.

d. The intended root operation is attempted using one approach but is converted to a different approach.

   Example:

   Laparoscopic cholecystectomy converted to an open cholecystectomy is coded as percutaneous endoscopic Inspection and open Resection.

Discontinued or incomplete procedures

B3.3. If the intended procedure is discontinued or otherwise not completed, code the procedure to the root operation performed. If a procedure is discontinued before any other root operation is performed, code the root operation Inspection of the body part or anatomical region inspected.

Example:

A planned aortic valve replacement procedure is discontinued after the initial thoracotomy and before any incision is made in the heart muscle, when the patient becomes hemodynamically unstable. This procedure is coded as an open Inspection of the mediastinum.

Biopsy procedures

B3.4a. Biopsy procedures are coded using the root operations Excision, Extraction, or Drainage and the qualifier Diagnostic.

Examples:

Fine needle aspiration biopsy of fluid in the lung is coded to the root operation Drainage with the qualifier Diagnostic.

Biopsy of bone marrow is coded to the root operation Extraction with the qualifier Diagnostic.

Lymph node sampling for biopsy is coded to the root operation Excision with the qualifier Diagnostic.

Biopsy followed by more definitive treatment

B3.4b. If a diagnostic Excision, Extraction, or Drainage procedure (biopsy) is followed by a more definitive procedure, such as Destruction, Excision or Resection at the same procedure site, both the biopsy and the more definitive treatment are coded.

Example:
Biopsy of breast followed by partial mastectomy at the same procedure site, both the biopsy and the partial mastectomy procedure are coded.

Overlapping body layers

B3.5. If root operations such as Excision, Extraction, Repair or Inspection are performed on overlapping layers of the musculoskeletal system, the body part specifying the deepest layer is coded.

Example:
Excisional debridement that includes skin and subcutaneous tissue and muscle is coded to the muscle body part.

Bypass procedures

B3.6a. Bypass procedures are coded by identifying the body part bypassed "from" and the body part bypassed "to." The fourth character body part specifies the body part bypassed from, and the qualifier specifies the body part bypassed to.

Example:
Bypass from stomach to jejunum, stomach is the body part and jejunum is the qualifier.

B3.6b. Coronary artery bypass procedures are coded differently than other bypass procedures as described in the previous guideline. Rather than identifying the body part bypassed from, the body part identifies the number of coronary arteries bypassed to, and the qualifier specifies the vessel bypassed from.

Example:
Aortocoronary artery bypass of the left anterior descending coronary artery and the obtuse marginal coronary artery is classified in the body part axis of classification as two coronary arteries, and the qualifier specifies the aorta as the body part bypassed from.

B3.6c. If multiple coronary arteries are bypassed, a separate procedure is coded for each coronary artery that uses a different device and/or qualifier.

Example:
Aortocoronary artery bypass and internal mammary coronary artery bypass are coded separately.

Control vs. more **specific** root operations

B3.7. The root operation Control is defined as, "Stopping, or attempting to stop, postprocedural or other acute bleeding." **Control is the root operation coded when the procedure performed to achieve hemostasis, beyond what would be considered integral to a procedure, utilizes techniques (e.g. cautery, application of substances or pressure, suturing or ligation or clipping of bleeding points at the site) that are not described by a more specific root operation definition, such as Bypass, Detachment, Excision, Extraction, Reposition, Replacement, or Resection. If a more specific root operation definition applies to the procedure performed, then the more specific root operation is coded instead of Control.**

Example:
Silver nitrate cautery to treat acute nasal bleeding is coded to the root operation Control.

Example:
Liquid embolization of the right internal iliac artery to treat acute hematoma by stopping blood flow is coded to the root operation Occlusion.

Example:
Suctioning of residual blood to achieve hemostasis during a transbronchial cryobiopsy is considered integral to the cryobiopsy procedure and is not coded separately.

Excision vs. Resection

B3.8. PCS contains specific body parts for anatomical subdivisions of a body part, such as lobes of the lungs or liver and regions of the intestine. Resection of the specific body part is coded whenever all of the body part is cut out or off, rather than coding Excision of a less specific body part.

Example:
Left upper lung lobectomy is coded to Resection of Upper Lung Lobe, Left rather than Excision of Lung, Left.

Excision for graft

B3.9. If an autograft is obtained from a different procedure site in order to complete the objective of the procedure, a separate procedure is coded, except when the seventh character qualifier value in the ICD-10-PCS table fully specifies the site from which the autograft was obtained.

Examples:
Coronary bypass with excision of saphenous vein graft, excision of saphenous vein is coded separately.

Replacement of breast with autologous deep inferior epigastric artery perforator (DIEP) flap, excision of the DIEP flap is not coded separately. The seventh character qualifier value Deep Inferior Epigastric Artery Perforator Flap in the Replacement table fully specifies the site of the autograft harvest.

Fusion procedures of the spine

B3.10a. The body part coded for a spinal vertebral joint(s) rendered immobile by a spinal fusion procedure is classified by the level of the spine (e.g. thoracic). There are distinct body part values for a single vertebral joint and for multiple vertebral joints at each spinal level.

Example:
Body part values specify Lumbar Vertebral Joint, Lumbar Vertebral Joints, 2 or More and Lumbosacral Vertebral Joint.

B3.10b. If multiple vertebral joints are fused, a separate procedure is coded for each vertebral joint that uses a different device and/or qualifier.

Example:
Fusion of lumbar vertebral joint, posterior approach, anterior column and fusion of lumbar vertebral joint, posterior approach, posterior column are coded separately.

B3.10c. Combinations of devices and materials are often used on a vertebral joint to render the joint immobile. When combinations of devices are used on the same vertebral joint, the device value coded for the procedure is as follows:

- If an interbody fusion device is used to render the joint immobile (containing bone graft or bone graft substitute), the procedure is coded with the device value Interbody Fusion Device

- If bone graft is the *only* device used to render the joint immobile, the procedure is coded with the device value Nonautologous Tissue Substitute or Autologous Tissue Substitute

- If a mixture of autologous and nonautologous bone graft (with or without biological or synthetic extenders or binders) is used to render the joint immobile, code the procedure with the device value Autologous Tissue Substitute

Examples:
Fusion of a vertebral joint using a cage style interbody fusion device containing morsellized bone graft is coded to the device Interbody Fusion Device.

Fusion of a vertebral joint using a bone dowel interbody fusion device made of cadaver bone and packed with a mixture of local morsellized bone and demineralized bone matrix is coded to the device Interbody Fusion Device.

Fusion of a vertebral joint using both autologous bone graft and bone bank bone graft is coded to the device Autologous Tissue Substitute.

Inspection procedures

B3.11a. Inspection of a body part(s) performed in order to achieve the objective of a procedure is not coded separately.

Example:
Fiberoptic bronchoscopy performed for irrigation of bronchus, only the irrigation procedure is coded.

B3.11b. If multiple tubular body parts are inspected, the most distal body part (the body part furthest from the starting point of the inspection) is coded. If multiple non-tubular body parts in a region are inspected, the body part that specifies the entire area inspected is coded.

Examples:
Cystoureteroscopy with inspection of bladder and ureters is coded to the ureter body part value.

Exploratory laparotomy with general inspection of abdominal contents is coded to the peritoneal cavity body part value.

B3.11c. When both an Inspection procedure and another procedure are performed on the same body part during the same episode, if the Inspection procedure is performed using a different approach than the other procedure, the Inspection procedure is coded separately.

Example:
Endoscopic Inspection of the duodenum is coded separately when open Excision of the duodenum is performed during the same procedural episode.

Occlusion vs. Restriction for vessel embolization procedures

B3.12. If the objective of an embolization procedure is to completely close a vessel, the root operation Occlusion is coded. If the objective of an embolization procedure is to narrow the lumen of a vessel, the root operation Restriction is coded.

Examples:
Tumor embolization is coded to the root operation Occlusion, because the objective of the procedure is to cut off the blood supply to the vessel.

Embolization of a cerebral aneurysm is coded to the root operation Restriction, because the objective of the procedure is not to close off the vessel entirely, but to narrow the lumen of the vessel at the site of the aneurysm where it is abnormally wide.

Release procedures

B3.13. In the root operation Release, the body part value coded is the body part being freed and not the tissue being manipulated or cut to free the body part.

Example:
Lysis of intestinal adhesions is coded to the specific intestine body part value.

Release vs. Division

B3.14. If the sole objective of the procedure is freeing a body part without cutting the body part, the root operation is Release. If the sole objective of the procedure is separating or transecting a body part, the root operation is Division.

Examples:
Freeing a nerve root from surrounding scar tissue to relieve pain is coded to the root operation Release.

Severing a nerve root to relieve pain is coded to the root operation Division.

Reposition for fracture treatment

B3.15. Reduction of a displaced fracture is coded to the root operation Reposition and the application of a cast or splint in conjunction with the Reposition procedure is not coded separately. Treatment of a nondisplaced fracture is coded to the procedure performed.

Examples:
Casting of a nondisplaced fracture is coded to the root operation Immobilization in the Placement section.

Putting a pin in a nondisplaced fracture is coded to the root operation Insertion.

Transplantation vs. Administration

B3.16. Putting in a mature and functioning living body part taken from another individual or animal is coded to the root operation Transplantation. Putting in autologous or nonautologous cells is coded to the Administration section.

Example:
Putting in autologous or nonautologous bone marrow, pancreatic islet cells or stem cells is coded to the Administration section.

Transfer procedures using multiple tissue layers

B3.17. The root operation Transfer contains qualifiers that can be used to specify when a transfer flap is composed of more than one tissue layer, such as a musculocutaneous flap. For procedures involving transfer of multiple tissue layers including skin, subcutaneous tissue, fascia or muscle, the procedure is coded to the body part value that describes the deepest tissue layer in the flap, and the qualifier can be used to describe the other tissue layer(s) in the transfer flap.

Example:
A musculocutaneous flap transfer is coded to the appropriate body part value in the body system Muscles, and the qualifier is used to describe the additional tissue layer(s) in the transfer flap.

Excision/Resection followed by replacement

B3.18. If an excision or resection of a body part is followed by a replacement procedure, code both procedures to identify each distinct objective, except when the excision or resection is considered integral and preparatory for the replacement procedure.

Examples:
Mastectomy followed by reconstruction, both resection and replacement of the breast are coded to fully capture the distinct objectives of the procedures performed.

Maxillectomy with obturator reconstruction, both excision and replacement of the maxilla are coded to fully capture the distinct objectives of the procedures performed.

Excisional debridement of tendon with skin graft, both the excision of the tendon and the replacement of the skin with a graft are coded to fully capture the distinct objectives of the procedures performed.

Esophagectomy followed by reconstruction with colonic interposition, both the resection and the transfer of the large intestine to function as the esophagus are coded to fully capture the distinct objectives of the procedures performed.

Examples:
Resection of a joint as part of a joint replacement procedure is considered integral and preparatory for the replacement of the joint and the resection is not coded separately.

Resection of a valve as part of a valve replacement procedure is considered integral and preparatory for the valve replacement and the resection is not coded separately.

B4. Body Part

General guidelines

B4.1a. If a procedure is performed on a portion of a body part that does not have a separate body part value, code the body part value corresponding to the whole body part.

> *Example:*
> A procedure performed on the alveolar process of the mandible is coded to the mandible body part.

B4.1b. If the prefix "peri" is combined with a body part to identify the site of the procedure, and the site of the procedure is not further specified, then the procedure is coded to the body part named. This guideline applies only when a more specific body part value is not available.

> *Examples:*
> A procedure site identified as perirenal is coded to the kidney body part when the site of the procedure is not further specified.
>
> A procedure site described in the documentation as peri-urethral, and the documentation also indicates that it is the vulvar tissue and not the urethral tissue that is the site of the procedure, then the procedure is coded to the vulva body part.
>
> A procedure site documented as involving the periosteum is coded to the corresponding bone body part.

B4.1c. If a procedure is performed on a continuous section of a tubular body part, code the body part value corresponding to the **anatomically most proximal (closest to the heart) portion of the tubular body part.**

> *Example:*
> A procedure performed on a continuous section of artery from the femoral artery to the external iliac artery with the point of entry at the femoral artery is coded to the external iliac body part.
>
> A procedure performed on a continuous section of artery from the femoral artery to the external iliac artery with the point of entry at the external iliac artery is also coded to the external iliac artery body part.

Branches of body parts

B4.2. Where a specific branch of a body part does not have its own body part value in PCS, the body part is typically coded to the closest proximal branch that has a specific body part value. In the cardiovascular body systems, if a general body part is available in the correct root operation table, and coding to a proximal branch would require assigning a code in a different body system, the procedure is coded using the general body part value.

> *Examples:*
> A procedure performed on the mandibular branch of the trigeminal nerve is coded to the trigeminal nerve body part value.
>
> Occlusion of the bronchial artery is coded to the body part value Upper Artery in the body system Upper Arteries, and not to the body part value Thoracic Aorta, Descending in the body system Heart and Great Vessels.

Bilateral body part values

B4.3. Bilateral body part values are available for a limited number of body parts. If the identical procedure is performed on contralateral body parts, and a bilateral body part value exists for that body part, a single procedure is coded using the bilateral body part value. If no bilateral body part value exists, each procedure is coded separately using the appropriate body part value.

> *Examples:*
> The identical procedure performed on both fallopian tubes is coded once using the body part value Fallopian Tube, Bilateral.
>
> The identical procedure performed on both knee joints is coded twice using the body part values Knee Joint, Right and Knee Joint, Left.

Coronary arteries

B4.4. The coronary arteries are classified as a single body part that is further specified by number of arteries treated. One procedure code specifying multiple arteries is used when the same procedure is performed, including the same device and qualifier values.

> *Examples:*
> Angioplasty of two distinct coronary arteries with placement of two stents is coded as Dilation of Coronary Artery, Two Arteries with Two Intraluminal Devices.
>
> Angioplasty of two distinct coronary arteries, one with stent placed and one without, is coded separately as Dilation of Coronary Artery, One Artery with Intraluminal Device, and Dilation of Coronary Artery, One Artery with no device.

Tendons, ligaments, bursae and fascia near a joint

B4.5. Procedures performed on tendons, ligaments, bursae and fascia supporting a joint are coded to the body part in the respective body system that is the focus of the procedure. Procedures performed on joint structures themselves are coded to the body part in the joint body systems.

> *Examples:*
> Repair of the anterior cruciate ligament of the knee is coded to the knee bursa and ligament body part in the bursae and ligaments body system.
>
> Knee arthroscopy with shaving of articular cartilage is coded to the knee joint body part in the Lower Joints body system.

Skin, subcutaneous tissue and fascia overlying a joint

B4.6. If a procedure is performed on the skin, subcutaneous tissue or fascia overlying a joint, the procedure is coded to the following body part:

- Shoulder is coded to Upper Arm
- Elbow is coded to Lower Arm
- Wrist is coded to Lower Arm
- Hip is coded to Upper Leg
- Knee is coded to Lower Leg
- Ankle is coded to Foot

Fingers and toes

B4.7. If a body system does not contain a separate body part value for fingers, procedures performed on the fingers are coded to the body part value for the hand. If a body system does not contain a separate body part value for toes, procedures performed on the toes are coded to the body part value for the foot.

> *Example:*
> Excision of finger muscle is coded to one of the hand muscle body part values in the Muscles body system.

Upper and lower intestinal tract

B4.8. In the Gastrointestinal body system, the general body part values Upper Intestinal Tract and Lower Intestinal Tract are provided as an option for the root operations **such as** Change, **Insertion,** Inspection, Removal and Revision. Upper Intestinal Tract includes the portion of the gastrointestinal tract from the esophagus down to and including the duodenum, and Lower Intestinal Tract includes the portion of the gastrointestinal tract from the jejunum down to and including the rectum and anus.

> *Example:*
> In the root operation Change table, change of a device in the jejunum is coded using the body part Lower Intestinal Tract.

B5. Approach

Open approach with percutaneous endoscopic assistance

B5.2a. Procedures performed using the open approach with percutaneous endoscopic assistance are coded to the approach Open.

> *Example:*
> Laparoscopic-assisted sigmoidectomy is coded to the approach Open.

Percutaneous endoscopic approach with extension of incision

B5.2b. Procedures performed using the percutaneous endoscopic approach, with incision or extension of an incision to assist in the removal of all or a portion of a body part or to anastomose a tubular body part to complete the procedure, are coded to the approach value Percutaneous Endoscopic.

> *Examples:*
> Laparoscopic sigmoid colectomy with extension of stapling port for removal of specimen and direct anastomosis is coded to the approach value percutaneous endoscopic.
>
> Laparoscopic nephrectomy with midline incision for removing the resected kidney is coded to the approach value percutaneous endoscopic.
>
> Robotic-assisted laparoscopic prostatectomy with extension of incision for removal of the resected prostate is coded to the approach value percutaneous endoscopic.

External approach

B5.3a. Procedures performed within an orifice on structures that are visible without the aid of any instrumentation are coded to the approach External.

> *Example:*
> Resection of tonsils is coded to the approach External.

B5.3b. Procedures performed indirectly by the application of external force through the intervening body layers are coded to the approach External.

> *Example:*
> Closed reduction of fracture is coded to the approach External.

Percutaneous procedure via device

B5.4. Procedures performed percutaneously via a device placed for the procedure are coded to the approach Percutaneous.

> *Example:*
> Fragmentation of kidney stone performed via percutaneous nephrostomy is coded to the approach Percutaneous.

B6. Device

General guidelines

B6.1a. A device is coded only if a device remains after the procedure is completed. If no device remains, the device value No Device is coded. In limited root operations, the classification provides the qualifier values Temporary and Intraoperative, for specific procedures involving clinically significant devices, where the purpose of the device is to be utilized for a brief duration during the procedure or current inpatient stay. If a device that is intended to remain after the procedure is completed requires removal before the end of the operative episode in which it was inserted (for example, the device size is inadequate or a complication occurs), both the insertion and removal of the device should be coded.

B6.1b. Materials such as sutures, ligatures, radiological markers and temporary post-operative wound drains are considered integral to the performance of a procedure and are not coded as devices.

B6.1c. Procedures performed on a device only and not on a body part are specified in the root operations Change, Irrigation, Removal and Revision, and are coded to the procedure performed.

> *Example:*
> Irrigation of percutaneous nephrostomy tube is coded to the root operation Irrigation of indwelling device in the Administration section.

Drainage device

B6.2. A separate procedure to put in a drainage device is coded to the root operation Drainage with the device value Drainage Device.

Obstetric Section Guidelines (section 1)

C. Obstetrics Section

Products of conception

C1. Procedures performed on the products of conception are coded to the Obstetrics section. Procedures performed on the pregnant female other than the products of conception are coded to the appropriate root operation in the Medical and Surgical section.

> *Examples:*
> Amniocentesis is coded to the products of conception body part in the Obstetrics section.
>
> Repair of obstetric urethral laceration is coded to the urethra body part in the Medical and Surgical section.

Procedures following delivery or abortion

C2. Procedures performed following a delivery or abortion for curettage of the endometrium or evacuation of retained products of conception are all coded in the Obstetrics section, to the root operation Extraction and the body part Products of Conception, Retained.

Diagnostic or therapeutic dilation and curettage performed during times other than the postpartum or post-abortion period are all coded in the Medical and Surgical section, to the root operation Extraction and the body part Endometrium.

Radiation Therapy Section Guidelines (section D)

D. Radiation Therapy Section

Brachytherapy

D1.a. Brachytherapy is coded to the modality Brachytherapy in the Radiation Therapy section. When a radioactive brachytherapy source is left in the body at the end of the procedure, it is coded separately to the root operation Insertion with the device value Radioactive Element.

Example:
Brachytherapy with implantation of a low dose rate brachytherapy source left in the body at the end of the procedure is coded to the applicable treatment site in section D, Radiation Therapy, with the modality Brachytherapy, the modality qualifier value Low Dose Rate, and the applicable isotope value and qualifier value. The implantation of the brachytherapy source is coded separately to the device value Radioactive Element in the appropriate Insertion table of the Medical and Surgical section. The Radiation Therapy section code identifies the specific modality and isotope of the brachytherapy, and the root operation Insertion code identifies the implantation of the brachytherapy source that remains in the body at the end of the procedure.

Exception:
Implantation of Cesium-131 brachytherapy seeds embedded in a collagen matrix to the treatment site after resection of brain tumor is coded to the root operation Insertion with the device value Radioactive Element, Cesium-131 Collagen Implant. The procedure is coded to the root operation Insertion only, because the device value identifies both the implantation of the radioactive element and a specific brachytherapy isotope that is not included in the Radiation Therapy section tables.

D1.b. A separate procedure to place a temporary applicator for delivering the brachytherapy is coded to the root operation Insertion and the device value Other Device.

Examples:
Intrauterine brachytherapy applicator placed as a separate procedure from the brachytherapy procedure is coded to Insertion of Other Device, and the brachytherapy is coded separately using the modality Brachytherapy in the Radiation Therapy section.

Intrauterine brachytherapy applicator placed concomitantly with delivery of the brachytherapy dose is coded with a single code using the modality Brachytherapy in the Radiation Therapy section.

New Technology Section Guidelines (section X)

E. New Technology Section

General guidelines

E1.a. Section X codes fully represent the specific procedure described in the code title, and do not require additional codes from other sections of ICD-10-PCS. When section X contains a code title which fully describes a specific new technology procedure, and it is the only procedure performed, only the section X code is reported for the procedure. There is no need to report an additional code in another section of ICD-10-PCS.

Example:
XW043A6 Introduction of **Cefiderocol** Anti-infective into Central Vein, Percutaneous Approach, New Technology Group **6**, can be coded to indicate that **Cefiderocol** Anti-infective was administered via a central vein. A separate code from table 3EØ in the Administration section of ICD-10-PCS is not coded in addition to this code.

E1.b. When multiple procedures are performed, New Technology section X codes are coded following the multiple procedures guideline.

Examples:
Dual filter cerebral embolic filtration used during transcatheter aortic valve replacement (TAVR), X2A5312 Cerebral Embolic Filtration, Dual Filter in Innominate Artery and Left Common Carotid Artery, Percutaneous Approach, New Technology Group 2, is coded for the cerebral embolic filtration, along with an ICD-10-PCS code for the TAVR procedure.

An extracorporeal flow reversal circuit for embolic neuroprotection placed during a transcarotid arterial revascularization procedure, a code from table X2A, Assistance of the Cardiovascular System is coded for the use of the extracorporeal flow reversal circuit, along with an ICD-10-PCS code for the transcarotid arterial revascularization procedure.

F. Selection of Principal Procedure
The following instructions should be applied in the selection of principal procedure and clarification on the importance of the relation to the principal diagnosis when more than one procedure is performed:

1. Procedure performed for definitive treatment of both principal diagnosis and secondary diagnosis

   a. Sequence procedure performed for definitive treatment most related to principal diagnosis as principal procedure.

2. Procedure performed for definitive treatment and diagnostic procedures performed for both principal diagnosis and secondary diagnosis.

   a. Sequence procedure performed for definitive treatment most related to principal diagnosis as principal procedure

3. A diagnostic procedure was performed for the principal diagnosis and a procedure is performed for definitive treatment of a secondary diagnosis.

   a. Sequence diagnostic procedure as principal procedure, since the procedure most related to the principal diagnosis takes precedence.

4. No procedures performed that are related to principal diagnosis; procedures performed for definitive treatment and diagnostic procedures were performed for secondary diagnosis

   a. Sequence procedure performed for definitive treatment of secondary diagnosis as principal procedure, since there are no procedures (definitive or nondefinitive treatment) related to principal diagnosis.

# #

3f (Aortic) Bioprosthesis valve *use* Zooplastic Tissue in Heart and Great Vessels

A

Abdominal aortic plexus *use* Abdominal Sympathetic Nerve
Abdominal esophagus *use* Esophagus, Lower
Abdominohysterectomy *see* Resection, Uterus ØUT9
Abdominoplasty
  see Alteration, Abdominal Wall ØWØF
  see Repair, Abdominal Wall ØWQF
  see Supplement, Abdominal Wall ØWUF
Abductor hallucis muscle
  use Foot Muscle, Left
  use Foot Muscle, Right
ABECMA® *use* Idecabtagene Vicleucel Immunotherapy
AbioCor® Total Replacement Heart *use* Synthetic Substitute
Ablation
  see Control bleeding in
  see Destruction
Abortion
  Abortifacient 10A07ZX
  Laminaria 10A07ZW
  Products of Conception 10AØ
  Vacuum 10A07Z6
Abrasion *see* Extraction
Absolute Pro Vascular (OTW) Self-Expanding Stent System *use* Intraluminal Device
Accelerate PhenoTest™ BC XXE5XN6
Accessory cephalic vein
  use Cephalic Vein, Left
  use Cephalic Vein, Right
Accessory obturator nerve *use* Lumbar Plexus
Accessory phrenic nerve *use* Phrenic Nerve
Accessory spleen *use* Spleen
Acculink (RX) Carotid Stent System *use* Intraluminal Device
Acellular Hydrated Dermis *use* Nonautologous Tissue Substitute
Acetabular cup *use* Liner in Lower Joints
Acetabulectomy
  see Excision, Lower Bones ØQB
  see Resection, Lower Bones ØQT
Acetabulofemoral joint
  use Hip Joint, Left
  use Hip Joint, Right
Acetabuloplasty
  see Repair, Lower Bones ØQQ
  see Replacement, Lower Bones ØQR
  see Supplement, Lower Bones ØQU
Achilles tendon
  use Lower Leg Tendon, Left
  use Lower Leg Tendon, Right
Achillorrhaphy *see* Repair, Tendons ØLQ
Achillotenotomy, achillotomy
  see Division, Tendons ØL8
  see Drainage, Tendons ØL9
Acoustic Pulse Thrombolysis *see* Fragmentation, Artery
Acromioclavicular ligament
  use Shoulder Bursa and Ligament, Left
  use Shoulder Bursa and Ligament, Right
Acromion (process)
  use Scapula, Left
  use Scapula, Right
Acromionectomy
  see Excision, Upper Joints ØRB
  see Resection, Upper Joints ØRT
Acromioplasty
  see Repair, Upper Joints ØRQ
  see Replacement, Upper Joints ØRR
  see Supplement, Upper Joints ØRU
ACTEMRA® *use* Tocilizumab
Activa PC neurostimulator *use* Stimulator Generator, Multiple Array in ØJH
Activa RC neurostimulator *use* Stimulator Generator, Multiple Array Rechargeable in ØJH
Activa SC neurostimulator *use* Stimulator Generator, Single Array in ØJH
Activities of Daily Living Assessment FØ2
Activities of Daily Living Treatment FØ8

ACUITY™ Steerable Lead
  use Cardiac Lead, Defibrillator in Ø2H
  use Cardiac Lead, Pacemaker in Ø2H
Acupuncture
  Breast
    Anesthesia 8EØH300
    No Qualifier 8EØH30Z
  Integumentary System
    Anesthesia 8EØH300
    No Qualifier 8EØH30Z
Adductor brevis muscle
  use Upper Leg Muscle, Left
  use Upper Leg Muscle, Right
Adductor hallucis muscle
  use Foot Muscle, Left
  use Foot Muscle, Right
Adductor longus muscle
  use Upper Leg Muscle, Left
  use Upper Leg Muscle, Right
Adductor magnus muscle
  use Upper Leg Muscle, Left
  use Upper Leg Muscle, Right
Adenohypophysis *use* Pituitary Gland
Adenoidectomy
  see Excision, Adenoids ØCBQ
  see Resection, Adenoids ØCTQ
Adenoidotomy *see* Drainage, Adenoids ØC9Q
Adhesiolysis *see* Release
Administration
  Blood products *see* Transfusion
  Other substance *see* Introduction of substance in or on
Adrenalectomy
  see Excision, Endocrine System ØGB
  see Resection, Endocrine System ØGT
Adrenalorrhaphy *see* Repair, Endocrine System ØGQ
Adrenalotomy *see* Drainage, Endocrine System ØG9
Advancement
  see Reposition
  see Transfer
Advisa (MRI) *use* Pacemaker, Dual Chamber in ØJH
AFX® Endovascular AAA System *use* Intraluminal Device
Aidoc Briefcase for PE (pulmonary embolism) XXE3X27
AIGISRx Antibacterial Envelope *use* Anti-Infective Envelope
Alar ligament of axis *use* Head and Neck Bursa and Ligament
Alfapump® system *use* Other Device
Alfieri Stitch Valvuloplasty *see* Restriction, Valve, Mitral Ø2VG
Alimentation *see* Introduction of substance in or on
ALPPS (Associating liver partition and portal vein ligation)
  see Division, Hepatobiliary System and Pancreas ØF8
  see Resection, Hepatobiliary System and Pancreas ØFT
Alteration
  Abdominal Wall ØWØF
  Ankle Region
    Left ØYØL
    Right ØYØK
  Arm
    Lower
      Left ØXØF
      Right ØXØD
    Upper
      Left ØXØ9
      Right ØXØ8
  Axilla
    Left ØXØ5
    Right ØXØ4
  Back
    Lower ØWØL
    Upper ØWØK
  Breast
    Bilateral ØHØV
    Left ØHØU
    Right ØHØT
  Buttock
    Left ØYØ1
    Right ØYØØ
  Chest Wall ØWØ8
  Ear
    Bilateral Ø9Ø2

Alteration — *continued*
  Ear — *continued*
    Left Ø9Ø1
    Right Ø9ØØ
  Elbow Region
    Left ØXØC
    Right ØXØB
  Extremity
    Lower
      Left ØYØB
      Right ØYØ9
    Upper
      Left ØXØ7
      Right ØXØ6
  Eyelid
    Lower
      Left Ø8ØR
      Right Ø8ØQ
    Upper
      Left Ø8ØP
      Right Ø8ØN
  Face ØWØ2
  Head ØWØØ
  Jaw
    Lower ØWØ5
    Upper ØWØ4
  Knee Region
    Left ØYØG
    Right ØYØF
  Leg
    Lower
      Left ØYØJ
      Right ØYØH
    Upper
      Left ØYØD
      Right ØYØC
  Lip
    Lower ØCØ1X
    Upper ØCØØX
  Nasal Mucosa and Soft Tissue Ø9ØK
  Neck ØWØ6
  Perineum
    Female ØWØN
    Male ØWØM
  Shoulder Region
    Left ØXØ3
    Right ØXØ2
  Subcutaneous Tissue and Fascia
    Abdomen ØJØ8
    Back ØJØ7
    Buttock ØJØ9
    Chest ØJØ6
    Face ØJØ1
    Lower Arm
      Left ØJØH
      Right ØJØG
    Lower Leg
      Left ØJØP
      Right ØJØN
    Neck
      Left ØJØ5
      Right ØJØ4
    Upper Arm
      Left ØJØF
      Right ØJØD
    Upper Leg
      Left ØJØM
      Right ØJØL
  Wrist Region
    Left ØXØH
    Right ØXØG
Alveolar process of mandible
  use Mandible, Left
  use Mandible, Right
Alveolar process of maxilla *use* Maxilla
Alveolectomy
  see Excision, Head and Facial Bones ØNB
  see Resection, Head and Facial Bones ØNT
Alveoloplasty
  see Repair, Head and Facial Bones ØNQ
  see Replacement, Head and Facial Bones ØNR
  see Supplement, Head and Facial Bones ØNU
Alveolotomy
  see Division, Head and Facial Bones ØN8
  see Drainage, Head and Facial Bones ØN9
Ambulatory cardiac monitoring 4A12X45
Amivantamab Monoclonal Antibody XWØ

Amniocentesis *see* Drainage, Products of Conception
1090
Amnioinfusion *see* Introduction of substance in or on,
Products of Conception 3E0E
Amnioscopy 10J08ZZ
Amniotomy *see* Drainage, Products of Conception 1090
AMPLATZER® Muscular VSD Occluder *use* Synthetic
Substitute
Amputation *see* Detachment
AMS 800® Urinary Control System *use* Artificial
Sphincter in Urinary System
Anal orifice *use* Anus
Analog radiography *see* Plain Radiography
Analog radiology *see* Plain Radiography
Anastomosis *see* Bypass
Anatomical snuffbox
  use Lower Arm and Wrist Muscle, Left
  use Lower Arm and Wrist Muscle, Right
Andexanet Alfa, Factor Xa Inhibitor Reversal Agent
  use Coagulation Factor Xa, Inactivated
Andexxa *use* Coagulation Factor Xa, Inactivated
AneuRx® AAA Advantage® *use* Intraluminal Device
Angiectomy
  see Excision, Heart and Great Vessels 02B
  see Excision, Lower Arteries 04B
  see Excision, Lower Veins 06B
  see Excision, Upper Arteries 03B
  see Excision, Upper Veins 05B
Angiocardiography
  Combined right and left heart *see* Fluoroscopy,
    Heart, Right and Left B216
  Left Heart *see* Fluoroscopy, Heart, Left B215
  Right Heart *see* Fluoroscopy, Heart, Right B214
  SPY system intravascular fluorescence *see* Monitor-
    ing, Physiological Systems 4A1
Angiography
  see Computerized Tomography (CT Scan), Artery
  see Fluoroscopy, Artery
  see Magnetic Resonance Imaging (MRI), Artery
  see Plain Radiography, Artery
Angioplasty
  see Dilation, Heart and Great Vessels 027
  see Dilation, Lower Arteries 047
  see Dilation, Upper Arteries 037
  see Repair, Heart and Great Vessels 02Q
  see Repair, Lower Arteries 04Q
  see Repair, Upper Arteries 03Q
  see Replacement, Heart and Great Vessels 02R
  see Replacement, Lower Arteries 04R
  see Replacement, Upper Arteries 03R
  see Supplement, Heart and Great Vessels 02U
  see Supplement, Lower Arteries 04U
  see Supplement, Upper Arteries 03U
Angiorrhaphy
  see Repair, Heart and Great Vessels 02Q
  see Repair, Lower Arteries 04Q
  see Repair, Upper Arteries 03Q
Angioscopy 02JY4ZZ, 03JY4ZZ, 04JY4ZZ
Angiotensin II *use* Synthetic Human Angiotensin II
Angiotripsy
  see Occlusion, Lower Arteries 04L
  see Occlusion, Upper Arteries 03L
Angular artery *use* Face Artery
Angular vein
  use Face Vein, Left
  use Face Vein, Right
Annular ligament
  use Elbow Bursa and Ligament, Left
  use Elbow Bursa and Ligament, Right
Annuloplasty
  see Repair, Heart and Great Vessels 02Q
  see Supplement, Heart and Great Vessels 02U
Annuloplasty ring *use* Synthetic Substitute
Anoplasty
  see Repair, Anus 0DQQ
  see Supplement, Anus 0DUQ
Anorectal junction *use* Rectum
Anoscopy 0DJD8ZZ
Ansa cervicalis *use* Cervical Plexus
Antabuse therapy HZ93ZZZ
Antebrachial fascia
  use Subcutaneous Tissue and Fascia, Left Lower
    Arm
  use Subcutaneous Tissue and Fascia, Right Lower
    Arm
Anterior cerebral artery *use* Intracranial Artery

Anterior cerebral vein *use* Intracranial Vein
Anterior choroidal artery *use* Intracranial Artery
Anterior circumflex humeral artery
  use Axillary Artery, Left
  use Axillary Artery, Right
Anterior communicating artery *use* Intracranial
  Artery
Anterior cruciate ligament (ACL)
  use Knee Bursa and Ligament, Left
  use Knee Bursa and Ligament, Right
Anterior crural nerve *use* Femoral Nerve
Anterior facial vein
  use Face Vein, Left
  use Face Vein, Right
Anterior intercostal artery
  use Internal Mammary Artery, Left
  use Internal Mammary Artery, Right
Anterior interosseous nerve *use* Median Nerve
Anterior lateral malleolar artery
  use Anterior Tibial Artery, Left
  use Anterior Tibial Artery, Right
Anterior lingual gland *use* Minor Salivary Gland
Anterior (pectoral) lymph node
  use Lymphatic, Left Axillary
  use Lymphatic, Right Axillary
Anterior medial malleolar artery
  use Anterior Tibial Artery, Left
  use Anterior Tibial Artery, Right
Anterior spinal artery
  use Vertebral Artery, Left
  use Vertebral Artery, Right
Anterior tibial recurrent artery
  use Anterior Tibial Artery, Left
  use Anterior Tibial Artery, Right
Anterior ulnar recurrent artery
  use Ulnar Artery, Left
  use Ulnar Artery, Right
Anterior vagal trunk *use* Vagus Nerve
Anterior vertebral muscle
  use Neck Muscle, Left
  use Neck Muscle, Right
Antibacterial Envelope (TYRX) (AIGISRx) *use* Anti-
  Infective Envelope
Antibiotic-eluting Bone Void Filler XW0V0P7
Antigen-free air conditioning *see* Atmospheric
  Control, Physiological Systems 6A0
Antihelix
  use External Ear, Bilateral
  use External Ear, Left
  use External Ear, Right
Antimicrobial envelope *use* Anti-Infective Envelope
Anti-SARS-CoV-2 hyperimmune globulin *use* Hyper-
  immune Globulin
Antitragus
  use External Ear, Bilateral
  use External Ear, Left
  use External Ear, Right
Antrostomy *see* Drainage, Ear, Nose, Sinus 099
Antrotomy *see* Drainage, Ear, Nose, Sinus 099
Antrum of Highmore
  use Maxillary Sinus, Left
  use Maxillary Sinus, Right
Aortic annulus *use* Aortic Valve
Aortic arch *use* Thoracic Aorta, Ascending/Arch
Aortic intercostal artery *use* Upper Artery
Aortography
  see Fluoroscopy, Lower Arteries B41
  see Fluoroscopy, Upper Arteries B31
  see Plain Radiography, Lower Arteries B40
  see Plain Radiography, Upper Arteries B30
Aortoplasty
  see Repair, Aorta, Abdominal 04Q0
  see Repair, Aorta, Thoracic, Ascending/Arch 02QX
  see Repair, Aorta, Thoracic, Descending 02QW
  see Replacement, Aorta, Abdominal 04R0
  see Replacement, Aorta, Thoracic, Ascending/Arch
    02RX
  see Replacement, Aorta, Thoracic, Descending
    02RW
  see Supplement, Aorta, Abdominal 04U0
  see Supplement, Aorta, Thoracic, Ascending/Arch
    02UX
  see Supplement, Aorta, Thoracic, Descending
    02UW
Apalutamide Antineoplastic XW0DXJ5

Apical (subclavicular) lymph node
  use Lymphatic, Left Axillary
  use Lymphatic, Right Axillary
**ApiFix® Minimally Invasive Deformity Correction
  (MID-C) System** *use* Posterior (Dynamic) Distrac-
  tion Device in New Technology
Apneustic center *use* Pons
Appendectomy
  see Excision, Appendix 0DBJ
  see Resection, Appendix 0DTJ
Appendicolysis *see* Release, Appendix 0DNJ
Appendicotomy *see* Drainage, Appendix 0D9J
Application *see* Introduction of substance in or on
aprevo™ *use* Interbody Fusion Device, Customizable
  in New Technology
Aquablation therapy, prostate XV508A4
Aquapheresis 6A550Z3
Aqueduct of Sylvius *use* Cerebral Ventricle
Aqueous humour
  use Anterior Chamber, Left
  use Anterior Chamber, Right
Arachnoid mater, intracranial *use* Cerebral Meninges
Arachnoid mater, spinal *use* Spinal Meninges
Arcuate artery
  use Foot Artery, Left
  use Foot Artery, Right
Areola
  use Nipple, Left
  use Nipple, Right
AROM (artificial rupture of membranes) 10907ZC
Arterial canal (duct) *use* Pulmonary Artery, Left
Arterial pulse tracing *see* Measurement, Arterial 4A03
Arteriectomy
  see Excision, Heart and Great Vessels 02B
  see Excision, Lower Arteries 04B
  see Excision, Upper Arteries 03B
Arteriography
  see Fluoroscopy, Heart B21
  see Fluoroscopy, Lower Arteries B41
  see Fluoroscopy, Upper Arteries B31
  see Plain Radiography, Heart B20
  see Plain Radiography, Lower Arteries B40
  see Plain Radiography, Upper Arteries B30
Arterioplasty
  see Repair, Heart and Great Vessels 02Q
  see Repair, Lower Arteries 04Q
  see Repair, Upper Arteries 03Q
  see Replacement, Heart and Great Vessels 02R
  see Replacement, Lower Arteries 04R
  see Replacement, Upper Arteries 03R
  see Supplement, Heart and Great Vessels 02U
  see Supplement, Lower Arteries 04U
  see Supplement, Upper Arteries 03U
Arteriorrhaphy
  see Repair, Heart and Great Vessels 02Q
  see Repair, Lower Arteries 04Q
  see Repair, Upper Arteries 03Q
Arterioscopy
  see Inspection, Artery, Lower 04JY
  see Inspection, Artery, Upper 03JY
  see Inspection, Great Vessel 02JY
Arthrectomy
  see Excision, Lower Joints 0SB
  see Excision, Upper Joints 0RB
  see Resection, Lower Joints 0ST
  see Resection, Upper Joints 0RT
Arthrocentesis
  see Drainage, Lower Joints 0S9
  see Drainage, Upper Joints 0R9
Arthrodesis
  see Fusion, Lower Joints 0SG
  see Fusion, Upper Joints 0RG
Arthrography
  see Plain Radiography, Non-Axial Lower Bones BQ0
  see Plain Radiography, Non-Axial Upper Bones BP0
  see Plain Radiography, Skull and Facial Bones BN0
Arthrolysis
  see Release, Lower Joints 0SN
  see Release, Upper Joints 0RN
Arthropexy
  see Repair, Lower Joints 0SQ
  see Repair, Upper Joints 0RQ
  see Reposition, Lower Joints 0SS
  see Reposition, Upper Joints 0RS
Arthroplasty
  see Repair, Lower Joints 0SQ

▽ Subterms under main terms may continue to next column or pag

throplasty — *continued*
see Repair, Upper Joints ØRQ
see Replacement, Lower Joints ØSR
see Replacement, Upper Joints ØRR
see Supplement, Lower Joints ØSU
see Supplement, Upper Joints ØRU
throplasty, radial head
see Replacement, Radius, Left ØPRJ
see Replacement, Radius, Right ØPRH
throscopy
see Inspection, Lower Joints ØSJ
see Inspection, Upper Joints ØRJ
throtomy
see Drainage, Lower Joints ØS9
see Drainage, Upper Joints ØR9
ticulating Spacer (Antibiotic) *use* Articulating
   Spacer in Lower Joints
tificial anal sphincter (AAS) *use* Artificial Sphincter
   in Gastrointestinal System
tificial bowel sphincter (neosphincter) *use* Artificial Sphincter in Gastrointestinal System
tificial Sphincter
Insertion of device in
   Anus ØDHQ
   Bladder ØटHB
   Bladder Neck ØटHC
   Urethra ØटHD
Removal of device from
   Anus ØDPQ
   Bladder ØटPB
   Urethra ØटPD
Revision of device in
   Anus ØDWQ
   Bladder ØटWB
   Urethra ØटWD
tificial urinary sphincter (AUS) *use* Artificial
   Sphincter in Urinary System
yepiglottic fold *use* Larynx
ytenoid cartilage *use* Larynx
ytenoid muscle
use Neck Muscle, Left
use Neck Muscle, Right
ytenoidectomy *see* Excision, Larynx ØCBS
ytenoidopexy *see* Repair, Larynx ØCQS
cenda Intrathecal Catheter *use* Infusion Device
cending aorta *use* Thoracic Aorta, Ascending/Arch
cending palatine artery *use* Face Artery
cending pharyngeal artery
use External Carotid Artery, Left
use External Carotid Artery, Right
cope™ Duodeno *see* New Technology, Hepatobiliary
   System and Pancreas XFJ
piration, fine needle
Fluid or gas *see* Drainage
Tissue biopsy
   see Excision
   see Extraction
sessment
Activities of daily living *see* Activities of Daily Living
   Assessment, Rehabilitation FØ2
Hearing *see* Hearing Assessment, Diagnostic Audi-
   ology F13
Hearing aid *see* Hearing Aid Assessment, Diagnos-
   tic Audiology F14
Intravascular perfusion, using indocyanine green
   (ICG) dye *see* Monitoring, Physiological Sys-
   tems 4A1
Motor function *see* Motor Function Assessment,
   Rehabilitation FØ1
Nerve function *see* Motor Function Assessment,
   Rehabilitation FØ1
Speech *see* Speech Assessment, Rehabilitation FØØ
Vestibular *see* Vestibular Assessment, Diagnostic
   Audiology F15
Vocational *see* Activities of Daily Living Treatment,
   Rehabilitation FØ8
sistance
Cardiac
   Continuous
      Balloon Pump 5AØ2210
      Impeller Pump 5AØ221D
      Other Pump 5AØ2216
      Pulsatile Compression 5AØ2215
   Intermittent
      Balloon Pump 5AØ2110
      Impeller Pump 5AØ211D
      Other Pump 5AØ2116

Assistance — *continued*
Cardiac — *continued*
   Intermittent — *continued*
      Pulsatile Compression 5AØ2115
   Circulatory
      Continuous
         Hyperbaric 5AØ5221
         Supersaturated 5AØ522C
      Intermittent
         Hyperbaric 5AØ5121
         Supersaturated 5AØ512C
   Respiratory
      24-96 Consecutive Hours
         Continuous Negative Airway Pressure
            5AØ9459
         Continuous Positive Airway Pressure
            5AØ9457
         High Nasal Flow/Velocity 5AØ945A
         Intermittent Negative Airway Pressure
            5AØ945B
         Intermittent Positive Airway Pressure
            5AØ9458
         No Qualifier 5AØ945Z
      Continuous, Filtration 5AØ920Z
      Greater than 96 Consecutive Hours
         Continuous Negative Airway Pressure
            5AØ9559
         Continuous Positive Airway Pressure
            5AØ9557
         High Nasal Flow/Velocity 5AØ955A
         Intermittent Negative Airway Pressure
            5AØ955B
         Intermittent Positive Airway Pressure
            5AØ9558
         No Qualifier 5AØ955Z
      Less than 24 Consecutive Hours
         Continuous Negative Airway Pressure
            5AØ9359
         Continuous Positive Airway Pressure
            5AØ9357
         High Nasal Flow/Velocity 5AØ935A
         Intermittent Negative Airway Pressure
            5AØ935B
         Intermittent Positive Airway Pressure
            5AØ9358
         No Qualifier 5AØ935Z
**Associating liver partition and portal vein ligation
   (ALPPS)**
see Division, Hepatobiliary System and Pancreas
   ØF8
see Resection, Hepatobiliary System and Pancreas
   ØFT
Assurant (Cobalt) stent *use* Intraluminal Device
Atezolizumab Antineoplastic XWØ
Atherectomy
see Extirpation, Heart and Great Vessels Ø2C
see Extirpation, Lower Arteries Ø4C
see Extirpation, Upper Arteries Ø3C
Atlantoaxial joint *use* Cervical Vertebral Joint
Atmospheric Control 6AØZ
AtriClip LAA Exclusion System *use* Extraluminal De-
   vice
Atrioseptoplasty
see Repair, Heart and Great Vessels Ø2Q
see Replacement, Heart and Great Vessels Ø2R
see Supplement, Heart and Great Vessels Ø2U
Atrioventricular node *use* Conduction Mechanism
Atrium dextrum cordis *use* Atrium, Right
Atrium pulmonale *use* Atrium, Left
Attain Ability® lead Ø2H
use Cardiac Lead, Defibrillator in Ø2H
use Cardiac Lead, Pacemaker in Ø2H
Attain Starfix® (OTW) lead
use Cardiac Lead, Defibrillator in Ø2H
use Cardiac Lead, Pacemaker in Ø2H
Audiology, diagnostic
see Hearing Aid Assessment, Diagnostic Audiology
   F14
see Hearing Assessment, Diagnostic Audiology
   F13
see Vestibular Assessment, Diagnostic Audiology
   F15
Audiometry *see* Hearing Assessment, Diagnostic Audiology F13
Auditory tube
use Eustachian Tube, Left
use Eustachian Tube, Right

Auerbach's (myenteric) plexus *use* Abdominal Sympathetic Nerve
Auricle
use
   use External Ear, Bilateral
   use External Ear, Left
   use External Ear, Right
Auricularis muscle *use* Head Muscle
Autograft *use* Autologous Tissue Substitute
Autologous artery graft
use Autologous Arterial Tissue in Heart and Great
   Vessels
use Autologous Arterial Tissue in Lower Arteries
use Autologous Arterial Tissue in Lower Veins
use Autologous Arterial Tissue in Upper Arteries
use Autologous Arterial Tissue in Upper Veins
Autologous vein graft
use Autologous Venous Tissue in Heart and Great
   Vessels
use Autologous Venous Tissue in Lower Arteries
use Autologous Venous Tissue in Lower Veins
use Autologous Venous Tissue in Upper Arteries
use Autologous Venous Tissue in Upper Veins
Automated Chest Compression (ACC) 5A1221J
AutoPulse® Resuscitation System 5A1221J
Autotransfusion *see* Transfusion
Autotransplant
Adrenal tissue *see* Reposition, Endocrine System
   ØGS
Kidney *see* Reposition, Urinary System ØTS
Pancreatic tissue *see* Reposition, Pancreas ØFSG
Parathyroid tissue *see* Reposition, Endocrine Sys-
   tem ØGS
Thyroid tissue *see* Reposition, Endocrine System
   ØGS
Tooth *see* Reattachment, Mouth and Throat ØCM
Avulsion *see* Extraction
AVYCAZ® (ceftazidime-avibactam) *use* Other Anti-
   infective
Axial Lumbar Interbody Fusion System *use* Inter-
   body Fusion Device in Lower Joints
AxiaLIF® System *use* Interbody Fusion Device in Lower
   Joints
Axicabtagene Ciloleucel *use* Axicabtagene Ciloleucel
   Immunotherapy
Axicabtagene Ciloleucel Immunotherapy XWØ
Axillary fascia
use Subcutaneous Tissue and Fascia, Left Upper
   Arm
use Subcutaneous Tissue and Fascia, Right Upper
   Arm
Axillary nerve *use* Brachial Plexus
AZEDRA® *use* Iobenguane I-131 Antineoplastic

B

BAK/C® Interbody Cervical Fusion System *use* Inter-
   body Fusion Device in Upper Joints
BAL (bronchial alveolar lavage), diagnostic *see*
   Drainage, Respiratory System ØB9
Balanoplasty
see Repair, Penis ØVQS
see Supplement, Penis ØVUS
Balloon atrial septostomy (BAS) Ø2163Z7
Balloon Pump
Continuous, Output 5AØ2210
Intermittent, Output 5AØ2110
Bamlanivimab Monoclonal Antibody XWØ
Bandage, Elastic *see* Compression
Banding
see Occlusion
see Restriction
Banding, esophageal varices *see* Occlusion, Vein,
   Esophageal Ø6L3
Banding, laparoscopic (adjustable) gastric
Initial procedure ØDV64CZ
Surgical correction *see* Revision of device in,
   Stomach ØDW6
Bard® Composix® Kugel® patch *use* Synthetic Substi-
   tute
Bard® Composix® (E/X) (LP) mesh *use* Synthetic
   Substitute
Bard® Dulex™ mesh *use* Synthetic Substitute
Bard® Ventralex™ hernia patch *use* Synthetic Substi-
   tute
Baricitinib XWØ

Barium swallow *see* Fluoroscopy, Gastrointestinal System BD1
Baroreflex Activation Therapy® (BAT®)
　use Stimulator Generator in Subcutaneous Tissue and Fascia
　use Stimulator Lead in Upper Arteries
Barricaid® Annular Closure Device (ACD) *use* Synthetic Substitute
Bartholin's (greater vestibular) gland *use* Vestibular Gland
Basal (internal) cerebral vein *use* Intracranial Vein
Basal metabolic rate (BMR) *see* Measurement, Physiological Systems 4A0Z
Basal nuclei *use* Basal Ganglia
Base of Tongue *use* Pharynx
Basilar artery *use* Intracranial Artery
Basis pontis *use* Pons
Beam Radiation
　Abdomen DW03
　　Intraoperative DW033Z0
　Adrenal Gland DG02
　　Intraoperative DG023Z0
　Bile Ducts DF02
　　Intraoperative DF023Z0
　Bladder DT02
　　Intraoperative DT023Z0
　Bone
　　Intraoperative DP0C3Z0
　　Other DP0C
　Bone Marrow D700
　　Intraoperative D7003Z0
　Brain D000
　　Intraoperative D0003Z0
　Brain Stem D001
　　Intraoperative D0013Z0
　Breast
　　Left DM00
　　　Intraoperative DM003Z0
　　Right DM01
　　　Intraoperative DM013Z0
　Bronchus DB01
　　Intraoperative DB013Z0
　Cervix DU01
　　Intraoperative DU013Z0
　Chest DW02
　　Intraoperative DW023Z0
　Chest Wall DB07
　　Intraoperative DB073Z0
　Colon DD05
　　Intraoperative DD053Z0
　Diaphragm DB08
　　Intraoperative DB083Z0
　Duodenum DD02
　　Intraoperative DD023Z0
　Ear D900
　　Intraoperative D9003Z0
　Esophagus DD00
　　Intraoperative DD003Z0
　Eye D800
　　Intraoperative D8003Z0
　Femur DP09
　　Intraoperative DP093Z0
　Fibula DP0B
　　Intraoperative DP0B3Z0
　Gallbladder DF01
　　Intraoperative DF013Z0
　Gland
　　Adrenal DG02
　　　Intraoperative DG023Z0
　　Parathyroid DG04
　　　Intraoperative DG043Z0
　　Pituitary DG00
　　　Intraoperative DG003Z0
　　Thyroid DG05
　　　Intraoperative DG053Z0
　Glands
　　Intraoperative D9063Z0
　　Salivary D906
　Head and Neck DW01
　　Intraoperative DW013Z0
　Hemibody DW04
　　Intraoperative DW043Z0
　Humerus DP06
　　Intraoperative DP063Z0
　Hypopharynx D903
　　Intraoperative D9033Z0
　Ileum DD04
　　Intraoperative DD043Z0

Beam Radiation — *continued*
　Jejunum DD03
　　Intraoperative DD033Z0
　Kidney DT00
　　Intraoperative DT003Z0
　Larynx D90B
　　Intraoperative D90B3Z0
　Liver DF00
　　Intraoperative DF003Z0
　Lung DB02
　　Intraoperative DB023Z0
　Lymphatics
　　Abdomen D706
　　　Intraoperative D7063Z0
　　Axillary D704
　　　Intraoperative D7043Z0
　　Inguinal D708
　　　Intraoperative D7083Z0
　　Neck D703
　　　Intraoperative D7033Z0
　　Pelvis D707
　　　Intraoperative D7073Z0
　　Thorax D705
　　　Intraoperative D7053Z0
　Mandible DP03
　　Intraoperative DP033Z0
　Maxilla DP02
　　Intraoperative DP023Z0
　Mediastinum DB06
　　Intraoperative DB063Z0
　Mouth D904
　　Intraoperative D9043Z0
　Nasopharynx D90D
　　Intraoperative D90D3Z0
　Neck and Head DW01
　　Intraoperative DW013Z0
　Nerve
　　Intraoperative D0073Z0
　　Peripheral D007
　Nose D901
　　Intraoperative D9013Z0
　Oropharynx D90F
　　Intraoperative D90F3Z0
　Ovary DU00
　　Intraoperative DU003Z0
　Palate
　　Hard D908
　　　Intraoperative D9083Z0
　　Soft D909
　　　Intraoperative D9093Z0
　Pancreas DF03
　　Intraoperative DF033Z0
　Parathyroid Gland DG04
　　Intraoperative DG043Z0
　Pelvic Bones DP08
　　Intraoperative DP083Z0
　Pelvic Region DW06
　　Intraoperative DW063Z0
　Pineal Body DG01
　　Intraoperative DG013Z0
　Pituitary Gland DG00
　　Intraoperative DG003Z0
　Pleura DB05
　　Intraoperative DB053Z0
　Prostate DV00
　　Intraoperative DV003Z0
　Radius DP07
　　Intraoperative DP073Z0
　Rectum DD07
　　Intraoperative DD073Z0
　Rib DP05
　　Intraoperative DP053Z0
　Sinuses D907
　　Intraoperative D9073Z0
　Skin
　　Abdomen DH08
　　　Intraoperative DH083Z0
　　Arm DH04
　　　Intraoperative DH043Z0
　　Back DH07
　　　Intraoperative DH073Z0
　　Buttock DH09
　　　Intraoperative DH093Z0
　　Chest DH06
　　　Intraoperative DH063Z0
　　Face DH02
　　　Intraoperative DH023Z0
　　Leg DH0B
　　　Intraoperative DH0B3Z0

Beam Radiation — *continued*
　Skin — *continued*
　　Neck DH03
　　　Intraoperative DH033Z0
　Skull DP00
　　Intraoperative DP003Z0
　Spinal Cord D006
　　Intraoperative D0063Z0
　Spleen D702
　　Intraoperative D7023Z0
　Sternum DP04
　　Intraoperative DP043Z0
　Stomach DD01
　　Intraoperative DD013Z0
　Testis DV01
　　Intraoperative DV013Z0
　Thymus D701
　　Intraoperative D7013Z0
　Thyroid Gland DG05
　　Intraoperative DG053Z0
　Tibia DP0B
　　Intraoperative DP0B3Z0
　Tongue D905
　　Intraoperative D9053Z0
　Trachea DB00
　　Intraoperative DB003Z0
　Ulna DP07
　　Intraoperative DP073Z0
　Ureter DT01
　　Intraoperative DT013Z0
　Urethra DT03
　　Intraoperative DT033Z0
　Uterus DU02
　　Intraoperative DU023Z0
　Whole Body DW05
　　Intraoperative DW053Z0
Bedside swallow F00ZJWZ
Berlin Heart Ventricular Assist Device *use* Implantable Heart Assist System in Heart and Great Vessels
Bezlotoxumab Monoclonal Antibody XW0
Biceps brachii muscle
　use Upper Arm Muscle, Left
　use Upper Arm Muscle, Right
Biceps femoris muscle
　use Upper Leg Muscle, Left
　use Upper Leg Muscle, Right
Bicipital aponeurosis
　use Subcutaneous Tissue and Fascia, Left Lower Arm
　use Subcutaneous Tissue and Fascia, Right Lower Arm
Bicuspid valve *use* Mitral Valve
Bili light therapy *see* Phototherapy, Skin 6A60
Bioactive embolization coil(s) *use* Intraluminal Device, Bioactive in Upper Arteries
Bioengineered Allogeneic Construct, Skin XHRPXF7
Biofeedback GZC9ZZZ
BioFire® FilmArray® Pneumonia Panel XXEBXQ6
Biopsy
　see Drainage with qualifier Diagnostic
　see Excision with qualifier Diagnostic
　see Extraction with qualifier Diagnostic
BiPAP *see* Assistance, Respiratory 5A09
Bisection *see* Division
Biventricular external heart assist system *use* Short-term External Heart Assist System in Heart and Great Vessels
Blepharectomy
　see Excision, Eye 08B
　see Resection, Eye 08T
Blepharoplasty
　see Repair, Eye 08Q
　see Replacement, Eye 08R
　see Reposition, Eye 08S
　see Supplement, Eye 08U
Blepharorrhaphy *see* Repair, Eye 08Q
Blepharotomy *see* Drainage, Eye 089
Blinatumomab *use* Other Antineoplastic
BLINCYTO® (blinatumomab) *use* Other Antineoplastic
Block, Nerve, anesthetic injection 3E0T3BZ
Blood glucose monitoring system *use* Monitoring Device
Blood pressure *see* Measurement, Arterial 4A03
BMR (basal metabolic rate) *see* Measurement, Physiological Systems 4A0Z

Bypass — *continued*
  Artery — *continued*
    Posterior Tibial — *continued*
      Right Ø41R
    Pulmonary
      Left Ø21R
      Right Ø21Q
    Pulmonary Trunk Ø21P
    Radial
      Left Ø31C
      Right Ø31B
    Splenic Ø414
    Subclavian
      Left Ø314Ø
      Right Ø313Ø
    Temporal
      Left Ø31TØ
      Right Ø31SØ
    Ulnar
      Left Ø31A
      Right Ø319
  Atrium
    Left Ø217
    Right Ø216
  Bladder ØT1B
  Cavity, Cranial ØW11ØJ
  Cecum ØD1H
  Cerebral Ventricle ØØ16
  Colon
    Ascending ØD1K
    Descending ØD1M
    Sigmoid ØD1N
    Transverse ØD1L
  Duct
    Common Bile ØF19
    Cystic ØF18
    Hepatic
      Common ØF17
      Left ØF16
      Right ØF15
    Lacrimal
      Left Ø81Y
      Right Ø81X
    Pancreatic ØF1D
      Accessory ØF1F
  Duodenum ØD19
  Ear
    Left Ø91EØ
    Right Ø91DØ
  Esophagus ØD15
    Lower ØD13
    Middle ØD12
    Upper ØD11
  Fallopian Tube
    Left ØU16
    Right ØU15
  Gallbladder ØF14
  Ileum ØD1B
  Intestine
    Large ØD1E
    Small ØD18
  Jejunum ØD1A
  Kidney Pelvis
    Left ØT14
    Right ØT13
  Pancreas ØF1G
  Pelvic Cavity ØW1J
  Peritoneal Cavity ØW1G
  Pleural Cavity
    Left ØW1B
    Right ØW19
  Spinal Canal ØØ1U
  Stomach ØD16
  Trachea ØB11
  Ureter
    Left ØT17
    Right ØT16
  Ureters, Bilateral ØT18
  Vas Deferens
    Bilateral ØV1Q
    Left ØV1P
    Right ØV1N
  Vein
    Axillary
      Left Ø518
      Right Ø517
    Azygos Ø51Ø
    Basilic
      Left Ø51C

Bypass — *continued*
  Vein
    Basilic — *continued*
      Right Ø51B
    Brachial
      Left Ø51A
      Right Ø519
    Cephalic
      Left Ø51F
      Right Ø51D
    Colic Ø617
    Common Iliac
      Left Ø61D
      Right Ø61C
    Esophageal Ø613
    External Iliac
      Left Ø61G
      Right Ø61F
    External Jugular
      Left Ø51Q
      Right Ø51P
    Face
      Left Ø51V
      Right Ø51T
    Femoral
      Left Ø61N
      Right Ø61M
    Foot
      Left Ø61V
      Right Ø61T
    Gastric Ø612
    Hand
      Left Ø51H
      Right Ø51G
    Hemiazygos Ø511
    Hepatic Ø614
    Hypogastric
      Left Ø61J
      Right Ø61H
    Inferior Mesenteric Ø616
    Innominate
      Left Ø514
      Right Ø513
    Internal Jugular
      Left Ø51N
      Right Ø51M
    Intracranial Ø51L
    Portal Ø618
    Renal
      Left Ø61B
      Right Ø619
    Saphenous
      Left Ø61Q
      Right Ø61P
    Splenic Ø611
    Subclavian
      Left Ø516
      Right Ø515
    Superior Mesenteric Ø615
    Vertebral
      Left Ø51S
      Right Ø51R
  Vena Cava
    Inferior Ø61Ø
    Superior Ø21V
  Ventricle
    Left Ø21L
    Right Ø21K

Bypass, cardiopulmonary 5A1221Z

C

Caesarean section *see* Extraction, Products of Conception 1ØDØ
Calcaneocuboid joint
  use Tarsal Joint, Left
  use Tarsal Joint, Right
Calcaneocuboid ligament
  use Foot Bursa and Ligament, Left
  use Foot Bursa and Ligament, Right
Calcaneofibular ligament
  use Ankle Bursa and Ligament, Left
  use Ankle Bursa and Ligament, Right
Calcaneus
  use Tarsal, Left
  use Tarsal, Right

Cannulation
  see Bypass
  see Dilation
  see Drainage
  see Irrigation
Canthorrhaphy *see* Repair, Eye Ø8Q
Canthotomy *see* Release, Eye Ø8N
Capitate bone
  use Carpal, Left
  use Carpal, Right
Caplacizumab XWØ
Capsulectomy, lens *see* Excision, Eye Ø8B
Capsulorrhaphy, joint
  see Repair, Lower Joints ØSQ
  see Repair, Upper Joints ØRQ
Caption Guidance system X2JAX47
Cardia *use* Esophagogastric Junction
Cardiac contractility modulation lead *use* Cardiac Lead in Heart and Great Vessels
Cardiac event recorder *use* Monitoring Device
Cardiac Lead
  Defibrillator
    Atrium
      Left Ø2H7
      Right Ø2H6
    Pericardium Ø2HN
    Vein, Coronary Ø2H4
    Ventricle
      Left Ø2HL
      Right Ø2HK
  Insertion of device in
    Atrium
      Left Ø2H7
      Right Ø2H6
    Pericardium Ø2HN
    Vein, Coronary Ø2H4
    Ventricle
      Left Ø2HL
      Right Ø2HK
  Pacemaker
    Atrium
      Left Ø2H7
      Right Ø2H6
    Pericardium Ø2HN
    Vein, Coronary Ø2H4
    Ventricle
      Left Ø2HL
      Right Ø2HK
  Removal of device from, Heart Ø2PA
  Revision of device in, Heart Ø2WA
Cardiac plexus *use* Thoracic Sympathetic Nerve
Cardiac Resynchronization Defibrillator Pulse Generator
  Abdomen ØJH8
  Chest ØJH6
Cardiac Resynchronization Pacemaker Pulse Generator
  Abdomen ØJH8
  Chest ØJH6
Cardiac resynchronization therapy (CRT) lead
  use Cardiac Lead, Defibrillator in Ø2H
  use Cardiac Lead, Pacemaker in Ø2H
Cardiac Rhythm Related Device
  Insertion of device in
    Abdomen ØJH8
    Chest ØJH6
  Removal of device from, Subcutaneous Tissue and Fascia, Trunk ØJPT
  Revision of device in, Subcutaneous Tissue and Fascia, Trunk ØJWT
Cardiocentesis *see* Drainage, Pericardial Cavity ØW9D
Cardioesophageal junction *use* Esophagogastric Junction
Cardiolysis *see* Release, Heart and Great Vessels Ø2N
CardioMEMS® pressure sensor *use* Monitoring Device, Pressure Sensor in Ø2H
Cardiomyotomy *see* Division, Esophagogastric Junction ØD84
Cardioplegia *see* Introduction of substance in or on, Heart 3EØ8
Cardiorrhaphy *see* Repair, Heart and Great Vessels Ø2Q
Cardioversion 5A22Ø4Z
Caregiver Training FØFZ
Carmat total artificial heart (TAH) *use* Biologic with Synthetic Substitute, Autoregulated Electrohydraulic in Ø2R

aroticotympanic artery
  use Internal Carotid Artery, Left
  use Internal Carotid Artery, Right
arotid glomus
  use Carotid Bodies, Bilateral
  use Carotid Body, Left
  use Carotid Body, Right
arotid sinus
  use Internal Carotid Artery, Left
  use Internal Carotid Artery, Right
arotid (artery) sinus (baroreceptor) lead *use*
  Stimulator Lead in Upper Arteries
arotid sinus nerve *use* Glossopharyngeal Nerve
arotid WALLSTENT® Monorail® Endoprosthesis
  use Intraluminal Device
arpectomy
  see Excision, Upper Bones ØPB
  see Resection, Upper Bones ØPT
arpometacarpal ligament
  use Hand Bursa and Ligament, Left
  use Hand Bursa and Ligament, Right
asirivimab (REGN10933) and Imdevimab (REGN10987) *use* REGN-COV2 Monoclonal Antibody
asting *see* Immobilization
AT scan *see* Computerized Tomography (CT Scan)
atheterization
  see Dilation
  see Drainage
  see Insertion of device in
  see Irrigation
  Heart *see* Measurement, Cardiac 4A02
  Umbilical vein, for infusion 06H033T
auda equina *use* Lumbar Spinal Cord
auterization
  see Destruction
  see Repair
avernous plexus *use* Head and Neck Sympathetic Nerve
BMA (Concentrated Bone Marrow Aspirate) *use* Concentrated Bone Marrow Aspirate
BMA (Concentrated Bone Marrow Aspirate) injection, intramuscular XK02303
D24Fc Immunomodulator XW0
ecectomy
  see Excision, Cecum ØDBH
  see Resection, Cecum ØDTH
ecocolostomy
  see Bypass, Gastrointestinal System 0D1
  see Drainage, Gastrointestinal System 0D9
ecopexy
  see Repair, Cecum ØDQH
  see Reposition, Cecum ØDSH
ecoplication *see* Restriction, Cecum ØDVH
ecorrhaphy *see* Repair, Cecum ØDQH
ecostomy
  see Bypass, Cecum ØD1H
  see Drainage, Cecum ØD9H
ecotomy *see* Drainage, Cecum ØD9H
efiderocol Anti-infective XW0
eftazidime-avibactam *use* Other Anti-infective
eftolozane/Tazobactam Anti-infective XW0
eliac ganglion *use* Abdominal Sympathetic Nerve
eliac lymph node *use* Lymphatic, Aortic
eliac (solar) plexus *use* Abdominal Sympathetic Nerve
eliac trunk *use* Celiac Artery
entral axillary lymph node
  use Lymphatic, Left Axillary
  use Lymphatic, Right Axillary
entral venous pressure *see* Measurement, Venous 4A04
entrimag® Blood Pump *use* Short-term External Heart Assist System in Heart and Great Vessels
ephalogram BN00ZZZ
ERAMENT® G *use* Antibiotic-eluting Bone Void Filler
eramic on ceramic bearing surface *use* Synthetic Substitute, Ceramic in ØSR
erclage *see* Restriction
erebral aqueduct (Sylvius) *use* Cerebral Ventricle
erebral Embolic Filtration
  Dual Filter X2A5312
  Extracorporeal Flow Reversal Circuit X2A
  Single Deflection Filter X2A6325
erebrum *use* Brain
ervical esophagus *use* Esophagus, Upper

Cervical facet joint
  use Cervical Vertebral Joint
  use Cervical Vertebral Joint, 2 or more
Cervical ganglion *use* Head and Neck Sympathetic Nerve
Cervical interspinous ligament *use* Head and Neck Bursa and Ligament
Cervical intertransverse ligament *use* Head and Neck Bursa and Ligament
Cervical Ligamentum Flavum *use* Head and Neck Bursa and Ligament
Cervical Lymph Node
  use Lymphatic, Left Neck
  use Lymphatic, Right Neck
Cervicectomy
  see Excision, Cervix ØUBC
  see Resection, Cervix ØUTC
Cervicothoracic facet joint *use* Cervicothoracic Vertebral Joint
Cesarean section *see* Extraction, Products of Conception 10D0
Cesium-131 Collagen Implant *use* Radioactive Element, Cesium-131 Collagen Implant in 00H
Change Device in
  Abdominal Wall ØW2FX
  Back
    Lower ØW2LX
    Upper ØW2KX
  Bladder ØT2BX
  Bone
    Facial ØN2WX
    Lower ØQ2YX
    Nasal ØN2BX
    Upper ØP2YX
  Bone Marrow 072TX
  Brain 0020X
  Breast
    Left ØH2UX
    Right ØH2TX
  Bursa and Ligament
    Lower ØM2YX
    Upper ØM2XX
  Cavity, Cranial ØW21X
  Chest Wall ØW28X
  Cisterna Chyli 072LX
  Diaphragm ØB2TX
  Duct
    Hepatobiliary ØF2BX
    Pancreatic ØF2DX
  Ear
    Left Ø92JX
    Right Ø92HX
  Epididymis and Spermatic Cord ØV2MX
  Extremity
    Lower
      Left ØY2BX
      Right ØY29X
    Upper
      Left ØX27X
      Right ØX26X
  Eye
    Left Ø821X
    Right Ø820X
  Face ØW22X
  Fallopian Tube ØU28X
  Gallbladder ØF24X
  Gland
    Adrenal ØG25X
    Endocrine ØG2SX
    Pituitary ØG20X
    Salivary ØC2AX
  Head ØW20X
  Intestinal Tract
    Lower ØD2DXUZ
    Upper ØD20XUZ
  Jaw
    Lower ØW25X
    Upper ØW24X
  Joint
    Lower ØS2YX
    Upper ØR2YX
  Kidney ØT25X
  Larynx ØC2SX
  Liver ØF20X
  Lung
    Left ØB2LX
    Right ØB2KX
  Lymphatic 072NX

Change Device in — *continued*
  Lymphatic — *continued*
    Thoracic Duct 072KX
  Mediastinum ØW2CX
  Mesentery ØD2VX
  Mouth and Throat ØC2YX
  Muscle
    Lower ØK2YX
    Upper ØK2XX
  Nasal Mucosa and Soft Tissue Ø92KX
  Neck ØW26X
  Nerve
    Cranial 002EX
    Peripheral 012YX
  Omentum ØD2UX
  Ovary ØU23X
  Pancreas ØF2GX
  Parathyroid Gland ØG2RX
  Pelvic Cavity ØW2JX
  Penis ØV2SX
  Pericardial Cavity ØW2DX
  Perineum
    Female ØW2NX
    Male ØW2MX
  Peritoneal Cavity ØW2GX
  Peritoneum ØD2WX
  Pineal Body ØG21X
  Pleura ØB2QX
  Pleural Cavity
    Left ØW2BX
    Right ØW29X
  Products of Conception 10207
  Prostate and Seminal Vesicles ØV24X
  Retroperitoneum ØW2HX
  Scrotum and Tunica Vaginalis ØV28X
  Sinus Ø92YX
  Skin ØH2PX
  Skull ØN20X
  Spinal Canal 002UX
  Spleen 072PX
  Subcutaneous Tissue and Fascia
    Head and Neck ØJ2SX
    Lower Extremity ØJ2WX
    Trunk ØJ2TX
    Upper Extremity ØJ2VX
  Tendon
    Lower ØL2YX
    Upper ØL2XX
  Testis ØV2DX
  Thymus 072MX
  Thyroid Gland ØG2KX
  Trachea ØB21
  Tracheobronchial Tree ØB20X
  Ureter ØT29X
  Urethra ØT2DX
  Uterus and Cervix ØU2DXHZ
  Vagina and Cul-de-sac ØU2HXGZ
  Vas Deferens ØV2RX
  Vulva ØU2MX
Change Device in or on
  Abdominal Wall 2W03X
  Anorectal 2Y03X5Z
  Arm
    Lower
      Left 2W0DX
      Right 2W0CX
    Upper
      Left 2W0BX
      Right 2W0AX
  Back 2W05X
  Chest Wall 2W04X
  Ear 2Y02X5Z
  Extremity
    Lower
      Left 2W0MX
      Right 2W0LX
    Upper
      Left 2W09X
      Right 2W08X
  Face 2W01X
  Finger
    Left 2W0KX
    Right 2W0JX
  Foot
    Left 2W0TX
    Right 2W0SX
  Genital Tract, Female 2Y04X5Z
  Hand
    Left 2W0FX

Change Device in or on — *continued*
  Hand — *continued*
    Right 2W0EX
  Head 2W00X
  Inguinal Region
    Left 2W07X
    Right 2W06X
  Leg
    Lower
      Left 2W0RX
      Right 2W0QX
    Upper
      Left 2W0PX
      Right 2W0NX
  Mouth and Pharynx 2Y00X5Z
  Nasal 2Y01X5Z
  Neck 2W02X
  Thumb
    Left 2W0HX
    Right 2W0GX
  Toe
    Left 2W0VX
    Right 2W0UX
  Urethra 2Y05X5Z
Chemoembolization *see* Introduction of substance in or on
Chemosurgery, Skin 3E00XTZ
Chemothalamectomy *see* Destruction, Thalamus 0059
Chemotherapy, Infusion for Cancer *see* Introduction of substance in or on
Chest compression (CPR), external
  Manual 5A12012
  Mechanical 5A1221J
Chest x-ray *see* Plain Radiography, Chest BW03
Chiropractic Manipulation
  Abdomen 9WB9X
  Cervical 9WB1X
  Extremities
    Lower 9WB6X
    Upper 9WB7X
  Head 9WB0X
  Lumbar 9WB3X
  Pelvis 9WB5X
  Rib Cage 9WB8X
  Sacrum 9WB4X
  Thoracic 9WB2X
Choana *use* Nasopharynx
Cholangiogram
  see Fluoroscopy, Hepatobiliary System and Pancreas BF1
  see Plain Radiography, Hepatobiliary System and Pancreas BF0
Cholecystectomy
  see Excision, Gallbladder 0FB4
  see Resection, Gallbladder 0FT4
Cholecystojejunostomy
  see Bypass, Hepatobiliary System and Pancreas 0F1
  see Drainage, Hepatobiliary System and Pancreas 0F9
Cholecystopexy
  see Repair, Gallbladder 0FQ4
  see Reposition, Gallbladder 0FS4
Cholecystoscopy 0FJ44ZZ
Cholecystostomy
  see Bypass, Gallbladder 0F14
  see Drainage, Gallbladder 0F94
Cholecystotomy *see* Drainage, Gallbladder 0F94
Choledochectomy
  see Excision, Hepatobiliary System and Pancreas 0FB
  see Resection, Hepatobiliary System and Pancreas 0FT
Choledocholithotomy *see* Extirpation, Duct, Common Bile 0FC9
Choledochoplasty
  see Repair, Hepatobiliary System and Pancreas 0FQ
  see Replacement, Hepatobiliary System and Pancreas 0FR
  see Supplement, Hepatobiliary System and Pancreas 0FU
Choledochoscopy 0FJB8ZZ
Choledochotomy *see* Drainage, Hepatobiliary System and Pancreas 0F9
Cholelithotomy *see* Extirpation, Hepatobiliary System and Pancreas 0FC
Chondrectomy
  see Excision, Lower Joints 0SB

Chondrectomy — *continued*
  see Excision, Upper Joints 0RB
  Knee *see* Excision, Lower Joints 0SB
  Semilunar cartilage *see* Excision, Lower Joints 0SB
Chondroglossus muscle *use* Tongue, Palate, Pharynx Muscle
Chorda tympani *use* Facial Nerve
Chordotomy *see* Division, Central Nervous System and Cranial Nerves 008
Choroid plexus *use* Cerebral Ventricle
Choroidectomy
  see Excision, Eye 08B
  see Resection, Eye 08T
Ciliary body
  use Eye, Left
  use Eye, Right
Ciliary ganglion *use* Head and Neck Sympathetic Nerve
Ciltacabtagene Autoleucel XW0
cilta-cel *use* Ciltacabtagene Autoleucel
Circle of Willis *use* Intracranial Artery
Circumcision 0VTTXZZ
Circumflex iliac artery
  use Femoral Artery, Left
  use Femoral Artery, Right
CivaSheet® *use* Radioactive Element
CivaSheet® Brachytherapy
  see Brachytherapy with qualifier Unidirectional Source
  see Insertion with device Radioactive Element
Clamp and rod internal fixation system (CRIF)
  use Internal Fixation Device in Lower Bones
  use Internal Fixation Device in Upper Bones
Clamping *see* Occlusion
Claustrum *use* Basal Ganglia
Claviculectomy
  see Excision, Upper Bones 0PB
  see Resection, Upper Bones 0PT
Claviculotomy
  see Division, Upper Bones 0P8
  see Drainage, Upper Bones 0P9
Clipping, aneurysm
  see Occlusion using Extraluminal Device
  see Restriction using Extraluminal Device
Clitorectomy, clitoridectomy
  see Excision, Clitoris 0UBJ
  see Resection, Clitoris 0UTJ
Clolar *use* Clofarabine
Closure
  see Occlusion
  see Repair
Clysis *see* Introduction of substance in or on
Coagulation *see* Destruction
Coagulation Factor Xa, inactivated XW0
Coagulation Factor Xa, (Recombinant) Inactivated *use* Coagulation Factor Xa, Inactivated
COALESCE® radiolucent interbody fusion device *use* Interbody Fusion Device, Radiolucent Porous in New Technology
CoAxia NeuroFlo catheter *use* Intraluminal Device
Cobalt/chromium head and polyethylene socket *use* Synthetic Substitute, Metal on Polyethylene in 0SR
Cobalt/chromium head and socket *use* Synthetic Substitute, Metal in 0SR
Coccygeal body *use* Coccygeal Glomus
Coccygeus muscle
  use Trunk Muscle, Left
  use Trunk Muscle, Right
Cochlea
  use Inner Ear, Left
  use Inner Ear, Right
Cochlear implant (CI), multiple channel (electrode) *use* Hearing Device, Multiple Channel Cochlear Prosthesis in 09H
Cochlear implant (CI), single channel (electrode) *use* Hearing Device, Single Channel Cochlear Prosthesis in 09H
Cochlear Implant Treatment F0BZ0
Cochlear nerve *use* Acoustic Nerve
COGNIS® CRT-D *use* Cardiac Resynchronization Defibrillator Pulse Generator in 0JH
COHERE® radiolucent interbody fusion device *use* Interbody Fusion Device, Radiolucent Porous in New Technology
Colectomy
  see Excision, Gastrointestinal System 0DB

Colectomy — *continued*
  see Resection, Gastrointestinal System 0DT
Collapse *see* Occlusion
Collection from
  Breast, Breast Milk 8E0HX62
  Indwelling Device
    Circulatory System
      Blood 8C02X6K
      Other Fluid 8C02X6L
    Nervous System
      Cerebrospinal Fluid 8C01X6J
      Other Fluid 8C01X6L
  Integumentary System, Breast Milk 8E0HX62
  Reproductive System, Male, Sperm 8E0VX63
Colocentesis *see* Drainage, Gastrointestinal System 0D9
Colofixation
  see Repair, Gastrointestinal System 0DQ
  see Reposition, Gastrointestinal System 0DS
Cololysis *see* Release, Gastrointestinal System 0DN
Colonic Z-Stent® *use* Intraluminal Device
Colonoscopy 0DJD8ZZ
Colopexy
  see Repair, Gastrointestinal System 0DQ
  see Reposition, Gastrointestinal System 0DS
Coloplication *see* Restriction, Gastrointestinal System 0DV
Coloproctectomy
  see Excision, Gastrointestinal System 0DB
  see Resection, Gastrointestinal System 0DT
Coloproctostomy
  see Bypass, Gastrointestinal System 0D1
  see Drainage, Gastrointestinal System 0D9
Colopuncture *see* Drainage, Gastrointestinal System 0D9
Colorrhaphy *see* Repair, Gastrointestinal System 0DQ
Colostomy
  see Bypass, Gastrointestinal System 0D1
  see Drainage, Gastrointestinal System 0D9
Colpectomy
  see Excision, Vagina 0UBG
  see Resection, Vagina 0UTG
Colpocentesis *see* Drainage, Vagina 0U9G
Colpopexy
  see Repair, Vagina 0UQG
  see Reposition, Vagina 0USG
Colpoplasty
  see Repair, Vagina 0UQG
  see Supplement, Vagina 0UUG
Colporrhaphy *see* Repair, Vagina 0UQG
Colposcopy 0UJH8ZZ
Columella *use* Nasal Mucosa and Soft Tissue
Common digital vein
  use Foot Vein, Left
  use Foot Vein, Right
Common facial vein
  use Face Vein, Left
  use Face Vein, Right
Common fibular nerve *use* Peroneal Nerve
Common hepatic artery *use* Hepatic Artery
Common iliac (subaortic) lymph node *use* Lymphatic, Pelvis
Common interosseous artery
  use Ulnar Artery, Left
  use Ulnar Artery, Right
Common peroneal nerve *use* Peroneal Nerve
Complete (SE) stent *use* Intraluminal Device
Compression
  see Restriction
  Abdominal Wall 2W13X
  Arm
    Lower
      Left 2W1DX
      Right 2W1CX
    Upper
      Left 2W1BX
      Right 2W1AX
  Back 2W15X
  Chest Wall 2W14X
  Extremity
    Lower
      Left 2W1MX
      Right 2W1LX
    Upper
      Left 2W19X
      Right 2W18X
  Face 2W11X

ompression — *continued*
Finger
　Left 2W1KX
　Right 2W1JX
Foot
　Left 2W1TX
　Right 2W1SX
Hand
　Left 2W1FX
　Right 2W1EX
Head 2W10X
Inguinal Region
　Left 2W17X
　Right 2W16X
Leg
　Lower
　　Left 2W1RX
　　Right 2W1QX
　Upper
　　Left 2W1PX
　　Right 2W1NX
Neck 2W12X
Thumb
　Left 2W1HX
　Right 2W1GX
Toe
　Left 2W1VX
　Right 2W1UX
omputer Assisted Procedure
Extremity
　Lower
　　No Qualifier 8E0YXBZ
　　With Computerized Tomography
　　　8E0YXBG
　　With Fluoroscopy 8E0YXBF
　　With Magnetic Resonance Imaging
　　　8E0YXBH
　Upper
　　No Qualifier 8E0XXBZ
　　With Computerized Tomography
　　　8E0XXBG
　　With Fluoroscopy 8E0XXBF
　　With Magnetic Resonance Imaging
　　　8E0XXBH
Head and Neck Region
　No Qualifier 8E09XBZ
　With Computerized Tomography 8E09XBG
　With Fluoroscopy 8E09XBF
　With Magnetic Resonance Imaging 8E09XBH
Trunk Region
　No Qualifier 8E0WXBZ
　With Computerized Tomography 8E0WXBG
　With Fluoroscopy 8E0WXBF
　With Magnetic Resonance Imaging 8E0WXBH
omputer-aided Assessment, Intracranial Vascular
　Activity XXE0X07
omputer-aided Guidance, Transthoracic
　Echocardiography X2JAX47
omputer-aided Mechanical Aspiration X2C
omputer-aided Triage and Notification, Pul-
　monary Artery Flow XXE3X27
omputer-assisted Intermittent Aspiration *see*
　New Technology, Cardiovascular System X2C
omputerized Tomography (CT Scan)
Abdomen BW20
　Chest and Pelvis BW25
Abdomen and Chest BW24
Abdomen and Pelvis BW21
Airway, Trachea BB2F
Ankle
　Left BQ2H
　Right BQ2G
Aorta
　Abdominal B420
　　Intravascular Optical Coherence
　　　B420Z2Z
　Thoracic B320
　　Intravascular Optical Coherence
　　　B320Z2Z
Arm
　Left BP2F
　Right BP2E
Artery
　Celiac B421
　　Intravascular Optical Coherence
　　　B421Z2Z
　Common Carotid
　　Bilateral B325

Computerized Tomography (CT Scan) — *continued*
Artery — *continued*
　Common Carotid — *continued*
　　Intravascular Optical Coherence
　　　B325Z2Z
　Coronary
　　Bypass Graft
　　　Intravascular Optical Coherence
　　　　B223Z2Z
　　　Multiple B223
　　Multiple B221
　　　Intravascular Optical Coherence
　　　　B221Z2Z
　Internal Carotid
　　Bilateral B328
　　Intravascular Optical Coherence
　　　B328Z2Z
　Intracranial B32R
　　Intravascular Optical Coherence
　　　B32RZ2Z
　Lower Extremity
　　Bilateral B42H
　　　Intravascular Optical Coherence
　　　　B42HZ2Z
　　Left B42G
　　　Intravascular Optical Coherence
　　　　B42GZ2Z
　　Right B42F
　　　Intravascular Optical Coherence
　　　　B42FZ2Z
　　Pelvic B42C
　　　Intravascular Optical Coherence
　　　　B42CZ2Z
　Pulmonary
　　Left B32T
　　　Intravascular Optical Coherence
　　　　B32TZ2Z
　　Right B32S
　　　Intravascular Optical Coherence
　　　　B32SZ2Z
　Renal
　　Bilateral B428
　　　Intravascular Optical Coherence
　　　　B428Z2Z
　　Transplant B42M
　　　Intravascular Optical Coherence
　　　　B42MZ2Z
　Superior Mesenteric B424
　　Intravascular Optical Coherence
　　　B424Z2Z
　Vertebral
　　Bilateral B32G
　　　Intravascular Optical Coherence
　　　　B32GZ2Z
Bladder BT20
Bone
　Facial BN25
　Temporal BN2F
Brain B020
Calcaneus
　Left BQ2K
　Right BQ2J
Cerebral Ventricle B028
Chest, Abdomen and Pelvis BW25
Chest and Abdomen BW24
Cisterna B027
Clavicle
　Left BP25
　Right BP24
Coccyx BR2F
Colon BD24
Ear B920
Elbow
　Left BP2H
　Right BP2G
Extremity
　Lower
　　Left BQ2S
　　Right BQ2R
　Upper
　　Bilateral BP2V
　　Left BP2U
　　Right BP2T
Eye
　Bilateral B827
　Left B826
　Right B825
Femur
　Left BQ24

Computerized Tomography (CT Scan) — *continued*
Femur — *continued*
　Right BQ23
Fibula
　Left BQ2C
　Right BQ2B
Finger
　Left BP2S
　Right BP2R
Foot
　Left BQ2M
　Right BQ2L
Forearm
　Left BP2K
　Right BP2J
Gland
　Adrenal, Bilateral BG22
　Parathyroid BG23
　Parotid, Bilateral B926
　Salivary, Bilateral B92D
　Submandibular, Bilateral B929
　Thyroid BG24
Hand
　Left BP2P
　Right BP2N
Hands and Wrists, Bilateral BP2Q
Head BW28
Head and Neck BW29
Heart
　Intravascular Optical Coherence B226Z2Z
　Right and Left B226
Hepatobiliary System, All BF2C
Hip
　Left BQ21
　Right BQ20
Humerus
　Left BP2B
　Right BP2A
Intracranial Sinus B522
　Intravascular Optical Coherence B522Z2Z
Joint
　Acromioclavicular, Bilateral BP23
　Finger
　　Left BP2DZZZ
　　Right BP2CZZZ
　Foot
　　Left BQ2Y
　　Right BQ2X
　Hand
　　Left BP2DZZZ
　　Right BP2CZZZ
　Sacroiliac BR2D
　Sternoclavicular
　　Bilateral BP22
　　Left BP21
　　Right BP20
　Temporomandibular, Bilateral BN29
　Toe
　　Left BQ2Y
　　Right BQ2X
Kidney
　Bilateral BT23
　Left BT22
　Right BT21
　Transplant BT29
Knee
　Left BQ28
　Right BQ27
Larynx B92J
Leg
　Left BQ2F
　Right BQ2D
Liver BF25
Liver and Spleen BF26
Lung, Bilateral BB24
Mandible BN26
Nasopharynx B92F
Neck BW2F
Neck and Head BW29
Orbit, Bilateral BN23
Oropharynx B92F
Pancreas BF27
Patella
　Left BQ2W
　Right BQ2V
Pelvic Region BW2G
Pelvis BR2C
　Chest and Abdomen BW25
Pelvis and Abdomen BW21

Computerized Tomography (CT Scan) — *continued*
  Pituitary Gland BØ29
  Prostate BV23
  Ribs
    Left BP2Y
    Right BP2X
  Sacrum BR2F
  Scapula
    Left BP27
    Right BP26
  Sella Turcica BØ29
  Shoulder
    Left BP29
    Right BP28
  Sinus
    Intracranial B522
      Intravascular Optical Coherence B522Z2Z
    Paranasal B922
  Skull BN2Ø
  Spinal Cord BØ2B
  Spine
    Cervical BR2Ø
    Lumbar BR29
    Thoracic BR27
  Spleen and Liver BF26
  Thorax BP2W
  Tibia
    Left BQ2C
    Right BQ2B
  Toe
    Left BQ2Q
    Right BQ2P
  Trachea BB2F
  Tracheobronchial Tree
    Bilateral BB29
    Left BB28
    Right BB27
  Vein
    Pelvic (Iliac)
      Left B52G
        Intravascular Optical Coherence B52GZ2Z
      Right B52F
        Intravascular Optical Coherence B52FZ2Z
    Pelvic (Iliac) Bilateral B52H
      Intravascular Optical Coherence B52HZ2Z
    Portal B52T
      Intravascular Optical Coherence B52TZ2Z
    Pulmonary
      Bilateral B52S
        Intravascular Optical Coherence B52SZ2Z
      Left B52R
        Intravascular Optical Coherence B52RZ2Z
      Right B52Q
        Intravascular Optical Coherence B52QZ2Z
    Renal
      Bilateral B52L
        Intravascular Optical Coherence B52LZ2Z
      Left B52K
        Intravascular Optical Coherence B52KZ2Z
      Right B52J
        Intravascular Optical Coherence B52JZ2Z
    Spanchnic B52T
      Intravascular Optical Coherence B52TZ2Z
  Vena Cava
    Inferior B529
      Intravascular Optical Coherence B529Z2Z
    Superior B528
      Intravascular Optical Coherence B528Z2Z
  Ventricle, Cerebral BØ28
  Wrist
    Left BP2M
    Right BP2L
Concentrated Bone Marrow Aspirate (CBMA) injection, intramuscular XKØ23Ø3

Concerto II CRT-D *use* Cardiac Resynchronization Defibrillator Pulse Generator in ØJH
Condylectomy
  see Excision, Head and Facial Bones ØNB
  see Excision, Lower Bones ØQB
  see Excision, Upper Bones ØPB
Condyloid process
  use Mandible, Left
  use Mandible, Right
Condylotomy
  see Division, Head and Facial Bones ØN8
  see Division, Lower Bones ØQ8
  see Division, Upper Bones ØP8
  see Drainage, Head and Facial Bones ØN9
  see Drainage, Lower Bones ØQ9
  see Drainage, Upper Bones ØP9
Condylysis
  see Release, Head and Facial Bones ØNN
  see Release, Lower Bones ØQN
  see Release, Upper Bones ØPN
Conization, cervix *see* Excision, Cervix ØUBC
Conjunctivoplasty
  see Repair, Eye Ø8Q
  see Replacement, Eye Ø8R
CONSERVE® PLUS Total Resurfacing Hip System *use* Resurfacing Device in Lower Joints
Construction
  Auricle, ear *see* Replacement, Ear, Nose, Sinus Ø9R
  Ileal conduit *see* Bypass, Urinary System ØT1
Consulta CRT-D *use* Cardiac Resynchronization Defibrillator Pulse Generator in ØJH
Consulta CRT-P *use* Cardiac Resynchronization Pacemaker Pulse Generator in ØJH
Contact Radiation
  Abdomen DWY37ZZ
  Adrenal Gland DGY27ZZ
  Bile Ducts DFY27ZZ
  Bladder DTY27ZZ
  Bone, Other DPYC7ZZ
  Brain DØY07ZZ
  Brain Stem DØY17ZZ
  Breast
    Left DMY07ZZ
    Right DMY17ZZ
  Bronchus DBY17ZZ
  Cervix DUY17ZZ
  Chest DWY27ZZ
  Chest Wall DBY77ZZ
  Colon DDY57ZZ
  Diaphragm DBY87ZZ
  Duodenum DDY27ZZ
  Ear D9Y07ZZ
  Esophagus DDY07ZZ
  Eye D8Y07ZZ
  Femur DPY97ZZ
  Fibula DPYB7ZZ
  Gallbladder DFY17ZZ
  Gland
    Adrenal DGY27ZZ
    Parathyroid DGY47ZZ
    Pituitary DGY07ZZ
    Thyroid DGY57ZZ
  Glands, Salivary D9Y67ZZ
  Head and Neck DWY17ZZ
  Hemibody DWY47ZZ
  Humerus DPY67ZZ
  Hypopharynx D9Y37ZZ
  Ileum DDY47ZZ
  Jejunum DDY37ZZ
  Kidney DTY07ZZ
  Larynx D9YB7ZZ
  Liver DFY07ZZ
  Lung DBY27ZZ
  Mandible DPY37ZZ
  Maxilla DPY27ZZ
  Mediastinum DBY67ZZ
  Mouth D9Y47ZZ
  Nasopharynx D9YD7ZZ
  Neck and Head DWY17ZZ
  Nerve, Peripheral DØY77ZZ
  Nose D9Y17ZZ
  Oropharynx D9YF7ZZ
  Ovary DUY07ZZ
  Palate
    Hard D9Y87ZZ
    Soft D9Y97ZZ
  Pancreas DFY37ZZ
  Parathyroid Gland DGY47ZZ

Contact Radiation — *continued*
  Pelvic Bones DPY87ZZ
  Pelvic Region DWY67ZZ
  Pineal Body DGY17ZZ
  Pituitary Gland DGY07ZZ
  Pleura DBY57ZZ
  Prostate DVY07ZZ
  Radius DPY77ZZ
  Rectum DDY77ZZ
  Rib DPY57ZZ
  Sinuses D9Y77ZZ
  Skin
    Abdomen DHY87ZZ
    Arm DHY47ZZ
    Back DHY77ZZ
    Buttock DHY97ZZ
    Chest DHY67ZZ
    Face DHY27ZZ
    Leg DHYB7ZZ
    Neck DHY37ZZ
  Skull DPY07ZZ
  Spinal Cord DØY67ZZ
  Sternum DPY47ZZ
  Stomach DDY17ZZ
  Testis DVY17ZZ
  Thyroid Gland DGY57ZZ
  Tibia DPYB7ZZ
  Tongue D9Y57ZZ
  Trachea DBY07ZZ
  Ulna DPY77ZZ
  Ureter DTY17ZZ
  Urethra DTY37ZZ
  Uterus DUY27ZZ
  Whole Body DWY57ZZ
ContaCT software (Measurement of intracranial arterial flow) 4AØ3X5D
CONTAK RENEWAL® 3 RF (HE) CRT-D *use* Cardiac Resynchronization Defibrillator Pulse Generator in ØJH
Contegra Pulmonary Valved Conduit *use* Zooplastic Tissue in Heart and Great Vessels
CONTEPO™ *use* Fosfomycin Anti-Infective
Continuous Glucose Monitoring (CGM) device *use* Monitoring Device
Continuous Negative Airway Pressure
  24-96 Consecutive Hours, Ventilation 5AØ9459
  Greater than 96 Consecutive Hours, Ventilation 5AØ9559
  Less than 24 Consecutive Hours, Ventilation 5AØ9359
Continuous Positive Airway Pressure
  24-96 Consecutive Hours, Ventilation 5AØ9457
  Greater than 96 Consecutive Hours, Ventilation 5AØ9557
  Less than 24 Consecutive Hours, Ventilation 5AØ9357
Continuous renal replacement therapy (CRRT) 5A1D90Z
Contraceptive Device
  Change device in, Uterus and Cervix ØU2DXHZ
  Insertion of device in
    Cervix ØUHC
    Subcutaneous Tissue and Fascia
      Abdomen ØJH8
      Chest ØJH6
      Lower Arm
        Left ØJHH
        Right ØJHG
      Lower Leg
        Left ØJHP
        Right ØJHN
      Upper Arm
        Left ØJHF
        Right ØJHD
      Upper Leg
        Left ØJHM
        Right ØJHL
    Uterus ØUH9
  Removal of device from
    Subcutaneous Tissue and Fascia
      Lower Extremity ØJPW
      Trunk ØJPT
      Upper Extremity ØJPV
    Uterus and Cervix ØUPD
  Revision of device in
    Subcutaneous Tissue and Fascia
      Lower Extremity ØJWW
      Trunk ØJWT

Cricothyroid artery
  use Thyroid Artery, Left
  use Thyroid Artery, Right
Cricothyroid muscle
  use Neck Muscle, Left
  use Neck Muscle, Right
Crisis Intervention GZ2ZZZZ
CRRT (Continuous renal replacement therapy)
  5A1D90Z
Crural fascia
  use Subcutaneous Tissue and Fascia, Left Upper
    Leg
  use Subcutaneous Tissue and Fascia, Right Upper
    Leg
Crushing, nerve
  Cranial *see* Destruction, Central Nervous System
    and Cranial Nerves 005
  Peripheral *see* Destruction, Peripheral Nervous
    System 015
Cryoablation *see* Destruction
Cryotherapy *see* Destruction
Cryptorchidectomy
  see Excision, Male Reproductive System 0VB
  see Resection, Male Reproductive System 0VT
Cryptorchiectomy
  see Excision, Male Reproductive System 0VB
  see Resection, Male Reproductive System 0VT
Cryptotomy
  see Division, Gastrointestinal System 0D8
  see Drainage, Gastrointestinal System 0D9
CT scan *see* Computerized Tomography (CT Scan)
CT sialogram *see* Computerized Tomography (CT Scan),
    Ear, Nose, Mouth and Throat B92
Cubital lymph node
  use Lymphatic, Left Upper Extremity
  use Lymphatic, Right Upper Extremity
Cubital nerve *use* Ulnar Nerve
Cuboid bone
  use Tarsal, Left
  use Tarsal, Right
Cuboideonavicular joint
  use Tarsal Joint, Left
  use Tarsal Joint, Right
Culdocentesis *see* Drainage, Cul-de-sac 0U9F
Culdoplasty
  see Repair, Cul-de-sac 0UQF
  see Supplement, Cul-de-sac 0UUF
Culdoscopy 0UJH8ZZ
Culdotomy *see* Drainage, Cul-de-sac 0U9F
Culmen *use* Cerebellum
Cultured epidermal cell autograft *use* Autologous
    Tissue Substitute
Cuneiform cartilage *use* Larynx
Cuneonavicular joint
  use Joint, Tarsal, Left
  use Joint, Tarsal, Right
Cuneonavicular ligament
  use Foot Bursa and Ligament, Left
  use Foot Bursa and Ligament, Right
Curettage
  see Excision
  see Extraction
Cutaneous (transverse) cervical nerve *use* Cervical
    Plexus
CVP (central venous pressure) *see* Measurement,
    Venous 4A04
Cyclodiathermy *see* Destruction, Eye 085
Cyclophotocoagulation *see* Destruction, Eye 085
CYPHER® Stent *use* Intraluminal Device, Drug-eluting
    in Heart and Great Vessels
Cystectomy
  see Excision, Bladder 0TBB
  see Resection, Bladder 0TTB
Cystocele repair *see* Repair, Subcutaneous Tissue and
    Fascia, Pelvic Region 0JQC
Cystography
  see Fluoroscopy, Urinary System BT1
  see Plain Radiography, Urinary System BT0
Cystolithotomy *see* Extirpation, Bladder 0TCB
Cystopexy
  see Repair, Bladder 0TQB
  see Reposition, Bladder 0TSB
Cystoplasty
  see Repair, Bladder 0TQB
  see Replacement, Bladder 0TRB
  see Supplement, Bladder 0TUB

Cystorrhaphy *see* Repair, Bladder 0TQB
Cystoscopy 0TJB8ZZ
Cystostomy *see* Bypass, Bladder 0T1B
Cystostomy Tube *use* Drainage Device
Cystotomy *see* Drainage, Bladder 0T9B
Cystourethrography
  see Fluoroscopy, Urinary System BT1
  see Plain Radiography, Urinary System BT0
Cystourethroplasty
  see Repair, Urinary System 0TQ
  see Replacement, Urinary System 0TR
  see Supplement, Urinary System 0TU
Cytarabine and Daunorubicin Liposome Antineo-
    plastic XW0

D

DBS lead *use* Neurostimulator Lead in Central Nervous
    System and Cranial Nerves
DeBakey Left Ventricular Assist Device *use* Im-
    plantable Heart Assist System in Heart and Great
    Vessels
Debridement
  Excisional *see* Excision
  Non-excisional *see* Extraction
Decompression, Circulatory 6A15
Decortication, lung
  see Extirpation, Respiratory System 0BC
  see Release, Respiratory System 0BN
Deep brain neurostimulator lead *use* Neurostimula-
    tor Lead in Central Nervous System and Cranial
    Nerves
Deep cervical fascia
  use Subcutaneous Tissue and Fascia, Left Neck
  use Subcutaneous Tissue and Fascia, Right Neck
Deep cervical vein
  use Vertebral Vein, Left
  use Vertebral Vein, Right
Deep circumflex iliac artery
  use External Iliac Artery, Left
  use External Iliac Artery, Right
Deep facial vein
  use Face Vein, Left
  use Face Vein, Right
Deep femoral artery
  use Femoral Artery, Left
  use Femoral Artery, Right
Deep femoral (profunda femoris) vein
  use Femoral Vein, Left
  use Femoral Vein, Right
Deep Inferior Epigastric Artery Perforator Flap
  Replacement
    Bilateral 0HRV077
    Left 0HRU077
    Right 0HRT077
  Transfer
    Left 0KXG
    Right 0KXF
Deep palmar arch
  use Hand Artery, Left
  use Hand Artery, Right
Deep transverse perineal muscle *use* Perineum
    Muscle
Deferential artery
  use Internal Iliac Artery, Left
  use Internal Iliac Artery, Right
Defibrillator Generator
  Abdomen 0JH8
  Chest 0JH6
Defibrotide Sodium Anticoagulant XW0
Defibtech Automated Chest Compression (ACC)
    device 5A1221J
Defitelio *use* Defibrotide Sodium Anticoagulant
Delivery
  Cesarean *see* Extraction, Products of Conception
    10D0
  Forceps *see* Extraction, Products of Conception
    10D0
  Manually assisted 10E0XZZ
  Products of Conception 10E0XZZ
  Vacuum assisted *see* Extraction, Products of Con-
    ception 10D0
Delta frame external fixator
  use External Fixation Device, Hybrid in 0PH
  use External Fixation Device, Hybrid in 0PS
  use External Fixation Device, Hybrid in 0QH

Delta frame external fixator — *continued*
  use External Fixation Device, Hybrid in 0QS
Delta III Reverse shoulder prosthesis *use* Synthetic
    Substitute, Reverse Ball and Socket in 0RR
Deltoid fascia
  use Subcutaneous Tissue and Fascia, Left Upper
    Arm
  use Subcutaneous Tissue and Fascia, Right Upper
    Arm
Deltoid ligament
  use Ankle Bursa and Ligament, Left
  use Ankle Bursa and Ligament, Right
Deltoid muscle
  use Shoulder Muscle, Left
  use Shoulder Muscle, Right
Deltopectoral (infraclavicular) lymph node
  use Lymphatic, Left Upper Extremity
  use Lymphatic, Right Upper Extremity
Denervation
  Cranial nerve *see* Destruction, Central Nervous
    System and Cranial Nerves 005
  Peripheral nerve *see* Destruction, Peripheral Ner-
    vous System 015
Dens *use* Cervical Vertebra
Densitometry
  Plain Radiography
    Femur
      Left BQ04ZZ1
      Right BQ03ZZ1
    Hip
      Left BQ01ZZ1
      Right BQ00ZZ1
    Spine
      Cervical BR00ZZ1
      Lumbar BR09ZZ1
      Thoracic BR07ZZ1
      Whole BR0GZZ1
  Ultrasonography
    Elbow
      Left BP4HZZ1
      Right BP4GZZ1
    Hand
      Left BP4PZZ1
      Right BP4NZZ1
    Shoulder
      Left BP49ZZ1
      Right BP48ZZ1
    Wrist
      Left BP4MZZ1
      Right BP4LZZ1
Denticulate (dentate) ligament *use* Spinal Meninges
Depressor anguli oris muscle *use* Facial Muscle
Depressor labii inferioris muscle *use* Facial Muscle
Depressor septi nasi muscle *use* Facial Muscle
Depressor supercilii muscle *use* Facial Muscle
Dermabrasion *see* Extraction, Skin and Breast 0HD
Dermis *use* Skin
Descending genicular artery
  use Femoral Artery, Left
  use Femoral Artery, Right
Destruction
  Acetabulum
    Left 0Q55
    Right 0Q54
  Adenoids 0C5Q
  Ampulla of Vater 0F5C
  Anal Sphincter 0D5R
  Anterior Chamber
    Left 08533ZZ
    Right 08523ZZ
  Anus 0D5Q
  Aorta
    Abdominal
    Thoracic
      Ascending/Arch 025X
      Descending 025W
  Aortic Body 0G5D
  Appendix 0D5J
  Artery
    Anterior Tibial
      Left 045Q
      Right 045P
    Axillary
      Left 0356
      Right 0355
    Brachial
      Left 0358
      Right 0357

Subterms under main terms may continue to next column or pag

Destruction — continued

Artery — continued
- Celiac Ø451
- Colic
  - Left Ø457
  - Middle Ø458
  - Right Ø456
- Common Carotid
  - Left Ø35J
  - Right Ø35H
- Common Iliac
  - Left Ø45D
  - Right Ø45C
- External Carotid
  - Left Ø35N
  - Right Ø35M
- External Iliac
  - Left Ø45J
  - Right Ø45H
- Face Ø35R
- Femoral
  - Left Ø45L
  - Right Ø45K
- Foot
  - Left Ø45W
  - Right Ø45V
- Gastric Ø452
- Hand
  - Left Ø35F
  - Right Ø35D
- Hepatic Ø453
- Inferior Mesenteric Ø45B
- Innominate Ø352
- Internal Carotid
  - Left Ø35L
  - Right Ø35K
- Internal Iliac
  - Left Ø45F
  - Right Ø45E
- Internal Mammary
  - Left Ø351
  - Right Ø350
- Intracranial Ø35G
- Lower Ø45Y
- Peroneal
  - Left Ø45U
  - Right Ø45T
- Popliteal
  - Left Ø45N
  - Right Ø45M
- Posterior Tibial
  - Left Ø45S
  - Right Ø45R
- Pulmonary
  - Left Ø25R
  - Right Ø25Q
- Pulmonary Trunk Ø25P
- Radial
  - Left Ø35C
  - Right Ø35B
- Renal
  - Left Ø45A
  - Right Ø459
- Splenic Ø454
- Subclavian
  - Left Ø354
  - Right Ø353
- Superior Mesenteric Ø455
- Temporal
  - Left Ø35T
  - Right Ø35S
- Thyroid
  - Left Ø35V
  - Right Ø35U
- Ulnar
  - Left Ø35A
  - Right Ø359
- Upper Ø35Y
- Vertebral
  - Left Ø35Q
  - Right Ø35P

Atrium
- Left Ø257
- Right Ø256

Auditory Ossicle
- Left Ø95A
- Right Ø959

Basal Ganglia ØØ58

Bladder ØT5B

Destruction — continued

Bladder Neck ØT5C

Bone
- Ethmoid
  - Left ØN5G
  - Right ØN5F
- Frontal ØN51
- Hyoid ØN5X
- Lacrimal
  - Left ØN5J
  - Right ØN5H
- Nasal ØN5B
- Occipital ØN57
- Palatine
  - Left ØN5L
  - Right ØN5K
- Parietal
  - Left ØN54
  - Right ØN53
- Pelvic
  - Left ØQ53
  - Right ØQ52
- Sphenoid ØN5C
- Temporal
  - Left ØN56
  - Right ØN55
- Zygomatic
  - Left ØN5N
  - Right ØN5M

Brain ØØ50

Breast
- Bilateral ØH5V
- Left ØH5U
- Right ØH5T

Bronchus
- Lingula ØB59
- Lower Lobe
  - Left ØB5B
  - Right ØB56
- Main
  - Left ØB57
  - Right ØB53
- Middle Lobe, Right ØB55
- Upper Lobe
  - Left ØB58
  - Right ØB54

Buccal Mucosa ØC54

Bursa and Ligament
- Abdomen
  - Left ØM5J
  - Right ØM5H
- Ankle
  - Left ØM5R
  - Right ØM5Q
- Elbow
  - Left ØM54
  - Right ØM53
- Foot
  - Left ØM5T
  - Right ØM5S
- Hand
  - Left ØM58
  - Right ØM57
- Head and Neck ØM50
- Hip
  - Left ØM5M
  - Right ØM5L
- Knee
  - Left ØM5P
  - Right ØM5N
- Lower Extremity
  - Left ØM5W
  - Right ØM5V
- Perineum ØM5K
- Rib(s) ØM5G
- Shoulder
  - Left ØM52
  - Right ØM51
- Spine
  - Lower ØM5D
  - Upper ØM5C
- Sternum ØM5F
- Upper Extremity
  - Left ØM5B
  - Right ØM59
- Wrist
  - Left ØM56
  - Right ØM55

Carina ØB52

Destruction — continued

Carotid Bodies, Bilateral ØG58

Carotid Body
- Left ØG56
- Right ØG57

Carpal
- Left ØP5N
- Right ØP5M

Cecum ØD5H

Cerebellum ØØ5C

Cerebral Hemisphere ØØ57

Cerebral Meninges ØØ51

Cerebral Ventricle ØØ56

Cervix ØU5C

Chordae Tendineae Ø259

Choroid
- Left Ø85B
- Right Ø85A

Cisterna Chyli Ø75L

Clavicle
- Left ØP5B
- Right ØP59

Clitoris ØU5J

Coccygeal Glomus ØG5B

Coccyx ØQ5S

Colon
- Ascending ØD5K
- Descending ØD5M
- Sigmoid ØD5N
- Transverse ØD5L

Conduction Mechanism Ø258

Conjunctiva
- Left Ø85TXZZ
- Right Ø85SXZZ

Cord
- Bilateral ØV5H
- Left ØV5G
- Right ØV5F

Cornea
- Left Ø859XZZ
- Right Ø858XZZ

Cul-de-sac ØU5F

Diaphragm ØB5T

Disc
- Cervical Vertebral ØR53
- Cervicothoracic Vertebral ØR55
- Lumbar Vertebral ØS52
- Lumbosacral ØS54
- Thoracic Vertebral ØR59
- Thoracolumbar Vertebral ØR5B

Duct
- Common Bile ØF59
- Cystic ØF58
- Hepatic
  - Common ØF57
  - Left ØF56
  - Right ØF55
- Lacrimal
  - Left Ø85Y
  - Right Ø85X
- Pancreatic ØF5D
  - Accessory ØF5F
- Parotid
  - Left ØC5C
  - Right ØC5B

Duodenum ØD59

Dura Mater ØØ52

Ear
- External
  - Left Ø951
  - Right Ø950
- External Auditory Canal
  - Left Ø954
  - Right Ø953
- Inner
  - Left Ø95E
  - Right Ø95D
- Middle
  - Left Ø956
  - Right Ø955

Endometrium ØU5B

Epididymis
- Bilateral ØV5L
- Left ØV5K
- Right ØV5J

Epiglottis ØC5R

Esophagogastric Junction ØD54

Esophagus ØD55
- Lower ØD53

Destruction — *continued*
- Esophagus — *continued*
  - Middle ØD52
  - Upper ØD51
- Eustachian Tube
  - Left Ø95G
  - Right Ø95F
- Eye
  - Left Ø851XZZ
  - Right Ø850XZZ
- Eyelid
  - Lower
    - Left Ø85R
    - Right Ø85Q
  - Upper
    - Left Ø85P
    - Right Ø85N
- Fallopian Tube
  - Left ØU56
  - Right ØU55
- Fallopian Tubes, Bilateral ØU57
- Femoral Shaft
  - Left ØQ59
  - Right ØQ58
- Femur
  - Lower
    - Left ØQ5C
    - Right ØQ5B
  - Upper
    - Left ØQ57
    - Right ØQ56
- Fibula
  - Left ØQ5K
  - Right ØQ5J
- Finger Nail ØH5QXZZ
- Gallbladder ØF54
- Gingiva
  - Lower ØC56
  - Upper ØC55
- Gland
  - Adrenal
    - Bilateral ØG54
    - Left ØG52
    - Right ØG53
  - Lacrimal
    - Left Ø85W
    - Right Ø85V
  - Minor Salivary ØC5J
  - Parotid
    - Left ØC59
    - Right ØC58
  - Pituitary ØG50
  - Sublingual
    - Left ØC5F
    - Right ØC5D
  - Submaxillary
    - Left ØC5H
    - Right ØC5G
  - Vestibular ØU5L
- Glenoid Cavity
  - Left ØP58
  - Right ØP57
- Glomus Jugulare ØG5C
- Humeral Head
  - Left ØP5D
  - Right ØP5C
- Humeral Shaft
  - Left ØP5G
  - Right ØP5F
- Hymen ØU5K
- Hypothalamus ØØ5A
- Ileocecal Valve ØD5C
- Ileum ØD5B
- Intestine
  - Large ØD5E
    - Left ØD5G
    - Right ØD5F
  - Small ØD58
- Iris
  - Left Ø85D3ZZ
  - Right Ø85C3ZZ
- Jejunum ØD5A
- Joint
  - Acromioclavicular
    - Left ØR5H
    - Right ØR5G
  - Ankle
    - Left ØS5G
    - Right ØS5F

Destruction — *continued*
- Joint — *continued*
  - Carpal
    - Left ØR5R
    - Right ØR5Q
  - Carpometacarpal
    - Left ØR5T
    - Right ØR5S
  - Cervical Vertebral ØR51
  - Cervicothoracic Vertebral ØR54
  - Coccygeal ØS56
  - Elbow
    - Left ØR5M
    - Right ØR5L
  - Finger Phalangeal
    - Left ØR5X
    - Right ØR5W
  - Hip
    - Left ØS5B
    - Right ØS59
  - Knee
    - Left ØS5D
    - Right ØS5C
  - Lumbar Vertebral ØS50
  - Lumbosacral ØS53
  - Metacarpophalangeal
    - Left ØR5V
    - Right ØR5U
  - Metatarsal-Phalangeal
    - Left ØS5N
    - Right ØS5M
  - Occipital-cervical ØR50
  - Sacrococcygeal ØS55
  - Sacroiliac
    - Left ØS58
    - Right ØS57
  - Shoulder
    - Left ØR5K
    - Right ØR5J
  - Sternoclavicular
    - Left ØR5F
    - Right ØR5E
  - Tarsal
    - Left ØS5J
    - Right ØS5H
  - Tarsometatarsal
    - Left ØS5L
    - Right ØS5K
  - Temporomandibular
    - Left ØR5D
    - Right ØR5C
  - Thoracic Vertebral ØR56
  - Thoracolumbar Vertebral ØR5A
  - Toe Phalangeal
    - Left ØS5Q
    - Right ØS5P
  - Wrist
    - Left ØR5P
    - Right ØR5N
- Kidney
  - Left ØT51
  - Right ØT50
- Kidney Pelvis
  - Left ØT54
  - Right ØT53
- Larynx ØC5S
- Lens
  - Left Ø85K3ZZ
  - Right Ø85J3ZZ
- Lip
  - Lower ØC51
  - Upper ØC50
- Liver ØF50
  - Left Lobe ØF52
  - Right Lobe ØF51
- Lung
  - Bilateral ØB5M
  - Left ØB5L
  - Lower Lobe
    - Left ØB5J
    - Right ØB5F
  - Middle Lobe, Right ØB5D
  - Right ØB5K
  - Upper Lobe
    - Left ØB5G
    - Right ØB5C
- Lung Lingula ØB5H
- Lymphatic
  - Aortic Ø75D

Destruction — *continued*
- Lymphatic — *continued*
  - Axillary
    - Left Ø756
    - Right Ø755
  - Head Ø750
  - Inguinal
    - Left Ø75J
    - Right Ø75H
  - Internal Mammary
    - Left Ø759
    - Right Ø758
  - Lower Extremity
    - Left Ø75G
    - Right Ø75F
  - Mesenteric Ø75B
  - Neck
    - Left Ø752
    - Right Ø751
  - Pelvis Ø75C
  - Thoracic Duct Ø75K
  - Thorax Ø757
  - Upper Extremity
    - Left Ø754
    - Right Ø753
- Mandible
  - Left ØN5V
  - Right ØN5T
- Maxilla ØN5R
- Medulla Oblongata ØØ5D
- Mesentery ØD5V
- Metacarpal
  - Left ØP5Q
  - Right ØP5P
- Metatarsal
  - Left ØQ5P
  - Right ØQ5N
- Muscle
  - Abdomen
    - Left ØK5L
    - Right ØK5K
  - Extraocular
    - Left Ø85M
    - Right Ø85L
  - Facial ØK51
  - Foot
    - Left ØK5W
    - Right ØK5V
  - Hand
    - Left ØK5D
    - Right ØK5C
  - Head ØK50
  - Hip
    - Left ØK5P
    - Right ØK5N
  - Lower Arm and Wrist
    - Left ØK5B
    - Right ØK59
  - Lower Leg
    - Left ØK5T
    - Right ØK5S
  - Neck
    - Left ØK53
    - Right ØK52
  - Papillary Ø25D
  - Perineum ØK5M
  - Shoulder
    - Left ØK56
    - Right ØK55
  - Thorax
    - Left ØK5J
    - Right ØK5H
  - Tongue, Palate, Pharynx ØK54
  - Trunk
    - Left ØK5G
    - Right ØK5F
  - Upper Arm
    - Left ØK58
    - Right ØK57
  - Upper Leg
    - Left ØK5R
    - Right ØK5Q
- Nasal Mucosa and Soft Tissue Ø95K
- Nasopharynx Ø95N
- Nerve
  - Abdominal Sympathetic Ø15M
  - Abducens ØØ5L
  - Accessory ØØ5R
  - Acoustic ØØ5N

▼ **Subterms under main terms may continue to next column or pag**

Destruction — continued
Nerve — continued
    Brachial Plexus 0153
    Cervical 0151
    Cervical Plexus 0150
    Facial 005M
    Femoral 015D
    Glossopharyngeal 005P
    Head and Neck Sympathetic 015K
    Hypoglossal 005S
    Lumbar 015B
    Lumbar Plexus 0159
    Lumbar Sympathetic 015N
    Lumbosacral Plexus 015A
    Median 0155
    Oculomotor 005H
    Olfactory 005F
    Optic 005G
    Peroneal 015H
    Phrenic 0152
    Pudendal 015C
    Radial 0156
    Sacral 015R
    Sacral Plexus 015Q
    Sacral Sympathetic 015P
    Sciatic 015F
    Thoracic 0158
    Thoracic Sympathetic 015L
    Tibial 015G
    Trigeminal 005K
    Trochlear 005J
    Ulnar 0154
    Vagus 005Q
Nipple
    Left 0H5X
    Right 0H5W
Omentum 0D5U
Orbit
    Left 0N5Q
    Right 0N5P
Ovary
    Bilateral 0U52
    Left 0U51
    Right 0U50
Palate
    Hard 0C52
    Soft 0C53
Pancreas 0F5G
Para-aortic Body 0G59
Paraganglion Extremity 0G5F
Parathyroid Gland 0G5R
    Inferior
        Left 0G5P
        Right 0G5N
    Multiple 0G5Q
    Superior
        Left 0G5M
        Right 0G5L
Patella
    Left 0Q5F
    Right 0Q5D
Penis 0V5S
Pericardium 025N
Peritoneum 0D5W
Phalanx
    Finger
        Left 0P5V
        Right 0P5T
    Thumb
        Left 0P5S
        Right 0P5R
    Toe
        Left 0Q5R
        Right 0Q5Q
Pharynx 0C5M
Pineal Body 0G51
Pleura
    Left 0B5P
    Right 0B5N
Pons 005B
Prepuce 0V5T
Prostate 0V50
    Robotic Waterjet Ablation XV508A4
Radius
    Left 0P5J
    Right 0P5H
Rectum 0D5P
Retina
    Left 085F3ZZ

Destruction — continued
Retina — continued
    Right 085E3ZZ
Retinal Vessel
    Left 085H3ZZ
    Right 085G3ZZ
Ribs
    1 to 2 0P51
    3 or More 0P52
Sacrum 0Q51
Scapula
    Left 0P56
    Right 0P55
Sclera
    Left 0857XZZ
    Right 0856XZZ
Scrotum 0V55
Septum
    Atrial 0255
    Nasal 095M
    Ventricular 025M
Sinus
    Accessory 095P
    Ethmoid
        Left 095V
        Right 095U
    Frontal
        Left 095T
        Right 095S
    Mastoid
        Left 095C
        Right 095B
    Maxillary
        Left 095R
        Right 095Q
    Sphenoid
        Left 095X
        Right 095W
Skin
    Abdomen 0H57XZ
    Back 0H56XZ
    Buttock 0H58XZ
    Chest 0H55XZ
    Ear
        Left 0H53XZ
        Right 0H52XZ
    Face 0H51XZ
    Foot
        Left 0H5NXZ
        Right 0H5MXZ
    Hand
        Left 0H5GXZ
        Right 0H5FXZ
    Inguinal 0H5AXZ
    Lower Arm
        Left 0H5EXZ
        Right 0H5DXZ
    Lower Leg
        Left 0H5LXZ
        Right 0H5KXZ
    Neck 0H54XZ
    Perineum 0H59XZ
    Scalp 0H50XZ
    Upper Arm
        Left 0H5CXZ
        Right 0H5BXZ
    Upper Leg
        Left 0H5JXZ
        Right 0H5HXZ
Skull 0N50
Spinal Cord
    Cervical 005W
    Lumbar 005Y
    Thoracic 005X
Spinal Meninges 005T
Spleen 075P
Sternum 0P50
Stomach 0D56
    Pylorus 0D57
Subcutaneous Tissue and Fascia
    Abdomen 0J58
    Back 0J57
    Buttock 0J59
    Chest 0J56
    Face 0J51
    Foot
        Left 0J5R
        Right 0J5Q

Destruction — continued
Subcutaneous Tissue and Fascia — continued
    Hand
        Left 0J5K
        Right 0J5J
    Lower Arm
        Left 0J5H
        Right 0J5G
    Lower Leg
        Left 0J5P
        Right 0J5N
    Neck
        Left 0J55
        Right 0J54
    Pelvic Region 0J5C
    Perineum 0J5B
    Scalp 0J50
    Upper Arm
        Left 0J5F
        Right 0J5D
    Upper Leg
        Left 0J5M
        Right 0J5L
Tarsal
    Left 0Q5M
    Right 0Q5L
Tendon
    Abdomen
        Left 0L5G
        Right 0L5F
    Ankle
        Left 0L5T
        Right 0L5S
    Foot
        Left 0L5W
        Right 0L5V
    Hand
        Left 0L58
        Right 0L57
    Head and Neck 0L50
    Hip
        Left 0L5K
        Right 0L5J
    Knee
        Left 0L5R
        Right 0L5Q
    Lower Arm and Wrist
        Left 0L56
        Right 0L55
    Lower Leg
        Left 0L5P
        Right 0L5N
    Perineum 0L5H
    Shoulder
        Left 0L52
        Right 0L51
    Thorax
        Left 0L5D
        Right 0L5C
    Trunk
        Left 0L5B
        Right 0L59
    Upper Arm
        Left 0L54
        Right 0L53
    Upper Leg
        Left 0L5M
        Right 0L5L
Testis
    Bilateral 0V5C
    Left 0V5B
    Right 0V59
Thalamus 0059
Thymus 075M
Thyroid Gland 0G5K
    Left Lobe 0G5G
    Right Lobe 0G5H
Tibia
    Left 0Q5H
    Right 0Q5G
Toe Nail 0H5RXZZ
Tongue 0C57
Tonsils 0C5P
Tooth
    Lower 0C5X
    Upper 0C5W
Trachea 0B51
Tunica Vaginalis
    Left 0V57

Destruction — *continued*
 Tunica Vaginalis — *continued*
  Right 0V56
 Turbinate, Nasal 095L
 Tympanic Membrane
  Left 0958
  Right 0957
 Ulna
  Left 0P5L
  Right 0P5K
 Ureter
  Left 0T57
  Right 0T56
 Urethra 0T5D
 Uterine Supporting Structure 0U54
 Uterus 0U59
 Uvula 0C5N
 Vagina 0U5G
 Valve
  Aortic 025F
  Mitral 025G
  Pulmonary 025H
  Tricuspid 025J
 Vas Deferens
  Bilateral 0V5Q
  Left 0V5P
  Right 0V5N
 Vein
  Axillary
   Left 0558
   Right 0557
  Azygos 0550
  Basilic
   Left 055C
   Right 055B
  Brachial
   Left 055A
   Right 0559
  Cephalic
   Left 055F
   Right 055D
  Colic 0657
  Common Iliac
   Left 065D
   Right 065C
  Coronary 0254
  Esophageal 0653
  External Iliac
   Left 065G
   Right 065F
  External Jugular
   Left 055Q
   Right 055P
  Face
   Left 055V
   Right 055T
  Femoral
   Left 065N
   Right 065M
  Foot
   Left 065V
   Right 065T
  Gastric 0652
  Hand
   Left 055H
   Right 055G
  Hemiazygos 0551
  Hepatic 0654
  Hypogastric
   Left 065J
   Right 065H
  Inferior Mesenteric 0656
  Innominate
   Left 0554
   Right 0553
  Internal Jugular
   Left 055N
   Right 055M
  Intracranial 055L
  Lower 065Y
  Portal 0658
  Pulmonary
   Left 025T
   Right 025S
  Renal
   Left 065B
   Right 0659
  Saphenous
   Left 065Q

Destruction — *continued*
 Vein — *continued*
  Saphenous — *continued*
   Right 065P
  Splenic 0651
  Subclavian
   Left 0556
   Right 0555
  Superior Mesenteric 0655
  Upper 055Y
  Vertebral
   Left 055S
   Right 055R
 Vena Cava
  Inferior 0650
  Superior 025V
 Ventricle
  Left 025L
  Right 025K
 Vertebra
  Cervical 0P53
  Lumbar 0Q50
  Thoracic 0P54
 Vesicle
  Bilateral 0V53
  Left 0V52
  Right 0V51
 Vitreous
  Left 08553ZZ
  Right 08543ZZ
 Vocal Cord
  Left 0C5V
  Right 0C5T
 Vulva 0U5M

Detachment
 Arm
  Lower
   Left 0X6F0Z
   Right 0X6D0Z
  Upper
   Left 0X690Z
   Right 0X680Z
 Elbow Region
  Left 0X6C0ZZ
  Right 0X6B0ZZ
 Femoral Region
  Left 0Y680ZZ
  Right 0Y670ZZ
 Finger
  Index
   Left 0X6P0Z
   Right 0X6N0Z
  Little
   Left 0X6W0Z
   Right 0X6V0Z
  Middle
   Left 0X6R0Z
   Right 0X6Q0Z
  Ring
   Left 0X6T0Z
   Right 0X6S0Z
 Foot
  Left 0Y6N0Z
  Right 0Y6M0Z
 Forequarter
  Left 0X610ZZ
  Right 0X600ZZ
 Hand
  Left 0X6K0Z
  Right 0X6J0Z
 Hindquarter
  Bilateral 0Y640ZZ
  Left 0Y630ZZ
  Right 0Y620ZZ
 Knee Region
  Left 0Y6G0ZZ
  Right 0Y6F0ZZ
 Leg
  Lower
   Left 0Y6J0Z
   Right 0Y6H0Z
  Upper
   Left 0Y6D0Z
   Right 0Y6C0Z
 Shoulder Region
  Left 0X630ZZ
  Right 0X620ZZ
 Thumb
  Left 0X6M0Z

Detachment — *continued*
 Thumb — *continued*
  Right 0X6L0Z
 Toe
  1st
   Left 0Y6Q0Z
   Right 0Y6P0Z
  2nd
   Left 0Y6S0Z
   Right 0Y6R0Z
  3rd
   Left 0Y6U0Z
   Right 0Y6T0Z
  4th
   Left 0Y6W0Z
   Right 0Y6V0Z
  5th
   Left 0Y6Y0Z
   Right 0Y6X0Z
Determination, Mental status GZ14ZZZ
Detorsion
 see Release
 see Reposition
Detoxification Services, for substance abuse
 HZ2ZZZZ
Device Fitting F0DZ
Diagnostic Audiology *see* Audiology, Diagnostic
Diagnostic imaging *see* Imaging, Diagnostic
Diagnostic radiology *see* Imaging, Diagnostic
Dialysis
 Hemodialysis *see* Performance, Urinary 5A1D
 Peritoneal 3E1M39Z
Diaphragma sellae *use* Dura Mater
Diaphragmatic pacemaker generator *use* Stimulator
 Generator in Subcutaneous Tissue and Fascia
Diaphragmatic Pacemaker Lead
 Insertion of device in, Diaphragm 0BHT
 Removal of device from, Diaphragm 0BPT
 Revision of device in, Diaphragm 0BWT
Digital radiography, plain *see* Plain Radiography
Dilation
 Ampulla of Vater 0F7C
 Anus 0D7Q
 Aorta
  Abdominal
  Thoracic
   Ascending/Arch 027X
   Descending 027W
 Artery
  Anterior Tibial
   Left 047Q
    Sustained Release Drug-eluting
     Intraluminal Device
     X27Q385
     Four or More X27Q3C5
     Three X27Q3B5
     Two X27Q395
   Right 047P
    Sustained Release Drug-eluting
     Intraluminal Device
     X27P385
     Four or More X27P3C5
     Three X27P3B5
     Two X27P395
  Axillary
   Left 0376
   Right 0375
  Brachial
   Left 0378
   Right 0377
  Celiac 0471
  Colic
   Left 0477
   Middle 0478
   Right 0476
  Common Carotid
   Left 037J
   Right 037H
  Common Iliac
   Left 047D
   Right 047C
  Coronary
   Four or More Arteries 0273
   One Artery 0270
   Three Arteries 0272
   Two Arteries 0271
  External Carotid
   Left 037N

Dilation — *continued*
  Vein — *continued*
    Hypogastric
      Left 067J
      Right 067H
    Inferior Mesenteric 0676
    Innominate
      Left 0574
      Right 0573
    Internal Jugular
      Left 057N
      Right 057M
    Intracranial 057L
    Lower 067Y
    Portal 0678
    Pulmonary
      Left 027T
      Right 027S
    Renal
      Left 067B
      Right 0679
    Saphenous
      Left 067Q
      Right 067P
    Splenic 0671
    Subclavian
      Left 0576
      Right 0575
    Superior Mesenteric 0675
    Upper 057Y
    Vertebral
      Left 057S
      Right 057R
  Vena Cava
    Inferior 0670
    Superior 027V
  Ventricle
    Left 027L
    Right 027K
Direct Lateral Interbody Fusion (DLIF) device *use*
  Interbody Fusion Device in Lower Joints
Disarticulation *see* Detachment
Discectomy, diskectomy
  see Excision, Lower Joints 0SB
  see Excision, Upper Joints 0RB
  see Resection, Lower Joints 0ST
  see Resection, Upper Joints 0RT
Discography
  see Fluoroscopy, Axial Skeleton, Except Skull and
    Facial Bones BR1
  see Plain Radiography, Axial Skeleton, Except Skull
    and Facial Bones BR0
Dismembered pyeloplasty *see* Repair, Kidney Pelvis
Distal humerus
  use Humeral Shaft, Left
  use Humeral Shaft, Right
Distal humerus, involving joint
  use Elbow Joint, Left
  use Elbow Joint, Right
Distal radioulnar joint
  use Wrist Joint, Left
  use Wrist Joint, Right
Diversion *see* Bypass
Diverticulectomy *see* Excision, Gastrointestinal System
  0DB
Division
  Acetabulum
    Left 0Q85
    Right 0Q84
  Anal Sphincter 0D8R
  Basal Ganglia 0088
  Bladder Neck 0T8C
  Bone
    Ethmoid
      Left 0N8G
      Right 0N8F
    Frontal 0N81
    Hyoid 0N8X
    Lacrimal
      Left 0N8J
      Right 0N8H
    Nasal 0N8B
    Occipital 0N87
    Palatine
      Left 0N8L
      Right 0N8K
    Parietal
      Left 0N84

Division — *continued*
  Bone
    Parietal — *continued*
      Right 0N83
    Pelvic
      Left 0Q83
      Right 0Q82
    Sphenoid 0N8C
    Temporal
      Left 0N86
      Right 0N85
    Zygomatic
      Left 0N8N
      Right 0N8M
  Brain 0080
  Bursa and Ligament
    Abdomen
      Left 0M8J
      Right 0M8H
    Ankle
      Left 0M8R
      Right 0M8Q
    Elbow
      Left 0M84
      Right 0M83
    Foot
      Left 0M8T
      Right 0M8S
    Hand
      Left 0M88
      Right 0M87
    Head and Neck 0M80
    Hip
      Left 0M8M
      Right 0M8L
    Knee
      Left 0M8P
      Right 0M8N
    Lower Extremity
      Left 0M8W
      Right 0M8V
    Perineum 0M8K
    Rib(s) 0M8G
    Shoulder
      Left 0M82
      Right 0M81
    Spine
      Lower 0M8D
      Upper 0M8C
    Sternum 0M8F
    Upper Extremity
      Left 0M8B
      Right 0M89
    Wrist
      Left 0M86
      Right 0M85
  Carpal
    Left 0P8N
    Right 0P8M
  Cerebral Hemisphere 0087
  Chordae Tendineae 0289
  Clavicle
    Left 0P8B
    Right 0P89
  Coccyx 0Q8S
  Conduction Mechanism 0288
  Esophagogastric Junction 0D84
  Femoral Shaft
    Left 0Q89
    Right 0Q88
  Femur
    Lower
      Left 0Q8C
      Right 0Q8B
    Upper
      Left 0Q87
      Right 0Q86
  Fibula
    Left 0Q8K
    Right 0Q8J
  Gland, Pituitary 0G80
  Glenoid Cavity
    Left 0P88
    Right 0P87
  Humeral Head
    Left 0P8D
    Right 0P8C
  Humeral Shaft
    Left 0P8G

Division — *continued*
  Humeral Shaft — *continued*
    Right 0P8F
  Hymen 0U8K
  Kidneys, Bilateral 0T82
  Liver 0F80
    Left Lobe 0F82
    Right Lobe 0F81
  Mandible
    Left 0N8V
    Right 0N8T
  Maxilla 0N8R
  Metacarpal
    Left 0P8Q
    Right 0P8P
  Metatarsal
    Left 0Q8P
    Right 0Q8N
  Muscle
    Abdomen
      Left 0K8L
      Right 0K8K
    Facial 0K81
    Foot
      Left 0K8W
      Right 0K8V
    Hand
      Left 0K8D
      Right 0K8C
    Head 0K80
    Hip
      Left 0K8P
      Right 0K8N
    Lower Arm and Wrist
      Left 0K8B
      Right 0K89
    Lower Leg
      Left 0K8T
      Right 0K8S
    Neck
      Left 0K83
      Right 0K82
    Papillary 028D
    Perineum 0K8M
    Shoulder
      Left 0K86
      Right 0K85
    Thorax
      Left 0K8J
      Right 0K8H
    Tongue, Palate, Pharynx 0K84
    Trunk
      Left 0K8G
      Right 0K8F
    Upper Arm
      Left 0K88
      Right 0K87
    Upper Leg
      Left 0K8R
      Right 0K8Q
  Nerve
    Abdominal Sympathetic 018M
    Abducens 008L
    Accessory 008R
    Acoustic 008N
    Brachial Plexus 0183
    Cervical 0181
    Cervical Plexus 0180
    Facial 008M
    Femoral 018D
    Glossopharyngeal 008P
    Head and Neck Sympathetic 018K
    Hypoglossal 008S
    Lumbar 018B
    Lumbar Plexus 0189
    Lumbar Sympathetic 018N
    Lumbosacral Plexus 018A
    Median 0185
    Oculomotor 008H
    Olfactory 008F
    Optic 008G
    Peroneal 018H
    Phrenic 0182
    Pudendal 018C
    Radial 0186
    Sacral 018R
    Sacral Plexus 018Q
    Sacral Sympathetic 018P
    Sciatic 018F

Division — *continued*
  Nerve — *continued*
    Thoracic 0188
    Thoracic Sympathetic 018L
    Tibial 018G
    Trigeminal 008K
    Trochlear 008J
    Ulnar 0184
    Vagus 008Q
  Orbit
    Left 0N8Q
    Right 0N8P
  Ovary
    Bilateral 0U82
    Left 0U81
    Right 0U80
  Pancreas 0F8G
  Patella
    Left 0Q8F
    Right 0Q8D
  Perineum, Female 0W8NXZZ
  Phalanx
    Finger
      Left 0P8V
      Right 0P8T
    Thumb
      Left 0P8S
      Right 0P8R
    Toe
      Left 0Q8R
      Right 0Q8Q
  Radius
    Left 0P8J
    Right 0P8H
  Ribs
    1 to 2 0P81
    3 or More 0P82
  Sacrum 0Q81
  Scapula
    Left 0P86
    Right 0P85
  Skin
    Abdomen 0H87XZZ
    Back 0H86XZZ
    Buttock 0H88XZZ
    Chest 0H85XZZ
    Ear
      Left 0H83XZZ
      Right 0H82XZZ
    Face 0H81XZZ
    Foot
      Left 0H8NXZZ
      Right 0H8MXZZ
    Hand
      Left 0H8GXZZ
      Right 0H8FXZZ
    Inguinal 0H8AXZZ
    Lower Arm
      Left 0H8EXZZ
      Right 0H8DXZZ
    Lower Leg
      Left 0H8LXZZ
      Right 0H8KXZZ
    Neck 0H84XZZ
    Perineum 0H89XZZ
    Scalp 0H80XZZ
    Upper Arm
      Left 0H8CXZZ
      Right 0H8BXZZ
    Upper Leg
      Left 0H8JXZZ
      Right 0H8HXZZ
  Skull 0N80
  Spinal Cord
    Cervical 008W
    Lumbar 008Y
    Thoracic 008X
  Sternum 0P80
  Stomach, Pylorus 0D87
  Subcutaneous Tissue and Fascia
    Abdomen 0J88
    Back 0J87
    Buttock 0J89
    Chest 0J86
    Face 0J81
    Foot
      Left 0J8R
      Right 0J8Q

Division — *continued*
  Subcutaneous Tissue and Fascia — *continued*
    Hand
      Left 0J8K
      Right 0J8J
    Head and Neck 0J8S
    Lower Arm
      Left 0J8H
      Right 0J8G
    Lower Extremity 0J8W
    Lower Leg
      Left 0J8P
      Right 0J8N
    Neck
      Left 0J85
      Right 0J84
    Pelvic Region 0J8C
    Perineum 0J8B
    Scalp 0J80
    Trunk 0J8T
    Upper Arm
      Left 0J8F
      Right 0J8D
    Upper Extremity 0J8V
    Upper Leg
      Left 0J8M
      Right 0J8L
  Tarsal
    Left 0Q8M
    Right 0Q8L
  Tendon
    Abdomen
      Left 0L8G
      Right 0L8F
    Ankle
      Left 0L8T
      Right 0L8S
    Foot
      Left 0L8W
      Right 0L8V
    Hand
      Left 0L88
      Right 0L87
    Head and Neck 0L80
    Hip
      Left 0L8K
      Right 0L8J
    Knee
      Left 0L8R
      Right 0L8Q
    Lower Arm and Wrist
      Left 0L86
      Right 0L85
    Lower Leg
      Left 0L8P
      Right 0L8N
    Perineum 0L8H
    Shoulder
      Left 0L82
      Right 0L81
    Thorax
      Left 0L8D
      Right 0L8C
    Trunk
      Left 0L8B
      Right 0L89
    Upper Arm
      Left 0L84
      Right 0L83
    Upper Leg
      Left 0L8M
      Right 0L8L
  Thyroid Gland Isthmus 0G8J
  Tibia
    Left 0Q8H
    Right 0Q8G
  Turbinate, Nasal 098L
  Ulna
    Left 0P8L
    Right 0P8K
  Uterine Supporting Structure 0U84
  Vertebra
    Cervical 0P83
    Lumbar 0Q80
    Thoracic 0P84
Doppler study *see* Ultrasonography
Dorsal digital nerve *use* Radial Nerve
Dorsal metacarpal vein
  use Hand Vein, Left

Dorsal metacarpal vein — *continued*
  use Hand Vein, Right
Dorsal metatarsal artery
  use Foot Artery, Left
  use Foot Artery, Right
Dorsal metatarsal vein
  use Foot Vein, Left
  use Foot Vein, Right
Dorsal root ganglion
  use Cervical Spinal Cord
  use Lumbar Spinal Cord
  use Spinal Cord
  use Thoracic Spinal Cord
Dorsal scapular artery
  use Subclavian Artery, Left
  use Subclavian Artery, Right
Dorsal scapular nerve *use* Brachial Plexus
Dorsal venous arch
  use Foot Vein, Left
  use Foot Vein, Right
Dorsalis pedis artery
  use Anterior Tibial Artery, Left
  use Anterior Tibial Artery, Right
DownStream® System 5A0512C, 5A0522C
Drainage
  Abdominal Wall 0W9F
  Acetabulum
    Left 0Q95
    Right 0Q94
  Adenoids 0C9Q
  Ampulla of Vater 0F9C
  Anal Sphincter 0D9R
  Ankle Region
    Left 0Y9L
    Right 0Y9K
  Anterior Chamber
    Left 0893
    Right 0892
  Anus 0D9Q
  Aorta, Abdominal 0490
  Aortic Body 0G9D
  Appendix 0D9J
  Arm
    Lower
      Left 0X9F
      Right 0X9D
    Upper
      Left 0X99
      Right 0X98
  Artery
    Anterior Tibial
      Left 049Q
      Right 049P
    Axillary
      Left 0396
      Right 0395
    Brachial
      Left 0398
      Right 0397
    Celiac 0491
    Colic
      Left 0497
      Middle 0498
      Right 0496
    Common Carotid
      Left 039J
      Right 039H
    Common Iliac
      Left 049D
      Right 049C
    External Carotid
      Left 039N
      Right 039M
    External Iliac
      Left 049J
      Right 049H
    Face 039R
    Femoral
      Left 049L
      Right 049K
    Foot
      Left 049W
      Right 049V
    Gastric 0492
    Hand
      Left 039F
      Right 039D
    Hepatic 0493

Drainage — *continued*
Artery — *continued*
Inferior Mesenteric 049B
Innominate 0392
Internal Carotid
Left 039L
Right 039K
Internal Iliac
Left 049F
Right 049E
Internal Mammary
Left 0391
Right 0390
Intracranial 039G
Lower 049Y
Peroneal
Left 049U
Right 049T
Popliteal
Left 049N
Right 049M
Posterior Tibial
Left 049S
Right 049R
Radial
Left 039C
Right 039B
Renal
Left 049A
Right 0499
Splenic 0494
Subclavian
Left 0394
Right 0393
Superior Mesenteric 0495
Temporal
Left 039T
Right 039S
Thyroid
Left 039V
Right 039U
Ulnar
Left 039A
Right 0399
Upper 039Y
Vertebral
Left 039Q
Right 039P
Auditory Ossicle
Left 099A
Right 0999
Axilla
Left 0X95
Right 0X94
Back
Lower 0W9L
Upper 0W9K
Basal Ganglia 0098
Bladder 0T9B
Bladder Neck 0T9C
Bone
Ethmoid
Left 0N9G
Right 0N9F
Frontal 0N91
Hyoid 0N9X
Lacrimal
Left 0N9J
Right 0N9H
Nasal 0N9B
Occipital 0N97
Palatine
Left 0N9L
Right 0N9K
Parietal
Left 0N94
Right 0N93
Pelvic
Left 0Q93
Right 0Q92
Sphenoid 0N9C
Temporal
Left 0N96
Right 0N95
Zygomatic
Left 0N9N
Right 0N9M
Bone Marrow 079T
Brain 0090

Drainage — *continued*
Breast
Bilateral 0H9V
Left 0H9U
Right 0H9T
Bronchus
Lingula 0B99
Lower Lobe
Left 0B9B
Right 0B96
Main
Left 0B97
Right 0B93
Middle Lobe, Right 0B95
Upper Lobe
Left 0B98
Right 0B94
Buccal Mucosa 0C94
Bursa and Ligament
Abdomen
Left 0M9J
Right 0M9H
Ankle
Left 0M9R
Right 0M9Q
Elbow
Left 0M94
Right 0M93
Foot
Left 0M9T
Right 0M9S
Hand
Left 0M98
Right 0M97
Head and Neck 0M90
Hip
Left 0M9M
Right 0M9L
Knee
Left 0M9P
Right 0M9N
Lower Extremity
Left 0M9W
Right 0M9V
Perineum 0M9K
Rib(s) 0M9G
Shoulder
Left 0M92
Right 0M91
Spine
Lower 0M9D
Upper 0M9C
Sternum 0M9F
Upper Extremity
Left 0M9B
Right 0M99
Wrist
Left 0M96
Right 0M95
Buttock
Left 0Y91
Right 0Y90
Carina 0B92
Carotid Bodies, Bilateral 0G98
Carotid Body
Left 0G96
Right 0G97
Carpal
Left 0P9N
Right 0P9M
Cavity, Cranial 0W91
Cecum 0D9H
Cerebellum 009C
Cerebral Hemisphere 0097
Cerebral Meninges 0091
Cerebral Ventricle 0096
Cervix 0U9C
Chest Wall 0W98
Choroid
Left 089B
Right 089A
Cisterna Chyli 079L
Clavicle
Left 0P9B
Right 0P99
Clitoris 0U9J
Coccygeal Glomus 0G9B
Coccyx 0Q9S

Drainage — *continued*
Colon
Ascending 0D9K
Descending 0D9M
Sigmoid 0D9N
Transverse 0D9L
Conjunctiva
Left 089T
Right 089S
Cord
Bilateral 0V9H
Left 0V9G
Right 0V9F
Cornea
Left 0899
Right 0898
Cul-de-sac 0U9F
Diaphragm 0B9T
Disc
Cervical Vertebral 0R93
Cervicothoracic Vertebral 0R95
Lumbar Vertebral 0S92
Lumbosacral 0S94
Thoracic Vertebral 0R99
Thoracolumbar Vertebral 0R9B
Duct
Common Bile 0F99
Cystic 0F98
Hepatic
Common 0F97
Left 0F96
Right 0F95
Lacrimal
Left 089Y
Right 089X
Pancreatic 0F9D
Accessory 0F9F
Parotid
Left 0C9C
Right 0C9B
Duodenum 0D99
Dura Mater 0092
Ear
External
Left 0991
Right 0990
External Auditory Canal
Left 0994
Right 0993
Inner
Left 099E
Right 099D
Middle
Left 0996
Right 0995
Elbow Region
Left 0X9C
Right 0X9B
Epididymis
Bilateral 0V9L
Left 0V9K
Right 0V9J
Epidural Space, Intracranial 0093
Epiglottis 0C9R
Esophagogastric Junction 0D94
Esophagus 0D95
Lower 0D93
Middle 0D92
Upper 0D91
Eustachian Tube
Left 099G
Right 099F
Extremity
Lower
Left 0Y9B
Right 0Y99
Upper
Left 0X97
Right 0X96
Eye
Left 0891
Right 0890
Eyelid
Lower
Left 089R
Right 089Q
Upper
Left 089P
Right 089N

▼ **Subterms under main terms may continue to next column or pag**

Drainage — *continued*
Face ØW92
Fallopian Tube
  Left ØU96
  Right ØU95
Fallopian Tubes, Bilateral ØU97
Femoral Region
  Left ØY98
  Right ØY97
Femoral Shaft
  Left ØQ99
  Right ØQ98
Femur
  Lower
    Left ØQ9C
    Right ØQ9B
  Upper
    Left ØQ97
    Right ØQ96
Fibula
  Left ØQ9K
  Right ØQ9J
Finger Nail ØH9Q
Foot
  Left ØY9N
  Right ØY9M
Gallbladder ØF94
Gingiva
  Lower ØC96
  Upper ØC95
Gland
  Adrenal
    Bilateral ØG94
    Left ØG92
    Right ØG93
  Lacrimal
    Left Ø89W
    Right Ø89V
  Minor Salivary ØC9J
  Parotid
    Left ØC99
    Right ØC98
  Pituitary ØG90
  Sublingual
    Left ØC9F
    Right ØC9D
  Submaxillary
    Left ØC9H
    Right ØC9G
  Vestibular ØU9L
Glenoid Cavity
  Left ØP98
  Right ØP97
Glomus Jugulare ØG9C
Hand
  Left ØX9K
  Right ØX9J
Head ØW90
Humeral Head
  Left ØP9D
  Right ØP9C
Humeral Shaft
  Left ØP9G
  Right ØP9F
Hymen ØU9K
Hypothalamus 009A
Ileocecal Valve ØD9C
Ileum ØD9B
Inguinal Region
  Left ØY96
  Right ØY95
Intestine
  Large ØD9E
    Left ØD9G
    Right ØD9F
  Small ØD98
Iris
  Left Ø89D
  Right Ø89C
Jaw
  Lower ØW95
  Upper ØW94
Jejunum ØD9A
Joint
  Acromioclavicular
    Left ØR9H
    Right ØR9G
  Ankle
    Left ØS9G

Drainage — *continued*
Joint — *continued*
  Ankle — *continued*
    Right ØS9F
  Carpal
    Left ØR9R
    Right ØR9Q
  Carpometacarpal
    Left ØR9T
    Right ØR9S
  Cervical Vertebral ØR91
  Cervicothoracic Vertebral ØR94
  Coccygeal ØS96
  Elbow
    Left ØR9M
    Right ØR9L
  Finger Phalangeal
    Left ØR9X
    Right ØR9W
  Hip
    Left ØS9B
    Right ØS99
  Knee
    Left ØS9D
    Right ØS9C
  Lumbar Vertebral ØS90
  Lumbosacral ØS93
  Metacarpophalangeal
    Left ØR9V
    Right ØR9U
  Metatarsal-Phalangeal
    Left ØS9N
    Right ØS9M
  Occipital-cervical ØR90
  Sacrococcygeal ØS95
  Sacroiliac
    Left ØS98
    Right ØS97
  Shoulder
    Left ØR9K
    Right ØR9J
  Sternoclavicular
    Left ØR9F
    Right ØR9E
  Tarsal
    Left ØS9J
    Right ØS9H
  Tarsometatarsal
    Left ØS9L
    Right ØS9K
  Temporomandibular
    Left ØR9D
    Right ØR9C
  Thoracic Vertebral ØR96
  Thoracolumbar Vertebral ØR9A
  Toe Phalangeal
    Left ØS9Q
    Right ØS9P
  Wrist
    Left ØR9P
    Right ØR9N
Kidney
  Left ØT91
  Right ØT90
Kidney Pelvis
  Left ØT94
  Right ØT93
Knee Region
  Left ØY9G
  Right ØY9F
Larynx ØC9S
Leg
  Lower
    Left ØY9J
    Right ØY9H
  Upper
    Left ØY9D
    Right ØY9C
Lens
  Left Ø89K
  Right Ø89J
Lip
  Lower ØC91
  Upper ØC90
Liver ØF90
  Left Lobe ØF92
  Right Lobe ØF91
Lung
  Bilateral ØB9M

Drainage — *continued*
Lung — *continued*
  Left ØB9L
  Lower Lobe
    Left ØB9J
    Right ØB9F
  Middle Lobe, Right ØB9D
  Right ØB9K
  Upper Lobe
    Left ØB9G
    Right ØB9C
Lung Lingula ØB9H
Lymphatic
  Aortic Ø79D
  Axillary
    Left Ø796
    Right Ø795
  Head Ø790
  Inguinal
    Left Ø79J
    Right Ø79H
  Internal Mammary
    Left Ø799
    Right Ø798
  Lower Extremity
    Left Ø79G
    Right Ø79F
  Mesenteric Ø79B
  Neck
    Left Ø792
    Right Ø791
  Pelvis Ø79C
  Thoracic Duct Ø79K
  Thorax Ø797
  Upper Extremity
    Left Ø794
    Right Ø793
Mandible
  Left ØN9V
  Right ØN9T
Maxilla ØN9R
Mediastinum ØW9C
Medulla Oblongata 009D
Mesentery ØD9V
Metacarpal
  Left ØP9Q
  Right ØP9P
Metatarsal
  Left ØQ9P
  Right ØQ9N
Muscle
  Abdomen
    Left ØK9L
    Right ØK9K
  Extraocular
    Left Ø89M
    Right Ø89L
  Facial ØK91
  Foot
    Left ØK9W
    Right ØK9V
  Hand
    Left ØK9D
    Right ØK9C
  Head ØK90
  Hip
    Left ØK9P
    Right ØK9N
  Lower Arm and Wrist
    Left ØK9B
    Right ØK99
  Lower Leg
    Left ØK9T
    Right ØK9S
  Neck
    Left ØK93
    Right ØK92
  Perineum ØK9M
  Shoulder
    Left ØK96
    Right ØK95
  Thorax
    Left ØK9J
    Right ØK9H
  Tongue, Palate, Pharynx ØK94
  Trunk
    Left ØK9G
    Right ØK9F

Drainage — continued
  Muscle — continued
    Upper Arm
      Left ØK98
      Right ØK97
    Upper Leg
      Left ØK9R
      Right ØK9Q
  Nasal Mucosa and Soft Tissue Ø99K
  Nasopharynx Ø99N
  Neck ØW96
  Nerve
    Abdominal Sympathetic Ø19M
    Abducens ØØ9L
    Accessory ØØ9R
    Acoustic ØØ9N
    Brachial Plexus Ø193
    Cervical Ø191
    Cervical Plexus Ø19Ø
    Facial ØØ9M
    Femoral Ø19D
    Glossopharyngeal ØØ9P
    Head and Neck Sympathetic Ø19K
    Hypoglossal ØØ9S
    Lumbar Ø19B
    Lumbar Plexus Ø199
    Lumbar Sympathetic Ø19N
    Lumbosacral Plexus Ø19A
    Median Ø195
    Oculomotor ØØ9H
    Olfactory ØØ9F
    Optic ØØ9G
    Peroneal Ø19H
    Phrenic Ø192
    Pudendal Ø19C
    Radial Ø196
    Sacral Ø19R
    Sacral Plexus Ø19Q
    Sacral Sympathetic Ø19P
    Sciatic Ø19F
    Thoracic Ø198
    Thoracic Sympathetic Ø19L
    Tibial Ø19G
    Trigeminal ØØ9K
    Trochlear ØØ9J
    Ulnar Ø194
    Vagus ØØ9Q
  Nipple
    Left ØH9X
    Right ØH9W
  Omentum ØD9U
  Oral Cavity and Throat ØW93
  Orbit
    Left ØN9Q
    Right ØN9P
  Ovary
    Bilateral ØU92
    Left ØU91
    Right ØU9Ø
  Palate
    Hard ØC92
    Soft ØC93
  Pancreas ØF9G
  Para-aortic Body ØG99
  Paraganglion Extremity ØG9F
  Parathyroid Gland ØG9R
    Inferior
      Left ØG9P
      Right ØG9N
    Multiple ØG9Q
    Superior
      Left ØG9M
      Right ØG9L
  Patella
    Left ØQ9F
    Right ØQ9D
  Pelvic Cavity ØW9J
  Penis ØV9S
  Pericardial Cavity ØW9D
  Perineum
    Female ØW9N
    Male ØW9M
  Peritoneal Cavity ØW9G
  Peritoneum ØD9W
  Phalanx
    Finger
      Left ØP9V
      Right ØP9T

Drainage — continued
  Phalanx — continued
    Thumb
      Left ØP9S
      Right ØP9R
    Toe
      Left ØQ9R
      Right ØQ9Q
  Pharynx ØC9M
  Pineal Body ØG91
  Pleura
    Left ØB9P
    Right ØB9N
  Pleural Cavity
    Left ØW9B
    Right ØW99
  Pons ØØ9B
  Prepuce ØV9T
  Products of Conception
    Amniotic Fluid
      Diagnostic 1Ø9Ø
      Therapeutic 1Ø9Ø
    Fetal Blood 1Ø9Ø
    Fetal Cerebrospinal Fluid 1Ø9Ø
    Fetal Fluid, Other 1Ø9Ø
    Fluid, Other 1Ø9Ø
  Prostate ØV9Ø
  Radius
    Left ØP9J
    Right ØP9H
  Rectum ØD9P
  Retina
    Left Ø89F
    Right Ø89E
  Retinal Vessel
    Left Ø89H
    Right Ø89G
  Retroperitoneum ØW9H
  Ribs
    1 to 2 ØP91
    3 or More ØP92
  Sacrum ØQ91
  Scapula
    Left ØP96
    Right ØP95
  Sclera
    Left Ø897
    Right Ø896
  Scrotum ØV95
  Septum, Nasal Ø99M
  Shoulder Region
    Left ØX93
    Right ØX92
  Sinus
    Accessory Ø99P
    Ethmoid
      Left Ø99V
      Right Ø99U
    Frontal
      Left Ø99T
      Right Ø99S
    Mastoid
      Left Ø99C
      Right Ø99B
    Maxillary
      Left Ø99R
      Right Ø99Q
    Sphenoid
      Left Ø99X
      Right Ø99W
  Skin
    Abdomen ØH97
    Back ØH96
    Buttock ØH98
    Chest ØH95
    Ear
      Left ØH93
      Right ØH92
    Face ØH91
    Foot
      Left ØH9N
      Right ØH9M
    Hand
      Left ØH9G
      Right ØH9F
    Inguinal ØH9A
    Lower Arm
      Left ØH9E
      Right ØH9D

Drainage — continued
  Skin — continued
    Lower Leg
      Left ØH9L
      Right ØH9K
    Neck ØH94
    Perineum ØH99
    Scalp ØH9Ø
    Upper Arm
      Left ØH9C
      Right ØH9B
    Upper Leg
      Left ØH9J
      Right ØH9H
  Skull ØN9Ø
  Spinal Canal ØØ9U
  Spinal Cord
    Cervical ØØ9W
    Lumbar ØØ9Y
    Thoracic ØØ9X
  Spinal Meninges ØØ9T
  Spleen Ø79P
  Sternum ØP9Ø
  Stomach ØD96
    Pylorus ØD97
  Subarachnoid Space, Intracranial ØØ95
  Subcutaneous Tissue and Fascia
    Abdomen ØJ98
    Back ØJ97
    Buttock ØJ99
    Chest ØJ96
    Face ØJ91
    Foot
      Left ØJ9R
      Right ØJ9Q
    Hand
      Left ØJ9K
      Right ØJ9J
    Lower Arm
      Left ØJ9H
      Right ØJ9G
    Lower Leg
      Left ØJ9P
      Right ØJ9N
    Neck
      Left ØJ95
      Right ØJ94
    Pelvic Region ØJ9C
    Perineum ØJ9B
    Scalp ØJ9Ø
    Upper Arm
      Left ØJ9F
      Right ØJ9D
    Upper Leg
      Left ØJ9M
      Right ØJ9L
  Subdural Space, Intracranial ØØ94
  Tarsal
    Left ØQ9M
    Right ØQ9L
  Tendon
    Abdomen
      Left ØL9G
      Right ØL9F
    Ankle
      Left ØL9T
      Right ØL9S
    Foot
      Left ØL9W
      Right ØL9V
    Hand
      Left ØL98
      Right ØL97
    Head and Neck ØL9Ø
    Hip
      Left ØL9K
      Right ØL9J
    Knee
      Left ØL9R
      Right ØL9Q
    Lower Arm and Wrist
      Left ØL96
      Right ØL95
    Lower Leg
      Left ØL9P
      Right ØL9N
    Perineum ØL9H
    Shoulder
      Left ØL92

Drainage — *continued*
  Tendon — *continued*
    Shoulder — *continued*
      Right 0L91
    Thorax
      Left 0L9D
      Right 0L9C
    Trunk
      Left 0L9B
      Right 0L99
    Upper Arm
      Left 0L94
      Right 0L93
    Upper Leg
      Left 0L9M
      Right 0L9L
  Testis
    Bilateral 0V9C
    Left 0V9B
    Right 0V99
  Thalamus 0099
  Thymus 079M
  Thyroid Gland 0G9K
    Left Lobe 0G9G
    Right Lobe 0G9H
  Tibia
    Left 0Q9H
    Right 0Q9G
  Toe Nail 0H9R
  Tongue 0C97
  Tonsils 0C9P
  Tooth
    Lower 0C9X
    Upper 0C9W
  Trachea 0B91
  Tunica Vaginalis
    Left 0V97
    Right 0V96
  Turbinate, Nasal 099L
  Tympanic Membrane
    Left 0998
    Right 0997
  Ulna
    Left 0P9L
    Right 0P9K
  Ureter
    Left 0T97
    Right 0T96
  Ureters, Bilateral 0T98
  Urethra 0T9D
  Uterine Supporting Structure 0U94
  Uterus 0U99
  Uvula 0C9N
  Vagina 0U9G
  Vas Deferens
    Bilateral 0V9Q
    Left 0V9P
    Right 0V9N
  Vein
    Axillary
      Left 0598
      Right 0597
    Azygos 0590
    Basilic
      Left 059C
      Right 059B
    Brachial
      Left 059A
      Right 0599
    Cephalic
      Left 059F
      Right 059D
    Colic 0697
    Common Iliac
      Left 069D
      Right 069C
    Esophageal 0693
    External Iliac
      Left 069G
      Right 069F
    External Jugular
      Left 059Q
      Right 059P
    Face
      Left 059V
      Right 059T
    Femoral
      Left 069N
      Right 069M

Drainage — *continued*
  Vein — *continued*
    Foot
      Left 069V
      Right 069T
    Gastric 0692
    Hand
      Left 059H
      Right 059G
    Hemiazygos 0591
    Hepatic 0694
    Hypogastric
      Left 069J
      Right 069H
    Inferior Mesenteric 0696
    Innominate
      Left 0594
      Right 0593
    Internal Jugular
      Left 059N
      Right 059M
    Intracranial 059L
    Lower 069Y
    Portal 0698
    Renal
      Left 069B
      Right 0699
    Saphenous
      Left 069Q
      Right 069P
    Splenic 0691
    Subclavian
      Left 0596
      Right 0595
    Superior Mesenteric 0695
    Upper 059Y
    Vertebral
      Left 059S
      Right 059R
  Vena Cava, Inferior 0690
  Vertebra
    Cervical 0P93
    Lumbar 0Q90
    Thoracic 0P94
  Vesicle
    Bilateral 0V93
    Left 0V92
    Right 0V91
  Vitreous
    Left 0895
    Right 0894
  Vocal Cord
    Left 0C9V
    Right 0C9T
  Vulva 0U9M
  Wrist Region
    Left 0X9H
    Right 0X9G

Dressing
  Abdominal Wall 2W23X4Z
  Arm
    Lower
      Left 2W2DX4Z
      Right 2W2CX4Z
    Upper
      Left 2W2BX4Z
      Right 2W2AX4Z
  Back 2W25X4Z
  Chest Wall 2W24X4Z
  Extremity
    Lower
      Left 2W2MX4Z
      Right 2W2LX4Z
    Upper
      Left 2W29X4Z
      Right 2W28X4Z
  Face 2W21X4Z
  Finger
    Left 2W2KX4Z
    Right 2W2JX4Z
  Foot
    Left 2W2TX4Z
    Right 2W2SX4Z
  Hand
    Left 2W2FX4Z
    Right 2W2EX4Z
  Head 2W20X4Z
  Inguinal Region
    Left 2W27X4Z

Dressing — *continued*
  Inguinal Region — *continued*
    Right 2W26X4Z
  Leg
    Lower
      Left 2W2RX4Z
      Right 2W2QX4Z
    Upper
      Left 2W2PX4Z
      Right 2W2NX4Z
  Neck 2W22X4Z
  Thumb
    Left 2W2HX4Z
    Right 2W2GX4Z
  Toe
    Left 2W2VX4Z
    Right 2W2UX4Z
Driver stent (RX) (OTW) *use* Intraluminal Device
Drotrecogin alfa, infusion *see* Introduction of Recombinant Human-activated Protein C
Duct of Santorini *use* Pancreatic Duct, Accessory
Duct of Wirsung *use* Pancreatic Duct
Ductogram, mammary *see* Plain Radiography, Skin, Subcutaneous Tissue and Breast BH0
Ductography, mammary *see* Plain Radiography, Skin, Subcutaneous Tissue and Breast BH0
Ductus deferens
  use Vas Deferens
  use Vas Deferens, Bilateral
  use Vas Deferens, Left
  use Vas Deferens, Right
Duodenal ampulla *use* Ampulla of Vater
Duodenectomy
  see Excision, Duodenum 0DB9
  see Resection, Duodenum 0DT9
Duodenocholedochotomy *see* Drainage, Gallbladder 0F94
Duodenocystostomy
  see Bypass, Gallbladder 0F14
  see Drainage, Gallbladder 0F94
Duodenoenterostomy
  see Bypass, Gastrointestinal System 0D1
  see Drainage, Gastrointestinal System 0D9
Duodenojejunal flexure *use* Jejunum
Duodenolysis *see* Release, Duodenum 0DN9
Duodenorrhaphy *see* Repair, Duodenum 0DQ9
Duodenoscopy, single-use (aScope™ Duodeno) (EXALT™ Model D) *see* New Technology, Hepatobiliary System and Pancreas XFJ
Duodenostomy
  see Bypass, Duodenum 0D19
  see Drainage, Duodenum 0D99
Duodenotomy *see* Drainage, Duodenum 0D99
Dura mater, intracranial *use* Dura Mater
Dura mater, spinal *use* Spinal Meninges
DuraGraft® Endothelial Damage Inhibitor *use* Endothelial Damage Inhibitor
DuraHeart Left Ventricular Assist System *use* Implantable Heart Assist System in Heart and Great Vessels
Dural venous sinus *use* Intracranial Vein
Durata® Defibrillation Lead *use* Cardiac Lead, Defibrillator in 02H
Durvalumab Antineoplastic XW0
DynaNail Mini®
  use Internal Fixation Device, Sustained Compression in 0RG
  use Internal Fixation Device, Sustained Compression in 0SG
DynaNail®
  use Internal Fixation Device, Sustained Compression in 0RG
  use Internal Fixation Device, Sustained Compression in 0SG
Dynesys® Dynamic Stabilization System
  use Spinal Stabilization Device, Pedicle-Based in 0RH
  use Spinal Stabilization Device, Pedicle-Based in 0SH

E

Earlobe
  use Ear, External, Bilateral
  use Ear, External, Left
  use Ear, External, Right

ECCO2R (Extracorporeal Carbon Dioxide Removal) 5A0920Z
Echocardiogram see Ultrasonography, Heart B24
Echography see Ultrasonography
EchoTip® Insight™ Portosystemic Pressure Gradient Measurement System 4A044B2
ECMO see Performance, Circulatory 5A15
ECMO, intraoperative see Performance, Circulatory 5A15A
Eculizumab XW0
EDWARDS INTUITY Elite valve system use Zooplastic Tissue, Rapid Deployment Technique in New Technology
EEG (electroencephalogram) see Measurement, Central Nervous 4A00
EGD (esophagogastroduodenoscopy) 0DJ08ZZ
Eighth cranial nerve use Acoustic Nerve
Ejaculatory duct
   use Vas Deferens
   use Vas Deferens, Bilateral
   use Vas Deferens, Left
   use Vas Deferens, Right
EKG (electrocardiogram) see Measurement, Cardiac 4A02
EKOS™ EkoSonic® Endovascular System see Fragmentation, Artery
Eladocagene exuparvovec XW0Q316
Electrical bone growth stimulator (EBGS)
   use Bone Growth Stimulator in Head and Facial Bones
   use Bone Growth Stimulator in Lower Bones
   use Bone Growth Stimulator in Upper Bones
Electrical muscle stimulation (EMS) lead use Stimulator Lead in Muscles
Electrocautery
   Destruction see Destruction
   Repair see Repair
Electroconvulsive Therapy
   Bilateral-Multiple Seizure GZB3ZZZ
   Bilateral-Single Seizure GZB2ZZZ
   Electroconvulsive Therapy, Other GZB4ZZZ
   Unilateral-Multiple Seizure GZB1ZZZ
   Unilateral-Single Seizure GZB0ZZZ
Electroencephalogram (EEG) see Measurement, Central Nervous 4A00
Electromagnetic Therapy
   Central Nervous 6A22
   Urinary 6A21
Electronic muscle stimulator lead use Stimulator Lead in Muscles
Electrophysiologic stimulation (EPS) see Measurement, Cardiac 4A02
Electroshock therapy see Electroconvulsive Therapy
Elevation, bone fragments, skull see Reposition, Head and Facial Bones 0NS
Eleventh cranial nerve use Accessory Nerve
Ellipsys® vascular access system see New Technology, Cardiovascular System X2K
E-Luminexx™ (Biliary) (Vascular) Stent use Intraluminal Device
Eluvia™ Drug-Eluting Vascular Stent System
   use Intraluminal Device, Sustained Release Drug-eluting in New Technology
   use Intraluminal Device, Sustained Release Drug-eluting, Two in New Technology
   use Intraluminal Device, Sustained Release Drug-eluting, Three in New Technology
   use Intraluminal Device, Sustained Release Drug-eluting, Four or More in New Technology
ELZONRIS™ use Tagraxofusp-erzs Antineoplastic
Embolectomy see Extirpation
Embolization
   see Occlusion
   see Restriction
Embolization coil(s) use Intraluminal Device
EMG (electromyogram) see Measurement, Musculoskeletal 4A0F
Encephalon use Brain
Endarterectomy
   see Extirpation, Lower Arteries 04C
   see Extirpation, Upper Arteries 03C
Endeavor® (III) (IV) (Sprint) Zotarolimus-eluting Coronary Stent System use Intraluminal Device, Drug-eluting in Heart and Great Vessels
EndoAVF procedure, using magnetic-guided radiofrequency see Bypass, Upper Arteries 031

EndoAVF procedure, using thermal resistance energy see New Technology, Cardiovascular System X2K
Endologix AFX® Endovascular AAA System use Intraluminal Device
EndoSure® sensor use Monitoring Device, Pressure Sensor in 02H
ENDOTAK RELIANCE® (G) Defibrillation Lead use Cardiac Lead, Defibrillator in 02H
Endothelial damage inhibitor, applied to vein graft XY0VX83
Endotracheal tube (cuffed) (double-lumen) use Intraluminal Device, Endotracheal Airway in Respiratory System
Endovascular fistula creation, using magnetic-guided radiofrequency see Bypass, Upper Arteries 031
Endovascular fistula creation, using thermal resistance energy see New Technology, Cardiovascular System X2K
Endurant® Endovascular Stent Graft use Intraluminal Device
Endurant® II AAA Stent Graft System use Intraluminal Device
Engineered Chimeric Antigen Receptor T-cell Immunotherapy
   Allogeneic XW0
   Autologous XW0
Enlargement
   see Dilation
   see Repair
EnRhythm use Pacemaker, Dual Chamber in 0JH
ENROUTE® Transcarotid Neuroprotection System see New Technology, Cardiovascular System X2A
ENSPRYNG™ use Satralizumab-mwge
Enterorrhaphy see Repair, Gastrointestinal System 0DQ
Enterra gastric neurostimulator use Stimulator Generator, Multiple Array in 0JH
Enucleation
   Eyeball see Resection, Eye 08T
   Eyeball with prosthetic implant see Replacement, Eye 08R
Ependyma use Cerebral Ventricle
Epicel® cultured epidermal autograft use Autologous Tissue Substitute
Epic™ Stented Tissue Valve (aortic) use Zooplastic Tissue in Heart and Great Vessels
Epidermis use Skin
Epididymectomy
   see Excision, Male Reproductive System 0VB
   see Resection, Male Reproductive System 0VT
Epididymoplasty
   see Repair, Male Reproductive System 0VQ
   see Supplement, Male Reproductive System 0VU
Epididymorrhaphy see Repair, Male Reproductive System 0VQ
Epididymotomy see Drainage, Male Reproductive System 0V9
Epidural space, spinal use Spinal Canal
Epiphysiodesis
   see Insertion of device in, Lower Bones 0QH
   see Insertion of device in, Upper Bones 0PH
   see Repair, Lower Bones 0QQ
   see Repair, Upper Bones 0PQ
Epiploic foramen use Peritoneum
Epiretinal Visual Prosthesis
   Left 08H105Z
   Right 08H005Z
Episiorrhaphy see Repair, Perineum, Female 0WQN
Episiotomy see Division, Perineum, Female 0W8N
Epithalamus use Thalamus
Epitrochlear lymph node
   use Lymphatic, Left Upper Extremity
   use Lymphatic, Right Upper Extremity
EPS (electrophysiologic stimulation) see Measurement, Cardiac 4A02
Eptifibatide, infusion see Introduction of Platelet Inhibitor
ERCP (endoscopic retrograde cholangiopancreatography) see Fluoroscopy, Hepatobiliary System and Pancreas BF1
Erdafitinib Antineoplastic XW0DXL5
Erector spinae muscle
   use Trunk Muscle, Left
   use Trunk Muscle, Right
ERLEADA™ use Apalutamide Antineoplastic

Esketamine Hydrochloride XW097M5
Esophageal artery use Upper Artery
Esophageal obturator airway (EOA) use Intraluminal Device, Airway in Gastrointestinal System
Esophageal plexus use Thoracic Sympathetic Nerve
Esophagectomy
   see Excision, Gastrointestinal System 0DB
   see Resection, Gastrointestinal System 0DT
Esophagocoloplasty
   see Repair, Gastrointestinal System 0DQ
   see Supplement, Gastrointestinal System 0DU
Esophagoenterostomy
   see Bypass, Gastrointestinal System 0D1
   see Drainage, Gastrointestinal System 0D9
Esophagoesophagostomy
   see Bypass, Gastrointestinal System 0D1
   see Drainage, Gastrointestinal System 0D9
Esophagogastrectomy
   see Excision, Gastrointestinal System 0DB
   see Resection, Gastrointestinal System 0DT
Esophagogastroduodenoscopy (EGD) 0DJ08ZZ
Esophagogastroplasty
   see Repair, Gastrointestinal System 0DQ
   see Supplement, Gastrointestinal System 0DU
Esophagogastroscopy 0DJ68ZZ
Esophagogastrostomy
   see Bypass, Gastrointestinal System 0D1
   see Drainage, Gastrointestinal System 0D9
Esophagojejunoplasty see Supplement, Gastrointestinal System 0DU
Esophagojejunostomy
   see Bypass, Gastrointestinal System 0D1
   see Drainage, Gastrointestinal System 0D9
Esophagomyotomy see Division, Esophagogastric Junction 0D84
Esophagoplasty
   see Repair, Gastrointestinal System 0DQ
   see Replacement, Esophagus 0DR5
   see Supplement, Gastrointestinal System 0DU
Esophagoplication see Restriction, Gastrointestinal System 0DV
Esophagorrhaphy see Repair, Gastrointestinal System 0DQ
Esophagoscopy 0DJ08ZZ
Esophagotomy see Drainage, Gastrointestinal System 0D9
Esteem® implantable hearing system use Hearing Device in Ear, Nose, Sinus
ESWL (extracorporeal shock wave lithotripsy) see Fragmentation
Etesevimab Monoclonal Antibody XW0
Ethmoidal air cell
   use Ethmoid Sinus, Left
   use Ethmoid Sinus, Right
Ethmoidectomy
   see Excision, Ear, Nose, Sinus 09B
   see Excision, Head and Facial Bones 0NB
   see Resection, Ear, Nose, Sinus 09T
   see Resection, Head and Facial Bones 0NT
Ethmoidotomy see Drainage, Ear, Nose, Sinus 099
Evacuation
   Hematoma see Extirpation
   Other Fluid see Drainage
Evera (XT) (S) (DR/VR) use Defibrillator Generator in 0JH
Everolimus-eluting coronary stent use Intraluminal Device, Drug-eluting in Heart and Great Vessels
Evisceration
   Eyeball see Resection, Eye 08T
   Eyeball with prosthetic implant see Replacement, Eye 08R
EXALT™ Model D Single-Use Duodenoscope see New Technology, Hepatobiliary System and Pancreas XFJ
Examination see Inspection
Exchange see Change device in
Excision
   Abdominal Wall 0WBF
   Acetabulum
      Left 0QB5
      Right 0QB4
   Adenoids 0CBQ
   Ampulla of Vater 0FBC
   Anal Sphincter 0DBR
   Ankle Region
      Left 0YBL
      Right 0YBK

Excision — *continued*
Anus ØDBQ
Aorta
　Abdominal
　　Thoracic
　　　Ascending/Arch Ø2BX
　　　Descending Ø2BW
Aortic Body ØGBD
Appendix ØDBJ
Arm
　Lower
　　Left ØXBF
　　Right ØXBD
　Upper
　　Left ØXB9
　　Right ØXB8
Artery
　Anterior Tibial
　　Left Ø4BQ
　　Right Ø4BP
　Axillary
　　Left Ø3B6
　　Right Ø3B5
　Brachial
　　Left Ø3B8
　　Right Ø3B7
　Celiac Ø4B1
　Colic
　　Left Ø4B7
　　Middle Ø4B8
　　Right Ø4B6
　Common Carotid
　　Left Ø3BJ
　　Right Ø3BH
　Common Iliac
　　Left Ø4BD
　　Right Ø4BC
　External Carotid
　　Left Ø3BN
　　Right Ø3BM
　External Iliac
　　Left Ø4BJ
　　Right Ø4BH
　Face Ø3BR
　Femoral
　　Left Ø4BL
　　Right Ø4BK
　Foot
　　Left Ø4BW
　　Right Ø4BV
　Gastric Ø4B2
　Hand
　　Left Ø3BF
　　Right Ø3BD
　Hepatic Ø4B3
　Inferior Mesenteric Ø4BB
　Innominate Ø3B2
　Internal Carotid
　　Left Ø3BL
　　Right Ø3BK
　Internal Iliac
　　Left Ø4BF
　　Right Ø4BE
　Internal Mammary
　　Left Ø3B1
　　Right Ø3BØ
　Intracranial Ø3BG
　Lower Ø4BY
　Peroneal
　　Left Ø4BU
　　Right Ø4BT
　Popliteal
　　Left Ø4BN
　　Right Ø4BM
　Posterior Tibial
　　Left Ø4BS
　　Right Ø4BR
　Pulmonary
　　Left Ø2BR
　　Right Ø2BQ
　Pulmonary Trunk Ø2BP
　Radial
　　Left Ø3BC
　　Right Ø3BB
　Renal
　　Left Ø4BA
　　Right Ø4B9
　Splenic Ø4B4

Excision — *continued*
Artery — *continued*
　Subclavian
　　Left Ø3B4
　　Right Ø3B3
　Superior Mesenteric Ø4B5
　Temporal
　　Left Ø3BT
　　Right Ø3BS
　Thyroid
　　Left Ø3BV
　　Right Ø3BU
　Ulnar
　　Left Ø3BA
　　Right Ø3B9
　Upper Ø3BY
　Vertebral
　　Left Ø3BQ
　　Right Ø3BP
Atrium
　Left Ø2B7
　Right Ø2B6
Auditory Ossicle
　Left Ø9BA
　Right Ø9B9
Axilla
　Left ØXB5
　Right ØXB4
Back
　Lower ØWBL
　Upper ØWBK
Basal Ganglia ØØB8
Bladder ØTBB
Bladder Neck ØTBC
Bone
　Ethmoid
　　Left ØNBG
　　Right ØNBF
　Frontal ØNB1
　Hyoid ØNBX
　Lacrimal
　　Left ØNBJ
　　Right ØNBH
　Nasal ØNBB
　Occipital ØNB7
　Palatine
　　Left ØNBL
　　Right ØNBK
　Parietal
　　Left ØNB4
　　Right ØNB3
　Pelvic
　　Left ØQB3
　　Right ØQB2
　Sphenoid ØNBC
　Temporal
　　Left ØNB6
　　Right ØNB5
　Zygomatic
　　Left ØNBN
　　Right ØNBM
Brain ØØBØ
Breast
　Bilateral ØHBV
　Left ØHBU
　Right ØHBT
　Supernumerary ØHBY
Bronchus
　Lingula ØBB9
　Lower Lobe
　　Left ØBBB
　　Right ØBB6
　Main
　　Left ØBB7
　　Right ØBB3
　Middle Lobe, Right ØBB5
　Upper Lobe
　　Left ØBB8
　　Right ØBB4
Buccal Mucosa ØCB4
Bursa and Ligament
　Abdomen
　　Left ØMBJ
　　Right ØMBH
　Ankle
　　Left ØMBR
　　Right ØMBQ
　Elbow
　　Left ØMB4

Excision — *continued*
Bursa and Ligament — *continued*
　Elbow — *continued*
　　Right ØMB3
　Foot
　　Left ØMBT
　　Right ØMBS
　Hand
　　Left ØMB8
　　Right ØMB7
　Head and Neck ØMBØ
　Hip
　　Left ØMBM
　　Right ØMBL
　Knee
　　Left ØMBP
　　Right ØMBN
　Lower Extremity
　　Left ØMBW
　　Right ØMBV
　Perineum ØMBK
　Rib(s) ØMBG
　Shoulder
　　Left ØMB2
　　Right ØMB1
　Spine
　　Lower ØMBD
　　Upper ØMBC
　Sternum ØMBF
　Upper Extremity
　　Left ØMBB
　　Right ØMB9
　Wrist
　　Left ØMB6
　　Right ØMB5
Buttock
　Left ØYB1
　Right ØYBØ
Carina ØBB2
Carotid Bodies, Bilateral ØGB8
Carotid Body
　Left ØGB6
　Right ØGB7
Carpal
　Left ØPBN
　Right ØPBM
Cecum ØDBH
Cerebellum ØØBC
Cerebral Hemisphere ØØB7
Cerebral Meninges ØØB1
Cerebral Ventricle ØØB6
Cervix ØUBC
Chest Wall ØWB8
Chordae Tendineae Ø2B9
Choroid
　Left Ø8BB
　Right Ø8BA
Cisterna Chyli Ø7BL
Clavicle
　Left ØPBB
　Right ØPB9
Clitoris ØUBJ
Coccygeal Glomus ØGBB
Coccyx ØQBS
Colon
　Ascending ØDBK
　Descending ØDBM
　Sigmoid ØDBN
　Transverse ØDBL
Conduction Mechanism Ø2B8
Conjunctiva
　Left Ø8BTXZ
　Right Ø8BSXZ
Cord
　Bilateral ØVBH
　Left ØVBG
　Right ØVBF
Cornea
　Left Ø8B9XZ
　Right Ø8B8XZ
Cul-de-sac ØUBF
Diaphragm ØBBT
Disc
　Cervical Vertebral ØRB3
　Cervicothoracic Vertebral ØRB5
　Lumbar Vertebral ØSB2
　Lumbosacral ØSB4
　Thoracic Vertebral ØRB9
　Thoracolumbar Vertebral ØRBB

Excision — *continued*
Duct
  Common Bile ØFB9
  Cystic ØFB8
  Hepatic
    Common ØFB7
    Left ØFB6
    Right ØFB5
  Lacrimal
    Left Ø8BY
    Right Ø8BX
  Pancreatic ØFBD
    Accessory ØFBF
  Parotid
    Left ØCBC
    Right ØCBB
Duodenum ØDB9
Dura Mater ØØB2
Ear
  External
    Left Ø9B1
    Right Ø9BØ
  External Auditory Canal
    Left Ø9B4
    Right Ø9B3
  Inner
    Left Ø9BE
    Right Ø9BD
  Middle
    Left Ø9B6
    Right Ø9B5
Elbow Region
  Left ØXBC
  Right ØXBB
Epididymis
  Bilateral ØVBL
  Left ØVBK
  Right ØVBJ
Epiglottis ØCBR
Esophagogastric Junction ØDB4
Esophagus ØDB5
  Lower ØDB3
  Middle ØDB2
  Upper ØDB1
Eustachian Tube
  Left Ø9BG
  Right Ø9BF
Extremity
  Lower
    Left ØYBB
    Right ØYB9
  Upper
    Left ØXB7
    Right ØXB6
Eye
  Left Ø8B1
  Right Ø8BØ
Eyelid
  Lower
    Left Ø8BR
    Right Ø8BQ
  Upper
    Left Ø8BP
    Right Ø8BN
Face ØWB2
Fallopian Tube
  Left ØUB6
  Right ØUB5
Fallopian Tubes, Bilateral ØUB7
Femoral Region
  Left ØYB8
  Right ØYB7
Femoral Shaft
  Left ØQB9
  Right ØQB8
Femur
  Lower
    Left ØQBC
    Right ØQBB
  Upper
    Left ØQB7
    Right ØQB6
Fibula
  Left ØQBK
  Right ØQBJ
Finger Nail ØHBQXZ
Floor of mouth *see* Excision, Oral Cavity and Throat ØWB3

Excision — *continued*
Foot
  Left ØYBN
  Right ØYBM
Gallbladder ØFB4
Gingiva
  Lower ØCB6
  Upper ØCB5
Gland
  Adrenal
    Bilateral ØGB4
    Left ØGB2
    Right ØGB3
  Lacrimal
    Left Ø8BW
    Right Ø8BV
  Minor Salivary ØCBJ
  Parotid
    Left ØCB9
    Right ØCB8
  Pituitary ØGBØ
  Sublingual
    Left ØCBF
    Right ØCBD
  Submaxillary
    Left ØCBH
    Right ØCBG
  Vestibular ØUBL
Glenoid Cavity
  Left ØPB8
  Right ØPB7
Glomus Jugulare ØGBC
Hand
  Left ØXBK
  Right ØXBJ
Head ØWBØ
Humeral Head
  Left ØPBD
  Right ØPBC
Humeral Shaft
  Left ØPBG
  Right ØPBF
Hymen ØUBK
Hypothalamus ØØBA
Ileocecal Valve ØDBC
Ileum ØDBB
Inguinal Region
  Left ØYB6
  Right ØYB5
Intestine
  Large ØDBE
    Left ØDBG
    Right ØDBF
  Small ØDB8
Iris
  Left Ø8BD3Z
  Right Ø8BC3Z
Jaw
  Lower ØWB5
  Upper ØWB4
Jejunum ØDBA
Joint
  Acromioclavicular
    Left ØRBH
    Right ØRBG
  Ankle
    Left ØSBG
    Right ØSBF
  Carpal
    Left ØRBR
    Right ØRBQ
  Carpometacarpal
    Left ØRBT
    Right ØRBS
  Cervical Vertebral ØRB1
  Cervicothoracic Vertebral ØRB4
  Coccygeal ØSB6
  Elbow
    Left ØRBM
    Right ØRBL
  Finger Phalangeal
    Left ØRBX
    Right ØRBW
  Hip
    Left ØSBB
    Right ØSB9
  Knee
    Left ØSBD
    Right ØSBC

Excision — *continued*
Joint — *continued*
  Lumbar Vertebral ØSBØ
  Lumbosacral ØSB3
  Metacarpophalangeal
    Left ØRBV
    Right ØRBU
  Metatarsal-Phalangeal
    Left ØSBN
    Right ØSBM
  Occipital-cervical ØRBØ
  Sacrococcygeal ØSB5
  Sacroiliac
    Left ØSB8
    Right ØSB7
  Shoulder
    Left ØRBK
    Right ØRBJ
  Sternoclavicular
    Left ØRBF
    Right ØRBE
  Tarsal
    Left ØSBJ
    Right ØSBH
  Tarsometatarsal
    Left ØSBL
    Right ØSBK
  Temporomandibular
    Left ØRBD
    Right ØRBC
  Thoracic Vertebral ØRB6
  Thoracolumbar Vertebral ØRBA
  Toe Phalangeal
    Left ØSBQ
    Right ØSBP
  Wrist
    Left ØRBP
    Right ØRBN
Kidney
  Left ØTB1
  Right ØTBØ
Kidney Pelvis
  Left ØTB4
  Right ØTB3
Knee Region
  Left ØYBG
  Right ØYBF
Larynx ØCBS
Leg
  Lower
    Left ØYBJ
    Right ØYBH
  Upper
    Left ØYBD
    Right ØYBC
Lens
  Left Ø8BK3Z
  Right Ø8BJ3Z
Lip
  Lower ØCB1
  Upper ØCBØ
Liver ØFBØ
  Left Lobe ØFB2
  Right Lobe ØFB1
Lung
  Bilateral ØBBM
  Left ØBBL
  Lower Lobe
    Left ØBBJ
    Right ØBBF
  Middle Lobe, Right ØBBD
  Right ØBBK
  Upper Lobe
    Left ØBBG
    Right ØBBC
Lung Lingula ØBBH
Lymphatic
  Aortic Ø7BD
  Axillary
    Left Ø7B6
    Right Ø7B5
  Head Ø7BØ
  Inguinal
    Left Ø7BJ
    Right Ø7BH
  Internal Mammary
    Left Ø7B9
    Right Ø7B8

Excision — *continued*
Lymphatic — *continued*
Lower Extremity
Left Ø7BG
Right Ø7BF
Mesenteric Ø7BB
Neck
Left Ø7B2
Right Ø7B1
Pelvis Ø7BC
Thoracic Duct Ø7BK
Thorax Ø7B7
Upper Extremity
Left Ø7B4
Right Ø7B3
Mandible
Left ØNBV
Right ØNBT
Maxilla ØNBR
Mediastinum ØWBC
Medulla Oblongata ØØBD
Mesentery ØDBV
Metacarpal
Left ØPBQ
Right ØPBP
Metatarsal
Left ØQBP
Right ØQBN
Muscle
Abdomen
Left ØKBL
Right ØKBK
Extraocular
Left Ø8BM
Right Ø8BL
Facial ØKB1
Foot
Left ØKBW
Right ØKBV
Hand
Left ØKBD
Right ØKBC
Head ØKBØ
Hip
Left ØKBP
Right ØKBN
Lower Arm and Wrist
Left ØKBB
Right ØKB9
Lower Leg
Left ØKBT
Right ØKBS
Neck
Left ØKB3
Right ØKB2
Papillary Ø2BD
Perineum ØKBM
Shoulder
Left ØKB6
Right ØKB5
Thorax
Left ØKBJ
Right ØKBH
Tongue, Palate, Pharynx ØKB4
Trunk
Left ØKBG
Right ØKBF
Upper Arm
Left ØKB8
Right ØKB7
Upper Leg
Left ØKBR
Right ØKBQ
Nasal Mucosa and Soft Tissue Ø9BK
Nasopharynx Ø9BN
Neck ØWB6
Nerve
Abdominal Sympathetic Ø1BM
Abducens ØØBL
Accessory ØØBR
Acoustic ØØBN
Brachial Plexus Ø1B3
Cervical Ø1B1
Cervical Plexus Ø1BØ
Facial ØØBM
Femoral Ø1BD
Glossopharyngeal ØØBP
Head and Neck Sympathetic Ø1BK
Hypoglossal ØØBS

Excision — *continued*
Nerve — *continued*
Lumbar Ø1BB
Lumbar Plexus Ø1B9
Lumbar Sympathetic Ø1BN
Lumbosacral Plexus Ø1BA
Median Ø1B5
Oculomotor ØØBH
Olfactory ØØBF
Optic ØØBG
Peroneal Ø1BH
Phrenic Ø1B2
Pudendal Ø1BC
Radial Ø1B6
Sacral Ø1BR
Sacral Plexus Ø1BQ
Sacral Sympathetic Ø1BP
Sciatic Ø1BF
Thoracic Ø1B8
Thoracic Sympathetic Ø1BL
Tibial Ø1BG
Trigeminal ØØBK
Trochlear ØØBJ
Ulnar Ø1B4
Vagus ØØBQ
Nipple
Left ØHBX
Right ØHBW
Omentum ØDBU
Oral Cavity and Throat ØWB3
Orbit
Left ØNBQ
Right ØNBP
Ovary
Bilateral ØUB2
Left ØUB1
Right ØUBØ
Palate
Hard ØCB2
Soft ØCB3
Pancreas ØFBG
Para-aortic Body ØGB9
Paraganglion Extremity ØGBF
Parathyroid Gland ØGBR
Inferior
Left ØGBP
Right ØGBN
Multiple ØGBQ
Superior
Left ØGBM
Right ØGBL
Patella
Left ØQBF
Right ØQBD
Penis ØVBS
Pericardium Ø2BN
Perineum
Female ØWBN
Male ØWBM
Peritoneum ØDBW
Phalanx
Finger
Left ØPBV
Right ØPBT
Thumb
Left ØPBS
Right ØPBR
Toe
Left ØQBR
Right ØQBQ
Pharynx ØCBM
Pineal Body ØGB1
Pleura
Left ØBBP
Right ØBBN
Pons ØØBB
Prepuce ØVBT
Prostate ØVBØ
Radius
Left ØPBJ
Right ØPBH
Rectum ØDBP
Retina
Left Ø8BF3Z
Right Ø8BE3Z
Retroperitoneum ØWBH
Ribs
1 to 2 ØPB1
3 or More ØPB2

Excision — *continued*
Sacrum ØQB1
Scapula
Left ØPB6
Right ØPB5
Sclera
Left Ø8B7XZ
Right Ø8B6XZ
Scrotum ØVB5
Septum
Atrial Ø2B5
Nasal Ø9BM
Ventricular Ø2BM
Shoulder Region
Left ØXB3
Right ØXB2
Sinus
Accessory Ø9BP
Ethmoid
Left Ø9BV
Right Ø9BU
Frontal
Left Ø9BT
Right Ø9BS
Mastoid
Left Ø9BC
Right Ø9BB
Maxillary
Left Ø9BR
Right Ø9BQ
Sphenoid
Left Ø9BX
Right Ø9BW
Skin
Abdomen ØHB7XZ
Back ØHB6XZ
Buttock ØHB8XZ
Chest ØHB5XZ
Ear
Left ØHB3XZ
Right ØHB2XZ
Face ØHB1XZ
Foot
Left ØIIBNXZ
Right ØHBMXZ
Hand
Left ØHBGXZ
Right ØHBFXZ
Inguinal ØHBAXZ
Lower Arm
Left ØHBEXZ
Right ØHBDXZ
Lower Leg
Left ØHBLXZ
Right ØHBKXZ
Neck ØHB4XZ
Perineum ØHB9XZ
Scalp ØHBØXZ
Upper Arm
Left ØHBCXZ
Right ØHBBXZ
Upper Leg
Left ØHBJXZ
Right ØHBHXZ
Skull ØNBØ
Spinal Cord
Cervical ØØBW
Lumbar ØØBY
Thoracic ØØBX
Spinal Meninges ØØBT
Spleen Ø7BP
Sternum ØPBØ
Stomach ØDB6
Pylorus ØDB7
Subcutaneous Tissue and Fascia
Abdomen ØJB8
Back ØJB7
Buttock ØJB9
Chest ØJB1
Face ØJB1
Foot
Left ØJBR
Right ØJBQ
Hand
Left ØJBK
Right ØJBJ
Lower Arm
Left ØJBH
Right ØJBG

Excision — *continued*
    Subcutaneous Tissue and Fascia — *continued*
        Lower Leg
            Left ØJBP
            Right ØJBN
        Neck
            Left ØJB5
            Right ØJB4
        Pelvic Region ØJBC
        Perineum ØJBB
        Scalp ØJBØ
        Upper Arm
            Left ØJBF
            Right ØJBD
        Upper Leg
            Left ØJBM
            Right ØJBL
    Tarsal
        Left ØQBM
        Right ØQBL
    Tendon
        Abdomen
            Left ØLBG
            Right ØLBF
        Ankle
            Left ØLBT
            Right ØLBS
        Foot
            Left ØLBW
            Right ØLBV
        Hand
            Left ØLB8
            Right ØLB7
        Head and Neck ØLBØ
        Hip
            Left ØLBK
            Right ØLBJ
        Knee
            Left ØLBR
            Right ØLBQ
        Lower Arm and Wrist
            Left ØLB6
            Right ØLB5
        Lower Leg
            Left ØLBP
            Right ØLBN
        Perineum ØLBH
        Shoulder
            Left ØLB2
            Right ØLB1
        Thorax
            Left ØLBD
            Right ØLBC
        Trunk
            Left ØLBB
            Right ØLB9
        Upper Arm
            Left ØLB4
            Right ØLB3
        Upper Leg
            Left ØLBM
            Right ØLBL
    Testis
        Bilateral ØVBC
        Left ØVBB
        Right ØVB9
    Thalamus ØØB9
    Thymus Ø7BM
    Thyroid Gland
        Left Lobe ØGBG
        Right Lobe ØGBH
    Thyroid Gland Isthmus ØGBJ
    Tibia
        Left ØQBH
        Right ØQBG
    Toe Nail ØHBRXZ
    Tongue ØCB7
    Tonsils ØCBP
    Tooth
        Lower ØCBX
        Upper ØCBW
    Trachea ØBB1
    Tunica Vaginalis
        Left ØVB7
        Right ØVB6
    Turbinate, Nasal Ø9BL
    Tympanic Membrane
        Left Ø9B8
        Right Ø9B7

Excision — *continued*
    Ulna
        Left ØPBL
        Right ØPBK
    Ureter
        Left ØTB7
        Right ØTB6
    Urethra ØTBD
    Uterine Supporting Structure ØUB4
    Uterus ØUB9
    Uvula ØCBN
    Vagina ØUBG
    Valve
        Aortic Ø2BF
        Mitral Ø2BG
        Pulmonary Ø2BH
        Tricuspid Ø2BJ
    Vas Deferens
        Bilateral ØVBQ
        Left ØVBP
        Right ØVBN
    Vein
        Axillary
            Left Ø5B8
            Right Ø5B7
        Azygos Ø5BØ
        Basilic
            Left Ø5BC
            Right Ø5BB
        Brachial
            Left Ø5BA
            Right Ø5B9
        Cephalic
            Left Ø5BF
            Right Ø5BD
        Colic Ø6B7
        Common Iliac
            Left Ø6BD
            Right Ø6BC
        Coronary Ø2B4
        Esophageal Ø6B3
        External Iliac
            Left Ø6BG
            Right Ø6BF
        External Jugular
            Left Ø5BQ
            Right Ø5BP
        Face
            Left Ø5BV
            Right Ø5BT
        Femoral
            Left Ø6BN
            Right Ø6BM
        Foot
            Left Ø6BV
            Right Ø6BT
        Gastric Ø6B2
        Hand
            Left Ø5BH
            Right Ø5BG
        Hemiazygos Ø5B1
        Hepatic Ø6B4
        Hypogastric
            Left Ø6BJ
            Right Ø6BH
        Inferior Mesenteric Ø6B6
        Innominate
            Left Ø5B4
            Right Ø5B3
        Internal Jugular
            Left Ø5BN
            Right Ø5BM
        Intracranial Ø5BL
        Lower Ø6BY
        Portal Ø6B8
        Pulmonary
            Left Ø2BT
            Right Ø2BS
        Renal
            Left Ø6BB
            Right Ø6B9
        Saphenous
            Left Ø6BQ
            Right Ø6BP
        Splenic Ø6B1
        Subclavian
            Left Ø5B6
            Right Ø5B5
        Superior Mesenteric Ø6B5

Excision — *continued*
    Vein — *continued*
        Upper Ø5BY
        Vertebral
            Left Ø5BS
            Right Ø5BR
    Vena Cava
        Inferior Ø6BØ
        Superior Ø2BV
    Ventricle
        Left Ø2BL
        Right Ø2BK
    Vertebra
        Cervical ØPB3
        Lumbar ØQBØ
        Thoracic ØPB4
    Vesicle
        Bilateral ØVB3
        Left ØVB2
        Right ØVB1
    Vitreous
        Left Ø8B53Z
        Right Ø8B43Z
    Vocal Cord
        Left ØCBV
        Right ØCBT
    Vulva ØUBM
    Wrist Region
        Left ØXBH
        Right ØXBG
EXCLUDER® AAA Endoprosthesis
    use Intraluminal Device
    use Intraluminal Device, Branched or Fenestrated,
        One or Two Arteries in Ø4V
    use Intraluminal Device, Branched or Fenestrated,
        Three or More Arteries in Ø4V
EXCLUDER® IBE Endoprosthesis *use* Intraluminal
    Device, Branched or Fenestrated, One or Two Ar-
    teries in Ø4V
Exclusion, Left atrial appendage (LAA) *see* Occlu-
    sion, Atrium, Left Ø2L7
Exercise, rehabilitation *see* Motor Treatment, Reha-
    bilitation FØ7
Exploration *see* Inspection
**Express® Biliary SD Monorail® Premounted Stent
    System** *use* Intraluminal Device
Express® (LD) Premounted Stent System *use* Intra-
    luminal Device
**Express® SD Renal Monorail® Premounted Stent
    System** *use* Intraluminal Device
Ex-PRESS™ mini glaucoma shunt *use* Synthetic
    Substitute
Extensor carpi radialis muscle
    use Lower Arm and Wrist Muscle, Left
    use Lower Arm and Wrist Muscle, Right
Extensor carpi ulnaris muscle
    use Lower Arm and Wrist Muscle, Left
    use Lower Arm and Wrist Muscle, Right
Extensor digitorum brevis muscle
    use Foot Muscle, Left
    use Foot Muscle, Right
Extensor digitorum longus muscle
    use Lower Leg Muscle, Left
    use Lower Leg Muscle, Right
Extensor hallucis brevis muscle
    use Foot Muscle, Left
    use Foot Muscle, Right
Extensor hallucis longus muscle
    use Lower Leg Muscle, Left
    use Lower Leg Muscle, Right
External anal sphincter *use* Anal Sphincter
External auditory meatus
    use External Auditory Canal, Left
    use External Auditory Canal, Right
External fixator
    use External Fixation Device in Head and Facial
        Bones
    use External Fixation Device in Lower Bones
    use External Fixation Device in Lower Joints
    use External Fixation Device in Upper Bones
    use External Fixation Device in Upper Joints
External maxillary artery *use* Face Artery
External naris *use* Nasal Mucosa and Soft Tissue
External oblique aponeurosis *use* Subcutaneous
    Tissue and Fascia, Trunk
External oblique muscle
    use Abdomen Muscle, Left

External oblique muscle — *continued*
  use Abdomen Muscle, Right
External popliteal nerve *use* Peroneal Nerve
External pudendal artery
  use Femoral Artery, Left
  use Femoral Artery, Right
External pudendal vein
  use Saphenous Vein, Left
  use Saphenous Vein, Right
External urethral sphincter *use* Urethra
Extirpation
  Acetabulum
    Left 0QC5
    Right 0QC4
  Adenoids 0CCQ
  Ampulla of Vater 0FCC
  Anal Sphincter 0DCR
  Anterior Chamber
    Left 08C3
    Right 08C2
  Anus 0DCQ
  Aorta
    Abdominal 04C0
    Thoracic
      Ascending/Arch 02CX
      Descending 02CW
  Aortic Body 0GCD
  Appendix 0DCJ
  Artery
    Anterior Tibial
      Left 04CQ
      Right 04CP
    Axillary
      Left 03C6
      Right 03C5
    Brachial
      Left 03C8
      Right 03C7
    Celiac 04C1
    Colic
      Left 04C7
      Middle 04C8
      Right 04C6
    Common Carotid
      Left 03CJ
      Right 03CH
    Common Iliac
      Left 04CD
      Right 04CC
    Coronary
      Four or More Arteries 02C3
      One Artery 02C0
      Three Arteries 02C2
      Two Arteries 02C1
    External Carotid
      Left 03CN
      Right 03CM
    External Iliac
      Left 04CJ
      Right 04CH
    Face 03CR
    Femoral
      Left 04CL
      Right 04CK
    Foot
      Left 04CW
      Right 04CV
    Gastric 04C2
    Hand
      Left 03CF
      Right 03CD
    Hepatic 04C3
    Inferior Mesenteric 04CB
    Innominate 03C2
    Internal Carotid
      Left 03CL
      Right 03CK
    Internal Iliac
      Left 04CF
      Right 04CE
    Internal Mammary
      Left 03C1
      Right 03C0
    Intracranial 03CG
    Lower 04CY
    Peroneal
      Left 04CU
      Right 04CT

Extirpation — *continued*
  Artery — *continued*
    Popliteal
      Left 04CN
      Right 04CM
    Posterior Tibial
      Left 04CS
      Right 04CR
    Pulmonary
      Left 02CR
      Right 02CQ
    Pulmonary Trunk 02CP
    Radial
      Left 03CC
      Right 03CB
    Renal
      Left 04CA
      Right 04C9
    Splenic 04C4
    Subclavian
      Left 03C4
      Right 03C3
    Superior Mesenteric 04C5
    Temporal
      Left 03CT
      Right 03CS
    Thyroid
      Left 03CV
      Right 03CU
    Ulnar
      Left 03CA
      Right 03C9
    Upper 03CY
    Vertebral
      Left 03CQ
      Right 03CP
  Atrium
    Left 02C7
    Right 02C6
  Auditory Ossicle
    Left 09CA
    Right 09C9
  Basal Ganglia 00C8
  Bladder 0TCB
  Bladder Neck 0TCC
  Bone
    Ethmoid
      Left 0NCG
      Right 0NCF
    Frontal 0NC1
    Hyoid 0NCX
    Lacrimal
      Left 0NCJ
      Right 0NCH
    Nasal 0NCB
    Occipital 0NC7
    Palatine
      Left 0NCL
      Right 0NCK
    Parietal
      Left 0NC4
      Right 0NC3
    Pelvic
      Left 0QC3
      Right 0QC2
    Sphenoid 0NCC
    Temporal
      Left 0NC6
      Right 0NC5
    Zygomatic
      Left 0NCN
      Right 0NCM
  Brain 00C0
  Breast
    Bilateral 0HCV
    Left 0HCU
    Right 0HCT
  Bronchus
    Lingula 0BC9
    Lower Lobe
      Left 0BCB
      Right 0BC6
    Main
      Left 0BC7
      Right 0BC3
    Middle Lobe, Right 0BC5
    Upper Lobe
      Left 0BC8
      Right 0BC4

Extirpation — *continued*
  Buccal Mucosa 0CC4
  Bursa and Ligament
    Abdomen
      Left 0MCJ
      Right 0MCH
    Ankle
      Left 0MCR
      Right 0MCQ
    Elbow
      Left 0MC4
      Right 0MC3
    Foot
      Left 0MCT
      Right 0MCS
    Hand
      Left 0MC8
      Right 0MC7
    Head and Neck 0MC0
    Hip
      Left 0MCM
      Right 0MCL
    Knee
      Left 0MCP
      Right 0MCN
    Lower Extremity
      Left 0MCW
      Right 0MCV
    Perineum 0MCK
    Rib(s) 0MCG
    Shoulder
      Left 0MC2
      Right 0MC1
    Spine
      Lower 0MCD
      Upper 0MCC
    Sternum 0MCF
    Upper Extremity
      Left 0MCB
      Right 0MC9
    Wrist
      Left 0MC6
      Right 0MC5
  Carina 0BC2
  Carotid Bodies, Bilateral 0GC8
  Carotid Body
    Left 0GC6
    Right 0GC7
  Carpal
    Left 0PCN
    Right 0PCM
  Cavity, Cranial 0WC1
  Cecum 0DCH
  Cerebellum 00CC
  Cerebral Hemisphere 00C7
  Cerebral Meninges 00C1
  Cerebral Ventricle 00C6
  Cervix 0UCC
  Chordae Tendineae 02C9
  Choroid
    Left 08CB
    Right 08CA
  Cisterna Chyli 07CL
  Clavicle
    Left 0PCB
    Right 0PC9
  Clitoris 0UCJ
  Coccygeal Glomus 0GCB
  Coccyx 0QCS
  Colon
    Ascending 0DCK
    Descending 0DCM
    Sigmoid 0DCN
    Transverse 0DCL
  Computer-aided Mechanical Aspiration X2C
  Conduction Mechanism 02C8
  Conjunctiva
    Left 08CTXZZ
    Right 08CSXZZ
  Cord
    Bilateral 0VCH
    Left 0VCG
    Right 0VCF
  Cornea
    Left 08C9XZZ
    Right 08C8XZZ
  Cul-de-sac 0UCF
  Diaphragm 0BCT

Extirpation — continued
  Disc
    Cervical Vertebral ØRC3
    Cervicothoracic Vertebral ØRC5
    Lumbar Vertebral ØSC2
    Lumbosacral ØSC4
    Thoracic Vertebral ØRC9
    Thoracolumbar Vertebral ØRCB
  Duct
    Common Bile ØFC9
    Cystic ØFC8
    Hepatic
      Common ØFC7
      Left ØFC6
      Right ØFC5
    Lacrimal
      Left 08CY
      Right 08CX
    Pancreatic ØFCD
      Accessory ØFCF
    Parotid
      Left ØCCC
      Right ØCCB
  Duodenum ØDC9
  Dura Mater 00C2
  Ear
    External
      Left 09C1
      Right 09C0
    External Auditory Canal
      Left 09C4
      Right 09C3
    Inner
      Left 09CE
      Right 09CD
    Middle
      Left 09C6
      Right 09C5
  Endometrium ØUCB
  Epididymis
    Bilateral ØVCL
    Left ØVCK
    Right ØVCJ
  Epidural Space, Intracranial 00C3
  Epiglottis ØCCR
  Esophagogastric Junction ØDC4
  Esophagus ØDC5
    Lower ØDC3
    Middle ØDC2
    Upper ØDC1
  Eustachian Tube
    Left 09CG
    Right 09CF
  Eye
    Left 08C1XZZ
    Right 08C0XZZ
  Eyelid
    Lower
      Left 08CR
      Right 08CQ
    Upper
      Left 08CP
      Right 08CN
  Fallopian Tube
    Left ØUC6
    Right ØUC5
  Fallopian Tubes, Bilateral ØUC7
  Femoral Shaft
    Left ØQC9
    Right ØQC8
  Femur
    Lower
      Left ØQCC
      Right ØQCB
    Upper
      Left ØQC7
      Right ØQC6
  Fibula
    Left ØQCK
    Right ØQCJ
  Finger Nail ØHCQXZZ
  Gallbladder ØFC4
  Gastrointestinal Tract ØWCP
  Genitourinary Tract ØWCR
  Gingiva
    Lower ØCC6
    Upper ØCC5

Extirpation — continued
  Gland
    Adrenal
      Bilateral ØGC4
      Left ØGC2
      Right ØGC3
    Lacrimal
      Left 08CW
      Right 08CV
    Minor Salivary ØCCJ
    Parotid
      Left ØCC9
      Right ØCC8
    Pituitary ØGC0
    Sublingual
      Left ØCCF
      Right ØCCD
    Submaxillary
      Left ØCCH
      Right ØCCG
    Vestibular ØUCL
  Glenoid Cavity
    Left ØPC8
    Right ØPC7
  Glomus Jugulare ØGCC
  Humeral Head
    Left ØPCD
    Right ØPCC
  Humeral Shaft
    Left ØPCG
    Right ØPCF
  Hymen ØUCK
  Hypothalamus 00CA
  Ileocecal Valve ØDCC
  Ileum ØDCB
  Intestine
    Large ØDCE
      Left ØDCG
      Right ØDCF
    Small ØDC8
  Iris
    Left 08CD
    Right 08CC
  Jaw
    Lower ØWC5
    Upper ØWC4
  Jejunum ØDCA
  Joint
    Acromioclavicular
      Left ØRCH
      Right ØRCG
    Ankle
      Left ØSCG
      Right ØSCF
    Carpal
      Left ØRCR
      Right ØRCQ
    Carpometacarpal
      Left ØRCT
      Right ØRCS
    Cervical Vertebral ØRC1
    Cervicothoracic Vertebral ØRC4
    Coccygeal ØSC6
    Elbow
      Left ØRCM
      Right ØRCL
    Finger Phalangeal
      Left ØRCX
      Right ØRCW
    Hip
      Left ØSCB
      Right ØSC9
    Knee
      Left ØSCD
      Right ØSCC
    Lumbar Vertebral ØSC0
    Lumbosacral ØSC3
    Metacarpophalangeal
      Left ØRCV
      Right ØRCU
    Metatarsal-Phalangeal
      Left ØSCN
      Right ØSCM
    Occipital-cervical ØRC0
    Sacrococcygeal ØSC5
    Sacroiliac
      Left ØSC8
      Right ØSC7

Extirpation — continued
  Joint — continued
    Shoulder
      Left ØRCK
      Right ØRCJ
    Sternoclavicular
      Left ØRCF
      Right ØRCE
    Tarsal
      Left ØSCJ
      Right ØSCH
    Tarsometatarsal
      Left ØSCL
      Right ØSCK
    Temporomandibular
      Left ØRCD
      Right ØRCC
    Thoracic Vertebral ØRC6
    Thoracolumbar Vertebral ØRCA
    Toe Phalangeal
      Left ØSCQ
      Right ØSCP
    Wrist
      Left ØRCP
      Right ØRCN
  Kidney
    Left ØTC1
    Right ØTC0
  Kidney Pelvis
    Left ØTC4
    Right ØTC3
  Larynx ØCCS
  Lens
    Left 08CK
    Right 08CJ
  Lip
    Lower ØCC1
    Upper ØCC0
  Liver ØFC0
    Left Lobe ØFC2
    Right Lobe ØFC1
  Lung
    Bilateral ØBCM
    Left ØBCL
    Lower Lobe
      Left ØBCJ
      Right ØBCF
    Middle Lobe, Right ØBCD
    Right ØBCK
    Upper Lobe
      Left ØBCG
      Right ØBCC
  Lung Lingula ØBCH
  Lymphatic
    Aortic 07CD
    Axillary
      Left 07C6
      Right 07C5
    Head 07C0
    Inguinal
      Left 07CJ
      Right 07CH
    Internal Mammary
      Left 07C9
      Right 07C8
    Lower Extremity
      Left 07CG
      Right 07CF
    Mesenteric 07CB
    Neck
      Left 07C2
      Right 07C1
    Pelvis 07CC
    Thoracic Duct 07CK
    Thorax 07C7
    Upper Extremity
      Left 07C4
      Right 07C3
  Mandible
    Left ØNCV
    Right ØNCT
  Maxilla ØNCR
  Mediastinum ØWCC
  Medulla Oblongata 00CD
  Mesentery ØDCV
  Metacarpal
    Left ØPCQ
    Right ØPCP

Extirpation — continued
 Metatarsal
  Left ØQCP
  Right ØQCN
 Muscle
  Abdomen
   Left ØKCL
   Right ØKCK
  Extraocular
   Left Ø8CM
   Right Ø8CL
  Facial ØKC1
  Foot
   Left ØKCW
   Right ØKCV
  Hand
   Left ØKCD
   Right ØKCC
  Head ØKCØ
  Hip
   Left ØKCP
   Right ØKCN
  Lower Arm and Wrist
   Left ØKCB
   Right ØKC9
  Lower Leg
   Left ØKCT
   Right ØKCS
  Neck
   Left ØKC3
   Right ØKC2
  Papillary Ø2CD
  Perineum ØKCM
  Shoulder
   Left ØKC6
   Right ØKC5
  Thorax
   Left ØKCJ
   Right ØKCH
  Tongue, Palate, Pharynx ØKC4
  Trunk
   Left ØKCG
   Right ØKCF
  Upper Arm
   Left ØKC8
   Right ØKC7
  Upper Leg
   Left ØKCR
   Right ØKCQ
 Nasal Mucosa and Soft Tissue Ø9CK
 Nasopharynx Ø9CN
 Nerve
  Abdominal Sympathetic Ø1CM
  Abducens ØØCL
  Accessory ØØCR
  Acoustic ØØCN
  Brachial Plexus Ø1C3
  Cervical Ø1C1
  Cervical Plexus Ø1CØ
  Facial ØØCM
  Femoral Ø1CD
  Glossopharyngeal ØØCP
  Head and Neck Sympathetic Ø1CK
  Hypoglossal ØØCS
  Lumbar Ø1CB
  Lumbar Plexus Ø1C9
  Lumbar Sympathetic Ø1CN
  Lumbosacral Plexus Ø1CA
  Median Ø1C5
  Oculomotor ØØCH
  Olfactory ØØCF
  Optic ØØCG
  Peroneal Ø1CH
  Phrenic Ø1C2
  Pudendal Ø1CC
  Radial Ø1C6
  Sacral Ø1CR
  Sacral Plexus Ø1CQ
  Sacral Sympathetic Ø1CP
  Sciatic Ø1CF
  Thoracic Ø1C8
  Thoracic Sympathetic Ø1CL
  Tibial Ø1CG
  Trigeminal ØØCK
  Trochlear ØØCJ
  Ulnar Ø1C4
  Vagus ØØCQ
 Nipple
  Left ØHCX

Extirpation — continued
 Nipple — continued
  Right ØHCW
 Omentum ØDCU
 Oral Cavity and Throat ØWC3
 Orbit
  Left ØNCQ
  Right ØNCP
 Orbital Atherectomy see Extirpation, Heart and
     Great Vessels Ø2C
 Ovary
  Bilateral ØUC2
  Left ØUC1
  Right ØUCØ
 Palate
  Hard ØCC2
  Soft ØCC3
 Pancreas ØFCG
 Para-aortic Body ØGC9
 Paraganglion Extremity ØGCF
 Parathyroid Gland ØGCR
  Inferior
   Left ØGCP
   Right ØGCN
  Multiple ØGCQ
  Superior
   Left ØGCM
   Right ØGCL
 Patella
  Left ØQCF
  Right ØQCD
 Pelvic Cavity ØWCJ
 Penis ØVCS
 Pericardial Cavity ØWCD
 Pericardium Ø2CN
 Peritoneal Cavity ØWCG
 Peritoneum ØDCW
 Phalanx
  Finger
   Left ØPCV
   Right ØPCT
  Thumb
   Left ØPCS
   Right ØPCR
  Toe
   Left ØQCR
   Right ØQCQ
 Pharynx ØCCM
 Pineal Body ØGC1
 Pleura
  Left ØBCP
  Right ØBCN
 Pleural Cavity
  Left ØWCB
  Right ØWC9
 Pons ØØCB
 Prepuce ØVCT
 Prostate ØVCØ
 Radius
  Left ØPCJ
  Right ØPCH
 Rectum ØDCP
 Respiratory Tract ØWCQ
 Retina
  Left Ø8CF
  Right Ø8CE
 Retinal Vessel
  Left Ø8CH
  Right Ø8CG
 Retroperitoneum ØWCH
 Ribs
  1 to 2 ØPC1
  3 or More ØPC2
 Sacrum ØQC1
 Scapula
  Left ØPC6
  Right ØPC5
 Sclera
  Left Ø8C7XZZ
  Right Ø8C6XZZ
 Scrotum ØVC5
 Septum
  Atrial Ø2C5
  Nasal Ø9CM
  Ventricular Ø2CM
 Sinus
  Accessory Ø9CP
  Ethmoid
   Left Ø9CV

Extirpation — continued
 Sinus — continued
  Ethmoid — continued
   Right Ø9CU
  Frontal
   Left Ø9CT
   Right Ø9CS
  Mastoid
   Left Ø9CC
   Right Ø9CB
  Maxillary
   Left Ø9CR
   Right Ø9CQ
  Sphenoid
   Left Ø9CX
   Right Ø9CW
 Skin
  Abdomen ØHC7XZZ
  Back ØHC6XZZ
  Buttock ØHC8XZZ
  Chest ØHC5XZZ
  Ear
   Left ØHC3XZZ
   Right ØHC2XZZ
  Face ØHC1XZZ
  Foot
   Left ØHCNXZZ
   Right ØHCMXZZ
  Hand
   Left ØHCGXZZ
   Right ØHCFXZZ
  Inguinal ØHCAXZZ
  Lower Arm
   Left ØHCEXZZ
   Right ØHCDXZZ
  Lower Leg
   Left ØHCLXZZ
   Right ØHCKXZZ
  Neck ØHC4XZZ
  Perineum ØHC9XZZ
  Scalp ØHCØXZZ
  Upper Arm
   Left ØHCCXZZ
   Right ØHCBXZZ
  Upper Leg
   Left ØHCJXZZ
   Right ØHCHXZZ
 Spinal Canal ØØCU
 Spinal Cord
  Cervical ØØCW
  Lumbar ØØCY
  Thoracic ØØCX
 Spinal Meninges ØØCT
 Spleen Ø7CP
 Sternum ØPCØ
 Stomach ØDC6
  Pylorus ØDC7
 Subarachnoid Space, Intracranial ØØC5
 Subcutaneous Tissue and Fascia
  Abdomen ØJC8
  Back ØJC7
  Buttock ØJC9
  Chest ØJC6
  Face ØJC1
  Foot
   Left ØJCR
   Right ØJCQ
  Hand
   Left ØJCK
   Right ØJCJ
  Lower Arm
   Left ØJCH
   Right ØJCG
  Lower Leg
   Left ØJCP
   Right ØJCN
  Neck
   Left ØJC5
   Right ØJC4
  Pelvic Region ØJCC
  Perineum ØJCB
  Scalp ØJCØ
  Upper Arm
   Left ØJCF
   Right ØJCD
  Upper Leg
   Left ØJCM
   Right ØJCL
 Subdural Space, Intracranial ØØC4

Extirpation — *continued*
Tarsal
  Left 0QCM
  Right 0QCL
Tendon
  Abdomen
    Left 0LCG
    Right 0LCF
  Ankle
    Left 0LCT
    Right 0LCS
  Foot
    Left 0LCW
    Right 0LCV
  Hand
    Left 0LC8
    Right 0LC7
  Head and Neck 0LC0
  Hip
    Left 0LCK
    Right 0LCJ
  Knee
    Left 0LCR
    Right 0LCQ
  Lower Arm and Wrist
    Left 0LC6
    Right 0LC5
  Lower Leg
    Left 0LCP
    Right 0LCN
  Perineum 0LCH
  Shoulder
    Left 0LC2
    Right 0LC1
  Thorax
    Left 0LCD
    Right 0LCC
  Trunk
    Left 0LCB
    Right 0LC9
  Upper Arm
    Left 0LC4
    Right 0LC3
  Upper Leg
    Left 0LCM
    Right 0LCL
Testis
  Bilateral 0VCC
  Left 0VCB
  Right 0VC9
Thalamus 00C9
Thymus 07CM
Thyroid Gland 0GCK
  Left Lobe 0GCG
  Right Lobe 0GCH
Tibia
  Left 0QCH
  Right 0QCG
Toe Nail 0HCRXZZ
Tongue 0CC7
Tonsils 0CCP
Tooth
  Lower 0CCX
  Upper 0CCW
Trachea 0BC1
Tunica Vaginalis
  Left 0VC7
  Right 0VC6
Turbinate, Nasal 09CL
Tympanic Membrane
  Left 09C8
  Right 09C7
Ulna
  Left 0PCL
  Right 0PCK
Ureter
  Left 0TC7
  Right 0TC6
Urethra 0TCD
Uterine Supporting Structure 0UC4
Uterus 0UC9
Uvula 0CCN
Vagina 0UCG
Valve
  Aortic 02CF
  Mitral 02CG
  Pulmonary 02CH
  Tricuspid 02CJ

Extirpation — *continued*
Vas Deferens
  Bilateral 0VCQ
  Left 0VCP
  Right 0VCN
Vein
  Axillary
    Left 05C8
    Right 05C7
  Azygos 05C0
  Basilic
    Left 05CC
    Right 05CB
  Brachial
    Left 05CA
    Right 05C9
  Cephalic
    Left 05CF
    Right 05CD
  Colic 06C7
  Common Iliac
    Left 06CD
    Right 06CC
  Coronary 02C4
  Esophageal 06C3
  External Iliac
    Left 06CG
    Right 06CF
  External Jugular
    Left 05CQ
    Right 05CP
  Face
    Left 05CV
    Right 05CT
  Femoral
    Left 06CN
    Right 06CM
  Foot
    Left 06CV
    Right 06CT
  Gastric 06C2
  Hand
    Left 05CH
    Right 05CG
  Hemiazygos 05C1
  Hepatic 06C4
  Hypogastric
    Left 06CJ
    Right 06CH
  Inferior Mesenteric 06C6
  Innominate
    Left 05C4
    Right 05C3
  Internal Jugular
    Left 05CN
    Right 05CM
  Intracranial 05CL
  Lower 06CY
  Portal 06C8
  Pulmonary
    Left 02CT
    Right 02CS
  Renal
    Left 06CB
    Right 06C9
  Saphenous
    Left 06CQ
    Right 06CP
  Splenic 06C1
  Subclavian
    Left 05C6
    Right 05C5
  Superior Mesenteric 06C5
  Upper 05CY
  Vertebral
    Left 05CS
    Right 05CR
Vena Cava
  Inferior 06C0
  Superior 02CV
Ventricle
  Left 02CL
  Right 02CK
Vertebra
  Cervical 0PC3
  Lumbar 0QC0
  Thoracic 0PC4
Vesicle
  Bilateral 0VC3

Extirpation — *continued*
Vesicle — *continued*
  Left 0VC2
  Right 0VC1
Vitreous
  Left 08C5
  Right 08C4
Vocal Cord
  Left 0CCV
  Right 0CCT
Vulva 0UCM
Extracorporeal Carbon Dioxide Removal (ECCO2R)
  5A0920Z
Extracorporeal shock wave lithotripsy *see* Fragmentation
Extracranial-intracranial bypass (EC-IC) *see* Bypass, Upper Arteries 031
Extraction
Acetabulum
  Left 0QD50ZZ
  Right 0QD40ZZ
Ampulla of Vater 0FDC
Anus 0DDQ
Appendix 0DDJ
Auditory Ossicle
  Left 09DA0ZZ
  Right 09D90ZZ
Bone
  Ethmoid
    Left 0NDG0ZZ
    Right 0NDF0ZZ
  Frontal 0ND10ZZ
  Hyoid 0NDX0ZZ
  Lacrimal
    Left 0NDJ0ZZ
    Right 0NDH0ZZ
  Nasal 0NDB0ZZ
  Occipital 0ND70ZZ
  Palatine
    Left 0NDL0ZZ
    Right 0NDK0ZZ
  Parietal
    Left 0ND40ZZ
    Right 0ND30ZZ
  Pelvic
    Left 0QD30ZZ
    Right 0QD20ZZ
  Sphenoid 0NDC0ZZ
  Temporal
    Left 0ND60ZZ
    Right 0ND50ZZ
  Zygomatic
    Left 0NDN0ZZ
    Right 0NDM0ZZ
Bone Marrow 07DT
  Iliac 07DR
  Sternum 07DQ
  Vertebral 07DS
Brain 00D0
Breast
  Bilateral 0HDV0ZZ
  Left 0HDU0ZZ
  Right 0HDT0ZZ
  Supernumerary 0HDY0ZZ
Bronchus
  Lingula 0BD9
  Lower Lobe
    Left 0BDB
    Right 0BD6
  Main
    Left 0BD7
    Right 0BD3
  Middle Lobe, Right 0BD5
  Upper Lobe
    Left 0BD8
    Right 0BD4
Bursa and Ligament
  Abdomen
    Left 0MDJ
    Right 0MDH
  Ankle
    Left 0MDR
    Right 0MDQ
  Elbow
    Left 0MD4
    Right 0MD3
  Foot
    Left 0MDT
    Right 0MDS

Extraction — *continued*
  Bursa and Ligament — *continued*
    Hand
      Left ØMD8
      Right ØMD7
    Head and Neck ØMDØ
    Hip
      Left ØMDM
      Right ØMDL
    Knee
      Left ØMDP
      Right ØMDN
    Lower Extremity
      Left ØMDW
      Right ØMDV
    Perineum ØMDK
    Rib(s) ØMDG
    Shoulder
      Left ØMD2
      Right ØMD1
    Spine
      Lower ØMDD
      Upper ØMDC
    Sternum ØMDF
    Upper Extremity
      Left ØMDB
      Right ØMD9
    Wrist
      Left ØMD6
      Right ØMD5
  Carina ØBD2
  Carpal
    Left ØPDNØZZ
    Right ØPDMØZZ
  Cecum ØDDH
  Cerebral Hemisphere ØØD7
  Cerebral Meninges ØØD1
  Cisterna Chyli Ø7DL
  Clavicle
    Left ØPDBØZZ
    Right ØPD9ØZZ
  Coccyx ØQDSØZZ
  Colon
    Ascending ØDDK
    Descending ØDDM
    Sigmoid ØDDN
    Transverse ØDDL
  Cornea
    Left Ø8D9XZ
    Right Ø8D8XZ
  Duct
    Common Bile ØFD9
    Cystic ØFD8
    Hepatic
      Common ØFD7
      Left ØFD6
      Right ØFD5
    Pancreatic ØFDD
      Accessory ØFDF
  Duodenum ØDD9
  Dura Mater ØØD2
  Endometrium ØUDB
  Esophagogastric Junction ØDD4
  Esophagus ØDD5
    Lower ØDD3
    Middle ØDD2
    Upper ØDD1
  Femoral Shaft
    Left ØQD9ØZZ
    Right ØQD8ØZZ
  Femur
    Lower
      Left ØQDCØZZ
      Right ØQDBØZZ
    Upper
      Left ØQD7ØZZ
      Right ØQD6ØZZ
  Fibula
    Left ØQDKØZZ
    Right ØQDJØZZ
  Finger Nail ØHDQXZZ
  Gallbladder ØFD4
  Glenoid Cavity
    Left ØPD8ØZZ
    Right ØPD7ØZZ
  Hair ØHDSXZZ
  Humeral Head
    Left ØPDDØZZ
    Right ØPDCØZZ

Extraction — *continued*
  Humeral Shaft
    Left ØPDGØZZ
    Right ØPDFØZZ
  Ileocecal Valve ØDDC
  Ileum ØDDB
  Intestine
    Large ØDDE
      Left ØDDG
      Right ØDDF
    Small ØDD8
  Jejunum ØDDA
  Kidney
    Left ØTD1
    Right ØTDØ
  Lens
    Left Ø8DK3ZZ
    Right Ø8DJ3ZZ
  Liver ØFDØ
    Left Lobe ØFD2
    Right Lobe ØFD1
  Lung
    Bilateral ØBDM
    Left ØBDL
    Lower Lobe
      Left ØBDJ
      Right ØBDF
    Middle Lobe, Right ØBDD
    Right ØBDK
    Upper Lobe
      Left ØBDG
      Right ØBDC
  Lung Lingula ØBDH
  Lymphatic
    Aortic Ø7DD
    Axillary
      Left Ø7D6
      Right Ø7D5
    Head Ø7DØ
    Inguinal
      Left Ø7DJ
      Right Ø7DH
    Internal Mammary
      Left Ø7D9
      Right Ø7D8
    Lower Extremity
      Left Ø7DG
      Right Ø7DF
    Mesenteric Ø7DB
    Neck
      Left Ø7D2
      Right Ø7D1
    Pelvis Ø7DC
    Thoracic Duct Ø7DK
    Thorax Ø7D7
    Upper Extremity
      Left Ø7D4
      Right Ø7D3
  Mandible
    Left ØNDVØZZ
    Right ØNDTØZZ
  Maxilla ØNDRØZZ
  Metacarpal
    Left ØPDQØZZ
    Right ØPDPØZZ
  Metatarsal
    Left ØQDPØZZ
    Right ØQDNØZZ
  Muscle
    Abdomen
      Left ØKDLØZZ
      Right ØKDKØZZ
    Facial ØKD1ØZZ
    Foot
      Left ØKDWØZZ
      Right ØKDVØZZ
    Hand
      Left ØKDDØZZ
      Right ØKDCØZZ
    Head ØKDØØZZ
    Hip
      Left ØKDPØZZ
      Right ØKDNØZZ
    Lower Arm and Wrist
      Left ØKDBØZZ
      Right ØKD9ØZZ
    Lower Leg
      Left ØKDTØZZ
      Right ØKDSØZZ

Extraction — *continued*
  Muscle — *continued*
    Neck
      Left ØKD3ØZZ
      Right ØKD2ØZZ
    Perineum ØKDMØZZ
    Shoulder
      Left ØKD6ØZZ
      Right ØKD5ØZZ
    Thorax
      Left ØKDJØZZ
      Right ØKDHØZZ
    Tongue, Palate, Pharynx ØKD4ØZZ
    Trunk
      Left ØKDGØZZ
      Right ØKDFØZZ
    Upper Arm
      Left ØKD8ØZZ
      Right ØKD7ØZZ
    Upper Leg
      Left ØKDRØZZ
      Right ØKDQØZZ
  Nerve
    Abdominal Sympathetic Ø1DM
    Abducens ØØDL
    Accessory ØØDR
    Acoustic ØØDN
    Brachial Plexus Ø1D3
    Cervical Ø1D1
    Cervical Plexus Ø1DØ
    Facial ØØDM
    Femoral Ø1DD
    Glossopharyngeal ØØDP
    Head and Neck Sympathetic Ø1DK
    Hypoglossal ØØDS
    Lumbar Ø1DB
    Lumbar Plexus Ø1D9
    Lumbar Sympathetic Ø1DN
    Lumbosacral Plexus Ø1DA
    Median Ø1D5
    Oculomotor ØØDH
    Olfactory ØØDF
    Optic ØØDG
    Peroneal Ø1DH
    Phrenic Ø1D2
    Pudendal Ø1DC
    Radial Ø1D6
    Sacral Ø1DR
    Sacral Plexus Ø1DQ
    Sacral Sympathetic Ø1DP
    Sciatic Ø1DF
    Thoracic Ø1D8
    Thoracic Sympathetic Ø1DL
    Tibial Ø1DG
    Trigeminal ØØDK
    Trochlear ØØDJ
    Ulnar Ø1D4
    Vagus ØØDQ
  Orbit
    Left ØNDQØZZ
    Right ØNDPØZZ
  Ova ØUDN
  Pancreas ØFDG
  Patella
    Left ØQDFØZZ
    Right ØQDDØZZ
  Phalanx
    Finger
      Left ØPDVØZZ
      Right ØPDTØZZ
    Thumb
      Left ØPDSØZZ
      Right ØPDRØZZ
    Toe
      Left ØQDRØZZ
      Right ØQDQØZZ
  Pleura
    Left ØBDP
    Right ØBDN
  Products of Conception
    Ectopic 1ØD2
    Extraperitoneal 1ØDØØZ2
    High 1ØDØØZØ
    High Forceps 1ØDØ7Z5
    Internal Version 1ØDØ7Z7
    Low 1ØDØØZ1
    Low Forceps 1ØDØ7Z3
    Mid Forceps 1ØDØ7Z4
    Other 1ØDØ7Z8

Extraction — *continued*
    Products of Conception — *continued*
        Retained 10D1
        Vacuum 10D07Z6
    Radius
        Left 0PDJ0ZZ
        Right 0PDH0ZZ
    Rectum 0DDP
    Ribs
        1 to 2 0PD10ZZ
        3 or More 0PD20ZZ
    Sacrum 0QD10ZZ
    Scapula
        Left 0PD60ZZ
        Right 0PD50ZZ
    Septum, Nasal 09DM
    Sinus
        Accessory 09DP
        Ethmoid
            Left 09DV
            Right 09DU
        Frontal
            Left 09DT
            Right 09DS
        Mastoid
            Left 09DC
            Right 09DB
        Maxillary
            Left 09DR
            Right 09DQ
        Sphenoid
            Left 09DX
            Right 09DW
    Skin
        Abdomen 0HD7XZZ
        Back 0HD6XZZ
        Buttock 0HD8XZZ
        Chest 0HD5XZZ
        Ear
            Left 0HD3XZZ
            Right 0HD2XZZ
        Face 0HD1XZZ
        Foot
            Left 0HDNXZZ
            Right 0HDMXZZ
        Hand
            Left 0HDGXZZ
            Right 0HDFXZZ
        Inguinal 0HDAXZZ
        Lower Arm
            Left 0HDEXZZ
            Right 0HDDXZZ
        Lower Leg
            Left 0HDLXZZ
            Right 0HDKXZZ
        Neck 0HD4XZZ
        Perineum 0HD9XZZ
        Scalp 0HD0XZZ
        Upper Arm
            Left 0HDCXZZ
            Right 0HDBXZZ
        Upper Leg
            Left 0HDJXZZ
            Right 0HDHXZZ
    Skull 0ND00ZZ
    Spinal Meninges 00DT
    Spleen 07DP
    Sternum 0PD00ZZ
    Stomach 0DD6
        Pylorus 0DD7
    Subcutaneous Tissue and Fascia
        Abdomen 0JD8
        Back 0JD7
        Buttock 0JD9
        Chest 0JD6
        Face 0JD1
        Foot
            Left 0JDR
            Right 0JDQ
        Hand
            Left 0JDK
            Right 0JDJ
        Lower Arm
            Left 0JDH
            Right 0JDG
        Lower Leg
            Left 0JDP
            Right 0JDN

Extraction — *continued*
    Subcutaneous Tissue and Fascia — *continued*
        Neck
            Left 0JD5
            Right 0JD4
        Pelvic Region 0JDC
        Perineum 0JDB
        Scalp 0JD0
        Upper Arm
            Left 0JDF
            Right 0JDD
        Upper Leg
            Left 0JDM
            Right 0JDL
    Tarsal
        Left 0QDM0ZZ
        Right 0QDL0ZZ
    Tendon
        Abdomen
            Left 0LDG0ZZ
            Right 0LDF0ZZ
        Ankle
            Left 0LDT0ZZ
            Right 0LDS0ZZ
        Foot
            Left 0LDW0ZZ
            Right 0LDV0ZZ
        Hand
            Left 0LD80ZZ
            Right 0LD70ZZ
        Head and Neck 0LD00ZZ
        Hip
            Left 0LDK0ZZ
            Right 0LDJ0ZZ
        Knee
            Left 0LDR0ZZ
            Right 0LDQ0ZZ
        Lower Arm and Wrist
            Left 0LD60ZZ
            Right 0LD50ZZ
        Lower Leg
            Left 0LDP0ZZ
            Right 0LDN0ZZ
        Perineum 0LDH0ZZ
        Shoulder
            Left 0LD20ZZ
            Right 0LD10ZZ
        Thorax
            Left 0LDD0ZZ
            Right 0LDC0ZZ
        Trunk
            Left 0LDB0ZZ
            Right 0LD90ZZ
        Upper Arm
            Left 0LD40ZZ
            Right 0LD30ZZ
        Upper Leg
            Left 0LDM0ZZ
            Right 0DLL0ZZ
    Thymus 07DM
    Tibia
        Left 0QDH0ZZ
        Right 0QDG0ZZ
    Toe Nail 0HDRXZZ
    Tooth
        Lower 0CDXXZ
        Upper 0CDWXZ
    Trachea 0BD1
    Turbinate, Nasal 09DL
    Tympanic Membrane
        Left 09D8
        Right 09D7
    Ulna
        Left 0PDL0ZZ
        Right 0PDK0ZZ
    Vein
        Basilic
            Left 05DC
            Right 05DB
        Brachial
            Left 05DA
            Right 05D9
        Cephalic
            Left 05DF
            Right 05DD
        Femoral
            Left 06DN
            Right 06DM

Extraction — *continued*
    Vein — *continued*
        Foot
            Left 06DV
            Right 06DT
        Hand
            Left 05DH
            Right 05DG
        Lower 06DY
        Saphenous
            Left 06DQ
            Right 06DP
        Upper 05DY
    Vertebra
        Cervical 0PD30ZZ
        Lumbar 0QD00ZZ
        Thoracic 0PD40ZZ
    Vocal Cord
        Left 0CDV
        Right 0CDT

Extradural space, intracranial *use* Epidural Space, Intracranial
Extradural space, spinal *use* Spinal Canal
EXtreme Lateral Interbody Fusion (XLIF) device *use* Interbody Fusion Device in Lower Joints

F

Face lift *see* Alteration, Face 0W02
Facet replacement spinal stabilization device
    use Spinal Stabilization Device, Facet Replacement in 0RH
    use Spinal Stabilization Device, Facet Replacement in 0SH
Facial artery *use* Face Artery
Factor Xa Inhibitor Reversal Agent, Andexanet Alfa *use* Coagulation Factor Xa, Inactivated
False vocal cord *use* Larynx
Falx cerebri *use* Dura Mater
Fascia lata
    use Subcutaneous Tissue and Fascia, Left Upper Leg
    use Subcutaneous Tissue and Fascia, Right Upper Leg
Fasciaplasty, fascioplasty
    see Repair, Subcutaneous Tissue and Fascia 0JQ
    see Replacement, Subcutaneous Tissue and Fascia 0JR
Fasciectomy *see* Excision, Subcutaneous Tissue and Fascia 0JB
Fasciorrhaphy *see* Repair, Subcutaneous Tissue and Fascia 0JQ
Fasciotomy
    see Division, Subcutaneous Tissue and Fascia 0J8
    see Drainage, Subcutaneous Tissue and Fascia 0J9
    see Release
Feeding Device
    Change device in
        Lower 0D2DXUZ
        Upper 0D20XUZ
    Insertion of device in
        Duodenum 0DH9
        Esophagus 0DH5
        Ileum 0DHB
        Intestine, Small 0DH8
        Jejunum 0DHA
        Stomach 0DH6
    Removal of device from
        Esophagus 0DP5
        Intestinal Tract
            Lower 0DPD
            Upper 0DP0
        Stomach 0DP6
    Revision of device in
        Intestinal Tract
            Lower 0DWD
            Upper 0DW0
        Stomach 0DW6
Femoral head
    use Upper Femur, Left
    use Upper Femur, Right
Femoral lymph node
    use Lymphatic, Left Lower Extremity
    use Lymphatic, Right Lower Extremity
Femoropatellar joint
    use Knee Joint, Left
    use Knee Joint, Left, Tibial Surface

Femoropatellar joint — *continued*
  use Knee Joint, Right
  use Knee Joint, Right, Femoral Surface
Femorotibial joint
  use Knee Joint, Left
  use Knee Joint, Left, Tibial Surface
  use Knee Joint, Right
  use Knee Joint, Right, Tibial Surface
FETROJA® *use* Cefiderocol Anti-infective
FGS (fluorescence-guided surgery) *see* Fluorescence
  Guided Procedure
Fibular artery
  use Peroneal Artery, Left
  use Peroneal Artery, Right
Fibular sesamoid
  use Metatarsal, Left
  use Metatarsal, Right
Fibularis brevis muscle
  use Lower Leg Muscle, Left
  use Lower Leg Muscle, Right
Fibularis longus muscle
  use Lower Leg Muscle, Left
  use Lower Leg Muscle, Right
Fifth cranial nerve *use* Trigeminal Nerve
Filum terminale *use* Spinal Meninges
Fimbriectomy
  see Excision, Female Reproductive System ØUB
  see Resection, Female Reproductive System ØUT
Fine needle aspiration
  Fluid or gas *see* Drainage
  Tissue biopsy
    see Excision
    see Extraction
First cranial nerve *use* Olfactory Nerve
First intercostal nerve *use* Brachial Plexus
Fistulization
  see Bypass
  see Drainage
  see Repair
Fitting
  Arch bars, for fracture reduction *see* Reposition,
    Mouth and Throat ØCS
  Arch bars, for immobilization *see* Immobilization,
    Face 2W31
  Artificial limb *see* Device Fitting, Rehabilitation
    FØD
  Hearing aid *see* Device Fitting, Rehabilitation FØD
  Ocular prosthesis FØDZ8UZ
  Prosthesis, limb *see* Device Fitting, Rehabilitation
    FØD
  Prosthesis, ocular FØDZ8UZ
Fixation, bone
  External, with fracture reduction *see* Reposition
  External, without fracture reduction *see* Insertion
  Internal, with fracture reduction *see* Reposition
  Internal, without fracture reduction *see* Insertion
FLAIR® Endovascular Stent Graft *use* Intraluminal
  Device
Flexible Composite Mesh *use* Synthetic Substitute
Flexor carpi radialis muscle
  use Lower Arm and Wrist Muscle, Left
  use Lower Arm and Wrist Muscle, Right
Flexor carpi ulnaris muscle
  use Lower Arm and Wrist Muscle, Left
  use Lower Arm and Wrist Muscle, Right
Flexor digitorum brevis muscle
  use Foot Muscle, Left
  use Foot Muscle, Right
Flexor digitorum longus muscle
  use Lower Leg Muscle, Left
  use Lower Leg Muscle, Right
Flexor hallucis brevis muscle
  use Foot Muscle, Left
  use Foot Muscle, Right
Flexor hallucis longus muscle
  use Lower Leg Muscle, Left
  use Lower Leg Muscle, Right
Flexor pollicis longus muscle
  use Lower Arm and Wrist Muscle, Left
  use Lower Arm and Wrist Muscle, Right
Flow Diverter embolization device *use* Intraluminal
  Device, Flow Diverter in Ø3V
FlowSense Noninvasive Thermal Sensor *see* Measurement, Central Nervous Cerebrospinal Fluid
  Shunt

Fluorescence Guided Procedure
  Extremity
    Lower 8EØY
    Upper 8EØX
  Head and Neck Region 8E09
    Aminolevulinic Acid 8E09ØEM
    No Qualifier 8E09ØEZ
  Trunk Region 8EØW
Fluorescent Pyrazine, Kidney XT25XE5
Fluoroscopy
  Abdomen and Pelvis BW11
  Airway, Upper BB1DZZZ
  Ankle
    Left BQ1H
    Right BQ1G
  Aorta
    Abdominal B41Ø
      Laser, Intraoperative B41Ø
    Thoracic B31Ø
      Laser, Intraoperative B31Ø
    Thoraco-Abdominal B31P
      Laser, Intraoperative B31P
  Aorta and Bilateral Lower Extremity Arteries B41D
    Laser, Intraoperative B41D
  Arm
    Left BP1FZZZ
    Right BP1EZZZ
  Artery
    Brachiocephalic-Subclavian
      Laser, Intraoperative B311
      Right B311
    Bronchial B31L
      Laser, Intraoperative B31L
    Bypass Graft, Other B21F
    Cervico-Cerebral Arch B31Q
      Laser, Intraoperative B31Q
    Common Carotid
      Bilateral B315
        Laser, Intraoperative B315
      Left B314
        Laser, Intraoperative B314
      Right B313
        Laser, Intraoperative B313
    Coronary
      Bypass Graft
        Multiple B213
          Laser, Intraoperative B213
        Single B212
          Laser, Intraoperative B212
      Multiple B211
        Laser, Intraoperative B211
      Single B21Ø
        Laser, Intraoperative B21Ø
    External Carotid
      Bilateral B31C
        Laser, Intraoperative B31C
      Left B31B
        Laser, Intraoperative B31B
      Right B319
        Laser, Intraoperative B319
    Hepatic B412
      Laser, Intraoperative B412
    Inferior Mesenteric B415
      Laser, Intraoperative B415
    Intercostal B31L
      Laser, Intraoperative B31L
    Internal Carotid
      Bilateral B318
        Laser, Intraoperative B318
      Left B317
        Laser, Intraoperative B317
      Right B316
        Laser, Intraoperative B316
    Internal Mammary Bypass Graft
      Left B218
      Right B217
    Intra-Abdominal
      Laser, Intraoperative B41B
      Other B41B
    Intracranial B31R
      Laser, Intraoperative B31R
    Lower
      Laser, Intraoperative B41J
      Other B41J
    Lower Extremity
      Bilateral and Aorta B41D
        Laser, Intraoperative B41D
      Left B41G
        Laser, Intraoperative B41G

Fluoroscopy — *continued*
  Artery — *continued*
    Lower Extremity — *continued*
      Right B41F
        Laser, Intraoperative B41F
    Lumbar B419
      Laser, Intraoperative B419
    Pelvic B41C
      Laser, Intraoperative B41C
    Pulmonary
      Left B31T
        Laser, Intraoperative B31T
      Right B31S
        Laser, Intraoperative B31S
    Pulmonary Trunk B31U
      Laser, Intraoperative B31U
    Renal
      Bilateral B418
        Laser, Intraoperative B418
      Left B417
        Laser, Intraoperative B417
      Right B416
        Laser, Intraoperative B416
    Spinal B31M
      Laser, Intraoperative B31M
    Splenic B413
      Laser, Intraoperative B413
    Subclavian
      Laser, Intraoperative B312
      Left B312
    Superior Mesenteric B414
      Laser, Intraoperative B414
    Upper
      Laser, Intraoperative B31N
      Other B31N
    Upper Extremity
      Bilateral B31K
        Laser, Intraoperative B31K
      Left B31J
        Laser, Intraoperative B31J
      Right B31H
        Laser, Intraoperative B31H
    Vertebral
      Bilateral B31G
        Laser, Intraoperative B31G
      Left B31F
        Laser, Intraoperative B31F
      Right B31D
        Laser, Intraoperative B31D
  Bile Duct BF1Ø
    Pancreatic Duct and Gallbladder BF14
  Bile Duct and Gallbladder BF13
  Biliary Duct BF11
  Bladder BT1Ø
    Kidney and Ureter BT14
    Left BT1F
    Right BT1D
  Bladder and Urethra BT1B
  Bowel, Small BD1
  Calcaneus
    Left BQ1KZZZ
    Right BQ1JZZZ
  Clavicle
    Left BP15ZZZ
    Right BP14ZZZ
  Coccyx BR1F
  Colon BD14
  Corpora Cavernosa BV1Ø
  Dialysis Fistula B51W
  Dialysis Shunt B51W
  Diaphragm BB16ZZZ
  Disc
    Cervical BR11
    Lumbar BR13
    Thoracic BR12
  Duodenum BD19
  Elbow
    Left BP1H
    Right BP1G
  Epiglottis B91G
  Esophagus BD11
  Extremity
    Lower BW1C
    Upper BW1J
  Facet Joint
    Cervical BR14
    Lumbar BR16
    Thoracic BR15

Fluoroscopy — *continued*
  Fallopian Tube
    Bilateral BU12
    Left BU11
    Right BU1Ø
  Fallopian Tube and Uterus BU18
  Femur
    Left BQ14ZZZ
    Right BQ13ZZZ
  Finger
    Left BP1SZZZ
    Right BP1RZZZ
  Foot
    Left BQ1MZZZ
    Right BQ1LZZZ
  Forearm
    Left BP1KZZZ
    Right BP1JZZZ
  Gallbladder BF12
    Bile Duct and Pancreatic Duct BF14
  Gallbladder and Bile Duct BF13
  Gastrointestinal, Upper BD1
  Hand
    Left BP1PZZZ
    Right BP1NZZZ
  Head and Neck BW19
  Heart
    Left B215
    Right B214
    Right and Left B216
  Hip
    Left BQ11
    Right BQ1Ø
  Humerus
    Left BP1BZZZ
    Right BP1AZZZ
  Ileal Diversion Loop BT1C
  Ileal Loop, Ureters and Kidney BT1G
  Intracranial Sinus B512
  Joint
    Acromioclavicular, Bilateral BP13ZZZ
    Finger
      Left BP1D
      Right BP1C
    Foot
      Left BQ1Y
      Right BQ1X
    Hand
      Left BP1D
      Right BP1C
    Lumbosacral BR1B
    Sacroiliac BR1D
    Sternoclavicular
      Bilateral BP12ZZZ
      Left BP11ZZZ
      Right BP1ØZZZ
    Temporomandibular
      Bilateral BN19
      Left BN18
      Right BN17
    Thoracolumbar BR18
    Toe
      Left BQ1Y
      Right BQ1X
  Kidney
    Bilateral BT13
    Ileal Loop and Ureter BT1G
    Left BT12
    Right BT11
    Ureter and Bladder BT14
      Left BT1F
      Right BT1D
  Knee
    Left BQ18
    Right BQ17
  Larynx B91J
  Leg
    Left BQ1FZZZ
    Right BQ1DZZZ
  Liver BF15
  Lung
    Bilateral BB14ZZZ
    Left BB13ZZZ
    Right BB12ZZZ
  Mediastinum BB1CZZZ
  Mouth BD1B
  Neck and Head BW19
  Oropharynx BD1B
  Pancreatic Duct BF1

Fluoroscopy — *continued*
  Pancreatic Duct — *continued*
    Gallbladder and Bile Buct BF14
  Patella
    Left BQ1WZZZ
    Right BQ1VZZZ
  Pelvis BR1C
  Pelvis and Abdomen BW11
  Pharynix B91G
  Ribs
    Left BP1YZZZ
    Right BP1XZZZ
  Sacrum BR1F
  Scapula
    Left BP17ZZZ
    Right BP16ZZZ
  Shoulder
    Left BP19
    Right BP18
  Sinus, Intracranial B512
  Spinal Cord BØ1B
  Spine
    Cervical BR1Ø
    Lumbar BR19
    Thoracic BR17
    Whole BR1G
  Sternum BR1H
  Stomach BD12
  Toe
    Left BQ1QZZZ
    Right BQ1PZZZ
  Tracheobronchial Tree
    Bilateral BB19YZZ
    Left BB18YZZ
    Right BB17YZZ
  Ureter
    Ileal Loop and Kidney BT1G
    Kidney and Bladder BT14
      Left BT1F
      Right BT1D
    Left BT17
    Right BT16
  Urethra BT15
  Urethra and Bladder BT1B
  Uterus BU16
  Uterus and Fallopian Tube BU18
  Vagina BU19
  Vasa Vasorum BV18
  Vein
    Cerebellar B511
    Cerebral B511
    Epidural B51Ø
    Jugular
      Bilateral B515
      Left B514
      Right B513
    Lower Extremity
      Bilateral B51D
      Left B51C
      Right B51B
    Other B51V
    Pelvic (Iliac)
      Left B51G
      Right B51F
    Pelvic (Iliac) Bilateral B51H
    Portal B51T
    Pulmonary
      Bilateral B51S
      Left B51R
      Right B51Q
    Renal
      Bilateral B51L
      Left B51K
      Right B51J
    Spanchnic B51T
    Subclavian
      Left B517
      Right B516
    Upper Extremity
      Bilateral B51P
      Left B51N
      Right B51M
  Vena Cava
    Inferior B519
    Superior B518
  Wrist
    Left BP1M
    Right BP1L

Fluoroscopy, laser intraoperative
  see Fluoroscopy, Heart B21
  see Fluoroscopy, Lower Arteries B41
  see Fluoroscopy, Upper Arteries B31
Flushing *see* Irrigation
Foley catheter *use* Drainage Device
Fontan completion procedure Stage II *see* Bypass, Vena Cava, Inferior Ø610
Foramen magnum *use* Occipital Bone
Foramen of Monro (intraventricular) *use* Cerebral Ventricle
Foreskin *use* Prepuce
Formula™ Balloon-Expandable Renal Stent System *use* Intraluminal Device
Fosfomycin Anti-infective XWØ
Fosfomycin injection *use* Fosfomycin Anti-infective
Fossa of Rosenmuller *use* Nasopharynx
Fourth cranial nerve *use* Trochlear Nerve
Fourth ventricle *use* Cerebral Ventricle
Fovea
  use Retina, Left
  use Retina, Right
Fragmentation
  Ampulla of Vater ØFFC
  Anus ØDFQ
  Appendix ØDFJ
  Artery
    Anterior Tibial
      Left Ø4FQ3Z
      Right Ø4FP3Z
    Axillary
      Left Ø3F63Z
      Right Ø3F53Z
    Brachial
      Left Ø3F83Z
      Right Ø3F73Z
    Common Iliac
      Left Ø4FD3Z
      Right Ø4FC3Z
    Coronary
      Four or More Arteries Ø2F33ZZ
      One Artery Ø2FØ3ZZ
      Three Arteries Ø2F23ZZ
      Two Arteries Ø2F13ZZ
    External Iliac
      Left Ø4FJ3Z
      Right Ø4FH3Z
    Femoral
      Left Ø4FL3Z
      Right Ø4FK3Z
    Innominate Ø3F23Z
    Internal Iliac
      Left Ø4FF3Z
      Right Ø4FE3Z
    Intracranial Ø3FG3Z
    Lower Ø4FY3Z
    Peroneal
      Left Ø4FU3Z
      Right Ø4FT3Z
    Popliteal
      Left Ø4FN3Z
      Right Ø4FM3Z
    Posterior Tibial
      Left Ø4FS3Z
      Right Ø4FR3Z
    Pulmonary
      Left Ø2FR3Z
      Right Ø2FQ3Z
    Pulmonary Trunk Ø2FP3Z
    Radial
      Left Ø3FC3Z
      Right Ø3FB3Z
    Subclavian
      Left Ø3F43Z
      Right Ø3F33Z
    Ulnar
      Left Ø3FA3Z
      Right Ø3F93Z
    Upper Ø3FY3Z
  Bladder ØTFB
  Bladder Neck ØTFC
  Bronchus
    Lingula ØBF9
    Lower Lobe
      Left ØBFB
      Right ØBF6
    Main
      Left ØBF7

Fragmentation — *continued*
  Bronchus — *continued*
    Main — *continued*
      Right ØBF3
    Middle Lobe, Right ØBF5
    Upper Lobe
      Left ØBF8
      Right ØBF4
  Carina ØBF2
  Cavity, Cranial ØWF1
  Cecum ØDFH
  Cerebral Ventricle ØØF6
  Colon
    Ascending ØDFK
    Descending ØDFM
    Sigmoid ØDFN
    Transverse ØDFL
  Duct
    Common Bile ØFF9
    Cystic ØFF8
    Hepatic
      Common ØFF7
      Left ØFF6
      Right ØFF5
    Pancreatic ØFFD
      Accessory ØFFF
    Parotid
      Left ØCFC
      Right ØCFB
  Duodenum ØDF9
  Epidural Space, Intracranial ØØF3
  Esophagus ØDF5
  Fallopian Tube
    Left ØUF6
    Right ØUF5
  Fallopian Tubes, Bilateral ØUF7
  Gallbladder ØFF4
  Gastrointestinal Tract ØWFP
  Genitourinary Tract ØWFR
  Ileum ØDFB
  Intestine
    Large ØDFE
      Left ØDFG
      Right ØDFF
    Small ØDF8
  Jejunum ØDFA
  Kidney Pelvis
    Left ØTF4
    Right ØTF3
  Mediastinum ØWFC
  Oral Cavity and Throat ØWF3
  Pelvic Cavity ØWFJ
  Pericardial Cavity ØWFD
  Pericardium Ø2FN
  Peritoneal Cavity ØWFG
  Pleural Cavity
    Left ØWFB
    Right ØWF9
  Rectum ØDFP
  Respiratory Tract ØWFQ
  Spinal Canal ØØFU
  Stomach ØDF6
  Subarachnoid Space, Intracranial ØØF5
  Subdural Space, Intracranial ØØF4
  Trachea ØBF1
  Ureter
    Left ØTF7
    Right ØTF6
  Urethra ØTFD
  Uterus ØUF9
  Vein
    Axillary
      Left Ø5F83Z
      Right Ø5F73Z
    Basilic
      Left Ø5FC3Z
      Right Ø5FB3Z
    Brachial
      Left Ø5FA3Z
      Right Ø5F93Z
    Cephalic
      Left Ø5FF3Z
      Right Ø5FD3Z
    Common Iliac
      Left Ø6FD3Z
      Right Ø6FC3Z
    External Iliac
      Left Ø6FG3Z
      Right Ø6FF3Z

Fragmentation — *continued*
  Vein — *continued*
    Femoral
      Left Ø6FN3Z
      Right Ø6FM3Z
    Hypogastric
      Left Ø6FJ3Z
      Right Ø6FH3Z
    Innominate
      Left Ø5F43Z
      Right Ø5F33Z
    Lower Ø6FY3Z
    Pulmonary
      Left Ø2FT3Z
      Right Ø2FS3Z
    Saphenous
      Left Ø6FQ3Z
      Right Ø6FP3Z
    Subclavian
      Left Ø5F63Z
      Right Ø5F53Z
    Upper Ø5FY3Z
  Vitreous
    Left Ø8F5
    Right Ø8F4
Fragmentation, Ultrasonic *see* Fragmentation, Artery
Freestyle (Stentless) Aortic Root Bioprosthesis *use*
  Zooplastic Tissue in Heart and Great Vessels
Frenectomy
  see Excision, Mouth and Throat ØCB
  see Resection, Mouth and Throat ØCT
Frenoplasty, frenuloplasty
  see Repair, Mouth and Throat ØCQ
  see Replacement, Mouth and Throat ØCR
  see Supplement, Mouth and Throat ØCU
Frenotomy
  see Drainage, Mouth and Throat ØC9
  see Release, Mouth and Throat ØCN
Frenulotomy
  see Drainage, Mouth and Throat ØC9
  see Release, Mouth and Throat ØCN
Frenulum labii inferioris *use* Lower Lip
Frenulum labii superioris *use* Upper Lip
Frenulum linguae *use* Tongue
Frenulumectomy
  see Excision, Mouth and Throat ØCB
  see Resection, Mouth and Throat ØCT
Frontal lobe *use* Cerebral Hemisphere
Frontal vein
  use Face Vein, Left
  use Face Vein, Right
Frozen elephant trunk (FET) technique, aortic arch
  replacement
  see New Technology, Cardiovascular System X2R
  see Replacement, Heart and Great Vessels Ø2R
Frozen elephant trunk (FET) technique, thoracic
  aorta restriction
  see New Technology, Cardiovascular System X2V
  see Restriction, Heart and Great Vessels Ø2V
FUJIFILM EP-7ØØØX System for Oxygen Saturation
  Endoscopic Imaging (OXEI) *see* New Technolo-
  gy, Gastrointestinal System XD2
Fulguration *see* Destruction
Fundoplication, gastroesophageal *see* Restriction,
  Esophagogastric Junction ØDV4
Fundus uteri *use* Uterus
Fusion
  Acromioclavicular
    Left ØRGH
    Right ØRGG
  Ankle
    Left ØSGG
    Right ØSGF
  Carpal
    Left ØRGR
    Right ØRGQ
  Carpometacarpal
    Left ØRGT
    Right ØRGS
  Cervical Vertebral ØRG1
    2 or more ØRG2
      Interbody Fusion Device
        Nanotextured Surface XRG2Ø92
        Radiolucent Porous XRG2ØF3
    Interbody Fusion Device
      Nanotextured Surface XRG1Ø92
      Radiolucent Porous XRG1ØF3

Fusion — *continued*
  Cervicothoracic Vertebral ØRG4
    Interbody Fusion Device
      Nanotextured Surface XRG4Ø92
      Radiolucent Porous XRG4ØF3
  Coccygeal ØSG6
  Elbow
    Left ØRGM
    Right ØRGL
  Finger Phalangeal
    Left ØRGX
    Right ØRGW
  Hip
    Left ØSGB
    Right ØSG9
  Knee
    Left ØSGD
    Right ØSGC
  Lumbar Vertebral ØSGØ
    2 or more ØSG1
      Interbody Fusion Device
        Customizable XRGC
        Nanotextured Surface XRGCØ92
        Radiolucent Porous XRGCØF3
    Interbody Fusion Device
      Customizable XRGB
      Nanotextured Surface XRGBØ92
      Radiolucent Porous XRGBØF3
  Lumbosacral ØSG3
    Interbody Fusion Device
      Customizable XRGD
      Nanotextured Surface XRGDØ92
      Radiolucent Porous XRGDØF3
  Metacarpophalangeal
    Left ØRGV
    Right ØRGU
  Metatarsal-Phalangeal
    Left ØSGN
    Right ØSGM
  Occipital-cervical ØRGØ
    Interbody Fusion Device
      Nanotextured Surface XRGØØ92
      Radiolucent Porous XRGØØF3
  Sacrococcygeal ØSG5
  Sacroiliac
    Left ØSG8
    Right ØSG7
  Shoulder
    Left ØRGK
    Right ØRGJ
  Sternoclavicular
    Left ØRGF
    Right ØRGE
  Tarsal
    Left ØSGJ
    Right ØSGH
  Tarsometatarsal
    Left ØSGL
    Right ØSGK
  Temporomandibular
    Left ØRGD
    Right ØRGC
  Thoracic Vertebral ØRG6
    2 to 7 ØRG7
      Interbody Fusion Device
        Nanotextured Surface XRG7Ø92
        Radiolucent Porous XRG7ØF3
    8 or more ØRG8
      Interbody Fusion Device
        Nanotextured Surface XRG8Ø92
        Radiolucent Porous XRG8ØF3
    Interbody Fusion Device
      Nanotextured Surface XRG6Ø92
      Radiolucent Porous XRG6ØF3
  Thoracolumbar Vertebral ØRGA
    Interbody Fusion Device
      Customizable XRGA
      Nanotextured Surface XRGAØ92
      Radiolucent Porous XRGAØF3
  Toe Phalangeal
    Left ØSGQ
    Right ØSGP
  Wrist
    Left ØRGP
    Right ØRGN
Fusion screw (compression) (lag) (locking)
  use Internal Fixation Device in Lower Joints
  use Internal Fixation Device in Upper Joints

G

Gait training see Motor Treatment, Rehabilitation F07
Galea aponeurotica use Subcutaneous Tissue and Fascia, Scalp
Gammaglobulin use Globulin
GammaTile™ use Radioactive Element, Cesium-131 Collagen Implant in 00H
GAMUNEX-C, for COVID-19 treatment use High-Dose Intravenous Immune Globulin
Ganglion impar (ganglion of Walther) use Sacral Sympathetic Nerve
Ganglionectomy
    Destruction of lesion see Destruction
    Excision of lesion see Excision
Gasserian ganglion use Trigeminal Nerve
Gastrectomy
    Partial see Excision, Stomach 0DB6
    Total see Resection, Stomach 0DT6
    Vertical (sleeve) see Excision, Stomach 0DB6
Gastric electrical stimulation (GES) lead use Stimulator Lead in Gastrointestinal System
Gastric lymph node use Lymphatic, Aortic
Gastric pacemaker lead use Stimulator Lead in Gastrointestinal System
Gastric plexus use Abdominal Sympathetic Nerve
Gastrocnemius muscle
    use Lower Leg Muscle, Left
    use Lower Leg Muscle, Right
Gastrocolic ligament use Omentum
Gastrocolic omentum use Omentum
Gastrocolostomy
    see Bypass, Gastrointestinal System 0D1
    see Drainage, Gastrointestinal System 0D9
Gastroduodenal artery use Hepatic Artery
Gastroduodenectomy
    see Excision, Gastrointestinal System 0DB
    see Resection, Gastrointestinal System 0DT
Gastroduodenoscopy 0DJ08ZZ
Gastroenteroplasty
    see Repair, Gastrointestinal System 0DQ
    see Supplement, Gastrointestinal System 0DU
Gastroenterostomy
    see Bypass, Gastrointestinal System 0D1
    see Drainage, Gastrointestinal System 0D9
Gastroesophageal (GE) junction use Esophagogastric Junction
Gastrogastrostomy
    see Bypass, Stomach 0D16
    see Drainage, Stomach 0D96
Gastrohepatic omentum use Omentum
Gastrojejunostomy
    see Bypass, Stomach 0D16
    see Drainage, Stomach 0D96
Gastrolysis see Release, Stomach 0DN6
Gastropexy
    see Repair, Stomach 0DQ6
    see Reposition, Stomach 0DS6
Gastrophrenic ligament use Omentum
Gastroplasty
    see Repair, Stomach 0DQ6
    see Supplement, Stomach 0DU6
Gastroplication see Restriction, Stomach 0DV6
Gastropylorectomy see Excision, Gastrointestinal System 0DB
Gastrorrhaphy see Repair, Stomach 0DQ6
Gastroscopy 0DJ68ZZ
Gastrosplenic ligament use Omentum
Gastrostomy
    see Bypass, Stomach 0D16
    see Drainage, Stomach 0D96
Gastrotomy see Drainage, Stomach 0D96
Gemellus muscle
    use Hip Muscle, Left
    use Hip Muscle, Right
Geniculate ganglion use Facial Nerve
Geniculate nucleus use Thalamus
Genioglossus muscle use Tongue, Palate, Pharynx Muscle
Genioplasty see Alteration, Jaw, Lower 0W05
Genitofemoral nerve use Lumbar Plexus
GIAPREZA™ use Synthetic Human Angiotensin II
Gilteritinib Antineoplastic XW0DXV5
Gingivectomy see Excision, Mouth and Throat 0CB

Gingivoplasty
    see Repair, Mouth and Throat 0CQ
    see Replacement, Mouth and Throat 0CR
    see Supplement, Mouth and Throat 0CU
Glans penis use Prepuce
Glenohumeral joint
    use Shoulder Joint, Left
    use Shoulder Joint, Right
Glenohumeral ligament
    use Shoulder Bursa and Ligament, Left
    use Shoulder Bursa and Ligament, Right
Glenoid fossa (of scapula)
    use Glenoid Cavity, Left
    use Glenoid Cavity, Right
Glenoid ligament (labrum)
    use Shoulder Joint, Left
    use Shoulder Joint, Right
Globus pallidus use Basal Ganglia
Glomectomy
    see Excision, Endocrine System 0GB
    see Resection, Endocrine System 0GT
Glossectomy
    see Excision, Tongue 0CB7
    see Resection, Tongue 0CT7
Glossoepiglottic fold use Epiglottis
Glossopexy
    see Repair, Tongue 0CQ7
    see Reposition, Tongue 0CS7
Glossoplasty
    see Repair, Tongue 0CQ7
    see Replacement, Tongue 0CR7
    see Supplement, Tongue 0CU7
Glossorrhaphy see Repair, Tongue 0CQ7
Glossotomy see Drainage, Tongue 0C97
Glottis use Larynx
Gluteal Artery Perforator Flap
    Replacement
        Bilateral 0HRV079
        Left 0HRU079
        Right 0HRT079
    Transfer
        Left 0KXG
        Right 0KXF
Gluteal lymph node use Lymphatic, Pelvis
Gluteal vein
    use Hypogastric Vein, Left
    use Hypogastric Vein, Right
Gluteus maximus muscle
    use Hip Muscle, Left
    use Hip Muscle, Right
Gluteus medius muscle
    use Hip Muscle, Left
    use Hip Muscle, Right
Gluteus minimus muscle
    use Hip Muscle, Left
    use Hip Muscle, Right
GORE EXCLUDER® AAA Endoprosthesis
    use Intraluminal Device
    use Intraluminal Device, Branched or Fenestrated, One or Two Arteries in 04V
    use Intraluminal Device, Branched or Fenestrated, Three or More Arteries in 04V
GORE EXCLUDER® IBE Endoprosthesis use Intraluminal Device, Branched or Fenestrated, One or Two Arteries in 04V
GORE TAG® Thoracic Endoprosthesis use Intraluminal Device
GORE® DUALMESH® use Synthetic Substitute
Gracilis muscle
    use Upper Leg Muscle, Left
    use Upper Leg Muscle, Right
Graft
    see Replacement
    see Supplement
Great auricular nerve use Cervical Plexus
Great cerebral vein use Intracranial Vein
Great(er) saphenous vein
    use Saphenous Vein, Left
    use Saphenous Vein, Right
Greater alar cartilage use Nasal Mucosa and Soft Tissue
Greater occipital nerve use Cervical Nerve
Greater Omentum use Omentum
Greater splanchnic nerve use Thoracic Sympathetic Nerve
Greater superficial petrosal nerve use Facial Nerve

Greater trochanter
    use Upper Femur, Left
    use Upper Femur, Right
Greater tuberosity
    use Humeral Head, Left
    use Humeral Head, Right
Greater vestibular (Bartholin's) gland use Vestibular Gland
Greater wing use Sphenoid Bone
GS-5734 use Remdesivir Anti-infective
Guedel airway use Intraluminal Device, Airway in Mouth and Throat
Guidance, catheter placement
    EKG see Measurement, Physiological Systems 4A0
    Fluoroscopy see Fluoroscopy, Veins B51
    Ultrasound see Ultrasonography, Veins B54

H

Hallux
    use 1st Toe, Left
    use 1st Toe, Right
Hamate bone
    use Carpal, Left
    use Carpal, Right
Hancock Bioprosthesis (aortic) (mitral) valve use Zooplastic Tissue in Heart and Great Vessels
Hancock Bioprosthetic Valved Conduit use Zooplastic Tissue in Heart and Great Vessels
Harmony™ transcatheter pulmonary valve (TPV) placement 02RH38M
Harvesting, Stem Cells see Pheresis, Circulatory 6A55
hdIVIG (high-dose intravenous immunoglobulin), for COVID-19 treatment use High-Dose Intravenous Immune Globulin
Head of fibula
    use Fibula, Left
    use Fibula, Right
Hearing Aid Assessment F14Z
Hearing Assessment F13Z
Hearing Device
    Bone Conduction
        Left 09HE
        Right 09HD
    Insertion of device in
        Left 0NH6
        Right 0NH5
    Multiple Channel Cochlear Prosthesis
        Left 09HE
        Right 09HD
    Removal of device from, Skull 0NP0
    Revision of device in, Skull 0NW0
    Single Channel Cochlear Prosthesis
        Left 09HE
        Right 09HD
Hearing Treatment F09Z
Heart Assist System
    Implantable
        Insertion of device in, Heart 02HA
        Removal of device from, Heart 02PA
        Revision of device in, Heart 02WA
    Short-term External
        Insertion of device in, Heart 02HA
        Removal of device from, Heart 02PA
        Revision of device in, Heart 02WA
HeartMate 3™ LVAS use Implantable Heart Assist System in Heart and Great Vessels
HeartMate II® Left Ventricular Assist Device (LVAD) use Implantable Heart Assist System in Heart and Great Vessels
HeartMate XVE® Left Ventricular Assist Device (LVAD) use Implantable Heart Assist System in Heart and Great Vessels
HeartMate® implantable heart assist system see Insertion of device in, Heart 02HA
Helix
    use Ear, External, Bilateral
    use Ear, External, Left
    use Ear, External, Right
Hematopoietic cell transplant (HCT) see Transfusion, Circulatory 302
Hemicolectomy see Resection, Gastrointestinal System 0DT
Hemicystectomy see Excision, Urinary System 0TB
Hemigastrectomy see Excision, Gastrointestinal System 0DB

▼ Subterms under main terms may continue to next column or pa[ge]

Hemiglossectomy *see* Excision, Mouth and Throat ØCB
Hemilaminectomy
   see Excision, Lower Bones ØQB
   see Excision, Upper Bones ØPB
Hemilaminotomy
   see Drainage, Lower Bones ØQ9
   see Drainage, Upper Bones ØP9
   see Excision, Lower Bones ØQB
   see Excision, Upper Bones ØPB
   see Release, Central Nervous System and Cranial
      Nerves ØØN
   see Release, Lower Bones ØQN
   see Release, Peripheral Nervous System Ø1N
   see Release, Upper Bones ØPN
Hemilaryngectomy *see* Excision, Larynx ØCBS
Hemimandibulectomy *see* Excision, Head and Facial
   Bones ØNB
Hemimaxillectomy *see* Excision, Head and Facial Bones
   ØNB
Hemipylorectomy *see* Excision, Gastrointestinal System ØDB
Hemispherectomy
   see Excision, Central Nervous System and Cranial
      Nerves ØØB
   see Resection, Central Nervous System and Cranial
      Nerves ØØT
Hemithyroidectomy
   see Excision, Endocrine System ØGB
   see Resection, Endocrine System ØGT
Hemodialysis *see* Performance, Urinary 5A1D
Hemolung® Respiratory Assist System (RAS)
   5A0920Z
Hemospray® Endoscopic Hemostat *use* Mineral-
   based Topical Hemostatic Agent
Hepatectomy
   see Excision, Hepatobiliary System and Pancreas
      ØFB
   see Resection, Hepatobiliary System and Pancreas
      ØFT
Hepatic artery proper *use* Hepatic Artery
Hepatic flexure *use* Transverse Colon
Hepatic lymph node *use* Lymphatic, Aortic
Hepatic plexus *use* Abdominal Sympathetic Nerve
Hepatic portal vein *use* Portal Vein
Hepaticoduodenostomy
   see Bypass, Hepatobiliary System and Pancreas
      ØF1
   see Drainage, Hepatobiliary System and Pancreas
      ØF9
Hepaticotomy *see* Drainage, Hepatobiliary System and
   Pancreas ØF9
Hepatocholedochostomy *see* Drainage, Duct, Common Bile ØF99
Hepatogastric ligament *use* Omentum
Hepatopancreatic ampulla *use* Ampulla of Vater
Hepatopexy
   see Repair, Hepatobiliary System and Pancreas ØFQ
   see Reposition, Hepatobiliary System and Pancreas
      ØFS
Hepatorrhaphy *see* Repair, Hepatobiliary System and
   Pancreas ØFQ
Hepatotomy *see* Drainage, Hepatobiliary System and
   Pancreas ØF9
Herculink (RX) Elite Renal Stent System *use* Intraluminal Device
Herniorrhaphy
   see Repair, Anatomical Regions, General ØWQ
   see Repair, Anatomical Regions, Lower Extremities
      ØYQ
   With synthetic substitute
      see Supplement, Anatomical Regions, General ØWU
      see Supplement, Anatomical Regions, Lower
         Extremities ØYU
HIG (hyperimmune globulin), for COVID-19 treatment *use* Hyperimmune Globulin
High-Dose Intravenous Immune Globulin, for COVID-19 treatment XW1
High-dose intravenous immunoglobulin (hdIVIG), for COVID-19 treatment *use* High-Dose Intravenous Immune Globulin
Hip (joint) liner *use* Liner in Lower Joints
HIPEC (hyperthermic intraperitoneal chemotherapy) 3E0M30Y
HIVIG (hyperimmune intravenous immunoglobulin), for COVID-19 treatment *use* Hyperimmune Globulin

Holter Monitoring 4A12X45
Holter valve ventricular shunt *use* Synthetic Substitute
Human angiotensin II, synthetic *use* Synthetic Human Angiotensin II
Humeroradial joint
   use Elbow Joint, Left
   use Elbow Joint, Right
Humeroulnar joint
   use Elbow Joint, Left
   use Elbow Joint, Right
Humerus, distal
   use Humeral Shaft, Left
   use Humeral Shaft, Right
Hydrocelectomy *see* Excision, Male Reproductive System ØVB
Hydrotherapy
   Assisted exercise in pool *see* Motor Treatment,
      Rehabilitation F07
   Whirlpool *see* Activities of Daily Living Treatment,
      Rehabilitation F08
Hymenectomy
   see Excision, Hymen ØUBK
   see Resection, Hymen ØUTK
Hymenoplasty
   see Repair, Hymen ØUQK
   see Supplement, Hymen ØUUK
Hymenorrhaphy *see* Repair, Hymen ØUQK
Hymenotomy
   see Division, Hymen ØU8K
   see Drainage, Hymen ØU9K
Hyoglossus muscle *use* Tongue, Palate, Pharynx Muscle
Hyoid artery
   use Thyroid Artery, Left
   use Thyroid Artery, Right
Hyperalimentation *see* Introduction of substance in or on
Hyperbaric oxygenation
   Decompression sickness treatment *see* Decompression, Circulatory 6A15
   Wound treatment *see* Assistance, Circulatory 5A05
Hyperimmune globulin *use* Globulin
Hyperimmune Globulin, for COVID-19 treatment XW1
Hyperimmune intravenous immunoglobulin (hIVIG), for COVID-19 treatment *use* Hyperimmune Globulin
Hyperthermia
   Radiation Therapy
      Abdomen DWY38ZZ
      Adrenal Gland DGY28ZZ
      Bile Ducts DFY28ZZ
      Bladder DTY28ZZ
      Bone Marrow D7Y08ZZ
      Bone, Other DPYC8ZZ
      Brain D0Y08ZZ
      Brain Stem D0Y18ZZ
      Breast
         Left DMY08ZZ
         Right DMY18ZZ
      Bronchus DBY18ZZ
      Cervix DUY18ZZ
      Chest DWY28ZZ
      Chest Wall DBY78ZZ
      Colon DDY58ZZ
      Diaphragm DBY88ZZ
      Duodenum DDY28ZZ
      Ear D9Y08ZZ
      Esophagus DDY08ZZ
      Eye D8Y08ZZ
      Femur DPY98ZZ
      Fibula DPYB8ZZ
      Gallbladder DFY18ZZ
      Gland
         Adrenal DGY28ZZ
         Parathyroid DGY48ZZ
         Pituitary DGY08ZZ
         Thyroid DGY58ZZ
      Glands, Salivary D9Y68ZZ
      Head and Neck DWY18ZZ
      Hemibody DWY48ZZ
      Humerus DPY68ZZ
      Hypopharynx D9Y38ZZ
      Ileum DDY48ZZ
      Jejunum DDY38ZZ
      Kidney DTY08ZZ
      Larynx D9YB8ZZ

Hyperthermia — *continued*
   Radiation Therapy — *continued*
      Liver DFY08ZZ
      Lung DBY28ZZ
      Lymphatics
         Abdomen D7Y68ZZ
         Axillary D7Y48ZZ
         Inguinal D7Y88ZZ
         Neck D7Y38ZZ
         Pelvis D7Y78ZZ
         Thorax D7Y58ZZ
      Mandible DPY38ZZ
      Maxilla DPY28ZZ
      Mediastinum DBY68ZZ
      Mouth D9Y48ZZ
      Nasopharynx D9YD8ZZ
      Neck and Head DWY18ZZ
      Nerve, Peripheral D0Y78ZZ
      Nose D9Y18ZZ
      Oropharynx D9YF8ZZ
      Ovary DUY08ZZ
      Palate
         Hard D9Y88ZZ
         Soft D9Y98ZZ
      Pancreas DFY38ZZ
      Parathyroid Gland DGY48ZZ
      Pelvic Bones DPY88ZZ
      Pelvic Region DWY68ZZ
      Pineal Body DGY18ZZ
      Pituitary Gland DGY08ZZ
      Pleura DBY58ZZ
      Prostate DVY08ZZ
      Radius DPY78ZZ
      Rectum DDY78ZZ
      Rib DPY58ZZ
      Sinuses D9Y78ZZ
      Skin
         Abdomen DHY88ZZ
         Arm DHY48ZZ
         Back DHY78ZZ
         Buttock DHY98ZZ
         Chest DHY68ZZ
         Face DHY28ZZ
         Leg DHYB8ZZ
         Neck DHY38ZZ
      Skull DPY08ZZ
      Spinal Cord D0Y68ZZ
      Spleen D7Y28ZZ
      Sternum DPY48ZZ
      Stomach DDY18ZZ
      Testis DVY18ZZ
      Thymus D7Y18ZZ
      Thyroid Gland DGY58ZZ
      Tibia DPYB8ZZ
      Tongue D9Y58ZZ
      Trachea DBY08ZZ
      Ulna DPY78ZZ
      Ureter DTY18ZZ
      Urethra DTY38ZZ
      Uterus DUY28ZZ
      Whole Body DWY58ZZ
   Whole Body 6A3Z
Hyperthermic Intraperitoneal Chemotherapy (HIPEC) 3E0M30Y
Hypnosis GZFZZZZ
Hypogastric artery
   use Internal Iliac Artery, Left
   use Internal Iliac Artery, Right
Hypopharynx *use* Pharynx
Hypophysectomy
   see Excision, Gland, Pituitary ØGBØ
   see Resection, Gland, Pituitary ØGTØ
Hypophysis *use* Pituitary Gland
Hypothalamotomy *see* Destruction, Thalamus 0059
Hypothenar muscle
   use Hand Muscle, Left
   use Hand Muscle, Right
Hypothermia, Whole Body 6A4Z
Hysterectomy
   Supracervical *see* Resection, Uterus ØUT9
   Total *see* Resection, Uterus ØUT9
Hysterolysis *see* Release, Uterus ØUN9
Hysteropexy
   see Repair, Uterus ØUQ9
   see Reposition, Uterus ØUS9
Hysteroplasty *see* Repair, Uterus ØUQ9
Hysterorrhaphy *see* Repair, Uterus ØUQ9
Hysteroscopy ØUJD8ZZ

Hysterotomy see Drainage, Uterus ØU99
Hysterotrachelectomy
   see Resection, Cervix ØUTC
   see Resection, Uterus ØUT9
Hysterotracheloplasty see Repair, Uterus ØUQ9
Hysterotrachelorrhaphy see Repair, Uterus ØUQ9

I

IABP (Intra-aortic balloon pump) see Assistance, Cardiac 5A02
IAEMT (Intraoperative anesthetic effect monitoring and titration) see Monitoring, Central Nervous 4A10
IASD® (InterAtrial Shunt Device), Corvia use Synthetic Substitute
Idarucizumab, Pradaxa® (dabigatran) reversal agent use Other Therapeutic Substance
Idecabtagene Vicleucel use Idecabtagene Vicleucel Immunotherapy
Idecabtagene Vicleucel Immunotherapy XWØ
Ide-cel use Idecabtagene Vicleucel Immunotherapy
IGIV-C, for COVID-19 treatment use Hyperimmune Globulin
IHD (Intermittent hemodialysis) 5A1D70Z
Ileal artery use Superior Mesenteric Artery
Ileectomy
   see Excision, Ileum ØDBB
   see Resection, Ileum ØDTB
Ileocolic artery use Superior Mesenteric Artery
Ileocolic vein use Colic Vein
Ileopexy
   see Repair, Ileum ØDQB
   see Reposition, Ileum ØDSB
Ileorrhaphy see Repair, Ileum ØDQB
Ileoscopy ØDJD8ZZ
Ileostomy
   see Bypass, Ileum ØD1B
   see Drainage, Ileum ØD9B
Ileotomy see Drainage, Ileum ØD9B
Ileoureterostomy see Bypass, Urinary System ØT1
Iliac crest
   use Pelvic Bone, Left
   use Pelvic Bone, Right
Iliac fascia
   use Subcutaneous Tissue and Fascia, Left Upper Leg
   use Subcutaneous Tissue and Fascia, Right Upper Leg
Iliac lymph node use Lymphatic, Pelvis
Iliacus muscle
   use Hip Muscle, Left
   use Hip Muscle, Right
Iliofemoral ligament
   use Hip Bursa and Ligament, Left
   use Hip Bursa and Ligament, Right
Iliohypogastric nerve use Lumbar Plexus
Ilioinguinal nerve use Lumbar Plexus
Iliolumbar artery
   use Internal Iliac Artery, Left
   use Internal Iliac Artery, Right
Iliolumbar ligament use Lower Spine Bursa and Ligament
Iliotibial tract (band)
   use Subcutaneous Tissue and Fascia, Left Upper Leg
   use Subcutaneous Tissue and Fascia, Right Upper Leg
Ilium
   use Pelvic Bone, Left
   use Pelvic Bone, Right
Ilizarov external fixator
   use External Fixation Device, Ring in ØPH
   use External Fixation Device, Ring in ØPS
   use External Fixation Device, Ring in ØQH
   use External Fixation Device, Ring in ØQS
Ilizarov-Vecklich device
   use External Fixation Device, Limb Lengthening in ØPH
   use External Fixation Device, Limb Lengthening in ØQH
Imaging, diagnostic
   see Computerized Tomography (CT Scan)
   see Fluoroscopy
   see Magnetic Resonance Imaging (MRI)
   see Plain Radiography

Imaging, diagnostic — continued
   see Ultrasonography
Imdevimab (REGN10987) and Casirivimab (REGN10933) use REGN-COV2 Monoclonal Antibody
IMFINZI® use Durvalumab Antineoplastic
Imipenem-cilastatin-relebactam Anti-infective XWØ
IMI/REL use Imipenem-cilastatin-relebactam Anti-infective
Immobilization
   Abdominal Wall 2W33X
   Arm
      Lower
         Left 2W3DX
         Right 2W3CX
      Upper
         Left 2W3BX
         Right 2W3AX
   Back 2W35X
   Chest Wall 2W34X
   Extremity
      Lower
         Left 2W3MX
         Right 2W3LX
      Upper
         Left 2W39X
         Right 2W38X
   Face 2W31X
   Finger
      Left 2W3KX
      Right 2W3JX
   Foot
      Left 2W3TX
      Right 2W3SX
   Hand
      Left 2W3FX
      Right 2W3EX
   Head 2W30X
   Inguinal Region
      Left 2W37X
      Right 2W36X
   Leg
      Lower
         Left 2W3RX
         Right 2W3QX
      Upper
         Left 2W3PX
         Right 2W3NX
   Neck 2W32X
   Thumb
      Left 2W3HX
      Right 2W3GX
   Toe
      Left 2W3VX
      Right 2W3UX
Immunization see Introduction of Serum, Toxoid, and Vaccine
Immunoglobulin use Globulin
Immunotherapy see Introduction of Immunotherapeutic Substance
Immunotherapy, antineoplastic
   Interferon see Introduction of Low-dose Interleukin-2
   Interleukin-2, high-dose see Introduction of High-dose Interleukin-2
   Interleukin-2, low-dose see Introduction of Low-dose Interleukin-2
   Monoclonal antibody see Introduction of Monoclonal Antibody
   Proleukin, high-dose see Introduction of High-dose Interleukin-2
   Proleukin, low-dose see Introduction of Low-dose Interleukin-2
Impella® heart pump use Short-term External Heart Assist System in Heart and Great Vessels
Impeller Pump
   Continuous, Output 5A0221D
   Intermittent, Output 5A0211D
Implantable cardioverter-defibrillator (ICD) use Defibrillator Generator in ØJH
Implantable drug infusion pump (anti-spasmodic) (chemotherapy) (pain) use Infusion Device, Pump in Subcutaneous Tissue and Fascia
Implantable glucose monitoring device use Monitoring Device
Implantable hemodynamic monitor (IHM) use Monitoring Device, Hemodynamic in ØJH

Implantable hemodynamic monitoring system (IHMS) use Monitoring Device, Hemodynamic in ØJH
Implantable Miniature Telescope™ (IMT) use Synthetic Substitute, Intraocular Telescope in Ø8R
Implantation
   see Insertion
   see Replacement
Implanted (venous)(access) port use Vascular Access Device, Totally Implantable in Subcutaneous Tissue and Fascia
IMV (intermittent mandatory ventilation) see Assistance, Respiratory 5A09
In Vitro Fertilization 8E0ZXY1
Incision, abscess see Drainage
Incudectomy
   see Excision, Ear, Nose, Sinus Ø9B
   see Resection, Ear, Nose, Sinus Ø9T
Incudopexy
   see Repair, Ear, Nose, Sinus Ø9Q
   see Reposition, Ear, Nose, Sinus Ø9S
Incus
   use Auditory Ossicle, Left
   use Auditory Ossicle, Right
Induction of labor
   Artificial rupture of membranes see Drainage, Pregnancy 1Ø9
   Oxytocin see Introduction of Hormone
InDura, intrathecal catheter (1P) (spinal) use Infusion Device
Inferior cardiac nerve use Thoracic Sympathetic Nerve
Inferior cerebellar vein use Intracranial Vein
Inferior cerebral vein use Intracranial Vein
Inferior epigastric artery
   use External Iliac Artery, Left
   use External Iliac Artery, Right
Inferior epigastric lymph node use Lymphatic, Pelvis
Inferior genicular artery
   use Popliteal Artery, Left
   use Popliteal Artery, Right
Inferior gluteal artery
   use Internal Iliac Artery, Left
   use Internal Iliac Artery, Right
Inferior gluteal nerve use Sacral Plexus
Inferior hypogastric plexus use Abdominal Sympathetic Nerve
Inferior labial artery use Face Artery
Inferior longitudinal muscle use Tongue, Palate, Pharynx Muscle
Inferior mesenteric ganglion use Abdominal Sympathetic Nerve
Inferior mesenteric lymph node use Lymphatic, Mesenteric
Inferior mesenteric plexus use Abdominal Sympathetic Nerve
Inferior oblique muscle
   use Extraocular Muscle, Left
   use Extraocular Muscle, Right
Inferior pancreaticoduodenal artery use Superior Mesenteric Artery
Inferior phrenic artery use Abdominal Aorta
Inferior rectus muscle
   use Extraocular Muscle, Left
   use Extraocular Muscle, Right
Inferior suprarenal artery
   use Renal Artery, Left
   use Renal Artery, Right
Inferior tarsal plate
   use Lower Eyelid, Left
   use Lower Eyelid, Right
Inferior thyroid vein
   use Innominate Vein, Left
   use Innominate Vein, Right
Inferior tibiofibular joint
   use Ankle Joint, Left
   use Ankle Joint, Right
Inferior turbinate use Nasal Turbinate
Inferior ulnar collateral artery
   use Brachial Artery, Left
   use Brachial Artery, Right
Inferior vesical artery
   use Internal Iliac Artery, Left
   use Internal Iliac Artery, Right
Infraauricular lymph node use Lymphatic, Head
Infraclavicular (deltopectoral) lymph node
   use Lymphatic, Left Upper Extremity

Infraclavicular (deltopectoral) lymph node —
continued
use Lymphatic, Right Upper Extremity
Infrahyoid muscle
use Neck Muscle, Left
use Neck Muscle, Right
Infraparotid lymph node *use* Lymphatic, Head
Infraspinatus fascia
use Subcutaneous Tissue and Fascia, Left Upper
Arm
use Subcutaneous Tissue and Fascia, Right Upper
Arm
Infraspinatus muscle
use Shoulder Muscle, Left
use Shoulder Muscle, Right
Infundibulopelvic ligament *use* Uterine Supporting
Structure
Infusion *see* Introduction of substance in or on
Infusion Device, Pump
Insertion of device in
Abdomen ØJH8
Back ØJH7
Chest ØJH6
Lower Arm
Left ØJHH
Right ØJHG
Lower Leg
Left ØJHP
Right ØJHN
Trunk ØJHT
Upper Arm
Left ØJHF
Right ØJHD
Upper Leg
Left ØJHM
Right ØJHL
Removal of device from
Lower Extremity ØJPW
Trunk ØJPT
Upper Extremity ØJPV
Revision of device in
Lower Extremity ØJWW
Trunk ØJWT
Upper Extremity ØJWV
Infusion, glucarpidase
Central Vein 3E043GQ
Peripheral Vein 3E033GQ
Inguinal canal
use Inguinal Region, Bilateral
use Inguinal Region, Left
use Inguinal Region, Right
Inguinal triangle
use Inguinal Region, Bilateral
use Inguinal Region, Left
use Inguinal Region, Right
Injection *see* Introduction of substance in or on
**Injection, Concentrated Bone Marrow Aspirate
(CBMA), intramuscular** XK02303
Injection reservoir, port *use* Vascular Access Device,
Totally Implantable in Subcutaneous Tissue and
Fascia
Injection reservoir, pump *use* Infusion Device, Pump
in Subcutaneous Tissue and Fascia
Insemination, artificial 3E0P7LZ
Insertion
Antimicrobial envelope *see* Introduction of Anti-
infective
Aqueous drainage shunt
see Bypass, Eye Ø81
see Drainage, Eye Ø89
Products of Conception 10H0
Spinal Stabilization Device
see Insertion of device in, Lower Joints ØSH
see Insertion of device in, Upper Joints ØRH
Insertion of device in
Abdominal Wall ØWHF
Acetabulum
Left ØQH5
Right ØQH4
Anal Sphincter ØDHR
Ankle Region
Left ØYHL
Right ØYHK
Anus ØDHQ
Aorta
Abdominal Ø4H0
Thoracic
Ascending/Arch Ø2HX

Insertion of device in — *continued*
Aorta — *continued*
Thoracic — *continued*
Descending Ø2HW
Arm
Lower
Left ØXHF
Right ØXHD
Upper
Left ØXH9
Right ØXH8
Artery
Anterior Tibial
Left Ø4HQ
Right Ø4HP
Axillary
Left Ø3H6
Right Ø3H5
Brachial
Left Ø3H8
Right Ø3H7
Celiac Ø4H1
Colic
Left Ø4H7
Middle Ø4H8
Right Ø4H6
Common Carotid
Left Ø3HJ
Right Ø3HH
Common Iliac
Left Ø4HD
Right Ø4HC
Coronary
Four or More Arteries Ø2H3
One Artery Ø2H0
Three Arteries Ø2H2
Two Arteries Ø2H1
External Carotid
Left Ø3HN
Right Ø3HM
External Iliac
Left Ø4HJ
Right Ø4HH
Face Ø3HR
Femoral
Left Ø4HL
Right Ø4HK
Foot
Left Ø4HW
Right Ø4HV
Gastric Ø4H2
Hand
Left Ø3HF
Right Ø3HD
Hepatic Ø4H3
Inferior Mesenteric Ø4HB
Innominate Ø3H2
Internal Carotid
Left Ø3HL
Right Ø3HK
Internal Iliac
Left Ø4HF
Right Ø4HE
Internal Mammary
Left Ø3H1
Right Ø3H0
Intracranial Ø3HG
Lower Ø4HY
Peroneal
Left Ø4HU
Right Ø4HT
Popliteal
Left Ø4HN
Right Ø4HM
Posterior Tibial
Left Ø4HS
Right Ø4HR
Pulmonary
Left Ø2HR
Right Ø2HQ
Pulmonary Trunk Ø2HP
Radial
Left Ø3HC
Right Ø3HB
Renal
Left Ø4HA
Right Ø4H9
Splenic Ø4H4

Insertion of device in — *continued*
Artery — *continued*
Subclavian
Left Ø3H4
Right Ø3H3
Superior Mesenteric Ø4H5
Temporal
Left Ø3HT
Right Ø3HS
Thyroid
Left Ø3HV
Right Ø3HU
Ulnar
Left Ø3HA
Right Ø3H9
Upper Ø3HY
Vertebral
Left Ø3HQ
Right Ø3HP
Atrium
Left Ø2H7
Right Ø2H6
Axilla
Left ØXH5
Right ØXH4
Back
Lower ØWHL
Upper ØWHK
Bladder ØTHB
Bladder Neck ØTHC
Bone
Ethmoid
Left ØNHG
Right ØNHF
Facial ØNHW
Frontal ØNH1
Hyoid ØNHX
Lacrimal
Left ØNHJ
Right ØNHH
Lower ØQHY
Nasal ØNHB
Occipital ØNH7
Palatine
Left ØNHL
Right ØNHK
Parietal
Left ØNH4
Right ØNH3
Pelvic
Left ØQH3
Right ØQH2
Sphenoid ØNHC
Temporal
Left ØNH6
Right ØNH5
Upper ØPHY
Zygomatic
Left ØNHN
Right ØNHM
Bone Marrow Ø7HT
Brain ØØH0
Breast
Bilateral ØHHV
Left ØHHU
Right ØHHT
Bronchus
Lingula ØBH9
Lower Lobe
Left ØBHB
Right ØBH6
Main
Left ØBH7
Right ØBH3
Middle Lobe, Right ØBH5
Upper Lobe
Left ØBH8
Right ØBH4
Bursa and Ligament
Lower ØMHY
Upper ØMHX
Buttock
Left ØYH1
Right ØYH0
Carpal
Left ØPHN
Right ØPHM
Cavity, Cranial ØWH1
Cerebral Ventricle ØØH6

Insertion of device in — *continued*
- Cervix 0UHC
- Chest Wall 0WH8
- Cisterna Chyli 07HL
- Clavicle
  - Left 0PHB
  - Right 0PH9
- Coccyx 0QHS
- Cul-de-sac 0UHF
- Diaphragm 0BHT
- Disc
  - Cervical Vertebral 0RH3
  - Cervicothoracic Vertebral 0RH5
  - Lumbar Vertebral 0SH2
  - Lumbosacral 0SH4
  - Thoracic Vertebral 0RH9
  - Thoracolumbar Vertebral 0RHB
- Duct
  - Hepatobiliary 0FHB
  - Pancreatic 0FHD
- Duodenum 0DH9
- Ear
  - Inner
    - Left 09HE
    - Right 09HD
  - Left 09HJ
  - Right 09HH
- Elbow Region
  - Left 0XHC
  - Right 0XHB
- Epididymis and Spermatic Cord 0VHM
- Esophagus 0DH5
- Extremity
  - Lower
    - Left 0YHB
    - Right 0YH9
  - Upper
    - Left 0XH7
    - Right 0XH6
- Eye
  - Left 08H1
  - Right 08H0
- Face 0WH2
- Fallopian Tube 0UH8
- Femoral Region
  - Left 0YH8
  - Right 0YH7
- Femoral Shaft
  - Left 0QH9
  - Right 0QH8
- Femur
  - Lower
    - Left 0QHC
    - Right 0QHB
  - Upper
    - Left 0QH7
    - Right 0QH6
- Fibula
  - Left 0QHK
  - Right 0QHJ
- Foot
  - Left 0YHN
  - Right 0YHM
- Gallbladder 0FH4
- Gastrointestinal Tract 0WHP
- Genitourinary Tract 0WHR
- Gland
  - Endocrine 0GHS
  - Salivary 0CHA
- Glenoid Cavity
  - Left 0PH8
  - Right 0PH7
- Hand
  - Left 0XHK
  - Right 0XHJ
- Head 0WH0
- Heart 02HA
- Humeral Head
  - Left 0PHD
  - Right 0PHC
- Humeral Shaft
  - Left 0PHG
  - Right 0PHF
- Ileum 0DHB
- Inguinal Region
  - Left 0YH6
  - Right 0YH5
- Intestinal Tract
  - Lower 0DHD

Insertion of device in — *continued*
- Intestinal Tract — *continued*
  - Upper 0DH0
- Intestine
  - Large 0DHE
  - Small 0DH8
- Jaw
  - Lower 0WH5
  - Upper 0WH4
- Jejunum 0DHA
- Joint
  - Acromioclavicular
    - Left 0RHH
    - Right 0RHG
  - Ankle
    - Left 0SHG
    - Right 0SHF
  - Carpal
    - Left 0RHR
    - Right 0RHQ
  - Carpometacarpal
    - Left 0RHT
    - Right 0RHS
  - Cervical Vertebral 0RH1
  - Cervicothoracic Vertebral 0RH4
  - Coccygeal 0SH6
  - Elbow
    - Left 0RHM
    - Right 0RHL
  - Finger Phalangeal
    - Left 0RHX
    - Right 0RHW
  - Hip
    - Left 0SHB
    - Right 0SH9
  - Knee
    - Left 0SHD
    - Right 0SHC
  - Lumbar Vertebral 0SH0
  - Lumbosacral 0SH3
  - Metacarpophalangeal
    - Left 0RHV
    - Right 0RHU
  - Metatarsal-Phalangeal
    - Left 0SHN
    - Right 0SHM
  - Occipital-cervical 0RH0
  - Sacrococcygeal 0SH5
  - Sacroiliac
    - Left 0SH8
    - Right 0SH7
  - Shoulder
    - Left 0RHK
    - Right 0RHJ
  - Sternoclavicular
    - Left 0RHF
    - Right 0RHE
  - Tarsal
    - Left 0SHJ
    - Right 0SHH
  - Tarsometatarsal
    - Left 0SHL
    - Right 0SHK
  - Temporomandibular
    - Left 0RHD
    - Right 0RHC
  - Thoracic Vertebral 0RH6
  - Thoracolumbar Vertebral 0RHA
  - Toe Phalangeal
    - Left 0SHQ
    - Right 0SHP
  - Wrist
    - Left 0RHP
    - Right 0RHN
- Kidney 0TH5
- Knee Region
  - Left 0YHG
  - Right 0YHF
- Larynx 0CHS
- Leg
  - Lower
    - Left 0YHJ
    - Right 0YHH
  - Upper
    - Left 0YHD
    - Right 0YHC
- Liver 0FH0
  - Left Lobe 0FH2
  - Right Lobe 0FH1

Insertion of device in — *continued*
- Lung
  - Left 0BHL
  - Right 0BHK
- Lymphatic 07HN
  - Thoracic Duct 07HK
- Mandible
  - Left 0NHV
  - Right 0NHT
- Maxilla 0NHR
- Mediastinum 0WHC
- Metacarpal
  - Left 0PHQ
  - Right 0PHP
- Metatarsal
  - Left 0QHP
  - Right 0QHN
- Mouth and Throat 0CHY
- Muscle
  - Lower 0KHY
  - Upper 0KHX
- Nasal Mucosa and Soft Tissue 09HK
- Nasopharynx 09HN
- Neck 0WH6
- Nerve
  - Cranial 00HE
  - Peripheral 01HY
- Nipple
  - Left 0HHX
  - Right 0HHW
- Oral Cavity and Throat 0WH3
- Orbit
  - Left 0NHQ
  - Right 0NHP
- Ovary 0UH3
- Pancreas 0FHG
- Patella
  - Left 0QHF
  - Right 0QHD
- Pelvic Cavity 0WHJ
- Penis 0VHS
- Pericardial Cavity 0WHD
- Pericardium 02HN
- Perineum
  - Female 0WHN
  - Male 0WHM
- Peritoneal Cavity 0WHG
- Phalanx
  - Finger
    - Left 0PHV
    - Right 0PHT
  - Thumb
    - Left 0PHS
    - Right 0PHR
  - Toe
    - Left 0QHR
    - Right 0QHQ
- Pleura 0BHQ
- Pleural Cavity
  - Left 0WHB
  - Right 0WH9
- Prostate 0VH0
- Prostate and Seminal Vesicles 0VH4
- Radius
  - Left 0PHJ
  - Right 0PHH
- Rectum 0DHP
- Respiratory Tract 0WHQ
- Retroperitoneum 0WHH
- Ribs
  - 1 to 2 0PH1
  - 3 or More 0PH2
- Sacrum 0QH1
- Scapula
  - Left 0PH6
  - Right 0PH5
- Scrotum and Tunica Vaginalis 0VH8
- Shoulder Region
  - Left 0XH3
  - Right 0XH2
- Sinus 09HY
- Skin 0HHPXYZ
- Skull 0NH0
- Spinal Canal 00HU
- Spinal Cord 00HV
- Spleen 07HP
- Sternum 0PH0
- Stomach 0DH6

Insertion of device in — *continued*
Subcutaneous Tissue and Fascia
  Abdomen ØJH8
  Back ØJH7
  Buttock ØJH9
  Chest ØJH6
  Face ØJH1
  Foot
    Left ØJHR
    Right ØJHQ
  Hand
    Left ØJHK
    Right ØJHJ
  Head and Neck ØJHS
  Lower Arm
    Left ØJHH
    Right ØJHG
  Lower Extremity ØJHW
  Lower Leg
    Left ØJHP
    Right ØJHN
  Neck
    Left ØJH5
    Right ØJH4
  Pelvic Region ØJHC
  Perineum ØJHB
  Scalp ØJHØ
  Trunk ØJHT
  Upper Arm
    Left ØJHF
    Right ØJHD
  Upper Extremity ØJHV
  Upper Leg
    Left ØJHM
    Right ØJHL
Tarsal
  Left ØQHM
  Right ØQHL
Tendon
  Lower ØLHY
  Upper ØLHX
Testis ØVHD
Thymus Ø7HM
Tibia
  Left ØQHH
  Right ØQHG
Tongue ØCH7
Trachea ØBH1
Tracheobronchial Tree ØBHØ
Ulna
  Left ØPHL
  Right ØPHK
Ureter ØTH9
Urethra ØTHD
Uterus ØUH9
Uterus and Cervix ØUHD
Vagina ØUHG
Vagina and Cul-de-sac ØUHH
Vas Deferens ØVHR
Vein
  Axillary
    Left Ø5H8
    Right Ø5H7
  Azygos Ø5HØ
  Basilic
    Left Ø5HC
    Right Ø5HB
  Brachial
    Left Ø5HA
    Right Ø5H9
  Cephalic
    Left Ø5HF
    Right Ø5HD
  Colic Ø6H7
  Common Iliac
    Left Ø6HD
    Right Ø6HC
  Coronary Ø2H4
  Esophageal Ø6H3
  External Iliac
    Left Ø6HG
    Right Ø6HF
  External Jugular
    Left Ø5HQ
    Right Ø5HP
  Face
    Left Ø5HV
    Right Ø5HT

Insertion of device in — *continued*
Vein — *continued*
  Femoral
    Left Ø6HN
    Right Ø6HM
  Foot
    Left Ø6HV
    Right Ø6HT
  Gastric Ø6H2
  Hand
    Left Ø5HH
    Right Ø5HG
  Hemiazygos Ø5H1
  Hepatic Ø6H4
  Hypogastric
    Left Ø6HJ
    Right Ø6HH
  Inferior Mesenteric Ø6H6
  Innominate
    Left Ø5H4
    Right Ø5H3
  Internal Jugular
    Left Ø5HN
    Right Ø5HM
  Intracranial Ø5HL
  Lower Ø6HY
  Portal Ø6H8
  Pulmonary
    Left Ø2HT
    Right Ø2HS
  Renal
    Left Ø6HB
    Right Ø6H9
  Saphenous
    Left Ø6HQ
    Right Ø6HP
  Splenic Ø6H1
  Subclavian
    Left Ø5H6
    Right Ø5H5
  Superior Mesenteric Ø6H5
  Upper Ø5HY
  Vertebral
    Left Ø5HS
    Right Ø5HR
Vena Cava
  Inferior Ø6HØ
  Superior Ø2HV
Ventricle
  Left Ø2HL
  Right Ø2HK
Vertebra
  Cervical ØPH3
  Lumbar ØQHØ
  Thoracic ØPH4
Wrist Region
  Left ØXHH
  Right ØXHG

Inspection
Abdominal Wall ØWJF
Ankle Region
  Left ØYJL
  Right ØYJK
Arm
  Lower
    Left ØXJF
    Right ØXJD
  Upper
    Left ØXJ9
    Right ØXJ8
Artery
  Lower Ø4JY
  Upper Ø3JY
Axilla
  Left ØXJ5
  Right ØXJ4
Back
  Lower ØWJL
  Upper ØWJK
Bladder ØTJB
Bone
  Facial ØNJW
  Lower ØQJY
  Nasal ØNJB
  Upper ØPJY
Bone Marrow Ø7JT
Brain ØØJØ
Breast
  Left ØHJU

Inspection — *continued*
Breast — *continued*
  Right ØHJT
Bursa and Ligament
  Lower ØMJY
  Upper ØMJX
Buttock
  Left ØYJ1
  Right ØYJØ
Cavity, Cranial ØWJ1
Chest Wall ØWJ8
Cisterna Chyli Ø7JL
Diaphragm ØBJT
Disc
  Cervical Vertebral ØRJ3
  Cervicothoracic Vertebral ØRJ5
  Lumbar Vertebral ØSJ2
  Lumbosacral ØSJ4
  Thoracic Vertebral ØRJ9
  Thoracolumbar Vertebral ØRJB
Duct
  Hepatobiliary ØFJB
  Pancreatic ØFJD
Ear
  Inner
    Left Ø9JE
    Right Ø9JD
  Left Ø9JJ
  Right Ø9JH
Elbow Region
  Left ØXJC
  Right ØXJB
Epididymis and Spermatic Cord ØVJM
Extremity
  Lower
    Left ØYJB
    Right ØYJ9
  Upper
    Left ØXJ7
    Right ØXJ6
Eye
  Left Ø8J1XZZ
  Right Ø8JØXZZ
Face ØWJ2
Fallopian Tube ØUJ8
Femoral Region
  Bilateral ØYJE
  Left ØYJ8
  Right ØYJ7
Finger Nail ØHJQXZZ
Foot
  Left ØYJN
  Right ØYJM
Gallbladder ØFJ4
Gastrointestinal Tract ØWJP
Genitourinary Tract ØWJR
Gland
  Adrenal ØGJ5
  Endocrine ØGJS
  Pituitary ØGJØ
  Salivary ØCJA
Great Vessel Ø2JY
Hand
  Left ØXJK
  Right ØXJJ
Head ØWJØ
Heart Ø2JA
Inguinal Region
  Bilateral ØYJA
  Left ØYJ6
  Right ØYJ5
Intestinal Tract
  Lower ØDJD
  Upper ØDJØ
Jaw
  Lower ØWJ5
  Upper ØWJ4
Joint
  Acromioclavicular
    Left ØRJH
    Right ØRJG
  Ankle
    Left ØSJG
    Right ØSJF
  Carpal
    Left ØRJR
    Right ØRJQ
  Carpometacarpal
    Left ØRJT

Internal pudendal vein
  use Hypogastric Vein, Left
  use Hypogastric Vein, Right
Internal thoracic artery
  use Internal Mammary Artery, Left
  use Internal Mammary Artery, Right
  use Subclavian Artery, Left
  use Subclavian Artery, Right
Internal urethral sphincter *use* Urethra
Interphalangeal (IP) joint
  use Finger Phalangeal Joint, Left
  use Finger Phalangeal Joint, Right
  use Toe Phalangeal Joint, Left
  use Toe Phalangeal Joint, Right
Interphalangeal ligament
  use Foot Bursa and Ligament, Left
  use Foot Bursa and Ligament, Right
  use Hand Bursa and Ligament, Left
  use Hand Bursa and Ligament, Right
Interrogation, cardiac rhythm related device
  Interrogation only *see* Measurement, Cardiac 4B02
  With cardiac function testing *see* Measurement,
    Cardiac 4A02
Interruption *see* Occlusion
Interspinalis muscle
  use Trunk Muscle, Left
  use Trunk Muscle, Right
Interspinous ligament, cervical *use* Head and Neck
  Bursa and Ligament
Interspinous ligament, lumbar *use* Lower Spine
  Bursa and Ligament
Interspinous ligament, thoracic *use* Upper Spine
  Bursa and Ligament
Interspinous process spinal stabilization device
  use Spinal Stabilization Device, Interspinous Pro-
    cess in 0RH
  use Spinal Stabilization Device, Interspinous Pro-
    cess in 0SH
InterStim® Therapy lead *use* Neurostimulator Lead
  in Peripheral Nervous System
InterStim™ II Therapy neurostimulator *use* Stimula-
  tor Generator, Single Array in 0JH
InterStim™ Micro Therapy neurostimulator *use*
  Stimulator Generator, Single Array Rechargeable
  in 0JH
Intertransversarius muscle
  use Trunk Muscle, Left
  use Trunk Muscle, Right
Intertransverse ligament, cervical *use* Head and
  Neck Bursa and Ligament
Intertransverse ligament, lumbar *use* Lower Spine
  Bursa and Ligament
Intertransverse ligament, thoracic *use* Upper Spine
  Bursa and Ligament
Interventricular foramen (Monro) *use* Cerebral
  Ventricle
Interventricular septum *use* Ventricular Septum
Intestinal lymphatic trunk *use* Cisterna Chyli
Intracranial Arterial Flow, Whole Blood mRNA
  XXE5XT7
Intraluminal Device
  Airway
    Esophagus 0DH5
    Mouth and Throat 0CHY
    Nasopharynx 09HN
  Bioactive
    Occlusion
      Common Carotid
        Left 03LJ
        Right 03LH
      External Carotid
        Left 03LN
        Right 03LM
      Internal Carotid
        Left 03LL
        Right 03LK
      Intracranial 03LG
      Vertebral
        Left 03LQ
        Right 03LP
    Restriction
      Common Carotid
        Left 03VJ
        Right 03VH
      External Carotid
        Left 03VN
        Right 03VM

Intraluminal Device — *continued*
  Bioactive — *continued*
    Restriction — *continued*
      Internal Carotid
        Left 03VL
        Right 03VK
      Intracranial 03VG
      Vertebral
        Left 03VQ
        Right 03VP
  Endobronchial Valve
    Lingula 0BH9
    Lower Lobe
      Left 0BHB
      Right 0BH6
    Main
      Left 0BH7
      Right 0BH3
    Middle Lobe, Right 0BH5
    Upper Lobe
      Left 0BH8
      Right 0BH4
  Endotracheal Airway
    Change device in, Trachea 0B21XEZ
    Insertion of device in, Trachea 0BH1
  Pessary
    Change device in, Vagina and Cul-de-sac
      0U2HXGZ
    Insertion of device in
      Cul-de-sac 0UHF
      Vagina 0UHG
Intramedullary (IM) rod (nail)
  use Internal Fixation Device, Intramedullary in
    Lower Bones
  use Internal Fixation Device, Intramedullary in
    Upper Bones
Intramedullary skeletal kinetic distractor (ISKD)
  use Internal Fixation Device, Intramedullary in
    Lower Bones
  use Internal Fixation Device, Intramedullary in
    Upper Bones
Intraocular Telescope
  Left 08RK30Z
  Right 08RJ30Z
Intraoperative Radiation Therapy (IORT)
  Anus DDY8CZZ
  Bile Ducts DFY2CZZ
  Bladder DTY2CZZ
  Brain D0Y0CZZ
  Brain Stem D0Y1CZZ
  Cervix DUY1CZZ
  Colon DDY5CZZ
  Duodenum DDY2CZZ
  Gallbladder DFY1CZZ
  Ileum DDY4CZZ
  Jejunum DDY3CZZ
  Kidney DTY0CZZ
  Larynx D9YBCZZ
  Liver DFY0CZZ
  Mouth D9Y4CZZ
  Nasopharynx D9YDCZZ
  Nerve, Peripheral D0Y7CZZ
  Ovary DUY0CZZ
  Pancreas DFY3CZZ
  Pharynx D9YCCZZ
  Prostate DVY0CZZ
  Rectum DDY7CZZ
  Spinal Cord D0Y6CZZ
  Stomach DDY1CZZ
  Ureter DTY1CZZ
  Urethra DTY3CZZ
  Uterus DUY2CZZ
Intra.OX 8E02XDZ
Intrauterine Device (IUD) *use* Contraceptive Device
  in Female Reproductive System
Intravascular fluorescence angiography (IFA) *see*
  Monitoring, Physiological Systems 4A1
Intravascular Lithotripsy (IVL) *see* Fragmentation
Intravascular ultrasound assisted thrombolysis
  see Fragmentation, Artery
Introduction of substance in or on
  Artery
    Central 3E06
      Analgesics 3E06
      Anesthetic, Intracirculatory 3E06
      Antiarrhythmic 3E06
      Anti-infective 3E06
      Anti-inflammatory 3E06

Introduction of substance in or on — *continued*
  Artery — *continued*
    Central — *continued*
      Antineoplastic 3E06
      Destructive Agent 3E06
      Diagnostic Substance, Other 3E06
      Electrolytic Substance 3E06
      Hormone 3E06
      Hypnotics 3E06
      Immunotherapeutic 3E06
      Nutritional Substance 3E06
      Platelet Inhibitor 3E06
      Radioactive Substance 3E06
      Sedatives 3E06
      Serum 3E06
      Thrombolytic 3E06
      Toxoid 3E06
      Vaccine 3E06
      Vasopressor 3E06
      Water Balance Substance 3E06
    Coronary 3E07
      Diagnostic Substance, Other 3E07
      Platelet Inhibitor 3E07
      Thrombolytic 3E07
    Peripheral 3E05
      Analgesics 3E05
      Anesthetic, Intracirculatory 3E05
      Antiarrhythmic 3E05
      Anti-infective 3E05
      Anti-inflammatory 3E05
      Antineoplastic 3E05
      Destructive Agent 3E05
      Diagnostic Substance, Other 3E05
      Electrolytic Substance 3E05
      Hormone 3E05
      Hypnotics 3E05
      Immunotherapeutic 3E05
      Nutritional Substance 3E05
      Platelet Inhibitor 3E05
      Radioactive Substance 3E05
      Sedatives 3E05
      Serum 3E05
      Thrombolytic 3E05
      Toxoid 3E05
      Vaccine 3E05
      Vasopressor 3E05
      Water Balance Substance 3E05
  Biliary Tract 3E0J
    Analgesics 3E0J
    Anesthetic Agent 3E0J
    Anti-infective 3E0J
    Anti-inflammatory 3E0J
    Antineoplastic 3E0J
    Destructive Agent 3E0J
    Diagnostic Substance, Other 3E0J
    Electrolytic Substance 3E0J
    Gas 3E0J
    Hypnotics 3E0J
    Islet Cells, Pancreatic 3E0J
    Nutritional Substance 3E0J
    Radioactive Substance 3E0J
    Sedatives 3E0J
    Water Balance Substance 3E0J
  Bone 3E0V
    Analgesics 3E0V3NZ
    Anesthetic Agent 3E0V3BZ
    Anti-infective 3E0V32
    Anti-inflammatory 3E0V33Z
    Antineoplastic 3E0V30
    Destructive Agent 3E0V3TZ
    Diagnostic Substance, Other 3E0V3KZ
    Electrolytic Substance 3E0V37Z
    Hypnotics 3E0V3NZ
    Nutritional Substance 3E0V36Z
    Radioactive Substance 3E0V3HZ
    Sedatives 3E0V3NZ
    Water Balance Substance 3E0V37Z
  Bone Marrow 3E0A3GC
    Antineoplastic 3E0A30
  Brain 3E0Q
    Analgesics 3E0Q
    Anesthetic Agent 3E0Q
    Anti-infective 3E0Q
    Anti-inflammatory 3E0Q
    Antineoplastic 3E0Q
    Destructive Agent 3E0Q
    Diagnostic Substance, Other 3E0Q
    Electrolytic Substance 3E0Q
    Gas 3E0Q

Introduction of substance in or on — *continued*
Brain — *continued*
  Hypnotics 3E0Q
  Nutritional Substance 3E0Q
  Radioactive Substance 3E0Q
  Sedatives 3E0Q
  Stem Cells
    Embryonic 3E0Q
    Somatic 3E0Q
  Water Balance Substance 3E0Q
Cranial Cavity 3E0Q
  Analgesics 3E0Q
  Anesthetic Agent 3E0Q
  Anti-infective 3E0Q
  Anti-inflammatory 3E0Q
  Antineoplastic 3E0Q
  Destructive Agent 3E0Q
  Diagnostic Substance, Other 3E0Q
  Electrolytic Substance 3E0Q
  Gas 3E0Q
  Hypnotics 3E0Q
  Nutritional Substance 3E0Q
  Radioactive Substance 3E0Q
  Sedatives 3E0Q
  Stem Cells
    Embryonic 3E0Q
    Somatic 3E0Q
  Water Balance Substance 3E0Q
Ear 3E0B
  Analgesics 3E0B
  Anesthetic Agent 3E0B
  Anti-infective 3E0B
  Anti-inflammatory 3E0B
  Antineoplastic 3E0B
  Destructive Agent 3E0B
  Diagnostic Substance, Other 3E0B
  Hypnotics 3E0B
  Radioactive Substance 3E0B
  Sedatives 3E0B
Epidural Space 3E0S3GC
  Analgesics 3E0S3NZ
  Anesthetic Agent 3E0S3BZ
  Anti-infective 3E0S32
  Anti-inflammatory 3E0S33Z
  Antineoplastic 3E0S30
  Destructive Agent 3E0S3TZ
  Diagnostic Substance, Other 3E0S3KZ
  Electrolytic Substance 3E0S37Z
  Gas 3E0S
  Hypnotics 3E0S3NZ
  Nutritional Substance 3E0S36Z
  Radioactive Substance 3E0S3HZ
  Sedatives 3E0S3NZ
  Water Balance Substance 3E0S37Z
Eye 3E0C
  Analgesics 3E0C
  Anesthetic Agent 3E0C
  Anti-infective 3E0C
  Anti-inflammatory 3E0C
  Antineoplastic 3E0C
  Destructive Agent 3E0C
  Diagnostic Substance, Other 3E0C
  Gas 3E0C
  Hypnotics 3E0C
  Pigment 3E0C
  Radioactive Substance 3E0C
  Sedatives 3E0C
Gastrointestinal Tract
  Lower 3E0H
    Analgesics 3E0H
    Anesthetic Agent 3E0H
    Anti-infective 3E0H
    Anti-inflammatory 3E0H
    Antineoplastic 3E0H
    Destructive Agent 3E0H
    Diagnostic Substance, Other 3E0H
    Electrolytic Substance 3E0H
    Gas 3E0H
    Hypnotics 3E0H
    Nutritional Substance 3E0H
    Radioactive Substance 3E0H
    Sedatives 3E0H
    Water Balance Substance 3E0H
  Upper 3E0G
    Analgesics 3E0G
    Anesthetic Agent 3E0G
    Anti-infective 3E0G
    Anti-inflammatory 3E0G
    Antineoplastic 3E0G

Introduction of substance in or on — *continued*
Gastrointestinal Tract — *continued*
  Upper — *continued*
    Destructive Agent 3E0G
    Diagnostic Substance, Other 3E0G
    Electrolytic Substance 3E0G
    Gas 3E0G
    Hypnotics 3E0G
    Nutritional Substance 3E0G
    Radioactive Substance 3E0G
    Sedatives 3E0G
    Water Balance Substance 3E0G
Genitourinary Tract 3E0K
  Analgesics 3E0K
  Anesthetic Agent 3E0K
  Anti-infective 3E0K
  Anti-inflammatory 3E0K
  Antineoplastic 3E0K
  Destructive Agent 3E0K
  Diagnostic Substance, Other 3E0K
  Electrolytic Substance 3E0K
  Gas 3E0K
  Hypnotics 3E0K
  Nutritional Substance 3E0K
  Radioactive Substance 3E0K
  Sedatives 3E0K
  Water Balance Substance 3E0K
Heart 3E08
  Diagnostic Substance, Other 3E08
  Platelet Inhibitor 3E08
  Thrombolytic 3E08
Joint 3E0U
  Analgesics 3E0U3NZ
  Anesthetic Agent 3E0U3BZ
  Anti-infective 3E0U
  Anti-inflammatory 3E0U33Z
  Antineoplastic 3E0U30
  Destructive Agent 3E0U3TZ
  Diagnostic Substance, Other 3E0U3KZ
  Electrolytic Substance 3E0U37Z
  Gas 3E0U3SF
  Hypnotics 3E0U3NZ
  Nutritional Substance 3E0U36Z
  Radioactive Substance 3E0U3HZ
  Sedatives 3E0U3NZ
  Water Balance Substance 3E0U37Z
Lymphatic 3E0W3GC
  Analgesics 3E0W3NZ
  Anesthetic Agent 3E0W3BZ
  Anti-infective 3E0W32
  Anti-inflammatory 3E0W33Z
  Antineoplastic 3E0W30
  Destructive Agent 3E0W3TZ
  Diagnostic Substance, Other 3E0W3KZ
  Electrolytic Substance 3E0W37Z
  Hypnotics 3E0W3NZ
  Nutritional Substance 3E0W36Z
  Radioactive Substance 3E0W3HZ
  Sedatives 3E0W3NZ
  Water Balance Substance 3E0W37Z
Mouth 3E0D
  Analgesics 3E0D
  Anesthetic Agent 3E0D
  Antiarrhythmic 3E0D
  Anti-infective 3E0D
  Anti-inflammatory 3E0D
  Antineoplastic 3E0D
  Destructive Agent 3E0D
  Diagnostic Substance, Other 3E0D
  Electrolytic Substance 3E0D
  Hypnotics 3E0D
  Nutritional Substance 3E0D
  Radioactive Substance 3E0D
  Sedatives 3E0D
  Serum 3E0D
  Toxoid 3E0D
  Vaccine 3E0D
  Water Balance Substance 3E0D
Mucous Membrane 3E00XGC
  Analgesics 3E00XNZ
  Anesthetic Agent 3E00XBZ
  Anti-infective 3E00X2
  Anti-inflammatory 3E00X3Z
  Antineoplastic 3E00X0
  Destructive Agent 3E00XTZ
  Diagnostic Substance, Other 3E00XKZ
  Hypnotics 3E00XNZ
  Pigment 3E00XMZ
  Sedatives 3E00XNZ

Introduction of substance in or on — *continued*
Mucous Membrane — *continued*
  Serum 3E00X4Z
  Toxoid 3E00X4Z
  Vaccine 3E00X4Z
Muscle 3E023GC
  Analgesics 3E023NZ
  Anesthetic Agent 3E023BZ
  Anti-infective 3E0232
  Anti-inflammatory 3E0233Z
  Antineoplastic 3E0230
  Destructive Agent 3E023TZ
  Diagnostic Substance, Other 3E023KZ
  Electrolytic Substance 3E0237Z
  Hypnotics 3E023NZ
  Nutritional Substance 3E0236Z
  Radioactive Substance 3E023HZ
  Sedatives 3E023NZ
  Serum 3E0234Z
  Toxoid 3E0234Z
  Vaccine 3E0234Z
  Water Balance Substance 3E0237Z
Nerve
  Cranial 3E0X3GC
    Anesthetic Agent 3E0X3BZ
    Anti-inflammatory 3E0X33Z
    Destructive Agent 3E0X3TZ
  Peripheral 3E0T3GC
    Anesthetic Agent 3E0T3BZ
    Anti-inflammatory 3E0T33Z
    Destructive Agent 3E0T3TZ
  Plexus 3E0T3GC
    Anesthetic Agent 3E0T3BZ
    Anti-inflammatory 3E0T33Z
    Destructive Agent 3E0T3TZ
Nose 3E09
  Analgesics 3E09
  Anesthetic Agent 3E09
  Anti-infective 3E09
  Anti-inflammatory 3E09
  Antineoplastic 3E09
  Destructive Agent 3E09
  Diagnostic Substance, Other 3E09
  Hypnotics 3E09
  Radioactive Substance 3E09
  Sedatives 3E09
  Serum 3E09
  Toxoid 3E09
  Vaccine 3E09
Pancreatic Tract 3E0J
  Analgesics 3E0J
  Anesthetic Agent 3E0J
  Anti-infective 3E0J
  Anti-inflammatory 3E0J
  Antineoplastic 3E0J
  Destructive Agent 3E0J
  Diagnostic Substance, Other 3E0J
  Electrolytic Substance 3E0J
  Gas 3E0J
  Hypnotics 3E0J
  Islet Cells, Pancreatic 3E0J
  Nutritional Substance 3E0J
  Radioactive Substance 3E0J
  Sedatives 3E0J
  Water Balance Substance 3E0J
Pericardial Cavity 3E0Y
  Analgesics 3E0Y3NZ
  Anesthetic Agent 3E0Y3BZ
  Anti-infective 3E0Y32
  Anti-inflammatory 3E0Y33Z
  Antineoplastic 3E0Y
  Destructive Agent 3E0Y3TZ
  Diagnostic Substance, Other 3E0Y3KZ
  Electrolytic Substance 3E0Y37Z
  Gas 3E0Y
  Hypnotics 3E0Y3NZ
  Nutritional Substance 3E0Y36Z
  Radioactive Substance 3E0Y3HZ
  Sedatives 3E0Y3NZ
  Water Balance Substance 3E0Y37Z
Peritoneal Cavity 3E0M
  Adhesion Barrier 3E0M
  Analgesics 3E0M3NZ
  Anesthetic Agent 3E0M3BZ
  Anti-infective 3E0M32
  Anti-inflammatory 3E0M33Z
  Antineoplastic 3E0M
  Destructive Agent 3E0M3TZ
  Diagnostic Substance, Other 3E0M3KZ

▼ Subterms under main terms may continue to next column or pa[ge]

Introduction of substance in or on — *continued*
  Peritoneal Cavity — *continued*
    Electrolytic Substance 3E0M37Z
    Gas 3E0M
    Hypnotics 3E0M3NZ
    Nutritional Substance 3E0M36Z
    Radioactive Substance 3E0M3HZ
    Sedatives 3E0M3NZ
    Water Balance Substance 3E0M37Z
  Pharynx 3E0D
    Analgesics 3E0D
    Anesthetic Agent 3E0D
    Antiarrhythmic 3E0D
    Anti-infective 3E0D
    Anti-inflammatory 3E0D
    Antineoplastic 3E0D
    Destructive Agent 3E0D
    Diagnostic Substance, Other 3E0D
    Electrolytic Substance 3E0D
    Hypnotics 3E0D
    Nutritional Substance 3E0D
    Radioactive Substance 3E0D
    Sedatives 3E0D
    Serum 3E0D
    Toxoid 3E0D
    Vaccine 3E0D
    Water Balance Substance 3E0D
  Pleural Cavity 3E0L
    Adhesion Barrier 3E0L
    Analgesics 3E0L3NZ
    Anesthetic Agent 3E0L3BZ
    Anti-infective 3E0L32
    Anti-inflammatory 3E0L33Z
    Antineoplastic 3E0L
    Destructive Agent 3E0L3TZ
    Diagnostic Substance, Other 3E0L3KZ
    Electrolytic Substance 3E0L37Z
    Gas 3E0L
    Hypnotics 3E0L3NZ
    Nutritional Substance 3E0L36Z
    Radioactive Substance 3E0L3HZ
    Sedatives 3E0L3NZ
    Water Balance Substance 3E0L37Z
  Products of Conception 3E0E
    Analgesics 3E0E
    Anesthetic Agent 3E0E
    Anti-infective 3E0E
    Anti-inflammatory 3E0E
    Antineoplastic 3E0E
    Destructive Agent 3E0E
    Diagnostic Substance, Other 3E0E
    Electrolytic Substance 3E0E
    Gas 3E0E
    Hypnotics 3E0E
    Nutritional Substance 3E0E
    Radioactive Substance 3E0E
    Sedatives 3E0E
    Water Balance Substance 3E0E
  Reproductive
    Female 3E0P
      Adhesion Barrier 3E0P
      Analgesics 3E0P
      Anesthetic Agent 3E0P
      Anti-infective 3E0P
      Anti-inflammatory 3E0P
      Antineoplastic 3E0P
      Destructive Agent 3E0P
      Diagnostic Substance, Other 3E0P
      Electrolytic Substance 3E0P
      Gas 3E0P
      Hormone 3E0P
      Hypnotics 3E0P
      Nutritional Substance 3E0P
      Ovum, Fertilized 3E0P
      Radioactive Substance 3E0P
      Sedatives 3E0P
      Sperm 3E0P
      Water Balance Substance 3E0P
    Male 3E0N
      Analgesics 3E0N
      Anesthetic Agent 3E0N
      Anti-infective 3E0N
      Anti-inflammatory 3E0N
      Antineoplastic 3E0N
      Destructive Agent 3E0N
      Diagnostic Substance, Other 3E0N
      Electrolytic Substance 3E0N
      Gas 3E0N
      Hypnotics 3E0N

Introduction of substance in or on — *continued*
  Reproductive — *continued*
    Male — *continued*
      Nutritional Substance 3E0N
      Radioactive Substance 3E0N
      Sedatives 3E0N
      Water Balance Substance 3E0N
  Respiratory Tract 3E0F
    Analgesics 3E0F
    Anesthetic Agent 3E0F
    Anti-infective 3E0F
    Anti-inflammatory 3E0F
    Antineoplastic 3E0F
    Destructive Agent 3E0F
    Diagnostic Substance, Other 3E0F
    Electrolytic Substance 3E0F
    Gas 3E0F
    Hypnotics 3E0F
    Nutritional Substance 3E0F
    Radioactive Substance 3E0F
    Sedatives 3E0F
    Water Balance Substance 3E0F
  Skin 3E00XGC
    Analgesics 3E00XNZ
    Anesthetic Agent 3E00XBZ
    Anti-infective 3E00X2
    Anti-inflammatory 3E00X3Z
    Antineoplastic 3E00X0
    Destructive Agent 3E00XTZ
    Diagnostic Substance, Other 3E00XKZ
    Hypnotics 3E00XNZ
    Pigment 3E00XMZ
    Sedatives 3E00XNZ
    Serum 3E00X4Z
    Toxoid 3E00X4Z
    Vaccine 3E00X4Z
  Spinal Canal 3E0R3GC
    Analgesics 3E0R3NZ
    Anesthetic Agent 3E0R3BZ
    Anti-infective 3E0R32
    Anti-inflammatory 3E0R33Z
    Antineoplastic 3E0R30
    Destructive Agent 3E0R3TZ
    Diagnostic Substance, Other 3E0R3KZ
    Electrolytic Substance 3E0R37Z
    Gas 3E0R
    Hypnotics 3E0R3NZ
    Nutritional Substance 3E0R36Z
    Radioactive Substance 3E0R3HZ
    Sedatives 3E0R3NZ
    Stem Cells
      Embryonic 3E0R
      Somatic 3E0R
    Water Balance Substance 3E0R37Z
  Subcutaneous Tissue 3E013GC
    Analgesics 3E013NZ
    Anesthetic Agent 3E013BZ
    Anti-infective 3E01
    Anti-inflammatory 3E0133Z
    Antineoplastic 3E0130
    Destructive Agent 3E013TZ
    Diagnostic Substance, Other 3E013KZ
    Electrolytic Substance 3E0137Z
    Hormone 3E013V
    Hypnotics 3E013NZ
    Nutritional Substance 3E0136Z
    Radioactive Substance 3E013HZ
    Sedatives 3E013NZ
    Serum 3E0134Z
    Toxoid 3E0134Z
    Vaccine 3E0134Z
    Water Balance Substance 3E0137Z
  Vein
    Central 3E04
      Analgesics 3E04
      Anesthetic, Intracirculatory 3E04
      Antiarrhythmic 3E04
      Anti-infective 3E04
      Anti-inflammatory 3E04
      Antineoplastic 3E04
      Destructive Agent 3E04
      Diagnostic Substance, Other 3E04
      Electrolytic Substance 3E04
      Hormone 3E04
      Hypnotics 3E04
      Immunotherapeutic 3E04
      Nutritional Substance 3E04
      Platelet Inhibitor 3E04
      Radioactive Substance 3E04

Introduction of substance in or on — *continued*
  Vein — *continued*
    Central — *continued*
      Sedatives 3E04
      Serum 3E04
      Thrombolytic 3E04
      Toxoid 3E04
      Vaccine 3E04
      Vasopressor 3E04
      Water Balance Substance 3E04
    Peripheral 3E03
      Analgesics 3E03
      Anesthetic, Intracirculatory 3E03
      Antiarrhythmic 3E03
      Anti-infective 3E03
      Anti-inflammatory 3E03
      Antineoplastic 3E03
      Destructive Agent 3E03
      Diagnostic Substance, Other 3E03
      Electrolytic Substance 3E03
      Hormone 3E03
      Hypnotics 3E03
      Immunotherapeutic 3E03
      Islet Cells, Pancreatic 3E03
      Nutritional Substance 3E03
      Platelet Inhibitor 3E03
      Radioactive Substance 3E03
      Sedatives 3E03
      Serum 3E03
      Thrombolytic 3E03
      Toxoid 3E03
      Vaccine 3E03
      Vasopressor 3E03
      Water Balance Substance 3E03

Intubation
  Airway
    see Insertion of device in, Esophagus 0DH5
    see Insertion of device in, Mouth and Throat 0CHY
    see Insertion of device in, Trachea 0BH1
  Drainage device *see* Drainage
  Feeding Device *see* Insertion of device in, Gastrointestinal System 0DH
INTUITY Elite valve system, EDWARDS *use* Zooplastic Tissue, Rapid Deployment Technique in New Technology
Iobenguane I-131 Antineoplastic XW0
Iobenguane I-131, High Specific Activity (HSA) *use* Iobenguane I-131 Antineoplastic
IPPB (intermittent positive pressure breathing) *see* Assistance, Respiratory 5A09
IRE (Irreversible Electroporation) *see* Destruction, Hepatobiliary System and Pancreas 0F5
Iridectomy
  see Excision, Eye 08B
  see Resection, Eye 08T
Iridoplasty
  see Repair, Eye 08Q
  see Replacement, Eye 08R
  see Supplement, Eye 08U
Iridotomy *see* Drainage, Eye 089
Irreversible Electroporation (IRE) *see* Destruction, Hepatobiliary System and Pancreas 0F5
Irrigation
  Biliary Tract, Irrigating Substance 3E1J
  Brain, Irrigating Substance 3E1Q38Z
  Cranial Cavity, Irrigating Substance 3E1Q38Z
  Ear, Irrigating Substance 3E1B
  Epidural Space, Irrigating Substance 3E1S38Z
  Eye, Irrigating Substance 3E1C
  Gastrointestinal Tract
    Lower, Irrigating Substance 3E1H
    Upper, Irrigating Substance 3E1G
  Genitourinary Tract, Irrigating Substance 3E1K
  Irrigating Substance 3C1ZX8Z
  Joint, Irrigating Substance 3E1U
  Mucous Membrane, Irrigating Substance 3E10
  Nose, Irrigating Substance 3E19
  Pancreatic Tract, Irrigating Substance 3E1J
  Pericardial Cavity, Irrigating Substance 3E1Y38Z
  Peritoneal Cavity
    Dialysate 3E1M39Z
    Irrigating Substance 3E1M
  Pleural Cavity, Irrigating Substance 3E1L38Z
  Reproductive
    Female, Irrigating Substance 3E1P
    Male, Irrigating Substance 3E1N
  Respiratory Tract, Irrigating Substance 3E1F

Irrigation — *continued*
Skin, Irrigating Substance 3E1Ø
Spinal Canal, Irrigating Substance 3E1R38Z
Isavuconazole (isavuconazonium sulfate) *use* Other Anti-infective
Ischiatic nerve *use* Sciatic Nerve
Ischiocavernosus muscle *use* Perineum Muscle
Ischiofemoral ligament
use Hip Bursa and Ligament, Left
use Hip Bursa and Ligament, Right
Ischium
use Pelvic Bone, Left
use Pelvic Bone, Right
ISC-REST kit
ISCDx XXE5XT7
QIAGEN Access Anti-SARS-CoV-2 Total Test XXE5XV7
QIAstat-Dx Respiratory SARS-CoV-2 Panel XXE97U7
Isolation 8EØZXY6
Isotope Administration, Other Radiation, Whole Body DWY5G
Itrel (3) (4) neurostimulator *use* Stimulator Generator, Single Array in ØJH

J

Jakafi® *use* Ruxolitinib
Jejunal artery *use* Superior Mesenteric Artery
Jejunectomy
see Excision, Jejunum ØDBA
see Resection, Jejunum ØDTA
Jejunocolostomy
see Bypass, Gastrointestinal System ØD1
see Drainage, Gastrointestinal System ØD9
Jejunopexy
see Repair, Jejunum ØDQA
see Reposition, Jejunum ØDSA
Jejunostomy
see Bypass, Jejunum ØD1A
see Drainage, Jejunum ØD9A
Jejunotomy *see* Drainage, Jejunum ØD9A
Joint fixation plate
use Internal Fixation Device in Lower Joints
use Internal Fixation Device in Upper Joints
Joint liner (insert) *use* Liner in Lower Joints
Joint spacer (antibiotic)
use Spacer in Lower Joints
use Spacer in Upper Joints
Jugular body *use* Glomus Jugulare
Jugular lymph node
use Lymphatic, Left Neck
use Lymphatic, Right Neck

K

Kappa *use* Pacemaker, Dual Chamber in ØJH
Kcentra *use* 4-Factor Prothrombin Complex Concentrate
Keratectomy, kerectomy
see Excision, Eye Ø8B
see Resection, Eye Ø8T
Keratocentesis *see* Drainage, Eye Ø89
Keratoplasty
see Repair, Eye Ø8Q
see Replacement, Eye Ø8R
see Supplement, Eye Ø8U
Keratotomy
see Drainage, Eye Ø89
see Repair, Eye Ø8Q
KEVZARA® *use* Sarilumab
Keystone Heart TriGuard 3™ CEPD (cerebral embolic protection device) X2A6325
Kirschner wire (K-wire)
use Internal Fixation Device in Head and Facial Bones
use Internal Fixation Device in Lower Bones
use Internal Fixation Device in Lower Joints
use Internal Fixation Device in Upper Bones
use Internal Fixation Device in Upper Joints
Knee (implant) insert *use* Liner in Lower Joints
KUB x-ray *see* Plain Radiography, Kidney, Ureter and Bladder BTØ4
Kuntscher nail
use Internal Fixation Device, Intramedullary in Lower Bones

Kuntscher nail — *continued*
use Internal Fixation Device, Intramedullary in Upper Bones
KYMRIAH® *use* Tisagenlecleucel Immunotherapy

L

Labia majora *use* Vulva
Labia minora *use* Vulva
Labial gland
use Lower Lip
use Upper Lip
Labiectomy
see Excision, Female Reproductive System ØUB
see Resection, Female Reproductive System ØUT
Lacrimal canaliculus
use Lacrimal Duct, Left
use Lacrimal Duct, Right
Lacrimal punctum
use Lacrimal Duct, Left
use Lacrimal Duct, Right
Lacrimal sac
use Lacrimal Duct, Left
use Lacrimal Duct, Right
LAGB (laparoscopic adjustable gastric banding)
Initial procedure ØDV64CZ
Surgical correction *see* Revision of device in, Stomach ØDW6
Laminectomy
see Excision, Lower Bones ØQB
see Excision, Upper Bones ØPB
see Release, Central Nervous System and Cranial Nerves ØØN
see Release, Peripheral Nervous System Ø1N
Laminotomy
see Drainage, Lower Bones ØQ9
see Drainage, Upper Bones ØP9
see Excision, Lower Bones ØQB
see Excision, Upper Bones ØPB
see Release, Central Nervous System and Cranial Nerves ØØN
see Release, Lower Bones ØQN
see Release, Peripheral Nervous System Ø1N
see Release, Upper Bones ØPN
Laparoscopic-assisted transanal pull-through
see Excision, Gastrointestinal System ØDB
see Resection, Gastrointestinal System ØDT
Laparoscopy *see* Inspection
Laparotomy
Drainage *see* Drainage, Peritoneal Cavity ØW9G
Exploratory *see* Inspection, Peritoneal Cavity ØWJG
LAP-BAND® adjustable gastric banding system *use* Extraluminal Device
Laryngectomy
see Excision, Larynx ØCBS
see Resection, Larynx ØCTS
Laryngocentesis *see* Drainage, Larynx ØC9S
Laryngogram *see* Fluoroscopy, Larynx B91J
Laryngopexy *see* Repair, Larynx ØCQS
Laryngopharynx *use* Pharynx
Laryngoplasty
see Repair, Larynx ØCQS
see Replacement, Larynx ØCRS
see Supplement, Larynx ØCUS
Laryngorrhaphy *see* Repair, Larynx ØCQS
Laryngoscopy ØCJS8ZZ
Laryngotomy *see* Drainage, Larynx ØC9S
Laser Interstitial Thermal Therapy
Adrenal Gland DGY2KZZ
Anus DDY8KZZ
Bile Ducts DFY2KZZ
Brain DØYØKZZ
Brain Stem DØY1KZZ
Breast
Left DMYØKZZ
Right DMY1KZZ
Bronchus DBY1KZZ
Chest Wall DBY7KZZ
Colon DDY5KZZ
Diaphragm DBY8KZZ
Duodenum DDY2KZZ
Esophagus DDYØKZZ
Gallbladder DFY1KZZ
Gland
Adrenal DGY2KZZ
Parathyroid DGY4KZZ

Laser Interstitial Thermal Therapy — *continued*
Gland — *continued*
Pituitary DGYØKZZ
Thyroid DGY5KZZ
Ileum DDY4KZZ
Jejunum DDY3KZZ
Liver DFYØKZZ
Lung DBY2KZZ
Mediastinum DBY6KZZ
Nerve, Peripheral DØY7KZZ
Pancreas DFY3KZZ
Parathyroid Gland DGY4KZZ
Pineal Body DGY1KZZ
Pituitary Gland DGYØKZZ
Pleura DBY5KZZ
Prostate DVYØKZZ
Rectum DDY7KZZ
Spinal Cord DØY6KZZ
Stomach DDY1KZZ
Thyroid Gland DGY5KZZ
Trachea DBYØKZZ
Lateral canthus
use Upper Eyelid, Left
use Upper Eyelid, Right
Lateral collateral ligament (LCL)
use Knee Bursa and Ligament, Left
use Knee Bursa and Ligament, Right
Lateral condyle of femur
use Lower Femur, Left
use Lower Femur, Right
Lateral condyle of tibia
use Tibia, Left
use Tibia, Right
Lateral cuneiform bone
use Tarsal, Left
use Tarsal, Right
Lateral epicondyle of femur
use Lower Femur, Left
use Lower Femur, Right
Lateral epicondyle of humerus
use Humeral Shaft, Left
use Humeral Shaft, Right
Lateral femoral cutaneous nerve *use* Lumbar Plexus
Lateral (brachial) lymph node
use Lymphatic, Left Axillary
use Lymphatic, Right Axillary
Lateral malleolus
use Fibula, Left
use Fibula, Right
Lateral meniscus
use Knee Joint, Left
use Knee Joint, Right
Lateral nasal cartilage *use* Nasal Mucosa and Soft Tissue
Lateral plantar artery
use Foot Artery, Left
use Foot Artery, Right
Lateral plantar nerve *use* Tibial Nerve
Lateral rectus muscle
use Extraocular Muscle, Left
use Extraocular Muscle, Right
Lateral sacral artery
use Internal Iliac Artery, Left
use Internal Iliac Artery, Right
Lateral sacral vein
use Hypogastric Vein, Left
use Hypogastric Vein, Right
Lateral sural cutaneous nerve *use* Peroneal Nerve
Lateral tarsal artery
use Foot Artery, Left
use Foot Artery, Right
Lateral temporomandibular ligament *use* Head and Neck Bursa and Ligament
Lateral thoracic artery
use Axillary Artery, Left
use Axillary Artery, Right
Latissimus dorsi muscle
use Trunk Muscle, Left
use Trunk Muscle, Right
Latissimus Dorsi Myocutaneous Flap
Replacement
Bilateral ØHRVØ75
Left ØHRUØ75
Right ØHRTØ75
Transfer
Left ØKXG
Right ØKXF

▽ Subterms under main terms may continue to next column or pa

Lavage
  see Irrigation
  Bronchial alveolar, diagnostic *see* Drainage, Respiratory System ØB9
Least splanchnic nerve *use* Thoracic Sympathetic Nerve
Lefamulin Anti-infective XWØ
Left ascending lumbar vein *use* Hemiazygos Vein
Left atrioventricular valve *use* Mitral Valve
Left auricular appendix *use* Atrium, Left
Left colic vein *use* Colic Vein
Left coronary sulcus *use* Heart, Left
Left gastric artery *use* Gastric Artery
Left gastroepiploic artery *use* Splenic Artery
Left gastroepiploic vein *use* Splenic Vein
Left inferior phrenic vein *use* Renal Vein, Left
Left inferior pulmonary vein *use* Pulmonary Vein, Left
Left jugular trunk *use* Thoracic Duct
Left lateral ventricle *use* Cerebral Ventricle
Left ovarian vein *use* Renal Vein, Left
Left second lumbar vein *use* Renal Vein, Left
Left subclavian trunk *use* Thoracic Duct
Left subcostal vein *use* Hemiazygos Vein
Left superior pulmonary vein *use* Pulmonary Vein, Left
Left suprarenal vein *use* Renal Vein, Left
Left testicular vein *use* Renal Vein, Left
Lengthening
  Bone, with device *see* Insertion of Limb Lengthening Device
  Muscle, by incision *see* Division, Muscles ØK8
  Tendon, by incision *see* Division, Tendons ØL8
Leptomeninges, intracranial *use* Cerebral Meninges
Leptomeninges, spinal *use* Spinal Meninges
Leronlimab Monoclonal Antibody XW013K6
Lesser alar cartilage *use* Nasal Mucosa and Soft Tissue
Lesser occipital nerve *use* Cervical Plexus
Lesser Omentum *use* Omentum
Lesser saphenous vein
  use Saphenous Vein, Left
  use Saphenous Vein, Right
Lesser splanchnic nerve *use* Thoracic Sympathetic Nerve
Lesser trochanter
  use Upper Femur, Left
  use Upper Femur, Right
Lesser tuberosity
  use Humeral Head, Left
  use Humeral Head, Right
Lesser wing *use* Sphenoid Bone
Leukopheresis, therapeutic *see* Pheresis, Circulatory 6A55
Levator anguli oris muscle *use* Facial Muscle
Levator ani muscle *use* Perineum Muscle
Levator labii superioris alaeque nasi muscle *use* Facial Muscle
Levator labii superioris muscle *use* Facial Muscle
Levator palpebrae superioris muscle
  use Upper Eyelid, Left
  use Upper Eyelid, Right
Levator scapulae muscle
  use Neck Muscle, Left
  use Neck Muscle, Right
Levator veli palatini muscle *use* Tongue, Palate, Pharynx Muscle
Levatores costarum muscle
  use Thorax Muscle, Left
  use Thorax Muscle, Right
Lifeline ARM Automated Chest Compression (ACC) device 5A1221J
LifeStent® (Flexstar) (XL) Vascular Stent System *use* Intraluminal Device
Lifileucel *use* Lifileucel Immunotherapy
Lifileucel Immunotherapy XWØ
Ligament of head of fibula
  use Knee Bursa and Ligament, Left
  use Knee Bursa and Ligament, Right
Ligament of the lateral malleolus
  use Ankle Bursa and Ligament, Left
  use Ankle Bursa and Ligament, Right
Ligamentum flavum, cervical *use* Head and Neck Bursa and Ligament
Ligamentum flavum, lumbar *use* Lower Spine Bursa and Ligament

Ligamentum flavum, thoracic *use* Upper Spine Bursa and Ligament
Ligation *see* Occlusion
Ligation, hemorrhoid *see* Occlusion, Lower Veins, Hemorrhoidal Plexus
Light Therapy GZJZZZZ
Liner
  Removal of device from
    Hip
      Left ØSPBØ9Z
      Right ØSP9Ø9Z
    Knee
      Left ØSPDØ9Z
      Right ØSPCØ9Z
  Revision of device in
    Hip
      Left ØSWBØ9Z
      Right ØSW9Ø9Z
    Knee
      Left ØSWDØ9Z
      Right ØSWCØ9Z
  Supplement
    Hip
      Left ØSUBØ9Z
        Acetabular Surface ØSUEØ9Z
        Femoral Surface ØSUSØ9Z
      Right ØSU9Ø9Z
        Acetabular Surface ØSUAØ9Z
        Femoral Surface ØSURØ9Z
    Knee
      Left ØSUDØ9
        Femoral Surface ØSUUØ9Z
        Tibial Surface ØSUWØ9Z
      Right ØSUCØ9
        Femoral Surface ØSUTØ9Z
        Tibial Surface ØSUVØ9Z
Lingual artery
  use External Carotid Artery, Left
  use External Carotid Artery, Right
Lingual tonsil *use* Pharynx
Lingulectomy, lung
  see Excision, Lung Lingula ØBBH
  see Resection, Lung Lingula ØBTH
Lisocabtagene Maraleucel *use* Lisocabtagene Maraleucel Immunotherapy
Lisocabtagene Maraleucel Immunotherapy XWØ
Lithoplasty *see* Fragmentation
Lithotripsy
  see Fragmentation
  With removal of fragments *see* Extirpation
LITT (laser interstitial thermal therapy) *see* Laser Interstitial Thermal Therapy
LIVIAN™ CRT-D *use* Cardiac Resynchronization Defibrillator Pulse Generator in ØJH
Lobectomy
  see Excision, Central Nervous System and Cranial Nerves ØØB
  see Excision, Endocrine System ØGB
  see Excision, Hepatobiliary System and Pancreas ØFB
  see Excision, Respiratory System ØBB
  see Resection, Endocrine System ØGT
  see Resection, Hepatobiliary System and Pancreas ØFT
  see Resection, Respiratory System ØBT
Lobotomy *see* Division, Brain ØØ8Ø
Localization
  see Imaging
  see Map
Locus ceruleus *use* Pons
Long thoracic nerve *use* Brachial Plexus
Loop ileostomy *see* Bypass, Ileum ØD1B
Loop recorder, implantable *use* Monitoring Device
Lower GI series *see* Fluoroscopy, Colon BD14
Lower Respiratory Fluid Nucleic Acid-base Microbial Detection XXEBXQ6
LTX Regional Anticoagulant *use* Nafamostat Anticoagulant
LUCAS® Chest Compression System 5A1221J
Lumbar artery *use* Abdominal Aorta
Lumbar facet joint *use* Lumbar Vertebral Joint
Lumbar ganglion *use* Lumbar Sympathetic Nerve
Lumbar lymph node *use* Lymphatic, Aortic
Lumbar lymphatic trunk *use* Cisterna Chyli
Lumbar splanchnic nerve *use* Lumbar Sympathetic Nerve
Lumbosacral facet joint *use* Lumbosacral Joint

Lumbosacral trunk *use* Lumbar Nerve
Lumpectomy *see* Excision
Lunate bone
  use Carpal, Left
  use Carpal, Right
Lunotriquetral ligament
  use Hand Bursa and Ligament, Left
  use Hand Bursa and Ligament, Right
Lurbinectedin XWØ
Lymphadenectomy
  see Excision, Lymphatic and Hemic Systems Ø7B
  see Resection, Lymphatic and Hemic Systems Ø7T
Lymphadenotomy *see* Drainage, Lymphatic and Hemic Systems Ø79
Lymphangiectomy
  see Excision, Lymphatic and Hemic Systems Ø7B
  see Resection, Lymphatic and Hemic Systems Ø7T
Lymphangiogram *see* Plain Radiography, Lymphatic System B7Ø
Lymphangioplasty
  see Repair, Lymphatic and Hemic Systems Ø7Q
  see Supplement, Lymphatic and Hemic Systems Ø7U
Lymphangiorrhaphy *see* Repair, Lymphatic and Hemic Systems Ø7Q
Lymphangiotomy *see* Drainage, Lymphatic and Hemic Systems Ø79
Lysis *see* Release

M

Macula XXE5XR7
  use Retina, Left
  use Retina, Right
MAGEC® Spinal Bracing and Distraction System *use* Magnetically Controlled Growth Rod(s) in New Technology
Magnet extraction, ocular foreign body *see* Extirpation, Eye Ø8C
Magnetic Resonance Imaging (MRI)
  Abdomen BW3Ø
  Ankle
    Left BQ3H
    Right BQ3G
  Aorta
    Abdominal B43Ø
    Thoracic B33Ø
  Arm
    Left BP3F
    Right BP3E
  Artery
    Celiac B431
    Cervico-Cerebral Arch B33Q
    Common Carotid, Bilateral B335
    Coronary
      Bypass Graft, Multiple B233
      Multiple B231
    Internal Carotid, Bilateral B338
    Intracranial B33R
    Lower Extremity
      Bilateral B43H
      Left B43G
      Right B43F
    Pelvic B43C
    Renal, Bilateral B438
    Spinal B33M
    Superior Mesenteric B434
    Upper Extremity
      Bilateral B33K
      Left B33J
      Right B33H
    Vertebral, Bilateral B33G
  Bladder BT3Ø
  Brachial Plexus BW3P
  Brain BØ3Ø
  Breast
    Bilateral BH32
    Left BH31
    Right BH3Ø
  Calcaneus
    Left BQ3K
    Right BQ3J
  Chest BW33Y
  Coccyx BR3F
  Connective Tissue
    Lower Extremity BL31
    Upper Extremity BL3Ø

Magnetic Resonance Imaging (MRI) — *continued*
Corpora Cavernosa BV3Ø
Disc
  Cervical BR31
  Lumbar BR33
  Thoracic BR32
Ear B93Ø
Elbow
  Left BP3H
  Right BP3G
Eye
  Bilateral B837
  Left B836
  Right B835
Femur
  Left BQ34
  Right BQ33
Fetal Abdomen BY33
Fetal Extremity BY35
Fetal Head BY3Ø
Fetal Heart BY31
Fetal Spine BY34
Fetal Thorax BY32
Fetus, Whole BY36
Foot
  Left BQ3M
  Right BQ3L
Forearm
  Left BP3K
  Right BP3J
Gland
  Adrenal, Bilateral BG32
  Parathyroid BG33
  Parotid, Bilateral B936
  Salivary, Bilateral B93D
  Submandibular, Bilateral B939
  Thyroid BG34
Head BW38
Heart, Right and Left B236
Hip
  Left BQ31
  Right BQ3Ø
Intracranial Sinus B532
Joint
  Finger
    Left BP3D
    Right BP3C
  Hand
    Left BP3D
    Right BP3C
  Temporomandibular, Bilateral BN39
Kidney
  Bilateral BT33
  Left BT32
  Right BT31
  Transplant BT39
Knee
  Left BQ38
  Right BQ37
Larynx B93J
Leg
  Left BQ3F
  Right BQ3D
Liver BF35
Liver and Spleen BF36
Lung Apices BB3G
Nasopharynx B93F
Neck BW3F
Nerve
  Acoustic BØ3C
  Brachial Plexus BW3P
Oropharynx B93F
Ovary
  Bilateral BU35
  Left BU34
  Right BU33
Ovary and Uterus BU3C
Pancreas BF37
Patella
  Left BQ3W
  Right BQ3V
Pelvic Region BW3G
Pelvis BR3C
Pituitary Gland BØ39
Plexus, Brachial BW3P
Prostate BV33
Retroperitoneum BW3H
Sacrum BR3F
Scrotum BV34

Magnetic Resonance Imaging (MRI) — *continued*
Sella Turcica BØ39
Shoulder
  Left BP39
  Right BP38
Sinus
  Intracranial B532
  Paranasal B932
Spinal Cord BØ3B
Spine
  Cervical BR3Ø
  Lumbar BR39
  Thoracic BR37
Spleen and Liver BF36
Subcutaneous Tissue
  Abdomen BH3H
  Extremity
    Lower BH3J
    Upper BH3F
  Head BH3D
  Neck BH3D
  Pelvis BH3H
  Thorax BH3G
Tendon
  Lower Extremity BL33
  Upper Extremity BL32
Testicle
  Bilateral BV37
  Left BV36
  Right BV35
Toe
  Left BQ3Q
  Right BQ3P
Uterus BU36
  Pregnant BU3B
Uterus and Ovary BU3C
Vagina BU39
Vein
  Cerebellar B531
  Cerebral B531
  Jugular, Bilateral B535
  Lower Extremity
    Bilateral B53D
    Left B53C
    Right B53B
  Other B53V
  Pelvic (Iliac) Bilateral B53H
  Portal B53T
  Pulmonary, Bilateral B53S
  Renal, Bilateral B53L
  Spanchnic B53T
  Upper Extremity
    Bilateral B53P
    Left B53N
    Right B53M
  Vena Cava
    Inferior B539
    Superior B538
Wrist
  Left BP3M
  Right BP3L
Magnetically Controlled Growth Rod(s)
Cervical XNS3
Lumbar XNSØ
Thoracic XNS4
Magnetic-guided radiofrequency endovascular fistula
Radial Artery, Left Ø31C3ZF
Radial Artery, Right Ø31B3ZF
Ulnar Artery, Left Ø31A3ZF
Ulnar Artery, Right Ø3193ZF
Malleotomy *see* Drainage, Ear, Nose, Sinus Ø99
Malleus
  use Auditory Ossicle, Left
  use Auditory Ossicle, Right
Mammaplasty, mammoplasty
  see Alteration, Skin and Breast ØHØ
  see Repair, Skin and Breast ØHQ
  see Replacement, Skin and Breast ØHR
  see Supplement, Skin and Breast ØHU
Mammary duct
  use Breast, Bilateral
  use Breast, Left
  use Breast, Right
Mammary gland
  use Breast, Bilateral
  use Breast, Left
  use Breast, Right

Mammectomy
  see Excision, Skin and Breast ØHB
  see Resection, Skin and Breast ØHT
Mammillary body *use* Hypothalamus
Mammography *see* Plain Radiography, Skin, Subcutaneous Tissue and Breast BHØ
Mammotomy *see* Drainage, Skin and Breast ØH9
Mandibular nerve *use* Trigeminal Nerve
Mandibular notch
  use Mandible, Left
  use Mandible, Right
Mandibulectomy
  see Excision, Head and Facial Bones ØNB
  see Resection, Head and Facial Bones ØNT
Manipulation
  Adhesions *see* Release
  Chiropractic *see* Chiropractic Manipulation
Manual removal, retained placenta *see* Extraction, Products of Conception, Retained 1ØD1
Manubrium *use* Sternum
Map
  Basal Ganglia ØØK8
  Brain ØØKØ
  Cerebellum ØØKC
  Cerebral Hemisphere ØØK7
  Conduction Mechanism Ø2K8
  Hypothalamus ØØKA
  Medulla Oblongata ØØKD
  Pons ØØKB
  Thalamus ØØK9
Mapping
  Doppler ultrasound *see* Ultrasonography
  Electrocardiogram only *see* Measurement, Cardiac 4AØ2
Mark IV Breathing Pacemaker System *use* Stimulator Generator in Subcutaneous Tissue and Fascia
Marsupialization
  see Drainage
  see Excision
Massage, cardiac
  External 5A12Ø12
  Open Ø2QAØZZ
Masseter muscle *use* Head Muscle
Masseteric fascia *use* Subcutaneous Tissue and Fascia, Face
Mastectomy
  see Excision, Skin and Breast ØHB
  see Resection, Skin and Breast ØHT
Mastoid air cells
  use Mastoid Sinus, Left
  use Mastoid Sinus, Right
Mastoid (postauricular) lymph node
  use Lymphatic, Left Neck
  use Lymphatic, Right Neck
Mastoid process
  use Temporal Bone, Left
  use Temporal Bone, Right
Mastoidectomy
  see Excision, Ear, Nose, Sinus Ø9B
  see Resection, Ear, Nose, Sinus Ø9T
Mastoidotomy *see* Drainage, Ear, Nose, Sinus Ø99
Mastopexy
  see Repair, Skin and Breast ØHQ
  see Reposition, Skin and Breast ØHS
Mastorrhaphy *see* Repair, Skin and Breast ØHQ
Mastotomy *see* Drainage, Skin and Breast ØH9
Maxillary artery
  use External Carotid Artery, Left
  use External Carotid Artery, Right
Maxillary nerve *use* Trigeminal Nerve
Maximo II DR (VR) *use* Defibrillator Generator in ØJH
Maximo II DR CRT-D *use* Cardiac Resynchronization Defibrillator Pulse Generator in ØJH
Measurement
  Arterial
    Flow
      Coronary 4AØ3
      Intracranial 4AØ3X5D
      Peripheral 4AØ3
      Pulmonary 4AØ3
    Pressure
      Coronary 4AØ3
      Peripheral 4AØ3
      Pulmonary 4AØ3
      Thoracic, Other 4AØ3
    Pulse
      Coronary 4AØ3

Measurement — *continued*
  Arterial — *continued*
    Pulse — *continued*
      Peripheral 4A03
      Pulmonary 4A03
    Saturation, Peripheral 4A03
    Sound, Peripheral 4A03
  Biliary
    Flow 4A0C
    Pressure 4A0C
  Cardiac
    Action Currents 4A02
    Defibrillator 4B02XTZ
    Electrical Activity 4A02
      Guidance 4A02X4A
      No Qualifier 4A02X4Z
    Output 4A02
    Pacemaker 4B02XSZ
    Rate 4A02
    Rhythm 4A02
    Sampling and Pressure
      Bilateral 4A02
      Left Heart 4A02
      Right Heart 4A02
    Sound 4A02
    Total Activity, Stress 4A02XM4
  Central Nervous
    Cerebrospinal Fluid Shunt, Wireless Sensor 4B00XW0
    Conductivity 4A00
    Electrical Activity 4A00
    Pressure 4A000BZ
      Intracranial 4A00
    Saturation, Intracranial 4A00
    Stimulator 4B00XVZ
    Temperature, Intracranial 4A00
  Circulatory, Volume 4A05XLZ
  Gastrointestinal
    Motility 4A0B
    Pressure 4A0B
    Secretion 4A0B
  Lower Respiratory Fluid Nucleic Acid-base Microbial Detection XXFBXQ6
  Lymphatic
    Flow 4A06
    Pressure 4A06
  Metabolism 4A0Z
  Musculoskeletal
    Contractility 4A0F
    Pressure 4A0F3BE
    Stimulator 4B0FXVZ
  Olfactory, Acuity 4A08X0Z
  Peripheral Nervous
    Conductivity
      Motor 4A01
      Sensory 4A01
    Electrical Activity 4A01
    Stimulator 4B01XVZ
  Positive Blood Culture Fluorescence Hybridization for Organism Identification, Concentration and Susceptibility XXE5XN6
  Products of Conception
    Cardiac
      Electrical Activity 4A0H
      Rate 4A0H
      Rhythm 4A0H
      Sound 4A0H
    Nervous
      Conductivity 4A0J
      Electrical Activity 4A0J
      Pressure 4A0J
  Respiratory
    Capacity 4A09
    Flow 4A09
    Pacemaker 4B09XSZ
    Rate 4A09
    Resistance 4A09
    Total Activity 4A09
    Volume 4A09
  Sleep 4A0ZXQZ
  Temperature 4A0Z
  Urinary
    Contractility 4A0D
    Flow 4A0D
    Pressure 4A0D
    Resistance 4A0D
    Volume 4A0D

Measurement — *continued*
  Venous
    Flow
      Central 4A04
      Peripheral 4A04
      Portal 4A04
      Pulmonary 4A04
    Pressure
      Central 4A04
      Peripheral 4A04
      Portal 4A04
      Pulmonary 4A04
    Pulse
      Central 4A04
      Peripheral 4A04
      Portal 4A04
      Pulmonary 4A04
    Saturation, Peripheral 4A04
  Visual
    Acuity 4A07X0Z
    Mobility 4A07X7Z
    Pressure 4A07XBZ
  Whole Blood Nucleic Acid-base Microbial Detection XXE5XM5
Meatoplasty, urethra *see* Repair, Urethra 0TQD
Meatotomy *see* Drainage, Urinary System 0T9
Mechanical chest compression (mCPR) 5A1221J
Mechanical Initial Specimen Diversion Technique Using Active Negative Pressure (blood collection) XXE5XR7
Mechanical ventilation *see* Performance, Respiratory 5A19
Medial canthus
  use Lower Eyelid, Left
  use Lower Eyelid, Right
Medial collateral ligament (MCL)
  use Knee Bursa and Ligament, Left
  use Knee Bursa and Ligament, Right
Medial condyle of femur
  use Lower Femur, Left
  use Lower Femur, Right
Medial condyle of tibia
  use Tibia, Left
  use Tibia, Right
Medial cuneiform bone
  use Tarsal, Left
  use Tarsal, Right
Medial epicondyle of femur
  use Lower Femur, Left
  use Lower Femur, Right
Medial epicondyle of humerus
  use Humeral Shaft, Left
  use Humeral Shaft, Right
Medial malleolus
  use Tibia, Left
  use Tibia, Right
Medial meniscus
  use Knee Joint, Left
  use Knee Joint, Right
Medial plantar artery
  use Foot Artery, Left
  use Foot Artery, Right
Medial plantar nerve *use* Tibial Nerve
Medial popliteal nerve *use* Tibial Nerve
Medial rectus muscle
  use Extraocular Muscle, Left
  use Extraocular Muscle, Right
Medial sural cutaneous nerve *use* Tibial Nerve
Median antebrachial vein
  use Basilic Vein, Left
  use Basilic Vein, Right
Median cubital vein
  use Basilic Vein, Left
  use Basilic Vein, Right
Median sacral artery *use* Abdominal Aorta
Mediastinal cavity *use* Mediastinum
Mediastinal lymph node *use* Lymphatic, Thorax
Mediastinal space *use* Mediastinum
Mediastinoscopy 0WJC4ZZ
Medication Management GZ3ZZZZ
  for substance abuse
    Antabuse HZ83ZZZ
    Bupropion HZ87ZZZ
    Clonidine HZ86ZZZ
    Levo-alpha-acetyl-methadol (LAAM) HZ82ZZZ
    Methadone Maintenance HZ81ZZZ

Medication Management — *continued*
  for substance abuse — *continued*
    Naloxone HZ85ZZZ
    Naltrexone HZ84ZZZ
    Nicotine Replacement HZ80ZZZ
    Other Replacement Medication HZ89ZZZ
    Psychiatric Medication HZ88ZZZ
Meditation 8E0ZXY5
Medtronic Endurant® II AAA stent graft system *use* Intraluminal Device
Meissner's (submucous) plexus *use* Abdominal Sympathetic Nerve
Melody® transcatheter pulmonary valve *use* Zooplastic Tissue in Heart and Great Vessels
Membranous urethra *use* Urethra
Meningeorrhaphy
  see Repair, Cerebral Meninges 00Q1
  see Repair, Spinal Meninges 00QT
Meniscectomy, knee
  see Excision, Joint, Knee, Left 0SBD
  see Excision, Joint, Knee, Right 0SBC
Mental foramen
  use Mandible, Left
  use Mandible, Right
Mentalis muscle *use* Facial Muscle
Mentoplasty *see* Alteration, Jaw, Lower 0W05
Meropenem-vaborbactam Anti-infective XW0
Mesenterectomy *see* Excision, Mesentery 0DBV
Mesenteriorrhaphy, mesenterorrhaphy *see* Repair, Mesentery 0DQV
Mesenteriplication *see* Repair, Mesentery 0DQV
Mesoappendix *use* Mesentery
Mesocolon *use* Mesentery
Metacarpal ligament
  use Hand Bursa and Ligament, Left
  use Hand Bursa and Ligament, Right
Metacarpophalangeal ligament
  use Hand Bursa and Ligament, Left
  use Hand Bursa and Ligament, Right
Metal on metal bearing surface *use* Synthetic Substitute, Metal in 0SR
Metatarsal ligament
  use Foot Bursa and Ligament, Left
  use Foot Bursa and Ligament, Right
Metatarsectomy
  see Excision, Lower Bones 0QB
  see Resection, Lower Bones 0QT
Metatarsophalangeal (MTP) joint
  use Metatarsal-Phalangeal Joint, Left
  use Metatarsal-Phalangeal Joint, Right
Metatarsophalangeal ligament
  use Foot Bursa and Ligament, Left
  use Foot Bursa and Ligament, Right
Metathalamus *use* Thalamus
Micro-Driver stent (RX) (OTW) *use* Intraluminal Device
MicroMed HeartAssist *use* Implantable Heart Assist System in Heart and Great Vessels
Micrus CERECYTE Microcoil *use* Intraluminal Device, Bioactive in Upper Arteries
Midcarpal joint
  use Carpal Joint, Left
  use Carpal Joint, Right
Middle cardiac nerve *use* Thoracic Sympathetic Nerve
Middle cerebral artery *use* Intracranial Artery
Middle cerebral vein *use* Intracranial Vein
Middle colic vein *use* Colic Vein
Middle genicular artery
  use Popliteal Artery, Left
  use Popliteal Artery, Right
Middle hemorrhoidal vein
  use Hypogastric Vein, Left
  use Hypogastric Vein, Right
Middle rectal artery
  use Internal Iliac Artery, Left
  use Internal Iliac Artery, Right
Middle suprarenal artery *use* Abdominal Aorta
Middle temporal artery
  use Temporal Artery, Left
  use Temporal Artery, Right
Middle turbinate *use* Nasal Turbinate
Mineral-based Topical Hemostatic Agent XW0
MIRODERM™ Biologic Wound Matrix *use* Skin Substitute, Porcine Liver Derived in New Technology
MitraClip valve repair system *use* Synthetic Substitute
Mitral annulus *use* Mitral Valve

Mitroflow® Aortic Pericardial Heart Valve *use* Zooplastic Tissue in Heart and Great Vessels
Mobilization, adhesions *see* Release
Molar gland *use* Buccal Mucosa
MolecuLight i:X® wound imaging *see* Other Imaging, Anatomical Regions BW5
Monitoring
Arterial
Flow
Coronary 4A13
Peripheral 4A13
Pulmonary 4A13
Pressure
Coronary 4A13
Peripheral 4A13
Pulmonary 4A13
Pulse
Coronary 4A13
Peripheral 4A13
Pulmonary 4A13
Saturation, Peripheral 4A13
Sound, Peripheral 4A13
Cardiac
Electrical Activity 4A12
Ambulatory 4A12X45
No Qualifier 4A12X4Z
Output 4A12
Rate 4A12
Rhythm 4A12
Sound 4A12
Total Activity, Stress 4A12XM4
Vascular Perfusion, Indocyanine Green Dye 4A12XSH
Central Nervous
Conductivity 4A10
Electrical Activity
Intraoperative 4A10
No Qualifier 4A10
Pressure 4A100BZ
Intracranial 4A10
Saturation, Intracranial 4A10
Temperature, Intracranial 4A10
Gastrointestinal
Motility 4A1B
Pressure 4A1B
Secretion 4A1B
Vascular Perfusion, Indocyanine Green Dye 4A1BXSH
Kidney, Fluorescent Pyrazine XT25XE5
Lymphatic
Flow
Indocyanine Green Dye 4A16
No Qualifier 4A16
Pressure 4A16
Oxygen Saturation Endoscopic Imaging (OXEI) XD2
Peripheral Nervous
Conductivity
Motor 4A11
Sensory 4A11
Electrical Activity
Intraoperative 4A11
No Qualifier 4A11
Products of Conception
Cardiac
Electrical Activity 4A1H
Rate 4A1H
Rhythm 4A1H
Sound 4A1H
Nervous
Conductivity 4A1J
Electrical Activity 4A1J
Pressure 4A1J
Respiratory
Capacity 4A19
Flow 4A19
Rate 4A19
Resistance 4A19
Volume 4A19
Skin and Breast, Vascular Perfusion, Indocyanine Green Dye 4A1GXSH
Sleep 4A1ZXQZ
Temperature 4A1Z
Urinary
Contractility 4A1D
Flow 4A1D
Pressure 4A1D
Resistance 4A1D
Volume 4A1D

Monitoring — *continued*
Venous
Flow
Central 4A14
Peripheral 4A14
Portal 4A14
Pulmonary 4A14
Pressure
Central 4A14
Peripheral 4A14
Portal 4A14
Pulmonary 4A14
Pulse
Central 4A14
Peripheral 4A14
Portal 4A14
Pulmonary 4A14
Saturation
Central 4A14
Portal 4A14
Pulmonary 4A14
Monitoring Device, Hemodynamic
Abdomen ØJH8
Chest ØJH6
Mosaic Bioprosthesis (aortic) (mitral) valve *use* Zooplastic Tissue in Heart and Great Vessels
Motor Function Assessment F01
Motor Treatment F07
MR Angiography
see Magnetic Resonance Imaging (MRI), Heart B23
see Magnetic Resonance Imaging (MRI), Lower Arteries B43
see Magnetic Resonance Imaging (MRI), Upper Arteries B33
MULTI-LINK (VISION) (MINI-VISION) (ULTRA) Coronary Stent System *use* Intraluminal Device
Multiple sleep latency test 4A0ZXQZ
Musculocutaneous nerve *use* Brachial Plexus
Musculopexy
see Repair, Muscles ØKQ
see Reposition, Muscles ØKS
Musculophrenic artery
use Internal Mammary Artery, Left
use Internal Mammary Artery, Right
Musculoplasty
see Repair, Muscles ØKQ
see Supplement, Muscles ØKU
Musculorrhaphy *see* Repair, Muscles ØKQ
Musculospiral nerve *use* Radial Nerve
Myectomy
see Excision, Muscles ØKB
see Resection, Muscles ØKT
Myelencephalon *use* Medulla Oblongata
Myelogram
CT *see* Computerized Tomography (CT Scan), Central Nervous System B02
MRI *see* Magnetic Resonance Imaging (MRI), Central Nervous System B03
Myenteric (Auerbach's) plexus *use* Abdominal Sympathetic Nerve
Myocardial Bridge Release *see* Release, Artery, Coronary
Myomectomy *see* Excision, Female Reproductive System ØUB
Myometrium *use* Uterus
Myopexy
see Repair, Muscles ØKQ
see Reposition, Muscles ØKS
Myoplasty
see Repair, Muscles ØKQ
see Supplement, Muscles ØKU
Myorrhaphy *see* Repair, Muscles ØKQ
Myoscopy *see* Inspection, Muscles ØKJ
Myotomy
see Division, Muscles ØK8
see Drainage, Muscles ØK9
Myringectomy
see Excision, Ear, Nose, Sinus Ø9B
see Resection, Ear, Nose, Sinus Ø9T
Myringoplasty
see Repair, Ear, Nose, Sinus Ø9Q
see Replacement, Ear, Nose, Sinus Ø9R
see Supplement, Ear, Nose, Sinus Ø9U
Myringostomy *see* Drainage, Ear, Nose, Sinus Ø99
Myringotomy *see* Drainage, Ear, Nose, Sinus Ø99

N

NA-1 (Nerinitide) *use* Nerinitide
Nafamostat Anticoagulant XY0YX37
Nail bed
use Finger Nail
use Toe Nail
Nail plate
use Finger Nail
use Toe Nail
nanoLOCK™ interbody fusion device *use* Interbody Fusion Device, Nanotextured Surface in New Technology
Narcosynthesis GZGZZZZ
Narsoplimab Monoclonal Antibody XW0
Nasal cavity *use* Nasal Mucosa and Soft Tissue
Nasal concha *use* Nasal Turbinate
Nasalis muscle *use* Facial Muscle
Nasolacrimal duct
use Lacrimal Duct, Left
use Lacrimal Duct, Right
Nasopharyngeal airway (NPA) *use* Intraluminal Device, Airway in Ear, Nose, Sinus
Navicular bone
use Tarsal, Left
use Tarsal, Right
Near Infrared Spectroscopy, Circulatory System 8E02
Neck of femur
use Upper Femur, Left
use Upper Femur, Right
Neck of humerus (anatomical) (surgical)
use Humeral Head, Left
use Humeral Head, Right
Neovasc Reducer™ *use* Reduction Device in New Technology
Nephrectomy
see Excision, Urinary System ØTB
see Resection, Urinary System ØTT
Nephrolithotomy *see* Extirpation, Urinary System ØTC
Nephrolysis *see* Release, Urinary System ØTN
Nephropexy
see Repair, Urinary System ØTQ
see Reposition, Urinary System ØTS
Nephroplasty
see Repair, Urinary System ØTQ
see Supplement, Urinary System ØTU
Nephropyeloureterostomy
see Bypass, Urinary System ØT1
see Drainage, Urinary System ØT9
Nephrorrhaphy *see* Repair, Urinary System ØTQ
Nephroscopy, transurethral ØTJ58ZZ
Nephrostomy
see Bypass, Urinary System ØT1
see Drainage, Urinary System ØT9
Nephrotomography
see Fluoroscopy, Urinary System BT1
see Plain Radiography, Urinary System BT0
Nephrotomy
see Division, Urinary System ØT8
see Drainage, Urinary System ØT9
Nerinitide XW0
Nerve conduction study
see Measurement, Central Nervous 4A00
see Measurement, Peripheral Nervous 4A01
Nerve Function Assessment F01
Nerve to the stapedius *use* Facial Nerve
Nesiritide *use* Human B-Type Natriuretic Peptide
Neurectomy
see Excision, Central Nervous System and Cranial Nerves 00B
see Excision, Peripheral Nervous System 01B
Neurexeresis
see Extraction, Central Nervous System and Cranial Nerves 00D
see Extraction, Peripheral Nervous System 01D
Neurohypophysis *use* Pituitary Gland
Neurolysis
see Release, Central Nervous System and Cranial Nerves 00N
see Release, Peripheral Nervous System 01N
Neuromuscular electrical stimulation (NEMS) lead *use* Stimulator Lead in Muscles
Neurophysiologic monitoring *see* Monitoring, Central Nervous 4A10

Neuroplasty
　see Repair, Central Nervous System and Cranial
　　Nerves 00Q
　see Repair, Peripheral Nervous System 01Q
　see Supplement, Central Nervous System and
　　Cranial Nerves 00U
　see Supplement, Peripheral Nervous System 01U
Neurorrhaphy
　see Repair, Central Nervous System and Cranial
　　Nerves 00Q
　see Repair, Peripheral Nervous System 01Q
Neurostimulator Generator
　Insertion of device in, Skull 0NH00NZ
　Removal of device from, Skull 0NP00NZ
　Revision of device in, Skull 0NW00NZ
Neurostimulator generator, multiple channel *use*
　Stimulator Generator, Multiple Array in 0JH
**Neurostimulator generator, multiple channel
　rechargeable** *use* Stimulator Generator, Multiple
　Array Rechargeable in 0JH
Neurostimulator generator, single channel *use*
　Stimulator Generator, Single Array in 0JH
**Neurostimulator generator, single channel
　rechargeable** *use* Stimulator Generator, Single
　Array Rechargeable in 0JH
Neurostimulator Lead
　Insertion of device in
　　Brain 00H0
　　Cerebral Ventricle 00H6
　　Nerve
　　　Cranial 00HE
　　　Peripheral 01HY
　　Spinal Canal 00HU
　　Spinal Cord 00HV
　　Vein
　　　Azygos 05H0
　　　Innominate
　　　　Left 05H4
　　　　Right 05H3
　Removal of device from
　　Brain 00P0
　　Cerebral Ventricle 00P6
　　Nerve
　　　Cranial 00PE
　　　Peripheral 01PY
　　Spinal Canal 00PU
　　Spinal Cord 00PV
　　Vein
　　　Azygos 05P0
　　　Innominate
　　　　Left 05P4
　　　　Right 05P3
　Revision of device in
　　Brain 00W0
　　Cerebral Ventricle 00W6
　　Nerve
　　　Cranial 00WE
　　　Peripheral 01WY
　　Spinal Canal 00WU
　　Spinal Cord 00WV
　　Vein
　　　Azygos 05W0
　　　Innominate
　　　　Left 05W4
　　　　Right 05W3
Neurostimulator Lead in Oropharynx XWHD7Q7
Neurotomy
　see Division, Central Nervous System and Cranial
　　Nerves 008
　see Division, Peripheral Nervous System 018
Neurotripsy
　see Destruction, Central Nervous System and Cra-
　　nial Nerves 005
　see Destruction, Peripheral Nervous System 015
Neutralization plate
　use Internal Fixation Device in Head and Facial
　　Bones
　use Internal Fixation Device in Lower Bones
　use Internal Fixation Device in Upper Bones
New Technology
　Amivantamab Monoclonal Antibody XW0
　Antibiotic-eluting Bone Void Filler XW0V0P7
　Aorta
　　Thoracic Arch using Branched Synthetic
　　　Substitute with Intraluminal Device
　　　X2RX0N7

New Technology — *continued*
　Aorta — *continued*
　　Thoracic Descending using Branched Synthet-
　　　ic Substitute with Intraluminal Device
　　　X2VW0N7
　Apalutamide Antineoplastic XW0DXJ5
　Atezolizumab Antineoplastic XW0
　Axicabtagene Ciloleucel Immunotherapy XW0
　Bamlanivimab Monoclonal Antibody XW0
　Baricitinib XW0
　Bezlotoxumab Monoclonal Antibody XW0
　Bioengineered Allogeneic Construct, Skin XHRPXF7
　Brexanolone XW0
　Brexucabtagene Autoleucel Immunotherapy XW0
　Bromelain-enriched Proteolytic Enzyme XW0
　Caplacizumab XW0
　CD24Fc Immunomodulator XW0
　Cefiderocol Anti-infective XW0
　Ceftolozane/Tazobactam Anti-infective XW0
　Cerebral Embolic Filtration
　　Dual Filter X2A5312
　　Extracorporeal Flow Reversal Circuit X2A
　　Single Deflection Filter X2A6325
　Ciltacabtagene Autoleucel XW0
　Coagulation Factor Xa, Inactivated XW0
　Computer-aided Assessment, Intracranial Vascular
　　Activity XXE0X07
　Computer-aided Guidance, Transthoracic
　　Echocardiography X2JAX47
　Computer-aided Mechanical Aspiration X2C
　Computer-aided Triage and Notification, Pul-
　　monary Artery Flow XXE3X27
　Concentrated Bone Marrow Aspirate XK02303
　Coronary Sinus, Reduction Device X2V73Q7
　COVID-19 Vaccine XW0
　COVID-19 Vaccine Dose 1 XW0
　COVID-19 Vaccine Dose 2 XW0
　Cytarabine and Daunorubicin Liposome Antineo-
　　plastic XW0
　Defibrotide Sodium Anticoagulant XW0
　Destruction, Prostate, Robotic Waterjet Ablation
　　XV508A4
　Dilation
　　Anterior Tibial
　　　Left
　　　　Sustained Release Drug-eluting
　　　　　Intraluminal Device
　　　　　X27Q385
　　　　Four or More X27Q3C5
　　　　Three X27Q3B5
　　　　Two X27Q395
　　　Right
　　　　Sustained Release Drug-eluting
　　　　　Intraluminal Device
　　　　　X27P385
　　　　Four or More X27P3C5
　　　　Three X27P3B5
　　　　Two X27P395
　　Femoral
　　　Left
　　　　Sustained Release Drug-eluting
　　　　　Intraluminal Device
　　　　　X27J385
　　　　Four or More X27J3C5
　　　　Three X27J3B5
　　　　Two X27J395
　　　Right
　　　　Sustained Release Drug-eluting
　　　　　Intraluminal Device
　　　　　X27H385
　　　　Four or More X27H3C5
　　　　Three X27H3B5
　　　　Two X27H395
　　Peroneal
　　　Left
　　　　Sustained Release Drug-eluting
　　　　　Intraluminal Device
　　　　　X27U385
　　　　Four or More X27U3C5
　　　　Three X27U3B5
　　　　Two X27U395
　　　Right
　　　　Sustained Release Drug-eluting
　　　　　Intraluminal Device
　　　　　X27T385
　　　　Four or More X27T3C5
　　　　Three X27T3B5
　　　　Two X27T395

New Technology — *continued*
　Dilation — *continued*
　　Popliteal
　　　Left Distal
　　　　Sustained Release Drug-eluting
　　　　　Intraluminal Device
　　　　　X27N385
　　　　Four or More X27N3C5
　　　　Three X27N3B5
　　　　Two X27N395
　　　Left Proximal
　　　　Sustained Release Drug-eluting
　　　　　Intraluminal Device
　　　　　X27L385
　　　　Four or More X27L3C5
　　　　Three X27L3B5
　　　　Two X27L395
　　　Right Distal
　　　　Sustained Release Drug-eluting
　　　　　Intraluminal Device
　　　　　X27M385
　　　　Four or More X27M3C5
　　　　Three X27M3B5
　　　　Two X27M395
　　　Right Proximal
　　　　Sustained Release Drug-eluting
　　　　　Intraluminal Device
　　　　　X27K385
　　　　Four or More X27K3C5
　　　　Three X27K3B5
　　　　Two X27K395
　　Posterior Tibial
　　　Left
　　　　Sustained Release Drug-eluting
　　　　　Intraluminal Device
　　　　　X27S385
　　　　Four or More X27S3C5
　　　　Three X27S3B5
　　　　Two X27S395
　　　Right
　　　　Sustained Release Drug-eluting
　　　　　Intraluminal Device
　　　　　X27R385
　　　　Four or More X27R3C5
　　　　Three X27R3B5
　　　　Two X27R395
　Durvalumab Antineoplastic XW0
　Eculizumab XW0
　Eladocagene exuparvovec XW0Q316
　Endothelial Damage Inhibitor XY0VX83
　Engineered Chimeric Antigen Receptor T-cell Im-
　　munotherapy
　　Allogeneic XW0
　　Autologous XW0
　Erdafitinib Antineoplastic XW0DXL5
　Esketamine Hydrochloride XW097M5
　Etesevimab Monoclonal Antibody XW0
　Fosfomycin Anti-infective XW0
　Fusion
　　Cervical Vertebral
　　　2 or more
　　　　Nanotextured Surface XRG2092
　　　　Radiolucent Porous XRG20F3
　　　Interbody Fusion Device
　　　　Nanotextured Surface XRG1092
　　　　Radiolucent Porous XRG10F3
　　Cervicothoracic Vertebral
　　　Nanotextured Surface XRG4092
　　　Radiolucent Porous XRG40F3
　　Lumbar Vertebral
　　　2 or more
　　　　Customizable XRGC
　　　　Nanotextured Surface XRGC092
　　　　Radiolucent Porous XRGC0F3
　　　Interbody Fusion Device
　　　　Customizable XRGB
　　　　Nanotextured Surface XRGB092
　　　　Radiolucent Porous XRGB0F3
　　Lumbosacral
　　　Customizable XRGD
　　　Nanotextured Surface XRGD092
　　　Radiolucent Porous XRGD0F3
　　Occipital-cervical
　　　Nanotextured Surface XRG0092
　　　Radiolucent Porous XRG00F3
　　Thoracic Vertebral
　　　2 to 7
　　　　Nanotextured Surface XRG7092
　　　　Radiolucent Porous XRG70F3

Oophorostomy see Drainage, Female Reproductive System ØU9
Oophorotomy
　see Division, Female Reproductive System ØU8
　see Drainage, Female Reproductive System ØU9
Oophorrhaphy see Repair, Female Reproductive System ØUQ
Open Pivot Aortic Valve Graft (AVG) use Synthetic Substitute
Open Pivot (mechanical) Valve use Synthetic Substitute
Ophthalmic artery use Intracranial Artery
Ophthalmic nerve use Trigeminal Nerve
Ophthalmic vein use Intracranial Vein
Opponensplasty
　Tendon replacement see Replacement, Tendons ØLR
　Tendon transfer see Transfer, Tendons ØLX
Optic chiasma use Optic Nerve
Optic disc
　use Retina, Left
　use Retina, Right
Optic foramen use Sphenoid Bone
Optical coherence tomography, intravascular see Computerized Tomography (CT Scan)
Optimizer™ III implantable pulse generator use Contractility Modulation Device in ØJH
Orbicularis oculi muscle
　use Upper Eyelid, Left
　use Upper Eyelid, Right
Orbicularis oris muscle use Facial Muscle
Orbital Atherectomy see Extirpation, Heart and Great Vessels Ø2C
Orbital fascia use Subcutaneous Tissue and Fascia, Face
Orbital portion of ethmoid bone
　use Orbit, Left
　use Orbit, Right
Orbital portion of frontal bone
　use Orbit, Left
　use Orbit, Right
Orbital portion of lacrimal bone
　use Orbit, Left
　use Orbit, Right
Orbital portion of maxilla
　use Orbit, Left
　use Orbit, Right
Orbital portion of palatine bone
　use Orbit, Left
　use Orbit, Right
Orbital portion of sphenoid bone
　use Orbit, Left
　use Orbit, Right
Orbital portion of zygomatic bone
　use Orbit, Left
　use Orbit, Right
Orchectomy, orchidectomy, orchiectomy
　see Excision, Male Reproductive System ØVB
　see Resection, Male Reproductive System ØVT
Orchidoplasty, orchioplasty
　see Repair, Male Reproductive System ØVQ
　see Replacement, Male Reproductive System ØVR
　see Supplement, Male Reproductive System ØVU
Orchidorrhaphy, orchiorrhaphy see Repair, Male Reproductive System ØVQ
Orchidotomy, orchiotomy, orchotomy see Drainage, Male Reproductive System ØV9
Orchiopexy
　see Repair, Male Reproductive System ØVQ
　see Reposition, Male Reproductive System ØVS
Oropharyngeal airway (OPA) use Intraluminal Device, Airway in Mouth and Throat
Oropharynx use Pharynx
Ossiculectomy
　see Excision, Ear, Nose, Sinus Ø9B
　see Resection, Ear, Nose, Sinus Ø9T
Ossiculotomy see Drainage, Ear, Nose, Sinus Ø99
Ostectomy
　see Excision, Head and Facial Bones ØNB
　see Excision, Lower Bones ØQB
　see Excision, Upper Bones ØPB
　see Resection, Head and Facial Bones ØNT
　see Resection, Lower Bones ØQT
　see Resection, Upper Bones ØPT
Osteoclasis
　see Division, Head and Facial Bones ØN8

Osteoclasis — continued
　see Division, Lower Bones ØQ8
　see Division, Upper Bones ØP8
Osteolysis
　see Release, Head and Facial Bones ØNN
　see Release, Lower Bones ØQN
　see Release, Upper Bones ØPN
Osteopathic Treatment
　Abdomen 7WØ9X
　Cervical 7WØ1X
　Extremity
　　Lower 7WØ6X
　　Upper 7WØ7X
　Head 7WØØX
　Lumbar 7WØ3X
　Pelvis 7WØ5X
　Rib Cage 7WØ8X
　Sacrum 7WØ4X
　Thoracic 7WØ2X
Osteopexy
　see Repair, Head and Facial Bones ØNQ
　see Repair, Lower Bones ØQQ
　see Repair, Upper Bones ØPQ
　see Reposition, Head and Facial Bones ØNS
　see Reposition, Lower Bones ØQS
　see Reposition, Upper Bones ØPS
Osteoplasty
　see Repair, Head and Facial Bones ØNQ
　see Repair, Lower Bones ØQQ
　see Repair, Upper Bones ØPQ
　see Replacement, Head and Facial Bones ØNR
　see Replacement, Lower Bones ØQR
　see Replacement, Upper Bones ØPR
　see Supplement, Head and Facial Bones ØNU
　see Supplement, Lower Bones ØQU
　see Supplement, Upper Bones ØPU
Osteorrhaphy
　see Repair, Head and Facial Bones ØNQ
　see Repair, Lower Bones ØQQ
　see Repair, Upper Bones ØPQ
Osteotomy, ostotomy
　see Division, Head and Facial Bones ØN8
　see Division, Lower Bones ØQ8
　see Division, Upper Bones ØP8
　see Drainage, Head and Facial Bones ØN9
　see Drainage, Lower Bones ØQ9
　see Drainage, Upper Bones ØP9
Other Imaging
　Bile Duct and Gallbladder, Indocyanine Green Dye, Intraoperative BF53200
　Bile Duct, Indocyanine Green Dye, Intraoperative BF50200
　Extremity
　　Lower BW5CZ1Z
　　Upper BW5JZ1Z
　Gallbladder and Bile Duct, Indocyanine Green Dye, Intraoperative BF53200
　Gallbladder, Indocyanine Green Dye, Intraoperative BF52200
　Head and Neck BW59Z1Z
　Hepatobiliary System, All, Indocyanine Green Dye, Intraoperative BF5C200
　Liver and Spleen, Indocyanine Green Dye, Intraoperative BF56200
　Liver, Indocyanine Green Dye, Intraoperative BF55200
　Neck and Head BW59Z1Z
　Pancreas, Indocyanine Green Dye, Intraoperative BF57200
　Spleen and Liver, Indocyanine Green Dye, Intraoperative BF56200
　Trunk BW52Z1Z
Other New Technology Monoclonal Antibody XWØ
Other New Technology Therapeutic Substance XWØ
Otic ganglion use Head and Neck Sympathetic Nerve
OTL-101 use Hematopoietic Stem/Progenitor Cells, Genetically Modified
OTL-103 use Hematopoietic Stem/Progenitor Cells, Genetically Modified
OTL-200 use Hematopoietic Stem/Progenitor Cells, Genetically Modified
Otoplasty
　see Repair, Ear, Nose, Sinus Ø9Q
　see Replacement, Ear, Nose, Sinus Ø9R
　see Supplement, Ear, Nose, Sinus Ø9U
Otoscopy see Inspection, Ear, Nose, Sinus Ø9J

Oval window
　use Middle Ear, Left
　use Middle Ear, Right
Ovarian artery use Abdominal Aorta
Ovarian ligament use Uterine Supporting Structure
Ovariectomy
　see Excision, Female Reproductive System ØUB
　see Resection, Female Reproductive System ØUT
Ovariocentesis see Drainage, Female Reproductive System ØU9
Ovariopexy
　see Repair, Female Reproductive System ØUQ
　see Reposition, Female Reproductive System ØUS
Ovariotomy
　see Division, Female Reproductive System ØU8
　see Drainage, Female Reproductive System ØU9
Ovatio™ CRT-D use Cardiac Resynchronization Defibrillator Pulse Generator in ØJH
Oversewing
　Gastrointestinal ulcer see Repair, Gastrointestinal System ØDQ
　Pleural bleb see Repair, Respiratory System ØBQ
Oviduct
　use Fallopian Tube, Left
　use Fallopian Tube, Right
Oximetry, Fetal pulse 10H073Z
OXINIUM use Synthetic Substitute, Oxidized Zirconium on Polyethylene in ØSR
Oxygen Saturation Endoscopic Imaging (OXEI) XD2
Oxygenation
　Extracorporeal membrane (ECMO) see Performance, Circulatory 5A15
　Hyperbaric see Assistance, Circulatory 5A05
　Supersaturated see Assistance, Circulatory 5A05

P

Pacemaker
　Dual Chamber
　　Abdomen ØJH8
　　Chest ØJH6
　Intracardiac
　　Insertion of device in
　　　Atrium
　　　　Left Ø2H7
　　　　Right Ø2H6
　　　Vein, Coronary Ø2H4
　　　Ventricle
　　　　Left Ø2HL
　　　　Right Ø2HK
　　Removal of device from, Heart Ø2PA
　　Revision of device in, Heart Ø2WA
　Single Chamber
　　Abdomen ØJH8
　　Chest ØJH6
　Single Chamber Rate Responsive
　　Abdomen ØJH8
　　Chest ØJH6
Packing
　Abdominal Wall 2W43X5Z
　Anorectal 2Y43X5Z
　Arm
　　Lower
　　　Left 2W4DX5Z
　　　Right 2W4CX5Z
　　Upper
　　　Left 2W4BX5Z
　　　Right 2W4AX5Z
　Back 2W45X5Z
　Chest Wall 2W44X5Z
　Ear 2Y42X5Z
　Extremity
　　Lower
　　　Left 2W4MX5Z
　　　Right 2W4LX5Z
　　Upper
　　　Left 2W49X5Z
　　　Right 2W48X5Z
　Face 2W41X5Z
　Finger
　　Left 2W4KX5Z
　　Right 2W4JX5Z
　Foot
　　Left 2W4TX5Z
　　Right 2W4SX5Z
　Genital Tract, Female 2Y44X5Z

acking — *continued*
Hand
Left 2W4FX5Z
Right 2W4EX5Z
Head 2W40X5Z
Inguinal Region
Left 2W47X5Z
Right 2W46X5Z
Leg
Lower
Left 2W4RX5Z
Right 2W4QX5Z
Upper
Left 2W4PX5Z
Right 2W4NX5Z
Mouth and Pharynx 2Y40X5Z
Nasal 2Y41X5Z
Neck 2W42X5Z
Thumb
Left 2W4HX5Z
Right 2W4GX5Z
Toe
Left 2W4VX5Z
Right 2W4UX5Z
Urethra 2Y45X5Z
aclitaxel-eluting coronary stent *use* Intraluminal
Device, Drug-eluting in Heart and Great Vessels
aclitaxel-eluting peripheral stent
use Intraluminal Device, Drug-eluting in Lower
Arteries
use Intraluminal Device, Drug-eluting in Upper
Arteries
alatine gland *use* Buccal Mucosa
alatine tonsil *use* Tonsils
alatine uvula *use* Uvula
alatoglossal muscle *use* Tongue, Palate, Pharynx
Muscle
alatopharyngeal muscle *use* Tongue, Palate, Pharynx Muscle
alatoplasty
see Repair, Mouth and Throat 0CQ
see Replacement, Mouth and Throat 0CR
see Supplement, Mouth and Throat 0CU
alatorrhaphy *see* Repair, Mouth and Throat 0CQ
Imar cutaneous nerve
use Median Nerve
use Radial Nerve
Imar (volar) digital vein
use Hand Vein, Left
use Hand Vein, Right
Imar fascia (aponeurosis)
use Subcutaneous Tissue and Fascia, Left Hand
use Subcutaneous Tissue and Fascia, Right Hand
Imar interosseous muscle
use Hand Muscle, Left
use Hand Muscle, Right
Imar (volar) metacarpal vein
use Hand Vein, Left
use Hand Vein, Right
Imar ulnocarpal ligament
use Wrist Bursa and Ligament, Left
use Wrist Bursa and Ligament, Right
maris longus muscle
use Lower Arm and Wrist Muscle, Left
use Lower Arm and Wrist Muscle, Right
ancreatectomy
see Excision, Pancreas 0FBG
see Resection, Pancreas 0FTG
ancreatic artery *use* Splenic Artery
ancreatic plexus *use* Abdominal Sympathetic Nerve
ancreatic vein *use* Splenic Vein
ancreaticoduodenostomy *see* Bypass, Hepatobiliary
System and Pancreas 0F1
ancreaticosplenic lymph node *use* Lymphatic,
Aortic
ancreatogram, endoscopic retrograde *see* Fluoroscopy, Pancreatic Duct BF18
ancreatolithotomy *see* Extirpation, Pancreas 0FCG
ancreatotomy
ee Division, Pancreas 0F8G
ee Drawage, Pancreas 0F9G
aniculectomy
ee Excision, Skin, Abdomen 0HB7
ee Excision, Subcutaneous Tissue and Fascia, Abdomen 0JB8
araaortic lymph node *use* Lymphatic, Aortic

Paracentesis
Eye *see* Drainage, Eye 089
Peritoneal Cavity *see* Drainage, Peritoneal Cavity
0W9G
Tympanum *see* Drainage, Ear, Nose, Sinus 099
Parapharyngeal space *use* Neck
Pararectal lymph node *use* Lymphatic, Mesenteric
Parasternal lymph node *use* Lymphatic, Thorax
Parathyroidectomy
see Excision, Endocrine System 0GB
see Resection, Endocrine System 0GT
Paratracheal lymph node *use* Lymphatic, Thorax
Paraurethral (Skene's) gland *use* Vestibular Gland
Parenteral nutrition, total *see* Introduction of Nutritional Substance
Parietal lobe *use* Cerebral Hemisphere
Parotid lymph node *use* Lymphatic, Head
Parotid plexus *use* Facial Nerve
Parotidectomy
see Excision, Mouth and Throat 0CB
see Resection, Mouth and Throat 0CT
Pars flaccida
use Tympanic Membrane, Left
use Tympanic Membrane, Right
Partial joint replacement
Hip *see* Replacement, Lower Joints 0SR
Knee *see* Replacement, Lower Joints 0SR
Shoulder *see* Replacement, Upper Joints 0RR
Partially absorbable mesh *use* Synthetic Substitute
Patch, blood, spinal 3E0R3GC
Patellapexy
see Repair, Lower Bones 0QQ
see Reposition, Lower Bones 0QS
Patellaplasty
see Repair, Lower Bones 0QQ
see Replacement, Lower Bones 0QR
see Supplement, Lower Bones 0QU
Patellar ligament
use Knee Bursa and Ligament, Left
use Knee Bursa and Ligament, Right
Patellar tendon
use Knee Tendon, Left
use Knee Tendon, Right
Patellectomy
see Excision, Lower Bones 0QB
see Resection, Lower Bones 0QT
Patellofemoral joint
use Knee Joint, Left
use Knee Joint, Left, Femoral Surface
use Knee Joint, Right
use Knee Joint, Right, Femoral Surface
**pAVF (percutaneous arteriovenous fistula), using
magnetic-guided radiofrequency** *see* Bypass,
Upper Arteries 031
**pAVF (percutaneous arteriovenous fistula), using
thermal resistance energy** *see* New Technology, Cardiovascular System X2K
Pectineus muscle
use Upper Leg Muscle, Left
use Upper Leg Muscle, Right
Pectoral fascia *use* Subcutaneous Tissue and Fascia,
Chest
Pectoral (anterior) lymph node
use Lymphatic Left, Axillary
use Lymphatic Right, Axillary
Pectoralis major muscle
use Thorax Muscle, Left
use Thorax Muscle, Right
Pectoralis minor muscle
use Thorax Muscle, Left
use Thorax Muscle, Right
Pedicle-based dynamic stabilization device
use Spinal Stabilization Device, Pedicle-Based in
0SH
use Spinal Stabilization Device, Pedicle-Based in
0RH
PEEP (positive end expiratory pressure) *see* Assistance, Respiratory 5A09
PEG (percutaneous endoscopic gastrostomy)
0DH63UZ
PEJ (percutaneous endoscopic jejunostomy)
0DHA3UZ
Pelvic splanchnic nerve
use Abdominal Sympathetic Nerve
use Sacral Sympathetic Nerve

Penectomy
see Excision, Male Reproductive System 0VB
see Resection, Male Reproductive System 0VT
Penile urethra *use* Urethra
Penumbra Indigo® Aspiration System *see* New
Technology, Cardiovascular System X2C
PERCEPT™ PC neurostimulator *use* Stimulator Generator, Multiple Array in 0JH
Perceval sutureless valve *use* Zooplastic Tissue, Rapid
Deployment Technique in New Technology
**Percutaneous endoscopic gastrojejunostomy
(PEG/J) tube** *use* Feeding Device in Gastrointestinal System
Percutaneous endoscopic gastrostomy (PEG) tube
use Feeding Device in Gastrointestinal System
Percutaneous nephrostomy catheter *use* Drainage
Device
**Percutaneous transluminal coronary angioplasty
(PTCA)** *see* Dilation, Heart and Great Vessels 027
Performance
Biliary
Multiple, Filtration 5A1C60Z
Single, Filtration 5A1C00Z
Cardiac
Continuous
Output 5A1221Z
Pacing 5A1223Z
Intermittent, Pacing 5A1213Z
Single, Output, Manual 5A12012
Circulatory
Continuous
Central Membrane 5A1522F
Peripheral Veno-arterial Membrane
5A1522G
Peripheral Veno-venous Membrane
5A1522H
Intraoperative
Central Membrane 5A15A2F
Peripheral Veno-arterial Membrane
5A15A2G
Peripheral Veno-venous Membrane
5A15A2H
Respiratory
24-96 Consecutive Hours, Ventilation
5A1945Z
Greater than 96 Consecutive Hours, Ventilation 5A1955Z
Less than 24 Consecutive Hours, Ventilation
5A1935Z
Single, Ventilation, Nonmechanical 5A19054
Urinary
Continuous, Greater than 18 hours per day,
Filtration 5A1D90Z
Intermittent, Less than 6 Hours Per Day, Filtration 5A1D70Z
Prolonged Intermittent, 6-18 hours per day,
Filtration 5A1D80Z
Perfusion *see* Introduction of substance in or on
Perfusion, donor organ
Heart 6AB50BZ
Kidney(s) 6ABT0BZ
Liver 6ABF0BZ
Lung(s) 6ABB0BZ
Pericardiectomy
see Excision, Pericardium 02BN
see Resection, Pericardium 02TN
Pericardiocentesis *see* Drainage, Pericardial Cavity
0W9D
Pericardiolysis *see* Release, Pericardium 02NN
Pericardiophrenic artery
use Internal Mammary Artery, Left
use Internal Mammary Artery, Right
Pericardioplasty
see Repair, Pericardium 02QN
see Replacement, Pericardium 02RN
see Supplement, Pericardium 02UN
Pericardiorrhaphy *see* Repair, Pericardium 02QN
Pericardiostomy *see* Drainage, Pericardial Cavity 0W9D
Pericardiotomy *see* Drainage, Pericardial Cavity 0W9D
Perimetrium *use* Uterus
**Peripheral Intravascular Lithotripsy (Peripheral
IVL)** *see* Fragmentation
Peripheral parenteral nutrition *see* Introduction of
Nutritional Substance
Peripherally inserted central catheter (PICC) *use*
Infusion Device
Peritoneal dialysis 3E1M39Z

Peritoneocentesis
 see Drainage, Peritoneal Cavity 0W9G
 see Drainage, Peritoneum 0D9W
Peritoneoplasty
 see Repair, Peritoneum 0DQW
 see Replacement, Peritoneum 0DRW
 see Supplement, Peritoneum 0DUW
Peritoneoscopy 0DJW4ZZ
Peritoneotomy *see* Drainage, Peritoneum 0D9W
Peritoneumectomy *see* Excision, Peritoneum 0DBW
Peroneus brevis muscle
 use Lower Leg Muscle, Left
 use Lower Leg Muscle, Right
Peroneus longus muscle
 use Lower Leg Muscle, Left
 use Lower Leg Muscle, Right
Pessary ring *use* Intraluminal Device, Pessary in Female
 Reproductive System
PET scan *see* Positron Emission Tomographic (PET)
 Imaging
Petrous part of temoporal bone
 use Temporal Bone, Left
 use Temporal Bone, Right
Phacoemulsification, lens
 With IOL implant *see* Replacement, Eye 08R
 Without IOL implant *see* Extraction, Eye 08D
Phagenyx® System XWHD7Q7
Phalangectomy
 see Excision, Lower Bones 0QB
 see Excision, Upper Bones 0PB
 see Resection, Lower Bones 0QT
 see Resection, Upper Bones 0PT
Phallectomy
 see Excision, Penis 0VBS
 see Resection, Penis 0VTS
Phalloplasty
 see Repair, Penis 0VQS
 see Supplement, Penis 0VUS
Phallotomy *see* Drainage, Penis 0V9S
Pharmacotherapy, for substance abuse
 Antabuse HZ93ZZZ
 Bupropion HZ97ZZZ
 Clonidine HZ96ZZZ
 Levo-alpha-acetyl-methadol (LAAM) HZ92ZZZ
 Methadone Maintenance HZ91ZZZ
 Naloxone HZ95ZZZ
 Naltrexone HZ94ZZZ
 Nicotine Replacement HZ90ZZZ
 Psychiatric Medication HZ98ZZZ
 Replacement Medication, Other HZ99ZZZ
Pharyngeal constrictor muscle *use* Tongue, Palate,
 Pharynx Muscle
Pharyngeal plexus *use* Vagus Nerve
Pharyngeal recess *use* Nasopharynx
Pharyngeal tonsil *use* Adenoids
Pharyngogram *see* Fluoroscopy, Pharynix B91G
Pharyngoplasty
 see Repair, Mouth and Throat 0CQ
 see Replacement, Mouth and Throat 0CR
 see Supplement, Mouth and Throat 0CU
Pharyngorrhaphy *see* Repair, Mouth and Throat 0CQ
Pharyngotomy *see* Drainage, Mouth and Throat 0C9
Pharyngotympanic tube
 use Eustachian Tube, Left
 use Eustachian Tube, Right
Pheresis
 Erythrocytes 6A55
 Leukocytes 6A55
 Plasma 6A55
 Platelets 6A55
 Stem Cells
 Cord Blood 6A55
 Hematopoietic 6A55
Phlebectomy
 see Excision, Lower Veins 06B
 see Excision, Upper Veins 05B
 see Extraction, Lower Veins 06D
 see Extraction, Upper Veins 05D
Phlebography
 see Plain Radiography, Veins B50
 Impedance 4A04X51
Phleborrhaphy
 see Repair, Lower Veins 06Q
 see Repair, Upper Veins 05Q
Phlebotomy
 see Drainage, Lower Veins 069
 see Drainage, Upper Veins 059

Photocoagulation
 For Destruction *see* Destruction
 For Repair *see* Repair
Photopheresis, therapeutic *see* Phototherapy, Circu-
 latory 6A65
Phototherapy
 Circulatory 6A65
 Skin 6A60
 Ultraviolet light *see* Ultraviolet Light Therapy,
 Physiological Systems 6A8
Phrenectomy, phrenoneurectomy *see* Excision,
 Nerve, Phrenic 01B2
Phrenemphraxis *see* Destruction, Nerve, Phrenic 0152
Phrenic nerve stimulator generator *use* Stimulator
 Generator in Subcutaneous Tissue and Fascia
Phrenic nerve stimulator lead *use* Diaphragmatic
 Pacemaker Lead in Respiratory System
Phreniclasis *see* Destruction, Nerve, Phrenic 0152
Phrenicoexeresis *see* Extraction, Nerve, Phrenic 01D2
Phrenicotomy *see* Division, Nerve, Phrenic 0182
Phrenicotripsy *see* Destruction, Nerve, Phrenic 0152
Phrenoplasty
 see Repair, Respiratory System 0BQ
 see Supplement, Respiratory System 0BU
Phrenotomy *see* Drainage, Respiratory System 0B9
Physiatry *see* Motor Treatment, Rehabilitation F07
Physical medicine *see* Motor Treatment, Rehabilitation
 F07
Physical therapy *see* Motor Treatment, Rehabilitation
 F07
PHYSIOMESH™ Flexible Composite Mesh *use* Syn-
 thetic Substitute
Pia mater, intracranial *use* Cerebral Meninges
Pia mater, spinal *use* Spinal Meninges
Pinealectomy
 see Excision, Pineal Body 0GB1
 see Resection, Pineal Body 0GT1
Pinealoscopy 0GJ14ZZ
Pinealotomy *see* Drainage, Pineal Body 0G91
Pinna
 use External Ear, Bilateral
 use External Ear, Left
 use External Ear, Right
Pipeline™ (Flex) embolization device *use* Intraluminal Device, Flow Diverter in 03V
Piriform recess (sinus) *use* Pharynx
Piriformis muscle
 use Hip Muscle, Left
 use Hip Muscle, Right
**PIRRT (Prolonged intermittent renal replacement
 therapy)** 5A1D80Z
Pisiform bone
 use Carpal, Left
 use Carpal, Right
Pisohamate ligament
 use Hand Bursa and Ligament, Left
 use Hand Bursa and Ligament, Right
Pisometacarpal ligament
 use Hand Bursa and Ligament, Left
 use Hand Bursa and Ligament, Right
Pituitectomy
 see Excision, Gland, Pituitary 0GB0
 see Resection, Gland, Pituitary 0GT0
Plain film radiology *see* Plain Radiography
Plain Radiography
 Abdomen BW00ZZZ
 Abdomen and Pelvis BW01ZZZ
 Abdominal Lymphatic
 Bilateral B701
 Unilateral B700
 Airway, Upper BB0DZZZ
 Ankle
 Left BQ0H
 Right BQ0G
 Aorta
 Abdominal B400
 Thoracic B300
 Thoraco-Abdominal B30P
 Aorta and Bilateral Lower Extremity Arteries B40D
 Arch
 Bilateral BN0DZZZ
 Left BN0CZZZ
 Right BN0BZZZ
 Arm
 Left BP0FZZZ
 Right BP0EZZZ

Plain Radiography — *continued*
 Artery
 Brachiocephalic-Subclavian, Right B301
 Bronchial B30L
 Bypass Graft, Other B20F
 Cervico-Cerebral Arch B30Q
 Common Carotid
 Bilateral B305
 Left B304
 Right B303
 Coronary
 Bypass Graft
 Multiple B203
 Single B202
 Multiple B201
 Single B200
 External Carotid
 Bilateral B30C
 Left B30B
 Right B309
 Hepatic B402
 Inferior Mesenteric B405
 Intercostal B30L
 Internal Carotid
 Bilateral B308
 Left B307
 Right B306
 Internal Mammary Bypass Graft
 Left B208
 Right B207
 Intra-Abdominal, Other B40B
 Intracranial B30R
 Lower Extremity
 Bilateral and Aorta B40D
 Left B40G
 Right B40F
 Lower, Other B40J
 Lumbar B409
 Pelvic B40C
 Pulmonary
 Left B30T
 Right B30S
 Renal
 Bilateral B408
 Left B407
 Right B406
 Transplant B40M
 Spinal B30M
 Splenic B403
 Subclavian, Left B302
 Superior Mesenteric B404
 Upper Extremity
 Bilateral B30K
 Left B30J
 Right B30H
 Upper, Other B30N
 Vertebral
 Bilateral B30G
 Left B30F
 Right B30D
 Bile Duct BF00
 Bile Duct and Gallbladder BF03
 Bladder BT00
 Kidney and Ureter BT04
 Bladder and Urethra BT0B
 Bone
 Facial BN05ZZZ
 Nasal BN04ZZZ
 Bones, Long, All BW0BZZZ
 Breast
 Bilateral BH02ZZZ
 Left BH01ZZZ
 Right BH00ZZZ
 Calcaneus
 Left BQ0KZZZ
 Right BQ0JZZZ
 Chest BW03ZZZ
 Clavicle
 Left BP05ZZZ
 Right BP04ZZZ
 Coccyx BR0FZZZ
 Corpora Cavernosa BV00
 Dialysis Fistula B50W
 Dialysis Shunt B50W
 Disc
 Cervical BR01
 Lumbar BR03
 Thoracic BR02

▽ **Subterms under main terms may continue to next column or p**

lain Radiography — *continued*
Duct
  Lacrimal
    Bilateral B8Ø2
    Left B8Ø1
    Right B8ØØ
  Mammary
    Multiple
      Left BHØ6
      Right BHØ5
    Single
      Left BHØ4
      Right BHØ3
Elbow
  Left BPØH
  Right BPØG
Epididymis
  Left BVØ2
  Right BVØ1
Extremity
  Lower BWØCZZZ
  Upper BWØJZZZ
Eye
  Bilateral B8Ø7ZZZ
  Left B8Ø6ZZZ
  Right B8Ø5ZZZ
Facet Joint
  Cervical BRØ4
  Lumbar BRØ6
  Thoracic BRØ5
Fallopian Tube
  Bilateral BUØ2
  Left BUØ1
  Right BUØØ
Fallopian Tube and Uterus BUØ8
Femur
  Left, Densitometry BQØ4ZZ1
  Right, Densitometry BQØ3ZZ1
Finger
  Left BPØSZZZ
  Right BPØRZZZ
Foot
  Left BQØMZZZ
  Right BQØLZZZ
Forearm
  Left BPØKZZZ
  Right BPØJZZZ
Gallbladder and Bile Duct BFØ3
Gland
  Parotid
    Bilateral B9Ø6
    Left B9Ø5
    Right B9Ø4
  Salivary
    Bilateral B9ØD
    Left B9ØC
    Right B9ØB
  Submandibular
    Bilateral B9Ø9
    Left B9Ø8
    Right B9Ø7
Hand
  Left BPØPZZZ
  Right BPØNZZZ
Heart
  Left B2Ø5
  Right B2Ø4
  Right and Left B2Ø6
Hepatobiliary System, All BFØC
Hip
  Left BQØ1
    Densitometry BQØ1ZZ1
  Right BQØØ
    Densitometry BQØØZZ1
Humerus
  Left BPØBZZZ
  Right BPØAZZZ
Ileal Diversion Loop BTØC
Intracranial Sinus B5Ø2
Joint
  Acromioclavicular, Bilateral BPØ3ZZZ
  Finger
    Left BPØD
    Right BPØC
  Foot
    Left BQØY
    Right BQØX
  Hand
    Left BPØD

Plain Radiography — *continued*
Joint — *continued*
  Hand — *continued*
    Right BPØC
  Lumbosacral BRØBZZZ
  Sacroiliac BRØD
  Sternoclavicular
    Bilateral BPØ2ZZZ
    Left BPØ1ZZZ
    Right BPØØZZZ
  Temporomandibular
    Bilateral BNØ9
    Left BNØ8
    Right BNØ7
  Thoracolumbar BRØ8ZZZ
  Toe
    Left BQØY
    Right BQØX
Kidney
  Bilateral BTØ3
  Left BTØ2
  Right BTØ1
  Ureter and Bladder BTØ4
Knee
  Left BQØ8
  Right BQØ7
Leg
  Left BQØFZZZ
  Right BQØDZZZ
Lymphatic
  Head B7Ø4
  Lower Extremity
    Bilateral B7ØB
    Left B7Ø9
    Right B7Ø8
  Neck B7Ø4
  Pelvic B7ØC
  Upper Extremity
    Bilateral B7Ø7
    Left B7Ø6
    Right B7Ø5
Mandible BNØ6ZZZ
Mastoid B9ØHZZZ
Nasopharynx B9ØF7ZZ
Optic Foramina
  Left B8Ø4ZZZ
  Right B8Ø3ZZZ
Orbit
  Bilateral BNØ3ZZZ
  Left BNØ2ZZZ
  Right BNØ1ZZZ
Oropharynx B9ØFZZZ
Patella
  Left BQØWZZZ
  Right BQØVZZZ
Pelvis BRØCZZZ
Pelvis and Abdomen BWØ1ZZZ
Prostate BVØ3
Retroperitoneal Lymphatic
  Bilateral B7Ø1
  Unilateral B7ØØ
Ribs
  Left BPØYZZZ
  Right BPØXZZZ
Sacrum BRØFZZZ
Scapula
  Left BPØ7ZZZ
  Right BPØ6ZZZ
Shoulder
  Left BPØ9
  Right BPØ8
Sinus
  Intracranial B5Ø2
  Paranasal B9Ø2ZZZ
Skull BNØØZZZ
Spinal Cord BØØB
Spine
  Cervical, Densitometry BRØØZZ1
  Lumbar, Densitometry BRØ9ZZ1
  Thoracic, Densitometry BRØ7ZZ1
  Whole, Densitometry BRØGZZ1
Sternum BRØHZZZ
Teeth
  All BNØJZZZ
  Multiple BNØHZZZ
Testicle
  Left BVØ6
  Right BVØ5

Plain Radiography — *continued*
Toe
  Left BQØQZZZ
  Right BQØPZZZ
Tooth, Single BNØGZZZ
Tracheobronchial Tree
  Bilateral BBØ9YZZ
  Left BBØ8YZZ
  Right BBØ7YZZ
Ureter
  Bilateral BTØ8
  Kidney and Bladder BTØ4
  Left BTØ7
  Right BTØ6
Urethra BTØ5
Urethra and Bladder BTØB
Uterus BUØ6
Uterus and Fallopian Tube BUØ8
Vagina BUØ9
Vasa Vasorum BVØ8
Vein
  Cerebellar B5Ø1
  Cerebral B5Ø1
  Epidural B5ØØ
  Jugular
    Bilateral B5Ø5
    Left B5Ø4
    Right B5Ø3
  Lower Extremity
    Bilateral B5ØD
    Left B5ØC
    Right B5ØB
  Other B5ØV
  Pelvic (Iliac)
    Left B5ØG
    Right B5ØF
  Pelvic (Iliac) Bilateral B5ØH
  Portal B5ØT
  Pulmonary
    Bilateral B5ØS
    Left B5ØR
    Right B5ØQ
  Renal
    Bilateral B5ØL
    Left B5ØK
    Right B5ØJ
  Spanchnic B5ØT
  Subclavian
    Left B5Ø7
    Right B5Ø6
  Upper Extremity
    Bilateral B5ØP
    Left B5ØN
    Right B5ØM
Vena Cava
  Inferior B5Ø9
  Superior B5Ø8
Whole Body BWØKZZZ
  Infant BWØMZZZ
Whole Skeleton BWØLZZZ
Wrist
  Left BPØM
  Right BPØL

Planar Nuclear Medicine Imaging
Abdomen CW1Ø
Abdomen and Chest CW14
Abdomen and Pelvis CW11
Anatomical Region, Other CW1ZZZZ
Anatomical Regions, Multiple CW1YYZZ
Bladder and Ureters CT1H
Bladder, Kidneys and Ureters CT13
Blood C713
Bone Marrow C71Ø
Brain CØ1Ø
Breast CH1YYZZ
  Bilateral CH12
  Left CH11
  Right CH1Ø
Bronchi and Lungs CB12
Central Nervous System CØ1YYZZ
Cerebrospinal Fluid CØ15
Chest CW13
Chest and Abdomen CW14
Chest and Neck CW16
Digestive System CD1YYZZ
Ducts, Lacrimal, Bilateral C819
Ear, Nose, Mouth and Throat C91YYZZ
Endocrine System CG1YYZZ

Planar Nuclear Medicine Imaging — *continued*
Extremity
  Lower CW1D
    Bilateral CP1F
    Left CP1D
    Right CP1C
  Upper CW1M
    Bilateral CP1B
    Left CP19
    Right CP18
Eye C81YYZZ
Gallbladder CF14
Gastrointestinal Tract CD17
  Upper CD15
Gland
  Adrenal, Bilateral CG14
  Parathyroid CG11
  Thyroid CG12
Glands, Salivary, Bilateral C91B
Head and Neck CW1B
Heart C21YYZZ
  Right and Left C216
Hepatobiliary System, All CF1C
Hepatobiliary System and Pancreas CF1YYZZ
Kidneys, Ureters and Bladder CT13
Liver CF15
Liver and Spleen CF16
Lungs and Bronchi CB12
Lymphatics
  Head C71J
  Head and Neck C715
  Lower Extremity C71P
  Neck C71K
  Pelvic C71D
  Trunk C71M
  Upper Chest C71L
  Upper Extremity C71N
Lymphatics and Hematologic System C71YYZZ
Musculoskeletal System
  All CP1Z
  Other CP1YYZZ
Myocardium C21G
Neck and Chest CW16
Neck and Head CW1B
Pancreas and Hepatobiliary System CF1YYZZ
Pelvic Region CW1J
Pelvis CP16
Pelvis and Abdomen CW11
Pelvis and Spine CP17
Reproductive System, Male CV1YYZZ
Respiratory System CB1YYZZ
Skin CH1YYZZ
Skull CP11
Spine CP15
Spine and Pelvis CP17
Spleen C712
Spleen and Liver CF16
Subcutaneous Tissue CH1YYZZ
Testicles, Bilateral CV19
Thorax CP14
Ureters and Bladder CT1H
Ureters, Kidneys and Bladder CT13
Urinary System CT1YYZZ
Veins C51YYZZ
  Central C51R
  Lower Extremity
    Bilateral C51D
    Left C51C
    Right C51B
  Upper Extremity
    Bilateral C51Q
    Left C51P
    Right C51N
Whole Body CW1N
Plantar digital vein
  use Foot Vein, Left
  use Foot Vein, Right
Plantar fascia (aponeurosis)
  use Subcutaneous Tissue and Fascia, Left Foot
  use Subcutaneous Tissue and Fascia, Right Foot
Plantar metatarsal vein
  use Foot Vein, Left
  use Foot Vein, Right
Plantar venous arch
  use Foot Vein, Left
  use Foot Vein, Right
Plaque Radiation
  Abdomen DWY3FZZ

Plaque Radiation — *continued*
Adrenal Gland DGY2FZZ
Anus DDY8FZZ
Bile Ducts DFY2FZZ
Bladder DTY2FZZ
Bone Marrow D7Y0FZZ
Bone, Other DPYCFZZ
Brain D0Y0FZZ
Brain Stem D0Y1FZZ
Breast
  Left DMY0FZZ
  Right DMY1FZZ
Bronchus DBY1FZZ
Cervix DUY1FZZ
Chest DWY2FZZ
Chest Wall DBY7FZZ
Colon DDY5FZZ
Diaphragm DBY8FZZ
Duodenum DDY2FZZ
Ear D9Y0FZZ
Esophagus DDY0FZZ
Eye D8Y0FZZ
Femur DPY9FZZ
Fibula DPYBFZZ
Gallbladder DFY1FZZ
Gland
  Adrenal DGY2FZZ
  Parathyroid DGY4FZZ
  Pituitary DGY0FZZ
  Thyroid DGY5FZZ
Glands, Salivary D9Y6FZZ
Head and Neck DWY1FZZ
Hemibody DWY4FZZ
Humerus DPY6FZZ
Ileum DDY4FZZ
Jejunum DDY3FZZ
Kidney DTY0FZZ
Larynx D9YBFZZ
Liver DFY0FZZ
Lung DBY2FZZ
Lymphatics
  Abdomen D7Y6FZZ
  Axillary D7Y4FZZ
  Inguinal D7Y8FZZ
  Neck D7Y3FZZ
  Pelvis D7Y7FZZ
  Thorax D7Y5FZZ
Mandible DPY3FZZ
Maxilla DPY2FZZ
Mediastinum DBY6FZZ
Mouth D9Y4FZZ
Nasopharynx D9YDFZZ
Neck and Head DWY1FZZ
Nerve, Peripheral D0Y7FZZ
Nose D9Y1FZZ
Ovary DUY0FZZ
Palate
  Hard D9Y8FZZ
  Soft D9Y9FZZ
Pancreas DFY3FZZ
Parathyroid Gland DGY4FZZ
Pelvic Bones DPY8FZZ
Pelvic Region DWY6FZZ
Pharynx D9YCFZZ
Pineal Body DGY1FZZ
Pituitary Gland DGY0FZZ
Pleura DBY5FZZ
Prostate DVY0FZZ
Radius DPY7FZZ
Rectum DDY7FZZ
Rib DPY5FZZ
Sinuses D9Y7FZZ
Skin
  Abdomen DHY8FZZ
  Arm DHY4FZZ
  Back DHY7FZZ
  Buttock DHY9FZZ
  Chest DHY6FZZ
  Face DHY2FZZ
  Foot DHYCFZZ
  Hand DHY5FZZ
  Leg DHYBFZZ
  Neck DHY3FZZ
Skull DPY0FZZ
Spinal Cord D0Y6FZZ
Spleen D7Y2FZZ
Sternum DPY4FZZ
Stomach DDY1FZZ
Testis DVY1FZZ

Plaque Radiation — *continued*
Thymus D7Y1FZZ
Thyroid Gland DGY5FZZ
Tibia DPYBFZZ
Tongue D9Y5FZZ
Trachea DBY0FZZ
Ulna DPY7FZZ
Ureter DTY1FZZ
Urethra DTY3FZZ
Uterus DUY2FZZ
Whole Body DWY5FZZ
Plasma, Convalescent (Nonautologous) XW1
Plasmapheresis, therapeutic *see* Pheresis, Physiological Systems 6A5
Plateletpheresis, therapeutic *see* Pheresis, Physiological Systems 6A5
Platysma muscle
  use Neck Muscle, Left
  use Neck Muscle, Right
Plazomicin Anti-infective XW0
Pleurectomy
  see Excision, Respiratory System 0BB
  see Resection, Respiratory System 0BT
Pleurocentesis *see* Drainage, Anatomical Regions, General 0W9
Pleurodesis, pleurosclerosis
  Chemical injection *see* Introduction of Substance in or on, Pleural Cavity 3E0L
  Surgical *see* Destruction, Respiratory System 0B5
Pleurolysis *see* Release, Respiratory System 0BN
Pleuroscopy 0BJQ4ZZ
Pleurotomy *see* Drainage, Respiratory System 0B9
Plica semilunaris
  use Conjunctiva, Left
  use Conjunctiva, Right
Plication *see* Restriction
Pneumectomy
  see Excision, Respiratory System 0BB
  see Resection, Respiratory System 0BT
Pneumocentesis *see* Drainage, Respiratory System 0B9
Pneumogastric nerve *use* Vagus Nerve
Pneumolysis *see* Release, Respiratory System 0BN
Pneumonectomy *see* Resection, Respiratory System 0BT
Pneumonolysis *see* Release, Respiratory System 0BN
Pneumonopexy
  see Repair, Respiratory System 0BQ
  see Reposition, Respiratory System 0BS
Pneumonorrhaphy *see* Repair, Respiratory System 0BQ
Pneumonotomy *see* Drainage, Respiratory System 0B
Pneumotaxic center *use* Pons
Pneumotomy *see* Drainage, Respiratory System 0B9
Pollicization *see* Transfer, Anatomical Regions, Upper Extremities 0XX
Polyclonal hyperimmune globulin *use* Globulin
Polyethylene socket *use* Synthetic Substitute, Polyethylene in 0SR
Polymethylmethacrylate (PMMA) *use* Synthetic Substitute
Polypectomy, gastrointestinal *see* Excision, Gastrointestinal System 0DB
Polypropylene mesh *use* Synthetic Substitute
Polysomnogram 4A1ZXQZ
Pontine tegmentum *use* Pons
Popliteal ligament
  use Knee Bursa and Ligament, Left
  use Knee Bursa and Ligament, Right
Popliteal lymph node
  use Lymphatic, Left Lower Extremity
  use Lymphatic, Right Lower Extremity
Popliteal vein
  use Femoral Vein, Left
  use Femoral Vein, Right
Popliteus muscle
  use Lower Leg Muscle, Left
  use Lower Leg Muscle, Right
Porcine (bioprosthetic) valve *use* Zooplastic Tissue in Heart and Great Vessels
Positive Blood Culture Fluorescence Hybridization for Organism Identification, Concentration and Susceptibility XXE5XN6
Positive end expiratory pressure *see* Performance, Respiratory 5A19
Positron Emission Tomographic (PET) Imaging
  Brain C030

⬇ Subterms under main terms may continue to next column or p

Pylorodiosis *see* Dilation, Stomach, Pylorus ØD77
Pylorogastrectomy
  see Excision, Gastrointestinal System ØDB
  see Resection, Gastrointestinal System ØDT
Pyloroplasty
  see Repair, Stomach, Pylorus ØDQ7
  see Supplement, Stomach, Pylorus ØDU7
Pyloroscopy ØDJ68ZZ
Pylorotomy *see* Drainage, Stomach, Pylorus ØD97
Pyramidalis muscle
  use Abdomen Muscle, Left
  use Abdomen Muscle, Right

Q

Quadrangular cartilage *use* Nasal Septum
Quadrant resection of breast *see* Excision, Skin and Breast ØHB
Quadrate lobe *use* Liver
Quadratus femoris muscle
  use Hip Muscle, Left
  use Hip Muscle, Right
Quadratus lumborum muscle
  use Trunk Muscle, Left
  use Trunk Muscle, Right
Quadratus plantae muscle
  use Foot Muscle, Left
  use Foot Muscle, Right
Quadriceps (femoris)
  use Upper Leg Muscle, Left
  use Upper Leg Muscle, Right
Quarantine 8EØZXY6

R

Radial artery arteriovenous fistula, using Thermal Resistance Energy X2K
Radial collateral carpal ligament
  use Wrist Bursa and Ligament, Left
  use Wrist Bursa and Ligament, Right
Radial collateral ligament
  use Elbow Bursa and Ligament, Left
  use Elbow Bursa and Ligament, Right
Radial notch
  use Ulna, Left
  use Ulna, Right
Radial recurrent artery
  use Radial Artery, Left
  use Radial Artery, Right
Radial vein
  use Brachial Vein, Left
  use Brachial Vein, Right
Radialis indicis
  use Hand Artery, Left
  use Hand Artery, Right
Radiation Therapy
  see Beam Radiation
  see Brachytherapy
  see Other Radiation
  see Stereotactic Radiosurgery
Radiation treatment *see* Radiation Therapy
Radiocarpal joint
  use Wrist Joint, Left
  use Wrist Joint, Right
Radiocarpal ligament
  use Wrist Bursa and Ligament, Left
  use Wrist Bursa and Ligament, Right
Radiography *see* Plain Radiography
Radiology, analog *see* Plain Radiography
Radiology, diagnostic *see* Imaging, Diagnostic
Radioulnar ligament
  use Wrist Bursa and Ligament, Left
  use Wrist Bursa and Ligament, Right
Range of motion testing *see* Motor Function Assessment, Rehabilitation FØ1
Rapid ASPECTS XXEØXØ7
REALIZE® Adjustable Gastric Band *use* Extraluminal Device
Reattachment
  Abdominal Wall ØWMFØZZ
  Ampulla of Vater ØFMC
  Ankle Region
    Left ØYMLØZZ
    Right ØYMKØZZ

Reattachment — *continued*
  Arm
    Lower
      Left ØXMFØZZ
      Right ØXMDØZZ
    Upper
      Left ØXM9ØZZ
      Right ØXM8ØZZ
  Axilla
    Left ØXM5ØZZ
    Right ØXM4ØZZ
  Back
    Lower ØWMLØZZ
    Upper ØWMKØZZ
  Bladder ØTMB
  Bladder Neck ØTMC
  Breast
    Bilateral ØHMVXZZ
    Left ØHMUXZZ
    Right ØHMTXZZ
  Bronchus
    Lingula ØBM9ØZZ
    Lower Lobe
      Left ØBMBØZZ
      Right ØBM6ØZZ
    Main
      Left ØBM7ØZZ
      Right ØBM3ØZZ
    Middle Lobe, Right ØBM5ØZZ
    Upper Lobe
      Left ØBM8ØZZ
      Right ØBM4ØZZ
  Bursa and Ligament
    Abdomen
      Left ØMMJ
      Right ØMMH
    Ankle
      Left ØMMR
      Right ØMMQ
    Elbow
      Left ØMM4
      Right ØMM3
    Foot
      Left ØMMT
      Right ØMMS
    Hand
      Left ØMM8
      Right ØMM7
    Head and Neck ØMMØ
    Hip
      Left ØMMM
      Right ØMML
    Knee
      Left ØMMP
      Right ØMMN
    Lower Extremity
      Left ØMMW
      Right ØMMV
    Perineum ØMMK
    Rib(s) ØMMG
    Shoulder
      Left ØMM2
      Right ØMM1
    Spine
      Lower ØMMD
      Upper ØMMC
    Sternum ØMMF
    Upper Extremity
      Left ØMMB
      Right ØMM9
    Wrist
      Left ØMM6
      Right ØMM5
  Buttock
    Left ØYM1ØZZ
    Right ØYMØØZZ
  Carina ØBM2ØZZ
  Cecum ØDMH
  Cervix ØUMC
  Chest Wall ØWM8ØZZ
  Clitoris ØUMJXZZ
  Colon
    Ascending ØDMK
    Descending ØDMM
    Sigmoid ØDMN
    Transverse ØDML
  Cord
    Bilateral ØVMH
    Left ØVMG

Reattachment — *continued*
  Cord — *continued*
    Right ØVMF
  Cul-de-sac ØUMF
  Diaphragm ØBMTØZZ
  Duct
    Common Bile ØFM9
    Cystic ØFM8
    Hepatic
      Common ØFM7
      Left ØFM6
      Right ØFM5
    Pancreatic ØFMD
      Accessory ØFMF
  Duodenum ØDM9
  Ear
    Left Ø9M1XZZ
    Right Ø9MØXZZ
  Elbow Region
    Left ØXMCØZZ
    Right ØXMBØZZ
  Esophagus ØDM5
  Extremity
    Lower
      Left ØYMBØZZ
      Right ØYM9ØZZ
    Upper
      Left ØXM7ØZZ
      Right ØXM6ØZZ
  Eyelid
    Lower
      Left Ø8MRXZZ
      Right Ø8MQXZZ
    Upper
      Left Ø8MPXZZ
      Right Ø8MNXZZ
  Face ØWM2ØZZ
  Fallopian Tube
    Left ØUM6
    Right ØUM5
  Fallopian Tubes, Bilateral ØUM7
  Femoral Region
    Left ØYM8ØZZ
    Right ØYM7ØZZ
  Finger
    Index
      Left ØXMPØZZ
      Right ØXMNØZZ
    Little
      Left ØXMWØZZ
      Right ØXMVØZZ
    Middle
      Left ØXMRØZZ
      Right ØXMQØZZ
    Ring
      Left ØXMTØZZ
      Right ØXMSØZZ
  Foot
    Left ØYMNØZZ
    Right ØYMMØZZ
  Forequarter
    Left ØXM1ØZZ
    Right ØXMØØZZ
  Gallbladder ØFM4
  Gland
    Left ØGM2
    Right ØGM3
  Hand
    Left ØXMKØZZ
    Right ØXMJØZZ
  Hindquarter
    Bilateral ØYM4ØZZ
    Left ØYM3ØZZ
    Right ØYM2ØZZ
  Hymen ØUMK
  Ileum ØDMB
  Inguinal Region
    Left ØYM6ØZZ
    Right ØYM5ØZZ
  Intestine
    Large ØDME
      Left ØDMG
      Right ØDMF
    Small ØDM8
  Jaw
    Lower ØWM5ØZZ
    Upper ØWM4ØZZ
  Jejunum ØDMA

▽ **Subterms under main terms may continue to next column or pa**

Reattachment — *continued*
  Kidney
    Left ØTM1
    Right ØTMØ
  Kidney Pelvis
    Left ØTM4
    Right ØTM3
  Kidneys, Bilateral ØTM2
  Knee Region
    Left ØYMGØZZ
    Right ØYMFØZZ
  Leg
    Lower
      Left ØYMJØZZ
      Right ØYMHØZZ
    Upper
      Left ØYMDØZZ
      Right ØYMCØZZ
  Lip
    Lower ØCM1ØZZ
    Upper ØCMØØZZ
  Liver ØFMØ
    Left Lobe ØFM2
    Right Lobe ØFM1
  Lung
    Left ØBMLØZZ
    Lower Lobe
      Left ØBMJØZZ
      Right ØBMFØZZ
    Middle Lobe, Right ØBMDØZZ
    Right ØBMKØZZ
    Upper Lobe
      Left ØBMGØZZ
      Right ØBMCØZZ
  Lung Lingula ØBMHØZZ
  Muscle
    Abdomen
      Left ØKML
      Right ØKMK
    Facial ØKM1
    Foot
      Left ØKMW
      Right ØKMV
    Hand
      Left ØKMD
      Right ØKMC
    Head ØKMØ
    Hip
      Left ØKMP
      Right ØKMN
    Lower Arm and Wrist
      Left ØKMB
      Right ØKM9
    Lower Leg
      Left ØKMT
      Right ØKMS
    Neck
      Left ØKM3
      Right ØKM2
    Perineum ØKMM
    Shoulder
      Left ØKM6
      Right ØKM5
    Thorax
      Left ØKMJ
      Right ØKMH
    Tongue, Palate, Pharynx ØKM4
    Trunk
      Left ØKMG
      Right ØKMF
    Upper Arm
      Left ØKM8
      Right ØKM7
    Upper Leg
      Left ØKMR
      Right ØKMQ
  Nasal Mucosa and Soft Tissue Ø9MKXZZ
  Neck ØWM6ØZZ
  Nipple
    Left ØHMXXZZ
    Right ØHMWXZZ
  Ovary
    Bilateral ØUM2
    Left ØUM1
    Right ØUMØ
  Palate, Soft ØCM3ØZZ
  Pancreas ØFMG
  Parathyroid Gland ØGMR

Reattachment — *continued*
  Parathyroid Gland — *continued*
    Inferior
      Left ØGMP
      Right ØGMN
    Multiple ØGMQ
    Superior
      Left ØGMM
      Right ØGML
  Penis ØVMSXZZ
  Perineum
    Female ØWMNØZZ
    Male ØWMMØZZ
  Rectum ØDMP
  Scrotum ØVM5XZZ
  Shoulder Region
    Left ØXM3ØZZ
    Right ØXM2ØZZ
  Skin
    Abdomen ØHM7XZZ
    Back ØHM6XZZ
    Buttock ØHM8XZZ
    Chest ØHM5XZZ
    Ear
      Left ØHM3XZZ
      Right ØHM2XZZ
    Face ØHM1XZZ
    Foot
      Left ØHMNXZZ
      Right ØHMMXZZ
    Hand
      Left ØHMGXZZ
      Right ØHMFXZZ
    Inguinal ØHMAXZZ
    Lower Arm
      Left ØHMEXZZ
      Right ØHMDXZZ
    Lower Leg
      Left ØHMLXZZ
      Right ØHMKXZZ
    Neck ØHM4XZZ
    Perineum ØHM9XZZ
    Scalp ØHMØXZZ
    Upper Arm
      Left ØHMCXZZ
      Right ØHMBXZZ
    Upper Leg
      Left ØHMJXZZ
      Right ØHMHXZZ
  Stomach ØDM6
  Tendon
    Abdomen
      Left ØLMG
      Right ØLMF
    Ankle
      Left ØLMT
      Right ØLMS
    Foot
      Left ØLMW
      Right ØLMV
    Hand
      Left ØLM8
      Right ØLM7
    Head and Neck ØLMØ
    Hip
      Left ØLMK
      Right ØLMJ
    Knee
      Left ØLMR
      Right ØLMQ
    Lower Arm and Wrist
      Left ØLM6
      Right ØLM5
    Lower Leg
      Left ØLMP
      Right ØLMN
    Perineum ØLMH
    Shoulder
      Left ØLM2
      Right ØLM1
    Thorax
      Left ØLMD
      Right ØLMC
    Trunk
      Left ØLMB
      Right ØLM9
    Upper Arm
      Left ØLM4
      Right ØLM3

Reattachment — *continued*
  Tendon — *continued*
    Upper Leg
      Left ØLMM
      Right ØLML
  Testis
    Bilateral ØVMC
    Left ØVMB
    Right ØVM9
  Thumb
    Left ØXMMØZZ
    Right ØXMLØZZ
  Thyroid Gland
    Left Lobe ØGMG
    Right Lobe ØGMH
  Toe
    1st
      Left ØYMQØZZ
      Right ØYMPØZZ
    2nd
      Left ØYMSØZZ
      Right ØYMRØZZ
    3rd
      Left ØYMUØZZ
      Right ØYMTØZZ
    4th
      Left ØYMWØZZ
      Right ØYMVØZZ
    5th
      Left ØYMYØZZ
      Right ØYMXØZZ
  Tongue ØCM7ØZZ
  Tooth
    Lower ØCMX
    Upper ØCMW
  Trachea ØBM1ØZZ
  Tunica Vaginalis
    Left ØVM7
    Right ØVM6
  Ureter
    Left ØTM7
    Right ØTM6
  Ureters, Bilateral ØTM8
  Urethra ØTMD
  Uterine Supporting Structure ØUM4
  Uterus ØUM9
  Uvula ØCMNØZZ
  Vagina ØUMG
  Vulva ØUMMXZZ
  Wrist Region
    Left ØXMHØZZ
    Right ØXMGØZZ

REBOA (resuscitative endovascular balloon occlusion of the aorta)
  Ø2LW3DJ
  Ø4LØ3DJ

Rebound HRD® (Hernia Repair Device) *use* Synthetic Substitute

RECELL® cell suspension autograft *see* Replacement, Skin and Breast ØHR

Recession
  see Repair
  see Reposition

Reclosure, disrupted abdominal wall ØWQFXZZ

Reconstruction
  see Repair
  see Replacement
  see Supplement

Rectectomy
  see Excision, Rectum ØDBP
  see Resection, Rectum ØDTP

Rectocele repair *see* Repair, Subcutaneous Tissue and Fascia, Pelvic Region ØJQC

Rectopexy
  see Repair, Gastrointestinal System ØDQ
  see Reposition, Gastrointestinal System ØDS

Rectoplasty
  see Repair, Gastrointestinal System ØDQ
  see Supplement, Gastrointestinal System ØDU

Rectorrhaphy *see* Repair, Gastrointestinal System ØDQ

Rectoscopy ØDJD8ZZ

Rectosigmoid junction *use* Sigmoid Colon

Rectosigmoidectomy
  see Excision, Gastrointestinal System ØDB
  see Resection, Gastrointestinal System ØDT

Rectostomy *see* Drainage, Rectum ØD9P

Rectotomy *see* Drainage, Rectum ØD9P

Rectus abdominis muscle
use Abdomen Muscle, Left
use Abdomen Muscle, Right
Rectus femoris muscle
use Upper Leg Muscle, Left
use Upper Leg Muscle, Right
Recurrent laryngeal nerve use Vagus Nerve
Reducer™ System use Reduction Device in New Technology
Reduction
Dislocation see Reposition
Fracture see Reposition
Intussusception, intestinal see Reposition, Gastrointestinal System ØDS
Mammoplasty see Excision, Skin and Breast ØHB
Prolapse see Reposition
Torsion see Reposition
Volvulus, gastrointestinal see Reposition, Gastrointestinal System ØDS
Reduction Device, Coronary Sinus X2V73Q7
Refusion see Fusion
REGN-COV2 Monoclonal Antibody XWØ
Rehabilitation
see Activities of Daily Living Assessment, Rehabilitation FØ2
see Activities of Daily Living Treatment, Rehabilitation FØ8
see Caregiver Training, Rehabilitation FØF
see Cochlear Implant Treatment, Rehabilitation FØB
see Device Fitting, Rehabilitation FØD
see Hearing Treatment, Rehabilitation FØ9
see Motor Function Assessment, Rehabilitation FØ1
see Motor Treatment, Rehabilitation FØ7
see Speech Assessment, Rehabilitation FØØ
see Speech Treatment, Rehabilitation FØ6
see Vestibular Treatment, Rehabilitation FØC
Reimplantation
see Reattachment
see Reposition
see Transfer
Reinforcement
see Repair
see Supplement
Relaxation, scar tissue see Release
Release
Acetabulum
Left ØQN5
Right ØQN4
Adenoids ØCNQ
Ampulla of Vater ØFNC
Anal Sphincter ØDNR
Anterior Chamber
Left Ø8N33ZZ
Right Ø8N23ZZ
Anus ØDNQ
Aorta
Abdominal Ø4NØ
Thoracic
Ascending/Arch Ø2NX
Descending Ø2NW
Aortic Body ØGND
Appendix ØDNJ
Artery
Anterior Tibial
Left Ø4NQ
Right Ø4NP
Axillary
Left Ø3N6
Right Ø3N5
Brachial
Left Ø3N8
Right Ø3N7
Celiac Ø4N1
Colic
Left Ø4N7
Middle Ø4N8
Right Ø4N6
Common Carotid
Left Ø3NJ
Right Ø3NH
Common Iliac
Left Ø4ND
Right Ø4NC
Coronary
Four or More Arteries Ø2N3

Release — continued
Artery — continued
Coronary — continued
One Artery Ø2NØ
Three Arteries Ø2N2
Two Arteries Ø2N1
External Carotid
Left Ø3NN
Right Ø3NM
External Iliac
Left Ø4NJ
Right Ø4NH
Face Ø3NR
Femoral
Left Ø4NL
Right Ø4NK
Foot
Left Ø4NW
Right Ø4NV
Gastric Ø4N2
Hand
Left Ø3NF
Right Ø3ND
Hepatic Ø4N3
Inferior Mesenteric Ø4NB
Innominate Ø3N2
Internal Carotid
Left Ø3NL
Right Ø3NK
Internal Iliac
Left Ø4NF
Right Ø4NE
Internal Mammary
Left Ø3N1
Right Ø3NØ
Intracranial Ø3NG
Lower Ø4NY
Peroneal
Left Ø4NU
Right Ø4NT
Popliteal
Left Ø4NN
Right Ø4NM
Posterior Tibial
Left Ø4NS
Right Ø4NR
Pulmonary
Left Ø2NR
Right Ø2NQ
Pulmonary Trunk Ø2NP
Radial
Left Ø3NC
Right Ø3NB
Renal
Left Ø4NA
Right Ø4N9
Splenic Ø4N4
Subclavian
Left Ø3N4
Right Ø3N3
Superior Mesenteric Ø4N5
Temporal
Left Ø3NT
Right Ø3NS
Thyroid
Left Ø3NV
Right Ø3NU
Ulnar
Left Ø3NA
Right Ø3N9
Upper Ø3NY
Vertebral
Left Ø3NQ
Right Ø3NP
Atrium
Left Ø2N7
Right Ø2N6
Auditory Ossicle
Left Ø9NA
Right Ø9N9
Basal Ganglia ØØN8
Bladder ØTNB
Bladder Neck ØTNC
Bone
Ethmoid
Left ØNNG
Right ØNNF
Frontal ØNN1
Hyoid ØNNX

Release — continued
Bone — continued
Lacrimal
Left ØNNJ
Right ØNNH
Nasal ØNNB
Occipital ØNN7
Palatine
Left ØNNL
Right ØNNK
Parietal
Left ØNN4
Right ØNN3
Pelvic
Left ØQN3
Right ØQN2
Sphenoid ØNNC
Temporal
Left ØNN6
Right ØNN5
Zygomatic
Left ØNNN
Right ØNNM
Brain ØØNØ
Breast
Bilateral ØHNV
Left ØHNU
Right ØHNT
Bronchus
Lingula ØBN9
Lower Lobe
Left ØBNB
Right ØBN6
Main
Left ØBN7
Right ØBN3
Middle Lobe, Right ØBN5
Upper Lobe
Left ØBN8
Right ØBN4
Buccal Mucosa ØCN4
Bursa and Ligament
Abdomen
Left ØMNJ
Right ØMNH
Ankle
Left ØMNR
Right ØMNQ
Elbow
Left ØMN4
Right ØMN3
Foot
Left ØMNT
Right ØMNS
Hand
Left ØMN8
Right ØMN7
Head and Neck ØMNØ
Hip
Left ØMNM
Right ØMNL
Knee
Left ØMNP
Right ØMNN
Lower Extremity
Left ØMNW
Right ØMNV
Perineum ØMNK
Rib(s) ØMNG
Shoulder
Left ØMN2
Right ØMN1
Spine
Lower ØMND
Upper ØMNC
Sternum ØMNF
Upper Extremity
Left ØMNB
Right ØMN9
Wrist
Left ØMN6
Right ØMN5
Carina ØBN2
Carotid Bodies, Bilateral ØGN8
Carotid Body
Left ØGN6
Right ØGN7
Carpal
Left ØPNN

Subterms under main terms may continue to next column or pa

Release — continued
  Carpal — continued
    Right ØPNM
  Cecum ØDNH
  Cerebellum ØØNC
  Cerebral Hemisphere ØØN7
  Cerebral Meninges ØØN1
  Cerebral Ventricle ØØN6
  Cervix ØUNC
  Chordae Tendineae Ø2N9
  Choroid
    Left Ø8NB
    Right Ø8NA
  Cisterna Chyli Ø7NL
  Clavicle
    Left ØPNB
    Right ØPN9
  Clitoris ØUNJ
  Coccygeal Glomus ØGNB
  Coccyx ØQNS
  Colon
    Ascending ØDNK
    Descending ØDNM
    Sigmoid ØDNN
    Transverse ØDNL
  Conduction Mechanism Ø2N8
  Conjunctiva
    Left Ø8NTXZZ
    Right Ø8NSXZZ
  Cord
    Bilateral ØVNH
    Left ØVNG
    Right ØVNF
  Cornea
    Left Ø8N9XZZ
    Right Ø8N8XZZ
  Cul-de-sac ØUNF
  Diaphragm ØBNT
  Disc
    Cervical Vertebral ØRN3
    Cervicothoracic Vertebral ØRN5
    Lumbar Vertebral ØSN2
    Lumbosacral ØSN4
    Thoracic Vertebral ØRN9
    Thoracolumbar Vertebral ØRNB
  Duct
    Common Bile ØFN9
    Cystic ØFN8
    Hepatic
      Common ØFN7
      Left ØFN6
      Right ØFN5
    Lacrimal
      Left Ø8NY
      Right Ø8NX
    Pancreatic ØFND
      Accessory ØFNF
    Parotid
      Left ØCNC
      Right ØCNB
  Duodenum ØDN9
  Dura Mater ØØN2
  Ear
    External
      Left Ø9N1
      Right Ø9NØ
    External Auditory Canal
      Left Ø9N4
      Right Ø9N3
    Inner
      Left Ø9NE
      Right Ø9ND
    Middle
      Left Ø9N6
      Right Ø9N5
  Epididymis
    Bilateral ØVNL
    Left ØVNK
    Right ØVNJ
  Epiglottis ØCNR
  Esophagogastric Junction ØDN4
  Esophagus ØDN5
    Lower ØDN3
    Middle ØDN2
    Upper ØDN1
  Eustachian Tube
    Left Ø9NG
    Right Ø9NF

Release — continued
  Eye
    Left Ø8N1XZZ
    Right Ø8NØXZZ
  Eyelid
    Lower
      Left Ø8NR
      Right Ø8NQ
    Upper
      Left Ø8NP
      Right Ø8NN
  Fallopian Tube
    Left ØUN6
    Right ØUN5
  Fallopian Tubes, Bilateral ØUN7
  Femoral Shaft
    Left ØQN9
    Right ØQN8
  Femur
    Lower
      Left ØQNC
      Right ØQNB
    Upper
      Left ØQN7
      Right ØQN6
  Fibula
    Left ØQNK
    Right ØQNJ
  Finger Nail ØHNQXZZ
  Gallbladder ØFN4
  Gingiva
    Lower ØCN6
    Upper ØCN5
  Gland
    Adrenal
      Bilateral ØGN4
      Left ØGN2
      Right ØGN3
    Lacrimal
      Left Ø8NW
      Right Ø8NV
    Minor Salivary ØCNJ
    Parotid
      Left ØCN9
      Right ØCN8
    Pituitary ØGNØ
    Sublingual
      Left ØCNF
      Right ØCND
    Submaxillary
      Left ØCNH
      Right ØCNG
    Vestibular ØUNL
  Glenoid Cavity
    Left ØPN8
    Right ØPN7
  Glomus Jugulare ØGNC
  Humeral Head
    Left ØPND
    Right ØPNC
  Humeral Shaft
    Left ØPNG
    Right ØPNF
  Hymen ØUNK
  Hypothalamus ØØNA
  Ileocecal Valve ØDNC
  Ileum ØDNB
  Intestine
    Large ØDNE
      Left ØDNG
      Right ØDNF
    Small ØDN8
  Iris
    Left Ø8ND3ZZ
    Right Ø8NC3ZZ
  Jejunum ØDNA
  Joint
    Acromioclavicular
      Left ØRNH
      Right ØRNG
    Ankle
      Left ØSNG
      Right ØSNF
    Carpal
      Left ØRNR
      Right ØRNQ
    Carpometacarpal
      Left ØRNT
      Right ØRNS

Release — continued
  Joint — continued
    Cervical Vertebral ØRN1
    Cervicothoracic Vertebral ØRN4
    Coccygeal ØSN6
    Elbow
      Left ØRNM
      Right ØRNL
    Finger Phalangeal
      Left ØRNX
      Right ØRNW
    Hip
      Left ØSNB
      Right ØSN9
    Knee
      Left ØSND
      Right ØSNC
    Lumbar Vertebral ØSNØ
    Lumbosacral ØSN3
    Metacarpophalangeal
      Left ØRNV
      Right ØRNU
    Metatarsal-Phalangeal
      Left ØSNN
      Right ØSNM
    Occipital-cervical ØRNØ
    Sacrococcygeal ØSN5
    Sacroiliac
      Left ØSN8
      Right ØSN7
    Shoulder
      Left ØRNK
      Right ØRNJ
    Sternoclavicular
      Left ØRNF
      Right ØRNE
    Tarsal
      Left ØSNJ
      Right ØSNH
    Tarsometatarsal
      Left ØSNL
      Right ØSNK
    Temporomandibular
      Left ØRND
      Right ØRNC
    Thoracic Vertebral ØRN6
    Thoracolumbar Vertebral ØRNA
    Toe Phalangeal
      Left ØSNQ
      Right ØSNP
    Wrist
      Left ØRNP
      Right ØRNN
  Kidney
    Left ØTN1
    Right ØTNØ
  Kidney Pelvis
    Left ØTN4
    Right ØTN3
  Larynx ØCNS
  Lens
    Left Ø8NK3ZZ
    Right Ø8NJ3ZZ
  Lip
    Lower ØCN1
    Upper ØCNØ
  Liver ØFNØ
    Left Lobe ØFN2
    Right Lobe ØFN1
  Lung
    Bilateral ØBNM
    Left ØBNL
    Lower Lobe
      Left ØBNJ
      Right ØBNF
    Middle Lobe, Right ØBND
    Right ØBNK
    Upper Lobe
      Left ØBNG
      Right ØBNC
  Lung Lingula ØBNH
  Lymphatic
    Aortic Ø7ND
    Axillary
      Left Ø7N6
      Right Ø7N5
    Head Ø7NØ
    Inguinal
      Left Ø7NJ

Release — *continued*
 Lymphatic — *continued*
  Inguinal — *continued*
   Right 07NH
  Internal Mammary
   Left 07N9
   Right 07N8
  Lower Extremity
   Left 07NG
   Right 07NF
  Mesenteric 07NB
  Neck
   Left 07N2
   Right 07N1
  Pelvis 07NC
  Thoracic Duct 07NK
  Thorax 07N7
  Upper Extremity
   Left 07N4
   Right 07N3
 Mandible
  Left 0NNV
  Right 0NNT
 Maxilla 0NNR
 Medulla Oblongata 00ND
 Mesentery 0DNV
 Metacarpal
  Left 0PNQ
  Right 0PNP
 Metatarsal
  Left 0QNP
  Right 0QNN
 Muscle
  Abdomen
   Left 0KNL
   Right 0KNK
  Extraocular
   Left 08NM
   Right 08NL
  Facial 0KN1
  Foot
   Left 0KNW
   Right 0KNV
  Hand
   Left 0KND
   Right 0KNC
  Head 0KN0
  Hip
   Left 0KNP
   Right 0KNN
  Lower Arm and Wrist
   Left 0KNB
   Right 0KN9
  Lower Leg
   Left 0KNT
   Right 0KNS
  Neck
   Left 0KN3
   Right 0KN2
  Papillary 02ND
  Perineum 0KNM
  Shoulder
   Left 0KN6
   Right 0KN5
  Thorax
   Left 0KNJ
   Right 0KNH
  Tongue, Palate, Pharynx 0KN4
  Trunk
   Left 0KNG
   Right 0KNF
  Upper Arm
   Left 0KN8
   Right 0KN7
  Upper Leg
   Left 0KNR
   Right 0KNQ
 Myocardial Bridge *see* Release, Artery, Coronary
 Nasal Mucosa and Soft Tissue 09NK
 Nasopharynx 09NN
 Nerve
  Abdominal Sympathetic 01NM
  Abducens 00NL
  Accessory 00NR
  Acoustic 00NN
  Brachial Plexus 01N3
  Cervical 01N1
  Cervical Plexus 01N0
  Facial 00NM

Release — *continued*
 Nerve — *continued*
  Femoral 01ND
  Glossopharyngeal 00NP
  Head and Neck Sympathetic 01NK
  Hypoglossal 00NS
  Lumbar 01NB
  Lumbar Plexus 01N9
  Lumbar Sympathetic 01NN
  Lumbosacral Plexus 01NA
  Median 01N5
  Oculomotor 00NH
  Olfactory 00NF
  Optic 00NG
  Peroneal 01NH
  Phrenic 01N2
  Pudendal 01NC
  Radial 01N6
  Sacral 01NR
  Sacral Plexus 01NQ
  Sacral Sympathetic 01NP
  Sciatic 01NF
  Thoracic 01N8
  Thoracic Sympathetic 01NL
  Tibial 01NG
  Trigeminal 00NK
  Trochlear 00NJ
  Ulnar 01N4
  Vagus 00NQ
 Nipple
  Left 0HNX
  Right 0HNW
 Omentum 0DNU
 Orbit
  Left 0NNQ
  Right 0NNP
 Ovary
  Bilateral 0UN2
  Left 0UN1
  Right 0UN0
 Palate
  Hard 0CN2
  Soft 0CN3
 Pancreas 0FNG
 Para-aortic Body 0GN9
 Paraganglion Extremity 0GNF
 Parathyroid Gland 0GNR
  Inferior
   Left 0GNP
   Right 0GNN
  Multiple 0GNQ
  Superior
   Left 0GNM
   Right 0GNL
 Patella
  Left 0QNF
  Right 0QND
 Penis 0VNS
 Pericardium 02NN
 Peritoneum 0DNW
 Phalanx
  Finger
   Left 0PNV
   Right 0PNT
  Thumb
   Left 0PNS
   Right 0PNR
  Toe
   Left 0QNR
   Right 0QNQ
 Pharynx 0CNM
 Pineal Body 0GN1
 Pleura
  Left 0BNP
  Right 0BNN
 Pons 00NB
 Prepuce 0VNT
 Prostate 0VN0
 Radius
  Left 0PNJ
  Right 0PNH
 Rectum 0DNP
 Retina
  Left 08NF3ZZ
  Right 08NE3ZZ
 Retinal Vessel
  Left 08NH3ZZ
  Right 08NG3ZZ

Release — *continued*
 Ribs
  1 to 2 0PN1
  3 or More 0PN2
 Sacrum 0QN1
 Scapula
  Left 0PN6
  Right 0PN5
 Sclera
  Left 08N7XZZ
  Right 08N6XZZ
 Scrotum 0VN5
 Septum
  Atrial 02N5
  Nasal 09NM
  Ventricular 02NM
 Sinus
  Accessory 09NP
  Ethmoid
   Left 09NV
   Right 09NU
  Frontal
   Left 09NT
   Right 09NS
  Mastoid
   Left 09NC
   Right 09NB
  Maxillary
   Left 09NR
   Right 09NQ
  Sphenoid
   Left 09NX
   Right 09NW
 Skin
  Abdomen 0HN7XZZ
  Back 0HN6XZZ
  Buttock 0HN8XZZ
  Chest 0HN5XZZ
  Ear
   Left 0HN3XZZ
   Right 0HN2XZZ
  Face 0HN1XZZ
  Foot
   Left 0HNNXZZ
   Right 0HNMXZZ
  Hand
   Left 0HNGXZZ
   Right 0HNFXZZ
  Inguinal 0HNAXZZ
  Lower Arm
   Left 0HNEXZZ
   Right 0HNDXZZ
  Lower Leg
   Left 0HNLXZZ
   Right 0HNKXZZ
  Neck 0HN4XZZ
  Perineum 0HN9XZZ
  Scalp 0HN0XZZ
  Upper Arm
   Left 0HNCXZZ
   Right 0HNBXZZ
  Upper Leg
   Left 0HNJXZZ
   Right 0HNHXZZ
 Spinal Cord
  Cervical 00NW
  Lumbar 00NY
  Thoracic 00NX
 Spinal Meninges 00NT
 Spleen 07NP
 Sternum 0PN0
 Stomach 0DN6
  Pylorus 0DN7
 Subcutaneous Tissue and Fascia
  Abdomen 0JN8
  Back 0JN7
  Buttock 0JN9
  Chest 0JN6
  Face 0JN1
  Foot
   Left 0JNR
   Right 0JNQ
  Hand
   Left 0JNK
   Right 0JNJ
  Lower Arm
   Left 0JNH
   Right 0JNG

Release — *continued*
  Subcutaneous Tissue and Fascia — *continued*
    Lower Leg
      Left ØJNP
      Right ØJNN
    Neck
      Left ØJN5
      Right ØJN4
    Pelvic Region ØJNC
    Perineum ØJNB
    Scalp ØJNØ
    Upper Arm
      Left ØJNF
      Right ØJND
    Upper Leg
      Left ØJNM
      Right ØJNL
  Tarsal
    Left ØQNM
    Right ØQNL
  Tendon
    Abdomen
      Left ØLNG
      Right ØLNF
    Ankle
      Left ØLNT
      Right ØLNS
    Foot
      Left ØLNW
      Right ØLNV
    Hand
      Left ØLN8
      Right ØLN7
    Head and Neck ØLNØ
    Hip
      Left ØLNK
      Right ØLNJ
    Knee
      Left ØLNR
      Right ØLNQ
    Lower Arm and Wrist
      Left ØLN6
      Right ØLN5
    Lower Leg
      Left ØLNP
      Right ØLNN
    Perineum ØLNH
    Shoulder
      Left ØLN2
      Right ØLN1
    Thorax
      Left ØLND
      Right ØLNC
    Trunk
      Left ØLNB
      Right ØLN9
    Upper Arm
      Left ØLN4
      Right ØLN3
    Upper Leg
      Left ØLNM
      Right ØLNL
  Testis
    Bilateral ØVNC
    Left ØVNB
    Right ØVN9
  Thalamus ØØN9
  Thymus Ø7NM
  Thyroid Gland ØGNK
    Left Lobe ØGNG
    Right Lobe ØGNH
  Tibia
    Left ØQNH
    Right ØQNG
  Toe Nail ØHNRXZZ
  Tongue ØCN7
  Tonsils ØCNP
  Tooth
    Lower ØCNX
    Upper ØCNW
  Trachea ØBN1
  Tunica Vaginalis
    Left ØVN7
    Right ØVN6
  Turbinate, Nasal Ø9NL
  Tympanic Membrane
    Left Ø9N8
    Right Ø9N7

Release — *continued*
  Ulna
    Left ØPNL
    Right ØPNK
  Ureter
    Left ØTN7
    Right ØTN6
  Urethra ØTND
  Uterine Supporting Structure ØUN4
  Uterus ØUN9
  Uvula ØCNN
  Vagina ØUNG
  Valve
    Aortic Ø2NF
    Mitral Ø2NG
    Pulmonary Ø2NH
    Tricuspid Ø2NJ
  Vas Deferens
    Bilateral ØVNQ
    Left ØVNP
    Right ØVNN
  Vein
    Axillary
      Left Ø5N8
      Right Ø5N7
    Azygos Ø5NØ
    Basilic
      Left Ø5NC
      Right Ø5NB
    Brachial
      Left Ø5NA
      Right Ø5N9
    Cephalic
      Left Ø5NF
      Right Ø5ND
    Colic Ø6N7
    Common Iliac
      Left Ø6ND
      Right Ø6NC
    Coronary Ø2N4
    Esophageal Ø6N3
    External Iliac
      Left Ø6NG
      Right Ø6NF
    External Jugular
      Left Ø5NQ
      Right Ø5NP
    Face
      Left Ø5NV
      Right Ø5NT
    Femoral
      Left Ø6NN
      Right Ø6NM
    Foot
      Left Ø6NV
      Right Ø6NT
    Gastric Ø6N2
    Hand
      Left Ø5NH
      Right Ø5NG
    Hemiazygos Ø5N1
    Hepatic Ø6N4
    Hypogastric
      Left Ø6NJ
      Right Ø6NH
    Inferior Mesenteric Ø6N6
    Innominate
      Left Ø5N4
      Right Ø5N3
    Internal Jugular
      Left Ø5NN
      Right Ø5NM
    Intracranial Ø5NL
    Lower Ø6NY
    Portal Ø6N8
    Pulmonary
      Left Ø2NT
      Right Ø2NS
    Renal
      Left Ø6NB
      Right Ø6N9
    Saphenous
      Left Ø6NQ
      Right Ø6NP
    Splenic Ø6N1
    Subclavian
      Left Ø5N6
      Right Ø5N5
    Superior Mesenteric Ø6N5

Release — *continued*
  Vein — *continued*
    Upper Ø5NY
    Vertebral
      Left Ø5NS
      Right Ø5NR
  Vena Cava
    Inferior Ø6NØ
    Superior Ø2NV
  Ventricle
    Left Ø2NL
    Right Ø2NK
  Vertebra
    Cervical ØPN3
    Lumbar ØQNØ
    Thoracic ØPN4
  Vesicle
    Bilateral ØVN3
    Left ØVN2
    Right ØVN1
  Vitreous
    Left Ø8N53ZZ
    Right Ø8N43ZZ
  Vocal Cord
    Left ØCNV
    Right ØCNT
  Vulva ØUNM
Relocation *see* Reposition
Remdesivir Anti-infective XWØ
Removal
  Abdominal Wall 2W53X
  Anorectal 2Y53X5Z
  Arm
    Lower
      Left 2W5DX
      Right 2W5CX
    Upper
      Left 2W5BX
      Right 2W5AX
  Back 2W55X
  Chest Wall 2W54X
  Ear 2Y52X5Z
  Extremity
    Lower
      Left 2W5MX
      Right 2W5LX
    Upper
      Left 2W59X
      Right 2W58X
  Face 2W51X
  Finger
    Left 2W5KX
    Right 2W5JX
  Foot
    Left 2W5TX
    Right 2W5SX
  Genital Tract, Female 2Y54X5Z
  Hand
    Left 2W5FX
    Right 2W5EX
  Head 2W50X
  Inguinal Region
    Left 2W57X
    Right 2W56X
  Leg
    Lower
      Left 2W5RX
      Right 2W5QX
    Upper
      Left 2W5PX
      Right 2W5NX
  Mouth and Pharynx 2Y5ØX5Z
  Nasal 2Y51X5Z
  Neck 2W52X
  Thumb
    Left 2W5HX
    Right 2W5GX
  Toe
    Left 2W5VX
    Right 2W5UX
  Urethra 2Y55X5Z
Removal of device from
  Abdominal Wall ØWPF
  Acetabulum
    Left ØQP5
    Right ØQP4
  Anal Sphincter ØDPR
  Anus ØDPQ

Removal of device from — *continued*
- Artery
  - Lower Ø4PY
  - Upper Ø3PY
- Back
  - Lower ØWPL
  - Upper ØWPK
- Bladder ØTPB
- Bone
  - Facial ØNPW
  - Lower ØQPY
  - Nasal ØNPB
  - Pelvic
    - Left ØQP3
    - Right ØQP2
  - Upper ØPPY
- Bone Marrow Ø7PT
- Brain ØØPØ
- Breast
  - Left ØHPU
  - Right ØHPT
- Bursa and Ligament
  - Lower ØMPY
  - Upper ØMPX
- Carpal
  - Left ØPPN
  - Right ØPPM
- Cavity, Cranial ØWP1
- Cerebral Ventricle ØØP6
- Chest Wall ØWP8
- Cisterna Chyli Ø7PL
- Clavicle
  - Left ØPPB
  - Right ØPP9
- Coccyx ØQPS
- Diaphragm ØBPT
- Disc
  - Cervical Vertebral ØRP3
  - Cervicothoracic Vertebral ØRP5
  - Lumbar Vertebral ØSP2
  - Lumbosacral ØSP4
  - Thoracic Vertebral ØRP9
  - Thoracolumbar Vertebral ØRPB
- Duct
  - Hepatobiliary ØFPB
  - Pancreatic ØFPD
- Ear
  - Inner
    - Left Ø9PJ
    - Right Ø9PD
  - Left Ø9PJ
  - Right Ø9PH
- Epididymis and Spermatic Cord ØVPM
- Esophagus ØDP5
- Extremity
  - Lower
    - Left ØYPB
    - Right ØYP9
  - Upper
    - Left ØXP7
    - Right ØXP6
- Eye
  - Left Ø8P1
  - Right Ø8PØ
- Face ØWP2
- Fallopian Tube ØUP8
- Femoral Shaft
  - Left ØQP9
  - Right ØQP8
- Femur
  - Lower
    - Left ØQPC
    - Right ØQPB
  - Upper
    - Left ØQP7
    - Right ØQP6
- Fibula
  - Left ØQPK
  - Right ØQPJ
- Finger Nail ØHPQX
- Gallbladder ØFP4
- Gastrointestinal Tract ØWPP
- Genitourinary Tract ØWPR
- Gland
  - Adrenal ØGP5
  - Endocrine ØGPS
  - Pituitary ØGPØ
  - Salivary ØCPA

Removal of device from — *continued*
- Glenoid Cavity
  - Left ØPP8
  - Right ØPP7
- Great Vessel Ø2PY
- Hair ØHPSX
- Head ØWPØ
- Heart Ø2PA
- Humeral Head
  - Left ØPPD
  - Right ØPPC
- Humeral Shaft
  - Left ØPPG
  - Right ØPPF
- Intestinal Tract
  - Lower ØDPD
  - Upper ØDPØ
- Jaw
  - Lower ØWP5
  - Upper ØWP4
- Joint
  - Acromioclavicular
    - Left ØRPH
    - Right ØRPG
  - Ankle
    - Left ØSPG
    - Right ØSPF
  - Carpal
    - Left ØRPR
    - Right ØRPQ
  - Carpometacarpal
    - Left ØRPT
    - Right ØRPS
  - Cervical Vertebral ØRP1
  - Cervicothoracic Vertebral ØRP4
  - Coccygeal ØSP6
  - Elbow
    - Left ØRPM
    - Right ØRPL
  - Finger Phalangeal
    - Left ØRPX
    - Right ØRPW
  - Hip
    - Left ØSPB
      - Acetabular Surface ØSPE
      - Femoral Surface ØSPS
    - Right ØSP9
      - Acetabular Surface ØSPA
      - Femoral Surface ØSPR
  - Knee
    - Left ØSPD
      - Femoral Surface ØSPU
      - Tibial Surface ØSPW
    - Right ØSPC
      - Femoral Surface ØSPT
      - Tibial Surface ØSPV
  - Lumbar Vertebral ØSPØ
  - Lumbosacral ØSP3
  - Metacarpophalangeal
    - Left ØRPV
    - Right ØRPU
  - Metatarsal-Phalangeal
    - Left ØSPN
    - Right ØSPM
  - Occipital-cervical ØRPØ
  - Sacrococcygeal ØSP5
  - Sacroiliac
    - Left ØSP8
    - Right ØSP7
  - Shoulder
    - Left ØRPK
    - Right ØRPJ
  - Sternoclavicular
    - Left ØRPF
    - Right ØRPE
  - Tarsal
    - Left ØSPJ
    - Right ØSPH
  - Tarsometatarsal
    - Left ØSPL
    - Right ØSPK
  - Temporomandibular
    - Left ØRPD
    - Right ØRPC
  - Thoracic Vertebral ØRP6
  - Thoracolumbar Vertebral ØRPA
  - Toe Phalangeal
    - Left ØSPQ
    - Right ØSPP

Removal of device from — *continued*
- Joint — *continued*
  - Wrist
    - Left ØRPP
    - Right ØRPN
- Kidney ØTP5
- Larynx ØCPS
- Lens
  - Left Ø8PK3
  - Right Ø8PJ3
- Liver ØFPØ
- Lung
  - Left ØBPL
  - Right ØBPK
- Lymphatic Ø7PN
  - Thoracic Duct Ø7PK
- Mediastinum ØWPC
- Mesentery ØDPV
- Metacarpal
  - Left ØPPQ
  - Right ØPPP
- Metatarsal
  - Left ØQPP
  - Right ØQPN
- Mouth and Throat ØCPY
- Muscle
  - Extraocular
    - Left Ø8PM
    - Right Ø8PL
  - Lower ØKPY
  - Upper ØKPX
- Nasal Mucosa and Soft Tissue Ø9PK
- Neck ØWP6
- Nerve
  - Cranial ØØPE
  - Peripheral Ø1PY
- Omentum ØDPU
- Ovary ØUP3
- Pancreas ØFPG
- Parathyroid Gland ØGPR
- Patella
  - Left ØQPF
  - Right ØQPD
- Pelvic Cavity ØWPJ
- Penis ØVPS
- Pericardial Cavity ØWPD
- Perineum
  - Female ØWPN
  - Male ØWPM
- Peritoneal Cavity ØWPG
- Peritoneum ØDPW
- Phalanx
  - Finger
    - Left ØPPV
    - Right ØPPT
  - Thumb
    - Left ØPPS
    - Right ØPPR
  - Toe
    - Left ØQPR
    - Right ØQPQ
- Pineal Body ØGP1
- Pleura ØBPQ
- Pleural Cavity
  - Left ØWPB
  - Right ØWP9
- Products of Conception 1ØPØ
- Prostate and Seminal Vesicles ØVP4
- Radius
  - Left ØPPJ
  - Right ØPPH
- Rectum ØDPP
- Respiratory Tract ØWPQ
- Retroperitoneum ØWPH
- Ribs
  - 1 to 2 ØPP1
  - 3 or More ØPP2
- Sacrum ØQP1
- Scapula
  - Left ØPP6
  - Right ØPP5
- Scrotum and Tunica Vaginalis ØVP8
- Sinus Ø9PY
- Skin ØHPPX
- Skull ØNPØ
- Spinal Canal ØØPU
- Spinal Cord ØØPV
- Spleen Ø7PP
- Sternum ØPPØ

▽ Subterms under main terms may continue to next column or

Removal of device from — continued
- Stomach ØDP6
- Subcutaneous Tissue and Fascia
  - Head and Neck ØJPS
  - Lower Extremity ØJPW
  - Trunk ØJPT
  - Upper Extremity ØJPV
- Tarsal
  - Left ØQPM
  - Right ØQPL
- Tendon
  - Lower ØLPY
  - Upper ØLPX
- Testis ØVPD
- Thymus Ø7PM
- Thyroid Gland ØGPK
- Tibia
  - Left ØQPH
  - Right ØQPG
- Toe Nail ØHPRX
- Trachea ØBP1
- Tracheobronchial Tree ØBPØ
- Tympanic Membrane
  - Left Ø9P8
  - Right Ø9P7
- Ulna
  - Left ØPPL
  - Right ØPPK
- Ureter ØTP9
- Urethra ØTPD
- Uterus and Cervix ØUPD
- Vagina and Cul-de-sac ØUPH
- Vas Deferens ØVPR
- Vein
  - Azygos Ø5PØ
  - Innominate
    - Left Ø5P4
    - Right Ø5P3
  - Lower Ø6PY
  - Upper Ø5PY
- Vertebra
  - Cervical ØPP3
  - Lumbar ØQPØ
  - Thoracic ØPP4
- Vulva ØUPM

enal calyx
- use Kidney
- use Kidney, Left
- use Kidney, Right
- use Kidneys, Bilateral

enal capsule
- use Kidney
- use Kidney, Left
- use Kidney, Right
- use Kidneys, Bilateral

enal cortex
- use Kidney
- use Kidney, Left
- use Kidney, Right
- use Kidneys, Bilateral

enal dialysis see Performance, Urinary 5A1D
enal nerve use Abdominal Sympathetic Nerve
enal plexus use Abdominal Sympathetic Nerve
enal segment
- use Kidney
- use Kidney, Left
- use Kidney, Right
- use Kidneys, Bilateral

nal segmental artery
- use Renal Artery, Left
- use Renal Artery, Right

opening, operative site
- Control of bleeding see Control bleeding in
- Inspection only see Inspection

pair
- Abdominal Wall ØWQF
- Acetabulum
  - Left ØQQ5
  - Right ØQQ4
- Adenoids ØCQQ
- Ampulla of Vater ØFQC
- Anal Sphincter ØDQR
- Ankle Region
  - Left ØYQL
  - Right ØYQK
- Anterior Chamber
  - Left Ø8Q33ZZ
  - Right Ø8Q23ZZ

Repair — continued
- Anus ØDQQ
- Aorta
  - Abdominal Ø4QØ
  - Thoracic
    - Ascending/Arch Ø2QX
    - Descending Ø2QW
- Aortic Body ØGQD
- Appendix ØDQJ
- Arm
  - Lower
    - Left ØXQF
    - Right ØXQD
  - Upper
    - Left ØXQ9
    - Right ØXQ8
- Artery
  - Anterior Tibial
    - Left Ø4QQ
    - Right Ø4QP
  - Axillary
    - Left Ø3Q6
    - Right Ø3Q5
  - Brachial
    - Left Ø3Q8
    - Right Ø3Q7
  - Celiac Ø4Q1
  - Colic
    - Left Ø4Q7
    - Middle Ø4Q8
    - Right Ø4Q6
  - Common Carotid
    - Left Ø3QJ
    - Right Ø3QH
  - Common Iliac
    - Left Ø4QD
    - Right Ø4QC
  - Coronary
    - Four or More Arteries Ø2Q3
    - One Artery Ø2QØ
    - Three Arteries Ø2Q2
    - Two Arteries Ø2Q1
  - External Carotid
    - Left Ø3QN
    - Right Ø3QM
  - External Iliac
    - Left Ø4QJ
    - Right Ø4QH
  - Face Ø3QR
  - Femoral
    - Left Ø4QL
    - Right Ø4QK
  - Foot
    - Left Ø4QW
    - Right Ø4QV
  - Gastric Ø4Q2
  - Hand
    - Left Ø3QF
    - Right Ø3QD
  - Hepatic Ø4Q3
  - Inferior Mesenteric Ø4QB
  - Innominate Ø3Q2
  - Internal Carotid
    - Left Ø3QL
    - Right Ø3QK
  - Internal Iliac
    - Left Ø4QF
    - Right Ø4QE
  - Internal Mammary
    - Left Ø3Q1
    - Right Ø3QØ
  - Intracranial Ø3QG
  - Lower Ø4QY
  - Peroneal
    - Left Ø4QU
    - Right Ø4QT
  - Popliteal
    - Left Ø4QN
    - Right Ø4QM
  - Posterior Tibial
    - Left Ø4QS
    - Right Ø4QR
  - Pulmonary
    - Left Ø2QR
    - Right Ø2QQ
  - Pulmonary Trunk Ø2QP
  - Radial
    - Left Ø3QC
    - Right Ø3QB

Repair — continued
- Artery — continued
  - Renal
    - Left Ø4QA
    - Right Ø4Q9
  - Splenic Ø4Q4
  - Subclavian
    - Left Ø3Q4
    - Right Ø3Q3
  - Superior Mesenteric Ø4Q5
  - Temporal
    - Left Ø3QT
    - Right Ø3QS
  - Thyroid
    - Left Ø3QV
    - Right Ø3QU
  - Ulnar
    - Left Ø3QA
    - Right Ø3Q9
  - Upper Ø3QY
  - Vertebral
    - Left Ø3QQ
    - Right Ø3QP
- Atrium
  - Left Ø2Q7
  - Right Ø2Q6
- Auditory Ossicle
  - Left Ø9QA
  - Right Ø9Q9
- Axilla
  - Left ØXQ5
  - Right ØXQ4
- Back
  - Lower ØWQL
  - Upper ØWQK
- Basal Ganglia ØØQ8
- Bladder ØTQB
- Bladder Neck ØTQC
- Bone
  - Ethmoid
    - Left ØNQG
    - Right ØNQF
  - Frontal ØNQ1
  - Hyoid ØNQX
  - Lacrimal
    - Left ØNQJ
    - Right ØNQH
  - Nasal ØNQB
  - Occipital ØNQ7
  - Palatine
    - Left ØNQL
    - Right ØNQK
  - Parietal
    - Left ØNQ4
    - Right ØNQ3
  - Pelvic
    - Left ØQQ3
    - Right ØQQ2
  - Sphenoid ØNQC
  - Temporal
    - Left ØNQ6
    - Right ØNQ5
  - Zygomatic
    - Left ØNQN
    - Right ØNQM
- Brain ØØQØ
- Breast
  - Bilateral ØHQV
  - Left ØHQU
  - Right ØHQT
  - Supernumerary ØHQY
- Bronchus
  - Lingula ØBQ9
  - Lower Lobe
    - Left ØBQB
    - Right ØBQ6
  - Main
    - Left ØBQ7
    - Right ØBQ3
  - Middle Lobe, Right ØBQ5
  - Upper Lobe
    - Left ØBQ8
    - Right ØBQ4
- Buccal Mucosa ØCQ4
- Bursa and Ligament
  - Abdomen
    - Left ØMQJ
    - Right ØMQH

Repair — *continued*
  Bursa and Ligament — *continued*
    Ankle
      Left ØMQR
      Right ØMQQ
    Elbow
      Left ØMQ4
      Right ØMQ3
    Foot
      Left ØMQT
      Right ØMQS
    Hand
      Left ØMQ8
      Right ØMQ7
    Head and Neck ØMQ0
    Hip
      Left ØMQM
      Right ØMQL
    Knee
      Left ØMQP
      Right ØMQN
    Lower Extremity
      Left ØMQW
      Right ØMQV
    Perineum ØMQK
    Rib(s) ØMQG
    Shoulder
      Left ØMQ2
      Right ØMQ1
    Spine
      Lower ØMQD
      Upper ØMQC
    Sternum ØMQF
    Upper Extremity
      Left ØMQB
      Right ØMQ9
    Wrist
      Left ØMQ6
      Right ØMQ5
  Buttock
    Left ØYQ1
    Right ØYQ0
  Carina ØBQ2
  Carotid Bodies, Bilateral ØGQ8
  Carotid Body
    Left ØGQ6
    Right ØGQ7
  Carpal
    Left ØPQN
    Right ØPQM
  Cecum ØDQH
  Cerebellum ØØQC
  Cerebral Hemisphere ØØQ7
  Cerebral Meninges ØØQ1
  Cerebral Ventricle ØØQ6
  Cervix ØUQC
  Chest Wall ØWQ8
  Chordae Tendineae Ø2Q9
  Choroid
    Left Ø8QB
    Right Ø8QA
  Cisterna Chyli Ø7QL
  Clavicle
    Left ØPQB
    Right ØPQ9
  Clitoris ØUQJ
  Coccygeal Glomus ØGQB
  Coccyx ØQQS
  Colon
    Ascending ØDQK
    Descending ØDQM
    Sigmoid ØDQN
    Transverse ØDQL
  Conduction Mechanism Ø2Q8
  Conjunctiva
    Left Ø8QTXZZ
    Right Ø8QSXZZ
  Cord
    Bilateral ØVQH
    Left ØVQG
    Right ØVQF
  Cornea
    Left Ø8Q9XZZ
    Right Ø8Q8XZZ
  Cul-de-sac ØUQF
  Diaphragm ØBQT
  Disc
    Cervical Vertebral ØRQ3
    Cervicothoracic Vertebral ØRQ5

Repair — *continued*
  Disc — *continued*
    Lumbar Vertebral ØSQ2
    Lumbosacral ØSQ4
    Thoracic Vertebral ØRQ9
    Thoracolumbar Vertebral ØRQB
  Duct
    Common Bile ØFQ9
    Cystic ØFQ8
    Hepatic
      Common ØFQ7
      Left ØFQ6
      Right ØFQ5
    Lacrimal
      Left Ø8QY
      Right Ø8QX
    Pancreatic ØFQD
      Accessory ØFQF
    Parotid
      Left ØCQC
      Right ØCQB
  Duodenum ØDQ9
  Dura Mater ØØQ2
  Ear
    External
      Bilateral Ø9Q2
      Left Ø9Q1
      Right Ø9Q0
    External Auditory Canal
      Left Ø9Q4
      Right Ø9Q3
    Inner
      Left Ø9QE
      Right Ø9QD
    Middle
      Left Ø9Q6
      Right Ø9Q5
  Elbow Region
    Left ØXQC
    Right ØXQB
  Epididymis
    Bilateral ØVQL
    Left ØVQK
    Right ØVQJ
  Epiglottis ØCQR
  Esophagogastric Junction ØDQ4
  Esophagus ØDQ5
    Lower ØDQ3
    Middle ØDQ2
    Upper ØDQ1
  Eustachian Tube
    Left Ø9QG
    Right Ø9QF
  Extremity
    Lower
      Left ØYQB
      Right ØYQ9
    Upper
      Left ØXQ7
      Right ØXQ6
  Eye
    Left Ø8Q1XZZ
    Right Ø8Q0XZZ
  Eyelid
    Lower
      Left Ø8QR
      Right Ø8QQ
    Upper
      Left Ø8QP
      Right Ø8QN
  Face ØWQ2
  Fallopian Tube
    Left ØUQ6
    Right ØUQ5
  Fallopian Tubes, Bilateral ØUQ7
  Femoral Region
    Bilateral ØYQE
    Left ØYQ8
    Right ØYQ7
  Femoral Shaft
    Left ØQQ9
    Right ØQQ8
  Femur
    Lower
      Left ØQQC
      Right ØQQB
    Upper
      Left ØQQ7
      Right ØQQ6

Repair — *continued*
  Fibula
    Left ØQQK
    Right ØQQJ
  Finger
    Index
      Left ØXQP
      Right ØXQN
    Little
      Left ØXQW
      Right ØXQV
    Middle
      Left ØXQR
      Right ØXQQ
    Ring
      Left ØXQT
      Right ØXQS
  Finger Nail ØHQQXZZ
  Floor of mouth *see* Repair, Oral Cavity and Throat ØWQ3
  Foot
    Left ØYQN
    Right ØYQM
  Gallbladder ØFQ4
  Gingiva
    Lower ØCQ6
    Upper ØCQ5
  Gland
    Adrenal
      Bilateral ØGQ4
      Left ØGQ2
      Right ØGQ3
    Lacrimal
      Left Ø8QW
      Right Ø8QV
    Minor Salivary ØCQJ
    Parotid
      Left ØCQ9
      Right ØCQ8
    Pituitary ØGQ0
    Sublingual
      Left ØCQF
      Right ØCQD
    Submaxillary
      Left ØCQH
      Right ØCQG
    Vestibular ØUQL
  Glenoid Cavity
    Left ØPQ8
    Right ØPQ7
  Glomus Jugulare ØGQC
  Hand
    Left ØXQK
    Right ØXQJ
  Head ØWQ0
  Heart Ø2QA
    Left Ø2QC
    Right Ø2QB
  Humeral Head
    Left ØPQD
    Right ØPQC
  Humeral Shaft
    Left ØPQG
    Right ØPQF
  Hymen ØUQK
  Hypothalamus ØØQA
  Ileocecal Valve ØDQC
  Ileum ØDQB
  Inguinal Region
    Bilateral ØYQA
    Left ØYQ6
    Right ØYQ5
  Intestine
    Large ØDQE
      Left ØDQG
      Right ØDQF
    Small ØDQ8
  Iris
    Left Ø8QD3ZZ
    Right Ø8QC3ZZ
  Jaw
    Lower ØWQ5
    Upper ØWQ4
  Jejunum ØDQA
  Joint
    Acromioclavicular
      Left ØRQH
      Right ØRQG

Repair — *continued*
 Phalanx — *continued*
  Thumb
   Left 0PQS
   Right 0PQR
  Toe
   Left 0QQR
   Right 0QQQ
 Pharynx 0CQM
 Pineal Body 0GQ1
 Pleura
  Left 0BQP
  Right 0BQN
 Pons 00QB
 Prepuce 0VQT
 Products of Conception 10Q0
 Prostate 0VQ0
 Radius
  Left 0PQJ
  Right 0PQH
 Rectum 0DQP
 Retina
  Left 08QF3ZZ
  Right 08QE3ZZ
 Retinal Vessel
  Left 08QH3ZZ
  Right 08QG3ZZ
 Ribs
  1 to 2 0PQ1
  3 or More 0PQ2
 Sacrum 0QQ1
 Scapula
  Left 0PQ6
  Right 0PQ5
 Sclera
  Left 08Q7XZZ
  Right 08Q6XZZ
 Scrotum 0VQ5
 Septum
  Atrial 02Q5
  Nasal 09QM
  Ventricular 02QM
 Shoulder Region
  Left 0XQ3
  Right 0XQ2
 Sinus
  Accessory 09QP
  Ethmoid
   Left 09QV
   Right 09QU
  Frontal
   Left 09QT
   Right 09QS
  Mastoid
   Left 09QC
   Right 09QB
  Maxillary
   Left 09QR
   Right 09QQ
  Sphenoid
   Left 09QX
   Right 09QW
 Skin
  Abdomen 0HQ7XZZ
  Back 0HQ6XZZ
  Buttock 0HQ8XZZ
  Chest 0HQ5XZZ
  Ear
   Left 0HQ3XZZ
   Right 0HQ2XZZ
  Face 0HQ1XZZ
  Foot
   Left 0HQNXZZ
   Right 0HQMXZZ
  Hand
   Left 0HQGXZZ
   Right 0HQFXZZ
  Inguinal 0HQAXZZ
  Lower Arm
   Left 0HQEXZZ
   Right 0HQDXZZ
  Lower Leg
   Left 0HQLXZZ
   Right 0HQKXZZ
  Neck 0HQ4XZZ
  Perineum 0HQ9XZZ
  Scalp 0HQ0XZZ
  Upper Arm
   Left 0HQCXZZ

Repair — *continued*
 Skin — *continued*
  Upper Arm — *continued*
   Right 0HQBXZZ
  Upper Leg
   Left 0HQJXZZ
   Right 0HQHXZZ
 Skull 0NQ0
 Spinal Cord
  Cervical 00QW
  Lumbar 00QY
  Thoracic 00QX
 Spinal Meninges 00QT
 Spleen 07QP
 Sternum 0PQ0
 Stomach 0DQ6
  Pylorus 0DQ7
 Subcutaneous Tissue and Fascia
  Abdomen 0JQ8
  Back 0JQ7
  Buttock 0JQ9
  Chest 0JQ6
  Face 0JQ1
  Foot
   Left 0JQR
   Right 0JQQ
  Hand
   Left 0JQK
   Right 0JQJ
  Lower Arm
   Left 0JQH
   Right 0JQG
  Lower Leg
   Left 0JQP
   Right 0JQN
  Neck
   Left 0JQ5
   Right 0JQ4
  Pelvic Region 0JQC
  Perineum 0JQB
  Scalp 0JQ0
  Upper Arm
   Left 0JQF
   Right 0JQD
  Upper Leg
   Left 0JQM
   Right 0JQL
 Tarsal
  Left 0QQM
  Right 0QQL
 Tendon
  Abdomen
   Left 0LQF
   Right 0LQF
  Ankle
   Left 0LQT
   Right 0LQS
  Foot
   Left 0LQW
   Right 0LQV
  Hand
   Left 0LQ8
   Right 0LQ7
  Head and Neck 0LQ0
  Hip
   Left 0LQK
   Right 0LQJ
  Knee
   Left 0LQR
   Right 0LQQ
  Lower Arm and Wrist
   Left 0LQ6
   Right 0LQ5
  Lower Leg
   Left 0LQP
   Right 0LQN
  Perineum 0LQH
  Shoulder
   Left 0LQ2
   Right 0LQ1
  Thorax
   Left 0LQD
   Right 0LQC
  Trunk
   Left 0LQB
   Right 0LQ9
  Upper Arm
   Left 0LQ4
   Right 0LQ3

Repair — *continued*
 Tendon — *continued*
  Upper Leg
   Left 0LQM
   Right 0LQL
 Testis
  Bilateral 0VQC
  Left 0VQB
  Right 0VQ9
 Thalamus 00Q9
 Thumb
  Left 0XQM
  Right 0XQL
 Thymus 07QM
 Thyroid Gland 0GQK
  Left Lobe 0GQG
  Right Lobe 0GQH
 Thyroid Gland Isthmus 0GQJ
 Tibia
  Left 0QQH
  Right 0QQG
 Toe
  1st
   Left 0YQQ
   Right 0YQP
  2nd
   Left 0YQS
   Right 0YQR
  3rd
   Left 0YQU
   Right 0YQT
  4th
   Left 0YQW
   Right 0YQV
  5th
   Left 0YQY
   Right 0YQX
 Toe Nail 0HQRXZZ
 Tongue 0CQ7
 Tonsils 0CQP
 Tooth
  Lower 0CQX
  Upper 0CQW
 Trachea 0BQ1
 Tunica Vaginalis
  Left 0VQ7
  Right 0VQ6
 Turbinate, Nasal 09QL
 Tympanic Membrane
  Left 09Q8
  Right 09Q7
 Ulna
  Left 0PQL
  Right 0PQK
 Ureter
  Left 0TQ7
  Right 0TQ6
 Urethra 0TQD
 Uterine Supporting Structure 0UQ4
 Uterus 0UQ9
 Uvula 0CQN
 Vagina 0UQG
 Valve
  Aortic 02QF
  Mitral 02QG
  Pulmonary 02QH
  Tricuspid 02QJ
 Vas Deferens
  Bilateral 0VQQ
  Left 0VQP
  Right 0VQN
 Vein
  Axillary
   Left 05Q8
   Right 05Q7
  Azygos 05Q0
  Basilic
   Left 05QC
   Right 05QB
  Brachial
   Left 05QA
   Right 05Q9
  Cephalic
   Left 05QF
   Right 05QD
  Colic 06Q7
  Common Iliac
   Left 06QD
   Right 06QC

Repair — *continued*
　Vein — *continued*
　　Coronary 02Q4
　　Esophageal 06Q3
　　External Iliac
　　　Left 06QG
　　　Right 06QF
　　External Jugular
　　　Left 05QQ
　　　Right 05QP
　　Face
　　　Left 05QV
　　　Right 05QT
　　Femoral
　　　Left 06QN
　　　Right 06QM
　　Foot
　　　Left 06QV
　　　Right 06QT
　　Gastric 06Q2
　　Hand
　　　Left 05QH
　　　Right 05QG
　　Hemiazygos 05Q1
　　Hepatic 06Q4
　　Hypogastric
　　　Left 06QJ
　　　Right 06QH
　　Inferior Mesenteric 06Q6
　　Innominate
　　　Left 05Q4
　　　Right 05Q3
　　Internal Jugular
　　　Left 05QN
　　　Right 05QM
　　Intracranial 05QL
　　Lower 06QY
　　Portal 06Q8
　　Pulmonary
　　　Left 02QT
　　　Right 02QS
　　Renal
　　　Left 06QB
　　　Right 06Q9
　　Saphenous
　　　Left 06QQ
　　　Right 06QP
　　Splenic 06Q1
　　Subclavian
　　　Left 05Q6
　　　Right 05Q5
　　Superior Mesenteric 06Q5
　　Upper 05QY
　　Vertebral
　　　Left 05QS
　　　Right 05QR
　Vena Cava
　　Inferior 06Q0
　　Superior 02QV
　Ventricle
　　Left 02QL
　　Right 02QK
　Vertebra
　　Cervical 0PQ3
　　Lumbar 0QQ0
　　Thoracic 0PQ4
　Vesicle
　　Bilateral 0VQ3
　　Left 0VQ2
　　Right 0VQ1
　Vitreous
　　Left 08Q53ZZ
　　Right 08Q43ZZ
　Vocal Cord
　　Left 0CQV
　　Right 0CQT
　Vulva 0UQM
　Wrist Region
　　Left 0XQH
　　Right 0XQG

Repair, obstetric laceration, periurethral 0UQMXZZ
Replacement
　Acetabulum
　　Left 0QR5
　　Right 0QR4
　Ampulla of Vater 0FRC
　Anal Sphincter 0DRR
　Aorta
　　Abdominal 04R0

Replacement — *continued*
　Aorta — *continued*
　　Thoracic
　　　Ascending/Arch 02RX
　　　Descending 02RW
　Artery
　　Anterior Tibial
　　　Left 04RQ
　　　Right 04RP
　　Axillary
　　　Left 03R6
　　　Right 03R5
　　Brachial
　　　Left 03R8
　　　Right 03R7
　　Celiac 04R1
　　Colic
　　　Left 04R7
　　　Middle 04R8
　　　Right 04R6
　　Common Carotid
　　　Left 03RJ
　　　Right 03RH
　　Common Iliac
　　　Left 04RD
　　　Right 04RC
　　External Carotid
　　　Left 03RN
　　　Right 03RM
　　External Iliac
　　　Left 04RJ
　　　Right 04RH
　　Face 03RR
　　Femoral
　　　Left 04RL
　　　Right 04RK
　　Foot
　　　Left 04RW
　　　Right 04RV
　　Gastric 04R2
　　Hand
　　　Left 03RF
　　　Right 03RD
　　Hepatic 04R3
　　Inferior Mesenteric 04RB
　　Innominate 03R2
　　Internal Carotid
　　　Left 03RL
　　　Right 03RK
　　Internal Iliac
　　　Left 04RF
　　　Right 04RE
　　Internal Mammary
　　　Left 03R1
　　　Right 03R0
　　Intracranial 03RG
　　Lower 04RY
　　Peroneal
　　　Left 04RU
　　　Right 04RT
　　Popliteal
　　　Left 04RN
　　　Right 04RM
　　Posterior Tibial
　　　Left 04RS
　　　Right 04RR
　　Pulmonary
　　　Left 02RR
　　　Right 02RQ
　　Pulmonary Trunk 02RP
　　Radial
　　　Left 03RC
　　　Right 03RB
　　Renal
　　　Left 04RA
　　　Right 04R9
　　Splenic 04R4
　　Subclavian
　　　Left 03R4
　　　Right 03R3
　　Superior Mesenteric 04R5
　　Temporal
　　　Left 03RT
　　　Right 03RS
　　Thyroid
　　　Left 03RV
　　　Right 03RU
　　Ulnar
　　　Left 03RA

Replacement — *continued*
　Artery — *continued*
　　Ulnar — *continued*
　　　Right 03R9
　　Upper 03RY
　　Vertebral
　　　Left 03RQ
　　　Right 03RP
　Atrium
　　Left 02R7
　　Right 02R6
　Auditory Ossicle
　　Left 09RA0
　　Right 09R90
　Bladder 0TRB
　Bladder Neck 0TRC
　Bone
　　Ethmoid
　　　Left 0NRG
　　　Right 0NRF
　　Frontal 0NR1
　　Hyoid 0NRX
　　Lacrimal
　　　Left 0NRJ
　　　Right 0NRH
　　Nasal 0NRB
　　Occipital 0NR7
　　Palatine
　　　Left 0NRL
　　　Right 0NRK
　　Parietal
　　　Left 0NR4
　　　Right 0NR3
　　Pelvic
　　　Left 0QR3
　　　Right 0QR2
　　Sphenoid 0NRC
　　Temporal
　　　Left 0NR6
　　　Right 0NR5
　　Zygomatic
　　　Left 0NRN
　　　Right 0NRM
　Breast
　　Bilateral 0HRV
　　Left 0HRU
　　Right 0HRT
　Bronchus
　　Lingula 0BR9
　　Lower Lobe
　　　Left 0BRB
　　　Right 0BR6
　　Main
　　　Left 0BR7
　　　Right 0BR3
　　Middle Lobe, Right 0BR5
　　Upper Lobe
　　　Left 0BR8
　　　Right 0BR4
　Buccal Mucosa 0CR4
　Bursa and Ligament
　　Abdomen
　　　Left 0MRJ
　　　Right 0MRH
　　Ankle
　　　Left 0MRR
　　　Right 0MRQ
　　Elbow
　　　Left 0MR4
　　　Right 0MR3
　　Foot
　　　Left 0MRT
　　　Right 0MRS
　　Hand
　　　Left 0MR8
　　　Right 0MR7
　　Head and Neck 0MR0
　　Hip
　　　Left 0MRM
　　　Right 0MRL
　　Knee
　　　Left 0MRP
　　　Right 0MRN
　　Lower Extremity
　　　Left 0MRW
　　　Right 0MRV
　　Perineum 0MRK
　　Rib(s) 0MRG

Replacement — *continued*
  Nerve — *continued*
    Olfactory 00RF
    Optic 00RG
    Peroneal 01RH
    Phrenic 01R2
    Pudendal 01RC
    Radial 01R6
    Sacral 01RR
    Sciatic 01RF
    Thoracic 01R8
    Tibial 01RG
    Trigeminal 00RK
    Trochlear 00RJ
    Ulnar 01R4
    Vagus 00RQ
  Nipple
    Left 0HRX
    Right 0HRW
  Omentum 0DRU
  Orbit
    Left 0NRQ
    Right 0NRP
  Palate
    Hard 0CR2
    Soft 0CR3
  Patella
    Left 0QRF
    Right 0QRD
  Pericardium 02RN
  Peritoneum 0DRW
  Phalanx
    Finger
      Left 0PRV
      Right 0PRT
    Thumb
      Left 0PRS
      Right 0PRR
    Toe
      Left 0QRR
      Right 0QRQ
  Pharynx 0CRM
  Radius
    Left 0PRJ
    Right 0PRH
  Retinal Vessel
    Left 08RH3
    Right 08RG3
  Ribs
    1 to 2 0PR1
    3 or More 0PR2
  Sacrum 0QR1
  Scapula
    Left 0PR6
    Right 0PR5
  Sclera
    Left 08R7X
    Right 08R6X
  Septum
    Atrial 02R5
    Nasal 09RM
    Ventricular 02RM
  Skin
    Abdomen 0HR7
    Back 0HR6
    Buttock 0HR8
    Chest 0HR5
    Ear
      Left 0HR3
      Right 0HR2
    Face 0HR1
    Foot
      Left 0HRN
      Right 0HRM
    Hand
      Left 0HRG
      Right 0HRF
    Inguinal 0HRA
    Lower Arm
      Left 0HRE
      Right 0HRD
    Lower Leg
      Left 0HRL
      Right 0HRK
    Neck 0HR4
    Perineum 0HR9
    Scalp 0HR0
    Upper Arm
      Left 0HRC

Replacement — *continued*
  Skin — *continued*
    Upper Arm — *continued*
      Right 0HRB
    Upper Leg
      Left 0HRJ
      Right 0HRH
  Skin Substitute, Porcine Liver Derived XHRPXL2
  Skull 0NR0
  Spinal Meninges 00RT
  Sternum 0PR0
  Subcutaneous Tissue and Fascia
    Abdomen 0JR8
    Back 0JR7
    Buttock 0JR9
    Chest 0JR6
    Face 0JR1
    Foot
      Left 0JRR
      Right 0JRQ
    Hand
      Left 0JRK
      Right 0JRJ
    Lower Arm
      Left 0JRH
      Right 0JRG
    Lower Leg
      Left 0JRP
      Right 0JRN
    Neck
      Left 0JR5
      Right 0JR4
    Pelvic Region 0JRC
    Perineum 0JRB
    Scalp 0JR0
    Upper Arm
      Left 0JRF
      Right 0JRD
    Upper Leg
      Left 0JRM
      Right 0JRL
  Tarsal
    Left 0QRM
    Right 0QRL
  Tendon
    Abdomen
      Left 0LRG
      Right 0LRF
    Ankle
      Left 0LRT
      Right 0LRS
    Foot
      Left 0LRW
      Right 0LRV
    Hand
      Left 0LR8
      Right 0LR7
    Head and Neck 0LR0
    Hip
      Left 0LRK
      Right 0LRJ
    Knee
      Left 0LRR
      Right 0LRQ
    Lower Arm and Wrist
      Left 0LR6
      Right 0LR5
    Lower Leg
      Left 0LRP
      Right 0LRN
    Perineum 0LRH
    Shoulder
      Left 0LR2
      Right 0LR1
    Thorax
      Left 0LRD
      Right 0LRC
    Trunk
      Left 0LRB
      Right 0LR9
    Upper Arm
      Left 0LR4
      Right 0LR3
    Upper Leg
      Left 0LRM
      Right 0LRL
  Testis
    Bilateral 0VRC0JZ
    Left 0VRB0JZ

Replacement — *continued*
  Testis — *continued*
    Right 0VR90JZ
  Thumb
    Left 0XRM
    Right 0XRL
  Tibia
    Left 0QRH
    Right 0QRG
  Toe Nail 0HRRX
  Tongue 0CR7
  Tooth
    Lower 0CRX
    Upper 0CRW
  Trachea 0BR1
  Turbinate, Nasal 09RL
  Tympanic Membrane
    Left 09R8
    Right 09R7
  Ulna
    Left 0PRL
    Right 0PRK
  Ureter
    Left 0TR7
    Right 0TR6
  Urethra 0TRD
  Uvula 0CRN
  Valve
    Aortic 02RF
    Mitral 02RG
    Pulmonary 02RH
    Tricuspid 02RJ
  Vein
    Axillary
      Left 05R8
      Right 05R7
    Azygos 05R0
    Basilic
      Left 05RC
      Right 05RB
    Brachial
      Left 05RA
      Right 05R9
    Cephalic
      Left 05RF
      Right 05RD
    Colic 06R7
    Common Iliac
      Left 06RD
      Right 06RC
    Esophageal 06R3
    External Iliac
      Left 06RG
      Right 06RF
    External Jugular
      Left 05RQ
      Right 05RP
    Face
      Left 05RV
      Right 05RT
    Femoral
      Left 06RN
      Right 06RM
    Foot
      Left 06RV
      Right 06RT
    Gastric 06R2
    Hand
      Left 05RH
      Right 05RG
    Hemiazygos 05R1
    Hepatic 06R4
    Hypogastric
      Left 06RJ
      Right 06RH
    Inferior Mesenteric 06R6
    Innominate
      Left 05R4
      Right 05R3
    Internal Jugular
      Left 05RN
      Right 05RM
    Intracranial 05RL
    Lower 06RY
    Portal 06R8
    Pulmonary
      Left 02RT
      Right 02RS

Replacement — *continued*
- Vein — *continued*
  - Renal
    - Left 06RB
    - Right 06R9
  - Saphenous
    - Left 06RQ
    - Right 06RP
  - Splenic 06R1
  - Subclavian
    - Left 05R6
    - Right 05R5
  - Superior Mesenteric 06R5
  - Upper 05RY
  - Vertebral
    - Left 05RS
    - Right 05RR
- Vena Cava
  - Inferior 06R0
  - Superior 02RV
- Ventricle
  - Left 02RL
  - Right 02RK
- Vertebra
  - Cervical 0PR3
  - Lumbar 0QR0
  - Thoracic 0PR4
- Vitreous
  - Left 08R53
  - Right 08R43
- Vocal Cord
  - Left 0CRV
  - Right 0CRT
- Zooplastic Tissue, Rapid Deployment Technique X2RF

Replacement, hip
- Partial or total *see* Replacement, Lower Joints 0SR
- Resurfacing only *see* Supplement, Lower Joints 0SU

Replantation *see* Reposition
Replantation, scalp *see* Reattachment, Skin, Scalp 0HM0

Reposition
- Acetabulum
  - Left 0QS5
  - Right 0QS4
- Ampulla of Vater 0FSC
- Anus 0DSQ
- Aorta
  - Abdominal 04S0
  - Thoracic
    - Ascending/Arch 02SX0ZZ
    - Descending 02SW0ZZ
- Artery
  - Anterior Tibial
    - Left 04SQ
    - Right 04SP
  - Axillary
    - Left 03S6
    - Right 03S5
  - Brachial
    - Left 03S8
    - Right 03S7
  - Celiac 04S1
  - Colic
    - Left 04S7
    - Middle 04S8
    - Right 04S6
  - Common Carotid
    - Left 03SJ
    - Right 03SH
  - Common Iliac
    - Left 04SD
    - Right 04SC
  - Coronary
    - One Artery 02S00ZZ
    - Two Arteries 02S10ZZ
  - External Carotid
    - Left 03SN
    - Right 03SM
  - External Iliac
    - Left 04SJ
    - Right 04SH
  - Face 03SR
  - Femoral
    - Left 04SL
    - Right 04SK
  - Foot
    - Left 04SW

Reposition — *continued*
- Artery — *continued*
  - Foot — *continued*
    - Right 04SV
  - Gastric 04S2
  - Hand
    - Left 03SF
    - Right 03SD
  - Hepatic 04S3
  - Inferior Mesenteric 04SB
  - Innominate 03S2
  - Internal Carotid
    - Left 03SL
    - Right 03SK
  - Internal Iliac
    - Left 04SF
    - Right 04SE
  - Internal Mammary
    - Left 03S1
    - Right 03S0
  - Intracranial 03SG
  - Lower 04SY
  - Peroneal
    - Left 04SU
    - Right 04ST
  - Popliteal
    - Left 04SN
    - Right 04SM
  - Posterior Tibial
    - Left 04SS
    - Right 04SR
  - Pulmonary
    - Left 02SR0ZZ
    - Right 02SQ0ZZ
  - Pulmonary Trunk 02SP0ZZ
  - Radial
    - Left 03SC
    - Right 03SB
  - Renal
    - Left 04SA
    - Right 04S9
  - Splenic 04S4
  - Subclavian
    - Left 03S4
    - Right 03S3
  - Superior Mesenteric 04S5
  - Temporal
    - Left 03ST
    - Right 03SS
  - Thyroid
    - Left 03SV
    - Right 03SU
  - Ulnar
    - Left 03SA
    - Right 03S9
  - Upper 03SY
  - Vertebral
    - Left 03SQ
    - Right 03SP
- Auditory Ossicle
  - Left 09SA
  - Right 09S9
- Bladder 0TSB
- Bladder Neck 0TSC
- Bone
  - Ethmoid
    - Left 0NSG
    - Right 0NSF
  - Frontal 0NS1
  - Hyoid 0NSX
  - Lacrimal
    - Left 0NSJ
    - Right 0NSH
  - Nasal 0NSB
  - Occipital 0NS7
  - Palatine
    - Left 0NSL
    - Right 0NSK
  - Parietal
    - Left 0NS4
    - Right 0NS3
  - Pelvic
    - Left 0QS3
    - Right 0QS2
  - Sphenoid 0NSC
  - Temporal
    - Left 0NS6
    - Right 0NS5

Reposition — *continued*
- Bone — *continued*
  - Zygomatic
    - Left 0NSN
    - Right 0NSM
- Breast
  - Bilateral 0HSV0ZZ
  - Left 0HSU0ZZ
  - Right 0HST0ZZ
- Bronchus
  - Lingula 0BS90ZZ
  - Lower Lobe
    - Left 0BSB0ZZ
    - Right 0BS60ZZ
  - Main
    - Left 0BS70ZZ
    - Right 0BS30ZZ
  - Middle Lobe, Right 0BS50ZZ
  - Upper Lobe
    - Left 0BS80ZZ
    - Right 0BS40ZZ
- Bursa and Ligament
  - Abdomen
    - Left 0MSJ
    - Right 0MSH
  - Ankle
    - Left 0MSR
    - Right 0MSQ
  - Elbow
    - Left 0MS4
    - Right 0MS3
  - Foot
    - Left 0MST
    - Right 0MSS
  - Hand
    - Left 0MS8
    - Right 0MS7
  - Head and Neck 0MS0
  - Hip
    - Left 0MSM
    - Right 0MSL
  - Knee
    - Left 0MSP
    - Right 0MSN
  - Lower Extremity
    - Left 0MSW
    - Right 0MSV
  - Perineum 0MSK
  - Rib(s) 0MSG
  - Shoulder
    - Left 0MS2
    - Right 0MS1
  - Spine
    - Lower 0MSD
    - Upper 0MSC
  - Sternum 0MSF
  - Upper Extremity
    - Left 0MSB
    - Right 0MS9
  - Wrist
    - Left 0MS6
    - Right 0MS5
- Carina 0BS20ZZ
- Carpal
  - Left 0PSN
  - Right 0PSM
- Cecum 0DSH
- Cervix 0USC
- Clavicle
  - Left 0PSB
  - Right 0PS9
- Coccyx 0QSS
- Colon
  - Ascending 0DSK
  - Descending 0DSM
  - Sigmoid 0DSN
  - Transverse 0DSL
- Cord
  - Bilateral 0VSH
  - Left 0VSG
  - Right 0VSF
- Cul-de-sac 0USF
- Diaphragm 0BST0ZZ
- Duct
  - Common Bile 0FS9
  - Cystic 0FS8
  - Hepatic
    - Common 0FS7
    - Left 0FS6

Reposition — *continued*
    Duct — *continued*
        Hepatic — *continued*
            Right ØFS5
        Lacrimal
            Left Ø8SY
            Right Ø8SX
        Pancreatic ØFSD
            Accessory ØFSF
        Parotid
            Left ØCSC
            Right ØCSB
    Duodenum ØDS9
    Ear
        Bilateral Ø9S2
        Left Ø9S1
        Right Ø9SØ
    Epiglottis ØCSR
    Esophagus ØDS5
    Eustachian Tube
        Left Ø9SG
        Right Ø9SF
    Eyelid
        Lower
            Left Ø8SR
            Right Ø8SQ
        Upper
            Left Ø8SP
            Right Ø8SN
    Fallopian Tube
        Left ØUS6
        Right ØUS5
    Fallopian Tubes, Bilateral ØUS7
    Femoral Shaft
        Left ØQS9
        Right ØQS8
    Femur
        Lower
            Left ØQSC
            Right ØQSB
        Upper
            Left ØQS7
            Right ØQS6
    Fibula
        Left ØQSK
        Right ØQSJ
    Gallbladder ØFS4
    Gland
        Adrenal
            Left ØGS2
            Right ØGS3
        Lacrimal
            Left Ø8SW
            Right Ø8SV
    Glenoid Cavity
        Left ØPS8
        Right ØPS7
    Hair ØHSSXZZ
    Humeral Head
        Left ØPSD
        Right ØPSC
    Humeral Shaft
        Left ØPSG
        Right ØPSF
    Ileum ØDSB
    Intestine
        Large ØDSE
        Small ØDS8
    Iris
        Left Ø8SD3ZZ
        Right Ø8SC3ZZ
    Jejunum ØDSA
    Joint
        Acromioclavicular
            Left ØRSH
            Right ØRSG
        Ankle
            Left ØSSG
            Right ØSSF
        Carpal
            Left ØRSR
            Right ØRSQ
        Carpometacarpal
            Left ØRST
            Right ØRSS
        Cervical Vertebral ØRS1
        Cervicothoracic Vertebral ØRS4
        Coccygeal ØSS6

Reposition — *continued*
    Joint — *continued*
        Elbow
            Left ØRSM
            Right ØRSL
        Finger Phalangeal
            Left ØRSV
            Right ØRSW
        Hip
            Left ØSSB
            Right ØSS9
        Knee
            Left ØSSD
            Right ØSSC
        Lumbar Vertebral ØSSØ
        Lumbosacral ØSS3
        Metacarpophalangeal
            Left ØRSV
            Right ØRSU
        Metatarsal-Phalangeal
            Left ØSSN
            Right ØSSM
        Occipital-cervical ØRSØ
        Sacrococcygeal ØSS5
        Sacroiliac
            Left ØSS8
            Right ØSS7
        Shoulder
            Left ØRSK
            Right ØRSJ
        Sternoclavicular
            Left ØRSF
            Right ØRSE
        Tarsal
            Left ØSSJ
            Right ØSSH
        Tarsometatarsal
            Left ØSSL
            Right ØSSK
        Temporomandibular
            Left ØRSD
            Right ØRSC
        Thoracic Vertebral ØRS6
        Thoracolumbar Vertebral ØRSA
        Toe Phalangeal
            Left ØSSQ
            Right ØSSP
        Wrist
            Left ØRSP
            Right ØRSN
    Kidney
        Left ØTS1
        Right ØTSØ
    Kidney Pelvis
        Left ØTS4
        Right ØTS3
    Kidneys, Bilateral ØTS2
    Lens
        Left Ø8SK3ZZ
        Right Ø8SJ3ZZ
    Lip
        Lower ØCS1
        Upper ØCSØ
    Liver ØFSØ
    Lung
        Left ØBSLØZZ
        Lower Lobe
            Left ØBSJØZZ
            Right ØBSFØZZ
        Middle Lobe, Right ØBSDØZZ
        Right ØBSKØZZ
        Upper Lobe
            Left ØBSGØZZ
            Right ØBSCØZZ
    Lung Lingula ØBSHØZZ
    Mandible
        Left ØNSV
        Right ØNST
    Maxilla ØNSR
    Metacarpal
        Left ØPSQ
        Right ØPSP
    Metatarsal
        Left ØQSP
        Right ØQSN
    Muscle
        Abdomen
            Left ØKSL
            Right ØKSK

Reposition — *continued*
    Muscle — *continued*
        Extraocular
            Left Ø8SM
            Right Ø8SL
        Facial ØKS1
        Foot
            Left ØKSW
            Right ØKSV
        Hand
            Left ØKSD
            Right ØKSC
        Head ØKSØ
        Hip
            Left ØKSP
            Right ØKSN
        Lower Arm and Wrist
            Left ØKSB
            Right ØKS9
        Lower Leg
            Left ØKST
            Right ØKSS
        Neck
            Left ØKS3
            Right ØKS2
        Perineum ØKSM
        Shoulder
            Left ØKS6
            Right ØKS5
        Thorax
            Left ØKSJ
            Right ØKSH
        Tongue, Palate, Pharynx ØKS4
        Trunk
            Left ØKSG
            Right ØKSF
        Upper Arm
            Left ØKS8
            Right ØKS7
        Upper Leg
            Left ØKSR
            Right ØKSQ
    Nasal Mucosa and Soft Tissue Ø9SK
    Nerve
        Abducens ØØSL
        Accessory ØØSR
        Acoustic ØØSN
        Brachial Plexus Ø1S3
        Cervical Ø1S1
        Cervical Plexus Ø1SØ
        Facial ØØSM
        Femoral Ø1SD
        Glossopharyngeal ØØSP
        Hypoglossal ØØSS
        Lumbar Ø1SB
        Lumbar Plexus Ø1S9
        Lumbosacral Plexus Ø1SA
        Median Ø1S5
        Oculomotor ØØSH
        Olfactory ØØSF
        Optic ØØSG
        Peroneal Ø1SH
        Phrenic Ø1S2
        Pudendal Ø1SC
        Radial Ø1S6
        Sacral Ø1SR
        Sacral Plexus Ø1SQ
        Sciatic Ø1SF
        Thoracic Ø1S8
        Tibial Ø1SG
        Trigeminal ØØSK
        Trochlear ØØSJ
        Ulnar Ø1S4
        Vagus ØØSQ
    Nipple
        Left ØHSXXZZ
        Right ØHSWXZZ
    Orbit
        Left ØNSQ
        Right ØNSP
    Ovary
        Bilateral ØUS2
        Left ØUS1
        Right ØUSØ
    Palate
        Hard ØCS2
        Soft ØCS3
    Pancreas ØFSG
    Parathyroid Gland ØGSR

Subterms under main terms may continue to next column or p

Resection — *continued*
  Joint — *continued*
    Toe Phalangeal — *continued*
      Right ØSTPØZZ
    Wrist
      Left ØRTPØZZ
      Right ØRTNØZZ
  Kidney
    Left ØTT1
    Right ØTTØ
  Kidney Pelvis
    Left ØTT4
    Right ØTT3
  Kidneys, Bilateral ØTT2
  Larynx ØCTS
  Lens
    Left Ø8TK3ZZ
    Right Ø8TJ3ZZ
  Lip
    Lower ØCT1
    Upper ØCTØ
  Liver ØFTØ
    Left Lobe ØFT2
    Right Lobe ØFT1
  Lung
    Bilateral ØBTM
    Left ØBTL
    Lower Lobe
      Left ØBTJ
      Right ØBTF
    Middle Lobe, Right ØBTD
    Right ØBTK
    Upper Lobe
      Left ØBTG
      Right ØBTC
  Lung Lingula ØBTH
  Lymphatic
    Aortic Ø7TD
    Axillary
      Left Ø7T6
      Right Ø7T5
    Head Ø7TØ
    Inguinal
      Left Ø7TJ
      Right Ø7TH
    Internal Mammary
      Left Ø7T9
      Right Ø7T8
    Lower Extremity
      Left Ø7TG
      Right Ø7TF
    Mesenteric Ø7TB
    Neck
      Left Ø7T2
      Right Ø7T1
    Pelvis Ø7TC
    Thoracic Duct Ø7TK
    Thorax Ø7T7
    Upper Extremity
      Left Ø7T4
      Right Ø7T3
  Mandible
    Left ØNTVØZZ
    Right ØNTTØZZ
  Maxilla ØNTRØZZ
  Metacarpal
    Left ØPTQØZZ
    Right ØPTPØZZ
  Metatarsal
    Left ØQTPØZZ
    Right ØQTNØZZ
  Muscle
    Abdomen
      Left ØKTL
      Right ØKTK
    Extraocular
      Left Ø8TM
      Right Ø8TL
    Facial ØKT1
    Foot
      Left ØKTW
      Right ØKTV
    Hand
      Left ØKTD
      Right ØKTC
    Head ØKTØ
    Hip
      Left ØKTP
      Right ØKTN

Resection — *continued*
  Muscle — *continued*
    Lower Arm and Wrist
      Left ØKTB
      Right ØKT9
    Lower Leg
      Left ØKTT
      Right ØKTS
    Neck
      Left ØKT3
      Right ØKT2
    Papillary Ø2TD
    Perineum ØKTM
    Shoulder
      Left ØKT6
      Right ØKT5
    Thorax
      Left ØKTJ
      Right ØKTH
    Tongue, Palate, Pharynx ØKT4
    Trunk
      Left ØKTG
      Right ØKTF
    Upper Arm
      Left ØKT8
      Right ØKT7
    Upper Leg
      Left ØKTR
      Right ØKTQ
  Nasal Mucosa and Soft Tissue Ø9TK
  Nasopharynx Ø9TN
  Nipple
    Left ØHTXXZZ
    Right ØHTWXZZ
  Omentum ØDTU
  Orbit
    Left ØNTQØZZ
    Right ØNTPØZZ
  Ovary
    Bilateral ØUT2
    Left ØUT1
    Right ØUTØ
  Palate
    Hard ØCT2
    Soft ØCT3
  Pancreas ØFTG
  Para-aortic Body ØGT9
  Paraganglion Extremity ØGTF
  Parathyroid Gland ØGTR
    Inferior
      Left ØGTP
      Right ØGTN
    Multiple ØGTQ
    Superior
      Left ØGTM
      Right ØGTL
  Patella
    Left ØQTFØZZ
    Right ØQTDØZZ
  Penis ØVTS
  Pericardium Ø2TN
  Phalanx
    Finger
      Left ØPTVØZZ
      Right ØPTTØZZ
    Thumb
      Left ØPTSØZZ
      Right ØPTRØZZ
    Toe
      Left ØQTRØZZ
      Right ØQTQØZZ
  Pharynx ØCTM
  Pineal Body ØGT1
  Prepuce ØVTT
  Products of Conception, Ectopic 1ØT2
  Prostate ØVTØ
  Radius
    Left ØPTJØZZ
    Right ØPTHØZZ
  Rectum ØDTP
  Ribs
    1 to 2 ØPT1ØZZ
    3 or More ØPT2ØZZ
  Scapula
    Left ØPT6ØZZ
    Right ØPT5ØZZ
  Scrotum ØVT5
  Septum
    Atrial Ø2T5

Resection — *continued*
  Septum — *continued*
    Nasal Ø9TM
    Ventricular Ø2TM
  Sinus
    Accessory Ø9TP
    Ethmoid
      Left Ø9TV
      Right Ø9TU
    Frontal
      Left Ø9TT
      Right Ø9TS
    Mastoid
      Left Ø9TC
      Right Ø9TB
    Maxillary
      Left Ø9TR
      Right Ø9TQ
    Sphenoid
      Left Ø9TX
      Right Ø9TW
  Spleen Ø7TP
  Sternum ØPTØØZZ
  Stomach ØDT6
    Pylorus ØDT7
  Tarsal
    Left ØQTMØZZ
    Right ØQTLØZZ
  Tendon
    Abdomen
      Left ØLTG
      Right ØLTF
    Ankle
      Left ØLTT
      Right ØLTS
    Foot
      Left ØLTW
      Right ØLTV
    Hand
      Left ØLT8
      Right ØLT7
    Head and Neck ØLTØ
    Hip
      Left ØLTK
      Right ØLTJ
    Knee
      Left ØLTR
      Right ØLTQ
    Lower Arm and Wrist
      Left ØLT6
      Right ØLT5
    Lower Leg
      Left ØLTP
      Right ØLTN
    Perineum ØLTH
    Shoulder
      Left ØLT2
      Right ØLT1
    Thorax
      Left ØLTD
      Right ØLTC
    Trunk
      Left ØLTB
      Right ØLT9
    Upper Arm
      Left ØLT4
      Right ØLT3
    Upper Leg
      Left ØLTM
      Right ØLTL
  Testis
    Bilateral ØVTC
    Left ØVTB
    Right ØVT9
  Thymus Ø7TM
  Thyroid Gland ØGTK
    Left Lobe ØGTG
    Right Lobe ØGTH
  Thyroid Gland Isthmus ØGTJ
  Tibia
    Left ØQTHØZZ
    Right ØQTGØZZ
  Toe Nail ØHTRXZZ
  Tongue ØCT7
  Tonsils ØCTP
  Tooth
    Lower ØCTXØZ
    Upper ØCTWØZ
  Trachea ØBT1

Resection — *continued*
Tunica Vaginalis
Left ØVT7
Right ØVT6
Turbinate, Nasal Ø9TL
Tympanic Membrane
Left Ø9T8
Right Ø9T7
Ulna
Left ØPTLØZZ
Right ØPTKØZZ
Ureter
Left ØTT7
Right ØTT6
Urethra ØTTD
Uterine Supporting Structure ØUT4
Uterus ØUT9
Uvula ØCTN
Vagina ØUTG
Valve, Pulmonary Ø2TH
Vas Deferens
Bilateral ØVTQ
Left ØVTP
Right ØVTN
Vesicle
Bilateral ØVT3
Left ØVT2
Right ØVT1
Vitreous
Left Ø8T53ZZ
Right Ø8T43ZZ
Vocal Cord
Left ØCTV
Right ØCTT
Vulva ØUTM
Resection, Left ventricular outflow tract obstruction (LVOT) *see* Dilation, Ventricle, Left Ø27L
Resection, Subaortic membrane (Left ventricular outflow tract obstruction) *see* Dilation, Ventricle, Left Ø27L
Restoration, Cardiac, Single, Rhythm 5A22Ø4Z
RestoreAdvanced neurostimulator (SureScan) (MRI Safe) *use* Stimulator Generator, Multiple Array Rechargeable in ØJH
RestoreSensor neurostimulator (SureScan) (MRI Safe) *use* Stimulator Generator, Multiple Array Rechargeable in ØJH
RestoreUltra neurostimulator (SureScan) (MRI Safe) *use* Stimulator Generator, Multiple Array Rechargeable in ØJH
Restriction
Ampulla of Vater ØFVC
Anus ØDVQ
Aorta
Abdominal Ø4VØ
Intraluminal Device, Branched or Fenestrated Ø4VØ
Thoracic
Ascending/Arch, Intraluminal Device, Branched or Fenestrated Ø2VX
Descending, Intraluminal Device, Branched or Fenestrated Ø2VW
Artery
Anterior Tibial
Left Ø4VQ
Right Ø4VP
Axillary
Left Ø3V6
Right Ø3V5
Brachial
Left Ø3V8
Right Ø3V7
Celiac Ø4V1
Colic
Left Ø4V7
Middle Ø4V8
Right Ø4V6
Common Carotid
Left Ø3VJ
Right Ø3VH
Common Iliac
Left Ø4VD
Right Ø4VC
External Carotid
Left Ø3VN
Right Ø3VM
External Iliac
Left Ø4VJ

Restriction — *continued*
Artery — *continued*
External Iliac — *continued*
Right Ø4VH
Face Ø3VR
Femoral
Left Ø4VL
Right Ø4VK
Foot
Left Ø4VW
Right Ø4VV
Gastric Ø4V2
Hand
Left Ø3VF
Right Ø3VD
Hepatic Ø4V3
Inferior Mesenteric Ø4VB
Innominate Ø3V2
Internal Carotid
Left Ø3VL
Right Ø3VK
Internal Iliac
Left Ø4VF
Right Ø4VE
Internal Mammary
Left Ø3V1
Right Ø3VØ
Intracranial Ø3VG
Lower Ø4VY
Peroneal
Left Ø4VU
Right Ø4VT
Popliteal
Left Ø4VN
Right Ø4VM
Posterior Tibial
Left Ø4VS
Right Ø4VR
Pulmonary
Left Ø2VR
Right Ø2VQ
Pulmonary Trunk Ø2VP
Radial
Left Ø3VC
Right Ø3VB
Renal
Left Ø4VA
Right Ø4V9
Splenic Ø4V4
Subclavian
Left Ø3V4
Right Ø3V3
Superior Mesenteric Ø4V5
Temporal
Left Ø3VT
Right Ø3VS
Thyroid
Left Ø3VV
Right Ø3VU
Ulnar
Left Ø3VA
Right Ø3V9
Upper Ø3VY
Vertebral
Left Ø3VQ
Right Ø3VP
Bladder ØTVB
Bladder Neck ØTVC
Bronchus
Lingula ØBV9
Lower Lobe
Left ØBVB
Right ØBV6
Main
Left ØBV7
Right ØBV3
Middle Lobe, Right ØBV5
Upper Lobe
Left ØBV8
Right ØBV4
Carina ØBV2
Cecum ØDVH
Cervix ØUVC
Cisterna Chyli Ø7VL
Colon
Ascending ØDVK
Descending ØDVM
Sigmoid ØDVN
Transverse ØDVL

Restriction — *continued*
Duct
Common Bile ØFV9
Cystic ØFV8
Hepatic
Common ØFV7
Left ØFV6
Right ØFV5
Lacrimal
Left Ø8VY
Right Ø8VX
Pancreatic ØFVD
Accessory ØFVF
Parotid
Left ØCVC
Right ØCVB
Duodenum ØDV9
Esophagogastric Junction ØDV4
Esophagus ØDV5
Lower ØDV3
Middle ØDV2
Upper ØDV1
Heart Ø2VA
Ileocecal Valve ØDVC
Ileum ØDVB
Intestine
Large ØDVE
Left ØDVG
Right ØDVF
Small ØDV8
Jejunum ØDVA
Kidney Pelvis
Left ØTV4
Right ØTV3
Lymphatic
Aortic Ø7VD
Axillary
Left Ø7V6
Right Ø7V5
Head Ø7VØ
Inguinal
Left Ø7VJ
Right Ø7VH
Internal Mammary
Left Ø7V9
Right Ø7V8
Lower Extremity
Left Ø7VG
Right Ø7VF
Mesenteric Ø7VB
Neck
Left Ø7V2
Right Ø7V1
Pelvis Ø7VC
Thoracic Duct Ø7VK
Thorax Ø7V7
Upper Extremity
Left Ø7V4
Right Ø7V3
Rectum ØDVP
Stomach ØDV6
Pylorus ØDV7
Trachea ØBV1
Ureter
Left ØTV7
Right ØTV6
Urethra ØTVD
Valve, Mitral Ø2VG
Vein
Axillary
Left Ø5V8
Right Ø5V7
Azygos Ø5VØ
Basilic
Left Ø5VC
Right Ø5VB
Brachial
Left Ø5VA
Right Ø5V9
Cephalic
Left Ø5VF
Right Ø5VD
Colic Ø6V7
Common Iliac
Left Ø6VD
Right Ø6VC
Esophageal Ø6V3
External Iliac
Left Ø6VG

Restriction — *continued*
  Vein — *continued*
    External Iliac — *continued*
      Right Ø6VF
    External Jugular
      Left Ø5VQ
      Right Ø5VP
    Face
      Left Ø5VV
      Right Ø5VT
    Femoral
      Left Ø6VN
      Right Ø6VM
    Foot
      Left Ø6VV
      Right Ø6VT
    Gastric Ø6V2
    Hand
      Left Ø5VH
      Right Ø5VG
    Hemiazygos Ø5V1
    Hepatic Ø6V4
    Hypogastric
      Left Ø6VJ
      Right Ø6VH
    Inferior Mesenteric Ø6V6
    Innominate
      Left Ø5V4
      Right Ø5V3
    Internal Jugular
      Left Ø5VN
      Right Ø5VM
    Intracranial Ø5VL
    Lower Ø6VY
    Portal Ø6V8
    Pulmonary
      Left Ø2VT
      Right Ø2VS
    Renal
      Left Ø6VB
      Right Ø6V9
    Saphenous
      Left Ø6VQ
      Right Ø6VP
    Splenic Ø6V1
    Subclavian
      Left Ø5V6
      Right Ø5V5
    Superior Mesenteric Ø6V5
    Upper Ø5VY
    Vertebral
      Left Ø5VS
      Right Ø5VR
  Vena Cava
    Inferior Ø6VØ
    Superior Ø2VV
  Ventricle, Left Ø2VL

Resurfacing Device
  Removal of device from
    Left ØSPBØBZ
    Right ØSP9ØBZ
  Revision of device in
    Left ØSWBØBZ
    Right ØSW9ØBZ
  Supplement
    Left ØSUBØBZ
      Acetabular Surface ØSUEØBZ
      Femoral Surface ØSUSØBZ
    Right ØSU9ØBZ
      Acetabular Surface ØSUAØBZ
      Femoral Surface ØSURØBZ

Resuscitation
  Cardiopulmonary *see* Assistance, Cardiac 5AØ2
  Cardioversion 5A22Ø4Z
  Defibrillation 5A22Ø4Z
  Endotracheal intubation *see* Insertion of device in, Trachea ØBH1
  External chest compression, manual 5A12Ø12
  External chest compression, mechanical 5A1221J
  Pulmonary 5A19Ø54

Resuscitative endovascular balloon occlusion of the aorta (REBOA)
  Ø2LW3DJ
  Ø4LØ3DJ

Resuture, Heart valve prosthesis *see* Revision of device in, Heart and Great Vessels Ø2W

Retained placenta, manual removal *see* Extraction, Products of Conception, Retained 1ØD1

Retraining
  Cardiac *see* Motor Treatment, Rehabilitation FØ7
  Vocational *see* Activities of Daily Living Treatment, Rehabilitation FØ8

Retrogasserian rhizotomy *see* Division, Nerve, Trigeminal ØØ8K

Retroperitoneal cavity *use* Retroperitoneum

Retroperitoneal lymph node *use* Lymphatic, Aortic

Retroperitoneal space *use* Retroperitoneum

Retropharyngeal lymph node
  use Lymphatic, Left Neck
  use Lymphatic, Right Neck

Retropharyngeal space *use* Neck

Retropubic space *use* Pelvic Cavity

Reveal (LINQ) (DX) (XT) *use* Monitoring Device

Reverse total shoulder replacement *see* Replacement, Upper Joints ØRR

Reverse® Shoulder Prosthesis *use* Synthetic Substitute, Reverse Ball and Socket in ØRR

Revision
  Correcting a portion of existing device *see* Revision of device in
  Removal of device without replacement *see* Removal of device from
  Replacement of existing device
    see Removal of device from
    see Root operation to place new device, e.g., Insertion, Replacement, Supplement

Revision of device in
  Abdominal Wall ØWWF
  Acetabulum
    Left ØQW5
    Right ØQW4
  Anal Sphincter ØDWR
  Anus ØDWQ
  Artery
    Lower Ø4WY
    Upper Ø3WY
  Auditory Ossicle
    Left Ø9WA
    Right Ø9W9
  Back
    Lower ØWWL
    Upper ØWWK
  Bladder ØTWB
  Bone
    Facial ØNWW
    Lower ØQWY
    Nasal ØNWB
    Pelvic
      Left ØQW3
      Right ØQW2
    Upper ØPWY
  Bone Marrow Ø7WT
  Brain ØØWØ
  Breast
    Left ØHWU
    Right ØHWT
  Bursa and Ligament
    Lower ØMWY
    Upper ØMWX
  Carpal
    Left ØPWN
    Right ØPWM
  Cavity, Cranial ØWW1
  Cerebral Ventricle ØØW6
  Chest Wall ØWW8
  Cisterna Chyli Ø7WL
  Clavicle
    Left ØPWB
    Right ØPW9
  Coccyx ØQWS
  Diaphragm ØBWT
  Disc
    Cervical Vertebral ØRW3
    Cervicothoracic Vertebral ØRW5
    Lumbar Vertebral ØSW2
    Lumbosacral ØSW4
    Thoracic Vertebral ØRW9
    Thoracolumbar Vertebral ØRWB
  Duct
    Hepatobiliary ØFWB
    Pancreatic ØFWD
  Ear
    Inner
      Left Ø9WE
      Right Ø9WD
    Left Ø9WJ

Revision of device in — *continued*
  Ear — *continued*
    Right Ø9WH
  Epididymis and Spermatic Cord ØVWM
  Esophagus ØDW5
  Extremity
    Lower
      Left ØYWB
      Right ØYW9
    Upper
      Left ØXW7
      Right ØXW6
  Eye
    Left Ø8W1
    Right Ø8WØ
  Face ØWW2
  Fallopian Tube ØUW8
  Femoral Shaft
    Left ØQW9
    Right ØQW8
  Femur
    Lower
      Left ØQWC
      Right ØQWB
    Upper
      Left ØQW7
      Right ØQW6
  Fibula
    Left ØQWK
    Right ØQWJ
  Finger Nail ØHWQX
  Gallbladder ØFW4
  Gastrointestinal Tract ØWWP
  Genitourinary Tract ØWWR
  Gland
    Adrenal ØGW5
    Endocrine ØGWS
    Pituitary ØGWØ
    Salivary ØCWA
  Glenoid Cavity
    Left ØPW8
    Right ØPW7
  Great Vessel Ø2WY
  Hair ØHWSX
  Head ØWWØ
  Heart Ø2WA
  Humeral Head
    Left ØPWD
    Right ØPWC
  Humeral Shaft
    Left ØPWG
    Right ØPWF
  Intestinal Tract
    Lower ØDWD
    Upper ØDWØ
  Intestine
    Large ØDWE
    Small ØDW8
  Jaw
    Lower ØWW5
    Upper ØWW4
  Joint
    Acromioclavicular
      Left ØRWH
      Right ØRWG
    Ankle
      Left ØSWG
      Right ØSWF
    Carpal
      Left ØRWR
      Right ØRWQ
    Carpometacarpal
      Left ØRWT
      Right ØRWS
    Cervical Vertebral ØRW1
    Cervicothoracic Vertebral ØRW4
    Coccygeal ØSW6
    Elbow
      Left ØRWM
      Right ØRWL
    Finger Phalangeal
      Left ØRWX
      Right ØRWW
    Hip
      Left ØSWB
        Acetabular Surface ØSWE
        Femoral Surface ØSWS
      Right ØSW9
        Acetabular Surface ØSWA

Revision of device in — *continued*
Joint — *continued*
  Hip — *continued*
    Right — *continued*
      Femoral Surface ØSWR
  Knee
    Left ØSWD
      Femoral Surface ØSWU
      Tibial Surface ØSWW
    Right ØSWC
      Femoral Surface ØSWT
      Tibial Surface ØSWV
  Lumbar Vertebral ØSWØ
  Lumbosacral ØSW3
  Metacarpophalangeal
    Left ØRWV
    Right ØRWU
  Metatarsal-Phalangeal
    Left ØSWN
    Right ØSWM
  Occipital-cervical ØRWØ
  Sacrococcygeal ØSW5
  Sacroiliac
    Left ØSW8
    Right ØSW7
  Shoulder
    Left ØRWK
    Right ØRWJ
  Sternoclavicular
    Left ØRWF
    Right ØRWE
  Tarsal
    Left ØSWJ
    Right ØSWH
  Tarsometatarsal
    Left ØSWL
    Right ØSWK
  Temporomandibular
    Left ØRWD
    Right ØRWC
  Thoracic Vertebral ØRW6
  Thoracolumbar Vertebral ØRWA
  Toe Phalangeal
    Left ØSWQ
    Right ØSWP
  Wrist
    Left ØRWP
    Right ØRWN
Kidney ØTW5
Larynx ØCWS
Lens
  Left Ø8WK
  Right Ø8WJ
Liver ØFWØ
Lung
  Left ØBWL
  Right ØBWK
Lymphatic Ø7WN
  Thoracic Duct Ø7WK
Mediastinum ØWWC
Mesentery ØDWV
Metacarpal
  Left ØPWQ
  Right ØPWP
Metatarsal
  Left ØQWP
  Right ØQWN
Mouth and Throat ØCWY
Muscle
  Extraocular
    Left Ø8WM
    Right Ø8WL
  Lower ØKWY
  Upper ØKWX
Nasal Mucosa and Soft Tissue Ø9WK
Neck ØWW6
Nerve
  Cranial ØØWE
  Peripheral Ø1WY
Omentum ØDWU
Ovary ØUW3
Pancreas ØFWG
Parathyroid Gland ØGWR
Patella
  Left ØQWF
  Right ØQWD
Pelvic Cavity ØWWJ
Penis ØVWS
Pericardial Cavity ØWWD

Revision of device in — *continued*
Perineum
  Female ØWWN
  Male ØWWM
Peritoneal Cavity ØWWG
Peritoneum ØDWW
Phalanx
  Finger
    Left ØPWV
    Right ØPWT
  Thumb
    Left ØPWS
    Right ØPWR
  Toe
    Left ØQWR
    Right ØQWQ
Pineal Body ØGW1
Pleura ØBWQ
Pleural Cavity
  Left ØWWB
  Right ØWW9
Prostate and Seminal Vesicles ØVW4
Radius
  Left ØPWJ
  Right ØPWH
Respiratory Tract ØWWQ
Retroperitoneum ØWWH
Ribs
  1 to 2 ØPW1
  3 or More ØPW2
Sacrum ØQW1
Scapula
  Left ØPW6
  Right ØPW5
Scrotum and Tunica Vaginalis ØVW8
Septum
  Atrial Ø2W5
  Ventricular Ø2WM
Sinus Ø9WY
Skin ØHWPX
Skull ØNWØ
Spinal Canal ØØWU
Spinal Cord ØØWV
Spleen Ø7WP
Sternum ØPWØ
Stomach ØDW6
Subcutaneous Tissue and Fascia
  Head and Neck ØJWS
  Lower Extremity ØJWW
  Trunk ØJWT
  Upper Extremity ØJWV
Tarsal
  Left ØQWM
  Right ØQWL
Tendon
  Lower ØLWY
  Upper ØLWX
Testis ØVWD
Thymus Ø7WM
Thyroid Gland ØGWK
Tibia
  Left ØQWH
  Right ØQWG
Toe Nail ØHWRX
Trachea ØBW1
Tracheobronchial Tree ØBWØ
Tympanic Membrane
  Left Ø9W8
  Right Ø9W7
Ulna
  Left ØPWL
  Right ØPWK
Ureter ØTW9
Urethra ØTWD
Uterus and Cervix ØUWD
Vagina and Cul-de-sac ØUWH
Valve
  Aortic Ø2WF
  Mitral Ø2WG
  Pulmonary Ø2WH
  Tricuspid Ø2WJ
Vas Deferens ØVWR
Vein
  Azygos Ø5WØ
  Innominate
    Left Ø5W4
    Right Ø5W3
  Lower Ø6WY
  Upper Ø5WY

Revision of device in — *continued*
Vertebra
  Cervical ØPW3
  Lumbar ØQWØ
  Thoracic ØPW4
Vulva ØUWM
Revo MRI™ SureScan® pacemaker *use* Pacemaker, Dual Chamber in ØJH
rhBMP-2 *use* Recombinant Bone Morphogenetic Protein
Rheos® System device *use* Stimulator Generator in Subcutaneous Tissue and Fascia
Rheos® System lead *use* Stimulator Lead in Upper Arteries
Rhinopharynx *use* Nasopharynx
Rhinoplasty
  see Alteration, Nasal Mucosa and Soft Tissue Ø9ØK
  see Repair, Nasal Mucosa and Soft Tissue Ø9QK
  see Replacement, Nasal Mucosa and Soft Tissue Ø9RK
  see Supplement, Nasal Mucosa and Soft Tissue Ø9UK
Rhinorrhaphy *see* Repair, Nasal Mucosa and Soft Tissue Ø9QK
Rhinoscopy Ø9JKXZZ
Rhizotomy
  see Division, Central Nervous System and Cranial Nerves ØØ8
  see Division, Peripheral Nervous System Ø18
Rhomboid major muscle
  use Trunk Muscle, Left
  use Trunk Muscle, Right
Rhomboid minor muscle
  use Trunk Muscle, Left
  use Trunk Muscle, Right
Rhythm electrocardiogram *see* Measurement, Cardiac 4AØ2
Rhytidectomy *see* Alteration, Face ØWØ2
Right ascending lumbar vein *use* Azygos Vein
Right atrioventricular valve *use* Tricuspid Valve
Right auricular appendix *use* Atrium, Right
Right colic vein *use* Colic Vein
Right coronary sulcus *use* Heart, Right
Right gastric artery *use* Gastric Artery
Right gastroepiploic vein *use* Superior Mesenteric Vein
Right inferior phrenic vein *use* Inferior Vena Cava
Right inferior pulmonary vein *use* Pulmonary Vein, Right
Right jugular trunk *use* Lymphatic, Right Neck
Right lateral ventricle *use* Cerebral Ventricle
Right lymphatic duct *use* Lymphatic, Right Neck
Right ovarian vein *use* Inferior Vena Cava
Right second lumbar vein *use* Inferior Vena Cava
Right subclavian trunk *use* Lymphatic, Right Neck
Right subcostal vein *use* Azygos Vein
Right superior pulmonary vein *use* Pulmonary Vein, Right
Right suprarenal vein *use* Inferior Vena Cava
Right testicular vein *use* Inferior Vena Cava
Rima glottidis *use* Larynx
Risorius muscle *use* Facial Muscle
RNS System lead *use* Neurostimulator Lead in Central Nervous System and Cranial Nerves
RNS system neurostimulator generator *use* Neurostimulator Generator in Head and Facial Bones
Robotic Assisted Procedure
  Extremity
    Lower 8EØY
    Upper 8EØX
  Head and Neck Region 8EØ9
  Trunk Region 8EØW
Robotic Waterjet Ablation, Destruction, Prostate XV5Ø8A4
Rotation of fetal head
  Forceps 1ØSØ7ZZ
  Manual 1ØSØXZZ
Round ligament of uterus *use* Uterine Supporting Structure
Round window
  use Inner Ear, Left
  use Inner Ear, Right
Roux-en-Y operation
  see Bypass, Gastrointestinal System ØD1
  see Bypass, Hepatobiliary System and Pancreas ØF1

Rupture

Adhesions *see* Release
Fluid collection *see* Drainage
Ruxolitinib XW0DXT5

S

Sacral ganglion *use* Sacral Sympathetic Nerve
Sacral lymph node *use* Lymphatic, Pelvis
Sacral nerve modulation (SNM) lead *use* Stimulator Lead in Urinary System
Sacral neuromodulation lead *use* Stimulator Lead in Urinary System
Sacral splanchnic nerve *use* Sacral Sympathetic Nerve
Sacrectomy *see* Excision, Lower Bones 0QB
Sacrococcygeal ligament *use* Lower Spine Bursa and Ligament
Sacrococcygeal symphysis *use* Sacrococcygeal Joint
Sacroiliac ligament *use* Lower Spine Bursa and Ligament
Sacrospinous ligament *use* Lower Spine Bursa and Ligament
Sacrotuberous ligament *use* Lower Spine Bursa and Ligament
Salpingectomy
see Excision, Female Reproductive System 0UB
see Resection, Female Reproductive System 0UT
Salpingolysis *see* Release, Female Reproductive System 0UN
Salpingopexy
see Repair, Female Reproductive System 0UQ
see Reposition, Female Reproductive System 0US
Salpingopharyngeus muscle *use* Tongue, Palate, Pharynx Muscle
Salpingoplasty
see Repair, Female Reproductive System 0UQ
see Supplement, Female Reproductive System 0UU
Salpingorrhaphy *see* Repair, Female Reproductive System 0UQ
Salpingoscopy 0UJ88ZZ
Salpingostomy *see* Drainage, Female Reproductive System 0U9
Salpingotomy *see* Drainage, Female Reproductive System 0U9
Salpinx
use Fallopian Tube, Left
use Fallopian Tube, Right
Saphenous nerve *use* Femoral Nerve
SAPIEN transcatheter aortic valve *use* Zooplastic Tissue in Heart and Great Vessels
Sarilumab XW0
SARS-CoV-2 Antibody Detection, Serum/Plasma Nanoparticle Fluorescence XXE5XV7
SARS-CoV-2 Polymerase Chain Reaction, Nasopharyngeal Fluid XXE97U7
Sartorius muscle
use Upper Leg Muscle, Left
use Upper Leg Muscle, Right
Satralizumab-mwge XW01397
SAVAL below-the-knee (BTK) drug-eluting stent system
use Intraluminal Device, Sustained Release Drug-eluting in New Technology
use Intraluminal Device, Sustained Release Drug-eluting, Two in New Technology
use Intraluminal Device, Sustained Release Drug-eluting, Three in New Technology
use Intraluminal Device, Sustained Release Drug-eluting, Four or More in New Technology
Scalene muscle
use Neck Muscle, Left
use Neck Muscle, Right
Scan
Computerized Tomography (CT) *see* Computerized Tomography (CT Scan)
Radioisotope *see* Planar Nuclear Medicine Imaging
Scaphoid bone
use Carpal, Left
use Carpal, Right
Scapholunate ligament
use Wrist Bursa and Ligament, Left
use Wrist Bursa and Ligament, Right
Scaphotrapezium ligament
use Hand Bursa and Ligament, Left
use Hand Bursa and Ligament, Right

Scapulectomy
see Excision, Upper Bones 0PB
see Resection, Upper Bones 0PT
Scapulopexy
see Repair, Upper Bones 0PQ
see Reposition, Upper Bones 0PS
Scarpa's (vestibular) ganglion *use* Acoustic Nerve
Sclerectomy *see* Excision, Eye 08B
Sclerotherapy, mechanical *see* Destruction
Sclerotherapy, via injection of sclerosing agent
see Introduction, Destructive Agent
Sclerotomy *see* Drainage, Eye 089
Scrotectomy
see Excision, Male Reproductive System 0VB
see Resection, Male Reproductive System 0VT
Scrotoplasty
see Repair, Male Reproductive System 0VQ
see Supplement, Male Reproductive System 0VU
Scrotorrhaphy *see* Repair, Male Reproductive System 0VQ
Scrototomy *see* Drainage, Male Reproductive System 0V9
Sebaceous gland *use* Skin
Second cranial nerve *use* Optic Nerve
Section, cesarean *see* Extraction, Pregnancy 10D
Secura (DR) (VR) *use* Defibrillator Generator in 0JH
Sella turcica *use* Sphenoid Bone
Semicircular canal
use Inner Ear, Left
use Inner Ear, Right
Semimembranosus muscle
use Upper Leg Muscle, Left
use Upper Leg Muscle, Right
Semitendinosus muscle
use Upper Leg Muscle, Left
use Upper Leg Muscle, Right
Sentinel™ Cerebral Protection System (CPS) X2A5312
Seprafilm *use* Adhesion Barrier
Septal cartilage *use* Nasal Septum
Septectomy
see Excision, Ear, Nose, Sinus 09B
see Excision, Heart and Great Vessels 02B
see Resection, Ear, Nose, Sinus 09T
see Resection, Heart and Great Vessels 02T
Septoplasty
see Repair, Ear, Nose, Sinus 09Q
see Repair, Heart and Great Vessels 02Q
see Replacement, Ear, Nose, Sinus 09R
see Replacement, Heart and Great Vessels 02R
see Reposition, Ear, Nose, Sinus 09S
see Supplement, Ear, Nose, Sinus 09U
see Supplement, Heart and Great Vessels 02U
Septostomy, balloon atrial 02163Z7
Septotomy *see* Drainage, Ear, Nose, Sinus 099
Sequestrectomy, bone *see* Extirpation
Serratus anterior muscle
use Thorax Muscle, Left
use Thorax Muscle, Right
Serratus posterior muscle
use Trunk Muscle, Left
use Trunk Muscle, Right
Seventh cranial nerve *use* Facial Nerve
Shapshot_NIR 8E02XDZ
Sheffield hybrid external fixator
use External Fixation Device, Hybrid in 0PH
use External Fixation Device, Hybrid in 0PS
use External Fixation Device, Hybrid in 0QH
use External Fixation Device, Hybrid in 0QS
Sheffield ring external fixator
use External Fixation Device, Ring in 0PH
use External Fixation Device, Ring in 0PS
use External Fixation Device, Ring in 0QH
use External Fixation Device, Ring in 0QS
Shirodkar cervical cerclage 0UVC7ZZ
Shock Wave Therapy, Musculoskeletal 6A93
Shockwave Intravascular Lithotripsy (Shockwave IVL) *see* Fragmentation
Short gastric artery *use* Splenic Artery
Shortening
see Excision
see Repair
see Reposition
Shunt creation *see* Bypass
Sialoadenectomy
Complete *see* Resection, Mouth and Throat 0CT

Sialoadenectomy — *continued*
Partial *see* Excision, Mouth and Throat 0CB
Sialodochoplasty
see Repair, Mouth and Throat 0CQ
see Replacement, Mouth and Throat 0CR
see Supplement, Mouth and Throat 0CU
Sialoectomy
see Excision, Mouth and Throat 0CB
see Resection, Mouth and Throat 0CT
Sialography *see* Plain Radiography, Ear, Nose, Mouth and Throat B90
Sialolithotomy *see* Extirpation, Mouth and Throat 0CC
S-ICD™ lead *use* Subcutaneous Defibrillator Lead in Subcutaneous Tissue and Fascia
Sigmoid artery *use* Inferior Mesenteric Artery
Sigmoid flexure *use* Sigmoid Colon
Sigmoid vein *use* Inferior Mesenteric Vein
Sigmoidectomy
see Excision, Gastrointestinal System 0DB
see Resection, Gastrointestinal System 0DT
Sigmoidorrhaphy *see* Repair, Gastrointestinal System 0DQ
Sigmoidoscopy 0DJD8ZZ
Sigmoidotomy *see* Drainage, Gastrointestinal System 0D9
Single lead pacemaker (atrium) (ventricle) *use* Pacemaker, Single Chamber in 0JH
Single lead rate responsive pacemaker (atrium) (ventricle) *use* Pacemaker, Single Chamber Rate Responsive in 0JH
Single-use Duodenoscope XFJ
Single-use Oversleeve with Intraoperative Colonic Irrigation XDPH8K7
Sinoatrial node *use* Conduction Mechanism
Sinogram
Abdominal Wall *see* Fluoroscopy, Abdomen and Pelvis BW11
Chest Wall *see* Plain Radiography, Chest BW03
Retroperitoneum *see* Fluoroscopy, Abdomen and Pelvis BW11
Sinus venosus *use* Atrium, Right
Sinusectomy
see Excision, Ear, Nose, Sinus 09B
see Resection, Ear, Nose, Sinus 09T
Sinusoscopy 09JY4ZZ
Sinusotomy *see* Drainage, Ear, Nose, Sinus 099
Sirolimus-eluting coronary stent *use* Intraluminal Device, Drug-eluting in Heart and Great Vessels
Sixth cranial nerve *use* Abducens Nerve
Size reduction, breast *see* Excision, Skin and Breast 0HB
SJM Biocor® Stented Valve System *use* Zooplastic Tissue in Heart and Great Vessels
Skene's (paraurethral) gland *use* Vestibular Gland
Skin Substitute, Porcine Liver Derived, Replacement XHRPXL2
Sling
Fascial, orbicularis muscle (mouth) *see* Supplement, Muscle, Facial 0KU1
Levator muscle, for urethral suspension *see* Reposition, Bladder Neck 0TSC
Pubococcygeal, for urethral suspension *see* Reposition, Bladder Neck 0TSC
Rectum *see* Reposition, Rectum 0DSP
Small bowel series *see* Fluoroscopy, Bowel, Small BD13
Small saphenous vein
use Saphenous Vein, Left
use Saphenous Vein, Right
Snapshot_NIR 8E02XDZ
Snaring, polyp, colon *see* Excision, Gastrointestinal System 0DB
Solar (celiac) plexus *use* Abdominal Sympathetic Nerve
Soleus muscle
use Lower Leg Muscle, Left
use Lower Leg Muscle, Right
Soliris® *use* Eculizumab
Spacer
Insertion of device in
Disc
Lumbar Vertebral 0SH2
Lumbosacral 0SH4
Joint
Acromioclavicular
Left 0RHH
Right 0RHG

Spacer — *continued*
Insertion of device in — *continued*
  Joint — *continued*
    Ankle
      Left ØSHG
      Right ØSHF
    Carpal
      Left ØRHR
      Right ØRHQ
    Carpometacarpal
      Left ØRHT
      Right ØRHS
    Cervical Vertebral ØRH1
    Cervicothoracic Vertebral ØRH4
    Coccygeal ØSH6
    Elbow
      Left ØRHM
      Right ØRHL
    Finger Phalangeal
      Left ØRHX
      Right ØRHW
    Hip
      Left ØSHB
      Right ØSH9
    Knee
      Left ØSHD
      Right ØSHC
    Lumbar Vertebral ØSHØ
    Lumbosacral ØSH3
    Metacarpophalangeal
      Left ØRHV
      Right ØRHU
    Metatarsal-Phalangeal
      Left ØSHN
      Right ØSHM
    Occipital-cervical ØRHØ
    Sacrococcygeal ØSH5
    Sacroiliac
      Left ØSH8
      Right ØSH7
    Shoulder
      Left ØRHK
      Right ØRHJ
    Sternoclavicular
      Left ØRHF
      Right ØRHE
    Tarsal
      Left ØSHJ
      Right ØSHH
    Tarsometatarsal
      Left ØSHL
      Right ØSHK
    Temporomandibular
      Left ØRHD
      Right ØRHC
    Thoracic Vertebral ØRH6
    Thoracolumbar Vertebral ØRHA
    Toe Phalangeal
      Left ØSHQ
      Right ØSHP
    Wrist
      Left ØRHP
      Right ØRHN
Removal of device from
  Acromioclavicular
    Left ØRPH
    Right ØRPG
  Ankle
    Left ØSPG
    Right ØSPF
  Carpal
    Left ØRPR
    Right ØRPQ
  Carpometacarpal
    Left ØRPT
    Right ØRPS
  Cervical Vertebral ØRP1
  Cervicothoracic Vertebral ØRP4
  Coccygeal ØSP6
  Elbow
    Left ØRPM
    Right ØRPL
  Finger Phalangeal
    Left ØRPX
    Right ØRPW
  Hip
    Left ØSPB
    Right ØSP9

Spacer — *continued*
Removal of device from — *continued*
  Knee
    Left ØSPD
    Right ØSPC
  Lumbar Vertebral ØSPØ
  Lumbosacral ØSP3
  Metacarpophalangeal
    Left ØRPV
    Right ØRPU
  Metatarsal-Phalangeal
    Left ØSPN
    Right ØSPM
  Occipital-cervical ØRPØ
  Sacrococcygeal ØSP5
  Sacroiliac
    Left ØSP8
    Right ØSP7
  Shoulder
    Left ØRPK
    Right ØRPJ
  Sternoclavicular
    Left ØRPF
    Right ØRPE
  Tarsal
    Left ØSPJ
    Right ØSPH
  Tarsometatarsal
    Left ØSPL
    Right ØSPK
  Temporomandibular
    Left ØRPD
    Right ØRPC
  Thoracic Vertebral ØRP6
  Thoracolumbar Vertebral ØRPA
  Toe Phalangeal
    Left ØSPQ
    Right ØSPP
  Wrist
    Left ØRPP
    Right ØRPN
Revision of device in
  Acromioclavicular
    Left ØRWH
    Right ØRWG
  Ankle
    Left ØSWG
    Right ØSWF
  Carpal
    Left ØRWR
    Right ØRWQ
  Carpometacarpal
    Left ØRWT
    Right ØRWS
  Cervical Vertebral ØRW1
  Cervicothoracic Vertebral ØRW4
  Coccygeal ØSW6
  Elbow
    Left ØRWM
    Right ØRWL
  Finger Phalangeal
    Left ØRWX
    Right ØRWW
  Hip
    Left ØSWB
    Right ØSW9
  Knee
    Left ØSWD
    Right ØSWC
  Lumbar Vertebral ØSWØ
  Lumbosacral ØSW3
  Metacarpophalangeal
    Left ØRWV
    Right ØRWU
  Metatarsal-Phalangeal
    Left ØSWN
    Right ØSWM
  Occipital-cervical ØRWØ
  Sacrococcygeal ØSW5
  Sacroiliac
    Left ØSW8
    Right ØSW7
  Shoulder
    Left ØRWK
    Right ØRWJ
  Sternoclavicular
    Left ØRWF
    Right ØRWE

Spacer — *continued*
Revision of device in — *continued*
  Tarsal
    Left ØSWJ
    Right ØSWH
  Tarsometatarsal
    Left ØSWL
    Right ØSWK
  Temporomandibular
    Left ØRWD
    Right ØRWC
  Thoracic Vertebral ØRW6
  Thoracolumbar Vertebral ØRWA
  Toe Phalangeal
    Left ØSWQ
    Right ØSWP
  Wrist
    Left ØRWP
    Right ØRWN
Spacer, Articulating (Antibiotic) *use* Articulating Spacer in Lower Joints
Spacer, Static (Antibiotic) *use* Spacer in Lower Joints
Spectroscopy
  Intravascular Near Infrared 8E023DZ
  Near Infrared *see* Physiological Systems and Anatomical Regions 8EØ
Speech Assessment FØØ
Speech therapy *see* Speech Treatment, Rehabilitation FØ6
Speech Treatment FØ6
Sphenoidectomy
  see Excision, Ear, Nose, Sinus Ø9B
  see Excision, Head and Facial Bones ØNB
  see Resection, Ear, Nose, Sinus Ø9T
  see Resection, Head and Facial Bones ØNT
Sphenoidotomy *see* Drainage, Ear, Nose, Sinus Ø99
Sphenomandibular ligament *use* Head and Neck Bursa and Ligament
Sphenopalatine (pterygopalatine) ganglion *use* Head and Neck Sympathetic Nerve
Sphincterorrhaphy, anal *see* Repair, Anal Sphincter ØDQR
Sphincterotomy, anal
  see Division, Anal Sphincter ØD8R
  see Drainage, Anal Sphincter ØD9R
Spinal cord neurostimulator lead *use* Neurostimulator Lead in Central Nervous System and Cranial Nerves
Spinal growth rods, magnetically controlled *use* Magnetically Controlled Growth Rod(s) in New Technology
Spinal nerve, cervical *use* Cervical Nerve
Spinal nerve, lumbar *use* Lumbar Nerve
Spinal nerve, sacral *use* Sacral Nerve
Spinal nerve, thoracic *use* Thoracic Nerve
Spinal Stabilization Device
  Facet Replacement
    Cervical Vertebral ØRH1
    Cervicothoracic Vertebral ØRH4
    Lumbar Vertebral ØSHØ
    Lumbosacral ØSH3
    Occipital-cervical ØRHØ
    Thoracic Vertebral ØRH6
    Thoracolumbar Vertebral ØRHA
  Interspinous Process
    Cervical Vertebral ØRH1
    Cervicothoracic Vertebral ØRH4
    Lumbar Vertebral ØSHØ
    Lumbosacral ØSH3
    Occipital-cervical ØRHØ
    Thoracic Vertebral ØRH6
    Thoracolumbar Vertebral ØRHA
  Pedicle-Based
    Cervical Vertebral ØRH1
    Cervicothoracic Vertebral ØRH4
    Lumbar Vertebral ØSHØ
    Lumbosacral ØSH3
    Occipital-cervical ØRHØ
    Thoracic Vertebral ØRH6
    Thoracolumbar Vertebral ØRHA
SpineJack® system *use* Synthetic Substitute, Mechanically Expandable (Paired) in New Technology
Spinous process
  use Cervical Vertebra
  use Lumbar Vertebra
  use Thoracic Vertebra
Spiral ganglion *use* Acoustic Nerve

Spiration IBV™ Valve System *use* Intraluminal Device, Endobronchial Valve in Respiratory System
Splenectomy
  see Excision, Lymphatic and Hemic Systems 07B
  see Resection, Lymphatic and Hemic Systems 07T
Splenic flexure *use* Transverse Colon
Splenic plexus *use* Abdominal Sympathetic Nerve
Splenius capitis muscle *use* Head Muscle
Splenius cervicis muscle
  use Neck Muscle, Left
  use Neck Muscle, Right
Splenolysis *see* Release, Lymphatic and Hemic Systems 07N
Splenopexy
  see Repair, Lymphatic and Hemic Systems 07Q
  see Reposition, Lymphatic and Hemic Systems 07S
Splenoplasty *see* Repair, Lymphatic and Hemic Systems 07Q
Splenorrhaphy *see* Repair, Lymphatic and Hemic Systems 07Q
Splenotomy *see* Drainage, Lymphatic and Hemic Systems 079
Splinting, musculoskeletal *see* Immobilization, Anatomical Regions 2W3
SPRAVATO™ *use* Esketamine Hydrochloride
SPY PINPOINT fluorescence imaging system
  see Monitoring, Physiological Systems 4A1
  see Other Imaging, Hepatobiliary System and Pancreas BF5
SPY system intraoperative fluorescence cholangiography *see* Other Imaging, Hepatobiliary System and Pancreas BF5
SPY system intravascular fluorescence angiography *see* Monitoring, Physiological Systems 4A1
Staged hepatectomy
  see Division, Hepatobiliary System and Pancreas 0F8
  see Resection, Hepatobiliary System and Pancreas 0FT
Stapedectomy
  see Excision, Ear, Nose, Sinus 09B
  see Resection, Ear, Nose, Sinus 09T
Stapediolysis *see* Release, Ear, Nose, Sinus 09N
Stapedioplasty
  see Repair, Ear, Nose, Sinus 09Q
  see Replacement, Ear, Nose, Sinus 09R
  see Supplement, Ear, Nose, Sinus 09U
Stapedotomy *see* Drainage, Ear, Nose, Sinus 099
Stapes
  use Auditory Ossicle, Left
  use Auditory Ossicle, Right
Static Spacer (Antibiotic) *use* Spacer in Lower Joints
STELARA® *use* Other New Technology Therapeutic Substance
Stellate ganglion *use* Head and Neck Sympathetic Nerve
Stem cell transplant *see* Transfusion, Circulatory 302
Stensen's duct
  use Parotid Duct, Left
  use Parotid Duct, Right
Stent, intraluminal (cardiovascular) (gastrointestinal) (hepatobiliary) (urinary) *use* Intraluminal Device
Stent retriever thrombectomy *see* Extirpation, Upper Arteries 03C
Stented tissue valve *use* Zooplastic Tissue in Heart and Great Vessels
Stereotactic Radiosurgery
  Abdomen DW23
  Adrenal Gland DG22
  Bile Ducts DF22
  Bladder DT22
  Bone Marrow D720
  Brain D020
  Brain Stem D021
  Breast
    Left DM20
    Right DM21
  Bronchus DB21
  Cervix DU21
  Chest DW22
  Chest Wall DB27
  Colon DD25
  Diaphragm DB28
  Duodenum DD22
  Ear D920
  Esophagus DD20

Stereotactic Radiosurgery — *continued*
  Eye D820
  Gallbladder DF21
  Gamma Beam
    Abdomen DW23JZZ
    Adrenal Gland DG22JZZ
    Bile Ducts DF22JZZ
    Bladder DT22JZZ
    Bone Marrow D720JZZ
    Brain D020JZZ
    Brain Stem D021JZZ
    Breast
      Left DM20JZZ
      Right DM21JZZ
    Bronchus DB21JZZ
    Cervix DU21JZZ
    Chest DW22JZZ
    Chest Wall DB27JZZ
    Colon DD25JZZ
    Diaphragm DB28JZZ
    Duodenum DD22JZZ
    Ear D920JZZ
    Esophagus DD20JZZ
    Eye D820JZZ
    Gallbladder DF21JZZ
    Gland
      Adrenal DG22JZZ
      Parathyroid DG24JZZ
      Pituitary DG20JZZ
      Thyroid DG25JZZ
    Glands, Salivary D926JZZ
    Head and Neck DW21JZZ
    Ileum DD24JZZ
    Jejunum DD23JZZ
    Kidney DT20JZZ
    Larynx D92BJZZ
    Liver DF20JZZ
    Lung DB22JZZ
    Lymphatics
      Abdomen D726JZZ
      Axillary D724JZZ
      Inguinal D728JZZ
      Neck D723JZZ
      Pelvis D727JZZ
      Thorax D725JZZ
    Mediastinum DB26JZZ
    Mouth D924JZZ
    Nasopharynx D92DJZZ
    Neck and Head DW21JZZ
    Nerve, Peripheral D027JZZ
    Nose D921JZZ
    Ovary DU20JZZ
    Palate
      Hard D928JZZ
      Soft D929JZZ
    Pancreas DF23JZZ
    Parathyroid Gland DG24JZZ
    Pelvic Region DW26JZZ
    Pharynx D92CJZZ
    Pineal Body DG21JZZ
    Pituitary Gland DG20JZZ
    Pleura DB25JZZ
    Prostate DV20JZZ
    Rectum DD27JZZ
    Sinuses D927JZZ
    Spinal Cord D026JZZ
    Spleen D722JZZ
    Stomach DD21JZZ
    Testis DV21JZZ
    Thymus D721JZZ
    Thyroid Gland DG25JZZ
    Tongue D925JZZ
    Trachea DB20JZZ
    Ureter DT21JZZ
    Urethra DT23JZZ
    Uterus DU22JZZ
  Gland
    Adrenal DG22
    Parathyroid DG24
    Pituitary DG20
    Thyroid DG25
  Glands, Salivary D926
  Head and Neck DW21
  Ileum DD24
  Jejunum DD23
  Kidney DT20
  Larynx D92B
  Liver DF20
  Lung DB22

Stereotactic Radiosurgery — *continued*
  Lymphatics
    Abdomen D726
    Axillary D724
    Inguinal D728
    Neck D723
    Pelvis D727
    Thorax D725
  Mediastinum DB26
  Mouth D924
  Nasopharynx D92D
  Neck and Head DW21
  Nerve, Peripheral D027
  Nose D921
  Other Photon
    Abdomen DW23DZZ
    Adrenal Gland DG22DZZ
    Bile Ducts DF22DZZ
    Bladder DT22DZZ
    Bone Marrow D720DZZ
    Brain D020DZZ
    Brain Stem D021DZZ
    Breast
      Left DM20DZZ
      Right DM21DZZ
    Bronchus DB21DZZ
    Cervix DU21DZZ
    Chest DW22DZZ
    Chest Wall DB27DZZ
    Colon DD25DZZ
    Diaphragm DB28DZZ
    Duodenum DD22DZZ
    Ear D920DZZ
    Esophagus DD20DZZ
    Eye D820DZZ
    Gallbladder DF21DZZ
    Gland
      Adrenal DG22DZZ
      Parathyroid DG24DZZ
      Pituitary DG20DZZ
      Thyroid DG25DZZ
    Glands, Salivary D926DZZ
    Head and Neck DW21DZZ
    Ileum DD24DZZ
    Jejunum DD23DZZ
    Kidney DT20DZZ
    Larynx D92BDZZ
    Liver DF20DZZ
    Lung DB22DZZ
    Lymphatics
      Abdomen D726DZZ
      Axillary D724DZZ
      Inguinal D728DZZ
      Neck D723DZZ
      Pelvis D727DZZ
      Thorax D725DZZ
    Mediastinum DB26DZZ
    Mouth D924DZZ
    Nasopharynx D92DDZZ
    Neck and Head DW21DZZ
    Nerve, Peripheral D027DZZ
    Nose D921DZZ
    Ovary DU20DZZ
    Palate
      Hard D928DZZ
      Soft D929DZZ
    Pancreas DF23DZZ
    Parathyroid Gland DG24DZZ
    Pelvic Region DW26DZZ
    Pharynx D92CDZZ
    Pineal Body DG21DZZ
    Pituitary Gland DG20DZZ
    Pleura DB25DZZ
    Prostate DV20DZZ
    Rectum DD27DZZ
    Sinuses D927DZZ
    Spinal Cord D026DZZ
    Spleen D722DZZ
    Stomach DD21DZZ
    Testis DV21DZZ
    Thymus D721DZZ
    Thyroid Gland DG25DZZ
    Tongue D925DZZ
    Trachea DB20DZZ
    Ureter DT21DZZ
    Urethra DT23DZZ
    Uterus DU22DZZ
  Ovary DU20

Stereotactic Radiosurgery — *continued*
  Palate
    Hard D928
    Soft D929
  Pancreas DF23
  Parathyroid Gland DG24
  Particulate
    Abdomen DW23HZZ
    Adrenal Gland DG22HZZ
    Bile Ducts DF22HZZ
    Bladder DT22HZZ
    Bone Marrow D720HZZ
    Brain D020HZZ
    Brain Stem D021HZZ
    Breast
      Left DM20HZZ
      Right DM21HZZ
    Bronchus DB21HZZ
    Cervix DU21HZZ
    Chest DW22HZZ
    Chest Wall DB27HZZ
    Colon DD25HZZ
    Diaphragm DB28HZZ
    Duodenum DD22HZZ
    Ear D920HZZ
    Esophagus DD20HZZ
    Eye D820HZZ
    Gallbladder DF21HZZ
    Gland
      Adrenal DG22HZZ
      Parathyroid DG24HZZ
      Pituitary DG20HZZ
      Thyroid DG25HZZ
    Glands, Salivary D926HZZ
    Head and Neck DW21HZZ
    Ileum DD24HZZ
    Jejunum DD23HZZ
    Kidney DT20HZZ
    Larynx D92BHZZ
    Liver DF20HZZ
    Lung DB22HZZ
    Lymphatics
      Abdomen D726HZZ
      Axillary D724HZZ
      Inguinal D728HZZ
      Neck D723HZZ
      Pelvis D727HZZ
      Thorax D725HZZ
    Mediastinum DB26HZZ
    Mouth D924HZZ
    Nasopharynx D92DHZZ
    Neck and Head DW21HZZ
    Nerve, Peripheral D027HZZ
    Nose D921HZZ
    Ovary DU20HZZ
    Palate
      Hard D928HZZ
      Soft D929HZZ
    Pancreas DF23HZZ
    Parathyroid Gland DG24HZZ
    Pelvic Region DW26HZZ
    Pharynx D92CHZZ
    Pineal Body DG21HZZ
    Pituitary Gland DG20HZZ
    Pleura DB25HZZ
    Prostate DV20HZZ
    Rectum DD27HZZ
    Sinuses D927HZZ
    Spinal Cord D026HZZ
    Spleen D722HZZ
    Stomach DD21HZZ
    Testis DV21HZZ
    Thymus D721HZZ
    Thyroid Gland DG25HZZ
    Tongue D925HZZ
    Trachea DB20HZZ
    Ureter DT21HZZ
    Urethra DT23HZZ
    Uterus DU22HZZ
  Pelvic Region DW26
  Pharynx D92C
  Pineal Body DG21
  Pituitary Gland DG20
  Pleura DB25
  Prostate DV20
  Rectum DD27
  Sinuses D927
  Spinal Cord D026
  Spleen D722

Stereotactic Radiosurgery — *continued*
  Stomach DD21
  Testis DV21
  Thymus D721
  Thyroid Gland DG25
  Tongue D925
  Trachea DB20
  Ureter DT21
  Urethra DT23
  Uterus DU22
Steripath® Micro™ Blood Collection System
  XXE5XR7
Sternoclavicular ligament
  use Shoulder Bursa and Ligament, Left
  use Shoulder Bursa and Ligament, Right
Sternocleidomastoid artery
  use Thyroid Artery, Left
  use Thyroid Artery, Right
Sternocleidomastoid muscle
  use Neck Muscle, Left
  use Neck Muscle, Right
Sternocostal ligament *use* Sternum Bursa and Ligament
Sternotomy
  see Division, Sternum 0P80
  see Drainage, Sternum 0P90
Stimulation, cardiac
  Cardioversion 5A2204Z
  Electrophysiologic testing *see* Measurement, Cardiac 4A02
Stimulator Generator
  Insertion of device in
    Abdomen 0JH8
    Back 0JH7
    Chest 0JH6
  Multiple Array
    Abdomen 0JH8
    Back 0JH7
    Chest 0JH6
  Multiple Array Rechargeable
    Abdomen 0JH8
    Back 0JH7
    Chest 0JH6
  Removal of device from, Subcutaneous Tissue and Fascia, Trunk 0JPT
  Revision of device in, Subcutaneous Tissue and Fascia, Trunk 0JWT
  Single Array
    Abdomen 0JH8
    Back 0JH7
    Chest 0JH6
  Single Array Rechargeable
    Abdomen 0JH8
    Back 0JH7
    Chest 0JH6
Stimulator Lead
  Insertion of device in
    Anal Sphincter 0DHR
    Artery
      Left 03HL
      Right 03HK
    Bladder 0THB
    Muscle
      Lower 0KHY
      Upper 0KHX
    Stomach 0DH6
    Ureter 0TH9
  Removal of device from
    Anal Sphincter 0DPR
    Artery, Upper 03PY
    Bladder 0TPB
    Muscle
      Lower 0KPY
      Upper 0KPX
    Stomach 0DP6
    Ureter 0TP9
  Revision of device in
    Anal Sphincter 0DWR
    Artery, Upper 03WY
    Bladder 0TWB
    Muscle
      Lower 0KWY
      Upper 0KWX
    Stomach 0DW6
    Ureter 0TW9
Stoma
  Excision
    Abdominal Wall 0WBFXZ2

Stoma — *continued*
  Excision — *continued*
    Neck 0WB6XZ2
  Repair
    Abdominal Wall 0WQFXZ2
    Neck 0WQ6XZ2
Stomatoplasty
  see Repair, Mouth and Throat 0CQ
  see Replacement, Mouth and Throat 0CR
  see Supplement, Mouth and Throat 0CU
Stomatorrhaphy *see* Repair, Mouth and Throat 0CQ
StrataGraft® *use* Bioengineered Allogeneic Construct
Stratos LV *use* Cardiac Resynchronization Pacemaker Pulse Generator in 0JH
Stress test 4A02XM4, 4A12XM4
Stripping *see* Extraction
Study
  Electrophysiologic stimulation, cardiac *see* Measurement, Cardiac 4A02
  Ocular motility 4A07X7Z
  Pulmonary airway flow measurement *see* Measurement, Respiratory 4A09
  Visual acuity 4A07X0Z
Styloglossus muscle *use* Tongue, Palate, Pharynx Muscle
Stylomandibular ligament *use* Head and Neck Bursa and Ligament
Stylopharyngeus muscle *use* Tongue, Palate, Pharynx Muscle
Subacromial bursa
  use Shoulder Bursa and Ligament, Left
  use Shoulder Bursa and Ligament, Right
Subaortic (common iliac) lymph node *use* Lymphatic, Pelvis
Subarachnoid space, spinal *use* Spinal Canal
Subclavicular (apical) lymph node
  use Lymphatic, Left Axillary
  use Lymphatic, Right Axillary
Subclavius muscle
  use Thorax Muscle, Left
  use Thorax Muscle, Right
Subclavius nerve *use* Brachial Plexus
Subcostal artery *use* Upper Artery
Subcostal muscle
  use Thorax Muscle, Left
  use Thorax Muscle, Right
Subcostal nerve *use* Thoracic Nerve
Subcutaneous Defibrillator Lead
  Insertion of device in, Subcutaneous Tissue and Fascia, Chest 0JH6
  Removal of device from, Subcutaneous Tissue and Fascia, Trunk 0JPT
  Revision of device in, Subcutaneous Tissue and Fascia, Trunk 0JWT
Subcutaneous injection reservoir, port *use* Vascular Access Device, Totally Implantable in Subcutaneous Tissue and Fascia
Subcutaneous injection reservoir, pump *use* Infusion Device, Pump in Subcutaneous Tissue and Fascia
Subdermal progesterone implant *use* Contraceptive Device in Subcutaneous Tissue and Fascia
Subdural space, spinal *use* Spinal Canal
Submandibular ganglion
  use Facial Nerve
  use Head and Neck Sympathetic Nerve
Submandibular gland
  use Submaxillary Gland, Left
  use Submaxillary Gland, Right
Submandibular lymph node *use* Lymphatic, Head
Submandibular space *use* Subcutaneous Tissue and Fascia, Face
Submaxillary ganglion *use* Head and Neck Sympathetic Nerve
Submaxillary lymph node *use* Lymphatic, Head
Submental artery *use* Face Artery
Submental lymph node *use* Lymphatic, Head
Submucous (Meissner's) plexus *use* Abdominal Sympathetic Nerve
Suboccipital nerve *use* Cervical Nerve
Suboccipital venous plexus
  use Vertebral Vein, Left
  use Vertebral Vein, Right
Subparotid lymph node *use* Lymphatic, Head
Subscapular aponeurosis
  use Subcutaneous Tissue and Fascia, Left Upper Arm

Subscapular aponeurosis — *continued*
  use Subcutaneous Tissue and Fascia, Right Upper Arm
Subscapular artery
  use Axillary Artery, Left
  use Axillary Artery, Right
Subscapular (posterior) lymph node
  use Lymphatic, Axillary, Left
  use Lymphatic, Axillary, Right
Subscapularis muscle
  use Shoulder Muscle, Left
  use Shoulder Muscle, Right
Substance Abuse Treatment
  Counseling
    Family, for substance abuse, Other Family Counseling HZ63ZZZ
    Group
      12-Step HZ43ZZZ
      Behavioral HZ41ZZZ
      Cognitive HZ40ZZZ
      Cognitive-Behavioral HZ42ZZZ
      Confrontational HZ48ZZZ
      Continuing Care HZ49ZZZ
      Infectious Disease
        Post-Test HZ4CZZZ
        Pre-Test HZ4CZZZ
      Interpersonal HZ44ZZZ
      Motivational Enhancement HZ47ZZZ
      Psychoeducation HZ46ZZZ
      Spiritual HZ4BZZZ
      Vocational HZ45ZZZ
    Individual
      12-Step HZ33ZZZ
      Behavioral HZ31ZZZ
      Cognitive HZ30ZZZ
      Cognitive-Behavioral HZ32ZZZ
      Confrontational HZ38ZZZ
      Continuing Care HZ39ZZZ
      Infectious Disease
        Post-Test HZ3CZZZ
        Pre-Test HZ3CZZZ
      Interpersonal HZ34ZZZ
      Motivational Enhancement HZ37ZZZ
      Psychoeducation HZ36ZZZ
      Spiritual HZ3BZZZ
      Vocational HZ35ZZZ
  Detoxification Services, for substance abuse HZ2ZZZZ
  Medication Management
    Antabuse HZ83ZZZ
    Bupropion HZ87ZZZ
    Clonidine HZ86ZZZ
    Levo-alpha-acetyl-methadol (LAAM) HZ82ZZZ
    Methadone Maintenance HZ81ZZZ
    Naloxone HZ85ZZZ
    Naltrexone HZ84ZZZ
    Nicotine Replacement HZ80ZZZ
    Other Replacement Medication HZ89ZZZ
    Psychiatric Medication HZ88ZZZ
  Pharmacotherapy
    Antabuse HZ93ZZZ
    Bupropion HZ97ZZZ
    Clonidine HZ96ZZZ
    Levo-alpha-acetyl-methadol (LAAM) HZ92ZZZ
    Methadone Maintenance HZ91ZZZ
    Naloxone HZ95ZZZ
    Naltrexone HZ94ZZZ
    Nicotine Replacement HZ90ZZZ
    Psychiatric Medication HZ98ZZZ
    Replacement Medication, Other HZ99ZZZ
  Psychotherapy
    12-Step HZ53ZZZ
    Behavioral HZ51ZZZ
    Cognitive HZ50ZZZ
    Cognitive-Behavioral HZ52ZZZ
    Confrontational HZ58ZZZ
    Interactive HZ55ZZZ
    Interpersonal HZ54ZZZ
    Motivational Enhancement HZ57ZZZ
    Psychoanalysis HZ5BZZZ
    Psychodynamic HZ5CZZZ
    Psychoeducation HZ56ZZZ
    Psychophysiological HZ5DZZZ
    Supportive HZ59ZZZ
Substantia nigra *use* Basal Ganglia

Subtalar (talocalcaneal) joint
  use Tarsal Joint, Left
  use Tarsal Joint, Right
Subtalar ligament
  use Foot Bursa and Ligament, Left
  use Foot Bursa and Ligament, Right
Subthalamic nucleus *use* Basal Ganglia
Suction curettage (D&C), nonobstetric *see* Extraction, Endometrium 0UDB
Suction curettage, obstetric post-delivery *see* Extraction, Products of Conception, Retained 10D1
Superficial circumflex iliac vein
  use Saphenous Vein, Left
  use Saphenous Vein, Right
Superficial epigastric artery
  use Femoral Artery, Left
  use Femoral Artery, Right
Superficial epigastric vein
  use Saphenous Vein, Left
  use Saphenous Vein, Right
Superficial Inferior Epigastric Artery Flap
  Replacement
    Bilateral 0HRV078
    Left 0HRU078
    Right 0HRT078
  Transfer
    Left 0KXG
    Right 0KXF
Superficial palmar arch
  use Hand Artery, Left
  use Hand Artery, Right
Superficial palmar venous arch
  use Hand Vein, Left
  use Hand Vein, Right
Superficial temporal artery
  use Temporal Artery, Left
  use Temporal Artery, Right
Superficial transverse perineal muscle *use* Perineum Muscle
Superior cardiac nerve *use* Thoracic Sympathetic Nerve
Superior cerebellar vein *use* Intracranial Vein
Superior cerebral vein *use* Intracranial Vein
Superior clunic (cluneal) nerve *use* Lumbar Nerve
Superior epigastric artery
  use Internal Mammary Artery, Left
  use Internal Mammary Artery, Right
Superior genicular artery
  use Popliteal Artery, Left
  use Popliteal Artery, Right
Superior gluteal artery
  use Internal Iliac Artery, Left
  use Internal Iliac Artery, Right
Superior gluteal nerve *use* Lumbar Plexus
Superior hypogastric plexus *use* Abdominal Sympathetic Nerve
Superior labial artery *use* Face Artery
Superior laryngeal artery
  use Thyroid Artery, Left
  use Thyroid Artery, Right
Superior laryngeal nerve *use* Vagus Nerve
Superior longitudinal muscle *use* Tongue, Palate, Pharynx Muscle
Superior mesenteric ganglion *use* Abdominal Sympathetic Nerve
Superior mesenteric lymph node *use* Lymphatic, Mesenteric
Superior mesenteric plexus *use* Abdominal Sympathetic Nerve
Superior oblique muscle
  use Extraocular Muscle, Left
  use Extraocular Muscle, Right
Superior olivary nucleus *use* Pons
Superior rectal artery *use* Inferior Mesenteric Artery
Superior rectal vein *use* Inferior Mesenteric Vein
Superior rectus muscle
  use Extraocular Muscle, Left
  use Extraocular Muscle, Right
Superior tarsal plate
  use Upper Eyelid, Left
  use Upper Eyelid, Right
Superior thoracic artery
  use Axillary Artery, Left
  use Axillary Artery, Right
Superior thyroid artery
  use External Carotid Artery, Left
  use External Carotid Artery, Right

Superior thyroid artery — *continued*
  use Thyroid Artery, Left
  use Thyroid Artery, Right
Superior turbinate *use* Nasal Turbinate
Superior ulnar collateral artery
  use Brachial Artery, Left
  use Brachial Artery, Right
Supersaturated Oxygen therapy 5A0512C, 5A0522C
Supplement
  Abdominal Wall 0WUF
  Acetabulum
    Left 0QU5
    Right 0QU4
  Ampulla of Vater 0FUC
  Anal Sphincter 0DUR
  Ankle Region
    Left 0YUL
    Right 0YUK
  Anus 0DUQ
  Aorta
    Abdominal 04U0
    Thoracic
      Ascending/Arch 02UX
      Descending 02UW
  Arm
    Lower
      Left 0XUF
      Right 0XUD
    Upper
      Left 0XU9
      Right 0XU8
  Artery
    Anterior Tibial
      Left 04UQ
      Right 04UP
    Axillary
      Left 03U6
      Right 03U5
    Brachial
      Left 03U8
      Right 03U7
    Celiac 04U1
    Colic
      Left 04U7
      Middle 04U8
      Right 04U6
    Common Carotid
      Left 03UJ
      Right 03UH
    Common Iliac
      Left 04UD
      Right 04UC
    Coronary
      Four or More Arteries 02U3
      One Artery 02U0
      Three Arteries 02U2
      Two Arteries 02U1
    External Carotid
      Left 03UN
      Right 03UM
    External Iliac
      Left 04UJ
      Right 04UH
    Face 03UR
    Femoral
      Left 04UL
      Right 04UK
    Foot
      Left 04UW
      Right 04UV
    Gastric 04U2
    Hand
      Left 03UF
      Right 03UD
    Hepatic 04U3
    Inferior Mesenteric 04UB
    Innominate 03U2
    Internal Carotid
      Left 03UL
      Right 03UK
    Internal Iliac
      Left 04UF
      Right 04UE
    Internal Mammary
      Left 03U1
      Right 03U0
    Intracranial 03UG
    Lower 04UY

Supplement — *continued*
Artery — *continued*
Peroneal
Left Ø4UU
Right Ø4UT
Popliteal
Left Ø4UN
Right Ø4UM
Posterior Tibial
Left Ø4US
Right Ø4UR
Pulmonary
Left Ø2UR
Right Ø2UQ
Pulmonary Trunk Ø2UP
Radial
Left Ø3UC
Right Ø3UB
Renal
Left Ø4UA
Right Ø4U9
Splenic Ø4U4
Subclavian
Left Ø3U4
Right Ø3U3
Superior Mesenteric Ø4U5
Temporal
Left Ø3UT
Right Ø3US
Thyroid
Left Ø3UV
Right Ø3UU
Ulnar
Left Ø3UA
Right Ø3U9
Upper Ø3UY
Vertebral
Left Ø3UQ
Right Ø3UP
Atrium
Left Ø2U7
Right Ø2U6
Auditory Ossicle
Left Ø9UA
Right Ø9U9
Axilla
Left ØXU5
Right ØXU4
Back
Lower ØWUL
Upper ØWUK
Bladder ØTUB
Bladder Neck ØTUC
Bone
Ethmoid
Left ØNUG
Right ØNUF
Frontal ØNU1
Hyoid ØNUX
Lacrimal
Left ØNUJ
Right ØNUH
Nasal ØNUB
Occipital ØNU7
Palatine
Left ØNUL
Right ØNUK
Parietal
Left ØNU4
Right ØNU3
Pelvic
Left ØQU3
Right ØQU2
Sphenoid ØNUC
Temporal
Left ØNU6
Right ØNU5
Zygomatic
Left ØNUN
Right ØNUM
Breast
Bilateral ØHUV
Left ØHUU
Right ØHUT
Bronchus
Lingula ØBU9
Lower Lobe
Left ØBUB
Right ØBU6

Supplement — *continued*
Bronchus — *continued*
Main
Left ØBU7
Right ØBU3
Middle Lobe, Right ØBU5
Upper Lobe
Left ØBU8
Right ØBU4
Buccal Mucosa ØCU4
Bursa and Ligament
Abdomen
Left ØMUJ
Right ØMUH
Ankle
Left ØMUR
Right ØMUQ
Elbow
Left ØMU4
Right ØMU3
Foot
Left ØMUT
Right ØMUS
Hand
Left ØMU8
Right ØMU7
Head and Neck ØMUØ
Hip
Left ØMUM
Right ØMUL
Knee
Left ØMUP
Right ØMUN
Lower Extremity
Left ØMUW
Right ØMUV
Perineum ØMUK
Rib(s) ØMUG
Shoulder
Left ØMU2
Right ØMU1
Spine
Lower ØMUD
Upper ØMUC
Sternum ØMUF
Upper Extremity
Left ØMUB
Right ØMU9
Wrist
Left ØMU6
Right ØMU5
Buttock
Left ØYU1
Right ØYUØ
Carina ØBU2
Carpal
Left ØPUN
Right ØPUM
Cecum ØDUH
Cerebral Meninges ØØU1
Cerebral Ventricle ØØU6
Chest Wall ØWU8
Chordae Tendineae Ø2U9
Cisterna Chyli Ø7UL
Clavicle
Left ØPUB
Right ØPU9
Clitoris ØUUJ
Coccyx ØQUS
Colon
Ascending ØDUK
Descending ØDUM
Sigmoid ØDUN
Transverse ØDUL
Cord
Bilateral ØVUH
Left ØVUG
Right ØVUF
Cornea
Left Ø8U9
Right Ø8U8
Cul-de-sac ØUUF
Diaphragm ØBUT
Disc
Cervical Vertebral ØRU3
Cervicothoracic Vertebral ØRU5
Lumbar Vertebral ØSU2
Lumbosacral ØSU4
Thoracic Vertebral ØRU9

Supplement — *continued*
Disc — *continued*
Thoracolumbar Vertebral ØRUB
Duct
Common Bile ØFU9
Cystic ØFU8
Hepatic
Common ØFU7
Left ØFU6
Right ØFU5
Lacrimal
Left Ø8UY
Right Ø8UX
Pancreatic ØFUD
Accessory ØFUF
Duodenum ØDU9
Dura Mater ØØU2
Ear
External
Bilateral Ø9U2
Left Ø9U1
Right Ø9UØ
Inner
Left Ø9UE
Right Ø9UD
Middle
Left Ø9U6
Right Ø9U5
Elbow Region
Left ØXUC
Right ØXUB
Epididymis
Bilateral ØVUL
Left ØVUK
Right ØVUJ
Epiglottis ØCUR
Esophagogastric Junction ØDU4
Esophagus ØDU5
Lower ØDU3
Middle ØDU2
Upper ØDU1
Extremity
Lower
Left ØYUB
Right ØYU9
Upper
Left ØXU7
Right ØXU6
Eye
Left Ø8U1
Right Ø8UØ
Eyelid
Lower
Left Ø8UR
Right Ø8UQ
Upper
Left Ø8UP
Right Ø8UN
Face ØWU2
Fallopian Tube
Left ØUU6
Right ØUU5
Fallopian Tubes, Bilateral ØUU7
Femoral Region
Bilateral ØYUE
Left ØYU8
Right ØYU7
Femoral Shaft
Left ØQU9
Right ØQU8
Femur
Lower
Left ØQUC
Right ØQUB
Upper
Left ØQU7
Right ØQU6
Fibula
Left ØQUK
Right ØQUJ
Finger
Index
Left ØXUP
Right ØXUN
Little
Left ØXUW
Right ØXUV
Middle
Left ØXUR

Supplement — *continued*
Finger — *continued*
Middle — *continued*
Right ØXUQ
Ring
Left ØXUT
Right ØXUS
Foot
Left ØYUN
Right ØYUM
Gingiva
Lower ØCU6
Upper ØCU5
Glenoid Cavity
Left ØPU8
Right ØPU7
Hand
Left ØXUK
Right ØXUJ
Head ØWUØ
Heart Ø2UA
Humeral Head
Left ØPUD
Right ØPUC
Humeral Shaft
Left ØPUG
Right ØPUF
Hymen ØUUK
Ileocecal Valve ØDUC
Ileum ØDUB
Inguinal Region
Bilateral ØYUA
Left ØYU6
Right ØYU5
Intestine
Large ØDUE
Left ØDUG
Right ØDUF
Small ØDU8
Iris
Left Ø8UD
Right Ø8UC
Jaw
Lower ØWU5
Upper ØWU4
Jejunum ØDUA
Joint
Acromioclavicular
Left ØRUH
Right ØRUG
Ankle
Left ØSUG
Right ØSUF
Carpal
Left ØRUR
Right ØRUQ
Carpometacarpal
Left ØRUT
Right ØRUS
Cervical Vertebral ØRU1
Cervicothoracic Vertebral ØRU4
Coccygeal ØSU6
Elbow
Left ØRUM
Right ØRUL
Finger Phalangeal
Left ØRUX
Right ØRUW
Hip
Left ØSUB
Acetabular Surface ØSUE
Femoral Surface ØSUS
Right ØSU9
Acetabular Surface ØSUA
Femoral Surface ØSUR
Knee
Left ØSUD
Femoral Surface ØSUUØ9Z
Tibial Surface ØSUWØ9Z
Right ØSUC
Femoral Surface ØSUTØ9Z
Tibial Surface ØSUVØ9Z
Lumbar Vertebral ØSUØ
Lumbosacral ØSU3
Metacarpophalangeal
Left ØRUV
Right ØRUU
Metatarsal-Phalangeal
Left ØSUN

Supplement — *continued*
Joint — *continued*
Metatarsal-Phalangeal — *continued*
Right ØSUM
Occipital-cervical ØRUØ
Sacrococcygeal ØSU5
Sacroiliac
Left ØSU8
Right ØSU7
Shoulder
Left ØRUK
Right ØRUJ
Sternoclavicular
Left ØRUF
Right ØRUE
Tarsal
Left ØSUJ
Right ØSUH
Tarsometatarsal
Left ØSUL
Right ØSUK
Temporomandibular
Left ØRUD
Right ØRUC
Thoracic Vertebral ØRU6
Thoracolumbar Vertebral ØRUA
Toe Phalangeal
Left ØSUQ
Right ØSUP
Wrist
Left ØRUP
Right ØRUN
Kidney Pelvis
Left ØTU4
Right ØTU3
Knee Region
Left ØYUG
Right ØYUF
Larynx ØCUS
Leg
Lower
Left ØYUJ
Right ØYUH
Upper
Left ØYUD
Right ØYUC
Lip
Lower ØCU1
Upper ØCUØ
Lymphatic
Aortic Ø7UD
Axillary
Left Ø7U6
Right Ø7U5
Head Ø7UØ
Inguinal
Left Ø7UJ
Right Ø7UH
Internal Mammary
Left Ø7U9
Right Ø7U8
Lower Extremity
Left Ø7UG
Right Ø7UF
Mesenteric Ø7UB
Neck
Left Ø7U2
Right Ø7U1
Pelvis Ø7UC
Thoracic Duct Ø7UK
Thorax Ø7U7
Upper Extremity
Left Ø7U4
Right Ø7U3
Mandible
Left ØNUV
Right ØNUT
Maxilla ØNUR
Mediastinum ØWUC
Mesentery ØDUV
Metacarpal
Left ØPUQ
Right ØPUP
Metatarsal
Left ØQUP
Right ØQUN
Muscle
Abdomen
Left ØKUL

Supplement — *continued*
Muscle — *continued*
Abdomen — *continued*
Right ØKUK
Extraocular
Left Ø8UM
Right Ø8UL
Facial ØKU1
Foot
Left ØKUW
Right ØKUV
Hand
Left ØKUD
Right ØKUC
Head ØKUØ
Hip
Left ØKUP
Right ØKUN
Lower Arm and Wrist
Left ØKUB
Right ØKU9
Lower Leg
Left ØKUT
Right ØKUS
Neck
Left ØKU3
Right ØKU2
Papillary Ø2UD
Perineum ØKUM
Shoulder
Left ØKU6
Right ØKU5
Thorax
Left ØKUJ
Right ØKUH
Tongue, Palate, Pharynx ØKU4
Trunk
Left ØKUG
Right ØKUF
Upper Arm
Left ØKU8
Right ØKU7
Upper Leg
Left ØKUR
Right ØKUQ
Nasal Mucosa and Soft Tissue Ø9UK
Nasopharynx Ø9UN
Neck ØWU6
Nerve
Abducens ØØUL
Accessory ØØUR
Acoustic ØØUN
Cervical Ø1U1
Facial ØØUM
Femoral Ø1UD
Glossopharyngeal ØØUP
Hypoglossal ØØUS
Lumbar Ø1UB
Median Ø1U5
Oculomotor ØØUH
Olfactory ØØUF
Optic ØØUG
Peroneal Ø1UH
Phrenic Ø1U2
Pudendal Ø1UC
Radial Ø1U6
Sacral Ø1UR
Sciatic Ø1UF
Thoracic Ø1U8
Tibial Ø1UG
Trigeminal ØØUK
Trochlear ØØUJ
Ulnar Ø1U4
Vagus ØØUQ
Nipple
Left ØHUX
Right ØHUW
Omentum ØDUU
Orbit
Left ØNUQ
Right ØNUP
Palate
Hard ØCU2
Soft ØCU3
Patella
Left ØQUF
Right ØQUD
Penis ØVUS
Pericardium Ø2UN

▼ **Subterms under main terms may continue to next column or pa**

Perineum
  Female ØWUN
  Male ØWUM
Peritoneum ØDUW
Phalanx
  Finger
    Left ØPUV
    Right ØPUT
  Thumb
    Left ØPUS
    Right ØPUR
  Toe
    Left ØQUR
    Right ØQUQ
Pharynx ØCUM
Prepuce ØVUT
Radius
  Left ØPUJ
  Right ØPUH
Rectum ØDUP
Retina
  Left Ø8UF
  Right Ø8UE
Retinal Vessel
  Left Ø8UH
  Right Ø8UG
Ribs
  1 to 2 ØPU1
  3 or More ØPU2
Sacrum ØQU1
Scapula
  Left ØPU6
  Right ØPU5
Scrotum ØVU5
Septum
  Atrial Ø2U5
  Nasal Ø9UM
  Ventricular Ø2UM
Shoulder Region
  Left ØXU3
  Right ØXU2
Sinus
  Accessory Ø9UP
  Ethmoid
    Left Ø9UV
    Right Ø9UU
  Frontal
    Left Ø9UT
    Right Ø9US
  Mastoid
    Left Ø9UC
    Right Ø9UB
  Maxillary
    Left Ø9UR
    Right Ø9UQ
  Sphenoid
    Left Ø9UX
    Right Ø9UW
Skull ØNUØ
Spinal Meninges ØØUT
Sternum ØPUØ
Stomach ØDU6
  Pylorus ØDU7
Subcutaneous Tissue and Fascia
  Abdomen ØJU8
  Back ØJU7
  Buttock ØJU9
  Chest ØJU6
  Face ØJU1
  Foot
    Left ØJUR
    Right ØJUQ
  Hand
    Left ØJUK
    Right ØJUJ
  Lower Arm
    Left ØJUH
    Right ØJUG
  Lower Leg
    Left ØJUP
    Right ØJUN
  Neck
    Left ØJU5
    Right ØJU4
  Pelvic Region ØJUC
  Perineum ØJUB
  Scalp ØJUØ

Subcutaneous Tissue and Fascia — continued
  Upper Arm
    Left ØJUF
    Right ØJUD
  Upper Leg
    Left ØJUM
    Right ØJUL
Tarsal
  Left ØQUM
  Right ØQUL
Tendon
  Abdomen
    Left ØLUG
    Right ØLUF
  Ankle
    Left ØLUT
    Right ØLUS
  Foot
    Left ØLUW
    Right ØLUV
  Hand
    Left ØLU8
    Right ØLU7
  Head and Neck ØLUØ
  Hip
    Left ØLUK
    Right ØLUJ
  Knee
    Left ØLUR
    Right ØLUQ
  Lower Arm and Wrist
    Left ØLU6
    Right ØLU5
  Lower Leg
    Left ØLUP
    Right ØLUN
  Perineum ØLUH
  Shoulder
    Left ØLU2
    Right ØLU1
  Thorax
    Left ØLUD
    Right ØLUC
  Trunk
    Left ØLUB
    Right ØLU9
  Upper Arm
    Left ØLU4
    Right ØLU3
  Upper Leg
    Left ØLUM
    Right ØLUL
Testis
  Bilateral ØVUCØ
  Left ØVUBØ
  Right ØVU9Ø
Thumb
  Left ØXUM
  Right ØXUL
Tibia
  Left ØQUH
  Right ØQUG
Toe
  1st
    Left ØYUQ
    Right ØYUP
  2nd
    Left ØYUS
    Right ØYUR
  3rd
    Left ØYUU
    Right ØYUT
  4th
    Left ØYUW
    Right ØYUV
  5th
    Left ØYUY
    Right ØYUX
Tongue ØCU7
Trachea ØBU1
Tunica Vaginalis
  Left ØVU7
  Right ØVU6
Turbinate, Nasal Ø9UL
Tympanic Membrane
  Left Ø9U8
  Right Ø9U7

Ulna
  Left ØPUL
  Right ØPUK
Ureter
  Left ØTU7
  Right ØTU6
Urethra ØTUD
Uterine Supporting Structure ØUU4
Uvula ØCUN
Vagina ØUUG
Valve
  Aortic Ø2UF
  Mitral Ø2UG
  Pulmonary Ø2UH
  Tricuspid Ø2UJ
Vas Deferens
  Bilateral ØVUQ
  Left ØVUP
  Right ØVUN
Vein
  Axillary
    Left Ø5U8
    Right Ø5U7
  Azygos Ø5UØ
  Basilic
    Left Ø5UC
    Right Ø5UB
  Brachial
    Left Ø5UA
    Right Ø5U9
  Cephalic
    Left Ø5UF
    Right Ø5UD
  Colic Ø6U7
  Common Iliac
    Left Ø6UD
    Right Ø6UC
  Esophageal Ø6U3
  External Iliac
    Left Ø6UG
    Right Ø6UF
  External Jugular
    Left Ø5UQ
    Right Ø5UP
  Face
    Left Ø5UV
    Right Ø5UT
  Femoral
    Left Ø6UN
    Right Ø6UM
  Foot
    Left Ø6UV
    Right Ø6UT
  Gastric Ø6U2
  Hand
    Left Ø5UH
    Right Ø5UG
  Hemiazygos Ø5U1
  Hepatic Ø6U4
  Hypogastric
    Left Ø6UJ
    Right Ø6UH
  Inferior Mesenteric Ø6U6
  Innominate
    Left Ø5U4
    Right Ø5U3
  Internal Jugular
    Left Ø5UN
    Right Ø5UM
  Intracranial Ø5UL
  Lower Ø6UY
  Portal Ø6U8
  Pulmonary
    Left Ø2UT
    Right Ø2US
  Renal
    Left Ø6UB
    Right Ø6U9
  Saphenous
    Left Ø6UQ
    Right Ø6UP
  Splenic Ø6U1
  Subclavian
    Left Ø5U6
    Right Ø5U5
  Superior Mesenteric Ø6U5
  Upper Ø5UY

Supplement — *continued*

Vein — *continued*

Vertebral

Left Ø5US

Right Ø5UR

Vena Cava

Inferior Ø6UØ

Superior Ø2UV

Ventricle

Left Ø2UL

Right Ø2UK

Vertebra

Cervical ØPU3

Lumbar ØQUØ

Mechanically Expandable (Paired) Synthetic Substitute XNUØ356

Thoracic ØPU4

Mechanically Expandable (Paired) Synthetic Substitute XNU4356

Vesicle

Bilateral ØVU3

Left ØVU2

Right ØVU1

Vocal Cord

Left ØCUV

Right ØCUT

Vulva ØUUM

Wrist Region

Left ØXUH

Right ØXUG

Supraclavicular (Virchow's) lymph node

use Lymphatic, Left Neck

use Lymphatic, Right Neck

Supraclavicular nerve *use* Cervical Plexus

Suprahyoid lymph node *use* Lymphatic, Head

Suprahyoid muscle

use Neck Muscle, Left

use Neck Muscle, Right

Suprainguinal lymph node *use* Lymphatic, Pelvis

Supraorbital vein

use Face Vein, Left

use Face Vein, Right

Suprarenal gland

use Adrenal Gland

use Adrenal Gland, Bilateral

use Adrenal Gland, Left

use Adrenal Gland, Right

Suprarenal plexus *use* Abdominal Sympathetic Nerve

Suprascapular nerve *use* Brachial Plexus

Supraspinatus fascia

use Subcutaneous Tissue and Fascia, Left Upper Arm

use Subcutaneous Tissue and Fascia, Right Upper Arm

Supraspinatus muscle

use Shoulder Muscle, Left

use Shoulder Muscle, Right

Supraspinous ligament

use Lower Spine Bursa and Ligament

use Upper Spine Bursa and Ligament

Suprasternal notch *use* Sternum

Supratrochlear lymph node

use Lymphatic, Left Upper Extremity

use Lymphatic, Right Upper Extremity

Sural artery

use Popliteal Artery, Left

use Popliteal Artery, Right

Surpass Streamline™ Flow Diverter *use* Intraluminal Device, Flow Diverter in Ø3V

Suspension

Bladder Neck *see* Reposition, Bladder Neck ØTSC

Kidney *see* Reposition, Urinary System ØTS

Urethra *see* Reposition, Urinary System ØTS

Urethrovesical *see* Reposition, Bladder Neck ØTSC

Uterus *see* Reposition, Uterus ØUS9

Vagina *see* Reposition, Vagina ØUSG

Sustained Release Drug-eluting Intraluminal Device

Dilation

Anterior Tibial

Left X27Q385

Right X27P385

Femoral

Left X27J385

Right X27H385

Peroneal

Left X27U385

Sustained Release Drug-eluting Intraluminal Device — *continued*

Dilation — *continued*

Peroneal — *continued*

Right X27T385

Popliteal

Left Distal X27N385

Left Proximal X27L385

Right Distal X27M385

Right Proximal X27K385

Posterior Tibial

Left X27S385

Right X27R385

Four or More

Anterior Tibial

Left X27Q3C5

Right X27P3C5

Femoral

Left X27J3C5

Right X27H3C5

Peroneal

Left X27U3C5

Right X27T3C5

Popliteal

Left Distal X27N3C5

Left Proximal X27L3C5

Right Distal X27M3C5

Right Proximal X27K3C5

Posterior Tibial

Left X27S3C5

Right X27R3C5

Three

Anterior Tibial

Left X27Q3B5

Right X27P3B5

Femoral

Left X27J3B5

Right X27H3B5

Peroneal

Left X27U3B5

Right X27T3B5

Popliteal

Left Distal X27N3B5

Left Proximal X27L3B5

Right Distal X27M3B5

Right Proximal X27K3B5

Posterior Tibial

Left X27S3B5

Right X27R3B5

Two

Anterior Tibial

Left X27Q395

Right X27P395

Femoral

Left X27J395

Right X27H395

Peroneal

Left X27U395

Right X27T395

Popliteal

Left Distal X27N395

Left Proximal X27L395

Right Distal X27M395

Right Proximal X27K395

Posterior Tibial

Left X27S395

Right X27R395

Suture

Laceration repair *see* Repair

Ligation *see* Occlusion

Suture Removal

Extremity

Lower 8EØYXY8

Upper 8EØXXY8

Head and Neck Region 8EØ9XY8

Trunk Region 8EØWXY8

Sutureless valve, Perceval *use* Zooplastic Tissue, Rapid Deployment Technique in New Technology

Sweat gland *use* Skin

Sympathectomy *see* Excision, Peripheral Nervous System Ø1B

SynCardia (temporary) total artificial heart (TAH) *use* Synthetic Substitute, Pneumatic in Ø2R

SynCardia Total Artificial Heart *use* Synthetic Substitute

Synchra CRT-P *use* Cardiac Resynchronization Pacemaker Pulse Generator in ØJH

SynchroMed pump *use* Infusion Device, Pump in Subcutaneous Tissue and Fascia

Synechiotomy, iris *see* Release, Eye Ø8N

Synovectomy

Lower joint *see* Excision, Lower Joints ØSB

Upper joint *see* Excision, Upper Joints ØRB

Synthetic Human Angiotensin II XWØ

Systemic Nuclear Medicine Therapy

Abdomen CW7Ø

Anatomical Regions, Multiple CW7YYZZ

Chest CW73

Thyroid CW7G

Whole Body CW7N

T

Tagraxofusp-erzs Antineoplastic XWØ

Takedown

Arteriovenous shunt *see* Removal of device from, Upper Arteries Ø3P

Arteriovenous shunt, with creation of new shunt *see* Bypass, Upper Arteries Ø31

Stoma

see Excision

see Reposition

Talent® Converter *use* Intraluminal Device

Talent® Occluder *use* Intraluminal Device

Talent® Stent Graft (abdominal) (thoracic) *use* Intraluminal Device

Talocalcaneal (subtalar) joint

use Tarsal Joint, Left

use Tarsal Joint, Right

Talocalcaneal ligament

use Foot Bursa and Ligament, Left

use Foot Bursa and Ligament, Right

Talocalcaneonavicular joint

use Tarsal Joint, Left

use Tarsal Joint, Right

Talocalcaneonavicular ligament

use Foot Bursa and Ligament, Left

use Foot Bursa and Ligament, Right

Talocrural joint

use Ankle Joint, Left

use Joint, Ankle, Right

Talofibular ligament

use Ankle Bursa and Ligament, Left

use Ankle Bursa and Ligament, Right

Talus bone

use Tarsal, Left

use Tarsal, Right

TandemHeart® System *use* Short-term External Heart Assist System in Heart and Great Vessels

Tarsectomy

see Excision, Lower Bones ØQB

see Resection, Lower Bones ØQT

Tarsometatarsal ligament

use Foot Bursa and Ligament, Left

use Foot Bursa and Ligament, Right

Tarsorrhaphy *see* Repair, Eye Ø8Q

Tattooing

Cornea 3EØCXMZ

Skin *see* Introduction of substance in or on, Skin 3EØØ

TAXUS® Liberté® Paclitaxel-eluting Coronary Stent System *use* Intraluminal Device, Drug-eluting in Heart and Great Vessels

TBNA (transbronchial needle aspiration)

Fluid or gas *see* Drainage, Respiratory System ØB9

Tissue biopsy *see* Extraction, Respiratory System ØBD

Tecartus™ *use* Brexucabtagene Autoleucel Immunotherapy

TECENTRIQ® *use* Atezolizumab Antineoplastic

Telemetry 4A12X4Z

Ambulatory 4A12X45

Temperature gradient study 4AØZXKZ

Temporal lobe *use* Cerebral Hemisphere

Temporalis muscle *use* Head Muscle

Temporoparietalis muscle *use* Head Muscle

Tendolysis *see* Release, Tendons ØLN

Tendonectomy

see Excision, Tendons ØLB

see Resection, Tendons ØLT

Tendonoplasty, tenoplasty

see Repair, Tendons ØLQ

see Replacement, Tendons ØLR

▽ **Subterms under main terms may continue to next column or pa**

Tendonoplasty, tenoplasty — *continued*
   see Supplement, Tendons ØLU
Tendorrhaphy *see* Repair, Tendons ØLQ
Tendototomy
   see Division, Tendons ØL8
   see Drainage, Tendons ØL9
Tenectomy, tenonectomy
   see Excision, Tendons ØLB
   see Resection, Tendons ØLT
Tenolysis *see* Release, Tendons ØLN
Tenontorrhaphy *see* Repair, Tendons ØLQ
Tenontotomy
   see Division, Tendons ØL8
   see Drainage, Tendons ØL9
Tenorrhaphy *see* Repair, Tendons ØLQ
Tenosynovectomy
   see Excision, Tendons ØLB
   see Resection, Tendons ØLT
Tenotomy
   see Division, Tendons ØL8
   see Drainage, Tendons ØL9
Tensor fasciae latae muscle
   use Hip Muscle, Left
   use Hip Muscle, Right
Tensor veli palatini muscle *use* Tongue, Palate,
   Pharynx Muscle
Tenth cranial nerve *use* Vagus Nerve
Tentorium cerebelli *use* Dura Mater
Teres major muscle
   use Shoulder Muscle, Left
   use Shoulder Muscle, Right
Teres minor muscle
   use Shoulder Muscle, Left
   use Shoulder Muscle, Right
Terlipressin XWØ
TERLIVAZ® *use* Terlipressin
Termination of pregnancy
   Aspiration curettage 10A07ZZ
   Dilation and curettage 10A07ZZ
   Hysterotomy 10A00ZZ
   Intra-amniotic injection 10A03ZZ
   Laminaria 10A07ZW
   Vacuum 10A07Z6
Testectomy
   see Excision, Male Reproductive System ØVB
   see Resection, Male Reproductive System ØVT
Testicular artery *use* Abdominal Aorta
Testing
   Glaucoma 4A07XBZ
   Hearing *see* Hearing Assessment, Diagnostic Audi-
      ology F13
   Mental health *see* Psychological Tests
   Muscle function, electromyography (EMG) *see*
      Measurement, Musculoskeletal 4A0F
   Muscle function, manual *see* Motor Function As-
      sessment, Rehabilitation F01
   Neurophysiologic monitoring, intra-operative *see*
      Monitoring, Physiological Systems 4A1
   Range of motion *see* Motor Function Assessment,
      Rehabilitation F01
   Vestibular function *see* Vestibular Assessment, Di-
      agnostic Audiology F15
Thalamectomy *see* Excision, Thalamus 00B9
Thalamotomy *see* Drainage, Thalamus 0099
Thenar muscle
   use Hand Muscle, Left
   use Hand Muscle, Right
Therapeutic Massage
   Musculoskeletal System 8E0KX1Z
   Reproductive System
      Prostate 8E0VX1C
      Rectum 8E0VX1D
Therapeutic occlusion coil(s) *use* Intraluminal Device
Thermography 4A0ZXKZ
Thermotherapy, prostate *see* Destruction, Prostate
   0V50
Third cranial nerve *use* Oculomotor Nerve
Third occipital nerve *use* Cervical Nerve
Third ventricle *use* Cerebral Ventricle
Thoracectomy *see* Excision, Anatomical Regions,
   General ØWB
Thoracentesis *see* Drainage, Anatomical Regions,
   General ØW9
Thoracic aortic plexus *use* Thoracic Sympathetic Nerve
Thoracic esophagus *use* Esophagus, Middle
Thoracic facet joint *use* Thoracic Vertebral Joint
Thoracic ganglion *use* Thoracic Sympathetic Nerve

Thoracoacromial artery
   use Axillary Artery, Left
   use Axillary Artery, Right
Thoracocentesis *see* Drainage, Anatomical Regions,
   General ØW9
Thoracolumbar facet joint *use* Thoracolumbar Verte-
   bral Joint
Thoracoplasty
   see Repair, Anatomical Regions, General ØWQ
   see Supplement, Anatomical Regions, General ØWU
Thoracostomy, for lung collapse *see* Drainage, Res-
   piratory System ØB9
Thoracostomy tube *use* Drainage Device
Thoracotomy *see* Drainage, Anatomical Regions,
   General ØW9
Thoraflex™ Hybrid device *use* Branched Synthetic
   Substitute with Intraluminal Device in New Tech-
   nology
Thoratec IVAD (Implantable Ventricular Assist
   Device) *use* Implantable Heart Assist System in
   Heart and Great Vessels
Thoratec Paracorporeal Ventricular Assist Device
   use Short-term External Heart Assist System in
   Heart and Great Vessels
Thrombectomy *see* Extirpation
Thrombolysis, Ultrasound assisted *see* Fragmenta-
   tion, Artery
Thymectomy
   see Excision, Lymphatic and Hemic Systems 07B
   see Resection, Lymphatic and Hemic Systems 07T
Thymopexy
   see Repair, Lymphatic and Hemic Systems 07Q
   see Reposition, Lymphatic and Hemic Systems 07S
Thymus gland *use* Thymus
Thyroarytenoid muscle
   use Neck Muscle, Left
   use Neck Muscle, Right
Thyrocervical trunk
   use Thyroid Artery, Left
   use Thyroid Artery, Right
Thyroid cartilage *use* Larynx
Thyroidectomy
   see Excision, Endocrine System ØGB
   see Resection, Endocrine System ØGT
Thyroidorrhaphy *see* Repair, Endocrine System ØGQ
Thyroidoscopy ØGJK4ZZ
Thyroidotomy *see* Drainage, Endocrine System ØG9
Tibial insert *use* Liner in Lower Joints
Tibial sesamoid
   use Metatarsal, Left
   use Metatarsal, Right
Tibialis anterior muscle
   use Lower Leg Muscle, Left
   use Lower Leg Muscle, Right
Tibialis posterior muscle
   use Lower Leg Muscle, Left
   use Lower Leg Muscle, Right
Tibiofemoral joint
   use Knee Joint, Left
   use Knee Joint, Right
   use Knee Joint, Tibial Surface, Left
   use Knee Joint, Tibial Surface, Right
Tibioperoneal trunk
   use Popliteal Artery, Left
   use Popliteal Artery, Right
Tisagenlecleucel *use* Tisagenlecleucel Immunotherapy
Tisagenlecleucel Immunotherapy XWØ
Tissue bank graft *use* Nonautologous Tissue Substitute
Tissue expander (inflatable) (injectable)
   use Tissue Expander in Skin and Breast
   use Tissue Expander in Subcutaneous Tissue and
      Fascia
Tissue Expander
   Insertion of device in
      Breast
         Bilateral ØHHV
         Left ØHHU
         Right ØHHT
      Nipple
         Left ØHHX
         Right ØHHW
      Subcutaneous Tissue and Fascia
         Abdomen ØJH8
         Back ØJH7
         Buttock ØJH9
         Chest ØJH6
         Face ØJH1

Tissue Expander — *continued*
   Insertion of device in — *continued*
      Subcutaneous Tissue and Fascia — *contin-*
         ued
         Foot
            Left ØJHR
            Right ØJHQ
         Hand
            Left ØJHK
            Right ØJHJ
         Lower Arm
            Left ØJHH
            Right ØJHG
         Lower Leg
            Left ØJHP
            Right ØJHN
         Neck
            Left ØJH5
            Right ØJH4
         Pelvic Region ØJHC
         Perineum ØJHB
         Scalp ØJHØ
         Upper Arm
            Left ØJHF
            Right ØJHD
         Upper Leg
            Left ØJHM
            Right ØJHL
   Removal of device from
      Breast
         Left ØHPU
         Right ØHPT
      Subcutaneous Tissue and Fascia
         Head and Neck ØJPS
         Lower Extremity ØJPW
         Trunk ØJPT
         Upper Extremity ØJPV
   Revision of device in
      Breast
         Left ØHWU
         Right ØHWT
      Subcutaneous Tissue and Fascia
         Head and Neck ØJWS
         Lower Extremity ØJWW
         Trunk ØJWT
         Upper Extremity ØJWV
Tissue Plasminogen Activator (tPA) (r-tPA) *use*
   Other Thrombolytic
Titanium Sternal Fixation System (TSFS)
   use Internal Fixation Device, Rigid Plate in ØPS
   use Internal Fixation Device, Rigid Plate in ØPH
Tocilizumab XWØ
Tomographic (Tomo) Nuclear Medicine Imaging
   Abdomen CW2Ø
   Abdomen and Chest CW24
   Abdomen and Pelvis CW21
   Anatomical Regions, Multiple CW2YYZZ
   Bladder, Kidneys and Ureters CT23
   Brain CØ2Ø
   Breast CH2YYZZ
      Bilateral CH22
      Left CH21
      Right CH2Ø
   Bronchi and Lungs CB22
   Central Nervous System CØ2YYZZ
   Cerebrospinal Fluid CØ25
   Chest CW23
   Chest and Abdomen CW24
   Chest and Neck CW26
   Digestive System CD2YYZZ
   Endocrine System CG2YYZZ
   Extremity
      Lower CW2D
         Bilateral CP2F
         Left CP2D
         Right CP2C
      Upper CW2M
         Bilateral CP2B
         Left CP29
         Right CP28
   Gallbladder CF24
   Gastrointestinal Tract CD27
   Gland, Parathyroid CG21
   Head and Neck CW2B
   Heart C22YYZZ
      Right and Left C226
   Hepatobiliary System and Pancreas CF2YYZZ
   Kidneys, Ureters and Bladder CT23
   Liver CF25

Transfer — *continued*
  Nerve — *continued*
    Trigeminal 00XK
    Trochlear 00XJ
    Ulnar 01X4
    Vagus 00XQ
  Palate, Soft 0CX3
  Prepuce 0VXT
  Skin
    Abdomen 0HX7XZZ
    Back 0HX6XZZ
    Buttock 0HX8XZZ
    Chest 0HX5XZZ
    Ear
      Left 0HX3XZZ
      Right 0HX2XZZ
    Face 0HX1XZZ
    Foot
      Left 0HXNXZZ
      Right 0HXMXZZ
    Hand
      Left 0HXGXZZ
      Right 0HXFXZZ
    Inguinal 0HXAXZZ
    Lower Arm
      Left 0HXEXZZ
      Right 0HXDXZZ
    Lower Leg
      Left 0HXLXZZ
      Right 0HXKXZZ
    Neck 0HX4XZZ
    Perineum 0HX9XZZ
    Scalp 0HX0XZZ
    Upper Arm
      Left 0HXCXZZ
      Right 0HXBXZZ
    Upper Leg
      Left 0HXJXZZ
      Right 0HXHXZZ
  Stomach 0DX6
  Subcutaneous Tissue and Fascia
    Abdomen 0JX8
    Back 0JX7
    Buttock 0JX9
    Chest 0JX6
    Face 0JX1
    Foot
      Left 0JXR
      Right 0JXQ
    Hand
      Left 0JXK
      Right 0JXJ
    Lower Arm
      Left 0JXH
      Right 0JXG
    Lower Leg
      Left 0JXP
      Right 0JXN
    Neck
      Left 0JX5
      Right 0JX4
    Pelvic Region 0JXC
    Perineum 0JXB
    Scalp 0JX0
    Upper Arm
      Left 0JXF
      Right 0JXD
    Upper Leg
      Left 0JXM
      Right 0JXL
  Tendon
    Abdomen
      Left 0LXG
      Right 0LXF
    Ankle
      Left 0LXT
      Right 0LXS
    Foot
      Left 0LXW
      Right 0LXV
    Hand
      Left 0LX8
      Right 0LX7
    Head and Neck 0LX0
    Hip
      Left 0LXK
      Right 0LXJ
    Knee
      Left 0LXR

Transfer — *continued*
  Tendon — *continued*
    Knee — *continued*
      Right 0LXQ
    Lower Arm and Wrist
      Left 0LX6
      Right 0LX5
    Lower Leg
      Left 0LXP
      Right 0LXN
    Perineum 0LXH
    Shoulder
      Left 0LX2
      Right 0LX1
    Thorax
      Left 0LXD
      Right 0LXC
    Trunk
      Left 0LXB
      Right 0LX9
    Upper Arm
      Left 0LX4
      Right 0LX3
    Upper Leg
      Left 0LXM
      Right 0LXL
  Tongue 0CX7
Transfusion
  Immunotherapy *see* New Technology, Anatomical
    Regions XW2
  Products of Conception
    Antihemophilic Factors 3027
    Blood
      Platelets 3027
      Red Cells 3027
        Frozen 3027
      White Cells 3027
      Whole 3027
    Factor IX 3027
    Fibrinogen 3027
    Globulin 3027
    Plasma
      Fresh 3027
      Frozen 3027
    Plasma Cryoprecipitate 3027
    Serum Albumin 3027
  Vein
    4-Factor Prothrombin Complex Concentrate
      30283B1
    Central
      Antihemophilic Factors 30243V
      Blood
        Platelets 30243R
        Red Cells 30243N
          Frozen 30243P
        White Cells 30243Q
        Whole 30243H
      Bone Marrow 30243G
      Factor IX 30243W
      Fibrinogen 30243T
      Globulin 30243S
      Hematopoietic Stem/Progenitor Cells
        (HSPC), Genetically Modified
        30243C0
      Pathogen Reduced Cryoprecipitated
        Fibrinogen Complex 30243D1
      Plasma
        Fresh 30243L
        Frozen 30243K
      Plasma Cryoprecipitate 30243M
      Serum Albumin 30243J
      Stem Cells
        Cord Blood 30243X
        Embryonic 30243AZ
        Hematopoietic 30243Y
        T-cell Depleted Hematopoietic
          30243U
    Peripheral
      Antihemophilic Factors 30233V
      Blood
        Platelets 30233R
        Red Cells 30233N
          Frozen 30233P
        White Cells 30233Q
        Whole 30233H
      Bone Marrow 30233G
      Factor IX 30233W
      Fibrinogen 30233T
      Globulin 30233S

Transfusion — *continued*
  Vein — *continued*
    Peripheral — *continued*
      Hematopoietic Stem/Progenitor Cells
        (HSPC), Genetically Modified
        30233C0
      Pathogen Reduced Cryoprecipitated
        Fibrinogen Complex 30233D1
      Plasma
        Fresh 30233L
        Frozen 30233K
      Plasma Cryoprecipitate 30233M
      Serum Albumin 30233J
      Stem Cells
        Cord Blood 30233X
        Embryonic 30233AZ
        Hematopoietic 30233Y
        T-cell Depleted Hematopoietic
          30233U
Transplant *see* Transplantation
Transplantation
  Bone marrow *see* Transfusion, Circulatory 302
  Esophagus 0DY50Z
  Face 0WY20Z
  Hand
    Left 0XYK0Z
    Right 0XYJ0Z
  Heart 02YA0Z
  Hematopoietic cell *see* Transfusion, Circulatory
    302
  Intestine
    Large 0DYE0Z
    Small 0DY80Z
  Kidney
    Left 0TY10Z
    Right 0TY00Z
  Liver 0FY00Z
  Lung
    Bilateral 0BYM0Z
    Left 0BYL0Z
    Lower Lobe
      Left 0BYJ0Z
      Right 0BYF0Z
    Middle Lobe, Right 0BYD0Z
    Right 0BYK0Z
    Upper Lobe
      Left 0BYG0Z
      Right 0BYC0Z
  Lung Lingula 0BYH0Z
  Ovary
    Left 0UY10Z
    Right 0UY00Z
  Pancreas 0FYG0Z
  Penis 0VYS0Z
  Products of Conception 10Y0
  Scrotum 0VY50Z
  Spleen 07YP0Z
  Stem cell *see* Transfusion, Circulatory 302
  Stomach 0DY60Z
  Thymus 07YM0Z
  Uterus 0UY90Z
Transposition
  see Bypass
  see Reposition
  see Transfer
Transversalis fascia *use* Subcutaneous Tissue and
  Fascia, Trunk
Transverse acetabular ligament
  use Hip Bursa and Ligament, Left
  use Hip Bursa and Ligament, Right
Transverse (cutaneous) cervical nerve *use* Cervical
  Plexus
Transverse facial artery
  use Temporal Artery, Left
  use Temporal Artery, Right
Transverse foramen *use* Cervical Vertebra
Transverse humeral ligament
  use Shoulder Bursa and Ligament, Left
  use Shoulder Bursa and Ligament, Right
Transverse ligament of atlas *use* Head and Neck
  Bursa and Ligament
Transverse process
  use Cervical Vertebra
  use Lumbar Vertebra
  use Thoracic Vertebra
Transverse Rectus Abdominis Myocutaneous Flap
  Replacement
    Bilateral 0HRV076

Transverse Rectus Abdominis Myocutaneous Flap — *continued*
  Replacement — *continued*
    Left ØHRUØ76
    Right ØHRTØ76
  Transfer
    Left ØKXL
    Right ØKXK
Transverse scapular ligament
  use Shoulder Bursa and Ligament, Left
  use Shoulder Bursa and Ligament, Right
Transverse thoracis muscle
  use Thorax Muscle, Left
  use Thorax Muscle, Right
Transversospinalis muscle
  use Trunk Muscle, Left
  use Trunk Muscle, Right
Transversus abdominis muscle
  use Abdomen Muscle, Left
  use Abdomen Muscle, Right
Trapezium bone
  use Carpal, Left
  use Carpal, Right
Trapezius muscle
  use Trunk Muscle, Left
  use Trunk Muscle, Right
Trapezoid bone
  use Carpal, Left
  use Carpal, Right
Triceps brachii muscle
  use Upper Arm Muscle, Left
  use Upper Arm Muscle, Right
Tricuspid annulus *use* Tricuspid Valve
Trifacial nerve *use* Trigeminal Nerve
Trifecta™ Valve (aortic) *use* Zooplastic Tissue in Heart and Great Vessels
Trigone of bladder *use* Bladder
TriGuard 3™ CEPD (cerebral embolic protection device) X2A6325
Trilaciclib XWØ
Trimming, excisional *see* Excision
Triquetral bone
  use Carpal, Left
  use Carpal, Right
Trochanteric bursa
  use Hip Bursa and Ligament, Left
  use Hip Bursa and Ligament, Right
TUMT (transurethral microwave thermotherapy of prostate) ØV5Ø7ZZ
TUNA (transurethral needle ablation of prostate) ØV5Ø7ZZ
Tunneled central venous catheter *use* Vascular Access Device, Tunneled in Subcutaneous Tissue and Fascia
Tunneled spinal (intrathecal) catheter *use* Infusion Device
Turbinectomy
  see Excision, Ear, Nose, Sinus Ø9B
  see Resection, Ear, Nose, Sinus Ø9T
Turbinoplasty
  see Repair, Ear, Nose, Sinus Ø9Q
  see Replacement, Ear, Nose, Sinus Ø9R
  see Supplement, Ear, Nose, Sinus Ø9U
Turbinotomy
  see Division, Ear, Nose, Sinus Ø98
  see Drainage, Ear, Nose, Sinus Ø99
TURP (transurethral resection of prostate) ØVBØ7ZZ
  see Excision, Prostate ØVBØ
  see Resection, Prostate ØVTØ
Twelfth cranial nerve *use* Hypoglossal Nerve
Two lead pacemaker *use* Pacemaker, Dual Chamber in ØJH
Tympanic cavity
  use Middle Ear, Left
  use Middle Ear, Right
Tympanic nerve *use* Glossopharyngeal Nerve
Tympanic part of temporal bone
  use Temporal Bone, Left
  use Temporal Bone, Right
Tympanogram *see* Hearing Assessment, Diagnostic Audiology F13
Tympanoplasty
  see Repair, Ear, Nose, Sinus Ø9Q
  see Replacement, Ear, Nose, Sinus Ø9R
  see Supplement, Ear, Nose, Sinus Ø9U

Tympanosympathectomy *see* Excision, Nerve, Head and Neck Sympathetic Ø1BK
Tympanotomy *see* Drainage, Ear, Nose, Sinus Ø99
TYRX Antibacterial Envelope *use* Anti-Infective Envelope

U

Ulnar collateral carpal ligament
  use Wrist Bursa and Ligament, Left
  use Wrist Bursa and Ligament, Right
Ulnar collateral ligament
  use Elbow Bursa and Ligament, Left
  use Elbow Bursa and Ligament, Right
Ulnar notch
  use Radius, Left
  use Radius, Right
Ulnar vein
  use Brachial Vein, Left
  use Brachial Vein, Right
Ultrafiltration
  Hemodialysis *see* Performance, Urinary 5A1D
  Therapeutic plasmapheresis *see* Pheresis, Circulatory 6A55
Ultraflex™ Precision Colonic Stent System *use* Intraluminal Device
ULTRAPRO Hernia System (UHS) *use* Synthetic Substitute
ULTRAPRO Partially Absorbable Lightweight Mesh *use* Synthetic Substitute
ULTRAPRO Plug *use* Synthetic Substitute
Ultrasonic osteogenic stimulator
  use Bone Growth Stimulator in Head and Facial Bones
  use Bone Growth Stimulator in Lower Bones
  use Bone Growth Stimulator in Upper Bones
Ultrasonography
  Abdomen BW4ØZZZ
  Abdomen and Pelvis BW41ZZZ
  Abdominal Wall BH49ZZZ
  Aorta
    Abdominal, Intravascular B44ØZZ3
    Thoracic, Intravascular B34ØZZ3
  Appendix BD48ZZZ
  Artery
    Brachiocephalic-Subclavian, Right, Intravascular B341ZZ3
    Celiac and Mesenteric, Intravascular B44KZZ3
    Common Carotid
      Bilateral, Intravascular B345ZZ3
      Left, Intravascular B344ZZ3
      Right, Intravascular B343ZZ3
    Coronary
      Multiple B241YZZ
        Intravascular B241ZZ3
        Transesophageal B241ZZ4
      Single B240YZZ
        Intravascular B24ØZZ3
        Transesophageal B24ØZZ4
    Femoral, Intravascular B44LZZ3
    Inferior Mesenteric, Intravascular B445ZZ3
    Internal Carotid
      Bilateral, Intravascular B348ZZ3
      Left, Intravascular B347ZZ3
      Right, Intravascular B346ZZ3
    Intra-Abdominal, Other, Intravascular B44BZZ3
    Intracranial, Intravascular B34RZZ3
    Lower Extremity
      Bilateral, Intravascular B44HZZ3
      Left, Intravascular B44GZZ3
      Right, Intravascular B44FZZ3
    Mesenteric and Celiac, Intravascular B44KZZ3
    Ophthalmic, Intravascular B34VZZ3
    Penile, Intravascular B44NZZ3
    Pulmonary
      Left, Intravascular B34TZZ3
      Right, Intravascular B34SZZ3
    Renal
      Bilateral, Intravascular B448ZZ3
      Left, Intravascular B447ZZ3
      Right, Intravascular B446ZZ3
    Subclavian, Left, Intravascular B342ZZ3
    Superior Mesenteric, Intravascular B444ZZ3
    Upper Extremity
      Bilateral, Intravascular B34KZZ3
      Left, Intravascular B34JZZ3

Ultrasonography — *continued*
  Artery — *continued*
    Upper Extremity — *continued*
      Right, Intravascular B34HZZ3
  Bile Duct BF4ØZZZ
  Bile Duct and Gallbladder BF43ZZZ
  Bladder BT4ØZZZ
    and Kidney BT4JZZZ
  Brain BØ4ØZZZ
  Breast
    Bilateral BH42ZZZ
    Left BH41ZZZ
    Right BH4ØZZZ
  Chest Wall BH4BZZZ
  Coccyx BR4FZZZ
  Connective Tissue
    Lower Extremity BL41ZZZ
    Upper Extremity BL4ØZZZ
  Duodenum BD49ZZZ
  Elbow
    Left, Densitometry BP4HZZ1
    Right, Densitometry BP4GZZ1
  Esophagus BD41ZZZ
  Extremity
    Lower BH48ZZZ
    Upper BH47ZZZ
  Eye
    Bilateral B847ZZZ
    Left B846ZZZ
    Right B845ZZZ
  Fallopian Tube
    Bilateral BU42
    Left BU41
    Right BU4Ø
  Fetal Umbilical Cord BY47ZZZ
  Fetus
    First Trimester, Multiple Gestation BY4BZZZ
    Second Trimester, Multiple Gestation BY4DZZZ
    Single
      First Trimester BY49ZZZ
      Second Trimester BY4CZZZ
      Third Trimester BY4FZZZ
    Third Trimester, Multiple Gestation BY4GZZZ
  Gallbladder BF42ZZZ
  Gallbladder and Bile Duct BF43ZZZ
  Gastrointestinal Tract BD47ZZZ
  Gland
    Adrenal
      Bilateral BG42ZZZ
      Left BG41ZZZ
      Right BG4ØZZZ
    Parathyroid BG43ZZZ
    Thyroid BG44ZZZ
  Hand
    Left, Densitometry BP4PZZ1
    Right, Densitometry BP4NZZ1
  Head and Neck BH4CZZZ
  Heart
    Left B245YZZ
      Intravascular B245ZZ3
      Transesophageal B245ZZ4
    Pediatric B24DYZZ
      Intravascular B24DZZ3
      Transesophageal B24DZZ4
    Right B244YZZ
      Intravascular B244ZZ3
      Transesophageal B244ZZ4
    Right and Left B246YZZ
      Intravascular B246ZZ3
      Transesophageal B246ZZ4
  Heart with Aorta B24BYZZ
    Intravascular B24BZZ3
    Transesophageal B24BZZ4
  Hepatobiliary System, All BF4CZZZ
  Hip
    Bilateral BQ42ZZZ
    Left BQ41ZZZ
    Right BQ4ØZZZ
  Kidney
    and Bladder BT4JZZZ
    Bilateral BT43ZZZ
    Left BT42ZZZ
    Right BT41ZZZ
    Transplant BT49ZZZ
  Knee
    Bilateral BQ49ZZZZ
    Left BQ48ZZZ
    Right BQ47ZZZ

▽ Subterms under main terms may continue to next column or ▶

Ultrasonography — *continued*
Liver BF45ZZZ
Liver and Spleen BF46ZZZ
Mediastinum BB4CZZZ
Neck BW4FZZZ
Ovary
  Bilateral BU45
  Left BU44
  Right BU43
Ovary and Uterus BU4C
Pancreas BF47ZZZ
Pelvic Region BW4GZZZ
Pelvis and Abdomen BW41ZZZ
Penis BV4BZZZ
Pericardium B24CYZZ
  Intravascular B24CZZ3
  Transesophageal B24CZZ4
Placenta BY48ZZZ
Pleura BB4BZZZ
Prostate and Seminal Vesicle BV49ZZZ
Rectum BD4CZZZ
Sacrum BR4FZZZ
Scrotum BV44ZZZ
Seminal Vesicle and Prostate BV49ZZZ
Shoulder
  Left, Densitometry BP49ZZ1
  Right, Densitometry BP48ZZ1
Spinal Cord B04BZZZ
Spine
  Cervical BR40ZZZ
  Lumbar BR49ZZZ
  Thoracic BR47ZZZ
Spleen and Liver BF46ZZZ
Stomach BD42ZZZ
Tendon
  Lower Extremity BL43ZZZ
  Upper Extremity BL42ZZZ
Ureter
  Bilateral BT48ZZZ
  Left BT47ZZZ
  Right BT46ZZZ
Urethra BT45ZZZ
Uterus BU46
Uterus and Ovary BU4C
Vein
  Jugular
    Left, Intravascular B544ZZ3
    Right, Intravascular B543ZZ3
  Lower Extremity
    Bilateral, Intravascular B54DZZ3
    Left, Intravascular B54CZZ3
    Right, Intravascular B54BZZ3
  Portal, Intravascular B54TZZ3
  Renal
    Bilateral, Intravascular B54LZZ3
    Left, Intravascular B54KZZ3
    Right, Intravascular B54JZZ3
  Spanchnic, Intravascular B54TZZ3
  Subclavian
    Left, Intravascular B547ZZ3
    Right, Intravascular B546ZZ3
  Upper Extremity
    Bilateral, Intravascular B54PZZ3
    Left, Intravascular B54NZZ3
    Right, Intravascular B54MZZ3
Vena Cava
  Inferior, Intravascular B549ZZ3
  Superior, Intravascular B548ZZ3
Wrist
  Left, Densitometry BP4MZZ1
  Right, Densitometry BP4LZZ1
Ultrasound bone healing system
use Bone Growth Stimulator in Head and Facial
  Bones
use Bone Growth Stimulator in Lower Bones
use Bone Growth Stimulator in Upper Bones
Ultrasound Therapy
Heart 6A75
No Qualifier 6A75
Vessels
  Head and Neck 6A75
  Other 6A75
  Peripheral 6A75
Ultraviolet Light Therapy, Skin 6A80
Umbilical artery
use Internal Iliac Artery, Left
use Internal Iliac Artery, Right
use Lower Artery

Uniplanar external fixator
use External Fixation Device, Monoplanar in 0PH
use External Fixation Device, Monoplanar in 0PS
use External Fixation Device, Monoplanar in 0QH
use External Fixation Device, Monoplanar in 0QS
Upper GI series *see* Fluoroscopy, Gastrointestinal, Upper BD15
Ureteral orifice
use Ureter
use Ureter, Left
use Ureter, Right
use Ureters, Bilateral
Ureterectomy
see Excision, Urinary System 0TB
see Resection, Urinary System 0TT
Ureterocolostomy *see* Bypass, Urinary System 0T1
Ureterocystostomy *see* Bypass, Urinary System 0T1
Ureteroenterostomy *see* Bypass, Urinary System 0T1
Ureteroileostomy *see* Bypass, Urinary System 0T1
Ureterolithotomy *see* Extirpation, Urinary System 0TC
Ureterolysis *see* Release, Urinary System 0TN
Ureteroneocystostomy
see Bypass, Urinary System 0T1
see Reposition, Urinary System 0TS
Ureteropelvic junction (UPJ)
use Kidney Pelvis, Left
use Kidney Pelvis, Right
Ureteropexy
see Repair, Urinary System 0TQ
see Reposition, Urinary System 0TS
Ureteroplasty
see Repair, Urinary System 0TQ
see Replacement, Urinary System 0TR
see Supplement, Urinary System 0TU
Ureteroplication *see* Restriction, Urinary System 0TV
Ureteropyelography *see* Fluoroscopy, Urinary System BT1
Ureterorrhaphy *see* Repair, Urinary System 0TQ
Ureteroscopy 0TJ98ZZ
Ureterostomy
see Bypass, Urinary System 0T1
see Drainage, Urinary System 0T9
Ureterotomy *see* Drainage, Urinary System 0T9
Ureteroureterostomy *see* Bypass, Urinary System 0T1
Ureterovesical orifice
use Ureter
use Ureter, Left
use Ureter, Right
use Ureters, Bilateral
Urethral catheterization, indwelling 0T9B70Z
Urethrectomy
see Excision, Urethra 0TBD
see Resection, Urethra 0TTD
Urethrolithotomy *see* Extirpation, Urethra 0TCD
Urethrolysis *see* Release, Urethra 0TND
Urethropexy
see Repair, Urethra 0TQD
see Reposition, Urethra 0TSD
Urethroplasty
see Repair, Urethra 0TQD
see Replacement, Urethra 0TRD
see Supplement, Urethra 0TUD
Urethrorrhaphy *see* Repair, Urethra 0TQD
Urethroscopy 0TJD8ZZ
Urethrotomy *see* Drainage, Urethra 0T9D
Uridine Triacetate XW0DX82
Urinary incontinence stimulator lead *use* Stimulator Lead in Urinary System
Urography *see* Fluoroscopy, Urinary System BT1
Ustekinumab *use* Other New Technology Therapeutic Substance
Uterine Artery
use Internal Iliac Artery, Left
use Internal Iliac Artery, Right
Uterine artery embolization (UAE) *see* Occlusion, Lower Arteries 04L
Uterine cornu *use* Uterus
Uterine tube
use Fallopian Tube, Left
use Fallopian Tube, Right
Uterine vein
use Hypogastric Vein, Left
use Hypogastric Vein, Right
Uvulectomy
see Excision, Uvula 0CBN
see Resection, Uvula 0CTN

Uvulorrhaphy *see* Repair, Uvula 0CQN
Uvulotomy *see* Drainage, Uvula 0C9N

V

Vabomere™ *use* Meropenem-vaborbactam Anti-infective
Vaccination *see* Introduction of Serum, Toxoid, and Vaccine
Vacuum extraction, obstetric 10D07Z6
Vaginal artery
use Internal Iliac Artery, Left
use Internal Iliac Artery, Right
Vaginal pessary *use* Intraluminal Device, Pessary in Female Reproductive System
Vaginal vein
use Hypogastric Vein, Left
use Hypogastric Vein, Right
Vaginectomy
see Excision, Vagina 0UBG
see Resection, Vagina 0UTG
Vaginofixation
see Repair, Vagina 0UQG
see Reposition, Vagina 0USG
Vaginoplasty
see Repair, Vagina 0UQG
see Supplement, Vagina 0UUG
Vaginorrhaphy *see* Repair, Vagina 0UQG
Vaginoscopy 0UJH8ZZ
Vaginotomy *see* Drainage, Female Reproductive System 0U9
Vagotomy *see* Division, Nerve, Vagus 008Q
Valiant Thoracic Stent Graft *use* Intraluminal Device
Valvotomy, valvulotomy
see Division, Heart and Great Vessels 028
see Release, Heart and Great Vessels 02N
Valvuloplasty
see Repair, Heart and Great Vessels 02Q
see Replacement, Heart and Great Vessels 02R
see Supplement, Heart and Great Vessels 02U
Valvuloplasty, Alfieri Stitch *see* Restriction, Valve, Mitral 02VG
Vascular Access Device
Totally Implantable
  Insertion of device in
    Abdomen 0JH8
    Chest 0JH6
    Lower Arm
      Left 0JHH
      Right 0JHG
    Lower Leg
      Left 0JHP
      Right 0JHN
    Upper Arm
      Left 0JHF
      Right 0JHD
    Upper Leg
      Left 0JHM
      Right 0JHL
  Removal of device from
    Lower Extremity 0JPW
    Trunk 0JPT
    Upper Extremity 0JPV
  Revision of device in
    Lower Extremity 0JWW
    Trunk 0JWT
    Upper Extremity 0JWV
Tunneled
  Insertion of device in
    Abdomen 0JH8
    Chest 0JH6
    Lower Arm
      Left 0JHH
      Right 0JHG
    Lower Leg
      Left 0JHP
      Right 0JHN
    Upper Arm
      Left 0JHF
      Right 0JHD
    Upper Leg
      Left 0JHM
      Right 0JHL
  Removal of device from
    Lower Extremity 0JPW
    Trunk 0JPT
    Upper Extremity 0JPV

Vascular Access Device — continued
Tunneled — *continued*
    Revision of device in
      Lower Extremity ØJWW
      Trunk ØJWT
      Upper Extremity ØJWV

Vasectomy *see* Excision, Male Reproductive System ØVB

Vasography
  see Fluoroscopy, Male Reproductive System BV1
  see Plain Radiography, Male Reproductive System BVØ

Vasoligation *see* Occlusion, Male Reproductive System ØVL

Vasorrhaphy *see* Repair, Male Reproductive System ØVQ

Vasostomy *see* Bypass, Male Reproductive System ØV1

Vasotomy
  Drainage *see* Drainage, Male Reproductive System ØV9
  With ligation *see* Occlusion, Male Reproductive System ØVL

Vasovasostomy *see* Repair, Male Reproductive System ØVQ

Vastus intermedius muscle
  use Upper Leg Muscle, Left
  use Upper Leg Muscle, Right

Vastus lateralis muscle
  use Upper Leg Muscle, Left
  use Upper Leg Muscle, Right

Vastus medialis muscle
  use Upper Leg Muscle, Left
  use Upper Leg Muscle, Right

VCG (vectorcardiogram) *see* Measurement, Cardiac 4AØ2

Vectra® Vascular Access Graft *use* Vascular Access Device, Tunneled in Subcutaneous Tissue and Fascia

Veklury *use* Remdesivir Anti-infective

Venclexta® *use* Venetoclax Antineoplastic

Venectomy
  see Excision, Lower Veins Ø6B
  see Excision, Upper Veins Ø5B

Venetoclax Antineoplastic XWØDXR5

Venography
  see Fluoroscopy, Veins B51
  see Plain Radiography, Veins B5Ø

Venorrhaphy
  see Repair, Lower Veins Ø6Q
  see Repair, Upper Veins Ø5Q

Venotripsy
  see Occlusion, Lower Veins Ø6L
  see Occlusion, Upper Veins Ø5L

Ventricular fold *use* Larynx

Ventriculoatriostomy *see* Bypass, Central Nervous System and Cranial Nerves ØØ1

Ventriculocisternostomy *see* Bypass, Central Nervous System and Cranial Nerves ØØ1

Ventriculogram, cardiac
  Combined left and right heart *see* Fluoroscopy, Heart, Right and Left B216
  Left ventricle *see* Fluoroscopy, Heart, Left B215
  Right ventricle *see* Fluoroscopy, Heart, Right B214

Ventriculopuncture, through previously implanted catheter 8CØ1X6J

Ventriculoscopy ØØJØ4ZZ

Ventriculostomy
  External drainage *see* Drainage, Cerebral Ventricle ØØ96
  Internal shunt *see* Bypass, Cerebral Ventricle ØØ16

Ventriculovenostomy *see* Bypass, Cerebral Ventricle ØØ16

Ventrio™ Hernia Patch *use* Synthetic Substitute

VEP (visual evoked potential) 4AØ7XØZ

Vermiform appendix *use* Appendix

Vermilion border
  use Lower Lip
  use Upper Lip

Versa *use* Pacemaker, Dual Chamber in ØJH

Version, obstetric
  External 1ØSØXZZ
  Internal 1ØSØ7ZZ

Vertebral arch
  use Cervical Vertebra
  use Lumbar Vertebra
  use Thoracic Vertebra

Vertebral body
  use Cervical Vertebra
  use Lumbar Vertebra
  use Thoracic Vertebra

Vertebral canal *use* Spinal Canal

Vertebral foramen
  use Cervical Vertebra
  use Lumbar Vertebra
  use Thoracic Vertebra

Vertebral lamina
  use Cervical Vertebra
  use Lumbar Vertebra
  use Thoracic Vertebra

Vertebral pedicle
  use Cervical Vertebra
  use Lumbar Vertebra
  use Thoracic Vertebra

Vesical vein
  use Hypogastric Vein, Left
  use Hypogastric Vein, Right

Vesicotomy *see* Drainage, Urinary System ØT9

Vesiculectomy
  see Excision, Male Reproductive System ØVB
  see Resection, Male Reproductive System ØVT

Vesiculogram, seminal *see* Plain Radiography, Male Reproductive System BVØ

Vesiculotomy *see* Drainage, Male Reproductive System ØV9

Vestibular Assessment F15Z

Vestibular (Scarpa's) ganglion *use* Acoustic Nerve

Vestibular nerve *use* Acoustic Nerve

Vestibular Treatment FØC

Vestibulocochlear nerve *use* Acoustic Nerve

VH-IVUS (virtual histology intravascular ultrasound) *see* Ultrasonography, Heart B24

Virchow's (supraclavicular) lymph node
  use Lymphatic, Left Neck
  use Lymphatic, Right Neck

Virtuoso (II) (DR) (VR) *use* Defibrillator Generator in ØJH

Vistogard(R) *use* Uridine Triacetate

Vitrectomy
  see Excision, Eye Ø8B
  see Resection, Eye Ø8T

Vitreous body
  use Vitreous, Left
  use Vitreous, Right

Viva (XT) (S) *use* Cardiac Resynchronization Defibrillator Pulse Generator in ØJH

Vocal fold
  use Vocal Cord, Left
  use Vocal Cord, Right

Vocational
  Assessment *see* Activities of Daily Living Assessment, Rehabilitation FØ2
  Retraining *see* Activities of Daily Living Treatment, Rehabilitation FØ8

Volar (palmar) digital vein
  use Hand Vein, Left
  use Hand Vein, Right

Volar (palmar) metacarpal vein
  use Hand Vein, Left
  use Hand Vein, Right

Vomer bone *use* Nasal Septum

Vomer of nasal septum *use* Nasal Bone

Voraxaze *use* Glucarpidase

Vulvectomy
  see Excision, Female Reproductive System ØUB
  see Resection, Female Reproductive System ØUT

V-Wave Interatrial Shunt System *use* Synthetic Substitute

VYXEOS™ *use* Cytarabine and Daunorubicin Liposome Antineoplastic

W

WALLSTENT® Endoprosthesis *use* Intraluminal Device

Washing *see* Irrigation

WavelinQ EndoAVF system
  Radial Artery, Left Ø31C3ZF
  Radial Artery, Right Ø31B3ZF
  Ulnar Artery, Left Ø31A3ZF
  Ulnar Artery, Right Ø3193ZF

Wedge resection, pulmonary *see* Excision, Respiratory System ØBB

Whole Blood Nucleic Acid-base Microbial Detection XXE5XM5

Window *see* Drainage

Wiring, dental 2W31X9Z

X

Xact Carotid Stent System *use* Intraluminal Device

XENLETA™ *use* Lefamulin Anti-infective

Xenograft *use* Zooplastic Tissue in Heart and Great Vessels

XIENCE Everolimus Eluting Coronary Stent System *use* Intraluminal Device, Drug-eluting in Heart and Great Vessels

Xiphoid process *use* Sternum

XLIF® System *use* Interbody Fusion Device in Lower Joints

XOSPATA® *use* Gilteritinib Antineoplastic

X-ray *see* Plain Radiography

X-STOP® Spacer
  use Spinal Stabilization Device, Interspinous Process in ØRH
  use Spinal Stabilization Device, Interspinous Process in ØSH

Y

Yescarta® *use* Axicabtagene Ciloleucel Immunotherapy

Yoga Therapy 8EØZXY4

Z

Zenith AAA Endovascular Graft *use* Intraluminal Device

Zenith Flex® AAA Endovascular Graft *use* Intraluminal Device

Zenith TX2® TAA Endovascular Graft *use* Intraluminal Device

Zenith® Fenestrated AAA Endovascular Graft
  use Intraluminal Device, Branched or Fenestrated, One or Two Arteries in Ø4V
  use Intraluminal Device, Branched or Fenestrated, Three or More Arteries in Ø4V

Zenith® Renu™ AAA Ancillary Graft *use* Intraluminal Device

ZEPZELCA™ *use* Lurbinectedin

ZERBAXA® *use* Ceftolozane/Tazobactam Anti-infective

Zilver® PTX® (paclitaxel) Drug-Eluting Peripheral Stent
  use Intraluminal Device, Drug-eluting in Lower Arteries
  use Intraluminal Device, Drug-eluting in Upper Arteries

Zimmer® NexGen® LPS Mobile Bearing Knee *use* Synthetic Substitute

Zimmer® NexGen® LPS-Flex Mobile Knee *use* Synthetic Substitute

ZINPLAVA™ *use* Bezlotoxumab Monoclonal Antibody

Zonule of Zinn
  use Lens, Left
  use Lens, Right

Zooplastic Tissue, Rapid Deployment Technique Replacement X2RF

Zotarolimus-eluting Coronary Stent *use* Intraluminal Device, Drug-eluting in Heart and Great Vessels

Z-plasty, skin for scar contracture *see* Release, Skin and Breast ØHN

ZULRESSO™ *use* Brexanolone

Zygomatic process of frontal bone *use* Frontal Bone

Zygomatic process of temporal bone
  use Temporal Bone, Left
  use Temporal Bone, Right

Zygomaticus muscle *use* Facial Muscle

Zyvox *use* Oxazolidinones

ICD-10-PCS Tables

Central Nervous System and Cranial Nerves 001–00X

Character Meanings

This Character Meaning table is provided as a guide to assist the user in the identification of character members that may be found in this section of code tables. It **SHOULD NOT** be used to build a PCS code.

Operation–Character 3		Body Part–Character 4		Approach–Character 5		Device–Character 6		Qualifier–Character 7	
1	Bypass	0	Brain	0	Open	0	Drainage Device	0	Nasopharynx
2	Change	1	Cerebral Meninges	3	Percutaneous	1	Radioactive Element	1	Mastoid Sinus
5	Destruction	2	Dura Mater	4	Percutaneous Endoscopic	2	Monitoring Device	2	Atrium
7	Dilation	3	Epidural Space, Intracranial	X	External	3	Infusion Device	3	Blood Vessel
8	Division	4	Subdural Space, Intracranial			4	Radioactive Element, Cesium-131 Collagen Implant	4	Pleural Cavity
9	Drainage	5	Subarachnoid Space, Intracranial			7	Autologous Tissue Substitute	5	Intestine
B	Excision	6	Cerebral Ventricle			J	Synthetic Substitute	6	Peritoneal Cavity
C	Extirpation	7	Cerebral Hemisphere			K	Nonautologous Tissue Substitute	7	Urinary Tract
D	Extraction	8	Basal Ganglia			M	Neurostimulator Lead	8	Bone Marrow
F	Fragmentation	9	Thalamus			Y	Other Device	9	Fallopian Tube
H	Insertion	A	Hypothalamus			Z	No Device	A	Subgaleal Space
J	Inspection	B	Pons					B	Cerebral Cisterns
K	Map	C	Cerebellum					F	Olfactory Nerve
N	Release	D	Medulla Oblongata					G	Optic Nerve
P	Removal	E	Cranial Nerve					H	Oculomotor Nerve
Q	Repair	F	Olfactory Nerve					J	Trochlear Nerve
R	Replacement	G	Optic Nerve					K	Trigeminal Nerve
S	Reposition	H	Oculomotor Nerve					L	Abducens Nerve
T	Resection	J	Trochlear Nerve					M	Facial Nerve
U	Supplement	K	Trigeminal Nerve					N	Acoustic Nerve
W	Revision	L	Abducens Nerve					P	Glossopharyngeal Nerve
X	Transfer	M	Facial Nerve					Q	Vagus Nerve
		N	Acoustic Nerve					R	Accessory Nerve
		P	Glossopharyngeal Nerve					S	Hypoglossal Nerve
		Q	Vagus Nerve					X	Diagnostic
		R	Accessory Nerve					Z	No Qualifier
		S	Hypoglossal Nerve						
		T	Spinal Meninges						
		U	Spinal Canal						
		V	Spinal Cord						
		W	Cervical Spinal Cord						
		X	Thoracic Spinal Cord						
		Y	Lumbar Spinal Cord						

AHA Coding Clinic for table 001

2021, 2Q, 19	Electromagnetic stealth guided ventriculoperitoneal shunt insertion with endoscopy
2019, 4Q, 21-22	Cerebral ventricle bypass Qualifier
2018, 4Q, 86	Placement of lumboatrial shunt
2017, 4Q, 39-41	Dilation and bypass of cerebral ventricle
2015, 2Q, 9	Revision of ventriculoperitoneal (VP) shunt
2013, 2Q, 36	Insertion of ventriculoperitoneal shunt with laparoscopic assistance

AHA Coding Clinic for table 005

2021, 2Q, 17	Dorsal root entry zone procedure

AHA Coding Clinic for table 007

2017, 4Q, 39-41	Dilation and bypass of cerebral ventricle

AHA Coding Clinic for table 009

2018, 4Q, 85	Externalization of lumboatrial shunt
2017, 1Q, 50	Failed lumbar puncture
2015, 3Q, 10	Open evacuation of subdural hematoma
2015, 3Q, 11	Percutaneous drainage of subdural hematoma
2015, 3Q, 12	Subdural evacuation portal system (SEPS) placement
2015, 3Q, 12	Placement of ventriculostomy catheter via burr hole
2015, 2Q, 30	Drainage of syrinx
2015, 1Q, 31	Intrathecal chemotherapy
2014, 1Q, 8	Diagnostic lumbar tap
2014, 1Q, 8	Lumbar drainage port aspiration

AHA Coding Clinic for table 00B

2017, 3Q, 17	Resection of schwannoma and placement of DuraGen and Lorenz cranial plating system
2016, 2Q, 12	Resection of malignant neoplasm of infratemporal fossa
2016, 2Q, 18	Amygdalohippocampectomy
2014, 4Q, 34	Resection of brain malignancy with implantation of chemotherapeutic wafer
2014, 3Q, 24	Repair of lipomyelomeningocele and tethered cord

AHA Coding Clinic for table 00C

2019, 3Q, 4	Evacuation of subdural hematoma and control of bleeding artery
2019, 2Q, 36	Evacuation of hematoma using NICO Brainpath® technology
2017, 4Q, 48	New and revised body part values - Extirpation spinal canal
2016, 2Q, 29	Decompressive craniectomy with cryopreservation and storage of bone flap
2015, 3Q, 10	Open evacuation of subdural hematoma
2015, 3Q, 11	Percutaneous drainage of subdural hematoma
2015, 3Q, 13	Evacuation of intracerebral hematoma

AHA Coding Clinic for table 00D

2015, 3Q, 13	Nonexcisional debridement of cranial wound with removal and replacement of hardware

AHA Coding Clinic for table 00H

2020, 4Q, 43-44	Insertion of radioactive element
2020, 2Q, 15	Ommaya Reservoir with Ventricular Catheter Placement
2020, 2Q, 16	Ommaya Reservoir Placement for Cerebrospinal Fluid Infusion Therapy
2017, 4Q, 30-31	Radiotherapeutic brain implant
2017, 3Q, 13	Implantation of bilateral neurostimulator electrodes
2014, 3Q, 19	End of life replacement of Baclofen pump

AHA Coding Clinic for table 00J

2021, 2Q, 19	Electromagnetic stealth guided ventriculoperitoneal shunt insertion with endoscopy
2019, 2Q, 36	Evacuation of hematoma using NICO Brainpath® technology
2017, 1Q, 50	Failed lumbar puncture

AHA Coding Clinic for table 00N

2019, 2Q, 19	Cervical spinal fusion, decompression and placement of interfacet stabilization device
2019, 1Q, 28	Decompressive laminectomy of both spinal cord and nerve roots
2018, 3Q, 30	Decompressive laminectomy (release of spinal cord versus release of spinal meninges)
2017, 3Q, 10	Repair of Chiari malformation
2017, 2Q, 23	Decompression of spinal cord and placement of instrumentation
2016, 2Q, 29	Decompressive craniectomy with cryopreservation and storage of bone flap
2015, 2Q, 20	Cervical laminoplasty
2015, 2Q, 21	Multiple decompressive cervical laminectomies
2015, 2Q, 34	Decompressive laminectomy
2014, 3Q, 24	Repair of lipomyelomeningocele and tethered cord

AHA Coding Clinic for table 00P

2014, 3Q, 19	End of life replacement of Baclofen pump

AHA Coding Clinic for table 00Q

2014, 3Q, 7	Hemi-cranioplasty for repair of cranial defect
2013, 3Q, 25	Fracture of frontal bone with repair and coagulation for hemostasis

AHA Coding Clinic for table 00S

2014, 4Q, 35	Reimplantation of buccal nerve

AHA Coding Clinic for table 00U

2018, 1Q, 9	Craniectomy with DuraGaurd placement
2017, 4Q, 62	Added and revised device values - Nerve substitutes
2017, 3Q, 10	Repair of Chiari malformation
2017, 3Q, 17	Resection of schwannoma and placement of DuraGen and Lorenz cranial plating system
2015, 4Q, 39	Dural patch graft
2014, 3Q, 24	Repair of lipomyelomeningocele and tethered cord

AHA Coding Clinic for table 00W

2018, 4Q, 86	Placement of lumboatrial shunt

Brain

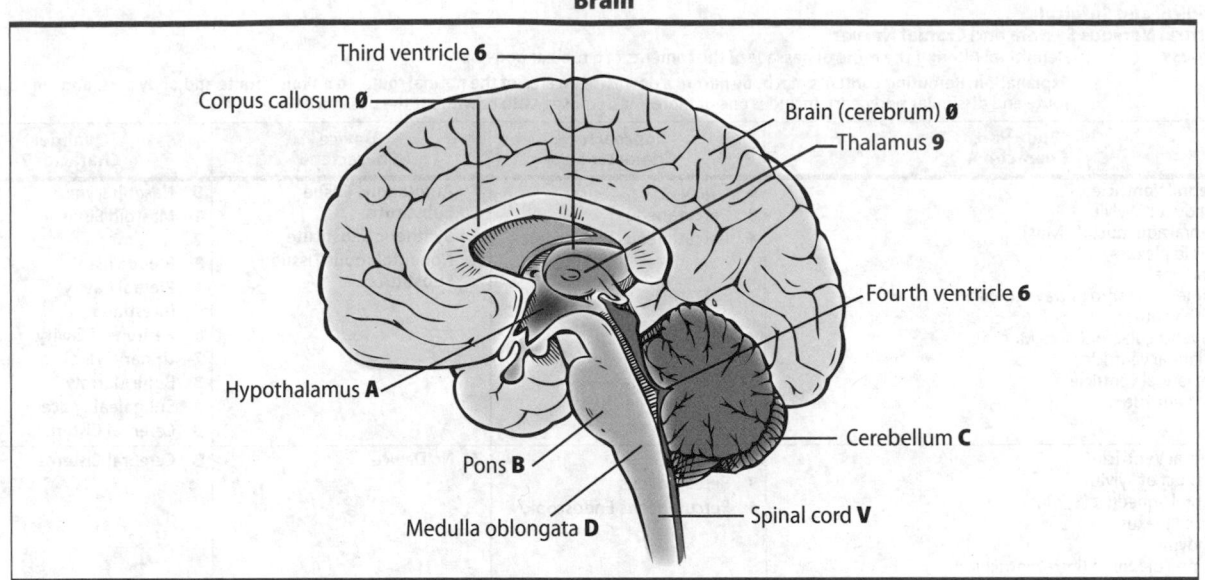

Third ventricle **6**
Corpus callosum **Ø**
Brain (cerebrum) **Ø**
Thalamus **9**
Fourth ventricle **6**
Hypothalamus **A**
Cerebellum **C**
Pons **B**
Medulla oblongata **D**
Spinal cord **V**

Cranial Nerves

Accessory nerve (XI) **R**
Hypoglossal nerve (XIII) **S**
Vagus nerve (X) **Q**
Glossopharyngeal nerve (IX) **P**
Vestibulocochlear nerve (VIII) **N**
Facial nerve (VII) **M**
Abducens nerve (VI) **L**
Trigeminal nerve (V) **K**
Trochlear nerve (IV) **J**
Oculomotor nerve (III) **H**
Optic nerve (II) **G**
Olfactory bulb (I) **F**
Pons **B**

Central Nervous System and Cranial Nerves

Ø   **Medical and Surgical**
Ø   **Central Nervous System and Cranial Nerves**
1   **Bypass**   Definition: Altering the route of passage of the contents of a tubular body part

           Explanation: Rerouting contents of a body part to a downstream area of the normal route, to a similar route and body part, or to an abnormal route and dissimilar body part. Includes one or more anastomoses, with or without the use of a device.

Body Part Character 4	Approach Character 5	Device Character 6	Qualifier Character 7

6 Cerebral Ventricle
  Aqueduct of Sylvius
  Cerebral aqueduct (Sylvius)
  Choroid plexus
  Ependyma
  Foramen of Monro (intraventricular)
  Fourth ventricle
  Interventricular foramen (Monro)
  Left lateral ventricle
  Right lateral ventricle
  Third ventricle
	Ø Open
	3 Percutaneous
	4 Percutaneous Endoscopic
		7 Autologous Tissue Substitute
		J Synthetic Substitute
		K Nonautologous Tissue Substitute
			Ø Nasopharynx
			1 Mastoid Sinus
			2 Atrium
			3 Blood Vessel
			4 Pleural Cavity
			5 Intestine
			6 Peritoneal Cavity
			7 Urinary Tract
			8 Bone Marrow
			A Subgaleal Space
			B Cerebral Cisterns

6 Cerebral Ventricle
  Aqueduct of Sylvius
  Cerebral aqueduct (Sylvius)
  Choroid plexus
  Ependyma
  Foramen of Monro (intraventricular)
  Fourth ventricle
  Interventricular foramen (Monro)
  Left lateral ventricle
  Right lateral ventricle
  Third ventricle
	Ø Open
	3 Percutaneous
	4 Percutaneous Endoscopic
		Z No Device	B Cerebral Cisterns

U Spinal Canal
  Epidural space, spinal
  Extradural space, spinal
  Subarachnoid space, spinal
  Subdural space, spinal
  Vertebral canal
	Ø Open
	3 Percutaneous
	4 Percutaneous Endoscopic
		7 Autologous Tissue Substitute
		J Synthetic Substitute
		K Nonautologous Tissue Substitute
			2 Atrium
			4 Pleural Cavity
			6 Peritoneal Cavity
			7 Urinary Tract
			9 Fallopian Tube

Ø   **Medical and Surgical**
Ø   **Central Nervous System and Cranial Nerves**
2   **Change**   Definition: Taking out or off a device from a body part and putting back an identical or similar device in or on the same body part without cutting or puncturing the skin or a mucous membrane

           Explanation: All CHANGE procedures are coded using the approach EXTERNAL

Body Part Character 4	Approach Character 5	Device Character 6	Qualifier Character 7

Ø Brain
  Cerebrum
  Corpus callosum
  Encephalon
E Cranial Nerve
U Spinal Canal
  Epidural space, spinal
  Extradural space, spinal
  Subarachnoid space, spinal
  Subdural space, spinal
  Vertebral canal
	X External	Ø Drainage Device
		Y Other Device
			Z No Qualifier

Non-OR   All body part, approach, device, and qualifier values

Ø   **Medical and Surgical**
Ø   **Central Nervous System and Cranial Nerves**
5   **Destruction**   Definition: Physical eradication of all or a portion of a body part by the direct use of energy, force, or a destructive agent
                 Explanation: None of the body part is physically taken out

Body Part Character 4		Approach Character 5	Device Character 6	Qualifier Character 7
Ø **Brain** Cerebrum Corpus callosum Encephalon	**H** **Oculomotor Nerve** Third cranial nerve **J** **Trochlear Nerve** Fourth cranial nerve	**Ø** Open **3** Percutaneous **4** Percutaneous Endoscopic	**Z** No Device	**Z** No Qualifier
1 **Cerebral Meninges** Arachnoid mater, intracranial Leptomeninges, intracranial Pia mater, intracranial	**K** **Trigeminal Nerve** Fifth cranial nerve Gasserian ganglion Mandibular nerve Maxillary nerve Ophthalmic nerve Trifacial nerve			
2 **Dura Mater** Diaphragma sellae Dura mater, intracranial Falx cerebri Tentorium cerebelli	**L** **Abducens Nerve** Sixth cranial nerve **M** **Facial Nerve** Chorda tympani Geniculate ganglion Greater superficial petrosal nerve Nerve to the stapedius Parotid plexus Posterior auricular nerve Seventh cranial nerve Submandibular ganglion			
6 **Cerebral Ventricle** Aqueduct of Sylvius Cerebral aqueduct (Sylvius) Choroid plexus Ependyma Foramen of Monro (intraventricular) Fourth ventricle Interventricular foramen (Monro) Left lateral ventricle Right lateral ventricle Third ventricle	**N** **Acoustic Nerve** Cochlear nerve Eighth cranial nerve Scarpa's (vestibular) ganglion Spiral ganglion Vestibular (Scarpa's) ganglion Vestibular nerve Vestibulocochlear nerve			
7 **Cerebral Hemisphere** Frontal lobe Occipital lobe Parietal lobe Temporal lobe	**P** **Glossopharyngeal Nerve** Carotid sinus nerve Ninth cranial nerve Tympanic nerve			
8 **Basal Ganglia** Basal nuclei Claustrum Corpus striatum Globus pallidus Substantia nigra Subthalamic nucleus	**Q** **Vagus Nerve** Anterior vagal trunk Pharyngeal plexus Pneumogastric nerve Posterior vagal trunk Pulmonary plexus Recurrent laryngeal nerve Superior laryngeal nerve Tenth cranial nerve			
9 **Thalamus** Epithalamus Geniculate nucleus Metathalamus Pulvinar	**R** **Accessory Nerve** Eleventh cranial nerve			
A **Hypothalamus** Mammillary body	**S** **Hypoglossal Nerve** Twelfth cranial nerve			
B **Pons** Apneustic center Basis pontis Locus ceruleus Pneumotaxic center Pontine tegmentum Superior olivary nucleus	**T** **Spinal Meninges** Arachnoid mater, spinal Denticulate (dentate) ligament Dura mater, spinal Filum terminale Leptomeninges, spinal Pia mater, spinal			
C **Cerebellum** Culmen	**W** **Cervical Spinal Cord** Dorsal root ganglion			
D **Medulla Oblongata** Myelencephalon	**X** **Thoracic Spinal Cord** Dorsal root ganglion			
F **Olfactory Nerve** First cranial nerve Olfactory bulb	**Y** **Lumbar Spinal Cord** Cauda equina Conus medullaris Dorsal root ganglion			
G **Optic Nerve** Optic chiasma Second cranial nerve				

Non-OR   ØØ5[F,G,H,J,K,L,M,N,P,Q,R,S][Ø,3,4]ZZ

Ø Medical and Surgical
Ø Central Nervous System and Cranial Nerves
7 Dilation   Definition: Expanding an orifice or the lumen of a tubular body part

Explanation: The orifice can be a natural orifice or an artificially created orifice. Accomplished by stretching a tubular body part using intraluminal pressure or by cutting part of the orifice or wall of the tubular body part.

Body Part Character 4	Approach Character 5	Device Character 6	Qualifier Character 7
6 Cerebral Ventricle Aqueduct of Sylvius Cerebral aqueduct (Sylvius) Choroid plexus Ependyma Foramen of Monro (intraventricular) Fourth ventricle Interventricular foramen (Monro) Left lateral ventricle Right lateral ventricle Third ventricle	**Ø** Open **3** Percutaneous **4** Percutaneous Endoscopic	**Z** No Device	**Z** No Qualifier

Ø Medical and Surgical
Ø Central Nervous System and Cranial Nerves
8 Division   Definition: Cutting into a body part, without draining fluids and/or gases from the body part, in order to separate or transect a body part

Explanation: All or a portion of the body part is separated into two or more portions

Body Part Character 4		Approach Character 5	Device Character 6	Qualifier Character 7
Ø Brain Cerebrum Corpus callosum Encephalon **7 Cerebral Hemisphere** Frontal lobe Occipital lobe Parietal lobe Temporal lobe **8 Basal Ganglia** Basal nuclei Claustrum Corpus striatum Globus pallidus Substantia nigra Subthalamic nucleus **F Olfactory Nerve** First cranial nerve Olfactory bulb **G Optic Nerve** Optic chiasma Second cranial nerve **H Oculomotor Nerve** Third cranial nerve **J Trochlear Nerve** Fourth cranial nerve **K Trigeminal Nerve** Fifth cranial nerve Gasserian ganglion Mandibular nerve Maxillary nerve Ophthalmic nerve Trifacial nerve **L Abducens Nerve** Sixth cranial nerve **M Facial Nerve** Chorda tympani Geniculate ganglion Greater superficial petrosal nerve Nerve to the stapedius Parotid plexus Posterior auricular nerve Seventh cranial nerve Submandibular ganglion	**N Acoustic Nerve** Cochlear nerve Eighth cranial nerve Scarpa's (vestibular) ganglion Spiral ganglion Vestibular (Scarpa's) ganglion Vestibular nerve Vestibulocochlear nerve **P Glossopharyngeal Nerve** Carotid sinus nerve Ninth cranial nerve Tympanic nerve **Q Vagus Nerve** Anterior vagal trunk Pharyngeal plexus Pneumogastric nerve Posterior vagal trunk Pulmonary plexus Recurrent laryngeal nerve Superior laryngeal nerve Tenth cranial nerve **R Accessory Nerve** Eleventh cranial nerve **S Hypoglossal Nerve** Twelfth cranial nerve **W Cervical Spinal Cord** Dorsal root ganglion **X Thoracic Spinal Cord** Dorsal root ganglion **Y Lumbar Spinal Cord** Cauda equina Conus medullaris Dorsal root ganglion	**Ø** Open **3** Percutaneous **4** Percutaneous Endoscopic	**Z** No Device	**Z** No Qualifier

Non-OR Procedure   DRG Non-OR Procedure   Valid OR Procedure   HAC Associated Procedure   Combination Only   New/Revised GREEN

Ø **Medical and Surgical**
Ø **Central Nervous System and Cranial Nerves**
9 **Drainage**　　　Definition: Taking or letting out fluids and/or gases from a body part
　　　　　　　　　Explanation: The qualifier DIAGNOSTIC is used to identify drainage procedures that are biopsies

Body Part Character 4		Approach Character 5	Device Character 6	Qualifier Character 7
Ø **Brain** 　Cerebrum 　Corpus callosum 　Encephalon 1 **Cerebral Meninges** 　Arachnoid mater, 　　intracranial 　Leptomeninges, 　　intracranial 　Pia mater, intracranial 2 **Dura Mater** 　Diaphragma sellae 　Dura mater, intracranial 　Falx cerebri 　Tentorium cerebelli 3 **Epidural Space,** **Intracranial** 　Extradural space, 　　intracranial 4 **Subdural Space,** **Intracranial** 5 **Subarachnoid Space,** **Intracranial** 6 **Cerebral Ventricle** 　Aqueduct of Sylvius 　Cerebral aqueduct 　　(Sylvius) 　Choroid plexus 　Ependyma 　Foramen of Monro 　　(intraventricular) 　Fourth ventricle 　Interventricular foramen 　　(Monro) 　Left lateral ventricle 　Right lateral ventricle 　Third ventricle 7 **Cerebral Hemisphere** 　Frontal lobe 　Occipital lobe 　Parietal lobe 　Temporal lobe 8 **Basal Ganglia** 　Basal nuclei 　Claustrum 　Corpus striatum 　Globus pallidus 　Substantia nigra 　Subthalamic nucleus 9 **Thalamus** 　Epithalamus 　Geniculate nucleus 　Metathalamus 　Pulvinar A **Hypothalamus** 　Mammillary body B **Pons** 　Apneustic center 　Basis pontis 　Locus ceruleus 　Pneumotaxic center 　Pontine tegmentum 　Superior olivary nucleus C **Cerebellum** 　Culmen D **Medulla Oblongata** 　Myelencephalon F **Olfactory Nerve** 　First cranial nerve 　Olfactory bulb	G **Optic Nerve** 　Optic chiasma 　Second cranial nerve H **Oculomotor Nerve** 　Third cranial nerve J **Trochlear Nerve** 　Fourth cranial nerve K **Trigeminal Nerve** 　Fifth cranial nerve 　Gasserian ganglion 　Mandibular nerve 　Maxillary nerve 　Ophthalmic nerve 　Trifacial nerve L **Abducens Nerve** 　Sixth cranial nerve M **Facial Nerve** 　Chorda tympani 　Geniculate ganglion 　Greater superficial petrosal 　　nerve 　Nerve to the stapedius 　Parotid plexus 　Posterior auricular nerve 　Seventh cranial nerve 　Submandibular ganglion N **Acoustic Nerve** 　Cochlear nerve 　Eighth cranial nerve 　Scarpa's (vestibular) ganglion 　Spiral ganglion 　Vestibular (Scarpa's) ganglion 　Vestibular nerve 　Vestibulocochlear nerve P **Glossopharyngeal Nerve** 　Carotid sinus nerve 　Ninth cranial nerve 　Tympanic nerve Q **Vagus Nerve** 　Anterior vagal trunk 　Pharyngeal plexus 　Pneumogastric nerve 　Posterior vagal trunk 　Pulmonary plexus 　Recurrent laryngeal nerve 　Superior laryngeal nerve 　Tenth cranial nerve R **Accessory Nerve** 　Eleventh cranial nerve S **Hypoglossal Nerve** 　Twelfth cranial nerve T **Spinal Meninges** 　Arachnoid mater, spinal 　Denticulate (dentate) 　　ligament 　Dura mater, spinal 　Filum terminale 　Leptomeninges, spinal 　Pia mater, spinal U **Spinal Canal** 　Epidural space, spinal 　Extradural space, spinal 　Subarachnoid space, spinal 　Subdural space, spinal 　Vertebral canal W **Cervical Spinal Cord** 　Dorsal root ganglion X **Thoracic Spinal Cord** 　Dorsal root ganglion Y **Lumbar Spinal Cord** 　Cauda equina 　Conus medullaris 　Dorsal root ganglion	Ø Open 3 Percutaneous 4 Percutaneous Endoscopic	Ø Drainage Device	Z No Qualifier

Non-OR	ØØ9[T,W,X,Y]3ØZ
Non-OR	ØØ9U[3,4]ØZ

ØØ9 Continued on next page

NC Noncovered Procedure　　LC Limited Coverage　　QA Questionable OB Admit　　NT New Tech Add-on　　⊞ Combination Member　　♂ Male　　♀ Female

ICD-10-PCS 2022　　　　　　　　　　　　　　　　　　　　　　　　　　　137

Central Nervous System and Cranial Nerves

Ø	Medical and Surgical		**ØØ9 Continued**
Ø	Central Nervous System and Cranial Nerves		
9	Drainage	Definition: Taking or letting out fluids and/or gases from a body part	
		Explanation: The qualifier DIAGNOSTIC is used to identify drainage procedures that are biopsies	

Body Part Character 4		Approach Character 5	Device Character 6	Qualifier Character 7
Ø **Brain** Cerebrum Corpus callosum Encephalon	G **Optic Nerve** Optic chiasma Second cranial nerve	Ø Open 3 Percutaneous 4 Percutaneous Endoscopic	Z No Device	X Diagnostic Z No Qualifier
1 **Cerebral Meninges** Arachnoid mater, intracranial Leptomeninges, intracranial Pia mater, intracranial	H **Oculomotor Nerve** Third cranial nerve J **Trochlear Nerve** Fourth cranial nerve K **Trigeminal Nerve** Fifth cranial nerve Gasserian ganglion			
2 **Dura Mater** Diaphragma sellae Dura mater, intracranial Falx cerebri Tentorium cerebelli	Mandibular nerve Maxillary nerve Ophthalmic nerve Trifacial nerve			
3 **Epidural Space, Intracranial** Extradural space, intracranial	L **Abducens Nerve** Sixth cranial nerve M **Facial Nerve** Chorda tympani Geniculate ganglion			
4 **Subdural Space, Intracranial**	Greater superficial petrosal nerve Nerve to the stapedius			
5 **Subarachnoid Space, Intracranial**	Parotid plexus Posterior auricular nerve			
6 **Cerebral Ventricle** Aqueduct of Sylvius Cerebral aqueduct (Sylvius) Choroid plexus Ependyma Foramen of Monro (intraventricular) Fourth ventricle Interventricular foramen (Monro) Left lateral ventricle Right lateral ventricle Third ventricle	Seventh cranial nerve Submandibular ganglion N **Acoustic Nerve** Cochlear nerve Eighth cranial nerve Scarpa's (vestibular) ganglion Spiral ganglion Vestibular (Scarpa's) ganglion Vestibular nerve Vestibulocochlear nerve			
7 **Cerebral Hemisphere** Frontal lobe Occipital lobe Parietal lobe Temporal lobe	P **Glossopharyngeal Nerve** Carotid sinus nerve Ninth cranial nerve Tympanic nerve			
8 **Basal Ganglia** Basal nuclei Claustrum Corpus striatum Globus pallidus Substantia nigra Subthalamic nucleus	Q **Vagus Nerve** Anterior vagal trunk Pharyngeal plexus Pneumogastric nerve Posterior vagal trunk Pulmonary plexus Recurrent laryngeal nerve Superior laryngeal nerve Tenth cranial nerve			
9 **Thalamus** Epithalamus Geniculate nucleus Metathalamus Pulvinar	R **Accessory Nerve** Eleventh cranial nerve S **Hypoglossal Nerve** Twelfth cranial nerve			
A **Hypothalamus** Mammillary body	T **Spinal Meninges** Arachnoid mater, spinal Denticulate (dentate) ligament			
B **Pons** Apneustic center Basis pontis Locus ceruleus Pneumotaxic center Pontine tegmentum Superior olivary nucleus	Dura mater, spinal Filum terminale Leptomeninges, spinal Pia mater, spinal U **Spinal Canal** Epidural space, spinal Extradural space, spinal Subarachnoid space, spinal Subdural space, spinal Vertebral canal			
C **Cerebellum** Culmen				
D **Medulla Oblongata** Myelencephalon	W **Cervical Spinal Cord** Dorsal root ganglion			
F **Olfactory Nerve** First cranial nerve Olfactory bulb	X **Thoracic Spinal Cord** Dorsal root ganglion Y **Lumbar Spinal Cord** Cauda equina Conus medullaris Dorsal root ganglion			

Non-OR   ØØ9[Ø,1,2,3,4,5,6,7,8,9,A,B,C,D,F,G,H,J,K,L,M,N,P,Q,R,S][3,4]ZX
Non-OR   ØØ9[T,W,X,Y]3Z[X,Z]
Non-OR   ØØ9U[3,4]Z[X,Z]

0 **Medical and Surgical**
0 **Central Nervous System and Cranial Nerves**
B **Excision** Definition: Cutting out or off, without replacement, a portion of a body part
Explanation: The qualifier DIAGNOSTIC is used to identify excision procedures that are biopsies

Body Part Character 4		Approach Character 5	Device Character 6	Qualifier Character 7
0 Brain Cerebrum Corpus callosum Encephalon	**H Oculomotor Nerve** Third cranial nerve	**0 Open** **3 Percutaneous** **4 Percutaneous Endoscopic**	**Z No Device**	**X Diagnostic** **Z No Qualifier**
1 Cerebral Meninges Arachnoid mater, intracranial Leptomeninges, intracranial Pia mater, intracranial	**J Trochlear Nerve** Fourth cranial nerve			
2 Dura Mater Diaphragma sellae Dura mater, intracranial Falx cerebri Tentorium cerebelli	**K Trigeminal Nerve** Fifth cranial nerve Gasserian ganglion Mandibular nerve Maxillary nerve Ophthalmic nerve Trifacial nerve			
6 Cerebral Ventricle Aqueduct of Sylvius Cerebral aqueduct (Sylvius) Choroid plexus Ependyma Foramen of Monro (intraventricular) Fourth ventricle Interventricular foramen (Monro) Left lateral ventricle Right lateral ventricle Third ventricle	**L Abducens Nerve** Sixth cranial nerve **M Facial Nerve** Chorda tympani Geniculate ganglion Greater superficial petrosal nerve Nerve to the stapedius Parotid plexus Posterior auricular nerve Seventh cranial nerve Submandibular ganglion			
7 Cerebral Hemisphere Frontal lobe Occipital lobe Parietal lobe Temporal lobe	**N Acoustic Nerve** Cochlear nerve Eighth cranial nerve Scarpa's (vestibular) ganglion Spiral ganglion Vestibular (Scarpa's) ganglion Vestibular nerve Vestibulocochlear nerve			
8 Basal Ganglia Basal nuclei Claustrum Corpus striatum Globus pallidus Substantia nigra Subthalamic nucleus	**P Glossopharyngeal Nerve** Carotid sinus nerve Ninth cranial nerve Tympanic nerve			
9 Thalamus Epithalamus Geniculate nucleus Metathalamus Pulvinar	**Q Vagus Nerve** Anterior vagal trunk Pharyngeal plexus Pneumogastric nerve Posterior vagal trunk Pulmonary plexus Recurrent laryngeal nerve Superior laryngeal nerve Tenth cranial nerve			
A Hypothalamus Mammillary body	**R Accessory Nerve** Eleventh cranial nerve			
B Pons Apneustic center Basis pontis Locus ceruleus Pneumotaxic center Pontine tegmentum Superior olivary nucleus	**S Hypoglossal Nerve** Twelfth cranial nerve **T Spinal Meninges** Arachnoid mater, spinal Denticulate (dentate) ligament Dura mater, spinal Filum terminale Leptomeninges, spinal Pia mater, spinal			
C Cerebellum Culmen	**W Cervical Spinal Cord** Dorsal root ganglion			
D Medulla Oblongata Myelencephalon	**X Thoracic Spinal Cord** Dorsal root ganglion			
F Olfactory Nerve First cranial nerve Olfactory bulb	**Y Lumbar Spinal Cord** Cauda equina Conus medullaris Dorsal root ganglion			
G Optic Nerve Optic chiasma Second cranial nerve				

Non-OR 00B[F,G,H,J,K,L,M,N,P,Q,R,S][3,4]ZX

Central Nervous System and Cranial Nerves

0   **Medical and Surgical**
0   **Central Nervous System and Cranial Nerves**
C   **Extirpation**   Definition: Taking or cutting out solid matter from a body part

Explanation: The solid matter may be an abnormal byproduct of a biological function or a foreign body; it may be imbedded in a body part or in the lumen of a tubular body part. The solid matter may or may not have been previously broken into pieces.

Body Part Character 4		Approach Character 5	Device Character 6	Qualifier Character 7

0 **Brain**
  Cerebrum
  Corpus callosum
  Encephalon
1 **Cerebral Meninges**
  Arachnoid mater,
    intracranial
  Leptomeninges,
    intracranial
  Pia mater, intracranial
2 **Dura Mater**
  Diaphragma sellae
  Dura mater, intracranial
  Falx cerebri
  Tentorium cerebelli
3 **Epidural Space,**
  Intracranial
  Extradural space,
    intracranial
4 **Subdural Space,**
  Intracranial
5 **Subarachnoid Space,**
  Intracranial
6 **Cerebral Ventricle**
  Aqueduct of Sylvius
  Cerebral aqueduct
    (Sylvius)
  Choroid plexus
  Ependyma
  Foramen of Monro
    (intraventricular)
  Fourth ventricle
  Interventricular foramen
    (Monro)
  Left lateral ventricle
  Right lateral ventricle
  Third ventricle
7 **Cerebral Hemisphere**
  Frontal lobe
  Occipital lobe
  Parietal lobe
  Temporal lobe
8 **Basal Ganglia**
  Basal nuclei
  Claustrum
  Corpus striatum
  Globus pallidus
  Substantia nigra
  Subthalamic nucleus
9 **Thalamus**
  Epithalamus
  Geniculate nucleus
  Metathalamus
  Pulvinar
A **Hypothalamus**
  Mammillary body
B **Pons**
  Apneustic center
  Basis pontis
  Locus ceruleus
  Pneumotaxic center
  Pontine tegmentum
  Superior olivary nucleus
C **Cerebellum**
  Culmen
D **Medulla Oblongata**
  Myelencephalon
F **Olfactory Nerve**
  First cranial nerve
  Olfactory bulb
	G **Optic Nerve**
	  Optic chiasma
	  Second cranial nerve
	H **Oculomotor Nerve**
	  Third cranial nerve
	J **Trochlear Nerve**
	  Fourth cranial nerve
	K **Trigeminal Nerve**
	  Fifth cranial nerve
	  Gasserian ganglion
	  Mandibular nerve
	  Maxillary nerve
	  Ophthalmic nerve
	  Trifacial nerve
	L **Abducens Nerve**
	  Sixth cranial nerve
	M **Facial Nerve**
	  Chorda tympani
	  Geniculate ganglion
	  Greater superficial petrosal
	    nerve
	  Nerve to the stapedius
	  Parotid plexus
	  Posterior auricular nerve
	  Seventh cranial nerve
	  Submandibular ganglion
	N **Acoustic Nerve**
	  Cochlear nerve
	  Eighth cranial nerve
	  Scarpa's (vestibular)
	    ganglion
	  Spiral ganglion
	  Vestibular (Scarpa's)
	    ganglion
	  Vestibular nerve
	  Vestibulocochlear nerve
	P **Glossopharyngeal Nerve**
	  Carotid sinus nerve
	  Ninth cranial nerve
	  Tympanic nerve
	Q **Vagus Nerve**
	  Anterior vagal trunk
	  Pharyngeal plexus
	  Pneumogastric nerve
	  Posterior vagal trunk
	  Pulmonary plexus
	  Recurrent laryngeal nerve
	  Superior laryngeal nerve
	  Tenth cranial nerve
	R **Accessory Nerve**
	  Eleventh cranial nerve
	S **Hypoglossal Nerve**
	  Twelfth cranial nerve
	T **Spinal Meninges**
	  Arachnoid mater, spinal
	  Denticulate (dentate)
	    ligament
	  Dura mater, spinal
	  Filum terminale
	  Leptomeninges, spinal
	  Pia mater, spinal
	U **Spinal Canal**
	W **Cervical Spinal Cord**
	  Dorsal root ganglion
	X **Thoracic Spinal Cord**
	  Dorsal root ganglion
	Y **Lumbar Spinal Cord**
	  Cauda equina
	  Conus medullaris
	  Dorsal root ganglion
		0 **Open**
		3 **Percutaneous**
		4 **Percutaneous Endoscopic**
			Z **No Device**	Z **No Qualifier**

Ø   **Medical and Surgical**
Ø   **Central Nervous System and Cranial Nerves**
D   **Extraction**   Definition: Pulling or stripping out or off all or a portion of a body part by the use of force
                       Explanation: The qualifier DIAGNOSTIC is used to identify extraction procedures that are biopsies

Body Part Character 4		Approach Character 5	Device Character 6	Qualifier Character 7

Ø Brain
  Cerebrum
  Corpus callosum
  Encephalon
1 **Cerebral Meninges**
  Arachnoid mater,
    intracranial
  Leptomeninges,
    intracranial
  Pia mater, intracranial
2 **Dura Mater**
  Diaphragma sellae
  Dura mater, intracranial
  Falx cerebri
  Tentorium cerebelli
7 Cerebral Hemisphere
  Frontal lobe
  Occipital lobe
  Parietal lobe
  Temporal lobe
F **Olfactory Nerve**
  First cranial nerve
  Olfactory bulb
G **Optic Nerve**
  Optic chiasma
  Second cranial nerve
H **Oculomotor Nerve**
  Third cranial nerve
J **Trochlear Nerve**
  Fourth cranial nerve
K **Trigeminal Nerve**
  Fifth cranial nerve
  Gasserian ganglion
  Mandibular nerve
  Maxillary nerve
  Ophthalmic nerve
  Trifacial nerve
L **Abducens Nerve**
  Sixth cranial nerve
	M **Facial Nerve**
	  Chorda tympani
	  Geniculate ganglion
	  Greater superficial petrosal
	    nerve
	  Nerve to the stapedius
	  Parotid plexus
	  Posterior auricular nerve
	  Seventh cranial nerve
	  Submandibular ganglion
	N **Acoustic Nerve**
	  Cochlear nerve
	  Eighth cranial nerve
	  Scarpa's (vestibular)
	    ganglion
	  Spiral ganglion
	  Vestibular (Scarpa's)
	    ganglion
	  Vestibular nerve
	  Vestibulocochlear nerve
	P **Glossopharyngeal Nerve**
	  Carotid sinus nerve
	  Ninth cranial nerve
	  Tympanic nerve
	Q **Vagus Nerve**
	  Anterior vagal trunk
	  Pharyngeal plexus
	  Pneumogastric nerve
	  Posterior vagal trunk
	  Pulmonary plexus
	  Recurrent laryngeal nerve
	  Superior laryngeal nerve
	  Tenth cranial nerve
	R **Accessory Nerve**
	  Eleventh cranial nerve
	S **Hypoglossal Nerve**
	  Twelfth cranial nerve
	T **Spinal Meninges**
	  Arachnoid mater, spinal
	  Denticulate (dentate)
	    ligament
	  Dura mater, spinal
	  Filum terminale
	  Leptomeninges, spinal
	  Pia mater, spinal
		Ø Open
		3 Percutaneous
		4 Percutaneous Endoscopic
			Z No Device	**Z** No Qualifier

0   **Medical and Surgical**
0   **Central Nervous System and Cranial Nerves**
F   **Fragmentation**   Definition: Breaking solid matter in a body part into pieces.

Explanation: Physical force (e.g., manual, ultrasonic) applied directly or indirectly is used to break the solid matter into pieces. The solid matter may be an abnormal byproduct of a biological function or a foreign body. The pieces of solid matter are not taken out.

Body Part Character 4	Approach Character 5	Device Character 6	Qualifier Character 7

3 **Epidural Space, Intracranial** NC
    Extradural space, intracranial
4 **Subdural Space, Intracranial** NC
5 **Subarachnoid Space, Intracranial** NC
6 **Cerebral Ventricle** NC
    Aqueduct of Sylvius
    Cerebral aqueduct (Sylvius)
    Choroid plexus
    Ependyma
    Foramen of Monro (intraventricular)
    Fourth ventricle
    Interventricular foramen (Monro)
    Left lateral ventricle
    Right lateral ventricle
    Third ventricle
U **Spinal Canal**
    Epidural space, spinal
    Extradural space, spinal
    Subarachnoid space, spinal
    Subdural space, spinal
    Vertebral canal
	0 Open
	3 Percutaneous
	4 Percutaneous Endoscopic
	X External
		Z No Device	**Z** No Qualifier

Non-OR	00F[3,4,5,6]XZZ
NC	00F[3,4,5,6]XZZ

0   **Medical and Surgical**
0   **Central Nervous System and Cranial Nerves**
H   **Insertion**   Definition: Putting in a nonbiological appliance that monitors, assists, performs, or prevents a physiological function but does not physically take the place of a body part

Explanation: None

Body Part Character 4	Approach Character 5	Device Character 6	Qualifier Character 7

0 **Brain** ⊞
    Cerebrum
    Corpus callosum
    Encephalon
	0 Open	**1** Radioactive Element
		2 Monitoring Device
		3 Infusion Device
		4 Radioactive Element, Cesium-131
		    Collagen Implant
		M Neurostimulator Lead
		Y Other Device
			Z No Qualifier

0 **Brain** ⊞
    Cerebrum
    Corpus callosum
    Encephalon
	3 Percutaneous
	4 Percutaneous Endoscopic
		1 Radioactive Element
		2 Monitoring Device
		3 Infusion Device
		M Neurostimulator Lead
		Y Other Device
			Z No Qualifier

6 **Cerebral Ventricle** ⊞
    Aqueduct of Sylvius
    Cerebral aqueduct (Sylvius)
    Choroid plexus
    Ependyma
    Foramen of Monro (intraventricular)
    Fourth ventricle Interventricular foramen
    (Monro)
    Left lateral ventricle
    Right lateral ventricle
    Third ventricle
E **Cranial Nerve** ⊞
U **Spinal Canal** ⊞
    Epidural space, spinal
    Extradural space, spinal
    Subarachnoid space, spinal
    Subdural space, spinal
    Vertebral canal
V **Spinal Cord** ⊞
    Dorsal root ganglion
	0 Open
	3 Percutaneous
	4 Percutaneous Endoscopic
		1 Radioactive Element
		2 Monitoring Device
		3 Infusion Device
		M Neurostimulator Lead
		Y Other Device
			Z No Qualifier

DRG Non-OR	00H004Z	**See Appendix L for Procedure Combinations**
Non-OR	00H[E,U,V]32Z	⊞ 00H00MZ
Non-OR	00H[E,U][3,4]YZ	⊞ 00H0[3,4]MZ
Non-OR	00H[U,V][0,3,4]3Z	⊞ 00H[6,E,U,V][0,3,4]MZ

Ø   **Medical and Surgical**
Ø   **Central Nervous System and Cranial Nerves**
J   **Inspection**   Definition: Visually and/or manually exploring a body part

           Explanation: Visual exploration may be performed with or without optical instrumentation. Manual exploration may be performed directly or through intervening body layers.

Body Part Character 4	Approach Character 5	Device Character 6	Qualifier Character 7

Ø **Brain**
    Cerebrum
    Corpus callosum
    Encephalon
E **Cranial Nerve**
U **Spinal Canal**
    Epidural space, spinal
    Extradural space, spinal
    Subarachnoid space, spinal
    Subdural space, spinal
    Vertebral canal
V **Spinal Cord**
    Dorsal root ganglion
	Ø Open
	3 Percutaneous
	4 Percutaneous Endoscopic
		Z No Device	Z No Qualifier

Non-OR	ØØJ[Ø,E,U,V]3ZZ

Ø   **Medical and Surgical**
Ø   **Central Nervous System and Cranial Nerves**
K   **Map**   Definition: Locating the route of passage of electrical impulses and/or locating functional areas in a body part

           Explanation: Applicable only to the cardiac conduction mechanism and the central nervous system

Body Part Character 4	Approach Character 5	Device Character 6	Qualifier Character 7

Ø **Brain**
    Cerebrum
    Corpus callosum
    Encephalon
7 **Cerebral Hemisphere**
    Frontal lobe
    Occipital lobe
    Parietal lobe
    Temporal lobe
8 **Basal Ganglia**
    Basal nuclei
    Claustrum
    Corpus striatum
    Globus pallidus
    Substantia nigra
    Subthalamic nucleus
9 **Thalamus**
    Epithalamus
    Geniculate nucleus
    Metathalamus
    Pulvinar
A **Hypothalamus**
    Mammillary body
B **Pons**
    Apneustic center
    Basis pontis
    Locus ceruleus
    Pneumotaxic center
    Pontine tegmentum
    Superior olivary nucleus
C **Cerebellum**
    Culmen
D **Medulla Oblongata**
    Myelencephalon
	Ø Open
	3 Percutaneous
	4 Percutaneous Endoscopic
		Z No Device	Z No Qualifier

Ø   Medical and Surgical
Ø   Central Nervous System and Cranial Nerves
N   Release   Definition: Freeing a body part from an abnormal physical constraint by cutting or by the use of force
                      Explanation: Some of the restraining tissue may be taken out but none of the body part is taken out

Body Part Character 4		Approach Character 5	Device Character 6	Qualifier Character 7

Ø Brain
 Cerebrum
 Corpus callosum
 Encephalon
 1 Cerebral Meninges
 Arachnoid mater,
    intracranial
 Leptomeninges,
    intracranial
 Pia mater, intracranial
 2 Dura Mater
 Diaphragma sellae
 Dura mater, intracranial
 Falx cerebri
 Tentorium cerebelli
 6 Cerebral Ventricle
 Aqueduct of Sylvius
 Cerebral aqueduct
    (Sylvius)
 Choroid plexus
 Ependyma
 Foramen of Monro
    (intraventricular)
 Fourth ventricle
 Interventricular foramen
    (Monro)
 Left lateral ventricle
 Right lateral ventricle
 Third ventricle
 7 Cerebral Hemisphere
 Frontal lobe
 Occipital lobe
 Parietal lobe
 Temporal lobe
 8 Basal Ganglia
 Basal nuclei
 Claustrum
 Corpus striatum
 Globus pallidus
 Substantia nigra
 Subthalamic nucleus
 9 Thalamus
 Epithalamus
 Geniculate nucleus
 Metathalamus
 Pulvinar
 A Hypothalamus
 Mammillary body
 B Pons
 Apneustic center
 Basis pontis
 Locus ceruleus
 Pneumotaxic center
 Pontine tegmentum
 Superior olivary nucleus
 C Cerebellum
 Culmen
 D Medulla Oblongata
 Myelencephalon
 F Olfactory Nerve
 First cranial nerve
 Olfactory bulb
 G Optic Nerve
 Optic chiasma
 Second cranial nerve
	H Oculomotor Nerve
	 Third cranial nerve
	 J Trochlear Nerve
	 Fourth cranial nerve
	 K Trigeminal Nerve
	 Fifth cranial nerve
	 Gasserian ganglion
	 Mandibular nerve
	 Maxillary nerve
	 Ophthalmic nerve
	 Trifacial nerve
	 L Abducens Nerve
	 Sixth cranial nerve
	 M Facial Nerve
	 Chorda tympani
	 Geniculate ganglion
	 Greater superficial petrosal
	    nerve
	 Nerve to the stapedius
	 Parotid plexus
	 Posterior auricular nerve
	 Seventh cranial nerve
	 Submandibular ganglion
	 N Acoustic Nerve
	 Cochlear nerve
	 Eighth cranial nerve
	 Scarpa's (vestibular)
	    ganglion
	 Spiral ganglion
	 Vestibular (Scarpa's)
	    ganglion
	 Vestibular nerve
	 Vestibulocochlear nerve
	 P Glossopharyngeal Nerve
	 Carotid sinus nerve
	 Ninth cranial nerve
	 Tympanic nerve
	 Q Vagus Nerve
	 Anterior vagal trunk
	 Pharyngeal plexus
	 Pneumogastric nerve
	 Posterior vagal trunk
	 Pulmonary plexus
	 Recurrent laryngeal nerve
	 Superior laryngeal nerve
	 Tenth cranial nerve
	 R Accessory Nerve
	 Eleventh cranial nerve
	 S Hypoglossal Nerve
	 Twelfth cranial nerve
	 T Spinal Meninges
	 Arachnoid mater, spinal
	 Denticulate (dentate)
	    ligament
	 Dura mater, spinal
	 Filum terminale
	 Leptomeninges, spinal
	 Pia mater, spinal
	 W Cervical Spinal Cord
	 Dorsal root ganglion
	 X Thoracic Spinal Cord
	 Dorsal root ganglion
	 Y Lumbar Spinal Cord
	 Cauda equina
	 Conus medullaris
	 Dorsal root ganglion
		Ø Open
		 3 Percutaneous
		 4 Percutaneous Endoscopic
			Z No Device	**Z No Qualifier**

Ø Medical and Surgical
Ø Central Nervous System and Cranial Nerves
P Removal   Definition: Taking out or off a device from a body part

Explanation: If a device is taken out and a similar device put in without cutting or puncturing the skin or mucous membrane, the procedure is coded to the root operation CHANGE. Otherwise, the procedure for taking out a device is coded to the root operation REMOVAL.

Body Part Character 4	Approach Character 5	Device Character 6	Qualifier Character 7
Ø Brain Cerebrum Corpus callosum Encephalon **V Spinal Cord** Dorsal root ganglion	**Ø** Open **3** Percutaneous **4** Percutaneous Endoscopic	**Ø** Drainage Device **2** Monitoring Device **3** Infusion Device **7** Autologous Tissue Substitute **J** Synthetic Substitute **K** Nonautologous Tissue Substitute **M** Neurostimulator Lead **Y** Other Device	**Z** No Qualifier
Ø Brain Cerebrum Corpus callosum Encephalon **V Spinal Cord** Dorsal root ganglion	**X** External	**Ø** Drainage Device **2** Monitoring Device **3** Infusion Device **M** Neurostimulator Lead	**Z** No Qualifier
6 Cerebral Ventricle Aqueduct of Sylvius Cerebral aqueduct (Sylvius) Choroid plexus Ependyma Foramen of Monro (intraventricular) Fourth ventricle Interventricular foramen (Monro) Left lateral ventricle Right lateral ventricle Third ventricle **U Spinal Canal** Epidural space, spinal Extradural space, spinal Subarachnoid space, spinal Subdural space, spinal Vertebral canal	**Ø** Open **3** Percutaneous **4** Percutaneous Endoscopic	**Ø** Drainage Device **2** Monitoring Device **3** Infusion Device **J** Synthetic Substitute **M** Neurostimulator Lead **Y** Other Device	**Z** No Qualifier
6 Cerebral Ventricle Aqueduct of Sylvius Cerebral aqueduct (Sylvius) Choroid plexus Ependyma Foramen of Monro (intraventricular) Fourth ventricle Interventricular foramen (Monro) Left lateral ventricle Right lateral ventricle Third ventricle **U Spinal Canal** Epidural space, spinal Extradural space, spinal Subarachnoid space, spinal Subdural space, spinal Vertebral canal	**X** External	**Ø** Drainage Device **2** Monitoring Device **3** Infusion Device **M** Neurostimulator Lead	**Z** No Qualifier
E Cranial Nerve	**Ø** Open **3** Percutaneous **4** Percutaneous Endoscopic	**Ø** Drainage Device **2** Monitoring Device **3** Infusion Device **7** Autologous Tissue Substitute **M** Neurostimulator Lead **Y** Other Device	**Z** No Qualifier
E Cranial Nerve	**X** External	**Ø** Drainage Device **2** Monitoring Device **3** Infusion Device **M** Neurostimulator Lead	**Z** No Qualifier

Non-OR	ØØP[Ø,V]3[Ø,2,3]Z
Non-OR	ØØP[Ø,V][3,4]YZ
Non-OR	ØØP[Ø,V]X[Ø,2,3,M]Z
Non-OR	ØØP[6,U]3[Ø,2,3]Z
Non-OR	ØØP[6,U][3,4]YZ
Non-OR	ØØP[6,U]X[Ø,2,3,M]Z
Non-OR	ØØPE3[Ø,2,3]Z
Non-OR	ØØPE[3,4]YZ
Non-OR	ØØPEX[Ø,2,3,M]Z

NC Noncovered Procedure   **LC** Limited Coverage   **QA** Questionable OB Admit   **NT** New Tech Add-on   ⊞ Combination Member   ♂ Male   ♀ Female

ICD-10-PCS 2022   145

Ø　Medical and Surgical
Ø　Central Nervous System and Cranial Nerves
Q　Repair　　　Definition: Restoring, to the extent possible, a body part to its normal anatomic structure and function

Explanation: Used only when the method to accomplish the repair is not one of the other root operations

Body Part Character 4		Approach Character 5	Device Character 6	Qualifier Character 7
Ø Brain 　Cerebrum 　Corpus callosum 　Encephalon **1 Cerebral Meninges** 　Arachnoid mater, 　　intracranial 　Leptomeninges, 　　intracranial 　Pia mater, intracranial **2 Dura Mater** 　Diaphragma sellae 　Dura mater, intracranial 　Falx cerebri 　Tentorium cerebelli **6 Cerebral Ventricle** 　Aqueduct of Sylvius 　Cerebral aqueduct 　　(Sylvius) 　Choroid plexus 　Ependyma 　Foramen of Monro 　　(intraventricular) 　Fourth ventricle 　Interventricular foramen 　　(Monro) 　Left lateral ventricle 　Right lateral ventricle 　Third ventricle **7 Cerebral Hemisphere** 　Frontal lobe 　Occipital lobe 　Parietal lobe 　Temporal lobe **8 Basal Ganglia** 　Basal nuclei 　Claustrum 　Corpus striatum 　Globus pallidus 　Substantia nigra 　Subthalamic nucleus **9 Thalamus** 　Epithalamus 　Geniculate nucleus 　Metathalamus 　Pulvinar **A Hypothalamus** 　Mammillary body **B Pons** 　Apneustic center 　Basis pontis 　Locus ceruleus 　Pneumotaxic center 　Pontine tegmentum 　Superior olivary nucleus **C Cerebellum** 　Culmen **D Medulla Oblongata** 　Myelencephalon **F Olfactory Nerve** 　First cranial nerve 　Olfactory bulb **G Optic Nerve** 　Optic chiasma 　Second cranial nerve	**H Oculomotor Nerve** 　Third cranial nerve **J Trochlear Nerve** 　Fourth cranial nerve **K Trigeminal Nerve** 　Fifth cranial nerve 　Gasserian ganglion 　Mandibular nerve 　Maxillary nerve 　Ophthalmic nerve 　Trifacial nerve **L Abducens Nerve** 　Sixth cranial nerve **M Facial Nerve** 　Chorda tympani 　Geniculate ganglion 　Greater superficial petrosal 　　nerve 　Nerve to the stapedius 　Parotid plexus 　Posterior auricular nerve 　Seventh cranial nerve 　Submandibular ganglion **N Acoustic Nerve** 　Cochlear nerve 　Eighth cranial nerve 　Scarpa's (vestibular) 　　ganglion 　Spiral ganglion 　Vestibular (Scarpa's) 　　ganglion 　Vestibular nerve 　Vestibulocochlear nerve **P Glossopharyngeal Nerve** 　Carotid sinus nerve 　Ninth cranial nerve 　Tympanic nerve **Q Vagus Nerve** 　Anterior vagal trunk 　Pharyngeal plexus 　Pneumogastric nerve 　Posterior vagal trunk 　Pulmonary plexus 　Recurrent laryngeal nerve 　Superior laryngeal nerve 　Tenth cranial nerve **R Accessory Nerve** 　Eleventh cranial nerve **S Hypoglossal Nerve** 　Twelfth cranial nerve **T Spinal Meninges** 　Arachnoid mater, spinal 　Denticulate (dentate) 　　ligament 　Dura mater, spinal 　Filum terminale 　Leptomeninges, spinal 　Pia mater, spinal **W Cervical Spinal Cord** 　Dorsal root ganglion **X Thoracic Spinal Cord** 　Dorsal root ganglion **Y Lumbar Spinal Cord** 　Cauda equina 　Conus medullaris 　Dorsal root ganglion	**Ø Open** **3 Percutaneous** **4 Percutaneous Endoscopic**	**Z No Device**	**Z No Qualifier**

Ø   Medical and Surgical
Ø   Central Nervous System and Cranial Nerves
R   Replacement   Definition: Putting in or on biological or synthetic material that physically takes the place and/or function of all or a portion of a body part

                     Explanation: The body part may have been taken out or replaced, or may be taken out, physically eradicated, or rendered nonfunctional during the REPLACEMENT procedure. A REMOVAL procedure is coded for taking out the device used in a previous replacement procedure.

Body Part Character 4		Approach Character 5	Device Character 6	Qualifier Character 7

1 Cerebral Meninges
  Arachnoid mater,
    intracranial
  Leptomeninges,
    intracranial
  Pia mater, intracranial
2 Dura Mater
  Diaphragma sellae
  Dura mater, intracranial
  Falx cerebri
  Tentorium cerebelli
6 Cerebral Ventricle
  Aqueduct of Sylvius
  Cerebral aqueduct
    (Sylvius)
  Choroid plexus
  Ependyma
  Foramen of Monro
    (intraventricular)
  Fourth ventricle
  Interventricular foramen
    (Monro)
  Left lateral ventricle
  Right lateral ventricle
  Third ventricle
F Olfactory Nerve
  First cranial nerve
  Olfactory bulb
G Optic Nerve
  Optic chiasma
  Second cranial nerve
H Oculomotor Nerve
  Third cranial nerve
J Trochlear Nerve
  Fourth cranial nerve
K Trigeminal Nerve
  Fifth cranial nerve
  Gasserian ganglion
  Mandibular nerve
  Maxillary nerve
  Ophthalmic nerve
  Trifacial nerve
L Abducens Nerve
  Sixth cranial nerve
	M Facial Nerve
	  Chorda tympani
	  Geniculate ganglion
	  Greater superficial petrosal
	    nerve
	  Nerve to the stapedius
	  Parotid plexus
	  Posterior auricular nerve
	  Seventh cranial nerve
	  Submandibular ganglion
	N Acoustic Nerve
	  Cochlear nerve
	  Eighth cranial nerve
	  Scarpa's (vestibular)
	    ganglion
	  Spiral ganglion
	  Vestibular (Scarpa's)
	    ganglion
	  Vestibular nerve
	  Vestibulocochlear nerve
	P Glossopharyngeal Nerve
	  Carotid sinus nerve
	  Ninth cranial nerve
	  Tympanic nerve
	Q Vagus Nerve
	  Anterior vagal trunk
	  Pharyngeal plexus
	  Pneumogastric nerve
	  Posterior vagal trunk
	  Pulmonary plexus
	  Recurrent laryngeal nerve
	  Superior laryngeal nerve
	  Tenth cranial nerve
	R Accessory Nerve
	  Eleventh cranial nerve
	S Hypoglossal Nerve
	  Twelfth cranial nerve
	T Spinal Meninges
	  Arachnoid mater, spinal
	  Denticulate (dentate)
	    ligament
	  Dura mater, spinal
	  Filum terminale
	  Leptomeninges, spinal
	  Pia mater, spinal
		Ø Open
		4 Percutaneous Endoscopic
			7 Autologous Tissue
			  Substitute
			J Synthetic Substitute
			K Nonautologous Tissue
			  Substitute
				Z No Qualifier

Central Nervous System and Cranial Nerves

0   **Medical and Surgical**
0   **Central Nervous System and Cranial Nerves**
S   **Reposition**   Definition: Moving to its normal location, or other suitable location, all or a portion of a body part

Explanation: The body part is moved to a new location from an abnormal location, or from a normal location where it is not functioning correctly. The body part may or may not be cut out or off to be moved to the new location.

Body Part Character 4		Approach Character 5	Device Character 6	Qualifier Character 7

F Olfactory Nerve
First cranial nerve
Olfactory bulb
G Optic Nerve
Optic chiasma
Second cranial nerve
H Oculomotor Nerve
Third cranial nerve
J Trochlear Nerve
Fourth cranial nerve
K Trigeminal Nerve
Fifth cranial nerve
Gasserian ganglion
Mandibular nerve
Maxillary nerve
Ophthalmic nerve
Trifacial nerve
L Abducens Nerve
Sixth cranial nerve
M Facial Nerve
Chorda tympani
Geniculate ganglion
Greater superficial petrosal
   nerve
Nerve to the stapedius
Parotid plexus
Posterior auricular nerve
Seventh cranial nerve
Submandibular ganglion
	N Acoustic Nerve
	Cochlear nerve
	Eighth cranial nerve
	Scarpa's (vestibular)
	   ganglion
	Spiral ganglion
	Vestibular (Scarpa's)
	   ganglion
	Vestibular nerve
	Vestibulocochlear nerve
	P Glossopharyngeal Nerve
	Carotid sinus nerve
	Ninth cranial nerve
	Tympanic nerve
	Q Vagus Nerve
	Anterior vagal trunk
	Pharyngeal plexus
	Pneumogastric nerve
	Posterior vagal trunk
	Pulmonary plexus
	Recurrent laryngeal nerve
	Superior laryngeal nerve
	Tenth cranial nerve
	R Accessory Nerve
	Eleventh cranial nerve
	S Hypoglossal Nerve
	Twelfth cranial nerve
	W Cervical Spinal Cord
	Dorsal root ganglion
	X Thoracic Spinal Cord
	Dorsal root ganglion
	Y Lumbar Spinal Cord
	Cauda equina
	Conus medullaris
	Dorsal root ganglion
		0 Open
		3 Percutaneous
		4 Percutaneous Endoscopic
			Z No Device	**Z** No Qualifier

0   **Medical and Surgical**
0   **Central Nervous System and Cranial Nerves**
T   **Resection**   Definition: Cutting out or off, without replacement, all of a body part

Explanation: None

Body Part Character 4	Approach Character 5	Device Character 6	Qualifier Character 7
7 Cerebral Hemisphere Frontal lobe Occipital lobe Parietal lobe Temporal lobe	**0** Open **3** Percutaneous **4** Percutaneous Endoscopic	**Z** No Device	**Z** No Qualifier

Ø   **Medical and Surgical**
Ø   **Central Nervous System and Cranial Nerves**
U   **Supplement**   Definition: Putting in or on biological or synthetic material that physically reinforces and/or augments the function of a portion of a body part

                 Explanation: The biological material is non-living, or is living and from the same individual. The body part may have been previously replaced, and the SUPPLEMENT procedure is performed to physically reinforce and/or augment the function of the replaced body part.

Body Part Character 4		Approach Character 5	Device Character 6	Qualifier Character 7

1   **Cerebral Meninges**
     Arachnoid mater,
        intracranial
     Leptomeninges,
        intracranial
     Pia mater, intracranial
2   **Dura Mater**
     Diaphragma sellae
     Dura mater, intracranial
     Falx cerebri
     Tentorium cerebelli
6   **Cerebral Ventricle**
     Aqueduct of Sylvius
     Cerebral aqueduct
        (Sylvius)
     Choroid plexus
     Ependyma
     Foramen of Monro
        (intraventricular)
     Fourth ventricle
     Interventricular foramen
        (Monro)
     Left lateral ventricle
     Right lateral ventricle
     Third ventricle
F   **Olfactory Nerve**
     First cranial nerve
     Olfactory bulb
G   **Optic Nerve**
     Optic chiasma
     Second cranial nerve
H   **Oculomotor Nerve**
     Third cranial nerve
J   **Trochlear Nerve**
     Fourth cranial nerve
K   **Trigeminal Nerve**
     Fifth cranial nerve
     Gasserian ganglion
     Mandibular nerve
     Maxillary nerve
     Ophthalmic nerve
     Trifacial nerve
L   **Abducens Nerve**
     Sixth cranial nerve
	M **Facial Nerve**
	     Chorda tympani
	     Geniculate ganglion
	     Greater superficial petrosal
	        nerve
	     Nerve to the stapedius
	     Parotid plexus
	     Posterior auricular nerve
	     Seventh cranial nerve
	     Submandibular ganglion
	N **Acoustic Nerve**
	     Cochlear nerve
	     Eighth cranial nerve
	     Scarpa's (vestibular)
	        ganglion
	     Spiral ganglion
	     Vestibular (Scarpa's)
	        ganglion
	     Vestibular nerve
	     Vestibulocochlear nerve
	P **Glossopharyngeal Nerve**
	     Carotid sinus nerve
	     Ninth cranial nerve
	     Tympanic nerve
	Q **Vagus Nerve**
	     Anterior vagal trunk
	     Pharyngeal plexus
	     Pneumogastric nerve
	     Posterior vagal trunk
	     Pulmonary plexus
	     Recurrent laryngeal nerve
	     Superior laryngeal nerve
	     Tenth cranial nerve
	R **Accessory Nerve**
	     Eleventh cranial nerve
	S **Hypoglossal Nerve**
	     Twelfth cranial nerve
	T **Spinal Meninges**
	     Arachnoid mater, spinal
	     Denticulate (dentate)
	        ligament
	     Dura mater, spinal
	     Filum terminale
	     Leptomeninges, spinal
	     Pia mater, spinal
		Ø Open
		3 Percutaneous
		4 Percutaneous Endoscopic
			7 Autologous Tissue
			     Substitute
			J Synthetic Substitute
			K Nonautologous Tissue
			     Substitute
				Z No Qualifier

NC Noncovered Procedure   **LC** Limited Coverage   **QA** Questionable OB Admit   **NT** New Tech Add-on   ⊞ Combination Member   ♂ Male   ♀ Female

ICD-10-PCS 2022   **149**

Central Nervous System and Cranial Nerves

Ø   **Medical and Surgical**
Ø   **Central Nervous System and Cranial Nerves**
W   **Revision**   Definition: Correcting, to the extent possible, a portion of a malfunctioning device or the position of a displaced device

                  Explanation: Revision can include correcting a malfunctioning or displaced device by taking out or putting in components of the device such as a screw or pin

Body Part Character 4	Approach Character 5	Device Character 6	Qualifier Character 7

Ø **Brain**
   Cerebrum
   Corpus callosum
   Encephalon
V **Spinal Cord**
   Dorsal root ganglion
	Ø Open
	3 Percutaneous
	4 Percutaneous Endoscopic
		Ø Drainage Device
		2 Monitoring Device
		3 Infusion Device
		7 Autologous Tissue Substitute
		J Synthetic Substitute
		K Nonautologous Tissue Substitute
		M Neurostimulator Lead
		Y Other Device
			Z No Qualifier

Ø **Brain**
   Cerebrum
   Corpus callosum
   Encephalon
V **Spinal Cord**
   Dorsal root ganglion
	X External	**Ø** Drainage Device
		2 Monitoring Device
		3 Infusion Device
		7 Autologous Tissue Substitute
		J Synthetic Substitute
		K Nonautologous Tissue Substitute
		M Neurostimulator Lead
			Z No Qualifier

6 **Cerebral Ventricle**
   Aqueduct of Sylvius
   Cerebral aqueduct (Sylvius)
   Choroid plexus
   Ependyma
   Foramen of Monro (intraventricular)
   Fourth ventricle
   Interventricular foramen (Monro)
   Left lateral ventricle
   Right lateral ventricle
   Third ventricle
U **Spinal Canal**
   Epidural space, spinal
   Extradural space, spinal
   Subarachnoid space, spinal
   Subdural space, spinal
   Vertebral canal
	Ø Open
	3 Percutaneous
	4 Percutaneous Endoscopic
		Ø Drainage Device
		2 Monitoring Device
		3 Infusion Device
		J Synthetic Substitute
		M Neurostimulator Lead
		Y Other Device
			Z No Qualifier

6 **Cerebral Ventricle**
   Aqueduct of Sylvius
   Cerebral aqueduct (Sylvius)
   Choroid plexus
   Ependyma
   Foramen of Monro (intraventricular)
   Fourth ventricle
   Interventricular foramen (Monro)
   Left lateral ventricle
   Right lateral ventricle
   Third ventricle
U **Spinal Canal**
   Epidural space, spinal
   Extradural space, spinal
   Subarachnoid space, spinal
   Subdural space, spinal
   Vertebral canal
	X External	**Ø** Drainage Device
		2 Monitoring Device
		3 Infusion Device
		J Synthetic Substitute
		M Neurostimulator Lead
			Z No Qualifier

E **Cranial Nerve**	**Ø** Open **3** Percutaneous **4** Percutaneous Endoscopic	**Ø** Drainage Device **2** Monitoring Device **3** Infusion Device **7** Autologous Tissue Substitute **M** Neurostimulator Lead **Y** Other Device	**Z** No Qualifier
E **Cranial Nerve**	**X** External	**Ø** Drainage Device **2** Monitoring Device **3** Infusion Device **7** Autologous Tissue Substitute **M** Neurostimulator Lead	**Z** No Qualifier

Non-OR   ØØW[Ø,V][3,4]YZ
Non-OR   ØØW[Ø,V]X[Ø,2,3,7,J,K,M]Z
Non-OR   ØØW[6,U][3,4]YZ
Non-OR   ØØW[6,U]X[Ø,2,3,J,M]Z
Non-OR   ØØWE[3,4]YZ
Non-OR   ØØWEX[Ø,2,3,7,M]Z

Non-OR Procedure   DRG Non-OR Procedure   Valid OR Procedure   HAC Associated Procedure   Combination Only   New/Revised GREEN

Ø   **Medical and Surgical**
Ø   **Central Nervous System and Cranial Nerves**
X   **Transfer**   Definition: Moving, without taking out, all or a portion of a body part to another location to take over the function of all or a portion of a body part
                  Explanation: The body part transferred remains connected to its vascular and nervous supply

Body Part Character 4	Approach Character 5	Device Character 6	Qualifier Character 7

F **Olfactory Nerve**
   First cranial nerve
   Olfactory bulb
G **Optic Nerve**
   Optic chiasma
   Second cranial nerve
H **Oculomotor Nerve**
   Third cranial nerve
J **Trochlear Nerve**
   Fourth cranial nerve
K **Trigeminal Nerve**
   Fifth cranial nerve
   Gasserian ganglion
   Mandibular nerve
   Maxillary nerve
   Ophthalmic nerve
   Trifacial nerve
L **Abducens Nerve**
   Sixth cranial nerve
M **Facial Nerve**
   Chorda tympani
   Geniculate ganglion
   Greater superficial petrosal nerve
   Nerve to the stapedius
   Parotid plexus
   Posterior auricular nerve
   Seventh cranial nerve
   Submandibular ganglion
N **Acoustic Nerve**
   Cochlear nerve
   Eighth cranial nerve
   Scarpa's (vestibular) ganglion
   Spiral ganglion
   Vestibular (Scarpa's) ganglion
   Vestibular nerve
   Vestibulocochlear nerve
P **Glossopharyngeal Nerve**
   Carotid sinus nerve
   Ninth cranial nerve
   Tympanic nerve
Q **Vagus Nerve**
   Anterior vagal trunk
   Pharyngeal plexus
   Pneumogastric nerve
   Posterior vagal trunk
   Pulmonary plexus
   Recurrent laryngeal nerve
   Superior laryngeal nerve
   Tenth cranial nerve
R **Accessory Nerve**
   Eleventh cranial nerve
S **Hypoglossal Nerve**
   Twelfth cranial nerve
	Ø Open
	4 Percutaneous Endoscopic
		Z No Device	**F** Olfactory Nerve
			G Optic Nerve
			H Oculomotor Nerve
			J Trochlear Nerve
			K Trigeminal Nerve
			L Abducens Nerve
			M Facial Nerve
			N Acoustic Nerve
			P Glossopharyngeal Nerve
			Q Vagus Nerve
			R Accessory Nerve
			S Hypoglossal Nerve

NC Noncovered Procedure   **LC** Limited Coverage   **QA** Questionable OB Admit   **NT** New Tech Add-on   ⊞ Combination Member   ♂ Male   ♀ Female

ICD-10-PCS 2022   151

Peripheral Nervous System Ø12–Ø1X

Character Meanings

This Character Meaning table is provided as a guide to assist the user in the identification of character members that may be found in this section of code tables. It **SHOULD NOT** be used to build a PCS code.

Operation–Character 3	Body Part–Character 4	Approach–Character 5	Device–Character 6	Qualifier–Character 7
2 Change	Ø Cervical Plexus	Ø Open	Ø Drainage Device	1 Cervical Nerve
5 Destruction	1 Cervical Nerve	3 Percutaneous	1 Radioactive Element	2 Phrenic Nerve
8 Division	2 Phrenic Nerve	4 Percutaneous Endoscopic	2 Monitoring Device	4 Ulnar Nerve
9 Drainage	3 Brachial Plexus	X External	7 Autologous Tissue Substitute	5 Median Nerve
B Excision	4 Ulnar Nerve		J Synthetic Substitute	6 Radial Nerve
C Extirpation	5 Median Nerve		K Nonautologous Tissue Substitute	8 Thoracic Nerve
D Extraction	6 Radial Nerve		M Neurostimulator Lead	B Lumbar Nerve
H Insertion	8 Thoracic Nerve		Y Other Device	C Perineal Nerve
J Inspection	9 Lumbar Plexus		Z No Device	D Femoral Nerve
N Release	A Lumbosacral Plexus			F Sciatic Nerve
P Removal	B Lumbar Nerve			G Tibial Nerve
Q Repair	C Pudendal Nerve			H Peroneal Nerve
R Replacement	D Femoral Nerve			X Diagnostic
S Reposition	F Sciatic Nerve			Z No Qualifier
U Supplement	G Tibial Nerve			
W Revision	H Peroneal Nerve			
X Transfer	K Head and Neck Sympathetic Nerve			
	L Thoracic Sympathetic Nerve			
	M Abdominal Sympathetic Nerve			
	N Lumbar Sympathetic Nerve			
	P Sacral Sympathetic Nerve			
	Q Sacral Plexus			
	R Sacral Nerve			
	Y Peripheral Nerve			

AHA Coding Clinic for table Ø1B
2018, 2Q, 22   Excision of synovial cyst
2017, 2Q, 19   Thoracic outlet decompression with sympathectomy

AHA Coding Clinic for table Ø1H
2020, 4Q, 43-44   Insertion of radioactive element

AHA Coding Clinic for table Ø1N
2019, 1Q, 28   Decompressive laminectomy of both spinal cord and nerve roots
2018, 2Q, 22   Excision of synovial cyst
2017, 2Q, 19   Thoracic outlet decompression with sympathectomy
2016, 2Q, 16   Decompressive laminectomy/foraminotomy and lumbar discectomy
2016, 2Q, 17   Removal of longitudinal ligament to decompress cervical nerve root
2016, 2Q, 23   Thoracic outlet syndrome and release of brachial plexus
2015, 2Q, 34   Decompressive laminectomy
2014, 3Q, 33   Radial fracture treatment with open reduction internal fixation, and release of carpal ligament

AHA Coding Clinic for table Ø1Q
2019, 3Q, 32   Breast reconstruction with neurotization

AHA Coding Clinic for table Ø1U
2019, 3Q, 32   Breast reconstruction with neurotization
2017, 4Q, 62   Added and revised device values - Nerve substitutes

Median and Ulnar Nerves

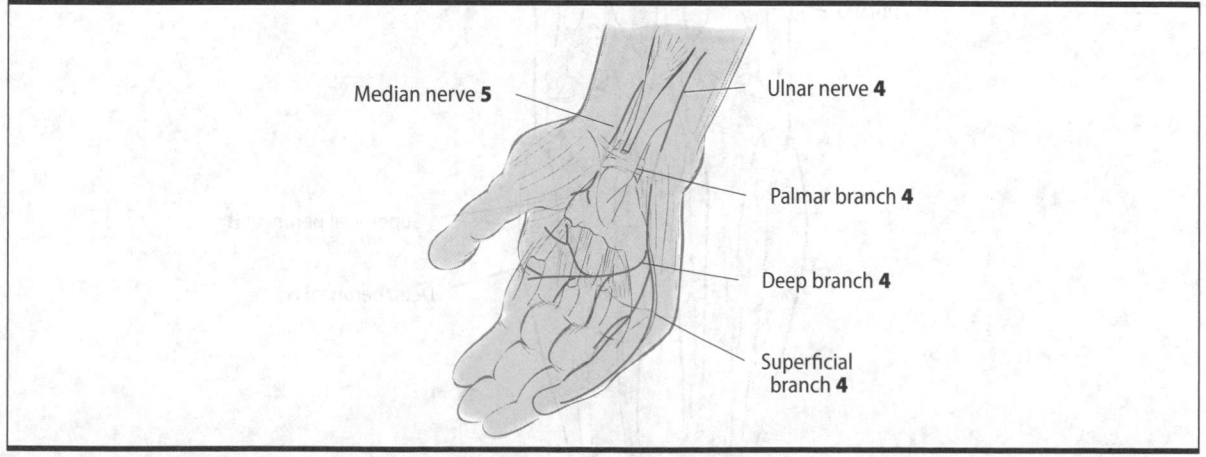

Median nerve **5**

Ulnar nerve **4**

Palmar branch **4**

Deep branch **4**

Superficial branch **4**

Peripheral Nervous System

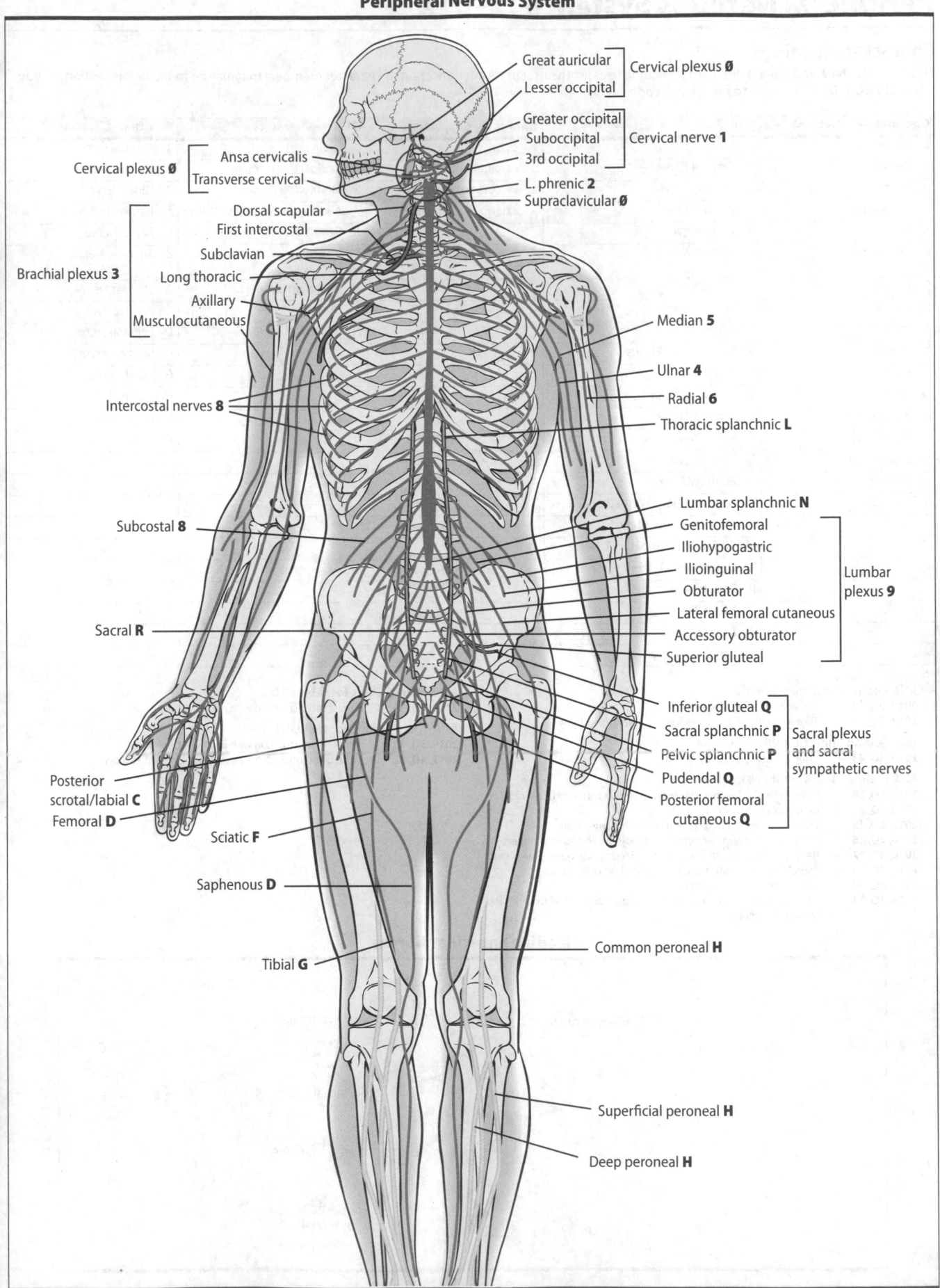

Great auricular
Lesser occipital
Cervical plexus **Ø**

Greater occipital
Suboccipital
3rd occipital
Cervical nerve **1**

Cervical plexus **Ø**
Ansa cervicalis
Transverse cervical
L. phrenic **2**
Supraclavicular **Ø**

Dorsal scapular
First intercostal
Subclavian
Brachial plexus **3**
Long thoracic
Axillary
Musculocutaneous

Median **5**

Ulnar **4**
Radial **6**
Thoracic splanchnic **L**

Intercostal nerves **8**

Lumbar splanchnic **N**
Genitofemoral
Iliohypogastric
Ilioinguinal
Lumbar plexus **9**
Obturator
Lateral femoral cutaneous
Accessory obturator
Superior gluteal

Subcostal **8**

Sacral **R**

Inferior gluteal **Q**
Sacral splanchnic **P**
Pelvic splanchnic **P**
Pudendal **Q**
Posterior femoral cutaneous **Q**
Sacral plexus and sacral sympathetic nerves

Posterior scrotal/labial **C**
Femoral **D**
Sciatic **F**

Saphenous **D**

Tibial **G**

Common peroneal **H**

Superficial peroneal **H**

Deep peroneal **H**

Ø   Medical and Surgical
1   Peripheral Nervous System
2   Change   Definition: Taking out or off a device from a body part and putting back an identical or similar device in or on the same body part without cutting or puncturing the skin or a mucous membrane
                Explanation: All CHANGE procedures are coded using the approach EXTERNAL

Body Part Character 4	Approach Character 5	Device Character 6	Qualifier Character 7
Y Peripheral Nerve	X External	Ø Drainage Device Y Other Device	Z No Qualifier

> Non-OR   All body part, approach, device, and qualifier values

Ø   Medical and Surgical
1   Peripheral Nervous System   Definition: Physical eradication of all or a portion of a body part by the direct use of energy, force, or a destructive agent
5   Destruction   Explanation: None of the body part is physically taken out

Body Part Character 4		Approach Character 5	Device Character 6	Qualifier Character 7

Ø   **Cervical Plexus**
    Ansa cervicalis
    Cutaneous (transverse) cervical nerve
    Great auricular nerve
    Lesser occipital nerve
    Supraclavicular nerve
    Transverse (cutaneous) cervical nerve
1   **Cervical Nerve**
    Greater occipital nerve
    Spinal nerve, cervical
    Suboccipital nerve
    Third occipital nerve
2   **Phrenic Nerve**
    Accessory phrenic nerve
3   **Brachial Plexus**
    Axillary nerve
    Dorsal scapular nerve
    First intercostal nerve
    Long thoracic nerve
    Musculocutaneous nerve
    Subclavius nerve
    Suprascapular nerve
4   **Ulnar Nerve**
    Cubital nerve
5   **Median Nerve**
    Anterior interosseous nerve
    Palmar cutaneous nerve
6   **Radial Nerve**
    Dorsal digital nerve
    Musculospiral nerve
    Palmar cutaneous nerve
    Posterior interosseous nerve
8   **Thoracic Nerve**
    Intercostal nerve
    Intercostobrachial nerve
    Spinal nerve, thoracic
    Subcostal nerve
9   **Lumbar Plexus**
    Accessory obturator nerve
    Genitofemoral nerve
    Iliohypogastric nerve
    Ilioinguinal nerve
    Lateral femoral cutaneous nerve
    Obturator nerve
    Superior gluteal nerve
A   **Lumbosacral Plexus**
B   **Lumbar Nerve**
    Lumbosacral trunk
    Spinal nerve, lumbar
    Superior clunic (cluneal) nerve
C   **Pudendal Nerve**
    Posterior labial nerve
    Posterior scrotal nerve
D   **Femoral Nerve**
    Anterior crural nerve
    Saphenous nerve
F   **Sciatic Nerve**
    Ischiatic nerve
G   **Tibial Nerve**
    Lateral plantar nerve
    Medial plantar nerve
    Medial popliteal nerve
    Medial sural cutaneous nerve
	H **Peroneal Nerve**
	    Common fibular nerve
	    Common peroneal nerve
	    External popliteal nerve
	    Lateral sural cutaneous nerve
	K **Head and Neck Sympathetic Nerve**
	    Cavernous plexus
	    Cervical ganglion
	    Ciliary ganglion
	    Internal carotid plexus
	    Otic ganglion
	    Pterygopalatine (sphenopalatine)
	      ganglion
	    Sphenopalatine (pterygopalatine)
	      ganglion
	    Stellate ganglion
	    Submandibular ganglion
	    Submaxillary ganglion
	L **Thoracic Sympathetic Nerve**
	    Cardiac plexus
	    Esophageal plexus
	    Greater splanchnic nerve
	    Inferior cardiac nerve
	    Least splanchnic nerve
	    Lesser splanchnic nerve
	    Middle cardiac nerve
	    Pulmonary plexus
	    Superior cardiac nerve
	    Thoracic aortic plexus
	    Thoracic ganglion
	M **Abdominal Sympathetic Nerve**
	    Abdominal aortic plexus
	    Auerbach's (myenteric) plexus
	    Celiac (solar) plexus
	    Celiac ganglion
	    Gastric plexus
	    Hepatic plexus
	    Inferior hypogastric plexus
	    Inferior mesenteric ganglion
	    Inferior mesenteric plexus
	    Meissner's (submucous) plexus
	    Myenteric (Auerbach's) plexus
	    Pancreatic plexus
	    Pelvic splanchnic nerve
	    Renal nerve
	    Renal plexus
	    Solar (celiac) plexus
	    Splenic plexus
	    Submucous (Meissner's) plexus
	    Superior hypogastric plexus
	    Superior mesenteric ganglion
	    Superior mesenteric plexus
	    Suprarenal plexus
	N **Lumbar Sympathetic Nerve**
	    Lumbar ganglion
	    Lumbar splanchnic nerve
	P **Sacral Sympathetic Nerve**
	    Ganglion impar (ganglion of
	      Walther)
	    Pelvic splanchnic nerve
	    Sacral ganglion
	    Sacral splanchnic nerve
	Q **Sacral Plexus**
	    Inferior gluteal nerve
	    Posterior femoral cutaneous nerve
	    Pudendal nerve
	R **Sacral Nerve**
	    Spinal nerve, sacral
		Ø Open
		3 Percutaneous
		4 Percutaneous
		    Endoscopic
			Z No Device	Z No Qualifier

> Non-OR   Ø15[Ø,2,3,4,5,6,9,A,C,D,F,G,H,Q][Ø,3,4]ZZ   Non-OR   Ø15[1,8,B,R]3ZZ

NC Noncovered Procedure   **LC** Limited Coverage   **QA** Questionable OB Admit   **NT** New Tech Add-on   ➕ Combination Member   ♂ Male   ♀ Female

Peripheral Nervous System *(left margin)*

Ø   **Medical and Surgical**
1   **Peripheral Nervous System**
8   **Division**   Definition: Cutting into a body part, without draining fluids and/or gases from the body part, in order to separate or transect a body part
                        Explanation: All or a portion of the body part is separated into two or more portions

Body Part Character 4		Approach Character 5	Device Character 6	Qualifier Character 7

Ø Cervical Plexus
  Ansa cervicalis
  Cutaneous (transverse) cervical
    nerve
  Great auricular nerve
  Lesser occipital nerve
  Supraclavicular nerve
  Transverse (cutaneous) cervical
    nerve
1 Cervical Nerve
  Greater occipital nerve
  Spinal nerve, cervical
  Suboccipital nerve
  Third occipital nerve
2 Phrenic Nerve
  Accessory phrenic nerve
3 Brachial Plexus
  Axillary nerve
  Dorsal scapular nerve
  First intercostal nerve
  Long thoracic nerve
  Musculocutaneous nerve
  Subclavius nerve
  Suprascapular nerve
4 Ulnar Nerve
  Cubital nerve
5 Median Nerve
  Anterior interosseous nerve
  Palmar cutaneous nerve
6 Radial Nerve
  Dorsal digital nerve
  Musculospiral nerve
  Palmar cutaneous nerve
  Posterior interosseous nerve
8 Thoracic Nerve
  Intercostal nerve
  Intercostobrachial nerve
  Spinal nerve, thoracic
  Subcostal nerve
9 Lumbar Plexus
  Accessory obturator nerve
  Genitofemoral nerve
  Iliohypogastric nerve
  Ilioinguinal nerve
  Lateral femoral cutaneous
    nerve
  Obturator nerve
  Superior gluteal nerve
A Lumbosacral Plexus
B Lumbar Nerve
  Lumbosacral trunk
  Spinal nerve, lumbar
  Superior clunic (cluneal) nerve
C Pudendal Nerve
  Posterior labial nerve
  Posterior scrotal nerve
D Femoral Nerve
  Anterior crural nerve
  Saphenous nerve
F Sciatic Nerve
  Ischiatic nerve
G Tibial Nerve
  Lateral plantar nerve
  Medial plantar nerve
  Medial popliteal nerve
  Medial sural cutaneous nerve
	H Peroneal Nerve
	  Common fibular nerve
	  Common peroneal nerve
	  External popliteal nerve
	  Lateral sural cutaneous nerve
	**K Head and Neck Sympathetic
	  Nerve**
	  Cavernous plexus
	  Cervical ganglion
	  Ciliary ganglion
	  Internal carotid plexus
	  Otic ganglion
	  Pterygopalatine
	    (sphenopalatine) ganglion
	  Sphenopalatine
	    (pterygopalatine) ganglion
	  Stellate ganglion
	  Submandibular ganglion
	  Submaxillary ganglion
	L Thoracic Sympathetic Nerve
	  Cardiac plexus
	  Esophageal plexus
	  Greater splanchnic nerve
	  Inferior cardiac nerve
	  Least splanchnic nerve
	  Lesser splanchnic nerve
	  Middle cardiac nerve
	  Pulmonary plexus
	  Superior cardiac nerve
	  Thoracic aortic plexus
	  Thoracic ganglion
	**M Abdominal Sympathetic
	  Nerve**
	  Abdominal aortic plexus
	  Auerbach's (myenteric) plexus
	  Celiac (solar) plexus
	  Celiac ganglion
	  Gastric plexus
	  Hepatic plexus
	  Inferior hypogastric plexus
	  Inferior mesenteric ganglion
	  Inferior mesenteric plexus
	  Meissner's (submucous) plexus
	  Myenteric (Auerbach's) plexus
	  Pancreatic plexus
	  Pelvic splanchnic nerve
	  Renal nerve
	  Renal plexus
	  Solar (celiac) plexus
	  Splenic plexus
	  Submucous (Meissner's) plexus
	  Superior hypogastric plexus
	  Superior mesenteric ganglion
	  Superior mesenteric plexus
	  Suprarenal plexus
	N Lumbar Sympathetic Nerve
	  Lumbar ganglion
	  Lumbar splanchnic nerve
	P Sacral Sympathetic Nerve
	  Ganglion impar (ganglion of
	    Walther)
	  Pelvic splanchnic nerve
	  Sacral ganglion
	  Sacral splanchnic nerve
	Q Sacral Plexus
	  Inferior gluteal nerve
	  Posterior femoral cutaneous
	    nerve
	  Pudendal nerve
	R Sacral Nerve
	  Spinal nerve, sacral
		Ø Open
		3 Percutaneous
		4 Percutaneous Endoscopic
			Z No Device	**Z No Qualifier**

Ø   **Medical and Surgical**
1   **Peripheral Nervous System**
9   **Drainage**   Definition: Taking or letting out fluids and/or gases from a body part
                Explanation: The qualifier DIAGNOSTIC is used to identify drainage procedures that are biopsies

Body Part Character 4		Approach Character 5	Device Character 6	Qualifier Character 7
Ø Cervical Plexus Ansa cervicalis Cutaneous (transverse) cervical nerve Great auricular nerve Lesser occipital nerve Supraclavicular nerve Transverse (cutaneous) cervical nerve **1 Cervical Nerve** Greater occipital nerve Spinal nerve, cervical Suboccipital nerve Third occipital nerve **2 Phrenic Nerve** Accessory phrenic nerve **3 Brachial Plexus** Axillary nerve Dorsal scapular nerve First intercostal nerve Long thoracic nerve Musculocutaneous nerve Subclavius nerve Suprascapular nerve **4 Ulnar Nerve** Cubital nerve **5 Median Nerve** Anterior interosseous nerve Palmar cutaneous nerve **6 Radial Nerve** Dorsal digital nerve Musculospiral nerve Palmar cutaneous nerve Posterior interosseous nerve **8 Thoracic Nerve** Intercostal nerve Intercostobrachial nerve Spinal nerve, thoracic Subcostal nerve **9 Lumbar Plexus** Accessory obturator nerve Genitofemoral nerve Iliohypogastric nerve Ilioinguinal nerve Lateral femoral cutaneous nerve Obturator nerve Superior gluteal nerve **A Lumbosacral Plexus** **B Lumbar Nerve** Lumbosacral trunk Spinal nerve, lumbar Superior clunic (cluneal) nerve **C Pudendal Nerve** Posterior labial nerve Posterior scrotal nerve **D Femoral Nerve** Anterior crural nerve Saphenous nerve **F Sciatic Nerve** Ischiatic nerve **G Tibial Nerve** Lateral plantar nerve Medial plantar nerve Medial popliteal nerve Medial sural cutaneous nerve	**H Peroneal Nerve** Common fibular nerve Common peroneal nerve External popliteal nerve Lateral sural cutaneous nerve **K Head and Neck Sympathetic Nerve** Cavernous plexus Cervical ganglion Ciliary ganglion Internal carotid plexus Otic ganglion Pterygopalatine (sphenopalatine) ganglion Sphenopalatine (pterygopalatine) ganglion Stellate ganglion Submandibular ganglion Submaxillary ganglion **L Thoracic Sympathetic Nerve** Cardiac plexus Esophageal plexus Greater splanchnic nerve Inferior cardiac nerve Least splanchnic nerve Lesser splanchnic nerve Middle cardiac nerve Pulmonary plexus Superior cardiac nerve Thoracic aortic plexus Thoracic ganglion **M Abdominal Sympathetic Nerve** Abdominal aortic plexus Auerbach's (myenteric) plexus Celiac (solar) plexus Celiac ganglion Gastric plexus Hepatic plexus Inferior hypogastric plexus Inferior mesenteric ganglion Inferior mesenteric plexus Meissner's (submucous) plexus Myenteric (Auerbach's) plexus Pancreatic plexus Pelvic splanchnic nerve Renal nerve Renal plexus Solar (celiac) plexus Splenic plexus Submucous (Meissner's) plexus Superior hypogastric plexus Superior mesenteric ganglion Superior mesenteric plexus Suprarenal plexus **N Lumbar Sympathetic Nerve** Lumbar ganglion Lumbar splanchnic nerve **P Sacral Sympathetic Nerve** Ganglion impar (ganglion of Walther) Pelvic splanchnic nerve Sacral ganglion Sacral splanchnic nerve **Q Sacral Plexus** Inferior gluteal nerve Posterior femoral cutaneous nerve Pudendal nerve **R Sacral Nerve** Spinal nerve, sacral	**Ø Open** **3 Percutaneous** **4 Percutaneous Endoscopic**	**Ø Drainage Device**	**Z No Qualifier**

Non-OR   Ø19[Ø,1,2,3,4,5,6,8,9,A,B,C,D,F,G,H,K,L,M,N,P,Q,R]3ØZ

Ø19 Continued on next page

019 Continued

0   **Medical and Surgical**
1   **Peripheral Nervous System**
9   **Drainage**   Definition: Taking or letting out fluids and/or gases from a body part

           Explanation: The qualifier DIAGNOSTIC is used to identify drainage procedures that are biopsies

Body Part Character 4		Approach Character 5	Device Character 6	Qualifier Character 7

0 **Cervical Plexus**
   Ansa cervicalis
   Cutaneous (transverse) cervical
      nerve
   Great auricular nerve
   Lesser occipital nerve
   Supraclavicular nerve
   Transverse (cutaneous) cervical
      nerve
1 **Cervical Nerve**
   Greater occipital nerve
   Spinal nerve, cervical
   Suboccipital nerve
   Third occipital nerve
2 **Phrenic Nerve**
   Accessory phrenic nerve
3 **Brachial Plexus**
   Axillary nerve
   Dorsal scapular nerve
   First intercostal nerve
   Long thoracic nerve
   Musculocutaneous nerve
   Subclavius nerve
   Suprascapular nerve
4 **Ulnar Nerve**
   Cubital nerve
5 **Median Nerve**
   Anterior interosseous nerve
   Palmar cutaneous nerve
6 **Radial Nerve**
   Dorsal digital nerve
   Musculospiral nerve
   Palmar cutaneous nerve
   Posterior interosseous nerve
8 **Thoracic Nerve**
   Intercostal nerve
   Intercostobrachial nerve
   Spinal nerve, thoracic
   Subcostal nerve
9 **Lumbar Plexus**
   Accessory obturator nerve
   Genitofemoral nerve
   Iliohypogastric nerve
   Ilioinguinal nerve
   Lateral femoral cutaneous
      nerve
   Obturator nerve
   Superior gluteal nerve
A **Lumbosacral Plexus**
B **Lumbar Nerve**
   Lumbosacral trunk
   Spinal nerve, lumbar
   Superior clunic (cluneal) nerve
C **Pudendal Nerve**
   Posterior labial nerve
   Posterior scrotal nerve
D **Femoral Nerve**
   Anterior crural nerve
   Saphenous nerve
F **Sciatic Nerve**
   Ischiatic nerve
G **Tibial Nerve**
   Lateral plantar nerve
   Medial plantar nerve
   Medial popliteal nerve
   Medial sural cutaneous nerve
	H **Peroneal Nerve**
	   Common fibular nerve
	   Common peroneal nerve
	   External popliteal nerve
	   Lateral sural cutaneous nerve
	K **Head and Neck Sympathetic
	   Nerve**
	   Cavernous plexus
	   Cervical ganglion
	   Ciliary ganglion
	   Internal carotid plexus
	   Otic ganglion
	   Pterygopalatine
	      (sphenopalatine) ganglion
	   Sphenopalatine
	      (pterygopalatine) ganglion
	   Stellate ganglion
	   Submandibular ganglion
	   Submaxillary ganglion
	L **Thoracic Sympathetic Nerve**
	   Cardiac plexus
	   Esophageal plexus
	   Greater splanchnic nerve
	   Inferior cardiac nerve
	   Least splanchnic nerve
	   Lesser splanchnic nerve
	   Middle cardiac nerve
	   Pulmonary plexus
	   Superior cardiac nerve
	   Thoracic aortic plexus
	   Thoracic ganglion
	M **Abdominal Sympathetic
	   Nerve**
	   Abdominal aortic plexus
	   Auerbach's (myenteric) plexus
	   Celiac (solar) plexus
	   Celiac ganglion
	   Gastric plexus
	   Hepatic plexus
	   Inferior hypogastric plexus
	   Inferior mesenteric ganglion
	   Inferior mesenteric plexus
	   Meissner's (submucous) plexus
	   Myenteric (Auerbach's) plexus
	   Pancreatic plexus
	   Pelvic splanchnic nerve
	   Renal nerve
	   Renal plexus
	   Solar (celiac) plexus
	   Splenic plexus
	   Submucous (Meissner's) plexus
	   Superior hypogastric plexus
	   Superior mesenteric ganglion
	   Superior mesenteric plexus
	   Suprarenal plexus
	N **Lumbar Sympathetic Nerve**
	   Lumbar ganglion
	   Lumbar splanchnic nerve
	P **Sacral Sympathetic Nerve**
	   Ganglion impar (ganglion of
	      Walther)
	   Pelvic splanchnic nerve
	   Sacral ganglion
	   Sacral splanchnic nerve
	Q **Sacral Plexus**
	   Inferior gluteal nerve
	   Posterior femoral cutaneous
	      nerve
	   Pudendal nerve
	R **Sacral Nerve**
	   Spinal nerve, sacral
		0 Open
		3 Percutaneous
		4 Percutaneous Endoscopic
			Z No Device	X Diagnostic
				Z No Qualifier

Non-OR   019[0,1,2,3,4,5,6,8,9,A,B,C,D,F,G,H,Q,R][3,4]ZX
Non-OR   019[0,1,2,3,4,5,6,8,9,A,B,C,D,F,G,H,K,L,M,N,P,Q,R]3ZZ

Non-OR Procedure   DRG Non-OR Procedure   Valid OR Procedure   HAC Associated Procedure   Combination Only   New/Revised GREEN

0   **Medical and Surgical**
1   **Peripheral Nervous System**
B   **Excision**   Definition: Cutting out or off, without replacement, a portion of a body part
                    Explanation: The qualifier DIAGNOSTIC is used to identify excision procedures that are biopsies

Body Part Character 4		Approach Character 5	Device Character 6	Qualifier Character 7

0   **Cervical Plexus**
    Ansa cervicalis
    Cutaneous (transverse) cervical
      nerve
    Great auricular nerve
    Lesser occipital nerve
    Supraclavicular nerve
    Transverse (cutaneous) cervical
      nerve
1   **Cervical Nerve**
    Greater occipital nerve
    Spinal nerve, cervical
    Suboccipital nerve
    Third occipital nerve
2   **Phrenic Nerve**
    Accessory phrenic nerve
3   **Brachial Plexus**
    Axillary nerve
    Dorsal scapular nerve
    First intercostal nerve
    Long thoracic nerve
    Musculocutaneous nerve
    Subclavius nerve
    Suprascapular nerve
4   **Ulnar Nerve**
    Cubital nerve
5   **Median Nerve**
    Anterior interosseous nerve
    Palmar cutaneous nerve
6   **Radial Nerve**
    Dorsal digital nerve
    Musculospiral nerve
    Palmar cutaneous nerve
    Posterior interosseous nerve
8   **Thoracic Nerve**
    Intercostal nerve
    Intercostobrachial nerve
    Spinal nerve, thoracic
    Subcostal nerve
9   **Lumbar Plexus**
    Accessory obturator nerve
    Genitofemoral nerve
    Iliohypogastric nerve
    Ilioinguinal nerve
    Lateral femoral cutaneous
      nerve
    Obturator nerve
    Superior gluteal nerve
A   **Lumbosacral Plexus**
B   **Lumbar Nerve**
    Lumbosacral trunk
    Spinal nerve, lumbar
    Superior clunic (cluneal) nerve
C   **Pudendal Nerve**
    Posterior labial nerve
    Posterior scrotal nerve
D   **Femoral Nerve**
    Anterior crural nerve
    Saphenous nerve
F   **Sciatic Nerve**
    Ischiatic nerve
G   **Tibial Nerve**
    Lateral plantar nerve
    Medial plantar nerve
    Medial popliteal nerve
    Medial sural cutaneous nerve
	H **Peroneal Nerve**
	    Common fibular nerve
	    Common peroneal nerve
	    External popliteal nerve
	    Lateral sural cutaneous nerve
	K **Head and Neck Sympathetic**
	    Nerve
	    Cavernous plexus
	    Cervical ganglion
	    Ciliary ganglion
	    Internal carotid plexus
	    Otic ganglion
	    Pterygopalatine
	      (sphenopalatine) ganglion
	    Sphenopalatine
	      (pterygopalatine) ganglion
	    Stellate ganglion
	    Submandibular ganglion
	    Submaxillary ganglion
	L **Thoracic Sympathetic**
	    Nerve
	    Cardiac plexus
	    Esophageal plexus
	    Greater splanchnic nerve
	    Inferior cardiac nerve
	    Least splanchnic nerve
	    Lesser splanchnic nerve
	    Middle cardiac nerve
	    Pulmonary plexus
	    Superior cardiac nerve
	    Thoracic aortic plexus
	    Thoracic ganglion
	M **Abdominal Sympathetic**
	    Nerve
	    Abdominal aortic plexus
	    Auerbach's (myenteric) plexus
	    Celiac (solar) plexus
	    Celiac ganglion
	    Gastric plexus
	    Hepatic plexus
	    Inferior hypogastric plexus
	    Inferior mesenteric ganglion
	    Inferior mesenteric plexus
	    Meissner's (submucous) plexus
	    Myenteric (Auerbach's) plexus
	    Pancreatic plexus
	    Pelvic splanchnic nerve
	    Renal nerve
	    Renal plexus
	    Solar (celiac) plexus
	    Splenic plexus
	    Submucous (Meissner's) plexus
	    Superior hypogastric plexus
	    Superior mesenteric ganglion
	    Superior mesenteric plexus
	    Suprarenal plexus
	N **Lumbar Sympathetic Nerve**
	    Lumbar ganglion
	    Lumbar splanchnic nerve
	P **Sacral Sympathetic Nerve**
	    Ganglion impar (ganglion of
	      Walther)
	    Pelvic splanchnic nerve
	    Sacral ganglion
	    Sacral splanchnic nerve
	Q **Sacral Plexus**
	    Inferior gluteal nerve
	    Posterior femoral cutaneous
	      nerve
	    Pudendal nerve
	R **Sacral Nerve**
	    Spinal nerve, sacral
		0 Open
		3 Percutaneous
		4 Percutaneous Endoscopic
			Z No Device	**X** Diagnostic
				Z No Qualifier

Non-OR   01B[0,1,2,3,4,5,6,8,9,A,B,C,D,F,G,H,Q,R][3,4]ZX

NC Noncovered Procedure   **LC** Limited Coverage   **OA** Questionable OB Admit   **NT** New Tech Add-on   ⊞ Combination Member   ♂ Male   ♀ Female

ICD-10-PCS 2022   159

Peripheral Nervous System

0   **Medical and Surgical**
1   **Peripheral Nervous System**
C   **Extirpation**   Definition: Taking or cutting out solid matter from a body part

Explanation: The solid matter may be an abnormal byproduct of a biological function or a foreign body; it may be imbedded in a body part or in the lumen of a tubular body part. The solid matter may or may not have been previously broken into pieces.

Body Part Character 4		Approach Character 5	Device Character 6	Qualifier Character 7

0 Cervical Plexus
Ansa cervicalis
Cutaneous (transverse) cervical
  nerve
Great auricular nerve
Lesser occipital nerve
Supraclavicular nerve
Transverse (cutaneous) cervical
  nerve
1 Cervical Nerve
Greater occipital nerve
Spinal nerve, cervical
Suboccipital nerve
Third occipital nerve
2 Phrenic Nerve
Accessory phrenic nerve
3 Brachial Plexus
Axillary nerve
Dorsal scapular nerve
First intercostal nerve
Long thoracic nerve
Musculocutaneous nerve
Subclavius nerve
Suprascapular nerve
4 Ulnar Nerve
Cubital nerve
5 Median Nerve
Anterior interosseous nerve
Palmar cutaneous nerve
6 Radial Nerve
Dorsal digital nerve
Musculospiral nerve
Palmar cutaneous nerve
Posterior interosseous nerve
8 Thoracic Nerve
Intercostal nerve
Intercostobrachial nerve
Spinal nerve, thoracic
Subcostal nerve
9 Lumbar Plexus
Accessory obturator nerve
Genitofemoral nerve
Iliohypogastric nerve
Ilioinguinal nerve
Lateral femoral cutaneous
  nerve
Obturator nerve
Superior gluteal nerve
A Lumbosacral Plexus
B Lumbar Nerve
Lumbosacral trunk
Spinal nerve, lumbar
Superior clunic (cluneal) nerve
C Pudendal Nerve
Posterior labial nerve
Posterior scrotal nerve
D Femoral Nerve
Anterior crural nerve
Saphenous nerve
F Sciatic Nerve
Ischiatic nerve
G Tibial Nerve
Lateral plantar nerve
Medial plantar nerve
Medial popliteal nerve
Medial sural cutaneous nerve
	H Peroneal Nerve
	Common fibular nerve
	Common peroneal nerve
	External popliteal nerve
	Lateral sural cutaneous nerve
	K Head and Neck Sympathetic
	Nerve
	Cavernous plexus
	Cervical ganglion
	Ciliary ganglion
	Internal carotid plexus
	Otic ganglion
	Pterygopalatine
	  (sphenopalatine) ganglion
	Sphenopalatine
	  (pterygopalatine) ganglion
	Stellate ganglion
	Submandibular ganglion
	Submaxillary ganglion
	L Thoracic Sympathetic Nerve
	Cardiac plexus
	Esophageal plexus
	Greater splanchnic nerve
	Inferior cardiac nerve
	Least splanchnic nerve
	Lesser splanchnic nerve
	Middle cardiac nerve
	Pulmonary plexus
	Superior cardiac nerve
	Thoracic aortic plexus
	Thoracic ganglion
	M Abdominal Sympathetic
	Nerve
	Abdominal aortic plexus
	Auerbach's (myenteric) plexus
	Celiac (solar) plexus
	Celiac ganglion
	Gastric plexus
	Hepatic plexus
	Inferior hypogastric plexus
	Inferior mesenteric ganglion
	Inferior mesenteric plexus
	Meissner's (submucous) plexus
	Myenteric (Auerbach's) plexus
	Pancreatic plexus
	Pelvic splanchnic nerve
	Renal nerve
	Renal plexus
	Solar (celiac) plexus
	Splenic plexus
	Submucous (Meissner's) plexus
	Superior hypogastric plexus
	Superior mesenteric ganglion
	Superior mesenteric plexus
	Suprarenal plexus
	N Lumbar Sympathetic Nerve
	Lumbar ganglion
	Lumbar splanchnic nerve
	P Sacral Sympathetic Nerve
	Ganglion impar (ganglion of
	  Walther)
	Pelvic splanchnic nerve
	Sacral ganglion
	Sacral splanchnic nerve
	Q Sacral Plexus
	Inferior gluteal nerve
	Posterior femoral cutaneous
	  nerve
	Pudendal nerve
	R Sacral Nerve
	Spinal nerve, sacral
		0 Open
		3 Percutaneous
		4 Percutaneous Endoscopic
			Z No Device	**Z No Qualifier**

Ø　Medical and Surgical
1　Peripheral Nervous System
D　Extraction　　　Definition: Pulling or stripping out or off all or a portion of a body part by the use of force
　　　　　　　　　　　Explanation: The qualifier DIAGNOSTIC is used to identify extraction procedures that are biopsies

Body Part Character 4		Approach Character 5	Device Character 6	Qualifier Character 7
Ø　Cervical Plexus 　　Ansa cervicalis 　　Cutaneous (transverse) cervical 　　　nerve 　　Great auricular nerve 　　Lesser occipital nerve 　　Supraclavicular nerve 　　Transverse (cutaneous) cervical 　　　nerve **1　Cervical Nerve** 　　Greater occipital nerve 　　Spinal nerve, cervical 　　Suboccipital nerve 　　Third occipital nerve **2　Phrenic Nerve** 　　Accessory phrenic nerve **3　Brachial Plexus** 　　Axillary nerve 　　Dorsal scapular nerve 　　First intercostal nerve 　　Long thoracic nerve 　　Musculocutaneous nerve 　　Subclavius nerve 　　Suprascapular nerve **4　Ulnar Nerve** 　　Cubital nerve **5　Median Nerve** 　　Anterior interosseous nerve 　　Palmar cutaneous nerve **6　Radial Nerve** 　　Dorsal digital nerve 　　Musculospiral nerve 　　Palmar cutaneous nerve 　　Posterior interosseous nerve **8　Thoracic Nerve** 　　Intercostal nerve 　　Intercostobrachial nerve 　　Spinal nerve, thoracic 　　Subcostal nerve **9　Lumbar Plexus** 　　Accessory obturator nerve 　　Genitofemoral nerve 　　Iliohypogastric nerve 　　Ilioinguinal nerve 　　Lateral femoral cutaneous nerve 　　Obturator nerve 　　Superior gluteal nerve **A　Lumbosacral Plexus** **B　Lumbar Nerve** 　　Lumbosacral trunk 　　Spinal nerve, lumbar 　　Superior clunic (cluneal) nerve **C　Pudendal Nerve]** 　　Posterior labial nerve 　　Posterior scrotal nerve **D　Femoral Nerve** 　　Anterior crural nerve 　　Saphenous nerve **F　Sciatic Nerve** 　　Ischiatic nerve **G　Tibial Nerve** 　　Lateral plantar nerve 　　Medial plantar nerve 　　Medial popliteal nerve 　　Medial sural cutaneous nerve	**H　Peroneal Nerve** 　　Common fibular nerve 　　Common peroneal nerve 　　External popliteal nerve 　　Lateral sural cutaneous nerve **K　Head and Neck Sympathetic** 　　**Nerve** 　　Cavernous plexus 　　Cervical ganglion 　　Ciliary ganglion 　　Internal carotid plexus 　　Otic ganglion 　　Pterygopalatine 　　　(sphenopalatine) ganglion 　　Sphenopalatine 　　　(pterygopalatine) ganglion 　　Stellate ganglion 　　Submandibular ganglion 　　Submaxillary ganglion **L　Thoracic Sympathetic Nerve** 　　Cardiac plexus 　　Esophageal plexus 　　Greater splanchnic nerve 　　Inferior cardiac nerve 　　Least splanchnic nerve 　　Lesser splanchnic nerve 　　Middle cardiac nerve 　　Pulmonary plexus 　　Superior cardiac nerve 　　Thoracic aortic plexus 　　Thoracic ganglion **M　Abdominal Sympathetic Nerve** 　　Abdominal aortic plexus 　　Auerbach's (myenteric) plexus 　　Celiac (solar) plexus 　　Celiac ganglion 　　Gastric plexus 　　Hepatic plexus 　　Inferior hypogastric plexus 　　Inferior mesenteric ganglion 　　Inferior mesenteric plexus 　　Meissner's (submucous) plexus 　　Myenteric (Auerbach's) plexus 　　Pancreatic plexus 　　Pelvic splanchnic nerve 　　Renal nerve 　　Renal plexus 　　Solar (celiac) plexus 　　Splenic plexus 　　Submucous (Meissner's) plexus 　　Superior hypogastric plexus 　　Superior mesenteric ganglion 　　Superior mesenteric plexus 　　Suprarenal plexus **N　Lumbar Sympathetic Nerve** 　　Lumbar ganglion 　　Lumbar splanchnic nerve **P　Sacral Sympathetic Nerve** 　　Ganglion impar (ganglion of 　　　Walther) 　　Pelvic splanchnic nerve 　　Sacral ganglion 　　Sacral splanchnic nerve **Q　Sacral Plexus** 　　Inferior gluteal nerve 　　Posterior femoral cutaneous 　　　nerve 　　Pudendal nerve **R　Sacral Nerve** 　　Spinal nerve, sacral	**Ø　Open** **3　Percutaneous** **4　Percutaneous Endoscopic**	**Z　No Device**	**Z　No Qualifier**

0　Medical and Surgical
1　Peripheral Nervous System
H　Insertion　Definition: Putting in a nonbiological appliance that monitors, assists, performs, or prevents a physiological function but does not physically take the place of a body part
　　　　　　　Explanation: None

Body Part Character 4	Approach Character 5	Device Character 6	Qualifier Character 7
Y　Peripheral Nerve　⊞	0　Open 3　Percutaneous 4　Percutaneous Endoscopic	1　Radioactive Element 2　Monitoring Device M　Neurostimulator Lead Y　Other Device	Z　No Qualifier

Non-OR	01HY31Z	
Non-OR	01HY[3,4]YZ	

See Appendix L for Procedure Combinations
　⊞　01HY[0,3,4]MZ

0　Medical and Surgical
1　Peripheral Nervous System
J　Inspection　Definition: Visually and/or manually exploring a body part
　　　　　　　Explanation: Visual exploration may be performed with or without optical instrumentation. Manual exploration may be performed directly or through intervening body layers.

Body Part Character 4	Approach Character 5	Device Character 6	Qualifier Character 7
Y　Peripheral Nerve	0　Open 3　Percutaneous 4　Percutaneous Endoscopic	Z　No Device	Z　No Qualifier

Non-OR	01JY3ZZ

Ø Medical and Surgical
1 Peripheral Nervous System
N Release   Definition: Freeing a body part from an abnormal physical constraint by cutting or by the use of force
                    Explanation: Some of the restraining tissue may be taken out but none of the body part is taken out

Body Part Character 4		Approach Character 5	Device Character 6	Qualifier Character 7
Ø Cervical Plexus Ansa cervicalis Cutaneous (transverse) cervical nerve Great auricular nerve Lesser occipital nerve Supraclavicular nerve Transverse (cutaneous) cervical nerve **1 Cervical Nerve** Greater occipital nerve Spinal nerve, cervical Suboccipital nerve Third occipital nerve **2 Phrenic Nerve** Accessory phrenic nerve **3 Brachial Plexus** Axillary nerve Dorsal scapular nerve First intercostal nerve Long thoracic nerve Musculocutaneous nerve Subclavius nerve Suprascapular nerve **4 Ulnar Nerve** Cubital nerve **5 Median Nerve** Anterior interosseous nerve Palmar cutaneous nerve **6 Radial Nerve** Dorsal digital nerve Musculospiral nerve Palmar cutaneous nerve Posterior interosseous nerve **8 Thoracic Nerve** Intercostal nerve Intercostobrachial nerve Spinal nerve, thoracic Subcostal nerve **9 Lumbar Plexus** Accessory obturator nerve Genitofemoral nerve Iliohypogastric nerve Ilioinguinal nerve Lateral femoral cutaneous nerve Obturator nerve Superior gluteal nerve **A Lumbosacral Plexus** **B Lumbar Nerve** Lumbosacral trunk Spinal nerve, lumbar Superior clunic (cluneal) nerve **C Pudendal Nerve** Posterior labial nerve Posterior scrotal nerve **D Femoral Nerve** Anterior crural nerve Saphenous nerve **F Sciatic Nerve** Ischiatic nerve **G Tibial Nerve** Lateral plantar nerve Medial plantar nerve Medial popliteal nerve Medial sural cutaneous nerve	**H Peroneal Nerve** Common fibular nerve Common peroneal nerve External popliteal nerve Lateral sural cutaneous nerve **K Head and Neck Sympathetic Nerve** Cavernous plexus Cervical ganglion Ciliary ganglion Internal carotid plexus Otic ganglion Pterygopalatine (sphenopalatine) ganglion Sphenopalatine (pterygopalatine) ganglion Stellate ganglion Submandibular ganglion Submaxillary ganglion **L Thoracic Sympathetic Nerve** Cardiac plexus Esophageal plexus Greater splanchnic nerve Inferior cardiac nerve Least splanchnic nerve Lesser splanchnic nerve Middle cardiac nerve Pulmonary plexus Superior cardiac nerve Thoracic aortic plexus Thoracic ganglion **M Abdominal Sympathetic Nerve** Abdominal aortic plexus Auerbach's (myenteric) plexus Celiac (solar) plexus Celiac ganglion Gastric plexus Hepatic plexus Inferior hypogastric plexus Inferior mesenteric ganglion Inferior mesenteric plexus Meissner's (submucous) plexus Myenteric (Auerbach's) plexus Pancreatic plexus Pelvic splanchnic nerve Renal nerve Renal plexus Solar (celiac) plexus Splenic plexus Submucous (Meissner's) plexus Superior hypogastric plexus Superior mesenteric ganglion Superior mesenteric plexus Suprarenal plexus **N Lumbar Sympathetic Nerve** Lumbar ganglion Lumbar splanchnic nerve **P Sacral Sympathetic Nerve** Ganglion impar (ganglion of Walther) Pelvic splanchnic nerve Sacral ganglion Sacral splanchnic nerve **Q Sacral Plexus** Inferior gluteal nerve Posterior femoral cutaneous nerve Pudendal nerve **R Sacral Nerve** Spinal nerve, sacral	**Ø Open** **3 Percutaneous** **4 Percutaneous Endoscopic**	**Z No Device**	**Z No Qualifier**

NC Noncovered Procedure   **LC** Limited Coverage   **QA** Questionable OB Admit   **NT** New Tech Add-on   ⊞ Combination Member   ♂ Male   ♀ Female

ICD-10-PCS 2022   163

Ø **Medical and Surgical**
1 **Peripheral Nervous System**
P **Removal**   Definition: Taking out or off a device from a body part

Explanation: If a device is taken out and a similar device put in without cutting or puncturing the skin or mucous membrane, the procedure is coded to the root operation CHANGE. Otherwise, the procedure for taking out a device is coded to the root operation REMOVAL.

Body Part Character 4	Approach Character 5	Device Character 6	Qualifier Character 7
Y Peripheral Nerve	Ø Open 3 Percutaneous 4 Percutaneous Endoscopic	Ø Drainage Device 2 Monitoring Device 7 Autologous Tissue Substitute M Neurostimulator Lead Y Other Device	Z No Qualifier
Y Peripheral Nerve	X External	Ø Drainage Device 2 Monitoring Device M Neurostimulator Lead	Z No Qualifier

Non-OR	Ø1PY3[Ø,2]Z
Non-OR	Ø1PY[3,4]YZ
Non-OR	Ø1PYX[Ø,2,M]Z

Ø **Medical and Surgical**
1 **Peripheral Nervous System**
Q **Repair**　　　　Definition: Restoring, to the extent possible, a body part to its normal anatomic structure and function
　　　　　　　　　　Explanation: Used only when the method to accomplish the repair is not one of the other root operations

Body Part Character 4		Approach Character 5	Device Character 6	Qualifier Character 7
Ø **Cervical Plexus** Ansa cervicalis Cutaneous (transverse) cervical nerve Great auricular nerve Lesser occipital nerve Supraclavicular nerve Transverse (cutaneous) cervical nerve **1** **Cervical Nerve** Greater occipital nerve Spinal nerve, cervical Suboccipital nerve Third occipital nerve **2** **Phrenic Nerve** Accessory phrenic nerve **3** **Brachial Plexus** Axillary nerve Dorsal scapular nerve First intercostal nerve Long thoracic nerve Musculocutaneous nerve Subclavius nerve Suprascapular nerve **4** **Ulnar Nerve** Cubital nerve **5** **Median Nerve** Anterior interosseous nerve Palmar cutaneous nerve **6** **Radial Nerve** Dorsal digital nerve Musculospiral nerve Palmar cutaneous nerve Posterior interosseous nerve **8** **Thoracic Nerve** Intercostal nerve Intercostobrachial nerve Spinal nerve, thoracic Subcostal nerve **9** **Lumbar Plexus** Accessory obturator nerve Genitofemoral nerve Iliohypogastric nerve Ilioinguinal nerve Lateral femoral cutaneous nerve Obturator nerve Superior gluteal nerve **A** **Lumbosacral Plexus** **B** **Lumbar Nerve** Lumbosacral trunk Spinal nerve, lumbar Superior clunic (cluneal) nerve **C** **Pudendal Nerve** Posterior labial nerve Posterior scrotal nerve **D** **Femoral Nerve** Anterior crural nerve Saphenous nerve **F** **Sciatic Nerve** Ischiatic nerve **G** **Tibial Nerve** Lateral plantar nerve Medial plantar nerve Medial popliteal nerve Medial sural cutaneous nerve	**H** **Peroneal Nerve** Common fibular nerve Common peroneal nerve External popliteal nerve Lateral sural cutaneous nerve **K** **Head and Neck Sympathetic Nerve** Cavernous plexus Cervical ganglion Ciliary ganglion Internal carotid plexus Otic ganglion Pterygopalatine (sphenopalatine) ganglion Sphenopalatine (pterygopalatine) ganglion Stellate ganglion Submandibular ganglion Submaxillary ganglion **L** **Thoracic Sympathetic Nerve** Cardiac plexus Esophageal plexus Greater splanchnic nerve Inferior cardiac nerve Least splanchnic nerve Lesser splanchnic nerve Middle cardiac nerve Pulmonary plexus Superior cardiac nerve Thoracic aortic plexus Thoracic ganglion **M** **Abdominal Sympathetic Nerve** Abdominal aortic plexus Auerbach's (myenteric) plexus Celiac (solar) plexus Celiac ganglion Gastric plexus Hepatic plexus Inferior hypogastric plexus Inferior mesenteric ganglion Inferior mesenteric plexus Meissner's (submucous) plexus Myenteric (Auerbach's) plexus Pancreatic plexus Pelvic splanchnic nerve Renal nerve Renal plexus Solar (celiac) plexus Splenic plexus Submucous (Meissner's) plexus Superior hypogastric plexus Superior mesenteric ganglion Superior mesenteric plexus Suprarenal plexus **N** **Lumbar Sympathetic Nerve** Lumbar ganglion Lumbar splanchnic nerve **P** **Sacral Sympathetic Nerve** Ganglion impar (ganglion of Walther) Pelvic splanchnic nerve Sacral ganglion Sacral splanchnic nerve **Q** **Sacral Plexus** Inferior gluteal nerve Posterior femoral cutaneous nerve Pudendal nerve **R** **Sacral Nerve** Spinal nerve, sacral	**Ø** Open **3** Percutaneous **4** Percutaneous Endoscopic	**Z** No Device	**Z** No Qualifier

Peripheral Nervous System

Ø   Medical and Surgical
1   Peripheral Nervous System
R   Replacement   Definition: Putting in or on biological or synthetic material that physically takes the place and/or function of all or a portion of a body part
Explanation: The body part may have been taken out or replaced, or may be taken out, physically eradicated, or rendered nonfunctional during the REPLACEMENT procedure. A REMOVAL procedure is coded for taking out the device used in a previous replacement procedure.

Body Part Character 4	Approach Character 5	Device Character 6	Qualifier Character 7

1 Cervical Nerve
   Greater occipital nerve
   Spinal nerve, cervical
   Suboccipital nerve
   Third occipital nerve
2 Phrenic Nerve
   Accessory phrenic nerve
4 Ulnar Nerve
   Cubital nerve
5 Median Nerve
   Anterior interosseous nerve
   Palmar cutaneous nerve
6 Radial Nerve
   Dorsal digital nerve
   Musculospiral nerve
   Palmar cutaneous nerve
   Posterior interosseous nerve
8 Thoracic Nerve
   Intercostal nerve
   Intercostobrachial nerve
   Spinal nerve, thoracic
   Subcostal nerve
B Lumbar Nerve
   Lumbosacral trunk
   Spinal nerve, lumbar
   Superior clunic (cluneal) nerve
C Pudendal Nerve
   Posterior labial nerve
   Posterior scrotal nerve
D Femoral Nerve
   Anterior crural nerve
   Saphenous nerve
F Sciatic Nerve
   Ischiatic nerve
G Tibial Nerve
   Lateral plantar nerve
   Medial plantar nerve
   Medial popliteal nerve
   Medial sural cutaneous nerve
H Peroneal Nerve
   Common fibular nerve
   Common peroneal nerve
   External popliteal nerve
   Lateral sural cutaneous nerve
R Sacral Nerve
   Spinal nerve, sacral
	Ø Open
	4 Percutaneous Endoscopic
		7 Autologous Tissue Substitute
		J Synthetic Substitute
		K Nonautologous Tissue Substitute
			Z No Qualifier

Peripheral Nervous System

Ø Medical and Surgical
1 Peripheral Nervous System
S Reposition   Definition: Moving to its normal location, or other suitable location, all or a portion of a body part

Explanation: The body part is moved to a new location from an abnormal location, or from a normal location where it is not functioning correctly. The body part may or may not be cut out or off to be moved to the new location.

Body Part Character 4	Approach Character 5	Device Character 6	Qualifier Character 7

Ø Cervical Plexus
    Ansa cervicalis
    Cutaneous (transverse) cervical nerve
    Great auricular nerve
    Lesser occipital nerve
    Supraclavicular nerve
    Transverse (cutaneous) cervical nerve
1 Cervical Nerve
    Greater occipital nerve
    Spinal nerve, cervical
    Suboccipital nerve
    Third occipital nerve
2 Phrenic Nerve
    Accessory phrenic nerve
3 Brachial Plexus
    Axillary nerve
    Dorsal scapular nerve
    First intercostal nerve
    Long thoracic nerve
    Musculocutaneous nerve
    Subclavius nerve
    Suprascapular nerve
4 Ulnar Nerve
    Cubital nerve
5 Median Nerve
    Anterior interosseous nerve
    Palmar cutaneous nerve
6 Radial Nerve
    Dorsal digital nerve
    Musculospiral nerve
    Palmar cutaneous nerve
    Posterior interosseous nerve
8 Thoracic Nerve
    Intercostal nerve
    Intercostobrachial nerve
    Spinal nerve, thoracic
    Subcostal nerve
9 Lumbar Plexus
    Accessory obturator nerve
    Genitofemoral nerve
    Iliohypogastric nerve
    Ilioinguinal nerve
    Lateral femoral cutaneous nerve
    Obturator nerve
    Superior gluteal nerve
A Lumbosacral Plexus
B Lumbar Nerve
    Lumbosacral trunk
    Spinal nerve, lumbar
    Superior clunic (cluneal) nerve
C Pudendal Nerve
    Posterior labial nerve
    Posterior scrotal nerve
D Femoral Nerve
    Anterior crural nerve
    Saphenous nerve
F Sciatic Nerve
    Ischiatic nerve
G Tibial Nerve
    Lateral plantar nerve
    Medial plantar nerve
    Medial popliteal nerve
    Medial sural cutaneous nerve
H Peroneal Nerve
    Common fibular nerve
    Common peroneal nerve
    External popliteal nerve
    Lateral sural cutaneous nerve
Q Sacral Plexus
    Inferior gluteal nerve
    Posterior femoral cutaneous nerve
    Pudendal nerve
R Sacral Nerve
    Spinal nerve, sacral
	Ø Open
	3 Percutaneous
	4 Percutaneous Endoscopic
		Z No Device	**Z No Qualifier**

NC Noncovered Procedure   **LC** Limited Coverage   **QA** Questionable OB Admit   **NT** New Tech Add-on   ⊞ Combination Member   ♂ Male   ♀ Female

Peripheral Nervous System

Ø Medical and Surgical
1 Peripheral Nervous System
U Supplement   Definition: Putting in or on biological or synthetic material that physically reinforces and/or augments the function of a portion of a body part

Explanation: The biological material is non-living, or is living and from the same individual. The body part may have been previously replaced, and the SUPPLEMENT procedure is performed to physically reinforce and/or augment the function of the replaced body part.

Body Part Character 4		Approach Character 5	Device Character 6	Qualifier Character 7
1	Cervical Nerve Greater occipital nerve Spinal nerve, cervical Suboccipital nerve Third occipital nerve	Ø Open 3 Percutaneous 4 Percutaneous Endoscopic	7 Autologous Tissue Substitute J Synthetic Substitute K Nonautologous Tissue Substitute	Z No Qualifier
2	Phrenic Nerve Accessory phrenic nerve			
4	Ulnar Nerve Cubital nerve			
5	Median Nerve Anterior interosseous nerve Palmar cutaneous nerve			
6	Radial Nerve Dorsal digital nerve Musculospiral nerve Palmar cutaneous nerve Posterior interosseous nerve			
8	Thoracic Nerve Intercostal nerve Intercostobrachial nerve Spinal nerve, thoracic Subcostal nerve			
B	Lumbar Nerve Lumbosacral trunk Spinal nerve, lumbar Superior clunic (cluneal) nerve			
C	Pudendal Nerve Posterior labial nerve Posterior scrotal nerve			
D	Femoral Nerve Anterior crural nerve Saphenous nerve			
F	Sciatic Nerve Ischiatic nerve			
G	Tibial Nerve Lateral plantar nerve Medial plantar nerve Medial popliteal nerve Medial sural cutaneous nerve			
H	Peroneal Nerve Common fibular nerve Common peroneal nerve External popliteal nerve Lateral sural cutaneous nerve			
R	Sacral Nerve Spinal nerve, sacral			

Ø Medical and Surgical
1 Peripheral Nervous System
W Revision   Definition: Correcting, to the extent possible, a portion of a malfunctioning device or the position of a displaced device

Explanation: Revision can include correcting a malfunctioning or displaced device by taking out or putting in components of the device such as a screw or pin

Body Part Character 4		Approach Character 5	Device Character 6	Qualifier Character 7
Y	Peripheral Nerve	Ø Open 3 Percutaneous 4 Percutaneous Endoscopic	Ø Drainage Device 2 Monitoring Device 7 Autologous Tissue Substitute M Neurostimulator Lead Y Other Device	Z No Qualifier
Y	Peripheral Nerve	X External	Ø Drainage Device 2 Monitoring Device 7 Autologous Tissue Substitute M Neurostimulator Lead	Z No Qualifier

Non-OR   Ø1WY[3,4]YZ
Non-OR   Ø1WYX[Ø,2,7,M]Z

Non-OR Procedure   DRG Non-OR Procedure   Valid OR Procedure   HAC Associated Procedure   Combination Only   New/Revised GREEN

Ø **Medical and Surgical**
1 **Peripheral Nervous System**
X **Transfer**   Definition: Moving, without taking out, all or a portion of a body part to another location to take over the function of all or a portion of a body part
                Explanation: The body part transferred remains connected to its vascular and nervous supply

Body Part Character 4	Approach Character 5	Device Character 6	Qualifier Character 7

1 **Cervical Nerve**
  Greater occipital nerve
  Spinal nerve, cervical
  Suboccipital nerve
  Third occipital nerve
2 **Phrenic Nerve**
  Accessory phrenic nerve
	Ø Open
	4 Percutaneous Endoscopic
		Z No Device	**1** Cervical Nerve
			2 Phrenic Nerve

4 **Ulnar Nerve**
  Cubital nerve
5 **Median Nerve**
  Anterior interosseous nerve
  Palmar cutaneous nerve
6 **Radial Nerve**
  Dorsal digital nerve
  Musculospiral nerve
  Palmar cutaneous nerve
  Posterior interosseous nerve
	Ø Open
	4 Percutaneous Endoscopic
		Z No Device	**4** Ulnar Nerve
			5 Median Nerve
			6 Radial Nerve

8 **Thoracic Nerve**
  Intercostal nerve
  Intercostobrachial nerve
  Spinal nerve, thoracic
  Subcostal nerve
	Ø Open
	4 Percutaneous Endoscopic
		Z No Device	**8** Thoracic Nerve

B **Lumbar Nerve**
  Lumbosacral trunk
  Spinal nerve, lumbar
  Superior clunic (cluneal) nerve
C **Pudendal Nerve**
  Posterior labial nerve
  Posterior scrotal nerve
	Ø Open
	4 Percutaneous Endoscopic
		Z No Device	**B** Lumbar Nerve
			C Perineal Nerve

D **Femoral Nerve**
  Anterior crural nerve
  Saphenous nerve
F **Sciatic Nerve**
  Ischiatic nerve
G **Tibial Nerve**
  Lateral plantar nerve
  Medial plantar nerve
  Medial popliteal nerve
  Medial sural cutaneous nerve
H **Peroneal Nerve**
  Common fibular nerve
  Common peroneal nerve
  External popliteal nerve
  Lateral sural cutaneous nerve
	Ø Open
	4 Percutaneous Endoscopic
		Z No Device	**D** Femoral Nerve
			F Sciatic Nerve
			G Tibial Nerve
			H Peroneal Nerve

Heart and Great Vessels Ø21–Ø2Y

Character Meanings

This Character Meaning table is provided as a guide to assist the user in the identification of character members that may be found in this section of code tables. It **SHOULD NOT** be used to build a PCS code.

Operation–Character 3	Body Part–Character 4	Approach–Character 5	Device–Character 6	Qualifier–Character 7
1 Bypass	Ø Coronary Artery, One Artery	Ø Open	Ø Monitoring Device, Pressure Sensor	Ø Allogeneic OR Ultrasonic
4 Creation	1 Coronary Artery, Two Arteries	3 Percutaneous	2 Monitoring Device	1 Syngeneic
5 Destruction	2 Coronary Artery, Three Arteries	4 Percutaneous Endoscopic	3 Infusion Device	2 Zooplastic OR Common Atrioventricular Valve
7 Dilation	3 Coronary Artery, Four or More Arteries	X External	4 Intraluminal Device, Drug-eluting	3 Coronary Artery
8 Division	4 Coronary Vein		5 Intraluminal Device, Drug-eluting, Two	4 Coronary Vein
B Excision	5 Atrial Septum		6 Intraluminal Device, Drug-eluting, Three	5 Coronary Circulation
C Extirpation	6 Atrium, Right		7 Intraluminal Device, Drug-eluting, Four or More OR Autologous Tissue Substitute	6 Bifurcation OR Atrium, Right
F Fragmentation	7 Atrium, Left		8 Zooplastic Tissue	7 Atrium, Left OR Orbital Atherectomy Technique
H Insertion	8 Conduction Mechanism		9 Autologous Venous Tissue	8 Internal Mammary, Right
J Inspection	9 Chordae Tendineae		A Autologous Arterial Tissue	9 Internal Mammary, Left
K Map	A Heart		C Extraluminal Device	A Innominate Artery
L Occlusion	B Heart, Right		D Intraluminal Device	B Subclavian
N Release	C Heart, Left		E Intraluminal Device, Two OR Intraluminal Device, Branched or Fenestrated, One or Two Arteries	C Thoracic Artery
P Removal	D Papillary Muscle		F Intraluminal Device, Three OR Intraluminal Device, Branched or Fenestrated, Three or More Arteries	D Carotid
Q Repair	F Aortic Valve		G Intraluminal Device, Four or More	E Atrioventricular Valve, Left
R Replacement	G Mitral Valve		J Synthetic Substitute OR Cardiac Lead, Pacemaker	F Abdominal Artery
S Reposition	H Pulmonary Valve		K Nonautologous Tissue Substitute OR Cardiac Lead, Defibrillator	G Atrioventricular Valve, Right OR Axillary Artery
T Resection	J Tricuspid Valve		L Biologic with Synthetic Substitute, Autoregulated Electrohydraulic	H Transapical OR Brachial Artery
U Supplement	K Ventricle, Right		M Cardiac Lead OR Synthetic Substitute, Pneumatic	J Truncal Valve OR Temporary OR Intraoperative
V Restriction	L Ventricle, Left		N Intracardiac Pacemaker	K Left Atrial Appendage
			Q Implantable Heart Assist System	L In Existing Conduit
			R Short-term External Heart Assist System	M Native Site
W Revision	M Ventricular Septum		T Intraluminal Device, Radioactive	P Pulmonary Trunk
Y Transplantation	N Pericardium		Y Other Device	Q Pulmonary Artery, Right
	P Pulmonary Trunk		Z No Device	R Pulmonary Artery, Left
	Q Pulmonary Artery, Right			S Pulmonary Vein, Right OR Biventricular
	R Pulmonary Artery, Left			T Pulmonary Vein, Left OR Ductus Arteriosus
	S Pulmonary Vein, Right			U Pulmonary Vein, Confluence
	T Pulmonary Vein, Left			V Lower Extremity Artery
	V Superior Vena Cava			W Aorta
	W Thoracic Aorta, Descending			X Diagnostic
	X Thoracic Aorta, Ascending/Arch			Z No Qualifier
	Y Great Vessel			

AHA Coding Clinic for table Ø21

2020, 4Q, 44-45	Atrium bypass qualifier
2020, 1Q, 24	Pulmonary artery unifocalization
2020, 1Q, 37	Bypass of ascending aorta to brachiocephalic artery
2019, 4Q, 23	Bypass thoracic aorta to innominate artery
2019, 3Q, 30	Aortic aneurysm repair with debranching of common carotid and brachiocephalic arteries
2018, 4Q, 45-46	Descending thoracic aorta bypass
2018, 3Q, 8	Coronary artery bypass graft surgery (revision versus total redo)
2018, 3Q, 26	Coronary artery bypass graft surgery with endarterectomy
2017, 4Q, 56	Added approach values - Percutaneous heart valve procedures
2017, 1Q, 19	Norwood Sano procedure
2016, 4Q, 80-81	Thoracic aorta, ascending/arch and descending
2016, 4Q, 82-83	Coronary artery, number of arteries
2016, 4Q, 102-109	Correction of congenital heart defects
2016, 4Q, 144	Repair of atrial septal defect and anomalous pulmonary venous return
2016, 4Q, 145	Modified Warden procedure for repair of septal defect and right partial anomalous pulmonary venous return
2016, 1Q, 27	Aortocoronary bypass graft utilizing Y-graft
2015, 4Q, 22, 24	Congenital heart corrective procedures
2015, 3Q, 16	Revision of previous truncus arteriosus surgery with ventricle to pulmonary artery conduit
2014, 3Q, 3	Blalock-Taussig shunt procedure
2014, 3Q, 8	Coronary artery bypass graft utilizing internal mammary as pedicle graft
2014, 3Q, 20	MAZE procedure performed with coronary artery bypass graft
2014, 3Q, 29	Fontan completion procedure stage II
2014, 3Q, 30	Creation of conduit from right ventricle to pulmonary artery
2014, 1Q, 10	Repair of thoracic aortic aneurysm & coronary artery bypass graft
2013, 2Q, 37	Coronary artery release performed during coronary artery bypass graft

AHA Coding Clinic for table Ø24

2016, 4Q, 101	Root operation Creation
2016, 4Q, 102-109	Correction of congenital heart defects

AHA Coding Clinic for table Ø25

2020, 1Q, 32	Ablation convergent procedure (catheter-based and thoracoscopic ablations)
2018, 3Q, 27	Alcohol septal ablation
2016, 4Q, 80-81	Thoracic aorta, ascending/arch and descending
2016, 3Q, 43-44	Peri-pulmonary catheter ablation
2016, 3Q, 44-45	Maze procedure
2016, 2Q, 17	Photodynamic therapy for treatment of malignant mesothelioma
2014, 4Q, 47	Catheter ablation of peripulmonary veins
2014, 3Q, 19	Ablation of ventricular tachycardia with Impella® support
2014, 3Q, 20	MAZE procedure performed with coronary artery bypass graft
2013, 2Q, 38	Catheter ablation to treat atrial fibrillation

AHA Coding Clinic for table Ø27

2018, 3Q, 7	Coronary brachytherapy with angioplasty
2018, 3Q, 10	Disruption of perma-catheter fibrin sheath via angioplasty of superior vena cava
2018, 2Q, 24	Coronary artery bifurcation
2017, 4Q, 32-33	Corrective surgery of left ventricular outflow tract obstruction
2016, 4Q, 80-81	Thoracic aorta, ascending/arch and descending
2016, 4Q, 82-83	Coronary artery, number of arteries
2016, 4Q, 84-85	Coronary Artery, number of stents
2016, 4Q, 86-88	Coronary and peripheral artery bifurcation
2016, 1Q, 16	Pulmonary valvotomy and dilation of annulus
2015, 4Q, 13	New Section X codes—New Technology procedures
2015, 3Q, 9	Failed attempt to treat coronary artery occlusion
2015, 3Q, 10	Coronary angioplasty with unsuccessful stent insertion
2015, 3Q, 16	Revision of previous truncus arteriosus surgery with ventricle to pulmonary artery conduit
2015, 2Q, 3-5	Coronary artery intervention site
2014, 2Q, 4	Coronary angioplasty of bypassed vessel

AHA Coding Clinic for table Ø2B

2019, 3Q, 32	Endomyocardial biopsy and right heart catheterization
2019, 2Q, 20	Pericardiectomy for constrictive pericarditis
2017, 1Q, 38	Mitral valve repair and chordae tendineae transfer
2016, 4Q, 80-81	Thoracic aorta, ascending/arch and descending
2015, 2Q, 23	Annuloplasty ring

AHA Coding Clinic for table Ø2C

2019, 4Q, 25	Coronary artery to root operation Supplement
2018, 3Q, 26	Coronary artery bypass graft surgery with endarterectomy
2018, 2Q, 24	Coronary artery bifurcation
2017, 2Q, 23	Thrombectomy via Fogarty catheter
2016, 4Q, 80-81	Thoracic aorta, ascending/arch and descending
2016, 4Q, 82-83	Coronary artery, number of arteries
2016, 4Q, 86-87	Coronary and peripheral artery bifurcation
2016, 2Q, 24	Repair/decalcification of mitral valve
2016, 2Q, 25	Aortic valve surgery with excision of calcium deposits

AHA Coding Clinic for table Ø2F

2020, 4Q, 45-49	New fragmentation tables
2020, 4Q, 49-50	Intravascular ultrasound assisted thrombolysis
2020, 4Q, 50	Intravascular lithotripsy

AHA Coding Clinic for table Ø2H

2021, 2Q, 23	Clarification of lead placement in bundle of HIS
2019, 4Q, 23-24	Coronary artery Body Part to root operation Insertion
2019, 3Q, 19	Insertion of left ventricular catheter
2019, 3Q, 23	Placement of pacemaker lead in Bundle of HIS
2019, 1Q, 24	Replacement of left ventricular assist device with retention of outflow graft
2018, 4Q, 94	Insertion and removal of failed Watchman™ device
2018, 2Q, 3-5	Intra-aortic balloon pump
2018, 2Q, 19	Pacing lead attached to automatic implantable cardioverter defibrillator
2017, 4Q, 42-45	Insertion of external heart assist devices
2017, 4Q, 63-64	Added and revised device values - Vascular access reservoir
2017, 4Q, 104	Placement of Watchman™ left atrial appendage device
2017, 3Q, 11	Placement of peripherally inserted central catheter using 3CG ECG technology
2017, 2Q, 24	Tunneled catheter versus totally implantable catheter
2017, 2Q, 26	Exchange of tunneled catheter
2017, 1Q, 10-11	External heart assist device
2016, 4Q, 80-81	Thoracic aorta, ascending/arch and descending
2016, 4Q, 95	Intracardiac pacemaker
2016, 4Q, 137-138	Heart assist device systems
2016, 2Q, 15	Removal and replacement of tunneled internal jugular catheter
2015, 4Q, 14	New Section X codes—New Technology procedures
2015, 4Q, 26-31	Vascular access devices
2015, 3Q, 35	Swan Ganz catheterization
2015, 2Q, 31	Leadless pacemaker insertion
2015, 2Q, 33	Totally implantable central venous access device (Port-a-Cath)
2013, 3Q, 18	Placement of peripherally inserted central catheter (PICC)

AHA Coding Clinic for table Ø2J

2015, 3Q, 9	Failed attempt to treat coronary artery occlusion

AHA Coding Clinic for table Ø2K

2020, 1Q, 32	Ablation convergent procedure (catheter-based and thoracoscopic ablations)

AHA Coding Clinic for table Ø2L

2018, 4Q, 94	Insertion and removal of failed Watchman™ device
2017, 4Q, 31	Resuscitative endovascular balloon occlusion of the aorta
2017, 4Q, 33-34	Occlusion/ligation of pulmonary trunk & right pulmonary artery
2016, 4Q, 102-109	Correction of congenital heart defects
2016, 2Q, 26	Embolization of pulmonary arteriovenous fistula
2015, 4Q, 23	Congenital heart corrective procedures
2014, 3Q, 20	MAZE procedure performed with coronary artery bypass graft

AHA Coding Clinic for table Ø2N

2019, 2Q, 13	Unroofing of anomalous coronary artery
2019, 2Q, 20	Pericardiectomy for constrictive pericarditis
2017, 4Q, 35	Release of myocardial bridge
2016, 4Q, 80-81	Thoracic aorta, ascending/arch and descending
2014, 3Q, 16	Repair of Tetralogy of Fallot

AHA Coding Clinic for table Ø2P

2019, 1Q, 24	Replacement of left ventricular assist device with retention of outflow graft
2018, 4Q, 52-54	Percutaneous extracorporeal membrane oxygenation
2018, 4Q, 85	Externalization of lumboatrial shunt
2018, 4Q, 94	Insertion and removal of failed Watchman™ device
2018, 2Q, 3-5	Intra-aortic balloon pump
2017, 4Q, 42-45	Insertion of external heart assist devices
2017, 4Q, 104	Placement of Watchman™ left atrial appendage device
2017, 3Q, 18	Intra-aortic balloon pump removal
2017, 2Q, 24	Tunneled catheter versus totally implantable catheter
2017, 2Q, 26	Exchange of tunneled catheter
2017, 1Q, 11	External heart assist device
2017, 1Q, 13	SynCardia total artificial heart
2016, 4Q, 95-96	Intracardiac pacemaker
2016, 4Q, 137-139	Heart assist device systems
2016, 3Q, 19	Nonoperative removal of peripherally inserted central catheter
2016, 2Q, 15	Removal and replacement of tunneled internal jugular catheter
2015, 4Q, 31	Vascular access devices
2015, 3Q, 33	Approach values for repositioning and removal of cardiac lead

AHA Coding Clinic for table Ø2Q

2018, 1Q, 12	Percutaneous balloon valvuloplasty & cardiac catheterization with ventriculogram
2017, 1Q, 18	Sutureless repair of pulmonary vein stenosis
2016, 4Q, 80-81	Thoracic aorta, ascending/arch and descending
2016, 4Q, 82-83	Coronary artery, number of arteries
2016, 4Q, 101	Root operation Creation
2016, 4Q, 102-109	Correction of congenital heart defects
2015, 4Q, 23	Congenital heart corrective procedures
2015, 3Q, 16	Vascular ring surgery and double aortic arch
2015, 2Q, 23	Annuloplasty ring
2013, 3Q, 26	Transcatheter replacement of heart valve (TAVR) with measurements

AHA Coding Clinic for table Ø2R

2020, 1Q, 25	Elephant trunk repair of aortic dissection
2019, 4Q, 24	Coronary artery Body Part to root operation Insertion
2019, 4Q, 46	Cerebral embolic filtration
2019, 3Q, 23	Replacement of atrioventricular valve
2019, 3Q, 24	Valve sparing aortic root replacement with modified Gleason Vascutek® graft to ascending aorta
2019, 1Q, 31	Transcatheter aortic valve in valve replacement
2018, 3Q, 11	Transcatheter aortic valve replacement via transaortic approach
2018, 1Q, 12	Percutaneous balloon valvuloplasty & cardiac catheterization with ventriculogram
2017, 4Q, 55-56	Added approach values - Percutaneous heart valve procedures
2017, 1Q, 13	SynCardia total artificial heart
2016, 4Q, 80-81	Thoracic aorta, ascending/arch and descending
2016, 3Q, 32	Transcatheter tricuspid valve replacement
2014, 1Q, 10	Repair of thoracic aortic aneurysm & coronary artery bypass graft

AHA Coding Clinic for table Ø2S

2016, 4Q, 80-81	Thoracic aorta, ascending/arch and descending
2016, 4Q, 82-83	Coronary artery, number of arteries
2016, 4Q, 102-109	Correction of congenital heart defects
2015, 4Q, 23	Congenital heart corrective procedures

AHA Coding Clinic for table Ø2U

2020, 4Q, 52	Transapical mitral valve repair with device
2020, 1Q, 24	Pulmonary artery unifocalization
2019, 4Q, 25	Coronary artery to root operation Supplement
2018, 1Q, 12	Percutaneous balloon valvuloplasty & cardiac catheterization with ventriculogram
2017, 4Q, 36	Alfieri stitch procedure
2017, 3Q, 7	Senning procedure (arterial switch)
2017, 1Q, 19	Norwood Sano procedure
2016, 4Q, 80-81	Thoracic aorta, ascending/arch and descending
2016, 4Q, 101	Root operation Creation
2016, 4Q, 102-109	Correction of congenital heart defects
2016, 2Q, 23	Repair of tetralogy of Fallot with autologous pericardial patch graft
2016, 2Q, 26	Aortic valve replacement with aortic root enlargement
2015, 4Q, 22-24	Congenital heart corrective procedures
2015, 3Q, 16	Revision of previous truncus arteriosus surgery with ventricle to pulmonary artery conduit
2015, 2Q, 23	Annuloplasty ring
2014, 3Q, 16	Repair of Tetralogy of Fallot

AHA Coding Clinic for table Ø2V

2020, 1Q, 25	Elephant trunk repair of aortic dissection
2017, 4Q, 35-36	Alfieri stitch procedure
2016, 4Q, 80-81	Thoracic aorta, ascending/arch and descending
2016, 4Q, 89-92	Branched and fenestrated endograft repair of aneurysms

AHA Coding Clinic for table Ø2W

2019, 1Q, 24	Replacement of left ventricular assist device with retention of outflow graft
2018, 3Q, 8	Coronary artery bypass graft surgery (revision versus total redo)
2018, 3Q, 9	Fibrin sheath stripping of malfunctioning port-a-cath
2018, 1Q, 17	Repositioning of Impella short-term external heart assist device
2017, 4Q, 42-45	Insertion of external heart assist devices
2017, 4Q, 55-56	Added approach values - Percutaneous heart valve procedures
2016, 4Q, 85	Coronary Artery, number of stents
2016, 4Q, 95-96	Intracardiac pacemaker
2015, 3Q, 32	Approach values for repositioning and removal of cardiac lead
2014, 3Q, 31	Closure of paravalvular leak using Amplatzer® vascular plug

AHA Coding Clinic for table Ø2Y

2013, 3Q, 18	Heart transplant surgery

Heart and Great Vessels (vertical, left margin)

Coronary Arteries

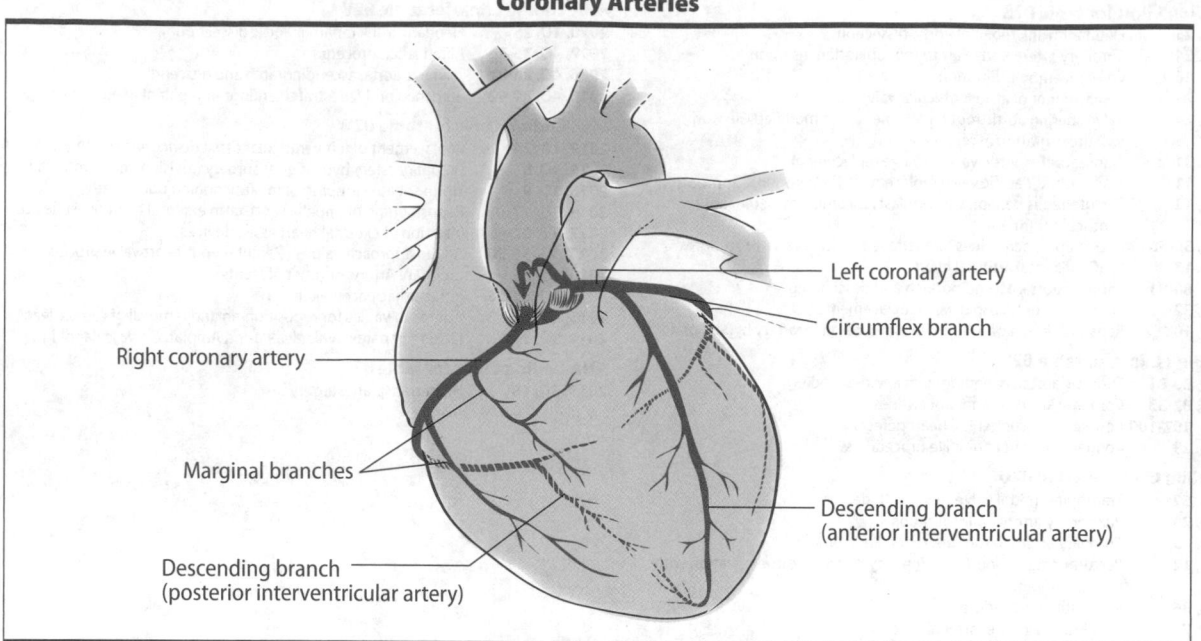

Left coronary artery

Circumflex branch

Right coronary artery

Marginal branches

Descending branch (anterior interventricular artery)

Descending branch (posterior interventricular artery)

Heart Anatomy

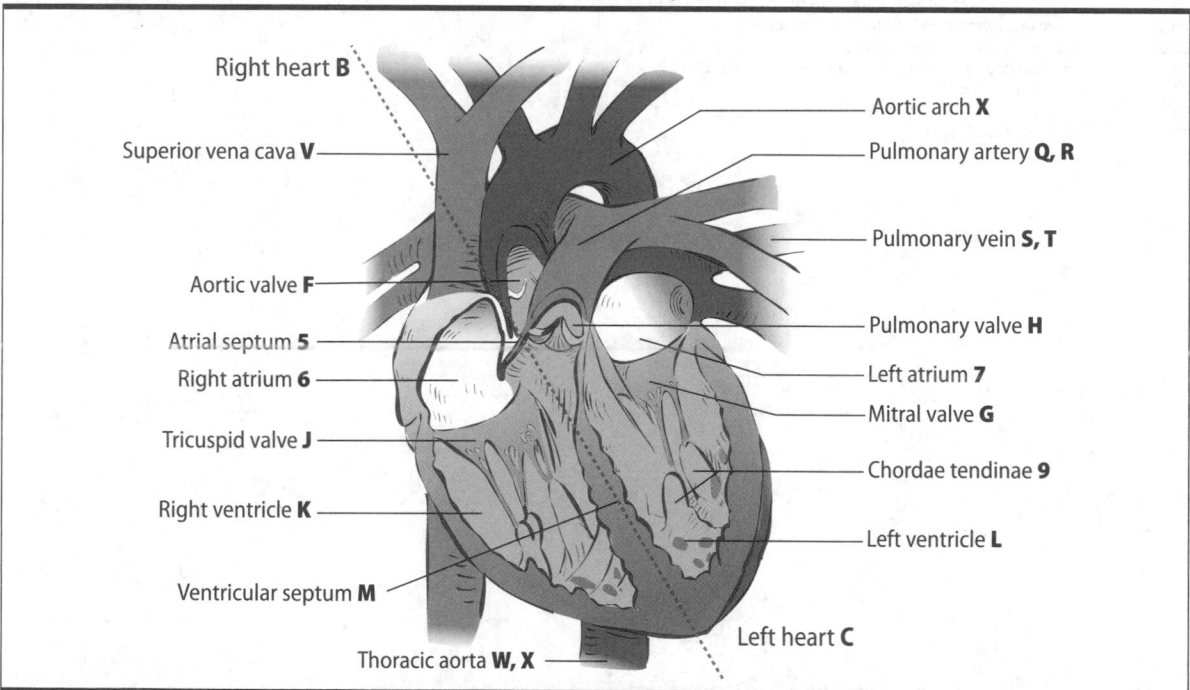

Right heart **B**

Aortic arch **X**

Superior vena cava **V**

Pulmonary artery **Q, R**

Pulmonary vein **S, T**

Aortic valve **F**

Pulmonary valve **H**

Atrial septum **5**

Left atrium **7**

Right atrium **6**

Mitral valve **G**

Tricuspid valve **J**

Chordae tendinae **9**

Right ventricle **K**

Left ventricle **L**

Ventricular septum **M**

Left heart **C**

Thoracic aorta **W, X**

Ø **Medical and Surgical**
2 **Heart and Great Vessels**
1 **Bypass**　　Definition: Altering the route of passage of the contents of a tubular body part
　　　　Explanation: Rerouting contents of a body part to a downstream area of the normal route, to a similar route and body part, or to an abnormal route and dissimilar body part. Includes one or more anastomoses, with or without the use of a device.

Body Part Character 4	Approach Character 5	Device Character 6	Qualifier Character 7
Ø Coronary Artery, One Artery 1 Coronary Artery, Two Arteries 2 Coronary Artery, Three Arteries 3 Coronary Artery, Four or More Arteries	Ø Open	8 Zooplastic Tissue 9 Autologous Venous Tissue A Autologous Arterial Tissue J Synthetic Substitute K Nonautologous Tissue Substitute	3 Coronary Artery 8 Internal Mammary, Right 9 Internal Mammary, Left C Thoracic Artery F Abdominal Artery W Aorta
Ø Coronary Artery, One Artery 1 Coronary Artery, Two Arteries 2 Coronary Artery, Three Arteries 3 Coronary Artery, Four or More Arteries	Ø Open	Z No Device	3 Coronary Artery 8 Internal Mammary, Right 9 Internal Mammary, Left C Thoracic Artery F Abdominal Artery
Ø Coronary Artery, One Artery 1 Coronary Artery, Two Arteries 2 Coronary Artery, Three Arteries 3 Coronary Artery, Four or More Arteries	3 Percutaneous	4 Intraluminal Device, Drug-eluting D Intraluminal Device	4 Coronary Vein
Ø Coronary Artery, One Artery 1 Coronary Artery, Two Arteries 2 Coronary Artery, Three Arteries 3 Coronary Artery, Four or More Arteries	4 Percutaneous Endoscopic	4 Intraluminal Device, Drug-eluting D Intraluminal Device	4 Coronary Vein
Ø Coronary Artery, One Artery 1 Coronary Artery, Two Arteries 2 Coronary Artery, Three Arteries 3 Coronary Artery, Four or More Arteries	4 Percutaneous Endoscopic	8 Zooplastic Tissue 9 Autologous Venous Tissue A Autologous Arterial Tissue J Synthetic Substitute K Nonautologous Tissue Substitute	3 Coronary Artery 8 Internal Mammary, Right 9 Internal Mammary, Left C Thoracic Artery F Abdominal Artery W Aorta
Ø Coronary Artery, One Artery 1 Coronary Artery, Two Arteries 2 Coronary Artery, Three Arteries 3 Coronary Artery, Four or More Arteries	4 Percutaneous Endoscopic	Z No Device	3 Coronary Artery 8 Internal Mammary, Right 9 Internal Mammary, Left C Thoracic Artery F Abdominal Artery
6 Atrium, Right Atrium dextrum cordis Right auricular appendix Sinus venosus	Ø Open 4 Percutaneous Endoscopic	8 Zooplastic Tissue 9 Autologous Venous Tissue A Autologous Arterial Tissue J Synthetic Substitute K Nonautologous Tissue Substitute	P Pulmonary Trunk Q Pulmonary Artery, Right R Pulmonary Artery, Left
6 Atrium, Right Atrium dextrum cordis Right auricular appendix Sinus venosus	Ø Open 4 Percutaneous Endoscopic	Z No Device	7 Atrium, Left P Pulmonary Trunk Q Pulmonary Artery, Right R Pulmonary Artery, Left
6 Atrium, Right Atrium dextrum cordis Right auricular appendix Sinus venosus	3 Percutaneous	Z No Device	7 Atrium, Left
7 Atrium, Left Atrium pulmonale Left auricular appendix	Ø Open 4 Percutaneous Endoscopic	8 Zooplastic Tissue 9 Autologous Venous Tissue A Autologous Arterial Tissue J Synthetic Substitute K Nonautologous Tissue Substitute Z No Device	P Pulmonary Trunk Q Pulmonary Artery, Right R Pulmonary Artery, Left S Pulmonary Vein, Right T Pulmonary Vein, Left U Pulmonary Vein, Confluence
7 Atrium, Left Atrium pulmonale Left auricular appendix	3 Percutaneous	J Synthetic Substitute	6 Atrium, Right
K Ventricle, Right Conus arteriosus L Ventricle, Left	Ø Open 4 Percutaneous Endoscopic	8 Zooplastic Tissue 9 Autologous Venous Tissue A Autologous Arterial Tissue J Synthetic Substitute K Nonautologous Tissue Substitute	P Pulmonary Trunk Q Pulmonary Artery, Right R Pulmonary Artery, Left

HAC　Ø21[Ø,1,2,3]Ø[8,9,A,J,K][3,8,9,C,F,W] when reported with SDx J98.51 or J98.59
HAC　Ø21[Ø,1,2,3]ØZ[3,8,9,C,F] when reported with SDx J98.51 or J98.59
HAC　Ø21[Ø,1,2,3]4[8,9,A,J,K][3,8,9,C,F,W] when reported with SDx J98.51 or J98.59
HAC　Ø21[Ø,1,2,3]4Z[3,8,9,C,F] when reported with SDx J98.51 or J98.59

Ø21 Continued on next page

NC Noncovered Procedure　LC Limited Coverage　QA Questionable OB Admit　NT New Tech Add-on　⊞ Combination Member　♂Male　♀Female

Ø21 Continued

Ø	Medical and Surgical
2	Heart and Great Vessels
1	Bypass

Definition: Altering the route of passage of the contents of a tubular body part

Explanation: Rerouting contents of a body part to a downstream area of the normal route, to a similar route and body part, or to an abnormal route and dissimilar body part. Includes one or more anastomoses, with or without the use of a device.

Body Part Character 4	Approach Character 5	Device Character 6	Qualifier Character 7
K Ventricle, Right Conus arteriosus L Ventricle, Left	Ø Open 4 Percutaneous Endoscopic	Z No Device	5 Coronary Circulation 8 Internal Mammary, Right 9 Internal Mammary, Left C Thoracic Artery F Abdominal Artery P Pulmonary Trunk Q Pulmonary Artery, Right R Pulmonary Artery, Left W Aorta

P Pulmonary Trunk
Q Pulmonary Artery, Right
R Pulmonary Artery, Left
  Arterial canal (duct)
  Botallo's duct
  Pulmoaortic canal
	Ø Open
	4 Percutaneous Endoscopic
		8 Zooplastic Tissue
		9 Autologous Venous Tissue
		A Autologous Arterial Tissue
		J Synthetic Substitute
		K Nonautologous Tissue Substitute
		Z No Device
			A Innominate Artery
			B Subclavian
			D Carotid

V Superior Vena Cava Precava	Ø Open 4 Percutaneous Endoscopic	8 Zooplastic Tissue 9 Autologous Venous Tissue A Autologous Arterial Tissue J Synthetic Substitute K Nonautologous Tissue Substitute Z No Device	P Pulmonary Trunk Q Pulmonary Artery, Right R Pulmonary Artery, Left S Pulmonary Vein, Right T Pulmonary Vein, Left U Pulmonary Vein, Confluence
W Thoracic Aorta, Descending	Ø Open	8 Zooplastic Tissue 9 Autologous Venous Tissue A Autologous Arterial Tissue J Synthetic Substitute K Nonautologous Tissue Substitute	A Innominate Artery B Subclavian D Carotid F Abdominal Artery G Axillary Artery H Brachial Artery P Pulmonary Trunk Q Pulmonary Artery, Right R Pulmonary Artery, Left V Lower Extremity Artery
W Thoracic Aorta, Descending	Ø Open	Z No Device	A Innominate Artery B Subclavian D Carotid P Pulmonary Trunk Q Pulmonary Artery, Right R Pulmonary Artery, Left
W Thoracic Aorta, Descending	4 Percutaneous Endoscopic	8 Zooplastic Tissue 9 Autologous Venous Tissue A Autologous Arterial Tissue J Synthetic Substitute K Nonautologous Tissue Substitute Z No Device	A Innominate Artery B Subclavian D Carotid P Pulmonary Trunk Q Pulmonary Artery, Right R Pulmonary Artery, Left

X Thoracic Aorta, Ascending/Arch
  Aortic arch
  Ascending aorta
	Ø Open
	4 Percutaneous Endoscopic
		8 Zooplastic Tissue
		9 Autologous Venous Tissue
		A Autologous Arterial Tissue
		J Synthetic Substitute
		K Nonautologous Tissue Substitute
		Z No Device
			A Innominate Artery
			B Subclavian
			D Carotid
			P Pulmonary Trunk
			Q Pulmonary Artery, Right
			R Pulmonary Artery, Left

Ø	Medical and Surgical
2	Heart and Great Vessels
4	Creation

Definition: Putting in or on biological or synthetic material to form a new body part that to the extent possible replicates the anatomic structure or function of an absent body part

Explanation: Used for gender reassignment surgery and corrective procedures in individuals with congenital anomalies

Body Part Character 4	Approach Character 5	Device Character 6	Qualifier Character 7
F Aortic Valve Aortic annulus	Ø Open	7 Autologous Tissue 8 Zooplastic Tissue J Synthetic Substitute K Nonautologous Tissue Substitute	J Truncal Valve

G Mitral Valve
  Bicuspid valve
  Left atrioventricular valve
  Mitral annulus
J Tricuspid Valve
  Right atrioventricular valve
  Tricuspid annulus
	Ø Open	7 Autologous Tissue
		8 Zooplastic Tissue
		J Synthetic Substitute
		K Nonautologous Tissue Substitute
			2 Common Atrioventricular Valve

Ø   Medical and Surgical
2   Heart and Great Vessels
5   Destruction   Definition: Physical eradication of all or a portion of a body part by the direct use of energy, force, or a destructive agent
                 Explanation: None of the body part is physically taken out

Body Part Character 4	Approach Character 5	Device Character 6	Qualifier Character 7
4 Coronary Vein	**Ø Open**	**Z No Device**	**Z No Qualifier**
5 Atrial Septum Interatrial septum	**3 Percutaneous** **4 Percutaneous Endoscopic**		

6   Atrium, Right
     Atrium dextrum cordis
     Right auricular appendix
     Sinus venosus			

8   Conduction Mechanism
     Atrioventricular node
     Bundle of His
     Bundle of Kent
     Sinoatrial node			

9 Chordae Tendineae			
D Papillary Muscle			
F Aortic Valve Aortic annulus			

G   Mitral Valve
     Bicuspid valve
     Left atrioventricular valve
     Mitral annulus			

H   Pulmonary Valve
     Pulmonary annulus
     Pulmonic valve			

J   Tricuspid Valve
     Right atrioventricular valve
     Tricuspid annulus			

K Ventricle, Right Conus arteriosus			
L Ventricle, Left			
M Ventricular Septum Interventricular septum			
N Pericardium			
P Pulmonary Trunk			
Q Pulmonary Artery, Right			

R   Pulmonary Artery, Left
     Arterial canal (duct)
     Botallo's duct
     Pulmoaortic canal			

S   Pulmonary Vein, Right
     Right inferior pulmonary vein
     Right superior pulmonary vein			

T   Pulmonary Vein, Left
     Left inferior pulmonary vein
     Left superior pulmonary vein			

V Superior Vena Cava Precava			
W Thoracic Aorta, Descending			

X   Thoracic Aorta, Ascending/Arch
     Aortic arch
     Ascending aorta			

7   Atrium, Left
     Atrium pulmonale
     Left auricular appendix
	Ø Open
	3 Percutaneous
	4 Percutaneous Endoscopic
		Z No Device	**K Left Atrial Appendage**
			Z No Qualifier

DRG Non-OR   Ø257[Ø,3,4]ZK

NC Noncovered Procedure   **LC** Limited Coverage   **QA** Questionable OB Admit   **NT** New Tech Add-on   ⊞ Combination Member   ♂ Male   ♀ Female

ICD-10-PCS 2022   177

Heart and Great Vessels

Ø	Medical and Surgical
2	Heart and Great Vessels
7	Dilation

Definition: Expanding an orifice or the lumen of a tubular body part

Explanation: The orifice can be a natural orifice or an artificially created orifice. Accomplished by stretching a tubular body part using intraluminal pressure or by cutting part of the orifice or wall of the tubular body part.

Body Part Character 4	Approach Character 5	Device Character 6	Qualifier Character 7

0 Coronary Artery, One Artery
1 Coronary Artery, Two Arteries
2 Coronary Artery, Three Arteries
3 Coronary Artery, Four or More Arteries
	0 Open
	3 Percutaneous
	4 Percutaneous Endoscopic
		4 Intraluminal Device,
		   Drug-eluting
		5 Intraluminal Device, Drug-eluting,
		   Two
		6 Intraluminal Device, Drug-eluting,
		   Three
		7 Intraluminal Device, Drug-eluting,
		   Four or More
		D Intraluminal Device
		E Intraluminal Device, Two
		F Intraluminal Device, Three
		G Intraluminal Device, Four or More
		T Intraluminal Device, Radioactive
		Z No Device
			6 Bifurcation
			Z No Qualifier

F Aortic Valve
   Aortic annulus
G Mitral Valve
   Bicuspid valve
   Left atrioventricular valve
   Mitral annulus
H Pulmonary Valve
   Pulmonary annulus
   Pulmonic valve
J Tricuspid Valve
   Right atrioventricular valve
   Tricuspid annulus
K Ventricle, Right
   Conus arteriosus
L Ventricle, Left
P Pulmonary Trunk
Q Pulmonary Artery, Right
S Pulmonary Vein, Right
   Right inferior pulmonary vein
   Right superior pulmonary vein
T Pulmonary Vein, Left
   Left inferior pulmonary vein
   Left superior pulmonary vein
V Superior Vena Cava
   Precava
W Thoracic Aorta, Descending
X Thoracic Aorta, Ascending/Arch
   Aortic arch
   Ascending aorta
	0 Open
	3 Percutaneous
	4 Percutaneous Endoscopic
		4 Intraluminal Device,
		   Drug-eluting
		D Intraluminal Device
		Z No Device
			Z No Qualifier

R Pulmonary Artery, Left
   Arterial canal (duct)
   Botallo's duct
   Pulmoaortic canal
	0 Open
	3 Percutaneous
	4 Percutaneous Endoscopic
		4 Intraluminal Device,
		   Drug-eluting
		D Intraluminal Device
		Z No Device
			T Ductus Arteriosus
			Z No Qualifier

Ø	Medical and Surgical
2	Heart and Great Vessels
8	Division

Definition: Cutting into a body part, without draining fluids and/or gases from the body part, in order to separate or transect a body part

Explanation: All or a portion of the body part is separated into two or more portions

Body Part Character 4	Approach Character 5	Device Character 6	Qualifier Character 7

8 Conduction Mechanism
   Atrioventricular node
   Bundle of His
   Bundle of Kent
   Sinoatrial node
9 Chordae Tendineae
D Papillary Muscle
	0 Open
	3 Percutaneous
	4 Percutaneous Endoscopic
		Z No Device	Z No Qualifier

0　Medical and Surgical
2　Heart and Great Vessels
B　Excision　　　Definition: Cutting out or off, without replacement, a portion of a body part
　　　　　　　　　　　Explanation: The qualifier DIAGNOSTIC is used to identify excision procedures that are biopsies

Body Part Character 4	Approach Character 5	Device Character 6	Qualifier Character 7
4　Coronary Vein	**0**　Open	**Z**　No Device	**X**　Diagnostic
5　Atrial Septum 　　Interatrial septum	**3**　Percutaneous		**Z**　No Qualifier
6　Atrium, Right 　　Atrium dextrum cordis 　　Right auricular appendix 　　Sinus venosus	**4**　Percutaneous Endoscopic		
8　Conduction Mechanism 　　Atrioventricular node 　　Bundle of His 　　Bundle of Kent 　　Sinoatrial node			
9　Chordae Tendineae			
D　Papillary Muscle			
F　Aortic Valve 　　Aortic annulus			
G　Mitral Valve 　　Bicuspid valve 　　Left atrioventricular valve 　　Mitral annulus			
H　Pulmonary Valve 　　Pulmonary annulus 　　Pulmonic valve			
J　Tricuspid Valve 　　Right atrioventricular valve 　　Tricuspid annulus			
K　Ventricle, Right　**NC** 　　Conus arteriosus			
L　Ventricle, Left　**NC**			
M　Ventricular Septum 　　Interventricular septum			
N　Pericardium			
P　Pulmonary Trunk			
Q　Pulmonary Artery, Right			
R　Pulmonary Artery, Left 　　Arterial canal (duct) 　　Botallo's duct 　　Pulmoaortic canal			
S　Pulmonary Vein, Right 　　Right inferior pulmonary vein 　　Right superior pulmonary vein			
T　Pulmonary Vein, Left 　　Left inferior pulmonary vein 　　Left superior pulmonary vein			
V　Superior Vena Cava 　　Precava			
W　Thoracic Aorta, Descending			
X　Thoracic Aorta, Ascending/Arch 　　Aortic arch 　　Ascending aorta			
7　Atrium, Left 　　Atrium pulmonale 　　Left auricular appendix	**0**　Open **3**　Percutaneous **4**　Percutaneous Endoscopic	**Z**　No Device	**K**　Left Atrial Appendage **X**　Diagnostic **Z**　No Qualifier

DRG Non-OR	02B7[0,3,4]ZK
Non-OR	02B[4,5,6,8,9,D,F,G,H,J,K,L,M][0,3,4]ZX
NC	02B[K,L][0,3,4]ZZ

NC Noncovered Procedure　　**LC** Limited Coverage　　**QA** Questionable OB Admit　　**NT** New Tech Add-on　　⊞ Combination Member　　♂ Male　　♀ Female

ICD-10-PCS 2022　　　　　　　　　　　　　　　　　　　　　　　　　　　　　　　　　　　　　　　**179**

Heart and Great Vessels

0 **Medical and Surgical**
2 **Heart and Great Vessels**
C **Extirpation**   Definition: Taking or cutting out solid matter from a body part

Explanation: The solid matter may be an abnormal byproduct of a biological function or a foreign body; it may be imbedded in a body part or in the lumen of a tubular body part. The solid matter may or may not have been previously broken into pieces.

Body Part Character 4	Approach Character 5	Device Character 6	Qualifier Character 7
0 **Coronary Artery, One Artery** **1** **Coronary Artery, Two Arteries** **2** **Coronary Artery, Three Arteries** **3** **Coronary Artery, Four or More Arteries**	**0** Open **4** Percutaneous Endoscopic	**Z** No Device	**6** Bifurcation **Z** No Qualifier
0 **Coronary Artery, One Artery** **1** **Coronary Artery, Two Arteries** **2** **Coronary Artery, Three Arteries** **3** **Coronary Artery, Four or More Arteries**	**3** Percutaneous	**Z** No Device	**6** Bifurcation **7** Orbital Atherectomy Technique **Z** No Qualifier
4 **Coronary Vein** **5** **Atrial Septum** Interatrial septum **6** **Atrium, Right** Atrium dextrum cordis Right auricular appendix Sinus venosus **7** **Atrium, Left** Atrium pulmonale Left auricular appendix **8** **Conduction Mechanism** Atrioventricular node Bundle of His Bundle of Kent Sinoatrial node **9** **Chordae Tendineae** **D** **Papillary Muscle** **F** **Aortic Valve** Aortic annulus **G** **Mitral Valve** Bicuspid valve Left atrioventricular valve Mitral annulus **H** **Pulmonary Valve** Pulmonary annulus Pulmonic valve **J** **Tricuspid Valve** Right atrioventricular valve Tricuspid annulus **K** **Ventricle, Right** Conus arteriosus **L** **Ventricle, Left** **M** **Ventricular Septum** Interventricular septum **N** **Pericardium** **P** **Pulmonary Trunk** **Q** **Pulmonary Artery, Right** **R** **Pulmonary Artery, Left** Arterial canal (duct) Botallo's duct Pulmoaortic canal **S** **Pulmonary Vein, Right** Right inferior pulmonary vein Right superior pulmonary vein **T** **Pulmonary Vein, Left** Left inferior pulmonary vein Left superior pulmonary vein **V** **Superior Vena Cava** Precava **W** **Thoracic Aorta, Descending** **X** **Thoracic Aorta, Ascending/Arch** Aortic arch Ascending aorta	**0** Open **3** Percutaneous **4** Percutaneous Endoscopic	**Z** No Device	**Z** No Qualifier

Non-OR Procedure   DRG Non-OR Procedure   Valid OR Procedure   HAC Associated Procedure   Combination Only   New/Revised GREEN

0   Medical and Surgical
2   Heart and Great Vessels
F   Fragmentation   Definition: Breaking solid matter in a body part into pieces

              Explanation: Physical force (e.g., manual, ultrasonic) applied directly or indirectly is used to break the solid matter into pieces. The solid matter may be an abnormal byproduct of a biological function or a foreign body. The pieces of solid matter are not taken out.

Body Part Character 4	Approach Character 5	Device Character 6	Qualifier Character 7
0 Coronary Artery, One Artery **1** Coronary Artery, Two Arteries **2** Coronary Artery, Three Arteries **3** Coronary Artery, Four or More Arteries	**3** Percutaneous	**Z** No Device	**Z** No Qualifier
N Pericardium `NC`	**0** Open **3** Percutaneous **4** Percutaneous Endoscopic **X** External	**Z** No Device	**Z** No Qualifier

P Pulmonary Trunk
Q Pulmonary Artery, Right
R Pulmonary Artery, Left
    Arterial canal (duct)
    Botallo's duct
    Pulmoaortic canal
S Pulmonary Vein, Right
    Right inferior pulmonary vein
    Right superior pulmonary vein
T Pulmonary Vein, Left
    Left inferior pulmonary vein
    Left superior pulmonary vein
	3 Percutaneous	**Z** No Device	**0** Ultrasonic
			Z No Qualifier

Non-OR   02FNXZZ
`NC`   02FNXZZ

`NC` Noncovered Procedure   `LC` Limited Coverage   `QA` Questionable OB Admit   `NT` New Tech Add-on   ⊞ Combination Member   ♂ Male   ♀ Female

Heart and Great Vessels (side tab)

0　Medical and Surgical
2　Heart and Great Vessels
H　Insertion　　Definition: Putting in a nonbiological appliance that monitors, assists, performs, or prevents a physiological function but does not physically take the place of a body part
　　　　　　　　Explanation: None

Body Part Character 4	Approach Character 5	Device Character 6	Qualifier Character 7
0　Coronary Artery, One Artery 1　Coronary Artery, Two Arteries 2　Coronary Artery, Three Arteries 3　Coronary Artery, Four or More Arteries	0　Open 3　Percutaneous 4　Percutaneous Endoscopic	D　Intraluminal Device Y　Other Device	Z　No Qualifier
4　Coronary Vein ⊞ 6　Atrium, Right ⊞ 　　Atrium dextrum cordis 　　Right auricular appendix 　　Sinus venosus 7　Atrium, Left ⊞ 　　Atrium pulmonale 　　Left auricular appendix K　Ventricle, Right ⊞ 　　Conus arteriosus L　Ventricle, Left ⊞	0　Open 3　Percutaneous 4　Percutaneous Endoscopic	0　Monitoring Device, Pressure Sensor 2　Monitoring Device 3　Infusion Device D　Intraluminal Device J　Cardiac Lead, Pacemaker K　Cardiac Lead, Defibrillator M　Cardiac Lead N　Intracardiac Pacemaker Y　Other Device	Z　No Qualifier
A　Heart　LC NC	0　Open 3　Percutaneous 4　Percutaneous Endoscopic	Q　Implantable Heart Assist System Y　Other Device	Z　No Qualifier
A　Heart ⊞	0　Open 3　Percutaneous 4　Percutaneous Endoscopic	R　Short-term External Heart Assist System	J　Intraoperative S　Biventricular Z　No Qualifier
N　Pericardium ⊞	0　Open 3　Percutaneous 4　Percutaneous Endoscopic	0　Monitoring Device, Pressure Sensor 2　Monitoring Device J　Cardiac Lead, Pacemaker K　Cardiac Lead, Defibrillator M　Cardiac Lead Y　Other Device	Z　No Qualifier
P　Pulmonary Trunk Q　Pulmonary Artery, Right R　Pulmonary Artery, Left 　　Arterial canal (duct) 　　Botallo's duct 　　Pulmoaortic canal S　Pulmonary Vein, Right 　　Right inferior pulmonary vein 　　Right superior pulmonary vein T　Pulmonary Vein, Left 　　Left inferior pulmonary vein 　　Left superior pulmonary vein V　Superior Vena Cava 　　Precava W　Thoracic Aorta, Descending	0　Open 3　Percutaneous 4　Percutaneous Endoscopic	0　Monitoring Device, Pressure Sensor 2　Monitoring Device 3　Infusion Device D　Intraluminal Device Y　Other Device	Z　No Qualifier
X　Thoracic Aorta, Ascending/Arch 　　Aortic arch 　　Ascending aorta	0　Open 3　Percutaneous 4　Percutaneous Endoscopic	0　Monitoring Device, Pressure Sensor 2　Monitoring Device 3　Infusion Device D　Intraluminal Device	Z　No Qualifier

DRG Non-OR	02H[4,6,7,K,L][0,3,4][J,M]Z	
DRG Non-OR	02HK32Z	
DRG Non-OR	02HN[0,3,4][J,M]Z	
Non-OR	02H[4,6,7,L]3[2,3]Z	
Non-OR	02H[6,7]3MZ	
Non-OR	02HK3[0,3]Z	
Non-OR	02HN32Z	
Non-OR	02HP[0,3,4][0,2,3]Z	
Non-OR	02H[Q,R][0,3,4][2,3]Z	
Non-OR	02H[S,T,V,W][0,3,4]3Z	
Non-OR	02H[S,T,V,W]32Z	
Non-OR	02HW[0,3]0Z	
Non-OR	02HX[0,3,4][0,3]Z	

HAC　02H43[J,K,M]Z when reported with SDx K68.11 or T81.40-T81.49, T82.6-T82.7 with 7th character A
HAC　02H[6,K]33Z when reported with SDx J95.811
HAC　02H[6,7]3[J,M]Z when reported with SDx K68.11 or T81.40-T81.49, T82.6-T82.7 with 7th character A
HAC　02H[K,L]3JZ when reported with SDx K68.11 or T81.40-T81.49, T82.6-T82.7 with 7th character A
HAC　02HN[0,3,4][J,M]Z when reported with SDx K68.11 or T81.40-T81.49, T82.6-T82.7 with 7th character A
HAC　02H[S,T,V][3,4]3Z when reported with SDx J95.811
LC　02HA0QZ
NC　02HA[3,4]QZ

See Appendix L for Procedure Combinations
⊞　02H[4,6,7,K,L][0,3,4][J,K,M]Z
⊞　02HA[0,4]R[S,Z]
⊞　02HA3RS
⊞　02HN[0,3,4][J,K,M]Z

Ø **Medical and Surgical**
2 **Heart and Great Vessels**
J **Inspection**   Definition: Visually and/or manually exploring a body part

          Explanation: Visual exploration may be performed with or without optical instrumentation. Manual exploration may be performed directly or through intervening body layers.

Body Part Character 4	Approach Character 5	Device Character 6	Qualifier Character 7
A Heart Y Great Vessel	Ø Open 3 Percutaneous 4 Percutaneous Endoscopic	Z No Device	Z No Qualifier

   Non-OR   02J[A,Y]3ZZ

Ø **Medical and Surgical**
2 **Heart and Great Vessels**
K **Map**   Definition: Locating the route of passage of electrical impulses and/or locating functional areas in a body part

          Explanation: Applicable only to the cardiac conduction mechanism and the central nervous system

Body Part Character 4	Approach Character 5	Device Character 6	Qualifier Character 7

8 Conduction Mechanism
   Atrioventricular node
   Bundle of His
   Bundle of Kent
   Sinoatrial node
	Ø Open
	3 Percutaneous
	4 Percutaneous Endoscopic
		Z No Device	Z No Qualifier

   DRG Non-OR   02K8[Ø,3,4]ZZ

Ø **Medical and Surgical**
2 **Heart and Great Vessels**
L **Occlusion**   Definition: Completely closing an orifice or the lumen of a tubular body part

          Explanation: The orifice can be a natural orifice or an artificially created orifice

Body Part Character 4	Approach Character 5	Device Character 6	Qualifier Character 7

7 Atrium, Left
   Atrium pulmonale
   Left auricular appendix
	Ø Open
	3 Percutaneous
	4 Percutaneous Endoscopic
		C Extraluminal Device
		D Intraluminal Device
		Z No Device
			K Left Atrial Appendage

H Pulmonary Valve
   Pulmonary annulus
   Pulmonic valve
P Pulmonary Trunk
Q Pulmonary Artery, Right
S Pulmonary Vein, Right
   Right inferior pulmonary vein
   Right superior pulmonary vein
T Pulmonary Vein, Left
   Left inferior pulmonary vein
   Left superior pulmonary vein
V Superior Vena Cava
   Precava
	Ø Open
	3 Percutaneous
	4 Percutaneous Endoscopic
		C Extraluminal Device
		D Intraluminal Device
		Z No Device
			Z No Qualifier

R Pulmonary Artery, Left
   Arterial canal (duct)
   Botallo's duct
   Pulmoaortic canal
	Ø Open
	3 Percutaneous
	4 Percutaneous Endoscopic
		C Extraluminal Device
		D Intraluminal Device
		Z No Device
			T Ductus Arteriosus
			Z No Qualifier

W Thoracic Aorta, Descending	3 Percutaneous	D Intraluminal Device	J Temporary

   DRG Non-OR   02L7[Ø,3,4][C,D,Z]K

Heart and Great Vessels

Ø **Medical and Surgical**
2 **Heart and Great Vessels**
N **Release**   Definition: Freeing a body part from an abnormal physical constraint by cutting or by the use of force
    Explanation: Some of the restraining tissue may be taken out but none of the body part is taken out

Body Part Character 4	Approach Character 5	Device Character 6	Qualifier Character 7
Ø Coronary Artery, One Artery	Ø Open	Z No Device	Z No Qualifier
1 Coronary Artery, Two Arteries	3 Percutaneous		
2 Coronary Artery, Three Arteries	4 Percutaneous Endoscopic		
3 Coronary Artery, Four or More Arteries			
4 Coronary Vein			
5 Atrial Septum Interatrial septum			
6 Atrium, Right Atrium dextrum cordis Right auricular appendix Sinus venosus			
7 Atrium, Left Atrium pulmonale Left auricular appendix			
8 Conduction Mechanism Atrioventricular node Bundle of His Bundle of Kent Sinoatrial node			
9 Chordae Tendineae			
D Papillary Muscle			
F Aortic Valve Aortic annulus			
G Mitral Valve Bicuspid valve Left atrioventricular valve Mitral annulus			
H Pulmonary Valve Pulmonary annulus Pulmonic valve			
J Tricuspid Valve Right atrioventricular valve Tricuspid annulus			
K Ventricle, Right Conus arteriosus			
L Ventricle, Left			
M Ventricular Septum Interventricular septum			
N Pericardium			
P Pulmonary Trunk			
Q Pulmonary Artery, Right			
R Pulmonary Artery, Left Arterial canal (duct) Botallo's duct Pulmoaortic canal			
S Pulmonary Vein, Right Right inferior pulmonary vein Right superior pulmonary vein			
T Pulmonary Vein, Left Left inferior pulmonary vein Left superior pulmonary vein			
V Superior Vena Cava Precava			
W Thoracic Aorta, Descending			
X Thoracic Aorta, Ascending/Arch Aortic arch Ascending aorta			

Ø2N–Ø2N

Non-OR Procedure   DRG Non-OR Procedure   Valid OR Procedure   HAC Associated Procedure   Combination Only   New/Revised GREEN
184   ICD-10-PCS 2022

0   **Medical and Surgical**
2   **Heart and Great Vessels**
P   **Removal**   Definition: Taking out or off a device from a body part

Explanation: If a device is taken out and a similar device put in without cutting or puncturing the skin or mucous membrane, the procedure is coded to the root operation CHANGE. Otherwise, the procedure for taking out a device is coded to the root operation REMOVAL.

Body Part Character 4	Approach Character 5	Device Character 6	Qualifier Character 7
A Heart	0 Open 3 Percutaneous 4 Percutaneous Endoscopic	2 Monitoring Device 3 Infusion Device 7 Autologous Tissue Substitute 8 Zooplastic Tissue C Extraluminal Device D Intraluminal Device J Synthetic Substitute K Nonautologous Tissue Substitute M Cardiac Lead N Intracardiac Pacemaker Q Implantable Heart Assist System Y Other Device	Z No Qualifier
A Heart ⊞	0 Open 3 Percutaneous 4 Percutaneous Endoscopic	R Short-term External Heart Assist System	S Biventricular Z No Qualifier
A Heart	X External	2 Monitoring Device 3 Infusion Device D Intraluminal Device M Cardiac Lead	Z No Qualifier
Y Great Vessel	0 Open 3 Percutaneous 4 Percutaneous Endoscopic	2 Monitoring Device 3 Infusion Device 7 Autologous Tissue Substitute 8 Zooplastic Tissue C Extraluminal Device D Intraluminal Device J Synthetic Substitute K Nonautologous Tissue Substitute Y Other Device	Z No Qualifier
Y Great Vessel	X External	2 Monitoring Device 3 Infusion Device D Intraluminal Device	Z No Qualifier

Non-OR 02PA3[2,3,D]Z	**See Appendix L for Procedure Combinations**
Non-OR 02PA[3,4]YZ	⊞ 02PA[0,3,4]RZ
Non-OR 02PAX[2,3,D,M]Z	
Non-OR 02PY3[2,3,D]Z	
Non-OR 02PY[3,4]YZ	
Non-OR 02PYX[2,3,D]Z	
HAC 02PA[0,3,4]MZ when reported with SDx K68.11 or T81.40-T81.49, T82.6- T82.7 with 7th character A	
HAC 02PAXMZ when reported with SDx K68.11 or T81.40-T81.49, T82.6-T82.7 with 7th character A	

NC Noncovered Procedure   **LC** Limited Coverage   **QA** Questionable OB Admit   **NT** New Tech Add-on   ⊞ Combination Member   ♂ Male   ♀ Female

ICD-10-PCS 2022   185

Heart and Great Vessels

- Ø   **Medical and Surgical**
- 2   **Heart and Great Vessels**
- Q   **Repair**   Definition: Restoring, to the extent possible, a body part to its normal anatomic structure and function

                            Explanation: Used only when the method to accomplish the repair is not one of the other root operations

Body Part Character 4	Approach Character 5	Device Character 6	Qualifier Character 7

Ø   **Coronary Artery, One Artery**
1   **Coronary Artery, Two Arteries**
2   **Coronary Artery, Three Arteries**
3   **Coronary Artery, Four or More**
      Arteries
4   **Coronary Vein**
5   **Atrial Septum**
      Interatrial septum
6   **Atrium, Right**
      Atrium dextrum cordis
      Right auricular appendix
      Sinus venosus
7   **Atrium, Left**
      Atrium pulmonale
      Left auricular appendix
8   **Conduction Mechanism**
      Atrioventricular node
      Bundle of His
      Bundle of Kent
      Sinoatrial node
9   **Chordae Tendineae**
A   **Heart**
B   **Heart, Right**
      Right coronary sulcus
C   **Heart, Left**
      Left coronary sulcus
      Obtuse margin
D   **Papillary Muscle**
H   **Pulmonary Valve**
      Pulmonary annulus
      Pulmonic valve
K   **Ventricle, Right**
      Conus arteriosus
L   **Ventricle, Left**
M   **Ventricular Septum**
      Interventricular septum
N   **Pericardium**
P   **Pulmonary Trunk**
Q   **Pulmonary Artery, Right**
R   **Pulmonary Artery, Left**
      Arterial canal (duct)
      Botallo's duct
      Pulmoaortic canal
S   **Pulmonary Vein, Right**
      Right inferior pulmonary vein
      Right superior pulmonary vein
T   **Pulmonary Vein, Left**
      Left inferior pulmonary vein
      Left superior pulmonary vein
V   **Superior Vena Cava**
      Precava
W   **Thoracic Aorta, Descending**
X   **Thoracic Aorta, Ascending/Arch**
      Aortic arch
      Ascending aorta
	Ø **Open**
	3 **Percutaneous**
	4 **Percutaneous Endoscopic**
		Z **No Device**	Z **No Qualifier**

F **Aortic Valve** Aortic annulus	Ø **Open** 3 **Percutaneous** 4 **Percutaneous Endoscopic**	Z **No Device**	J **Truncal Valve** Z **No Qualifier**

G   **Mitral Valve**
      Bicuspid valve
      Left atrioventricular valve
      Mitral annulus
	Ø **Open**
	3 **Percutaneous**
	4 **Percutaneous Endoscopic**
		Z **No Device**	E **Atrioventricular Valve, Left**
			Z **No Qualifier**

J   **Tricuspid Valve**
      Right atrioventricular valve
      Tricuspid annulus
	Ø **Open**
	3 **Percutaneous**
	4 **Percutaneous Endoscopic**
		Z **No Device**	G **Atrioventricular Valve, Right**
			Z **No Qualifier**

Ø   **Medical and Surgical**
2   **Heart and Great Vessels**
R   **Replacement**   Definition: Putting in or on biological or synthetic material that physically takes the place and/or function of all or a portion of a body part

Explanation: The body part may have been taken out or replaced, or may be taken out, physically eradicated, or rendered nonfunctional during the REPLACEMENT procedure. A REMOVAL procedure is coded for taking out the device used in a previous replacement procedure.

Body Part — Character 4	Approach — Character 5	Device — Character 6	Qualifier — Character 7
5 Atrial Septum Interatrial septum **6 Atrium, Right** Atrium dextrum cordis Right auricular appendix Sinus venosus **7 Atrium, Left** Atrium pulmonale Left auricular appendix **9 Chordae Tendineae** **D Papillary Muscle** **K Ventricle, Right** LC NC ⊞ Conus arteriosus **L Ventricle, Left** LC NC ⊞ **M Ventricular Septum** Interventricular septum **N Pericardium** **P Pulmonary Trunk** **Q Pulmonary Artery, Right** **R Pulmonary Artery, Left** Arterial canal (duct) Botallo's duct Pulmoaortic canal **S Pulmonary Vein, Right** Right inferior pulmonary vein Right superior pulmonary vein **T Pulmonary Vein, Left** Left inferior pulmonary vein Left superior pulmonary vein **V Superior Vena Cava** Precava **W Thoracic Aorta, Descending** **X Thoracic Aorta, Ascending/Arch** Aortic arch Ascending aorta	**Ø Open** **4 Percutaneous Endoscopic**	**7 Autologous Tissue Substitute** **8 Zooplastic Tissue** **J Synthetic Substitute** **K Nonautologous Tissue Substitute**	**Z No Qualifier**
A Heart	**Ø Open**	**L Biologic with Synthetic Substitute, Autoregulated Electrohydraulic** **M Synthetic Substitute, Pneumatic**	**Z No Qualifier**
F Aortic Valve Aortic annulus **G Mitral Valve** Bicuspid valve Left atrioventricular valve Mitral annulus **J Tricuspid Valve** Right atrioventricular valve Tricuspid annulus	**Ø Open** **4 Percutaneous Endoscopic**	**7 Autologous Tissue Substitute** **8 Zooplastic Tissue** **J Synthetic Substitute** **K Nonautologous Tissue Substitute**	**Z No Qualifier**
F Aortic Valve Aortic annulus **G Mitral Valve** Bicuspid valve Left atrioventricular valve Mitral annulus **J Tricuspid Valve** Right atrioventricular valve Tricuspid annulus	**3 Percutaneous**	**7 Autologous Tissue Substitute** **8 Zooplastic Tissue** **J Synthetic Substitute** **K Nonautologous Tissue Substitute**	**H Transapical** **Z No Qualifier**
H Pulmonary Valve Pulmonary annulus Pulmonic valve	**Ø Open** **4 Percutaneous Endoscopic**	**7 Autologous Tissue Substitute** **8 Zooplastic Tissue** **J Synthetic Substitute** **K Nonautologous Tissue Substitute**	**Z No Qualifier**
H Pulmonary Valve Pulmonary annulus Pulmonic valve	**3 Percutaneous**	**7 Autologous Tissue Substitute** **J Synthetic Substitute** **K Nonautologous Tissue Substitute**	**H Transapical** **Z No Qualifier**
H Pulmonary Valve Pulmonary annulus Pulmonic valve	**3 Percutaneous**	**8 Zooplastic Tissue**	**H Transapical** **L In Existing Conduit** **M Native Site** **Z No Qualifier**

LC   Ø2RKØJZ with Ø2RLØJZ with diagnosis code ZØØ.6
NC   Ø2RKØJZ with Ø2RLØJZ without diagnosis code ZØØ.6

See Appendix L for Procedure Combinations
⊞   Ø2R[K,L]ØJZ

Ø   **Medical and Surgical**
2   **Heart and Great Vessels**
S   **Reposition**   Definition: Moving to its normal location, or other suitable location, all or a portion of a body part

                 Explanation: The body part is moved to a new location from an abnormal location, or from a normal location where it is not functioning correctly. The body part may or may not be cut out or off to be moved to the new location.

Body Part Character 4	Approach Character 5	Device Character 6	Qualifier Character 7

Ø   Coronary Artery, One Artery
1   Coronary Artery, Two Arteries
P   Pulmonary Trunk
Q   Pulmonary Artery, Right
R   Pulmonary Artery, Left
     Arterial canal (duct)
     Botallo's duct
     Pulmoaortic canal
S   Pulmonary Vein, Right
     Right inferior pulmonary vein
     Right superior pulmonary vein
T   Pulmonary Vein, Left
     Left inferior pulmonary vein
     Left superior pulmonary vein
V   Superior Vena Cava
     Precava
W   Thoracic Aorta, Descending
X   Thoracic Aorta, Ascending/Arch
     Aortic arch
     Ascending aorta
	Ø Open	**Z** No Device	**Z** No Qualifier

Ø   **Medical and Surgical**
2   **Heart and Great Vessels**
T   **Resection**   Definition: Cutting out or off, without replacement, all of a body part

                 Explanation: None

Body Part Character 4	Approach Character 5	Device Character 6	Qualifier Character 7

5   Atrial Septum
     Interatrial septum
8   Conduction Mechanism
     Atrioventricular node
     Bundle of His
     Bundle of Kent
     Sinoatrial node
9   Chordae Tendineae
D   Papillary Muscle
H   Pulmonary Valve
     Pulmonary annulus
     Pulmonic valve
M   Ventricular Septum
     Interventricular septum
N   Pericardium
	Ø Open
	3 Percutaneous
	4 Percutaneous Endoscopic
		Z No Device	**Z** No Qualifier

Ø Medical and Surgical
2 Heart and Great Vessels
U Supplement   Definition: Putting in or on biological or synthetic material that physically reinforces and/or augments the function of a portion of a body part

Explanation: The biological material is non-living, or is living and from the same individual. The body part may have been previously replaced, and the SUPPLEMENT procedure is performed to physically reinforce and/or augment the function of the replaced body part.

Body Part Character 4	Approach Character 5	Device Character 6	Qualifier Character 7

Ø Coronary Artery, One Artery
1 Coronary Artery, Two Arteries
2 Coronary Artery, Three Arteries
3 Coronary Artery, Four or More Arteries
5 Atrial Septum
  Interatrial septum
6 Atrium, Right
  Atrium dextrum cordis
  Right auricular appendix
  Sinus venosus
7 Atrium, Left
  Atrium pulmonale
  Left auricular appendix
9 Chordae Tendineae
A Heart
D Papillary Muscle
H Pulmonary Valve
  Pulmonary annulus
  Pulmonic valve
K Ventricle, Right
  Conus arteriosus
L Ventricle, Left
M Ventricular Septum
  Interventricular septum
N Pericardium
P Pulmonary Trunk
Q Pulmonary Artery, Right
R Pulmonary Artery, Left
  Arterial canal (duct)
  Botallo's duct
  Pulmoaortic canal
S Pulmonary Vein, Right
  Right inferior pulmonary vein
  Right superior pulmonary vein
T Pulmonary Vein, Left
  Left inferior pulmonary vein
  Left superior pulmonary vein
V Superior Vena Cava
  Precava
W Thoracic Aorta, Descending
X Thoracic Aorta, Ascending/Arch
  Aortic arch
  Ascending aorta
	Ø Open
	3 Percutaneous
	4 Percutaneous Endoscopic
		7 Autologous Tissue Substitute
		8 Zooplastic Tissue
		J Synthetic Substitute
		K Nonautologous Tissue Substitute
			Z No Qualifier

F Aortic Valve Aortic annulus	Ø Open 3 Percutaneous 4 Percutaneous Endoscopic	7 Autologous Tissue Substitute 8 Zooplastic Tissue J Synthetic Substitute K Nonautologous Tissue Substitute	J Truncal Valve Z No Qualifier

G Mitral Valve
  Bicuspid valve
  Left atrioventricular valve
  Mitral annulus
	Ø Open
	4 Percutaneous Endoscopic
		7 Autologous Tissue Substitute
		8 Zooplastic Tissue
		J Synthetic Substitute
		K Nonautologous Tissue Substitute
			E Atrioventricular Valve, Left
			Z No Qualifier

G Mitral Valve
  Bicuspid valve
  Left atrioventricular valve
  Mitral annulus
	3 Percutaneous	7 Autologous Tissue Substitute
		8 Zooplastic Tissue
		K Nonautologous Tissue Substitute
			E Atrioventricular Valve, Left
			Z No Qualifier

G Mitral Valve
  Bicuspid valve
  Left atrioventricular valve
  Mitral annulus
	3 Percutaneous	J Synthetic Substitute	E Atrioventricular Valve, Left
			H Transapical
			Z No Qualifier

J Tricuspid Valve
  Right atrioventricular valve
  Tricuspid annulus
	Ø Open
	3 Percutaneous
	4 Percutaneous Endoscopic
		7 Autologous Tissue Substitute
		8 Zooplastic Tissue
		J Synthetic Substitute
		K Nonautologous Tissue Substitute
			G Atrioventricular Valve, Right
			Z No Qualifier

DRG Non-OR   Ø2U7[3,4]JZ

Heart and Great Vessels

0   **Medical and Surgical**
2   **Heart and Great Vessels**
V   **Restriction**   Definition: Partially closing an orifice or the lumen of a tubular body part
                Explanation: The orifice can be a natural orifice or an artificially created orifice

Body Part Character 4	Approach Character 5	Device Character 6	Qualifier Character 7
A Heart	**Ø** Open **3** Percutaneous **4** Percutaneous Endoscopic	**C** Extraluminal Device **Z** No Device	**Z** No Qualifier
G Mitral Valve Bicuspid valve Left atrioventricular valve Mitral annulus	**Ø** Open **3** Percutaneous **4** Percutaneous Endoscopic	**Z** No Device	**Z** No Qualifier
L Ventricle, Left **P Pulmonary Trunk** **Q Pulmonary Artery, Right** **S Pulmonary Vein, Right** Right inferior pulmonary vein Right superior pulmonary vein **T Pulmonary Vein, Left** Left inferior pulmonary vein Left superior pulmonary vein **V Superior Vena Cava** Precava	**Ø** Open **3** Percutaneous **4** Percutaneous Endoscopic	**C** Extraluminal Device **D** Intraluminal Device **Z** No Device	**Z** No Qualifier
R Pulmonary Artery, Left Arterial canal (duct) Botallo's duct Pulmoaortic canal	**Ø** Open **3** Percutaneous **4** Percutaneous Endoscopic	**C** Extraluminal Device **D** Intraluminal Device **Z** No Device	**T** Ductus Arteriosus **Z** No Qualifier
W Thoracic Aorta, Descending **X Thoracic Aorta, Ascending/Arch** Aortic arch Ascending aorta	**Ø** Open **3** Percutaneous **4** Percutaneous Endoscopic	**C** Extraluminal Device **D** Intraluminal Device **E** Intraluminal Device, Branched or Fenestrated, One or Two Arteries **F** Intraluminal Device, Branched or Fenestrated, Three or More Arteries **Z** No Device	**Z** No Qualifier

Ø **Medical and Surgical**
2 **Heart and Great Vessels**
W **Revision** Definition: Correcting, to the extent possible, a portion of a malfunctioning device or the position of a displaced device
Explanation: Revision can include correcting a malfunctioning or displaced device by taking out or putting in components of the device such as a screw or pin

Body Part Character 4	Approach Character 5	Device Character 6	Qualifier Character 7
5 Atrial Septum Interatrial septum **M Ventricular Septum** Interventricular septum	**Ø** Open **4** Percutaneous Endoscopic	**J** Synthetic Substitute	**Z** No Qualifier
A Heart LC NC ⊞	**Ø** Open **3** Percutaneous **4** Percutaneous Endoscopic	**2** Monitoring Device **3** Infusion Device **7** Autologous Tissue Substitute **8** Zooplastic Tissue **C** Extraluminal Device **D** Intraluminal Device **J** Synthetic Substitute **K** Nonautologous Tissue Substitute **M** Cardiac Lead **N** Intracardiac Pacemaker **Q** Implantable Heart Assist System **Y** Other Device	**Z** No Qualifier
A Heart ⊞	**Ø** Open **3** Percutaneous **4** Percutaneous Endoscopic	**R** Short-term External Heart Assist System	**S** Biventricular **Z** No Qualifier
A Heart	**X** External	**2** Monitoring Device **3** Infusion Device **7** Autologous Tissue Substitute **8** Zooplastic Tissue **C** Extraluminal Device **D** Intraluminal Device **J** Synthetic Substitute **K** Nonautologous Tissue Substitute **M** Cardiac Lead **N** Intracardiac Pacemaker **Q** Implantable Heart Assist System	**Z** No Qualifier
A Heart	**X** External	**R** Short-term External Heart Assist System	**S** Biventricular **Z** No Qualifier
F Aortic Valve Aortic annulus **G Mitral Valve** Bicuspid valve Left atrioventricular valve Mitral annulus **H Pulmonary Valve** Pulmonary annulus Pulmonic valve **J Tricuspid Valve** Right atrioventricular valve Tricuspid annulus	**Ø** Open **3** Percutaneous **4** Percutaneous Endoscopic	**7** Autologous Tissue Substitute **8** Zooplastic Tissue **J** Synthetic Substitute **K** Nonautologous Tissue Substitute	**Z** No Qualifier
Y Great Vessel	**Ø** Open **3** Percutaneous **4** Percutaneous Endoscopic	**2** Monitoring Device **3** Infusion Device **7** Autologous Tissue Substitute **8** Zooplastic Tissue **C** Extraluminal Device **D** Intraluminal Device **J** Synthetic Substitute **K** Nonautologous Tissue Substitute **Y** Other Device	**Z** No Qualifier
Y Great Vessel	**X** External	**2** Monitoring Device **3** Infusion Device **7** Autologous Tissue Substitute **8** Zooplastic Tissue **C** Extraluminal Device **D** Intraluminal Device **J** Synthetic Substitute **K** Nonautologous Tissue Substitute	**Z** No Qualifier

Non-OR	Ø2WA3[2,3,D]Z	
Non-OR	Ø2WA[3,4]YZ	
Non-OR	Ø2WAX[2,3,7,8,C,D,J,K,M,N,Q]Z	
Non-OR	Ø2WAXRZ	
Non-OR	Ø2WY3[2,3,D]Z	
Non-OR	Ø2WY[3,4]YZ	
Non-OR	Ø2WYX[2,3,7,8,C,D,J,K]Z	

HAC Ø2WA[Ø,3,4]MZ when reported with T81.4Ø–T81.49, T82.6–T82.7 with 7th character A
LC Ø2WAØ[J,Q]Z
NC Ø2WA[3,4]QZ

See Appendix L for Procedure Combinations
⊞ Ø2WA[Ø,3,4]QZ
⊞ Ø2WA[Ø,3,4]RZ

Heart and Great Vessels

Ø   **Medical and Surgical**
2   **Heart and Great Vessels**
Y   **Transplantation**   Definition: Putting in or on all or a portion of a living body part taken from another individual or animal to physically take the place and/or function of all or a portion of a similar body part

                    Explanation: The native body part may or may not be taken out, and the transplanted body part may take over all or a portion of its function

Body Part Character 4	Approach Character 5	Device Character 6	Qualifier Character 7
A Heart LC	Ø Open	Z No Device	Ø Allogeneic 1 Syngeneic 2 Zooplastic

LC   Ø2YAØZ[Ø,1,2]

Upper Arteries Ø31–Ø3W

Character Meanings

This Character Meaning table is provided as a guide to assist the user in the identification of character members that may be found in this section of code tables. It **SHOULD NOT** be used to build a PCS code.

Operation–Character 3	Body Part–Character 4	Approach–Character 5	Device–Character 6	Qualifier–Character 7
1 Bypass	Ø Internal Mammary Artery, Right	Ø Open	Ø Drainage Device	Ø Upper Arm Artery, Right OR Ultrasonic
5 Destruction	1 Internal Mammary Artery, Left	3 Percutaneous	2 Monitoring Device	1 Upper Arm Artery, Left OR Drug-Coated Balloon
7 Dilation	2 Innominate Artery	4 Percutaneous Endoscopic	3 Infusion Device	2 Upper Arm Artery, Bilateral
9 Drainage	3 Subclavian Artery, Right	X External	4 Intraluminal Device, Drug-eluting	3 Lower Arm Artery, Right
B Excision	4 Subclavian Artery, Left		5 Intraluminal Device, Drug-eluting, Two	4 Lower Arm Artery, Left
C Extirpation	5 Axillary Artery, Right		6 Intraluminal Device, Drug-eluting, Three	5 Lower Arm Artery, Bilateral
F Fragmentation	6 Axillary Artery, Left		7 Intraluminal Device, Drug-eluting, Four or More OR Autologous Tissue Substitute	6 Upper Leg Artery, Right
H Insertion	7 Brachial Artery, Right		9 Autologous Venous Tissue	7 Upper Leg Artery, Left OR Stent Retriever
J Inspection	8 Brachial Artery, Left		A Autologous Arterial Tissue	8 Upper Leg Artery, Bilateral
L Occlusion	9 Ulnar Artery, Right		B Intraluminal Device, Bioactive	9 Lower Leg Artery, Right
N Release	A Ulnar Artery, Left		C Extraluminal Device	B Lower Leg Artery, Left
P Removal	B Radial Artery, Right		D Intraluminal Device	C Lower Leg Artery, Bilateral
Q Repair	C Radial Artery, Left		E Intraluminal Device, Two	D Upper Arm Vein
R Replacement	D Hand Artery, Right		F Intraluminal Device, Three	F Lower Arm Vein
S Reposition	F Hand Artery, Left		G Intraluminal Device, Four or More	G Intracranial Artery
U Supplement	G Intracranial Artery		H Intraluminal Device, Flow Diverter	J Extracranial Artery, Right
V Restriction	H Common Carotid Artery, Right		J Synthetic Substitute	K Extracranial Artery, Left
W Revision	J Common Carotid Artery, Left		K Nonautologous Tissue Substitute	M Pulmonary Artery, Right
	K Internal Carotid Artery, Right		M Stimulator Lead	N Pulmonary Artery, Left
	L Internal Carotid Artery, Left		Y Other Device	T Abdominal Artery
	M External Carotid Artery, Right		Z No Device	V Superior Vena Cava
	N External Carotid Artery, Left			W Lower Extremity Vein
	P Vertebral Artery, Right			X Diagnostic
	Q Vertebral Artery, Left			Y Upper Artery
	R Face Artery			Z No Qualifier
	S Temporal Artery, Right			
	T Temporal Artery, Left			
	U Thyroid Artery, Right			
	V Thyroid Artery, Left			
	Y Upper Artery			

AHA Coding Clinic for table Ø31

2019, 4Q, 26	Upper artery bypass Qualifier
2019, 4Q, 26	Percutaneous approach upper artery bypass
2017, 4Q, 64-65	New qualifier values - Left to right carotid bypass
2017, 2Q, 22	Carotid artery to subclavian artery transposition
2017, 1Q, 31	Left to right common carotid artery bypass
2016, 3Q, 37	Insertion of arteriovenous graft using HeRO device
2016, 3Q, 39	Revision of arteriovenous graft
2013, 4Q, 125	Stage II cephalic vein transposition (superficialization) of arteriovenous fistula
2013, 1Q, 27	Creation of radial artery fistula

AHA Coding Clinic for table Ø37

2020, 4Q, 70-71	Cerebral embolic filtration extracorporeal flow reversal circuit
2019, 4Q, 27	Bifurcation Qualifier
2019, 3Q, 29	Transcarotid arterial catheterization
2018, 2Q, 24	Coronary artery bifurcation
2016, 4Q, 86	Peripheral artery, number of stents
2016, 4Q, 86-87	Coronary and peripheral artery bifurcation
2015, 1Q, 32	Deployment of stent for herniated/migrated coil in basilar artery

AHA Coding Clinic for table Ø3B

2016, 2Q, 12	Resection of malignant neoplasm of infratemporal fossa

AHA Coding Clinic for table Ø3C

2021, 2Q, 13	Thromboendarterectomy with deconstruction of internal carotid artery
2020, 3Q, 38	Thrombectomy of arteriovenous fistula with angioplasty and stent placement
2019, 4Q, 27	Bifurcation Qualifier
2018, 4Q, 47-48	Endovascular thrombectomy with stent retriever
2018, 2Q, 24	Coronary artery bifurcation
2017, 4Q, 64-65	New qualifier values - Left to right carotid bypass
2017, 2Q, 23	Thrombectomy via Fogarty catheter
2016, 4Q, 86-87	Coronary and peripheral artery bifurcation
2016, 2Q, 11	Carotid endarterectomy with patch angioplasty
2015, 1Q, 29	Discontinued carotid endarterectomy

AHA Coding Clinic for table Ø3F

2020, 4Q, 45-49	New fragmentation tables
2020, 4Q, 49-50	Intravascular ultrasound assisted thrombolysis
2020, 4Q, 50	Intravascular lithotripsy

AHA Coding Clinic for table Ø3H

2020, 1Q, 25	Elephant trunk repair of aortic dissection
2016, 2Q, 32	Arterial catheter placement

AHA Coding Clinic for table Ø3J

2021, 1Q, 16	Placement of Sentinel™ embolic protection device with deployment of single filter
2015, 1Q, 29	Discontinued carotid endarterectomy

AHA Coding Clinic for table Ø3L

2021, 2Q, 13	Thromboendarterectomy with deconstruction of internal carotid artery
2016, 2Q, 30	Clipping (occlusion) of cerebral artery, decompressive craniectomy and storage of bone flap in abdominal wall
2014, 4Q, 20	Control of epistaxis
2014, 4Q, 37	Endovascular embolization of arteriovenous malformation using Onyx-18 liquid

AHA Coding Clinic for table Ø3Q

2017, 1Q, 31	Left to right common carotid artery bypass

AHA Coding Clinic for table Ø3S

2017, 2Q, 22	Carotid artery to subclavian artery transposition
2015, 3Q, 27	Moyamoya disease and hemispheric pial synagiosis with craniotomy

AHA Coding Clinic for table Ø3U

2019, 1Q, 22	Cerebral artery fusiform aneurysm repair via wrapping
2016, 2Q, 11	Carotid endarterectomy with patch angioplasty

AHA Coding Clinic for table Ø3V

2019, 4Q, 27-28	Aneurysm treatment using flow diverter stent
2019, 1Q, 22	Cerebral artery fusiform aneurysm repair via wrapping
2016, 1Q, 19	Embolization of superior hypophyseal aneurysm using stent-assisted coil

AHA Coding Clinic for table Ø3W

2016, 3Q, 39	Revision of arteriovenous graft
2015, 1Q, 32	Deployment of stent for herniated/migrated coil in basilar artery

Upper Arteries

Middle temporal **S, T**
Transverse facial **S, T**
Superficial temporal **S, T**
Face **R**
External carotid **M, N**
Internal carotid **K, L**
Common carotid **H, J**
Superior thyroid **U, V**
Vertebral **P, Q**
Inferior thyroid **U, V**
Subclavian **3, 4**
Innominate **2**
Axillary **5, 6**
Internal thoracic (mammary) **Ø, 1**
Brachial **7, 8**
Radial **B, C**
Ulnar **9, A**
Deep palmar arch **D, F**
Superficial palmar arch **D, F**

Head and Neck Arteries

Middle cerebral **G**
Anterior cerebral **G**
Posterior communicating **G**
Anterior communicating **G**
Posterior cerebral **G**
Ophthalmic **G**
Basilar **G**
Internal carotid **K,L**
External carotid **M,N**
Vertebral **P,Q**
Common carotid **H,J**

Upper Arteries

Ø	Medical and Surgical
3	Upper Arteries
1	Bypass

Definition: Altering the route of passage of the contents of a tubular body part

Explanation: Rerouting contents of a body part to a downstream area of the normal route, to a similar route and body part, or to an abnormal route and dissimilar body part. Includes one or more anastomoses, with or without the use of a device.

Body Part Character 4	Approach Character 5	Device Character 6	Qualifier Character 7
2 Innominate Artery Brachiocephalic artery Brachiocephalic trunk	Ø Open	9 Autologous Venous Tissue A Autologous Arterial Tissue J Synthetic Substitute K Nonautologous Tissue Substitute Z No Device	Ø Upper Arm Artery, Right 1 Upper Arm Artery, Left 2 Upper Arm Artery, Bilateral 3 Lower Arm Artery, Right 4 Lower Arm Artery, Left 5 Lower Arm Artery, Bilateral 6 Upper Leg Artery, Right 7 Upper Leg Artery, Left 8 Upper Leg Artery, Bilateral 9 Lower Leg Artery, Right B Lower Leg Artery, Left C Lower Leg Artery, Bilateral D Upper Arm Vein F Lower Arm Vein J Extracranial Artery, Right K Extracranial Artery, Left W Lower Extremity Vein
3 Subclavian Artery, Right Costocervical trunk Dorsal scapular artery Internal thoracic artery **4 Subclavian Artery, Left** *See 3 Subclavian Artery, Right*	Ø Open	9 Autologous Venous Tissue A Autologous Arterial Tissue J Synthetic Substitute K Nonautologous Tissue Substitute Z No Device	Ø Upper Arm Artery, Right 1 Upper Arm Artery, Left 2 Upper Arm Artery, Bilateral 3 Lower Arm Artery, Right 4 Lower Arm Artery, Left 5 Lower Arm Artery, Bilateral 6 Upper Leg Artery, Right 7 Upper Leg Artery, Left 8 Upper Leg Artery, Bilateral 9 Lower Leg Artery, Right B Lower Leg Artery, Left C Lower Leg Artery, Bilateral D Upper Arm Vein F Lower Arm Vein J Extracranial Artery, Right K Extracranial Artery, Left M Pulmonary Artery, Right N Pulmonary Artery, Left W Lower Extremity Vein
5 Axillary Artery, Right Anterior circumflex humeral artery Lateral thoracic artery Posterior circumflex humeral artery Subscapular artery Superior thoracic artery Thoracoacromial artery **6 Axillary Artery, Left** *See 5 Axillary Artery, Right*	Ø Open	9 Autologous Venous Tissue A Autologous Arterial Tissue J Synthetic Substitute K Nonautologous Tissue Substitute Z No Device	Ø Upper Arm Artery, Right 1 Upper Arm Artery, Left 2 Upper Arm Artery, Bilateral 3 Lower Arm Artery, Right 4 Lower Arm Artery, Left 5 Lower Arm Artery, Bilateral 6 Upper Leg Artery, Right 7 Upper Leg Artery, Left 8 Upper Leg Artery, Bilateral 9 Lower Leg Artery, Right B Lower Leg Artery, Left C Lower Leg Artery, Bilateral D Upper Arm Vein F Lower Arm Vein J Extracranial Artery, Right K Extracranial Artery, Left T Abdominal Artery V Superior Vena Cava W Lower Extremity Vein
7 Brachial Artery, Right Inferior ulnar collateral artery Profunda brachii Superior ulnar collateral artery	Ø Open	9 Autologous Venous Tissue A Autologous Arterial Tissue J Synthetic Substitute K Nonautologous Tissue Substitute Z No Device	Ø Upper Arm Artery, Right 3 Lower Arm Artery, Right D Upper Arm Vein F Lower Arm Vein V Superior Vena Cava W Lower Extremity Vein
7 Brachial Artery, Right Inferior ulnar collateral artery Profunda brachii Superior ulnar collateral artery	3 Percutaneous	Z No Device	F Lower Arm Vein

Ø31 Continued on next page

Ø Medical and Surgical
3 Upper Arteries
1 Bypass

Ø31 Continued

Definition: Altering the route of passage of the contents of a tubular body part

Explanation: Rerouting contents of a body part to a downstream area of the normal route, to a similar route and body part, or to an abnormal route and dissimilar body part. Includes one or more anastomoses, with or without the use of a device.

Body Part Character 4	Approach Character 5	Device Character 6	Qualifier Character 7
8 Brachial Artery, Left Inferior ulnar collateral artery Profunda brachii Superior ulnar collateral artery	Ø Open	9 Autologous Venous Tissue A Autologous Arterial Tissue J Synthetic Substitute K Nonautologous Tissue Substitute Z No Device	1 Upper Arm Artery, Left 4 Lower Arm Artery, Left D Upper Arm Vein F Lower Arm Vein V Superior Vena Cava W Lower Extremity Vein
8 Brachial Artery, Left Inferior ulnar collateral artery Profunda brachii Superior ulnar collateral artery	3 Percutaneous	Z No Device	F Lower Arm Vein
9 Ulnar Artery, Right Anterior ulnar recurrent artery Common interosseous artery Posterior ulnar recurrent artery **B Radial Artery, Right** Radial recurrent artery	Ø Open	9 Autologous Venous Tissue A Autologous Arterial Tissue J Synthetic Substitute K Nonautologous Tissue Substitute Z No Device	3 Lower Arm Artery, Right F Lower Arm Vein
9 Ulnar Artery, Right Anterior ulnar recurrent artery Common interosseous artery Posterior ulnar recurrent artery **B Radial Artery, Right** Radial recurrent artery	3 Percutaneous	Z No Device	F Lower Arm Vein
A Ulnar Artery, Left Anterior ulnar recurrent artery Common interosseous artery Posterior ulnar recurrent artery **C Radial Artery, Left** Radial recurrent artery	Ø Open	9 Autologous Venous Tissue A Autologous Arterial Tissue J Synthetic Substitute K Nonautologous Tissue Substitute Z No Device	4 Lower Arm Artery, Left F Lower Arm Vein
A Ulnar Artery, Left Anterior ulnar recurrent artery Common interosseous artery Posterior ulnar recurrent artery **C Radial Artery, Left** Radial recurrent artery	3 Percutaneous	Z No Device	F Lower Arm Vein

G Intracranial Artery
Anterior cerebral artery
Anterior choroidal artery
Anterior communicating artery
Basilar artery
Circle of Willis
Internal carotid artery, intracranial
   portion
Middle cerebral artery
Ophthalmic artery
Posterior cerebral artery
Posterior communicating artery
Posterior inferior cerebellar artery
   (PICA)
S Temporal Artery, Right
Middle temporal artery
Superficial temporal artery
Transverse facial artery
T Temporal Artery, Left
See S Temporal Artery, Right
	Ø Open	9 Autologous Venous Tissue
		A Autologous Arterial Tissue
		J Synthetic Substitute
		K Nonautologous Tissue Substitute
		Z No Device
			G Intracranial Artery

H Common Carotid Artery, Right **J Common Carotid Artery, Left**	Ø Open	9 Autologous Venous Tissue A Autologous Arterial Tissue J Synthetic Substitute K Nonautologous Tissue Substitute Z No Device	G Intracranial Artery J Extracranial Artery, Right K Extracranial Artery, Left Y Upper Artery

Ø31 Continued on next page

NC Noncovered Procedure   LC Limited Coverage   QA Questionable OB Admit   NT New Tech Add-on   ⊞ Combination Member   ♂ Male   ♀ Female

Ø   **Medical and Surgical**   *Ø31 Continued*
3   **Upper Arteries**
1   **Bypass**   Definition: Altering the route of passage of the contents of a tubular body part

                     Explanation: Rerouting contents of a body part to a downstream area of the normal route, to a similar route and body part, or to an abnormal route and dissimilar body part. Includes one or more anastomoses, with or without the use of a device.

Body Part Character 4	Approach Character 5	Device Character 6	Qualifier Character 7

K   **Internal Carotid Artery, Right**
    Caroticotympanic artery
    Carotid sinus
L   **Internal Carotid Artery, Left**
    Caroticotympanic artery
    Carotid sinus
M   **External Carotid Artery, Right**
    Ascending pharyngeal artery
    Internal maxillary artery
    Lingual artery
    Maxillary artery
    Occipital artery
    Posterior auricular artery
    Superior thyroid artery
N   **External Carotid Artery, Left**
    Ascending pharyngeal artery
    Internal maxillary artery
    Lingual artery
    Maxillary artery
    Occipital artery
    Posterior auricular artery
    Superior thyroid artery
	Ø Open	**9** Autologous Venous Tissue
		A Autologous Arterial Tissue
		J Synthetic Substitute
		K Nonautologous Tissue Substitute
		Z No Device
			J Extracranial Artery, Right
			K Extracranial Artery, Left

Ø　Medical and Surgical
3　Upper Arteries
5　Destruction　　Definition: Physical eradication of all or a portion of a body part by the direct use of energy, force, or a destructive agent
　　　　　　　　　　　　Explanation: None of the body part is physically taken out

Body Part Character 4		Approach Character 5	Device Character 6	Qualifier Character 7
Ø Internal Mammary Artery, Right Anterior intercostal artery Internal thoracic artery Musculophrenic artery Pericardiophrenic artery Superior epigastric artery **1 Internal Mammary Artery, Left** *See Ø Internal Mammary Artery, Right* **2 Innominate Artery** Brachiocephalic artery Brachiocephalic trunk **3 Subclavian Artery, Right** Costocervical trunk Dorsal scapular artery Internal thoracic artery **4 Subclavian Artery, Left** *See 3 Subclavian Artery, Right* **5 Axillary Artery, Right** Anterior circumflex humeral artery Lateral thoracic artery Posterior circumflex humeral artery Subscapular artery Superior thoracic artery Thoracoacromial artery **6 Axillary Artery, Left** *See 5 Axillary Artery, Right* **7 Brachial Artery, Right** Inferior ulnar collateral artery Profunda brachii Superior ulnar collateral artery **8 Brachial Artery, Left** *See 7 Brachial Artery, Right* **9 Ulnar Artery, Right** Anterior ulnar recurrent artery Common interosseous artery Posterior ulnar recurrent artery **A Ulnar Artery, Left** *See 9 Ulnar Artery, Right* **B Radial Artery, Right** Radial recurrent artery **C Radial Artery, Left** *See B Radial Artery, Right* **D Hand Artery, Right** Deep palmar arch Princeps pollicis artery Radialis indicis Superficial palmar arch **F Hand Artery, Left** *See D Hand Artery, Right* **G Intracranial Artery** Anterior cerebral artery Anterior choroidal artery Anterior communicating artery Basilar artery Circle of Willis Internal carotid artery, intracranial portion Middle cerebral artery Ophthalmic artery Posterior cerebral artery Posterior communicating artery Posterior inferior cerebellar artery (PICA)	**H Common Carotid Artery, Right** **J Common Carotid Artery, Left** **K Internal Carotid Artery, Right** Caroticotympanic artery Carotid sinus **L Internal Carotid Artery, Left** *See K Internal Carotid Artery, Right* **M External Carotid Artery, Right** Ascending pharyngeal artery Internal maxillary artery Lingual artery Maxillary artery Occipital artery Posterior auricular artery Superior thyroid artery **N External Carotid Artery, Left** *See M External Carotid Artery, Right* **P Vertebral Artery, Right** Anterior spinal artery Posterior spinal artery **Q Vertebral Artery, Left** *See P Vertebral Artery, Right* **R Face Artery** Angular artery Ascending palatine artery External maxillary artery Facial artery Inferior labial artery Submental artery Superior labial artery **S Temporal Artery, Right** Middle temporal artery Superficial temporal artery Transverse facial artery **T Temporal Artery, Left** *See S Temporal Artery, Right* **U Thyroid Artery, Right** Cricothyroid artery Hyoid artery Sternocleidomastoid artery Superior laryngeal artery Superior thyroid artery Thyrocervical trunk **V Thyroid Artery, Left** *See U Thyroid Artery, Right* **Y Upper Artery** Aortic intercostal artery Bronchial artery Esophageal artery Subcostal artery	**Ø Open** **3 Percutaneous** **4 Percutaneous Endoscopic**	**Z No Device**	**Z No Qualifier**

NC Noncovered Procedure　　**LC** Limited Coverage　　**OA** Questionable OB Admit　　**NT** New Tech Add-on　　⊞ Combination Member　　♂ Male　　♀ Female

ICD-10-PCS 2022　　　199

Ø35–Ø35

Ø   Medical and Surgical
3   Upper Arteries
7   Dilation

Definition: Expanding an orifice or the lumen of a tubular body part

Explanation: The orifice can be a natural orifice or an artificially created orifice. Accomplished by stretching a tubular body part using intraluminal pressure or by cutting part of the orifice or wall of the tubular body part.

Body Part Character 4		Approach Character 5	Device Character 6	Qualifier Character 7
0 Internal Mammary Artery, Right Anterior intercostal artery Internal thoracic artery Musculophrenic artery Pericardiophrenic artery Superior epigastric artery **1 Internal Mammary Artery, Left** *See 0 Internal Mammary Artery, Right* **2 Innominate Artery** Brachiocephalic artery Brachiocephalic trunk **3 Subclavian Artery, Right** Costocervical trunk Dorsal scapular artery Internal thoracic artery **4 Subclavian Artery, Left** *See 3 Subclavian Artery, Right* **5 Axillary Artery, Right** Anterior circumflex humeral artery Lateral thoracic artery Posterior circumflex humeral artery Subscapular artery Superior thoracic artery Thoracoacromial artery	**6 Axillary Artery, Left** *See 5 Axillary Artery, Right* **7 Brachial Artery, Right** Inferior ulnar collateral artery Profunda brachii Superior ulnar collateral artery **8 Brachial Artery, Left** *See 7 Brachial Artery, Right* **9 Ulnar Artery, Right** Anterior ulnar recurrent artery Common interosseous artery Posterior ulnar recurrent artery **A Ulnar Artery, Left** *See 9 Ulnar Artery, Right* **B Radial Artery, Right** Radial recurrent artery **C Radial Artery, Left** *See B Radial Artery, Right*	**0 Open** **3 Percutaneous** **4 Percutaneous Endoscopic**	**4 Intraluminal Device, Drug-eluting** **5 Intraluminal Device, Drug-eluting, Two** **6 Intraluminal Device, Drug-eluting, Three** **7 Intraluminal Device, Drug-eluting, Four or More** **E Intraluminal Device, Two** **F Intraluminal Device, Three** **G Intraluminal Device, Four or More**	**Z No Qualifier**
0 Internal Mammary Artery, Right Anterior intercostal artery Internal thoracic artery Musculophrenic artery Pericardiophrenic artery Superior epigastric artery **1 Internal Mammary Artery, Left** *See 0 Internal Mammary Artery, Right* **2 Innominate Artery** Brachiocephalic artery Brachiocephalic trunk **3 Subclavian Artery, Right** Costocervical trunk Dorsal scapular artery Internal thoracic artery **4 Subclavian Artery, Left** *See 3 Subclavian Artery, Right* **5 Axillary Artery, Right** Anterior circumflex humeral artery Lateral thoracic artery Posterior circumflex humeral artery Subscapular artery Superior thoracic artery Thoracoacromial artery	**6 Axillary Artery, Left** *See 5 Axillary Artery, Right* **7 Brachial Artery, Right** Inferior ulnar collateral artery Profunda brachii Superior ulnar collateral artery **8 Brachial Artery, Left** *See 7 Brachial Artery, Right* **9 Ulnar Artery, Right** Anterior ulnar recurrent artery Common interosseous artery Posterior ulnar recurrent artery **A Ulnar Artery, Left** *See 9 Ulnar Artery, Right* **B Radial Artery, Right** Radial recurrent artery **C Radial Artery, Left** *See B Radial Artery, Right*	**0 Open** **3 Percutaneous** **4 Percutaneous Endoscopic**	**D Intraluminal Device** **Z No Device**	**1 Drug-Coated Balloon** **Z No Qualifier**

Ø37 Continued on next page

Non-OR Procedure   DRG Non-OR Procedure   Valid OR Procedure   HAC Associated Procedure   Combination Only   New/Revised GREEN

Ø   **Medical and Surgical**   *Ø37 Continued*
3   **Upper Arteries**
7   **Dilation**   Definition: Expanding an orifice or the lumen of a tubular body part

                          Explanation: The orifice can be a natural orifice or an artificially created orifice. Accomplished by stretching a tubular body part using intraluminal pressure or by cutting part of the orifice or wall of the tubular body part.

Body Part Character 4		Approach Character 5	Device Character 6	Qualifier Character 7

D **Hand Artery, Right**
   Deep palmar arch
   Princeps pollicis artery
   Radialis indicis
   Superficial palmar arch
F **Hand Artery, Left**
   See D Hand Artery, Right
G **Intracranial Artery** NC
   Anterior cerebral artery
   Anterior choroidal artery
   Anterior communicating artery
   Basilar artery
   Circle of Willis
   Internal carotid artery,
     intracranial portion
   Middle cerebral artery
   Ophthalmic artery
   Posterior cerebral artery
   Posterior communicating
     artery
   Posterior inferior cerebellar
     artery (PICA)
H **Common Carotid Artery,**
   Right
J **Common Carotid Artery, Left**
K **Internal Carotid Artery, Right**
   Caroticotympanic artery
   Carotid sinus
L **Internal Carotid Artery, Left**
   See K Internal Carotid Artery,
     Right
M **External Carotid Artery, Right**
   Ascending pharyngeal artery
   Internal maxillary artery
   Lingual artery
   Maxillary artery
   Occipital artery
   Posterior auricular artery
   Superior thyroid artery
	N **External Carotid Artery, Left**
	   See M External Carotid Artery,
	     Right
	P **Vertebral Artery, Right**
	   Anterior spinal artery
	   Posterior spinal artery
	Q **Vertebral Artery, Left**
	   See P Vertebral Artery, Right
	R **Face Artery**
	   Angular artery
	   Ascending palatine artery
	   External maxillary artery
	   Facial artery
	   Inferior labial artery
	   Submental artery
	   Superior labial artery
	S **Temporal Artery, Right**
	   Middle temporal artery
	   Superficial temporal artery
	   Transverse facial artery
	T **Temporal Artery, Left**
	   See S Temporal Artery, Right
	U **Thyroid Artery, Right**
	   Cricothyroid artery
	   Hyoid artery
	   Sternocleidomastoid artery
	   Superior laryngeal artery
	   Superior thyroid artery
	   Thyrocervical trunk
	V **Thyroid Artery, Left**
	   See U Thyroid Artery, Right
	Y **Upper Artery**
	   Aortic intercostal artery
	   Bronchial artery
	   Esophageal artery
	   Subcostal artery
		Ø Open
		3 Percutaneous
		4 Percutaneous Endoscopic
			4 Intraluminal Device,
			   Drug-eluting
			5 Intraluminal Device, Drug-
			   eluting, Two
			6 Intraluminal Device, Drug-
			   eluting, Three
			7 Intraluminal Device, Drug-
			   eluting, Four or More
			D Intraluminal Device
			E Intraluminal Device, Two
			F Intraluminal Device, Three
			G Intraluminal Device, Four
			   or More
			Z No Device
				Z No Qualifier

NC   Ø37G[3,4]ZZ

NC Noncovered Procedure   LC Limited Coverage   QA Questionable OB Admit   NT New Tech Add-on   ⊞ Combination Member   ♂ Male   ♀ Female

ICD-10-PCS 2022   **201**

Ø37–Ø37

Upper Arteries

Ø   **Medical and Surgical**
3   **Upper Arteries**
9   **Drainage**   Definition: Taking or letting out fluids and/or gases from a body part

Explanation: The qualifier DIAGNOSTIC is used to identify drainage procedures that are biopsies

Body Part Character 4		Approach Character 5	Device Character 6	Qualifier Character 7
Ø Internal Mammary Artery, Right	**H Common Carotid Artery, Right**	**Ø Open**	**Ø Drainage Device**	**Z No Qualifier**
Anterior intercostal artery	**J Common Carotid Artery, Left**	**3 Percutaneous**		
Internal thoracic artery	**K Internal Carotid Artery, Right**	**4 Percutaneous Endoscopic**		
Musculophrenic artery	Caroticotympanic artery			
Pericardiophrenic artery	Carotid sinus			
Superior epigastric artery	**L Internal Carotid Artery, Left**			
1 Internal Mammary Artery, Left	*See K Internal Carotid Artery, Right*			
See Ø Internal Mammary Artery, Right above	**M External Carotid Artery, Right**			
2 Innominate Artery	Ascending pharyngeal artery			
Brachiocephalic artery	Internal maxillary artery			
Brachiocephalic trunk	Lingual artery			
3 Subclavian Artery, Right	Maxillary artery			
Costocervical trunk	Occipital artery			
Dorsal scapular artery	Posterior auricular artery			
Internal thoracic artery	Superior thyroid artery			
4 Subclavian Artery, Left	**N External Carotid Artery, Left**			
See 3 Subclavian Artery, Right	*See M External Carotid Artery, Right*			
5 Axillary Artery, Right	**P Vertebral Artery, Right**			
Anterior circumflex humeral artery	Anterior spinal artery			
Lateral thoracic artery	Posterior spinal artery			
Posterior circumflex humeral artery	**Q Vertebral Artery, Left**			
Subscapular artery	*See P Vertebral Artery, Right*			
Superior thoracic artery	**R Face Artery**			
Thoracoacromial artery	Angular artery			
6 Axillary Artery, Left	Ascending palatine artery			
See 5 Axillary Artery, Right	External maxillary artery			
7 Brachial Artery, Right	Facial artery			
Inferior ulnar collateral artery	Inferior labial artery			
Profunda brachii	Submental artery			
Superior ulnar collateral artery	Superior labial artery			
8 Brachial Artery, Left	**S Temporal Artery, Right**			
See 7 Brachial Artery, Right	Middle temporal artery			
9 Ulnar Artery, Right	Superficial temporal artery			
Anterior ulnar recurrent artery	Transverse facial artery			
Common interosseous artery	**T Temporal Artery, Left**			
Posterior ulnar recurrent artery	*See S Temporal Artery, Right*			
A Ulnar Artery, Left	**U Thyroid Artery, Right**			
See 9 Ulnar Artery, Right	Cricothyroid artery			
B Radial Artery, Right	Hyoid artery			
Radial recurrent artery	Sternocleidomastoid artery			
C Radial Artery, Left	Superior laryngeal artery			
See B Radial Artery, Right	Superior thyroid artery			
D Hand Artery, Right	Thyrocervical trunk			
Deep palmar arch	**V Thyroid Artery, Left**			
Princeps pollicis artery	*See U Thyroid Artery, Right*			
Radialis indicis	**Y Upper Artery**			
Superficial palmar arch	Aortic intercostal artery			
F Hand Artery, Left	Bronchial artery			
See D Hand Artery, Right	Esophageal artery			
G Intracranial Artery	Subcostal artery			
Anterior cerebral artery				
Anterior choroidal artery				
Anterior communicating artery				
Basilar artery				
Circle of Willis				
Internal carotid artery, intracranial portion				
Middle cerebral artery				
Ophthalmic artery				
Posterior cerebral artery				
Posterior communicating artery				
Posterior inferior cerebellar artery (PICA)				

Non-OR   Ø39[Ø,1,2,3,4,5,6,7,8,9,A,B,C,D,F,G,H,J,K,L,M,N,P,Q,R,S,T,U,V,Y][Ø,3,4]ØZ

Ø39 Continued on next page

Non-OR Procedure   DRG Non-OR Procedure   Valid OR Procedure   HAC Associated Procedure   Combination Only   New/Revised GREEN

Ø   **Medical and Surgical**   ***Ø39 Continued***
3   **Upper Arteries**
9   **Drainage**   Definition: Taking or letting out fluids and/or gases from a body part
                         Explanation: The qualifier DIAGNOSTIC is used to identify drainage procedures that are biopsies

Body Part Character 4		Approach Character 5	Device Character 6	Qualifier Character 7
Ø Internal Mammary Artery, Right Anterior intercostal artery Internal thoracic artery Musculophrenic artery Pericardiophrenic artery Superior epigastric artery **1 Internal Mammary Artery, Left** *See Ø Internal Mammary Artery, Right* **2 Innominate Artery** Brachiocephalic artery Brachiocephalic trunk **3 Subclavian Artery, Right** Costocervical trunk Dorsal scapular artery Internal thoracic artery **4 Subclavian Artery, Left** *See 3 Subclavian Artery, Right* **5 Axillary Artery, Right** Anterior circumflex humeral artery Lateral thoracic artery Posterior circumflex humeral artery Subscapular artery Superior thoracic artery Thoracoacromial artery **6 Axillary Artery, Left** *See 5 Axillary Artery, Right* **7 Brachial Artery, Right** Inferior ulnar collateral artery Profunda brachii Superior ulnar collateral artery **8 Brachial Artery, Left** *See 7 Brachial Artery, Right* **9 Ulnar Artery, Right** Anterior ulnar recurrent artery Common interosseous artery Posterior ulnar recurrent artery **A Ulnar Artery, Left** *See 9 Ulnar Artery, Right* **B Radial Artery, Right** Radial recurrent artery **C Radial Artery, Left** *See B Radial Artery, Right* **D Hand Artery, Right** Deep palmar arch Princeps pollicis artery Radialis indicis Superficial palmar arch **F Hand Artery, Left** *See D Hand Artery, Right* **G Intracranial Artery** Anterior cerebral artery Anterior choroidal artery Anterior communicating artery Basilar artery Circle of Willis Internal carotid artery, intracranial portion Middle cerebral artery Ophthalmic artery Posterior cerebral artery Posterior communicating artery Posterior inferior cerebellar artery (PICA)	**H Common Carotid Artery, Right** **J Common Carotid Artery, Left** **K Internal Carotid Artery, Right** Caroticotympanic artery Carotid sinus **L Internal Carotid Artery, Left** *See K Internal Carotid Artery, Right* **M External Carotid Artery, Right** Ascending pharyngeal artery Internal maxillary artery Lingual artery Maxillary artery Occipital artery Posterior auricular artery Superior thyroid artery **N External Carotid Artery, Left** *See M External Carotid Artery, Right* **P Vertebral Artery, Right** Anterior spinal artery Posterior spinal artery **Q Vertebral Artery, Left** *See P Vertebral Artery, Right* **R Face Artery** Angular artery Ascending palatine artery External maxillary artery Facial artery Inferior labial artery Submental artery Superior labial artery **S Temporal Artery, Right** Middle temporal artery Superficial temporal artery Transverse facial artery **T Temporal Artery, Left** *See S Temporal Artery, Right* **U Thyroid Artery, Right** Cricothyroid artery Hyoid artery Sternocleidomastoid artery Superior laryngeal artery Superior thyroid artery Thyrocervical trunk **V Thyroid Artery, Left** *See U Thyroid Artery, Right* **Y Upper Artery** Aortic intercostal artery Bronchial artery Esophageal artery Subcostal artery	**Ø Open** **3 Percutaneous** **4 Percutaneous Endoscopic**	**Z No Device**	**X Diagnostic** **Z No Qualifier**

Non-OR   Ø39[Ø,1,2,3,4,5,6,7,8,9,A,B,C,D,F,G,H,J,K,L,M,N,P,Q,R,S,T,U,V,Y]3ZX
Non-OR   Ø39[Ø,1,2,3,4,5,6,7,8,9,A,B,C,D,F,G,H,J,K,L,M,N,P,Q,R,S,T,U,V,Y][Ø,3,4]ZZ

NC Noncovered Procedure   **LC** Limited Coverage   **QA** Questionable OB Admit   **NT** New Tech Add-on   ⊞ Combination Member   ♂ Male   ♀ Female

ICD-10-PCS 2022   203

Ø39–Ø39

Upper Arteries

0   Medical and Surgical
3   Upper Arteries
B   Excision

Definition: Cutting out or off, without replacement, a portion of a body part
Explanation: The qualifier DIAGNOSTIC is used to identify excision procedures that are biopsies

Body Part Character 4		Approach Character 5	Device Character 6	Qualifier Character 7
0 Internal Mammary Artery, Right	**H Common Carotid Artery, Right**	**0** Open	**Z** No Device	**X** Diagnostic
Anterior intercostal artery	**J Common Carotid Artery, Left**	**3** Percutaneous		**Z** No Qualifier
Internal thoracic artery	**K Internal Carotid Artery, Right**	**4** Percutaneous Endoscopic		
Musculophrenic artery	Caroticotympanic artery			
Pericardiophrenic artery	Carotid sinus			
Superior epigastric artery	**L Internal Carotid Artery, Left**			
1 Internal Mammary Artery, Left	*See K Internal Carotid Artery, Right*			
See 0 Internal Mammary Artery, Right	**M External Carotid Artery, Right**			
2 Innominate Artery	Ascending pharyngeal artery			
Brachiocephalic artery	Internal maxillary artery			
Brachiocephalic trunk	Lingual artery			
3 Subclavian Artery, Right	Maxillary artery			
Costocervical trunk	Occipital artery			
Dorsal scapular artery	Posterior auricular artery			
Internal thoracic artery	Superior thyroid artery			
4 Subclavian Artery, Left	**N External Carotid Artery, Left**			
See 3 Subclavian Artery, Right	*See M External Carotid Artery, Right*			
5 Axillary Artery, Right	**P Vertebral Artery, Right**			
Anterior circumflex humeral artery	Anterior spinal artery			
Lateral thoracic artery	Posterior spinal artery			
Posterior circumflex humeral artery	**Q Vertebral Artery, Left**			
Subscapular artery	*See P Vertebral Artery, Right*			
Superior thoracic artery	**R Face Artery**			
Thoracoacromial artery	Angular artery			
6 Axillary Artery, Left	Ascending palatine artery			
See 5 Axillary Artery, Right	External maxillary artery			
7 Brachial Artery, Right	Facial artery			
Inferior ulnar collateral artery	Inferior labial artery			
Profunda brachii	Submental artery			
Superior ulnar collateral artery	Superior labial artery			
8 Brachial Artery, Left	**S Temporal Artery, Right**			
See 7 Brachial Artery, Right	Middle temporal artery			
9 Ulnar Artery, Right	Superficial temporal artery			
Anterior ulnar recurrent artery	Transverse facial artery			
Common interosseous artery	**T Temporal Artery, Left**			
Posterior ulnar recurrent artery	*See S Temporal Artery, Right*			
A Ulnar Artery, Left	**U Thyroid Artery, Right**			
See 9 Ulnar Artery, Right	Cricothyroid artery			
B Radial Artery, Right	Hyoid artery			
Radial recurrent artery	Sternocleidomastoid artery			
C Radial Artery, Left	Superior laryngeal artery			
See B Radial Artery, Right	Superior thyroid artery			
D Hand Artery, Right	Thyrocervical trunk			
Deep palmar arch	**V Thyroid Artery, Left**			
Princeps pollicis artery	*See U Thyroid Artery, Right*			
Radialis indicis	**Y Upper Artery**			
Superficial palmar arch	Aortic intercostal artery			
F Hand Artery, Left	Bronchial artery			
See D Hand Artery, Right	Esophageal artery			
G Intracranial Artery	Subcostal artery			
Anterior cerebral artery				
Anterior choroidal artery				
Anterior communicating artery				
Basilar artery				
Circle of Willis				
Internal carotid artery, intracranial portion				
Middle cerebral artery				
Ophthalmic artery				
Posterior cerebral artery				
Posterior communicating artery				
Posterior inferior cerebellar artery (PICA)				

Ø Medical and Surgical
3 Upper Arteries
C Extirpation   Definition: Taking or cutting out solid matter from a body part

Explanation: The solid matter may be an abnormal byproduct of a biological function or a foreign body; it may be imbedded in a body part or in the lumen of a tubular body part. The solid matter may or may not have been previously broken into pieces.

Body Part Character 4		Approach Character 5	Device Character 6	Qualifier Character 7
Ø Internal Mammary Artery, Right Anterior intercostal artery Internal thoracic artery Musculophrenic artery Pericardiophrenic artery Superior epigastric artery **1 Internal Mammary Artery, Left** *See Ø Internal Mammary Artery, Right* **2 Innominate Artery** Brachiocephalic artery Brachiocephalic trunk **3 Subclavian Artery, Right** Costocervical trunk Dorsal scapular artery Internal thoracic artery **4 Subclavian Artery, Left** *See 3 Subclavian Artery, Right* **5 Axillary Artery, Right** Anterior circumflex humeral artery Lateral thoracic artery Posterior circumflex humeral artery Subscapular artery Superior thoracic artery Thoracoacromial artery **6 Axillary Artery, Left** *See 5 Axillary Artery, Right* **7 Brachial Artery, Right** Inferior ulnar collateral artery Profunda brachii Superior ulnar collateral artery **8 Brachial Artery, Left** *See 7 Brachial Artery, Right* **9 Ulnar Artery, Right** Anterior ulnar recurrent artery Common interosseous artery Posterior ulnar recurrent artery	**A Ulnar Artery, Left** *See 9 Ulnar Artery, Right* **B Radial Artery, Right** Radial recurrent artery **C Radial Artery, Left** *See B Radial Artery, Right* **D Hand Artery, Right** Deep palmar arch Princeps pollicis artery Radialis indicis Superficial palmar arch **F Hand Artery, Left** *See D Hand Artery, Right* **R Face Artery** Angular artery Ascending palatine artery External maxillary artery Facial artery Inferior labial artery Submental artery Superior labial artery **S Temporal Artery, Right** Middle temporal artery Superficial temporal artery Transverse facial artery **T Temporal Artery, Left** *See S Temporal Artery, Right* **U Thyroid Artery, Right** Cricothyroid artery Hyoid artery Sternocleidomastoid artery Superior laryngeal artery Superior thyroid artery Thyrocervical trunk **V Thyroid Artery, Left** *See U Thyroid Artery, Right* **Y Upper Artery** Aortic intercostal artery Bronchial artery Esophageal artery Subcostal artery	**Ø Open** **3 Percutaneous** **4 Percutaneous Endoscopic**	**Z No Device**	**Z No Qualifier**
G Intracranial Artery Anterior cerebral artery Anterior choroidal artery Anterior communicating artery Basilar artery Circle of Willis Internal carotid artery, intracranial portion Middle cerebral artery Ophthalmic artery Posterior cerebral artery Posterior communicating artery Posterior inferior cerebellar artery (PICA) **H Common Carotid Artery, Right** **J Common Carotid Artery, Left** **K Internal Carotid Artery, Right** Caroticotympanic artery Carotid sinus	**L Internal Carotid Artery, Left** *See K Internal Carotid Artery, Right* **M External Carotid Artery, Right** Ascending pharyngeal artery Internal maxillary artery Lingual artery Maxillary artery Occipital artery Posterior auricular artery Superior thyroid artery **N External Carotid Artery, Left** *See M External Carotid Artery, Right* **P Vertebral Artery, Right** Anterior spinal artery Posterior spinal artery **Q Vertebral Artery, Left** *See P Vertebral Artery, Right*	**Ø Open** **4 Percutaneous Endoscopic**	**Z No Device**	**Z No Qualifier**

Ø3C Continued on next page

NC Noncovered Procedure   **LC** Limited Coverage   **QA** Questionable OB Admit   **NT** New Tech Add-on   ⊞ Combination Member   ♂ Male   ♀ Female

ICD-10-PCS 2022   205

Ø3C–Ø3C

Ø   Medical and Surgical   *03C Continued*
3   Upper Arteries
C   Extirpation   Definition: Taking or cutting out solid matter from a body part

Explanation: The solid matter may be an abnormal byproduct of a biological function or a foreign body; it may be imbedded in a body part or in the lumen of a tubular body part. The solid matter may or may not have been previously broken into pieces.

Body Part Character 4		Approach Character 5	Device Character 6	Qualifier Character 7

G Intracranial Artery
Anterior cerebral artery
Anterior choroidal artery
Anterior communicating
  artery
Basilar artery
Circle of Willis
Internal carotid artery,
  intracranial portion
Middle cerebral artery
Ophthalmic artery
Posterior cerebral artery
Posterior communicating
  artery
Posterior inferior cerebellar
  artery (PICA)
H Common Carotid Artery,
Right
J Common Carotid Artery, Left
K Internal Carotid Artery, Right
Caroticotympanic artery
Carotid sinus
	L Internal Carotid Artery, Left
	See K Internal Carotid Artery,
	Right
	M External Carotid Artery, Right
	Ascending pharyngeal artery
	Internal maxillary artery
	Lingual artery
	Maxillary artery
	Occipital artery
	Posterior auricular artery
	Superior thyroid artery
	N External Carotid Artery, Left
	See M External Carotid Artery,
	Right
	P Vertebral Artery, Right
	Anterior spinal artery
	Posterior spinal artery
	Q Vertebral Artery, Left
	See P Vertebral Artery, Right
		3 Percutaneous	**Z No Device**	**7 Stent Retriever**
				Z No Qualifier

Ø   Medical and Surgical
3   Upper Arteries
F   Fragmentation   Definition: Breaking solid matter in a body part into pieces

Explanation: Physical force (e.g., manual, ultrasonic) applied directly or indirectly is used to break the solid matter into pieces. The solid matter may be an abnormal byproduct of a biological function or a foreign body. The pieces of solid matter are not taken out.

Body Part Character 4		Approach Character 5	Device Character 6	Qualifier Character 7

2 Innominate Artery
Brachiocephalic artery
Brachiocephalic trunk
3 Subclavian Artery, Right
Costocervical trunk
Dorsal scapular artery
Internal thoracic artery
4 Subclavian Artery, Left
See 3 Subclavian Artery, Right
5 Axillary Artery, Right
Anterior circumflex humeral
  artery
Lateral thoracic artery
Posterior circumflex humeral
  artery
Subscapular artery
Superior thoracic artery
Thoracoacromial artery
6 Axillary Artery, Left
See 5 Axillary Artery, Right
7 Brachial Artery, Right
Inferior ulnar collateral artery
Profunda brachii
Superior ulnar collateral artery
8 Brachial Artery, Left
See 7 Brachial Artery, Right
	9 Ulnar Artery, Right
	Anterior ulnar recurrent artery
	Common interosseous artery
	Posterior ulnar recurrent artery
	A Ulnar Artery, Left
	See 9 Ulnar Artery, Right
	B Radial Artery, Right
	Radial recurrent artery
	C Radial Artery, Left
	See B Radial Artery, Right
	G Intracranial Artery
	Anterior cerebral artery
	Anterior choroidal artery
	Anterior communicating artery
	Basilar artery
	Circle of Willis
	Internal carotid artery,
	  intracranial portion
	Middle cerebral artery
	Ophthalmic artery
	Posterior cerebral artery
	Posterior communicating
	  artery
	Posterior inferior cerebellar
	  artery (PICA)
	Y Upper Artery
	Aortic intercostal artery
	Bronchial artery
	Esophageal artery
	Subcostal artery
		3 Percutaneous	**Z No Device**	**Ø Ultrasonic**
				Z No Qualifier

Ø   Medical and Surgical
3   Upper Arteries
H   Insertion   Definition: Putting in a nonbiological appliance that monitors, assists, performs, or prevents a physiological function but does not physically take the place of a body part
                   Explanation: None

Body Part Character 4		Approach Character 5	Device Character 6	Qualifier Character 7
Ø **Internal Mammary Artery, Right** Anterior intercostal artery Internal thoracic artery Musculophrenic artery Pericardiophrenic artery Superior epigastric artery **1** **Internal Mammary Artery, Left** *See Ø Internal Mammary Artery, Right* **2** **Innominate Artery** Brachiocephalic artery Brachiocephalic trunk **3** **Subclavian Artery, Right** Costocervical trunk Dorsal scapular artery Internal thoracic artery **4** **Subclavian Artery, Left** *See 3 Subclavian Artery, Right* **5** **Axillary Artery, Right** Anterior circumflex humeral artery Lateral thoracic artery Posterior circumflex humeral artery Subscapular artery Superior thoracic artery Thoracoacromial artery **6** **Axillary Artery, Left** *See 5 Axillary Artery, Right* **7** **Brachial Artery, Right** Inferior ulnar collateral artery Profunda brachii Superior ulnar collateral artery **8** **Brachial Artery, Left** *See 7 Brachial Artery, Right* **9** **Ulnar Artery, Right** Anterior ulnar recurrent artery Common interosseous artery Posterior ulnar recurrent artery **A** **Ulnar Artery, Left** *See 9 Ulnar Artery, Right* **B** **Radial Artery, Right** Radial recurrent artery **C** **Radial Artery, Left** *See B Radial Artery, Right* **D** **Hand Artery, Right** Deep palmar arch Princeps pollicis artery Radialis indicis Superficial palmar arch **F** **Hand Artery, Left** *See D Hand Artery, Right*	**G** **Intracranial Artery** Anterior cerebral artery Anterior choroidal artery Anterior communicating artery Basilar artery Circle of Willis Internal carotid artery, intracranial portion Middle cerebral artery Ophthalmic artery Posterior cerebral artery Posterior communicating artery Posterior inferior cerebellar artery (PICA) **H** **Common Carotid Artery, Right** **J** **Common Carotid Artery, Left** **M** **External Carotid Artery, Right** Ascending pharyngeal artery Internal maxillary artery Lingual artery Maxillary artery Occipital artery Posterior auricular artery Superior thyroid artery **N** **External Carotid Artery, Left** *See M External Carotid Artery, Right* **P** **Vertebral Artery, Right** Anterior spinal artery Posterior spinal artery **Q** **Vertebral Artery, Left** *See P Vertebral Artery, Right* **R** **Face Artery** Angular artery Ascending palatine artery External maxillary artery Facial artery Inferior labial artery Submental artery Superior labial artery **S** **Temporal Artery, Right** Middle temporal artery Superficial temporal artery Transverse facial artery **T** **Temporal Artery, Left** *See S Temporal Artery, Right* **U** **Thyroid Artery, Right** Cricothyroid artery Hyoid artery Sternocleidomastoid artery Superior laryngeal artery Superior thyroid artery Thyrocervical trunk **V** **Thyroid Artery, Left** *See U Thyroid Artery, Right*	**Ø** Open **3** Percutaneous **4** Percutaneous Endoscopic	**3** Infusion Device **D** Intraluminal Device	**Z** No Qualifier
K **Internal Carotid Artery, Right** Caroticotympanic artery Carotid sinus **L** **Internal Carotid Artery, Left** *See K Internal Carotid Artery, Right*		**Ø** Open **3** Percutaneous **4** Percutaneous Endoscope	**3** Infusion Device **D** Intraluminal Device **M** Stimulator Lead **NT**	**Z** No Qualifier
Y **Upper Artery** Aortic intercostal artery Bronchial artery Esophageal artery Subcostal artery		**Ø** Open **3** Percutaneous **4** Percutaneous Endoscopic	**2** Monitoring Device **3** Infusion Device **D** Intraluminal Device **Y** Other Device	**Z** No Qualifier

Non-OR	Ø3H[Ø,1,2,3,4,5,6,7,8,9,A,B,C,D,F,G,H,J,M,N,P,Q,R,S,T,U,V][Ø,3,4]3Z
Non-OR	Ø3H[K,L][Ø,3,4]3Z
Non-OR	Ø3HY[Ø,3,4]3Z
Non-OR	Ø3HY32Z
Non-OR	Ø3HY[3,4]YZ
NT	Ø3HK3MZ or Ø3HL3MZ in combination with ØJH6ØMZ *See Appendix H for applicable device trade name*

NC Noncovered Procedure   **LC** Limited Coverage   **QA** Questionable OB Admit   **NT** New Tech Add-on   ⊞ Combination Member   ♂ Male   ♀ Female

ICD-10-PCS 2022   **207**

Ø3H–Ø3H

Ø   **Medical and Surgical**
3   **Upper Arteries**
J   **Inspection**   Definition: Visually and/or manually exploring a body part

Explanation: Visual exploration may be performed with or without optical instrumentation. Manual exploration may be performed directly or through intervening body layers.

Body Part Character 4	Approach Character 5	Device Character 6	Qualifier Character 7

Y   **Upper Artery**
     Aortic intercostal artery
     Bronchial artery
     Esophageal artery
     Subcostal artery
	Ø Open
	3 Percutaneous
	4 Percutaneous Endoscopic
	X External
		Z No Device	**Z** No Qualifier

Non-OR   03JY[3,4,X]ZZ

0   **Medical and Surgical**
3   **Upper Arteries**
L   **Occlusion**   Definition: Completely closing an orifice or the lumen of a tubular body part
                     Explanation: The orifice can be a natural orifice or an artificially created orifice

Body Part Character 4		Approach Character 5	Device Character 6	Qualifier Character 7
0 Internal Mammary Artery, Right Anterior intercostal artery Internal thoracic artery Musculophrenic artery Pericardiophrenic artery Superior epigastric artery **1 Internal Mammary Artery, Left** *See 0 Internal Mammary Artery, Left* **2 Innominate Artery** Brachiocephalic artery Brachiocephalic trunk **3 Subclavian Artery, Right** Costocervical trunk Dorsal scapular artery Internal thoracic artery **4 Subclavian Artery, Left** *See 3 Subclavian Artery, Right* **5 Axillary Artery, Right** Anterior circumflex humeral artery Lateral thoracic artery Posterior circumflex humeral artery Subscapular artery Superior thoracic artery Thoracoacromial artery **6 Axillary Artery, Left** *See 5 Axillary Artery, Right* **7 Brachial Artery, Right** Inferior ulnar collateral artery Profunda brachii Superior ulnar collateral artery **8 Brachial Artery, Left** *See 7 Brachial Artery, Right* **9 Ulnar Artery, Right** Anterior ulnar recurrent artery Common interosseous artery Posterior ulnar recurrent artery	**A Ulnar Artery, Left** *See 9 Ulnar Artery, Right* **B Radial Artery, Right** Radial recurrent artery **C Radial Artery, Left** *See B Radial Artery, Right* **D Hand Artery, Right** Deep palmar arch Princeps pollicis artery Radialis indicis Superficial palmar arch **F Hand Artery, Left** *See D Hand Artery, Right* **R Face Artery** Angular artery Ascending palatine artery External maxillary artery Facial artery Inferior labial artery Submental artery Superior labial artery **S Temporal Artery, Right** Middle temporal artery Superficial temporal artery Transverse facial artery **T Temporal Artery, Left** *See S Temporal Artery, Right* **U Thyroid Artery, Right** Cricothyroid artery Hyoid artery Sternocleidomastoid artery Superior laryngeal artery Superior thyroid artery Thyrocervical trunk **V Thyroid Artery, Left** *See U Thyroid Artery, Right* **Y Upper Artery** Aortic intercostal artery Bronchial artery Esophageal artery Subcostal artery	**0 Open** **3 Percutaneous** **4 Percutaneous Endoscopic**	**C Extraluminal Device** **D Intraluminal Device** **Z No Device**	**Z No Qualifier**
G Intracranial Artery Anterior cerebral artery Anterior choroidal artery Anterior communicating artery Basilar artery Circle of Willis Internal carotid artery, intracranial portion Middle cerebral artery Ophthalmic artery Posterior cerebral artery Posterior communicating artery Posterior inferior cerebellar artery (PICA) **H Common Carotid Artery, Right** **J Common Carotid Artery, Left** **K Internal Carotid Artery, Right** Caroticotympanic artery Carotid sinus	**L Internal Carotid Artery, Left** *See K Internal Carotid Artery, Right* **M External Carotid Artery, Right** Ascending pharyngeal artery Internal maxillary artery Lingual artery Maxillary artery Occipital artery Posterior auricular artery Superior thyroid artery **N External Carotid Artery, Left** *See M External Carotid Artery, Right* **P Vertebral Artery, Right** Anterior spinal artery Posterior spinal artery **Q Vertebral Artery, Left** *See P Vertebral Artery, Right*	**0 Open** **3 Percutaneous** **4 Percutaneous Endoscopic**	**B Intraluminal Device, Bioactive** **C Extraluminal Device** **D Intraluminal Device** **Z No Device**	**Z No Qualifier**

NC Noncovered Procedure   **LC** Limited Coverage   **QA** Questionable OB Admit   **NT** New Tech Add-on   ⊞ Combination Member   ♂ Male   ♀ Female

ICD-10-PCS 2022   **209**

03L–03L

Ø   **Medical and Surgical**
3   **Upper Arteries**
N   **Release**   Definition: Freeing a body part from an abnormal physical constraint by cutting or by the use of force
                         Explanation: Some of the restraining tissue may be taken out but none of the body part is taken out

Body Part Character 4		Approach Character 5	Device Character 6	Qualifier Character 7

Ø **Internal Mammary Artery, Right**
    Anterior intercostal artery
    Internal thoracic artery
    Musculophrenic artery
    Pericardiophrenic artery
    Superior epigastric artery
1 **Internal Mammary Artery, Left**
    See Ø Internal Mammary Artery, Right
2 **Innominate Artery**
    Brachiocephalic artery
    Brachiocephalic trunk
3 **Subclavian Artery, Right**
    Costocervical trunk
    Dorsal scapular artery
    Internal thoracic artery
4 **Subclavian Artery, Left**
    See 3 Subclavian Artery, Right
5 **Axillary Artery, Right**
    Anterior circumflex humeral artery
    Lateral thoracic artery
    Posterior circumflex humeral artery
    Subscapular artery
    Superior thoracic artery
    Thoracoacromial artery
6 **Axillary Artery, Left**
    See 5 Axillary Artery, Right
7 **Brachial Artery, Right**
    Inferior ulnar collateral artery
    Profunda brachii
    Superior ulnar collateral artery
8 **Brachial Artery, Left**
    See 7 Brachial Artery, Right
9 **Ulnar Artery, Right**
    Anterior ulnar recurrent artery
    Common interosseous artery
    Posterior ulnar recurrent artery
A **Ulnar Artery, Left**
    See 9 Ulnar Artery, Right
B **Radial Artery, Right**
    Radial recurrent artery
C **Radial Artery, Left**
    See B Radial Artery, Right
D **Hand Artery, Right**
    Deep palmar arch
    Princeps pollicis artery
    Radialis indicis
    Superficial palmar arch
F **Hand Artery, Left**
    See D Hand Artery, Right
G **Intracranial Artery**
    Anterior cerebral artery
    Anterior choroidal artery
    Anterior communicating artery
    Basilar artery
    Circle of Willis
    Internal carotid artery, intracranial portion
    Middle cerebral artery
    Ophthalmic artery
    Posterior cerebral artery
    Posterior communicating artery
    Posterior inferior cerebellar artery (PICA)
	H **Common Carotid Artery, Right**
	J **Common Carotid Artery, Left**
	K **Internal Carotid Artery, Right**
	    Caroticotympanic artery
	    Carotid sinus
	L **Internal Carotid Artery, Left**
	    See K Internal Carotid Artery, Right
	M **External Carotid Artery, Right**
	    Ascending pharyngeal artery
	    Internal maxillary artery
	    Lingual artery
	    Maxillary artery
	    Occipital artery
	    Posterior auricular artery
	    Superior thyroid artery
	N **External Carotid Artery, Left**
	    See M External Carotid Artery, Right
	P **Vertebral Artery, Right**
	    Anterior spinal artery
	    Posterior spinal artery
	Q **Vertebral Artery, Left**
	    See P Vertebral Artery, Right
	R **Face Artery**
	    Angular artery
	    Ascending palatine artery
	    External maxillary artery
	    Facial artery
	    Inferior labial artery
	    Submental artery
	    Superior labial artery
	S **Temporal Artery, Right**
	    Middle temporal artery
	    Superficial temporal artery
	    Transverse facial artery
	T **Temporal Artery, Left**
	    See S Temporal Artery, Right
	U **Thyroid Artery, Right**
	    Cricothyroid artery
	    Hyoid artery
	    Sternocleidomastoid artery
	    Superior laryngeal artery
	    Superior thyroid artery
	    Thyrocervical trunk
	V **Thyroid Artery, Left**
	    See U Thyroid Artery, Right
	Y **Upper Artery**
	    Aortic intercostal artery
	    Bronchial artery
	    Esophageal artery
	    Subcostal artery
		Ø Open
		3 Percutaneous
		4 Percutaneous Endoscopic
			Z No Device	**Z** No Qualifier

Non-OR Procedure   DRG Non-OR Procedure   Valid OR Procedure   HAC Associated Procedure   Combination Only   New/Revised GREEN

0 Medical and Surgical
3 Upper Arteries
P Removal   Definition: Taking out or off a device from a body part

Explanation: If a device is taken out and a similar device put in without cutting or puncturing the skin or mucous membrane, the procedure is coded to the root operation CHANGE. Otherwise, the procedure for taking out a device is coded to the root operation REMOVAL.

Body Part Character 4	Approach Character 5	Device Character 6	Qualifier Character 7

Y Upper Artery
  Aortic intercostal artery
  Bronchial artery
  Esophageal artery
  Subcostal artery
	0 Open
	3 Percutaneous
	4 Percutaneous Endoscopic
		0 Drainage Device
		2 Monitoring Device
		3 Infusion Device
		7 Autologous Tissue Substitute
		C Extraluminal Device
		D Intraluminal Device
		J Synthetic Substitute
		K Nonautologous Tissue Substitute
		M Stimulator Lead
		Y Other Device
			Z No Qualifier

Y Upper Artery
  Aortic intercostal artery
  Bronchial artery
  Esophageal artery
  Subcostal artery
	X External	**0** Drainage Device
		2 Monitoring Device
		3 Infusion Device
		D Intraluminal Device
		M Stimulator Lead
			Z No Qualifier

Non-OR   03PY3[0,2,3,D]Z
Non-OR   03PY[3,4]YZ
Non-OR   03PYX[0,2,3,D,M]Z

0   Medical and Surgical
3   Upper Arteries
Q   Repair   Definition: Restoring, to the extent possible, a body part to its normal anatomic structure and function
                  Explanation: Used only when the method to accomplish the repair is not one of the other root operations

Body Part Character 4		Approach Character 5	Device Character 6	Qualifier Character 7
0 Internal Mammary Artery, Right Anterior intercostal artery Internal thoracic artery Musculophrenic artery Pericardiophrenic artery Superior epigastric artery **1 Internal Mammary Artery, Left** *See 0 Internal Mammary Artery, Right* **2 Innominate Artery** Brachiocephalic artery Brachiocephalic trunk **3 Subclavian Artery, Right** Costocervical trunk Dorsal scapular artery Internal thoracic artery **4 Subclavian Artery, Left** *See 3 Subclavian Artery, Right* **5 Axillary Artery, Right** Anterior circumflex humeral artery Lateral thoracic artery Posterior circumflex humeral artery Subscapular artery Superior thoracic artery Thoracoacromial artery **6 Axillary Artery, Left** *See 5 Axillary Artery, Right* **7 Brachial Artery, Right** Inferior ulnar collateral artery Profunda brachii Superior ulnar collateral artery **8 Brachial Artery, Left** *See 7 Brachial Artery, Right* **9 Ulnar Artery, Right** Anterior ulnar recurrent artery Common interosseous artery Posterior ulnar recurrent artery **A Ulnar Artery, Left** *See 9 Ulnar Artery, Right* **B Radial Artery, Right** Radial recurrent artery **C Radial Artery, Left** *See B Radial Artery, Right* **D Hand Artery, Right** Deep palmar arch Princeps pollicis artery Radialis indicis Superficial palmar arch **F Hand Artery, Left** *See D Hand Artery, Right* **G Intracranial Artery** Anterior cerebral artery Anterior choroidal artery Anterior communicating artery Basilar artery Circle of Willis Internal carotid artery, intracranial portion Middle cerebral artery Ophthalmic artery Posterior cerebral artery Posterior communicating artery Posterior inferior cerebellar artery (PICA)	**H Common Carotid Artery, Right** **J Common Carotid Artery, Left** **K Internal Carotid Artery, Right** Caroticotympanic artery Carotid sinus **L Internal Carotid Artery, Left** *See K Internal Carotid Artery, Right* **M External Carotid Artery, Right** Ascending pharyngeal artery Internal maxillary artery Lingual artery Maxillary artery Occipital artery Posterior auricular artery Superior thyroid artery **N External Carotid Artery, Left** *See M External Carotid Artery, Right* **P Vertebral Artery, Right** Anterior spinal artery Posterior spinal artery **Q Vertebral Artery, Left** *See P Vertebral Artery, Right* **R Face Artery** Angular artery Ascending palatine artery External maxillary artery Facial artery Inferior labial artery Submental artery Superior labial artery **S Temporal Artery, Right** Middle temporal artery Superficial temporal artery Transverse facial artery **T Temporal Artery, Left** *See S Temporal Artery, Right* **U Thyroid Artery, Right** Cricothyroid artery Hyoid artery Sternocleidomastoid artery Superior laryngeal artery Superior thyroid artery Thyrocervical trunk **V Thyroid Artery, Left** *See U Thyroid Artery, Right* **Y Upper Artery** Aortic intercostal artery Bronchial artery Esophageal artery Subcostal artery	**0 Open** **3 Percutaneous** **4 Percutaneous Endoscopic**	**Z No Device**	**Z No Qualifier**

Upper Arteries

Ø	Medical and Surgical
3	Upper Arteries
R	Replacement

Definition: Putting in or on biological or synthetic material that physically takes the place and/or function of all or a portion of a body part

Explanation: The body part may have been taken out or replaced, or may be taken out, physically eradicated, or rendered nonfunctional during the REPLACEMENT procedure. A REMOVAL procedure is coded for taking out the device used in a previous replacement procedure.

Body Part — Character 4		Approach — Character 5	Device — Character 6	Qualifier — Character 7
Ø Internal Mammary Artery, Right Anterior intercostal artery Internal thoracic artery Musculophrenic artery Pericardiophrenic artery Superior epigastric artery **1 Internal Mammary Artery, Left** *See Ø Internal Mammary Artery, Right* **2 Innominate Artery** Brachiocephalic artery Brachiocephalic trunk **3 Subclavian Artery, Right** Costocervical trunk Dorsal scapular artery Internal thoracic artery **4 Subclavian Artery, Left** *See 3 Subclavian Artery, Right* **5 Axillary Artery, Right** Anterior circumflex humeral artery Lateral thoracic artery Posterior circumflex humeral artery Subscapular artery Superior thoracic artery Thoracoacromial artery **6 Axillary Artery, Left** *See 5 Axillary Artery, Right* **7 Brachial Artery, Right** Inferior ulnar collateral artery Profunda brachii Superior ulnar collateral artery **8 Brachial Artery, Left** *See 7 Brachial Artery, Right* **9 Ulnar Artery, Right** Anterior ulnar recurrent artery Common interosseous artery Posterior ulnar recurrent artery **A Ulnar Artery, Left** *See 9 Ulnar Artery, Right* **B Radial Artery, Right** Radial recurrent artery **C Radial Artery, Left** *See B Radial Artery, Right* **D Hand Artery, Right** Deep palmar arch Princeps pollicis artery Radialis indicis Superficial palmar arch **F Hand Artery, Left** *See D Hand Artery, Right* **G Intracranial Artery** Anterior cerebral artery Anterior choroidal artery Anterior communicating artery Basilar artery Circle of Willis Internal carotid artery, intracranial portion Middle cerebral artery Ophthalmic artery Posterior cerebral artery Posterior communicating artery Posterior inferior cerebellar artery (PICA)	**H Common Carotid Artery, Right** **J Common Carotid Artery, Left** **K Internal Carotid Artery, Right** Caroticotympanic artery Carotid sinus **L Internal Carotid Artery, Left** *See K Internal Carotid Artery, Right* **M External Carotid Artery, Right** Ascending pharyngeal artery Internal maxillary artery Lingual artery Maxillary artery Occipital artery Posterior auricular artery Superior thyroid artery **N External Carotid Artery, Left** *See M External Carotid Artery, Right* **P Vertebral Artery, Right** Anterior spinal artery Posterior spinal artery **Q Vertebral Artery, Left** *See P Vertebral Artery, Right* **R Face Artery** Angular artery Ascending palatine artery External maxillary artery Facial artery Inferior labial artery Submental artery Superior labial artery **S Temporal Artery, Right** Middle temporal artery Superficial temporal artery Transverse facial artery **T Temporal Artery, Left** *See S Temporal Artery, Right* **U Thyroid Artery, Right** Cricothyroid artery Hyoid artery Sternocleidomastoid artery Superior laryngeal artery Superior thyroid artery Thyrocervical trunk **V Thyroid Artery, Left** *See U Thyroid Artery, Right* **Y Upper Artery** Aortic intercostal artery Bronchial artery Esophageal artery Subcostal artery	**Ø Open** **4 Percutaneous Endoscopic**	**7 Autologous Tissue Substitute** **J Synthetic Substitute** **K Nonautologous Tissue Substitute**	**Z No Qualifier**

Ø   Medical and Surgical
3   Upper Arteries
S   Reposition

Definition: Moving to its normal location, or other suitable location, all or a portion of a body part

Explanation: The body part is moved to a new location from an abnormal location, or from a normal location where it is not functioning correctly. The body part may or may not be cut out or off to be moved to the new location.

Body Part Character 4		Approach Character 5	Device Character 6	Qualifier Character 7
Ø Internal Mammary Artery, Right	**H Common Carotid Artery, Right**	**Ø Open**	**Z No Device**	**Z No Qualifier**

Body Part — Character 4:

Ø Internal Mammary Artery, Right
  Anterior intercostal artery
  Internal thoracic artery
  Musculophrenic artery
  Pericardiophrenic artery
  Superior epigastric artery
1 Internal Mammary Artery, Left
  See Ø Internal Mammary Artery, Right
2 Innominate Artery
  Brachiocephalic artery
  Brachiocephalic trunk
3 Subclavian Artery, Right
  Costocervical trunk
  Dorsal scapular artery
  Internal thoracic artery
4 Subclavian Artery, Left
  See 3 Subclavian Artery, Right
5 Axillary Artery, Right
  Anterior circumflex humeral artery
  Lateral thoracic artery
  Posterior circumflex humeral artery
  Subscapular artery
  Superior thoracic artery
  Thoracoacromial artery
6 Axillary Artery, Left
  See 5 Axillary Artery, Right
7 Brachial Artery, Right
  Inferior ulnar collateral artery
  Profunda brachii
  Superior ulnar collateral artery
8 Brachial Artery, Left
  See 7 Brachial Artery, Right
9 Ulnar Artery, Right
  Anterior ulnar recurrent artery
  Common interosseous artery
  Posterior ulnar recurrent artery
A Ulnar Artery, Left
  See 9 Ulnar Artery, Right
B Radial Artery, Right
  Radial recurrent artery
C Radial Artery, Left
  See B Radial Artery, Right
D Hand Artery, Right
  Deep palmar arch
  Princeps pollicis artery
  Radialis indicis
  Superficial palmar arch
F Hand Artery, Left
  See D Hand Artery, Right
G Intracranial Artery
  Anterior cerebral artery
  Anterior choroidal artery
  Anterior communicating artery
  Basilar artery
  Circle of Willis
  Internal carotid artery, intracranial portion
  Middle cerebral artery
  Ophthalmic artery
  Posterior cerebral artery
  Posterior communicating artery
  Posterior inferior cerebellar artery (PICA)

H Common Carotid Artery, Right
J Common Carotid Artery, Left
K Internal Carotid Artery, Right
  Caroticotympanic artery
  Carotid sinus
L Internal Carotid Artery, Left
  See K Internal Carotid Artery, Right
M External Carotid Artery, Right
  Ascending pharyngeal artery
  Internal maxillary artery
  Lingual artery
  Maxillary artery
  Occipital artery
  Posterior auricular artery
  Superior thyroid artery
N External Carotid Artery, Left
  See M External Carotid Artery, Right
P Vertebral Artery, Right
  Anterior spinal artery
  Posterior spinal artery
Q Vertebral Artery, Left
  See P Vertebral Artery, Right
R Face Artery
  Angular artery
  Ascending palatine artery
  External maxillary artery
  Facial artery
  Inferior labial artery
  Submental artery
  Superior labial artery
S Temporal Artery, Right
  Middle temporal artery
  Superficial temporal artery
  Transverse facial artery
T Temporal Artery, Left
  See S Temporal Artery, Right
U Thyroid Artery, Right
  Cricothyroid artery
  Hyoid artery
  Sternocleidomastoid artery
  Superior laryngeal artery
  Superior thyroid artery
  Thyrocervical trunk
V Thyroid Artery, Left
  See U Thyroid Artery, Right
Y Upper Artery
  Aortic intercostal artery
  Bronchial artery
  Esophageal artery
  Subcostal artery

Approach — Character 5:
Ø Open
3 Percutaneous
4 Percutaneous Endoscopic

Device — Character 6:
Z No Device

Qualifier — Character 7:
Z No Qualifier

Ø   Medical and Surgical
3   Upper Arteries
U   Supplement   Definition: Putting in or on biological or synthetic material that physically reinforces and/or augments the function of a portion of a body part

Explanation: The biological material is non-living, or is living and from the same individual. The body part may have been previously replaced, and the SUPPLEMENT procedure is performed to physically reinforce and/or augment the function of the replaced body part.

Body Part Character 4		Approach Character 5	Device Character 6	Qualifier Character 7
Ø Internal Mammary Artery, Right Anterior intercostal artery Internal thoracic artery Musculophrenic artery Pericardiophrenic artery Superior epigastric artery	**H Common Carotid Artery, Right**	**Ø Open** **3 Percutaneous** **4 Percutaneous Endoscopic**	**7 Autologous Tissue Substitute** **J Synthetic Substitute** **K Nonautologous Tissue Substitute**	**Z No Qualifier**
1 Internal Mammary Artery, Left *See Ø Internal Mammary Artery, Right*	**J Common Carotid Artery, Left** **K Internal Carotid Artery, Right** Caroticotympanic artery Carotid sinus			
2 Innominate Artery Brachiocephalic artery Brachiocephalic trunk	**L Internal Carotid Artery, Left** *See K Internal Carotid Artery, Right*			
3 Subclavian Artery, Right Costocervical trunk Dorsal scapular artery Internal thoracic artery	**M External Carotid Artery, Right** Ascending pharyngeal artery Internal maxillary artery Lingual artery Maxillary artery Occipital artery			
4 Subclavian Artery, Left *See 3 Subclavian Artery, Right*	Posterior auricular artery Superior thyroid artery			
5 Axillary Artery, Right Anterior circumflex humeral artery Lateral thoracic artery Posterior circumflex humeral artery Subscapular artery Superior thoracic artery Thoracoacromial artery	**N External Carotid Artery, Left** *See M External Carotid Artery, Right* **P Vertebral Artery, Right** Anterior spinal artery Posterior spinal artery **Q Vertebral Artery, Left** *See P Vertebral Artery, Right*			
6 Axillary Artery, Left *See 5 Axillary Artery, Right*	**R Face Artery** Angular artery Ascending palatine artery External maxillary artery			
7 Brachial Artery, Right Inferior ulnar collateral artery Profunda brachii Superior ulnar collateral artery	Facial artery Inferior labial artery Submental artery Superior labial artery			
8 Brachial Artery, Left *See 7 Brachial Artery, Right*	**S Temporal Artery, Right** Middle temporal artery Superficial temporal artery Transverse facial artery			
9 Ulnar Artery, Right Anterior ulnar recurrent artery Common interosseous artery Posterior ulnar recurrent artery	**T Temporal Artery, Left** *See S Temporal Artery, Right* **U Thyroid Artery, Right** Cricothyroid artery Hyoid artery			
A Ulnar Artery, Left *See 9 Ulnar Artery, Right*	Sternocleidomastoid artery Superior laryngeal artery Superior thyroid artery Thyrocervical trunk			
B Radial Artery, Right Radial recurrent artery	**V Thyroid Artery, Left** *See U Thyroid Artery, Right*			
C Radial Artery, Left *See B Radial Artery, Right*	**Y Upper Artery** Aortic intercostal artery			
D Hand Artery, Right Deep palmar arch Princeps pollicis artery Radialis indicis Superficial palmar arch	Bronchial artery Esophageal artery Subcostal artery			
F Hand Artery, Left *See D Hand Artery, Right*				
G Intracranial Artery Anterior cerebral artery Anterior choroidal artery Anterior communicating artery Basilar artery Circle of Willis Internal carotid artery, intracranial portion Middle cerebral artery Ophthalmic artery Posterior cerebral artery Posterior communicating artery Posterior inferior cerebellar artery (PICA)				

Upper Arteries

Ø   **Medical and Surgical**
3   **Upper Arteries**
V   **Restriction**   Definition: Partially closing an orifice or the lumen of a tubular body part

Explanation: The orifice can be a natural orifice or an artificially created orifice

Body Part Character 4		Approach Character 5	Device Character 6	Qualifier Character 7
Ø **Internal Mammary Artery, Right** Anterior intercostal artery Internal thoracic artery Musculophrenic artery Pericardiophrenic artery Superior epigastric artery 1 **Internal Mammary Artery, Left** *See Ø Internal Mammary Artery, Right* 2 **Innominate Artery** Brachiocephalic artery Brachiocephalic trunk 3 **Subclavian Artery, Right** Costocervical trunk Dorsal scapular artery Internal thoracic artery 4 **Subclavian Artery, Left** *See 3 Subclavian Artery, Right* 5 **Axillary Artery, Right** Anterior circumflex humeral artery Lateral thoracic artery Posterior circumflex humeral artery Subscapular artery Superior thoracic artery Thoracoacromial artery 6 **Axillary Artery, Left** *See 5 Axillary Artery, Right* 7 **Brachial Artery, Right** Inferior ulnar collateral artery Profunda brachii Superior ulnar collateral artery 8 **Brachial Artery, Left** *See 7 Brachial Artery, Right* 9 **Ulnar Artery, Right** Anterior ulnar recurrent artery Common interosseous artery Posterior ulnar recurrent artery A **Ulnar Artery, Left** *See 9 Ulnar Artery, Right*	B **Radial Artery, Right** Radial recurrent artery C **Radial Artery, Left** *See B Radial Artery, Right* D **Hand Artery, Right** Deep palmar arch Princeps pollicis artery Radialis indicis Superficial palmar arch F **Hand Artery, Left** *See D Hand Artery, Right* R **Face Artery** Angular artery Ascending palatine artery External maxillary artery Facial artery Inferior labial artery Submental artery Superior labial artery S **Temporal Artery, Right** Middle temporal artery Superficial temporal artery Transverse facial artery T **Temporal Artery, Left** *See S Temporal Artery, Right* U **Thyroid Artery, Right** Cricothyroid artery Hyoid artery Sternocleidomastoid artery Superior laryngeal artery Superior thyroid artery Thyrocervical trunk V **Thyroid Artery, Left** *See U Thyroid Artery, Right* Y **Upper Artery** Aortic intercostal artery Bronchial artery Esophageal artery Subcostal artery	Ø Open 3 Percutaneous 4 Percutaneous Endoscopic	C Extraluminal Device D Intraluminal Device Z No Device	Z No Qualifier
G **Intracranial Artery** Anterior cerebral artery Anterior choroidal artery Anterior communicating artery Basilar artery Circle of Willis Internal carotid artery, intracranial portion Middle cerebral artery Ophthalmic artery Posterior cerebral artery Posterior communicating artery Posterior inferior cerebellar artery (PICA) H **Common Carotid Artery, Right** J **Common Carotid Artery, Left** K **Internal Carotid Artery, Right** Caroticotympanic artery Carotid sinus	L **Internal Carotid Artery, Left** *See K Internal Carotid Artery, Right* M **External Carotid Artery, Right** Ascending pharyngeal artery Internal maxillary artery Lingual artery Maxillary artery Occipital artery Posterior auricular artery Superior thyroid artery N **External Carotid Artery, Left** *See M External Carotid Artery, Right* P **Vertebral Artery, Right** Anterior spinal artery Posterior spinal artery Q **Vertebral Artery, Left** *See P Vertebral Artery, Right*	Ø Open 3 Percutaneous 4 Percutaneous Endoscopic	B Intraluminal Device, Bioactive C Extraluminal Device D Intraluminal Device H Intraluminal Device, Flow Diverter Z No Device	Z No Qualifier

0 Medical and Surgical
3 Upper Arteries
W Revision

Definition: Correcting, to the extent possible, a portion of a malfunctioning device or the position of a displaced device
Explanation: Revision can include correcting a malfunctioning or displaced device by taking out or putting in components of the device such as a screw or pin

Body Part Character 4	Approach Character 5	Device Character 6	Qualifier Character 7

Y Upper Artery
  Aortic intercostal artery
  Bronchial artery
  Esophageal artery
  Subcostal artery
	0 Open
	3 Percutaneous
	4 Percutaneous Endoscopic
		0 Drainage Device
		2 Monitoring Device
		3 Infusion Device
		7 Autologous Tissue Substitute
		C Extraluminal Device
		D Intraluminal Device
		J Synthetic Substitute
		K Nonautologous Tissue Substitute
		M Stimulator Lead
		Y Other Device
			Z No Qualifier

Y Upper Artery
  Aortic intercostal artery
  Bronchial artery
  Esophageal artery
  Subcostal artery
	X External	0 Drainage Device
		2 Monitoring Device
		3 Infusion Device
		7 Autologous Tissue Substitute
		C Extraluminal Device
		D Intraluminal Device
		J Synthetic Substitute
		K Nonautologous Tissue Substitute
		M Stimulator Lead
			Z No Qualifier

Non-OR 03WY3[0,2,3,D]Z
Non-OR 03WY[3,4]YZ
Non-OR 03WYX[0,2,3,7,C,D,J,K,M]Z

Lower Arteries Ø41–Ø4W

Character Meanings

This Character Meaning table is provided as a guide to assist the user in the identification of character members that may be found in this section of code tables. It **SHOULD NOT** be used to build a PCS code.

Operation–Character 3	Body Part–Character 4	Approach–Character 5	Device–Character 6	Qualifier–Character 7
1 Bypass	Ø Abdominal Aorta	Ø Open	Ø Drainage Device	Ø Abdominal Aorta OR Ultrasonic
5 Destruction	1 Celiac Artery	3 Percutaneous	1 Radioactive Element	1 Celiac Artery OR Drug-Coated Balloon
7 Dilation	2 Gastric Artery	4 Percutaneous Endoscopic	2 Monitoring Device	2 Mesenteric Artery
9 Drainage	3 Hepatic Artery	X External	3 Infusion Device	3 Renal Artery, Right
B Excision	4 Splenic Artery		4 Intraluminal Device, Drug-eluting	4 Renal Artery, Left
C Extirpation	5 Superior Mesenteric Artery		5 Intraluminal Device, Drug-eluting, Two	5 Renal Artery, Bilateral
F Fragmentation	6 Colic Artery, Right		6 Intraluminal Device, Drug-eluting, Three	6 Common Iliac Artery, Right
H Insertion	7 Colic Artery, Left		7 Intraluminal Device, Drug-eluting, Four or More OR Autologous Tissue Substitute	7 Common Iliac Artery, Left
J Inspection	8 Colic Artery, Middle		9 Autologous Venous Tissue	8 Common Iliac Arteries, Bilateral
L Occlusion	9 Renal Artery, Right		A Autologous Arterial Tissue	9 Internal Iliac Artery, Right
N Release	A Renal Artery, Left		C Extraluminal Device	B Internal Iliac Artery, Left
P Removal	B Inferior Mesenteric Artery		D Intraluminal Device	C Internal Iliac Arteries, Bilateral
Q Repair	C Common Iliac Artery, Right		E Intraluminal Device, Two OR Intraluminal Device, Branched or Fenestrated, One or Two Arteries	D External Iliac Artery, Right
R Replacement	D Common Iliac Artery, Left		F Intraluminal Device, Three OR Intraluminal Device, Branched or Fenestrated, Three or More Arteries	F External Iliac Artery, Left
S Reposition	E Internal Iliac Artery, Right		G Intraluminal Device, Four or More	G External Iliac Arteries, Bilateral
U Supplement	F Internal Iliac Artery, Left		J Synthetic Substitute	H Femoral Artery, Right
V Restriction	H External Iliac Artery, Right		K Nonautologous Tissue Substitute	J Femoral Artery, Left OR Temporary
W Revision	J External Iliac Artery, Left		Y Other Device	K Femoral Arteries, Bilateral
	K Femoral Artery, Right		Z No Device	L Popliteal Artery
	L Femoral Artery, Left			M Peroneal Artery
	M Popliteal Artery, Right			N Posterior Tibial Artery
	N Popliteal Artery, Left			P Foot Artery
	P Anterior Tibial Artery, Right			Q Lower Extremity Artery
	Q Anterior Tibial Artery, Left			R Lower Artery
	R Posterior Tibial Artery, Right			S Lower Extremity Vein
	S Posterior Tibial Artery, Left			T Uterine Artery, Right
	T Peroneal Artery, Right			U Uterine Artery, Left
	U Peroneal Artery, Left			X Diagnostic
	V Foot Artery, Right			Z No Qualifier
	W Foot Artery, Left			
	Y Lower Artery			

AHA Coding Clinic for table Ø41

2019, 1Q, 23	Endovascular repair of shaggy aorta and deployment of chimney stent grafts
2018, 3Q, 25	Femoral artery to tibioperoneal trunk bypass
2017, 4Q, 46-47	New and revised body part values - Bypass hepatic artery to renal artery
2017, 3Q, 5	Femoral artery to posterior tibial artery bypass using autologous and synthetic grafts
2017, 3Q, 16	Abdominal aortic debranching with bypass of external iliac artery to bilateral renal arteries and superior mesenteric artery
2017, 1Q, 32	Peroneal artery to dorsalis pedis artery bypass using saphenous vein graft
2016, 2Q, 18	Femoral-tibial artery bypass and saphenous vein graft
2015, 3Q, 28	Bilateral renal artery bypass

AHA Coding Clinic for table Ø47

2020, 4Q, 50	Intravascular lithotripsy
2019, 4Q, 27	Bifurcation Qualifier
2019, 2Q, 14	Revision of occluded femoral-popliteal bypass graft
2018, 2Q, 24	Coronary artery bifurcation
2016, 4Q, 86	Peripheral artery, number of stents
2016, 4Q, 86-88	Coronary and peripheral artery bifurcation
2016, 3Q, 39	Infrarenal abdominal aortic aneurysm repair with iliac graft extension
2015, 4Q, 4-7, 15	Drug-coated balloon angioplasty in peripheral vessels
2015, 3Q, 9	Aborted endovascular stenting of superficial femoral artery

AHA Coding Clinic for table Ø4C

2021, 1Q, 15	Iliofemoral endarterectomy and furthest point of entry
2019, 4Q, 27	Bifurcation Qualifier
2019, 1Q, 23	Endovascular repair of shaggy aorta and deployment of chimney stent grafts
2018, 2Q, 24	Coronary artery bifurcation
2017, 2Q, 23	Thrombectomy via Fogarty catheter
2016, 4Q, 86-88	Coronary and peripheral artery bifurcation
2016, 1Q, 31	Iliofemoral endarterectomy with patch repair
2015, 1Q, 29	Discontinued carotid endarterectomy
2015, 1Q, 36	Percutaneous mechanical thrombectomy of femoropopliteal bypass graft

AHA Coding Clinic for table Ø4F

2020, 4Q, 45-49	New fragmentation tables
2020, 4Q, 49-50	Intravascular ultrasound assisted thrombolysis
2020, 4Q, 50-51	Intravascular lithotripsy

AHA Coding Clinic for table Ø4H

2019, 3Q, 20	Removal and revision of ECMO component
2019, 1Q, 23	Endovascular repair of shaggy aorta and deployment of chimney stent grafts
2017, 1Q, 30	Insertion of umbilical artery catheter

AHA Coding Clinic for table Ø4L

2020, 3Q, 43	Staged laparoscopic gastric conduit and placement of feeding tube
2018, 2Q, 18	Transverse rectus abdominis myocutaneous (TRAM) delay
2017, 4Q, 31	Resuscitative endovascular balloon occlusion of the aorta
2015, 2Q, 27	Uterine artery embolization using Gelfoam
2014, 3Q, 26	Coil embolization of gastroduodenal artery with chemoembolization of hepatic artery
2014, 1Q, 24	Endovascular embolization for gastrointestinal bleeding

AHA Coding Clinic for table Ø4N

2015, 2Q, 28	Release and replacement of celiac artery

AHA Coding Clinic for table Ø4P

2019, 3Q, 20	Removal and revision of ECMO component

AHA Coding Clinic for table Ø4Q

2014, 1Q, 21	Repair of femoral artery pseudoaneurysm

AHA Coding Clinic for table Ø4R

2019, 1Q, 22	Abdominal aortic aneurysm repair using tube graft
2015, 2Q, 28	Release and replacement of celiac artery

AHA Coding Clinic for table Ø4U

2019, 1Q, 22	Abdominal aortic aneurysm repair using tube graft
2016, 2Q, 18	Femoral-tibial artery bypass and saphenous vein graft
2016, 1Q, 31	Iliofemoral endarterectomy with patch repair
2014, 4Q, 37	Bovine patch arterioplasty
2014, 1Q, 22	Repair of pseudoaneurysm of femoral-popliteal bypass graft

AHA Coding Clinic for table Ø4V

2019, 4Q, 27	Bifurcation Qualifier
2019, 1Q, 22	Abdominal aortic aneurysm repair using tube graft
2018, 2Q, 24	Coronary artery bifurcation
2016, 4Q, 86-87	Coronary and peripheral artery bifurcation
2016, 4Q, 89-93	Branched and fenestrated endograft repair of aneurysms
2016, 3Q, 39	Infrarenal abdominal aortic aneurysm repair with iliac graft extension
2014, 1Q, 9	Endovascular repair of abdominal aortic aneurysm

AHA Coding Clinic for table Ø4W

2020, 3Q, 5	Types of endoleaks following endovascular aneurysm repair
2019, 2Q, 14	Revision of occluded femoral-popliteal bypass graft
2015, 1Q, 36	Revision of femoropopliteal bypass graft
2014, 1Q, 9	Endovascular repair of endoleak
2014, 1Q, 22	Repair of pseudoaneurysm of femoral-popliteal bypass graft

Lower Arteries

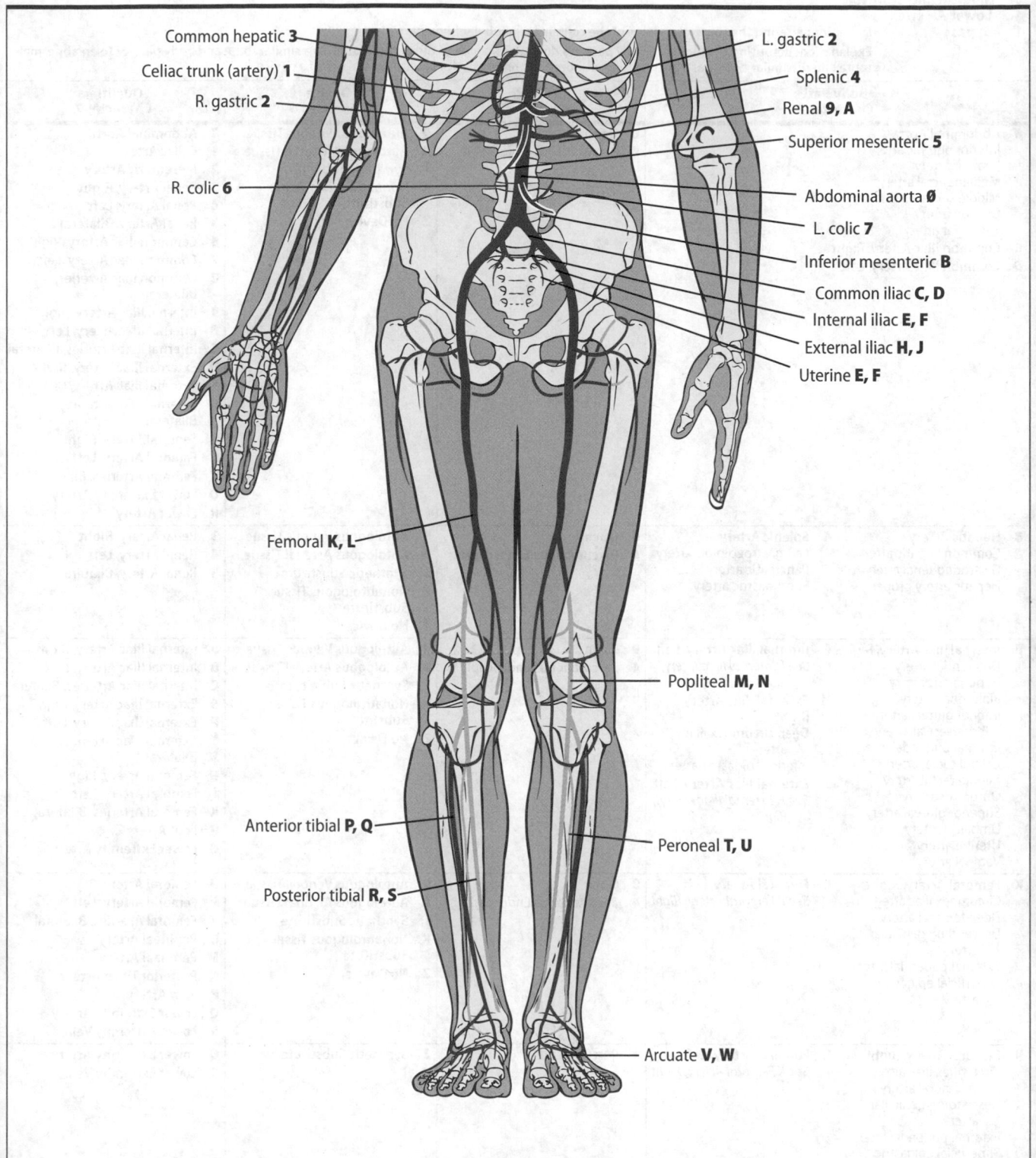

Common hepatic **3**
Celiac trunk (artery) **1**
R. gastric **2**
R. colic **6**

L. gastric **2**
Splenic **4**
Renal **9, A**
Superior mesenteric **5**
Abdominal aorta **Ø**
L. colic **7**
Inferior mesenteric **B**
Common iliac **C, D**
Internal iliac **E, F**
External iliac **H, J**
Uterine **E, F**

Femoral **K, L**

Popliteal **M, N**

Anterior tibial **P, Q**
Peroneal **T, U**
Posterior tibial **R, S**

Arcuate **V, W**

Lower Arteries

Ø   Medical and Surgical
4   Lower Arteries
1   Bypass   Definition: Altering the route of passage of the contents of a tubular body part

Explanation: Rerouting contents of a body part to a downstream area of the normal route, to a similar route and body part, or to an abnormal route and dissimilar body part. Includes one or more anastomoses, with or without the use of a device.

Body Part Character 4	Approach Character 5	Device Character 6	Qualifier Character 7

Ø Abdominal Aorta
   Inferior phrenic artery
   Lumbar artery
   Median sacral artery
   Middle suprarenal artery
   Ovarian artery
   Testicular artery
C Common Iliac Artery, Right
D Common Iliac Artery, Left
	Ø Open
	4 Percutaneous Endoscopic
		9 Autologous Venous Tissue
		A Autologous Arterial Tissue
		J Synthetic Substitute
		K Nonautologous Tissue Substitute
		Z No Device
			Ø Abdominal Aorta
			1 Celiac Artery
			2 Mesenteric Artery
			3 Renal Artery, Right
			4 Renal Artery, Left
			5 Renal Artery, Bilateral
			6 Common Iliac Artery, Right
			7 Common Iliac Artery, Left
			8 Common Iliac Arteries, Bilateral
			9 Internal Iliac Artery, Right
			B Internal Iliac Artery, Left
			C Internal Iliac Arteries, Bilateral
			D External Iliac Artery, Right
			F External Iliac Artery, Left
			G External Iliac Arteries, Bilateral
			H Femoral Artery, Right
			J Femoral Artery, Left
			K Femoral Arteries, Bilateral
			Q Lower Extremity Artery
			R Lower Artery

3 Hepatic Artery
   Common hepatic artery
   Gastroduodenal artery
   Hepatic artery proper
4 Splenic Artery
   Left gastroepiploic artery
   Pancreatic artery
   Short gastric artery
	Ø Open
	4 Percutaneous Endoscopic
		9 Autologous Venous Tissue
		A Autologous Arterial Tissue
		J Synthetic Substitute
		K Nonautologous Tissue Substitute
		Z No Device
			3 Renal Artery, Right
			4 Renal Artery, Left
			5 Renal Artery, Bilateral

E Internal Iliac Artery, Right
   Deferential artery
   Hypogastric artery
   Iliolumbar artery
   Inferior gluteal artery
   Inferior vesical artery
   Internal pudendal artery
   Lateral sacral artery
   Middle rectal artery
   Obturator artery
   Superior gluteal artery
   Umbilical artery
   Uterine artery
   Vaginal artery
F Internal Iliac Artery, Left
   See E Internal Iliac Artery, Right
H External Iliac Artery, Right
   Deep circumflex iliac artery
   Inferior epigastric artery
J External Iliac Artery, Left
   See H External Iliac Artery, Right
	Ø Open
	4 Percutaneous Endoscopic
		9 Autologous Venous Tissue
		A Autologous Arterial Tissue
		J Synthetic Substitute
		K Nonautologous Tissue Substitute
		Z No Device
			9 Internal Iliac Artery, Right
			B Internal Iliac Artery, Left
			C Internal Iliac Arteries, Bilateral
			D External Iliac Artery, Right
			F External Iliac Artery, Left
			G External Iliac Arteries, Bilateral
			H Femoral Artery, Right
			J Femoral Artery, Left
			K Femoral Arteries, Bilateral
			P Foot Artery
			Q Lower Extremity Artery

K Femoral Artery, Right
   Circumflex iliac artery
   Deep femoral artery
   Descending genicular artery
   External pudendal artery
   Superficial epigastric artery
L Femoral Artery, Left
   See K Femoral Artery, Right
	Ø Open
	4 Percutaneous Endoscopic
		9 Autologous Venous Tissue
		A Autologous Arterial Tissue
		J Synthetic Substitute
		K Nonautologous Tissue Substitute
		Z No Device
			H Femoral Artery, Right
			J Femoral Artery, Left
			K Femoral Arteries, Bilateral
			L Popliteal Artery
			M Peroneal Artery
			N Posterior Tibial Artery
			P Foot Artery
			Q Lower Extremity Artery
			S Lower Extremity Vein

K Femoral Artery, Right
   Circumflex iliac artery
   Deep femoral artery
   Descending genicular artery
   External pudendal artery
   Superficial epigastric artery
L Femoral Artery, Left
   See K Femoral Artery, Right
	3 Percutaneous	**J Synthetic Substitute**	**Q Lower Extremity Artery**
			S Lower Extremity Vein

M Popliteal Artery, Right
   Inferior genicular artery
   Middle genicular artery
   Superior genicular artery
   Sural artery
   Tibioperoneal trunk
N Popliteal Artery, Left
   See M Popliteal Artery, Right
	Ø Open
	4 Percutaneous Endoscopic
		9 Autologous Venous Tissue
		A Autologous Arterial Tissue
		J Synthetic Substitute
		K Nonautologous Tissue Substitute
		Z No Device
			L Popliteal Artery
			M Peroneal Artery
			P Foot Artery
			Q Lower Extremity Artery
			S Lower Extremity Vein

Ø41 Continued on next page

Ø Medical and Surgical
4 Lower Arteries
1 Bypass

041 Continued

Definition: Altering the route of passage of the contents of a tubular body part

Explanation: Rerouting contents of a body part to a downstream area of the normal route, to a similar route and body part, or to an abnormal route and dissimilar body part. Includes one or more anastomoses, with or without the use of a device.

Body Part Character 4		Approach Character 5	Device Character 6	Qualifier Character 7
M Popliteal Artery, Right Inferior genicular artery Middle genicular artery Superior genicular artery Sural artery Tibioperoneal trunk	**N Popliteal Artery, Left** *See M Popliteal Artery, Right*	**3** Percutaneous	**J** Synthetic Substitute	**Q** Lower Extremity Artery **S** Lower Extremity Vein
P Anterior Tibial Artery, Right Anterior lateral malleolar artery Anterior medial malleolar artery Anterior tibial recurrent artery Dorsalis pedis artery Posterior tibial recurrent artery	**Q Anterior Tibial Artery, Left** *See P Anterior Tibial Artery, Right* **R Posterior Tibial Artery, Right** **S Posterior Tibial Artery, Left**	**Ø** Open **3** Percutaneous **4** Percutaneous Endoscopic	**J** Synthetic Substitute	**Q** Lower Extremity Artery **S** Lower Extremity Vein
T Peroneal Artery, Right Fibular artery **U Peroneal Artery, Left** *See T Peroneal Artery, Right*	**V Foot Artery, Right** Arcuate artery Dorsal metatarsal artery Lateral plantar artery Lateral tarsal artery Medial plantar artery **W Foot Artery, Left** *See V Foot Artery, Right*	**Ø** Open **4** Percutaneous Endoscopic	**9** Autologous Venous Tissue **A** Autologous Arterial Tissue **J** Synthetic Substitute **K** Nonautologous Tissue Substitute **Z** No Device	**P** Foot Artery **Q** Lower Extremity Artery **S** Lower Extremity Vein
T Peroneal Artery, Right Fibular artery **U Peroneal Artery, Left** *See T Peroneal Artery, Right*	**V Foot Artery, Right** Arcuate artery Dorsal metatarsal artery Lateral plantar artery Lateral tarsal artery Medial plantar artery **W Foot Artery, Left** *See V Foot Artery, Right*	**3** Percutaneous	**J** Synthetic Substitute	**Q** Lower Extremity Artery **S** Lower Extremity Vein

NC Noncovered Procedure   LC Limited Coverage   QA Questionable OB Admit   NT New Tech Add-on   ⊞ Combination Member   ♂Male   ♀Female

ICD-10-PCS 2022   223

041–041

0   **Medical and Surgical**
4   **Lower Arteries**
5   **Destruction**   Definition: Physical eradication of all or a portion of a body part by the direct use of energy, force, or a destructive agent

                                Explanation: None of the body part is physically taken out

Body Part Character 4		Approach Character 5	Device Character 6	Qualifier Character 7

0   **Abdominal Aorta**
     Inferior phrenic artery
     Lumbar artery
     Median sacral artery
     Middle suprarenal artery
     Ovarian artery
     Testicular artery
1   **Celiac Artery**
     Celiac trunk
2   **Gastric Artery**
     Left gastric artery
     Right gastric artery
3   **Hepatic Artery**
     Common hepatic artery
     Gastroduodenal artery
     Hepatic artery proper
4   **Splenic Artery**
     Left gastroepiploic artery
     Pancreatic artery
     Short gastric artery
5   **Superior Mesenteric Artery**
     Ileal artery
     Ileocolic artery
     Inferior pancreaticoduodenal
       artery
     Jejunal artery
6   **Colic Artery, Right**
7   **Colic Artery, Left**
8   **Colic Artery, Middle**
9   **Renal Artery, Right**
     Inferior suprarenal artery
     Renal segmental artery
A   **Renal Artery, Left**
     See 9 Renal Artery, Right
B   **Inferior Mesenteric Artery**
     Sigmoid artery
     Superior rectal artery
C   **Common Iliac Artery, Right**
D   **Common Iliac Artery, Left**
E   **Internal Iliac Artery, Right**
     Deferential artery
     Hypogastric artery
     Iliolumbar artery
     Inferior gluteal artery
     Inferior vesical artery
     Internal pudendal artery
     Lateral sacral artery
     Middle rectal artery
     Obturator artery
     Superior gluteal artery
     Umbilical artery
     Uterine artery
     Vaginal artery
	F **Internal Iliac Artery, Left**
	     See E Internal Iliac Artery, Right
	H **External Iliac Artery, Right**
	     Deep circumflex iliac artery
	     Inferior epigastric artery
	J **External Iliac Artery, Left**
	     See H External Iliac Artery, Right
	K **Femoral Artery, Right**
	     Circumflex iliac artery
	     Deep femoral artery
	     Descending genicular artery
	     External pudendal artery
	     Superficial epigastric artery
	L **Femoral Artery, Left**
	     See K Femoral Artery, Right
	M **Popliteal Artery, Right**
	     Inferior genicular artery
	     Middle genicular artery
	     Superior genicular artery
	     Sural artery
	     Tibioperoneal trunk
	N **Popliteal Artery, Left**
	     See M Popliteal Artery, Right
	P **Anterior Tibial Artery, Right**
	     Anterior lateral malleolar
	       artery
	     Anterior medial malleolar
	       artery
	     Anterior tibial recurrent artery
	     Dorsalis pedis artery
	     Posterior tibial recurrent artery
	Q **Anterior Tibial Artery, Left**
	     See P Anterior Tibial Artery,
	       Right
	R **Posterior Tibial Artery, Right**
	S **Posterior Tibial Artery, Left**
	T **Peroneal Artery, Right**
	     Fibular artery
	U **Peroneal Artery, Left**
	     See T Peroneal Artery, Right
	V **Foot Artery, Right**
	     Arcuate artery
	     Dorsal metatarsal artery
	     Lateral plantar artery
	     Lateral tarsal artery
	     Medial plantar artery
	W **Foot Artery, Left**
	     See V Foot Artery, Right
	Y **Lower Artery**
	     Umbilical artery
		0 Open
		3 Percutaneous
		4 Percutaneous Endoscopic
			Z No Device	**Z** No Qualifier

Ø   Medical and Surgical
4   Lower Arteries
7   Dilation   Definition: Expanding an orifice or the lumen of a tubular body part

Explanation: The orifice can be a natural orifice or an artificially created orifice. Accomplished by stretching a tubular body part using intraluminal pressure or by cutting part of the orifice or wall of the tubular body part.

Body Part Character 4		Approach Character 5	Device Character 6	Qualifier Character 7
Ø Abdominal Aorta Inferior phrenic artery Lumbar artery Median sacral artery Middle suprarenal artery Ovarian artery Testicular artery **1 Celiac Artery** Celiac trunk **2 Gastric Artery** Left gastric artery Right gastric artery **3 Hepatic Artery** Common hepatic artery Gastroduodenal artery Hepatic artery proper **4 Splenic Artery** Left gastroepiploic artery Pancreatic artery Short gastric artery **5 Superior Mesenteric Artery** Ileal artery Ileocolic artery Inferior pancreaticoduodenal artery Jejunal artery **6 Colic Artery, Right** **7 Colic Artery, Left** **8 Colic Artery, Middle** **9 Renal Artery, Right** Inferior suprarenal artery Renal segmental artery **A Renal Artery, Left** *See 9 Renal Artery, Right* **B Inferior Mesenteric Artery** Sigmoid artery Superior rectal artery **C Common Iliac Artery, Right** **D Common Iliac Artery, Left** **E Internal Iliac Artery, Right** Deferential artery Hypogastric artery Iliolumbar artery Inferior gluteal artery Inferior vesical artery Internal pudendal artery Lateral sacral artery Middle rectal artery Obturator artery Superior gluteal artery Umbilical artery Uterine artery Vaginal artery	**F Internal Iliac Artery, Left** *See E Internal Iliac Artery, Right* **H External Iliac Artery, Right** Deep circumflex iliac artery Inferior epigastric artery **J External Iliac Artery, Left** *See H External Iliac Artery, Right* **K Femoral Artery, Right** Circumflex iliac artery Deep femoral artery Descending genicular artery External pudendal artery Superficial epigastric artery **L Femoral Artery, Left** *See K Femoral Artery, Right* **M Popliteal Artery, Right** Inferior genicular artery Middle genicular artery Superior genicular artery Sural artery Tibioperoneal trunk **N Popliteal Artery, Left** *See M Popliteal Artery, Right* **P Anterior Tibial Artery, Right** Anterior lateral malleolar artery Anterior medial malleolar artery Anterior tibial recurrent artery Dorsalis pedis artery Posterior tibial recurrent artery **Q Anterior Tibial Artery, Left** *See P Anterior Tibial Artery, Right* **R Posterior Tibial Artery, Right** **S Posterior Tibial Artery, Left** **T Peroneal Artery, Right** Fibular artery **U Peroneal Artery, Left** *See T Peroneal Artery, Right* **V Foot Artery, Right** Arcuate artery Dorsal metatarsal artery Lateral plantar artery Lateral tarsal artery Medial plantar artery **W Foot Artery, Left** *See V Foot Artery, Right* **Y Lower Artery** Umbilical artery	**Ø** Open **3** Percutaneous **4** Percutaneous Endoscopic	**4** Intraluminal Device, Drug-eluting **D** Intraluminal Device **Z** No Device	**1** Drug-Coated Balloon **Z** No Qualifier

Ø47 Continued on next page

NC Noncovered Procedure   **LC** Limited Coverage   **QA** Questionable OB Admit   **NT** New Tech Add-on   ⊞ Combination Member   ♂ Male   ♀ Female

ICD-10-PCS 2022   225

047–047

0   **Medical and Surgical**   *047 Continued*
4   **Lower Arteries**
7   **Dilation**

Definition: Expanding an orifice or the lumen of a tubular body part

Explanation: The orifice can be a natural orifice or an artificially created orifice. Accomplished by stretching a tubular body part using intraluminal pressure or by cutting part of the orifice or wall of the tubular body part.

Body Part Character 4		Approach Character 5	Device Character 6	Qualifier Character 7

0 Abdominal Aorta
  Inferior phrenic artery
  Lumbar artery
  Median sacral artery
  Middle suprarenal artery
  Ovarian artery
  Testicular artery
1 Celiac Artery
  Celiac trunk
2 Gastric Artery
  Left gastric artery
  Right gastric artery
3 Hepatic Artery
  Common hepatic artery
  Gastroduodenal artery
  Hepatic artery proper
4 Splenic Artery
  Left gastroepiploic artery
  Pancreatic artery
  Short gastric artery
5 Superior Mesenteric Artery
  Ileal artery
  Ileocolic artery
  Inferior pancreaticoduodenal
    artery
  Jejunal artery
6 Colic Artery, Right
7 Colic Artery, Left
8 Colic Artery, Middle
9 Renal Artery, Right
  Inferior suprarenal artery
  Renal segmental artery
A Renal Artery, Left
  See 9 Renal Artery, Right
B Inferior Mesenteric Artery
  Sigmoid artery
  Superior rectal artery
C Common Iliac Artery, Right
D Common Iliac Artery, Left
E Internal Iliac Artery, Right
  Deferential artery
  Hypogastric artery
  Iliolumbar artery
  Inferior gluteal artery
  Inferior vesical artery
  Internal pudendal artery
  Lateral sacral artery
  Middle rectal artery
  Obturator artery
  Superior gluteal artery
  Umbilical artery
  Uterine artery
  Vaginal artery
	F Internal Iliac Artery, Left
	  See E Internal Iliac Artery, Right
	H External Iliac Artery, Right
	  Deep circumflex iliac artery
	  Inferior epigastric artery
	J External Iliac Artery, Left
	  See H External Iliac Artery, Right
	K Femoral Artery, Right
	  Circumflex iliac artery
	  Deep femoral artery
	  Descending genicular artery
	  External pudendal artery
	  Superficial epigastric artery
	L Femoral Artery, Left
	  See K Femoral Artery, Right
	M Popliteal Artery, Right
	  Inferior genicular artery
	  Middle genicular artery
	  Superior genicular artery
	  Sural artery
	  Tibioperoneal trunk
	N Popliteal Artery, Left
	  See M Popliteal Artery, Right
	P Anterior Tibial Artery, Right
	  Anterior lateral malleolar
	    artery
	  Anterior medial malleolar
	    artery
	  Anterior tibial recurrent artery
	  Dorsalis pedis artery
	  Posterior tibial recurrent artery
	Q Anterior Tibial Artery, Left
	  *See P Anterior Tibial Artery,
	    Right*
	R Posterior Tibial Artery, Right
	S Posterior Tibial Artery, Left
	T Peroneal Artery, Right
	  Fibular artery
	U Peroneal Artery, Left
	  See T Peroneal Artery, Right
	V Foot Artery, Right
	  Arcuate artery
	  Dorsal metatarsal artery
	  Lateral plantar artery
	  Lateral tarsal artery
	  Medial plantar artery
	W Foot Artery, Left
	  See V Foot Artery, Right
	Y Lower Artery
	  Umbilical artery
		0 Open
		3 Percutaneous
		4 Percutaneous Endoscopic
			5 Intraluminal Device, Drug-
			  eluting, Two
			6 Intraluminal Device, Drug-
			  eluting, Three
			7 Intraluminal Device, Drug-
			  eluting, Four or More
			E Intraluminal Device, Two
			F Intraluminal Device, Three
			G Intraluminal Device, Four
			  or More
				Z No Qualifier

Ø **Medical and Surgical**
4 **Lower Arteries**
9 **Drainage**   Definition: Taking or letting out fluids and/or gases from a body part
                        Explanation: The qualifier DIAGNOSTIC is used to identify drainage procedures that are biopsies

Body Part Character 4		Approach Character 5	Device Character 6	Qualifier Character 7

Ø **Abdominal Aorta**
  Inferior phrenic artery
  Lumbar artery
  Median sacral artery
  Middle suprarenal artery
  Ovarian artery
  Testicular artery
1 **Celiac Artery**
  Celiac trunk
2 **Gastric Artery**
  Left gastric artery
  Right gastric artery
3 **Hepatic Artery**
  Common hepatic artery
  Gastroduodenal artery
  Hepatic artery proper
4 **Splenic Artery**
  Left gastroepiploic artery
  Pancreatic artery
  Short gastric artery
5 **Superior Mesenteric Artery**
  Ileal artery
  Ileocolic artery
  Inferior pancreaticoduodenal
    artery
  Jejunal artery
6 **Colic Artery, Right**
7 **Colic Artery, Left**
8 **Colic Artery, Middle**
9 **Renal Artery, Right**
  Inferior suprarenal artery
  Renal segmental artery
A **Renal Artery, Left**
  See 9 Renal Artery, Right
B **Inferior Mesenteric Artery**
  Sigmoid artery
  Superior rectal artery
C **Common Iliac Artery, Right**
D **Common Iliac Artery, Left**
E **Internal Iliac Artery, Right**
  Deferential artery
  Hypogastric artery
  Iliolumbar artery
  Inferior gluteal artery
  Inferior vesical artery
  Internal pudendal artery
  Lateral sacral artery
  Middle rectal artery
  Obturator artery
  Superior gluteal artery
  Umbilical artery
  Uterine artery
  Vaginal artery
	F **Internal Iliac Artery, Left**
	  See E Internal Iliac Artery, Right
	H **External Iliac Artery, Right**
	  Deep circumflex iliac artery
	  Inferior epigastric artery
	J **External Iliac Artery, Left**
	  See H External Iliac Artery, Right
	K **Femoral Artery, Right**
	  Circumflex iliac artery
	  Deep femoral artery
	  Descending genicular artery
	  External pudendal artery
	  Superficial epigastric artery
	L **Femoral Artery, Left**
	  See K Femoral Artery, Right
	M **Popliteal Artery, Right**
	  Inferior genicular artery
	  Middle genicular artery
	  Superior genicular artery
	  Sural artery
	  Tibioperoneal trunk
	N **Popliteal Artery, Left**
	  See M Popliteal Artery, Right
	P **Anterior Tibial Artery, Right**
	  Anterior lateral malleolar
	    artery
	  Anterior medial malleolar
	    artery
	  Anterior tibial recurrent artery
	  Dorsalis pedis artery
	  Posterior tibial recurrent artery
	Q **Anterior Tibial Artery, Left**
	  See P Anterior Tibial Artery,
	    Right
	R **Posterior Tibial Artery, Right**
	S **Posterior Tibial Artery, Left**
	T **Peroneal Artery, Right**
	  Fibular artery
	U **Peroneal Artery, Left**
	  See T Peroneal Artery, Right
	V **Foot Artery, Right**
	  Arcuate artery
	  Dorsal metatarsal artery
	  Lateral plantar artery
	  Lateral tarsal artery
	  Medial plantar artery
	W **Foot Artery, Left**
	  See V Foot Artery, Right
	Y **Lower Artery**
	  Umbilical artery
		Ø Open
		3 Percutaneous
		4 Percutaneous Endoscopic
			Ø Drainage Device	Z No Qualifier

Non-OR   Ø49[Ø,1,2,3,4,5,6,7,8,9,A,B,C,D,E,F,H,J,K,L,M,N,P,Q,R,S,T,U,V,W,Y][Ø,3,4]ØZ

Ø49 Continued on next page

NC Noncovered Procedure   LC Limited Coverage   QA Questionable OB Admit   NT New Tech Add-on   ⊞ Combination Member   ♂ Male   ♀ Female

Lower Arteries

Ø Medical and Surgical
4 Lower Arteries
9 Drainage

Ø49 Continued

Definition: Taking or letting out fluids and/or gases from a body part
Explanation: The qualifier DIAGNOSTIC is used to identify drainage procedures that are biopsies

Body Part Character 4		Approach Character 5	Device Character 6	Qualifier Character 7

Ø **Abdominal Aorta**
  Inferior phrenic artery
  Lumbar artery
  Median sacral artery
  Middle suprarenal artery
  Ovarian artery
  Testicular artery
1 **Celiac Artery**
  Celiac trunk
2 **Gastric Artery**
  Left gastric artery
  Right gastric artery
3 **Hepatic Artery**
  Common hepatic artery
  Gastroduodenal artery
  Hepatic artery proper
4 **Splenic Artery**
  Left gastroepiploic artery
  Pancreatic artery
  Short gastric artery
5 **Superior Mesenteric Artery**
  Ileal artery
  Ileocolic artery
  Inferior pancreaticoduodenal
    artery
  Jejunal artery
6 **Colic Artery, Right**
7 **Colic Artery, Left**
8 **Colic Artery, Middle**
9 **Renal Artery, Right**
  Inferior suprarenal artery
  Renal segmental artery
A **Renal Artery, Left**
  See 9 Renal Artery, Right
B **Inferior Mesenteric Artery**
  Sigmoid artery
  Superior rectal artery
C **Common Iliac Artery, Right**
D **Common Iliac Artery, Left**
E **Internal Iliac Artery, Right**
  Deferential artery
  Hypogastric artery
  Iliolumbar artery
  Inferior gluteal artery
  Inferior vesical artery
  Internal pudendal artery
  Lateral sacral artery
  Middle rectal artery
  Obturator artery
  Superior gluteal artery
  Umbilical artery
  Uterine artery
  Vaginal artery
	F **Internal Iliac Artery, Left**
	  See E Internal Iliac Artery, Right
	H **External Iliac Artery, Right**
	  Deep circumflex iliac artery
	  Inferior epigastric artery
	J **External Iliac Artery, Left**
	  See H External Iliac Artery, Right
	K **Femoral Artery, Right**
	  Circumflex iliac artery
	  Deep femoral artery
	  Descending genicular artery
	  External pudendal artery
	  Superficial epigastric artery
	L **Femoral Artery, Left**
	  See K Femoral Artery, Right
	M **Popliteal Artery, Right**
	  Inferior genicular artery
	  Middle genicular artery
	  Superior genicular artery
	  Sural artery
	  Tibioperoneal trunk
	N **Popliteal Artery, Left**
	  See M Popliteal Artery, Right
	P **Anterior Tibial Artery, Right**
	  Anterior lateral malleolar
	    artery
	  Anterior medial malleolar
	    artery
	  Anterior tibial recurrent artery
	  Dorsalis pedis artery
	  Posterior tibial recurrent artery
	Q **Anterior Tibial Artery, Left**
	  *See P Anterior Tibial Artery,
	    Right*
	R **Posterior Tibial Artery, Right**
	S **Posterior Tibial Artery, Left**
	T **Peroneal Artery, Right**
	  Fibular artery
	U **Peroneal Artery, Left**
	  See T Peroneal Artery, Right
	V **Foot Artery, Right**
	  Arcuate artery
	  Dorsal metatarsal artery
	  Lateral plantar artery
	  Lateral tarsal artery
	  Medial plantar artery
	W **Foot Artery, Left**
	  See V Foot Artery, Right
	Y **Lower Artery**
	  Umbilical artery
		Ø Open
		3 Percutaneous
		4 Percutaneous Endoscopic
			Z No Device	X Diagnostic
				Z No Qualifier

Non-OR Ø49[Ø,1,2,3,4,5,6,7,8,9,A,B,C,D,E,F,H,J,K,L,M,N,P,Q,R,S,T,U,V,W,Y]3ZX
Non-OR Ø49[Ø,1,2,3,4,5,6,7,8,9,A,B,C,D,E,F,H,J,K,L,M,N,P,Q,R,S,T,U,V,W,Y][Ø,3,4]ZZ

Ø **Medical and Surgical**
4 **Lower Arteries**
B **Excision**   Definition: Cutting out or off, without replacement, a portion of a body part
     Explanation: The qualifier DIAGNOSTIC is used to identify excision procedures that are biopsies

Body Part — Character 4		Approach — Character 5	Device — Character 6	Qualifier — Character 7
Ø Abdominal Aorta Inferior phrenic artery Lumbar artery Median sacral artery Middle suprarenal artery Ovarian artery Testicular artery **1 Celiac Artery** Celiac trunk **2 Gastric Artery** Left gastric artery Right gastric artery **3 Hepatic Artery** Common hepatic artery Gastroduodenal artery Hepatic artery proper **4 Splenic Artery** Left gastroepiploic artery Pancreatic artery Short gastric artery **5 Superior Mesenteric Artery** Ileal artery Ileocolic artery Inferior pancreaticoduodenal artery Jejunal artery **6 Colic Artery, Right** **7 Colic Artery, Left** **8 Colic Artery, Middle** **9 Renal Artery, Right** Inferior suprarenal artery Renal segmental artery **A Renal Artery, Left** *See 9 Renal Artery, Right* **B Inferior Mesenteric Artery** Sigmoid artery Superior rectal artery **C Common Iliac Artery, Right** **D Common Iliac Artery, Left** **E Internal Iliac Artery, Right** Deferential artery Hypogastric artery Iliolumbar artery Inferior gluteal artery Inferior vesical artery Internal pudendal artery Lateral sacral artery Middle rectal artery Obturator artery Superior gluteal artery Umbilical artery Uterine artery Vaginal artery	**F Internal Iliac Artery, Left** *See E Internal Iliac Artery, Right* **H External Iliac Artery, Right** Deep circumflex iliac artery Inferior epigastric artery **J External Iliac Artery, Left** *See H External Iliac Artery, Right* **K Femoral Artery, Right** Circumflex iliac artery Deep femoral artery Descending genicular artery External pudendal artery Superficial epigastric artery **L Femoral Artery, Left** *See K Femoral Artery, Right* **M Popliteal Artery, Right** Inferior genicular artery Middle genicular artery Superior genicular artery Sural artery Tibioperoneal trunk **N Popliteal Artery, Left** *See M Popliteal Artery, Right* **P Anterior Tibial Artery, Right** Anterior lateral malleolar artery Anterior medial malleolar artery Anterior tibial recurrent artery Dorsalis pedis artery Posterior tibial recurrent artery **Q Anterior Tibial Artery, Left** *See P Anterior Tibial Artery, Right* **R Posterior Tibial Artery, Right** **S Posterior Tibial Artery, Left** **T Peroneal Artery, Right** Fibular artery **U Peroneal Artery, Left** *See T Peroneal Artery, Right* **V Foot Artery, Right** Arcuate artery Dorsal metatarsal artery Lateral plantar artery Lateral tarsal artery Medial plantar artery **W Foot Artery, Left** *See V Foot Artery, Right* **Y Lower Artery** Umbilical artery	**Ø Open** **3 Percutaneous** **4 Percutaneous Endoscopic**	**Z No Device**	**X Diagnostic** **Z No Qualifier**

NC Noncovered Procedure · LC Limited Coverage · QA Questionable OB Admit · NT New Tech Add-on · ⊞ Combination Member · ♂Male · ♀Female

ICD-10-PCS 2022 · 04B–04B · 229

Lower Arteries

0   **Medical and Surgical**
4   **Lower Arteries**
C   **Extirpation**   Definition: Taking or cutting out solid matter from a body part

Explanation: The solid matter may be an abnormal byproduct of a biological function or a foreign body; it may be imbedded in a body part or in the lumen of a tubular body part. The solid matter may or may not have been previously broken into pieces.

Body Part Character 4		Approach Character 5	Device Character 6	Qualifier Character 7

0 **Abdominal Aorta**
   Inferior phrenic artery
   Lumbar artery
   Median sacral artery
   Middle suprarenal artery
   Ovarian artery
   Testicular artery
1 **Celiac Artery**
   Celiac trunk
2 **Gastric Artery**
   Left gastric artery
   Right gastric artery
3 **Hepatic Artery**
   Common hepatic artery
   Gastroduodenal artery
   Hepatic artery proper
4 **Splenic Artery**
   Left gastroepiploic artery
   Pancreatic artery
   Short gastric artery
5 **Superior Mesenteric Artery**
   Ileal artery
   Ileocolic artery
   Inferior pancreaticoduodenal
     artery
   Jejunal artery
6 **Colic Artery, Right**
7 **Colic Artery, Left**
8 **Colic Artery, Middle**
9 **Renal Artery, Right**
   Inferior suprarenal artery
   Renal segmental artery
A **Renal Artery, Left**
   See 9 Renal Artery, Right
B **Inferior Mesenteric Artery**
   Sigmoid artery
   Superior rectal artery
C **Common Iliac Artery, Right**
D **Common Iliac Artery, Left**
E **Internal Iliac Artery, Right**
   Deferential artery
   Hypogastric artery
   Iliolumbar artery
   Inferior gluteal artery
   Inferior vesical artery
   Internal pudendal artery
   Lateral sacral artery
   Middle rectal artery
   Obturator artery
   Superior gluteal artery
   Umbilical artery
   Uterine artery
   Vaginal artery
	F **Internal Iliac Artery, Left**
	   See E Internal Iliac Artery, Right
	H **External Iliac Artery, Right**
	   Deep circumflex iliac artery
	   Inferior epigastric artery
	J **External Iliac Artery, Left**
	   See H External Iliac Artery, Right
	K **Femoral Artery, Right**
	   Circumflex iliac artery
	   Deep femoral artery
	   Descending genicular artery
	   External pudendal artery
	   Superficial epigastric artery
	L **Femoral Artery, Left**
	   See K Femoral Artery, Right
	M **Popliteal Artery, Right**
	   Inferior genicular artery
	   Middle genicular artery
	   Superior genicular artery
	   Sural artery
	   Tibioperoneal trunk
	N **Popliteal Artery, Left**
	   See M Popliteal Artery, Right
	P **Anterior Tibial Artery, Right**
	   Anterior lateral malleolar artery
	   Anterior medial malleolar artery
	   Anterior tibial recurrent artery
	   Dorsalis pedis artery
	   Posterior tibial recurrent artery
	Q **Anterior Tibial Artery, Left**
	   See P Anterior Tibial Artery,
	    Right
	R **Posterior Tibial Artery, Right**
	S **Posterior Tibial Artery, Left**
	T **Peroneal Artery, Right**
	   Fibular artery
	U **Peroneal Artery, Left**
	   See T Peroneal Artery, Right
	V **Foot Artery, Right**
	   Arcuate artery
	   Dorsal metatarsal artery
	   Lateral plantar artery
	   Lateral tarsal artery
	   Medial plantar artery
	W **Foot Artery, Left**
	   See V Foot Artery, Right
	Y **Lower Artery**
	   Umbilical artery
		0 Open
		3 Percutaneous
		4 Percutaneous Endoscopic
			Z No Device	**Z** No Qualifier

Ø Medical and Surgical
4 Lower Arteries
F Fragmentation Definition: Breaking solid matter in a body part into pieces
　　　　　　　　　　Explanation: Physical force (e.g., manual, ultrasonic) applied directly or indirectly is used to break the solid matter into pieces. The solid matter may be an abnormal byproduct of a biological function or a foreign body. The pieces of solid matter are not taken out.

Body Part Character 4	Approach Character 5	Device Character 6	Qualifier Character 7
C Common Iliac Artery, Right	**3 Percutaneous**	**Z No Device**	**Ø Ultrasonic**
D Common Iliac Artery, Left			**Z No Qualifier**
E Internal Iliac Artery, Right Deferential artery Hypogastric artery Iliolumbar artery Inferior gluteal artery Inferior vesical artery Internal pudendal artery Lateral sacral artery Middle rectal artery Obturator artery Superior gluteal artery Umbilical artery Uterine artery Vaginal artery			
F Internal Iliac Artery, Left *See* E Internal Iliac Artery, Right			
H External Iliac Artery, Right Deep circumflex iliac artery Inferior epigastric artery			
J External Iliac Artery, Left *See* H External Iliac Artery, Right			
K Femoral Artery, Right Circumflex iliac artery Deep femoral artery Descending genicular artery External pudendal artery Superficial epigastric artery			
L Femoral Artery, Left *See* K Femoral Artery, Right			
M Popliteal Artery, Right Inferior genicular artery Middle genicular artery Superior genicular artery Sural artery Tibioperoneal trunk			
N Popliteal Artery, Left *See* M Popliteal Artery, Right			
P Anterior Tibial Artery, Right Anterior lateral malleolar artery Anterior medial malleolar artery Anterior tibial recurrent artery Dorsalis pedis artery Posterior tibial recurrent artery			
Q Anterior Tibial Artery, Left *See* P Anterior Tibial Artery, Right			
R Posterior Tibial Artery, Right			
S Posterior Tibial Artery, Left			
T Peroneal Artery, Right Fibular artery			
U Peroneal Artery, Left *See* T Peroneal Artery, Right			
Y Lower Artery Umbilical artery			

Lower Arteries

Ø **Medical and Surgical**
4 **Lower Arteries**
H **Insertion**

Definition: Putting in a nonbiological appliance that monitors, assists, performs, or prevents a physiological function but does not physically take the place of a body part
Explanation: None

Body Part Character 4		Approach Character 5	Device Character 6	Qualifier Character 7
Ø **Abdominal Aorta** Inferior phrenic artery Lumbar artery Median sacral artery Middle suprarenal artery Ovarian artery Testicular artery		**Ø** Open **3** Percutaneous **4** Percutaneous Endoscopic	**2** Monitoring Device **3** Infusion Device **D** Intraluminal Device	**Z** No Qualifier

1 **Celiac Artery**
Celiac trunk
2 **Gastric Artery**
Left gastric artery
Right gastric artery
3 **Hepatic Artery**
Common hepatic artery
Gastroduodenal artery
Hepatic artery proper
4 **Splenic Artery**
Left gastroepiploic artery
Pancreatic artery
Short gastric artery
5 **Superior Mesenteric Artery**
Ileal artery
Ileocolic artery
Inferior pancreaticoduodenal
    artery
Jejunal artery
6 **Colic Artery, Right**
7 **Colic Artery, Left**
8 **Colic Artery, Middle**
9 **Renal Artery, Right**
Inferior suprarenal artery
Renal segmental artery
A **Renal Artery, Left**
See 9 Renal Artery, Right
B **Inferior Mesenteric Artery**
Sigmoid artery
Superior rectal artery
C **Common Iliac Artery, Right**
D **Common Iliac Artery, Left**
E **Internal Iliac Artery, Right**
Deferential artery
Hypogastric artery
Iliolumbar artery
Inferior gluteal artery
Inferior vesical artery
Internal pudendal artery
Lateral sacral artery
Middle rectal artery
Obturator artery
Superior gluteal artery
Umbilical artery
Uterine artery
Vaginal artery
	F **Internal Iliac Artery, Left**
	See E Internal Iliac Artery, Right
	H **External Iliac Artery, Right**
	Deep circumflex iliac artery
	Inferior epigastric artery
	J **External Iliac Artery, Left**
	See H External Iliac Artery, Right
	K **Femoral Artery, Right**
	Circumflex iliac artery
	Deep femoral artery
	Descending genicular artery
	External pudendal artery
	Superficial epigastric artery
	L **Femoral Artery, Left**
	See K Femoral Artery, Right
	M **Popliteal Artery, Right**
	Inferior genicular artery
	Middle genicular artery
	Superior genicular artery
	Sural artery
	Tibioperoneal trunk
	N **Popliteal Artery, Left**
	See M Popliteal Artery, Right
	P **Anterior Tibial Artery, Right**
	Anterior lateral malleolar artery
	Anterior medial malleolar artery
	Anterior tibial recurrent artery
	Dorsalis pedis artery
	Posterior tibial recurrent artery
	Q **Anterior Tibial Artery, Left**
	See P Anterior Tibial Artery,
	    Right
	R **Posterior Tibial Artery, Right**
	S **Posterior Tibial Artery, Left**
	T **Peroneal Artery, Right**
	Fibular artery
	U **Peroneal Artery, Left**
	See T Peroneal Artery, Right
	V **Foot Artery, Right**
	Arcuate artery
	Dorsal metatarsal artery
	Lateral plantar artery
	Lateral tarsal artery
	Medial plantar artery
	W **Foot Artery, Left**
	See V Foot Artery, Right
		Ø Open
		3 Percutaneous
		4 Percutaneous Endoscopic
			3 Infusion Device
			D Intraluminal Device
				Z No Qualifier

Y **Lower Artery** Umbilical artery		**Ø** Open **3** Percutaneous **4** Percutaneous Endoscopic	**2** Monitoring Device **3** Infusion Device **D** Intraluminal Device **Y** Other Device	**Z** No Qualifier

Non-OR   Ø4HØ[Ø,3,4][2,3]Z
Non-OR   Ø4H[1,2,3,4,5,6,7,8,9,A,B,C,D,E,F,H,J,K,L,M,N,P,Q,R,S,T,U,V,W][Ø,3,4]3Z
Non-OR   Ø4HY32Z
Non-OR   Ø4HY[Ø,3,4]3Z
Non-OR   Ø4HY[3,4]YZ

Ø   **Medical and Surgical**
4   **Lower Arteries**
J   **Inspection**   Definition: Visually and/or manually exploring a body part

Explanation: Visual exploration may be performed with or without optical instrumentation. Manual exploration may be performed directly or through intervening body layers.

Body Part Character 4	Approach Character 5	Device Character 6	Qualifier Character 7
Y Lower Artery Umbilical artery	**Ø** Open **3** Percutaneous **4** Percutaneous Endoscopic **X** External	**Z** No Device	**Z** No Qualifier

Non-OR   Ø4JY[3,4,X]ZZ

Ø   **Medical and Surgical**
4   **Lower Arteries**
L   **Occlusion**   Definition: Completely closing an orifice or the lumen of a tubular body part

Explanation: The orifice can be a natural orifice or an artificially created orifice

Body Part Character 4	Approach Character 5	Device Character 6	Qualifier Character 7

Ø   Abdominal Aorta
     Inferior phrenic artery
     Lumbar artery
     Median sacral artery
     Middle suprarenal artery
     Ovarian artery
     Testicular artery
	Ø Open
	4 Percutaneous Endoscopic
		C Extraluminal Device
		D Intraluminal Device
		Z No Device
			Z No Qualifier

Ø   Abdominal Aorta
     Inferior phrenic artery
     Lumbar artery
     Median sacral artery
     Middle suprarenal artery
     Ovarian artery
     Testicular artery
	3 Percutaneous	**C** Extraluminal Device
		Z No Device
			Z No Qualifier

Ø   Abdominal Aorta
     Inferior phrenic artery
     Lumbar artery
     Median sacral artery
     Middle suprarenal artery
     Ovarian artery
     Testicular artery
	3 Percutaneous	**D** Intraluminal Device	**J** Temporary
			Z No Qualifier

Ø4L Continued on next page

Lower Arteries (side tab)

Ø   Medical and Surgical
4   Lower Arteries
L   Occlusion

Ø4L Continued

Definition: Completely closing an orifice or the lumen of a tubular body part

Explanation: The orifice can be a natural orifice or an artificially created orifice

Body Part Character 4		Approach Character 5	Device Character 6	Qualifier Character 7

1 Celiac Artery
  Celiac trunk
2 Gastric Artery
  Left gastric artery
  Right gastric artery
3 Hepatic Artery
  Common hepatic artery
  Gastroduodenal artery
  Hepatic artery proper
4 Splenic Artery
  Left gastroepiploic artery
  Pancreatic artery
  Short gastric artery
5 Superior Mesenteric Artery
  Ileal artery
  Ileocolic artery
  Inferior pancreaticoduodenal
    artery
  Jejunal artery
6 Colic Artery, Right
7 Colic Artery, Left
8 Colic Artery, Middle
9 Renal Artery, Right
  Inferior suprarenal artery
  Renal segmental artery
A Renal Artery, Left
  See 9 Renal Artery, Right
B Inferior Mesenteric Artery
  Sigmoid artery
  Superior rectal artery
C Common Iliac Artery, Right
D Common Iliac Artery, Left
H External Iliac Artery, Right
  Deep circumflex iliac artery
  Inferior epigastric artery
J External Iliac Artery, Left
  See H External Iliac Artery, Right
	K Femoral Artery, Right
	  Circumflex iliac artery
	  Deep femoral artery
	  Descending genicular artery
	  External pudendal artery
	  Superficial epigastric artery
	L Femoral Artery, Left
	  See K Femoral Artery, Right
	M Popliteal Artery, Right
	  Inferior genicular artery
	  Middle genicular artery
	  Superior genicular artery
	  Sural artery
	  Tibioperoneal trunk
	N Popliteal Artery, Left
	  See M Popliteal Artery, Right
	P Anterior Tibial Artery, Right
	  Anterior lateral malleolar
	    artery
	  Anterior medial malleolar
	    artery
	  Anterior tibial recurrent artery
	  Dorsalis pedis artery
	  Posterior tibial recurrent artery
	Q Anterior Tibial Artery, Left
	  *See P Anterior Tibial Artery,
	   Right*
	R Posterior Tibial Artery, Right
	S Posterior Tibial Artery, Left
	T Peroneal Artery, Right
	  Fibular artery
	U Peroneal Artery, Left
	  See T Peroneal Artery, Right
	V Foot Artery, Right
	  Arcuate artery
	  Dorsal metatarsal artery
	  Lateral plantar artery
	  Lateral tarsal artery
	  Medial plantar artery
	W Foot Artery, Left
	  See V Foot Artery, Right
	Y Lower Artery
	  Umbilical artery
		Ø Open
		3 Percutaneous
		4 Percutaneous Endoscopic
			C Extraluminal Device
			D Intraluminal Device
			Z No Device
				Z No Qualifier

E Internal Iliac Artery, Right
  Deferential artery
  Hypogastric artery
  Iliolumbar artery
  Inferior gluteal artery
  Inferior vesical artery
  Internal pudendal artery
  Lateral sacral artery
  Middle rectal artery
  Obturator artery
  Superior gluteal artery
  Umbilical artery
  Uterine artery
  Vaginal artery
		Ø Open
		3 Percutaneous
		4 Percutaneous Endoscopic
			C Extraluminal Device
			D Intraluminal Device
			Z No Device
				T Uterine Artery, Right ♀
				Z No Qualifier

F Internal Iliac Artery, Left
  Deferential artery
  Hypogastric artery
  Iliolumbar artery
  Inferior gluteal artery
  Inferior vesical artery
  Internal pudendal artery
  Lateral sacral artery
  Middle rectal artery
  Obturator artery
  Superior gluteal artery
  Umbilical artery
  Uterine Artery
  Vaginal artery
		Ø Open
		3 Percutaneous
		4 Percutaneous Endoscopic
			C Extraluminal Device
			D Intraluminal Device
			Z No Device
				U Uterine Artery, Left ♀
				Z No Qualifier

♀   Ø4LE[Ø,3,4][C,D,Z]T
♀   Ø4LF[Ø,3,4][C,D,Z]U

Ø   **Medical and Surgical**
4   **Lower Arteries**
N   **Release**

Definition: Freeing a body part from an abnormal physical constraint by cutting or by the use of force

Explanation: Some of the restraining tissue may be taken out but none of the body part is taken out

Body Part Character 4		Approach Character 5	Device Character 6	Qualifier Character 7
Ø **Abdominal Aorta** Inferior phrenic artery Lumbar artery Median sacral artery Middle suprarenal artery Ovarian artery Testicular artery **1** **Celiac Artery** Celiac trunk **2** **Gastric Artery** Left gastric artery Right gastric artery **3** **Hepatic Artery** Common hepatic artery Gastroduodenal artery Hepatic artery proper **4** **Splenic Artery** Left gastroepiploic artery Pancreatic artery Short gastric artery **5** **Superior Mesenteric Artery** Ileal artery Ileocolic artery Inferior pancreaticoduodenal artery Jejunal artery **6** **Colic Artery, Right** **7** **Colic Artery, Left** **8** **Colic Artery, Middle** **9** **Renal Artery, Right** Inferior suprarenal artery Renal segmental artery **A** **Renal Artery, Left** *See 9 Renal Artery, Right* **B** **Inferior Mesenteric Artery** Sigmoid artery Superior rectal artery **C** **Common Iliac Artery, Right** **D** **Common Iliac Artery, Left** **E** **Internal Iliac Artery, Right** Deferential artery Hypogastric artery Iliolumbar artery Inferior gluteal artery Inferior vesical artery Internal pudendal artery Lateral sacral artery Middle rectal artery Obturator artery Superior gluteal artery Umbilical artery Uterine artery Vaginal artery	**F** **Internal Iliac Artery, Left** *See E Internal Iliac Artery, Right* **H** **External Iliac Artery, Right** Deep circumflex iliac artery Inferior epigastric artery **J** **External Iliac Artery, Left** *See H External Iliac Artery, Right* **K** **Femoral Artery, Right** Circumflex iliac artery Deep femoral artery Descending genicular artery External pudendal artery Superficial epigastric artery **L** **Femoral Artery, Left** *See K Femoral Artery, Right* **M** **Popliteal Artery, Right** Inferior genicular artery Middle genicular artery Superior genicular artery Sural artery Tibioperoneal trunk **N** **Popliteal Artery, Left** *See M Popliteal Artery, Right* **P** **Anterior Tibial Artery, Right** Anterior lateral malleolar artery Anterior medial malleolar artery Anterior tibial recurrent artery Dorsalis pedis artery Posterior tibial recurrent artery **Q** **Anterior Tibial Artery, Left** *See P Anterior Tibial Artery, Right* **R** **Posterior Tibial Artery, Right** **S** **Posterior Tibial Artery, Left** **T** **Peroneal Artery, Right** Fibular artery **U** **Peroneal Artery, Left** *See T Peroneal Artery, Right* **V** **Foot Artery, Right** Arcuate artery Dorsal metatarsal artery Lateral plantar artery Lateral tarsal artery Medial plantar artery **W** **Foot Artery, Left** *See V Foot Artery, Right* **Y** **Lower Artery** Umbilical artery	**Ø** Open **3** Percutaneous **4** Percutaneous Endoscopic	**Z** No Device	**Z** No Qualifier

NC Noncovered Procedure   **LC** Limited Coverage   **QA** Questionable OB Admit   **NT** New Tech Add-on   ⊞ Combination Member   ♂ Male   ♀ Female

ICD-10-PCS 2022   **235**

Ø4N–Ø4N

Ø   Medical and Surgical
4   Lower Arteries
P   Removal

Definition: Taking out or off a device from a body part

Explanation: If a device is taken out and a similar device put in without cutting or puncturing the skin or mucous membrane, the procedure is coded to the root operation CHANGE. Otherwise, the procedure for taking out a device is coded to the root operation REMOVAL.

Body Part Character 4	Approach Character 5	Device Character 6	Qualifier Character 7

Y Lower Artery
    Umbilical artery
	Ø Open
	3 Percutaneous
	4 Percutaneous Endoscopic
		Ø Drainage Device
		2 Monitoring Device
		3 Infusion Device
		7 Autologous Tissue
		    Substitute
		C Extraluminal Device
		D Intraluminal Device
		J Synthetic Substitute
		K Nonautologous Tissue
		    Substitute
		Y Other Device
			Z No Qualifier

Y Lower Artery Umbilical artery	X External	Ø Drainage Device 1 Radioactive Element 2 Monitoring Device 3 Infusion Device D Intraluminal Device	Z No Qualifier

Non-OR	Ø4PY3[Ø,2,3,D]Z
Non-OR	Ø4PY[3,4]YZ
Non-OR	Ø4PYX[Ø,1,2,3,D]Z

Ø   **Medical and Surgical**
4   **Lower Arteries**
Q   **Repair**   Definition: Restoring, to the extent possible, a body part to its normal anatomic structure and function
                 Explanation: Used only when the method to accomplish the repair is not one of the other root operations

Body Part Character 4		Approach Character 5	Device Character 6	Qualifier Character 7

Ø **Abdominal Aorta**
    Inferior phrenic artery
    Lumbar artery
    Median sacral artery
    Middle suprarenal artery
    Ovarian artery
    Testicular artery
1 **Celiac Artery**
    Celiac trunk
2 **Gastric Artery**
    Left gastric artery
    Right gastric artery
3 **Hepatic Artery**
    Common hepatic artery
    Gastroduodenal artery
    Hepatic artery proper
4 **Splenic Artery**
    Left gastroepiploic artery
    Pancreatic artery
    Short gastric artery
5 **Superior Mesenteric Artery**
    Ileal artery
    Ileocolic artery
    Inferior pancreaticoduodenal
       artery
    Jejunal artery
6 **Colic Artery, Right**
7 **Colic Artery, Left**
8 **Colic Artery, Middle**
9 **Renal Artery, Right**
    Inferior suprarenal artery
    Renal segmental artery
A **Renal Artery, Left**
    See 9 Renal Artery, Right
B **Inferior Mesenteric Artery**
    Sigmoid artery
    Superior rectal artery
C **Common Iliac Artery, Right**
D **Common Iliac Artery, Left**
E **Internal Iliac Artery, Right**
    Deferential artery
    Hypogastric artery
    Iliolumbar artery
    Inferior gluteal artery
    Inferior vesical artery
    Internal pudendal artery
    Lateral sacral artery
    Middle rectal artery
    Obturator artery
    Superior gluteal artery
    Umbilical artery
    Uterine artery
    Vaginal artery
	F **Internal Iliac Artery, Left**
	    See E Internal Iliac Artery,
	    Right
	H **External Iliac Artery, Right**
	    Deep circumflex iliac artery
	    Inferior epigastric artery
	J **External Iliac Artery, Left**
	    See H External Iliac Artery,
	    Right
	K **Femoral Artery, Right**
	    Circumflex iliac artery
	    Deep femoral artery
	    Descending genicular artery
	    External pudendal artery
	    Superficial epigastric artery
	L **Femoral Artery, Left**
	    See K Femoral Artery, Right
	M **Popliteal Artery, Right**
	    Inferior genicular artery
	    Middle genicular artery
	    Superior genicular artery
	    Sural artery
	    Tibioperoneal trunk
	N **Popliteal Artery, Left**
	    See M Popliteal Artery, Right
	P **Anterior Tibial Artery, Right**
	    Anterior lateral malleolar
	       artery
	    Anterior medial malleolar
	       artery
	    Anterior tibial recurrent
	       artery
	    Dorsalis pedis artery
	    Posterior tibial recurrent
	       artery
	Q **Anterior Tibial Artery, Left**
	    See P Anterior Tibial Artery,
	    Right
	R **Posterior Tibial Artery,**
	    Right
	S **Posterior Tibial Artery, Left**
	T **Peroneal Artery, Right**
	    Fibular artery
	U **Peroneal Artery, Left**
	    See T Peroneal Artery, Right
	V **Foot Artery, Right**
	    Arcuate artery
	    Dorsal metatarsal artery
	    Lateral plantar artery
	    Lateral tarsal artery
	    Medial plantar artery
	W **Foot Artery, Left**
	    See V Foot Artery, Right
	Y **Lower Artery**
	    Umbilical artery
		Ø Open
		3 Percutaneous
		4 Percutaneous Endoscopic
			Z No Device	**Z** No Qualifier

NC Noncovered Procedure   **LC** Limited Coverage   **QA** Questionable OB Admit   **NT** New Tech Add-on   ⊞ Combination Member   ♂ Male   ♀ Female

ICD-10-PCS 2022   **237**

0   Medical and Surgical
4   Lower Arteries
R   Replacement   Definition: Putting in or on biological or synthetic material that physically takes the place and/or function of all or a portion of a body part

Explanation: The body part may have been taken out or replaced, or may be taken out, physically eradicated, or rendered nonfunctional during the REPLACEMENT procedure. A REMOVAL procedure is coded for taking out the device used in a previous replacement procedure.

Body Part Character 4		Approach Character 5	Device Character 6	Qualifier Character 7

0 Abdominal Aorta
 Inferior phrenic artery
 Lumbar artery
 Median sacral artery
 Middle suprarenal artery
 Ovarian artery
 Testicular artery
 1 Celiac Artery
 Celiac trunk
 2 Gastric Artery
 Left gastric artery
 Right gastric artery
 3 Hepatic Artery
 Common hepatic artery
 Gastroduodenal artery
 Hepatic artery proper
 4 Splenic Artery
 Left gastroepiploic artery
 Pancreatic artery
 Short gastric artery
 5 Superior Mesenteric Artery
 Ileal artery
 Ileocolic artery
 Inferior pancreaticoduodenal
    artery
 Jejunal artery
 6 Colic Artery, Right
 7 Colic Artery, Left
 8 Colic Artery, Middle
 9 Renal Artery, Right
 Inferior suprarenal artery
 Renal segmental artery
 A Renal Artery, Left
 See 9 Renal Artery, Right
 B Inferior Mesenteric Artery
 Sigmoid artery
 Superior rectal artery
 C Common Iliac Artery, Right
 D Common Iliac Artery, Left
 E Internal Iliac Artery, Right
 Deferential artery
 Hypogastric artery
 Iliolumbar artery
 Inferior gluteal artery
 Inferior vesical artery
 Internal pudendal artery
 Lateral sacral artery
 Middle rectal artery
 Obturator artery
 Superior gluteal artery
 Umbilical artery
 Uterine artery
 Vaginal artery
	F Internal Iliac Artery, Left
	 See E Internal Iliac Artery, Right
	 H External Iliac Artery, Right
	 Deep circumflex iliac artery
	 Inferior epigastric artery
	 J External Iliac Artery, Left
	 See H External Iliac Artery, Right
	 K Femoral Artery, Right
	 Circumflex iliac artery
	 Deep femoral artery
	 Descending genicular artery
	 External pudendal artery
	 Superficial epigastric artery
	 L Femoral Artery, Left
	 See K Femoral Artery, Right
	 M Popliteal Artery, Right
	 Inferior genicular artery
	 Middle genicular artery
	 Superior genicular artery
	 Sural artery
	 Tibioperoneal trunk
	 N Popliteal Artery, Left
	 See M Popliteal Artery, Right
	 P Anterior Tibial Artery, Right
	 Anterior lateral malleolar
	    artery
	 Anterior medial malleolar
	    artery
	 Anterior tibial recurrent artery
	 Dorsalis pedis artery
	 Posterior tibial recurrent artery
	 Q Anterior Tibial Artery, Left
	 See P Anterior Tibial Artery, Right
	 R Posterior Tibial Artery, Right
	 S Posterior Tibial Artery, Left
	 T Peroneal Artery, Right
	 Fibular artery
	 U Peroneal Artery, Left
	 See T Peroneal Artery, Right
	 V Foot Artery, Right
	 Arcuate artery
	 Dorsal metatarsal artery
	 Lateral plantar artery
	 Lateral tarsal artery
	 Medial plantar artery
	 W Foot Artery, Left
	 See V Foot Artery, Right
	 Y Lower Artery
	 Umbilical artery
		0 Open
		 4 Percutaneous Endoscopic
			7 Autologous Tissue
			 Substitute
			 J Synthetic Substitute
			 K Nonautologous Tissue
			 Substitute
				Z No Qualifier

Ø   Medical and Surgical
4   Lower Arteries
S   Reposition   Definition: Moving to its normal location, or other suitable location, all or a portion of a body part

Explanation: The body part is moved to a new location from an abnormal location, or from a normal location where it is not functioning correctly. The body part may or may not be cut out or off to be moved to the new location.

Body Part Character 4		Approach Character 5	Device Character 6	Qualifier Character 7

Ø Abdominal Aorta
Inferior phrenic artery
Lumbar artery
Median sacral artery
Middle suprarenal artery
Ovarian artery
Testicular artery
1 Celiac Artery
Celiac trunk
2 Gastric Artery
Left gastric artery
Right gastric artery
3 Hepatic Artery
Common hepatic artery
Gastroduodenal artery
Hepatic artery proper
4 Splenic Artery
Left gastroepiploic artery
Pancreatic artery
Short gastric artery
5 Superior Mesenteric Artery
Ileal artery
Ileocolic artery
Inferior pancreaticoduodenal
   artery
Jejunal artery
6 Colic Artery, Right
7 Colic Artery, Left
8 Colic Artery, Middle
9 Renal Artery, Right
Inferior suprarenal artery
Renal segmental artery
A Renal Artery, Left
See 9 Renal Artery, Right
B Inferior Mesenteric Artery
Sigmoid artery
Superior rectal artery
C Common Iliac Artery, Right
D Common Iliac Artery, Left
E Internal Iliac Artery, Right
Deferential artery
Hypogastric artery
Iliolumbar artery
Inferior gluteal artery
Inferior vesical artery
Internal pudendal artery
Lateral sacral artery
Middle rectal artery
Obturator artery
Superior gluteal artery
Umbilical artery
Uterine artery
Vaginal artery
	F Internal Iliac Artery, Left
	See E Internal Iliac Artery, Right
	H External Iliac Artery, Right
	Deep circumflex iliac artery
	Inferior epigastric artery
	J External Iliac Artery, Left
	See H External Iliac Artery, Right
	K Femoral Artery, Right
	Circumflex iliac artery
	Deep femoral artery
	Descending genicular artery
	External pudendal artery
	Superficial epigastric artery
	L Femoral Artery, Left
	See K Femoral Artery, Right
	M Popliteal Artery, Right
	Inferior genicular artery
	Middle genicular artery
	Superior genicular artery
	Sural artery
	Tibioperoneal trunk
	N Popliteal Artery, Left
	See M Popliteal Artery, Right
	P Anterior Tibial Artery, Right
	Anterior lateral malleolar
	   artery
	Anterior medial malleolar
	   artery
	Anterior tibial recurrent artery
	Dorsalis pedis artery
	Posterior tibial recurrent artery
	Q Anterior Tibial Artery, Left
	*See P Anterior Tibial Artery,
	   Right*
	R Posterior Tibial Artery, Right
	S Posterior Tibial Artery, Left
	T Peroneal Artery, Right
	Fibular artery
	U Peroneal Artery, Left
	See T Peroneal Artery, Right
	V Foot Artery, Right
	Arcuate artery
	Dorsal metatarsal artery
	Lateral plantar artery
	Lateral tarsal artery
	Medial plantar artery
	W Foot Artery, Left
	See V Foot Artery, Right
	Y Lower Artery
	Umbilical artery
		Ø Open
		3 Percutaneous
		4 Percutaneous Endoscopic
			Z No Device	**Z No Qualifier**

NC Noncovered Procedure   LC Limited Coverage   QA Questionable OB Admit   NT New Tech Add-on   ⊞ Combination Member   ♂ Male   ♀ Female

ICD-10-PCS 2022   239

04S–04S

Lower Arteries

0   **Medical and Surgical**
4   **Lower Arteries**
U   **Supplement**   Definition: Putting in or on biological or synthetic material that physically reinforces and/or augments the function of a portion of a body part
                        Explanation: The biological material is non-living, or is living and from the same individual. The body part may have been previously replaced, and the SUPPLEMENT procedure is performed to physically reinforce and/or augment the function of the replaced body part.

Body Part Character 4		Approach Character 5	Device Character 6	Qualifier Character 7

0 **Abdominal Aorta**
    Inferior phrenic artery
    Lumbar artery
    Median sacral artery
    Middle suprarenal artery
    Ovarian artery
    Testicular artery
1 **Celiac Artery**
    Celiac trunk
2 **Gastric Artery**
    Left gastric artery
    Right gastric artery
3 **Hepatic Artery**
    Common hepatic artery
    Gastroduodenal artery
    Hepatic artery proper
4 **Splenic Artery**
    Left gastroepiploic artery
    Pancreatic artery
    Short gastric artery
5 **Superior Mesenteric Artery**
    Ileal artery
    Ileocolic artery
    Inferior pancreaticoduodenal
       artery
    Jejunal artery
6 **Colic Artery, Right**
7 **Colic Artery, Left**
8 **Colic Artery, Middle**
9 **Renal Artery, Right**
    Inferior suprarenal artery
    Renal segmental artery
A **Renal Artery, Left**
    See 9 Renal Artery, Right
B **Inferior Mesenteric Artery**
    Sigmoid artery
    Superior rectal artery
C **Common Iliac Artery, Right**
D **Common Iliac Artery, Left**
E **Internal Iliac Artery, Right**
    Deferential artery
    Hypogastric artery
    Iliolumbar artery
    Inferior gluteal artery
    Inferior vesical artery
    Internal pudendal artery
    Lateral sacral artery
    Middle rectal artery
    Obturator artery
    Superior gluteal artery
    Umbilical artery
    Uterine artery
    Vaginal artery
	F **Internal Iliac Artery, Left**
	    See E Internal Iliac Artery, Right
	H **External Iliac Artery, Right**
	    Deep circumflex iliac artery
	    Inferior epigastric artery
	J **External Iliac Artery, Left**
	    See H External Iliac Artery, Right
	K **Femoral Artery, Right**
	    Circumflex iliac artery
	    Deep femoral artery
	    Descending genicular artery
	    External pudendal artery
	    Superficial epigastric artery
	L **Femoral Artery, Left**
	    See K Femoral Artery, Right
	M **Popliteal Artery, Right**
	    Inferior genicular artery
	    Middle genicular artery
	    Superior genicular artery
	    Sural artery
	    Tibioperoneal trunk
	N **Popliteal Artery, Left**
	    See M Popliteal Artery, Right
	P **Anterior Tibial Artery, Right**
	    Anterior lateral malleolar
	       artery
	    Anterior medial malleolar
	       artery
	    Anterior tibial recurrent artery
	    Dorsalis pedis artery
	    Posterior tibial recurrent artery
	Q **Anterior Tibial Artery, Left**
	    See P Anterior Tibial Artery,
	      Right
	R **Posterior Tibial Artery, Right**
	S **Posterior Tibial Artery, Left**
	T **Peroneal Artery, Right**
	    Fibular artery
	U **Peroneal Artery, Left**
	    See T Peroneal Artery, Right
	V **Foot Artery, Right**
	    Arcuate artery
	    Dorsal metatarsal artery
	    Lateral plantar artery
	    Lateral tarsal artery
	    Medial plantar artery
	W **Foot Artery, Left**
	    See V Foot Artery, Right
	Y **Lower Artery**
	    Umbilical artery
		0 Open
		3 Percutaneous
		4 Percutaneous Endoscopic
			7 Autologous Tissue
			    Substitute
			J Synthetic Substitute
			K Nonautologous Tissue
			    Substitute
				Z No Qualifier

Ø **Medical and Surgical**
4 **Lower Arteries**
V **Restriction** — Definition: Partially closing an orifice or the lumen of a tubular body part
　　　　　　　　　Explanation: The orifice can be a natural orifice or an artificially created orifice

Body Part Character 4		Approach Character 5	Device Character 6	Qualifier Character 7
Ø **Abdominal Aorta** Inferior phrenic artery Lumbar artery Median sacral artery Middle suprarenal artery Ovarian artery Testicular artery		**Ø** Open **3** Percutaneous **4** Percutaneous Endoscopic	**C** Extraluminal Device **E** Intraluminal Device, Branched or Fenestrated, One or Two Arteries **F** Intraluminal Device, Branched or Fenestrated, Three or More Arteries **Z** No Device	**Z** No Qualifier
Ø **Abdominal Aorta** Inferior phrenic artery Lumbar artery Median sacral artery Middle suprarenal artery Ovarian artery Testicular artery		**Ø** Open **3** Percutaneous **4** Percutaneous Endoscopic	**D** Intraluminal Device	**J** Temporary **Z** No Qualifier
1 **Celiac Artery** Celiac trunk **2** **Gastric Artery** Left gastric artery Right gastric artery **3** **Hepatic Artery** Common hepatic artery Gastroduodenal artery Hepatic artery proper **4** **Splenic Artery** Left gastroepiploic artery Pancreatic artery Short gastric artery **5** **Superior Mesenteric Artery** Ileal artery Ileocolic artery Inferior pancreaticoduodenal artery Jejunal artery **6** **Colic Artery, Right** **7** **Colic Artery, Left** **8** **Colic Artery, Middle** **9** **Renal Artery, Right** Inferior suprarenal artery Renal segmental artery **A** **Renal Artery, Left** *See 9 Renal Artery, Right* **B** **Inferior Mesenteric Artery** Sigmoid artery Superior rectal artery **E** **Internal Iliac Artery, Right** Deferential artery Hypogastric artery Iliolumbar artery Inferior gluteal artery Inferior vesical artery Internal pudendal artery Lateral sacral artery Middle rectal artery Obturator artery Superior gluteal artery Umbilical artery Uterine artery Vaginal artery **F** **Internal Iliac Artery, Left** *See E Internal Iliac Artery, Right*	**H** **External Iliac Artery, Right** Deep circumflex iliac artery Inferior epigastric artery **J** **External Iliac Artery, Left** *See H External Iliac Artery, Right* **K** **Femoral Artery, Right** Circumflex iliac artery Deep femoral artery Descending genicular artery External pudendal artery Superficial epigastric artery **L** **Femoral Artery, Left** *See K Femoral Artery, Right* **M** **Popliteal Artery, Right** Inferior genicular artery Middle genicular artery Superior genicular artery Sural artery Tibioperoneal trunk **N** **Popliteal Artery, Left** *See M Popliteal Artery, Right* **P** **Anterior Tibial Artery, Right** Anterior lateral malleolar artery Anterior medial malleolar artery Anterior tibial recurrent artery Dorsalis pedis artery Posterior tibial recurrent artery **Q** **Anterior Tibial Artery, Left** *See P Anterior Tibial Artery, Right* **R** **Posterior Tibial Artery, Right** **S** **Posterior Tibial Artery, Left** **T** **Peroneal Artery, Right** Fibular artery **U** **Peroneal Artery, Left** *See T Peroneal Artery, Right* **V** **Foot Artery, Right** Arcuate artery Dorsal metatarsal artery Lateral plantar artery Lateral tarsal artery Medial plantar artery **W** **Foot Artery, Left** *See V Foot Artery, Right* **Y** **Lower Artery** Umbilical artery	**Ø** Open **3** Percutaneous **4** Percutaneous Endoscopic	**C** Extraluminal Device **D** Intraluminal Device **Z** No Device	**Z** No Qualifier
C **Common Iliac Artery, Right** **D** **Common Iliac Artery, Left**		**Ø** Open **3** Percutaneous **4** Percutaneous Endoscopic	**C** Extraluminal Device **D** Intraluminal Device **E** Intraluminal Device, Branched or Fenestrated, One or Two Arteries **Z** No Device	**Z** No Qualifier

NC Noncovered Procedure　　**LC** Limited Coverage　　**QA** Questionable OB Admit　　**NT** New Tech Add-on　　⊞ Combination Member　　♂ Male　　♀ Female

ICD-10-PCS 2022　　　　　　　　　　　　　　　　　　　　　　　　　　　　　　　　　　　　**241**

04V–04V

Lower Arteries

0 **Medical and Surgical**
4 **Lower Arteries**
W **Revision**　　Definition: Correcting, to the extent possible, a portion of a malfunctioning device or the position of a displaced device

Explanation: Revision can include correcting a malfunctioning or displaced device by taking out or putting in components of the device such as a screw or pin

Body Part Character 4	Approach Character 5	Device Character 6	Qualifier Character 7
Y **Lower Artery** Umbilical artery	**0** Open **3** Percutaneous **4** Percutaneous Endoscopic	**0** Drainage Device **2** Monitoring Device **3** Infusion Device **7** Autologous Tissue Substitute **C** Extraluminal Device **D** Intraluminal Device **J** Synthetic Substitute **K** Nonautologous Tissue Substitute **Y** Other Device	**Z** No Qualifier
Y **Lower Artery** Umbilical artery	**X** External	**0** Drainage Device **2** Monitoring Device **3** Infusion Device **7** Autologous Tissue Substitute **C** Extraluminal Device **D** Intraluminal Device **J** Synthetic Substitute **K** Nonautologous Tissue Substitute	**Z** No Qualifier

Non-OR　04WY3[0,2,3,D]Z
Non-OR　04WY[3,4]YZ
Non-OR　04WYX[0,2,3,7,C,D,J,K]Z

Upper Veins Ø51–Ø5W

Character Meanings

This Character Meaning table is provided as a guide to assist the user in the identification of character members that may be found in this section of code tables. It **SHOULD NOT** be used to build a PCS code.

Operation–Character 3		Body Part–Character 4		Approach–Character 5		Device–Character 6		Qualifier–Character 7	
1	Bypass	Ø	Azygos Vein	Ø	Open	Ø	Drainage Device	Ø	Ultrasonic
5	Destruction	1	Hemiazygos Vein	3	Percutaneous	2	Monitoring Device	1	Drug-Coated Balloon
7	Dilation	3	Innominate Vein, Right	4	Percutaneous Endoscopic	3	Infusion Device	X	Diagnostic
9	Drainage	4	Innominate Vein, Left	X	External	7	Autologous Tissue Substitute	Y	Upper Vein
B	Excision	5	Subclavian Vein, Right			9	Autologous Venous Tissue	Z	No Qualifier
C	Extirpation	6	Subclavian Vein, Left			A	Autologous Arterial Tissue		
D	Extraction	7	Axillary Vein, Right			C	Extraluminal Device		
F	Fragmentation	8	Axillary Vein, Left			D	Intraluminal Device		
H	Insertion	9	Brachial Vein, Right			J	Synthetic Substitute		
J	Inspection	A	Brachial Vein, Left			K	Nonautologous Tissue Substitute		
L	Occlusion	B	Basilic Vein, Right			M	Neurostimulator Lead		
N	Release	C	Basilic Vein, Left			Y	Other Device		
P	Removal	D	Cephalic Vein, Right			Z	No Device		
Q	Repair	F	Cephalic Vein, Left						
R	Replacement	G	Hand Vein, Right						
S	Reposition	H	Hand Vein, Left						
U	Supplement	L	Intracranial Vein						
V	Restriction	M	Internal Jugular Vein, Right						
W	Revision	N	Internal Jugular Vein, Left						
		P	External Jugular Vein, Right						
		Q	External Jugular Vein, Left						
		R	Vertebral Vein, Right						
		S	Vertebral Vein, Left						
		T	Face Vein, Right						
		V	Face Vein, Left						
		Y	Upper Vein						

AHA Coding Clinic for table Ø51
2020, 1Q, 28   Free flap microvascular breast reconstruction
2017, 3Q, 15   Bypass of innominate vein to atrial appendage

AHA Coding Clinic for table Ø57
2020, 3Q, 38   Thrombectomy of arteriovenous fistula with angioplasty and stent placement

AHA Coding Clinic for table Ø59
2018, 3Q, 7   Catheter placement for treatment of congestive heart failure

AHA Coding Clinic for table Ø5B
2021, 2Q, 15   Excision of pituitary macroadenoma within cavernous sinus
2020, 3Q, 40   Excision of ulceration of arteriovenous fistula
2020, 1Q, 24   Resection of vascular malformation, likely cavernoma
2016, 2Q, 12   Resection of malignant neoplasm of infratemporal fossa

AHA Coding Clinic for table Ø5C
2020, 3Q, 37   Repair of aneurysm of arteriovenous fistula with endovenectomy
2020, 3Q, 38   Thrombectomy of arteriovenous fistula with angioplasty and stent placement

AHA Coding Clinic for table Ø5F
2020, 4Q, 45-49   New fragmentation tables
2020, 4Q, 49-50   Intravascular ultrasound assisted thrombolysis
2020, 4Q, 50   Intravascular lithotripsy

AHA Coding Clinic for table Ø5H
2016, 4Q, 97-98   Phrenic neurostimulator

AHA Coding Clinic for table Ø5P
2016, 4Q, 97-98   Phrenic neurostimulator

AHA Coding Clinic for table Ø5Q
2017, 3Q, 15   Bypass of innominate vein to atrial appendage

AHA Coding Clinic for table Ø5S
2013, 4Q, 125   Stage II cephalic vein transposition (superficialization) of arteriovenous fistula

AHA Coding Clinic for table Ø5V
2020, 3Q, 37   Repair of aneurysm of arteriovenous fistula with endovenectomy

AHA Coding Clinic for table Ø5W
2016, 4Q, 97-98   Phrenic neurostimulator

Head and Neck Veins

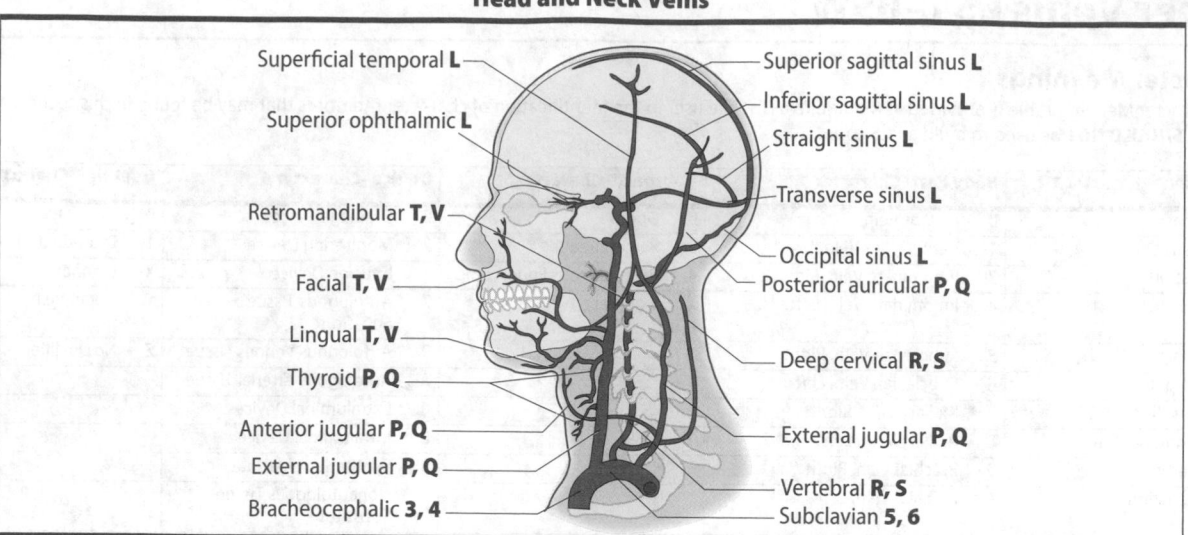

Superficial temporal **L**
Superior ophthalmic **L**
Retromandibular **T, V**
Facial **T, V**
Lingual **T, V**
Thyroid **P, Q**
Anterior jugular **P, Q**
External jugular **P, Q**
Bracheocephalic **3, 4**

Superior sagittal sinus **L**
Inferior sagittal sinus **L**
Straight sinus **L**
Transverse sinus **L**
Occipital sinus **L**
Posterior auricular **P, Q**
Deep cervical **R, S**
External jugular **P, Q**
Vertebral **R, S**
Subclavian **5, 6**

Upper Veins

Superficial temporal **L**
Vertebral **R, S**
Internal jugular **M, N**
External jugular **P, Q**
Subclavian **5, 6**
Innominate **3, 4**
Azygos **Ø**
Axillary **7,8**
Hemiazygos **1**
Brachial **9, A**
Cephalic **D, F**
Basilic **B, C**
Radial **9, A**
Ulnar **9, A**
Digital **G, H**

Ø   Medical and Surgical
5   Upper Veins
1   Bypass   Definition: Altering the route of passage of the contents of a tubular body part

           Explanation: Rerouting contents of a body part to a downstream area of the normal route, to a similar route and body part, or to an abnormal route and dissimilar body part. Includes one or more anastomoses, with or without the use of a device.

Body Part Character 4	Approach Character 5	Device Character 6	Qualifier Character 7
Ø Azygos Vein Right ascending lumbar vein Right subcostal vein **1 Hemiazygos Vein** Left ascending lumbar vein Left subcostal vein **3 Innominate Vein, Right** Brachiocephalic vein Inferior thyroid vein **4 Innominate Vein, Left** *See 3 Innominate Vein, Right* **5 Subclavian Vein, Right** **6 Subclavian Vein, Left** **7 Axillary Vein, Right** **8 Axillary Vein, Left** **9 Brachial Vein, Right** Radial vein Ulnar vein **A Brachial Vein, Left** *See 9 Brachial Vein, Right* **B Basilic Vein, Right** Median antebrachial vein Median cubital vein **C Basilic Vein, Left** *See B Basilic Vein, Right* **D Cephalic Vein, Right** Accessory cephalic vein **F Cephalic Vein, Left** *See D Cephalic Vein, Right* **G Hand Vein, Right** Dorsal metacarpal vein Palmar (volar) digital vein Palmar (volar) metacarpal vein Superficial palmar venous arch Volar (palmar) digital vein Volar (palmar) metacarpal vein **H Hand Vein, Left** *See G Hand Vein, Right* **L Intracranial Vein** Anterior cerebral vein Basal (internal) cerebral vein Dural venous sinus Great cerebral vein Inferior cerebellar vein Inferior cerebral vein Internal (basal) cerebral vein Middle cerebral vein Ophthalmic vein Superior cerebellar vein Superior cerebral vein **M Internal Jugular Vein, Right** **N Internal Jugular Vein, Left** **P External Jugular Vein, Right** Posterior auricular vein **Q External Jugular Vein, Left** *See P External Jugular Vein, Right* **R Vertebral Vein, Right** Deep cervical vein Suboccipital venous plexus **S Vertebral Vein, Left** *See R Vertebral Vein, Right* **T Face Vein, Right** Angular vein Anterior facial vein Common facial vein Deep facial vein Frontal vein Posterior facial (retromandibular) vein Supraorbital vein **V Face Vein, Left** *See T Face Vein, Right*	**Ø Open** **4 Percutaneous Endoscopic**	**7 Autologous Tissue Substitute** **9 Autologous Venous Tissue** **A Autologous Arterial Tissue** **J Synthetic Substitute** **K Nonautologous Tissue Substitute** **Z No Device**	**Y Upper Vein**

NC Noncovered Procedure   **LC** Limited Coverage   **QA** Questionable OB Admit   **NT** New Tech Add-on   ⊞ Combination Member   ♂ Male   ♀ Female

Upper Veins

0   **Medical and Surgical**
5   **Upper Veins**
5   **Destruction**   Definition: Physical eradication of all or a portion of a body part by the direct use of energy, force, or a destructive agent
                 Explanation: None of the body part is physically taken out

Body Part Character 4	Approach Character 5	Device Character 6	Qualifier Character 7

0   **Azygos Vein**
     Right ascending lumbar vein
     Right subcostal vein
1   **Hemiazygos Vein**
     Left ascending lumbar vein
     Left subcostal vein
3   **Innominate Vein, Right**
     Brachiocephalic vein
     Inferior thyroid vein
4   **Innominate Vein, Left**
     See 3 Innominate Vein, Right
5   **Subclavian Vein, Right**
6   **Subclavian Vein, Left**
7   **Axillary Vein, Right**
8   **Axillary Vein, Left**
9   **Brachial Vein, Right**
     Radial vein
     Ulnar vein
A   **Brachial Vein, Left**
     See 9 Brachial Vein, Right
B   **Basilic Vein, Right**
     Median antebrachial vein
     Median cubital vein
C   **Basilic Vein, Left**
     See B Basilic Vein, Right
D   **Cephalic Vein, Right**
     Accessory cephalic vein
F   **Cephalic Vein, Left**
     See D Cephalic Vein, Right
G   **Hand Vein, Right**
     Dorsal metacarpal vein
     Palmar (volar) digital vein
     Palmar (volar) metacarpal vein
     Superficial palmar venous arch
     Volar (palmar) digital vein
     Volar (palmar) metacarpal vein
H   **Hand Vein, Left**
     See G Hand Vein, Right
L   **Intracranial Vein**
     Anterior cerebral vein
     Basal (internal) cerebral vein
     Dural venous sinus
     Great cerebral vein
     Inferior cerebellar vein
     Inferior cerebral vein
     Internal (basal) cerebral vein
     Middle cerebral vein
     Ophthalmic vein
     Superior cerebellar vein
     Superior cerebral vein
M   **Internal Jugular Vein, Right**
N   **Internal Jugular Vein, Left**
P   **External Jugular Vein, Right**
     Posterior auricular vein
Q   **External Jugular Vein, Left**
     See P External Jugular Vein, Right
R   **Vertebral Vein, Right**
     Deep cervical vein
     Suboccipital venous plexus
S   **Vertebral Vein, Left**
     See R Vertebral Vein, Right
T   **Face Vein, Right**
     Angular vein
     Anterior facial vein
     Common facial vein
     Deep facial vein
     Frontal vein
     Posterior facial (retromandibular) vein
     Supraorbital vein
V   **Face Vein, Left**
     See T Face Vein, Right
Y   **Upper Vein**
	0 Open
	3 Percutaneous
	4 Percutaneous Endoscopic
		Z No Device	**Z** No Qualifier

Ø   Medical and Surgical
5   Upper Veins
7   Dilation   Definition: Expanding an orifice or the lumen of a tubular body part

                 Explanation: The orifice can be a natural orifice or an artificially created orifice. Accomplished by stretching a tubular body part using intraluminal pressure or by cutting part of the orifice or wall of the tubular body part.

Body Part Character 4	Approach Character 5	Device Character 6	Qualifier Character 7

Ø   Azygos Vein
    Right ascending lumbar vein
    Right subcostal vein
1   Hemiazygos Vein
    Left ascending lumbar vein
    Left subcostal vein
G   Hand Vein, Right
    Dorsal metacarpal vein
    Palmar (volar) digital vein
    Palmar (volar) metacarpal vein
    Superficial palmar venous arch
    Volar (palmar) digital vein
    Volar (palmar) metacarpal vein
H   Hand Vein, Left
    See G Hand Vein, Right
L   Intracranial Vein `NC`
    Anterior cerebral vein
    Basal (internal) cerebral vein
    Dural venous sinus
    Great cerebral vein
    Inferior cerebellar vein
    Inferior cerebral vein
    Internal (basal) cerebral vein
    Middle cerebral vein
    Ophthalmic vein
    Superior cerebellar vein
    Superior cerebral vein
M   Internal Jugular Vein, Right
N   Internal Jugular Vein, Left
P   External Jugular Vein, Right
    Posterior auricular vein
Q   External Jugular Vein, Left
    See P External Jugular Vein, Right
R   Vertebral Vein, Right
    Deep cervical vein
    Suboccipital venous plexus
S   Vertebral Vein, Left
    See R Vertebral Vein, Right
T   Face Vein, Right
    Angular vein
    Anterior facial vein
    Common facial vein
    Deep facial vein
    Frontal vein
    Posterior facial (retromandibular) vein
    Supraorbital vein
V   Face Vein, Left
    See T Face Vein, Right
Y   Upper Vein
	Ø Open
	3 Percutaneous
	4 Percutaneous Endoscopic
		D Intraluminal Device
		Z No Device
			Z No Qualifier

3   Innominate Vein, Right
    Brachiocephalic vein
    Inferior thyroid vein
4   Innominate Vein, Left
    See 3 Innominate Vein, Right
5   Subclavian Vein, Right
6   Subclavian Vein, Left
7   Axillary Vein, Right
8   Axillary Vein, Left
9   Brachial Vein, Right
    Radial vein
    Ulnar vein
A   Brachial Vein, Left
    See 9 Brachial Vein, Right
B   Basilic Vein, Right
    Median antebrachial vein
    Median cubital vein
C   Basilic Vein, Left
    See B Basilic Vein, Right
D   Cephalic Vein, Right
    Accessory cephalic vein
F   Cephalic Vein, Left
    See D Cephalic Vein, Right
	Ø Open
	3 Percutaneous
	4 Percutaneous Endoscopic
		D Intraluminal Device
		Z No Device
			1 Drug-Coated Balloon
			Z No Qualifier

`NC`   Ø57L[3,4]ZZ

`NC` Noncovered Procedure   `LC` Limited Coverage   `QA` Questionable OB Admit   `NT` New Tech Add-on   ⊞ Combination Member   ♂ Male   ♀ Female

Upper Veins

Ø　Medical and Surgical
5　Upper Veins
9　Drainage　　Definition: Taking or letting out fluids and/or gases from a body part
　　　　　　　　　　Explanation: The qualifier DIAGNOSTIC is used to identify drainage procedures that are biopsies

Body Part Character 4		Approach Character 5	Device Character 6	Qualifier Character 7
Ø **Azygos Vein** 　Right ascending lumbar vein 　Right subcostal vein 1 **Hemiazygos Vein** 　Left ascending lumbar vein 　Left subcostal vein 3 **Innominate Vein, Right** 　Brachiocephalic vein 　Inferior thyroid vein 4 **Innominate Vein, Left** 　*See 3 Innominate Vein, Right* 5 **Subclavian Vein, Right** 6 **Subclavian Vein, Left** 7 **Axillary Vein, Right** 8 **Axillary Vein, Left** 9 **Brachial Vein, Right** 　Radial vein 　Ulnar vein A **Brachial Vein, Left** 　*See 9 Brachial Vein, Right* B **Basilic Vein, Right** 　Median antebrachial vein 　Median cubital vein C **Basilic Vein, Left** 　*See B Basilic Vein, Right* D **Cephalic Vein, Right** 　Accessory cephalic vein F **Cephalic Vein, Left** 　*See D Cephalic Vein, Right* G **Hand Vein, Right** 　Dorsal metacarpal vein 　Palmar (volar) digital vein 　Palmar (volar) metacarpal vein 　Superficial palmar venous arch 　Volar (palmar) digital vein 　Volar (palmar) metacarpal vein	H **Hand Vein, Left** 　*See G Hand Vein, Right* L **Intracranial Vein** 　Anterior cerebral vein 　Basal (internal) cerebral vein 　Dural venous sinus 　Great cerebral vein 　Inferior cerebellar vein 　Inferior cerebral vein 　Internal (basal) cerebral vein 　Middle cerebral vein 　Ophthalmic vein 　Superior cerebellar vein 　Superior cerebral vein M **Internal Jugular Vein, Right** N **Internal Jugular Vein, Left** P **External Jugular Vein, Right** 　Posterior auricular vein Q **External Jugular Vein, Left** 　*See P External Jugular Vein, Right* R **Vertebral Vein, Right** 　Deep cervical vein 　Suboccipital venous plexus S **Vertebral Vein, Left** 　*See R Vertebral Vein, Right* T **Face Vein, Right** 　Angular vein 　Anterior facial vein 　Common facial vein 　Deep facial vein 　Frontal vein 　Posterior facial 　　(retromandibular) vein 　Supraorbital vein V **Face Vein, Left** 　*See T Face Vein, Right* Y **Upper Vein**	Ø **Open** 3 **Percutaneous** 4 **Percutaneous Endoscopic**	Ø **Drainage Device**	Z **No Qualifier**
Ø **Azygos Vein** 　Right ascending lumbar vein 　Right subcostal vein 1 **Hemiazygos Vein** 　Left ascending lumbar vein 　Left subcostal vein 3 **Innominate Vein, Right** 　Brachiocephalic vein 　Inferior thyroid vein 4 **Innominate Vein, Left** 　*See 3 Innominate Vein, Right* 5 **Subclavian Vein, Right** 6 **Subclavian Vein, Left** 7 **Axillary Vein, Right** 8 **Axillary Vein, Left** 9 **Brachial Vein, Right** 　Radial vein 　Ulnar vein A **Brachial Vein, Left** 　*See 9 Brachial Vein, Right* B **Basilic Vein, Right** 　Median antebrachial vein 　Median cubital vein C **Basilic Vein, Left** 　*See B Basilic Vein, Right* D **Cephalic Vein, Right** 　Accessory cephalic vein F **Cephalic Vein, Left** 　*See D Cephalic Vein, Right* G **Hand Vein, Right** 　Dorsal metacarpal vein 　Palmar (volar) digital vein 　Palmar (volar) metacarpal vein 　Superficial palmar venous arch 　Volar (palmar) digital vein 　Volar (palmar) metacarpal vein	H **Hand Vein, Left** 　*See G Hand Vein, Right* L **Intracranial Vein** 　Anterior cerebral vein 　Basal (internal) cerebral vein 　Dural venous sinus 　Great cerebral vein 　Inferior cerebellar vein 　Inferior cerebral vein 　Internal (basal) cerebral vein 　Middle cerebral vein 　Ophthalmic vein 　Superior cerebellar vein 　Superior cerebral vein M **Internal Jugular Vein, Right** N **Internal Jugular Vein, Left** P **External Jugular Vein, Right** 　Posterior auricular vein Q **External Jugular Vein, Left** 　*See P External Jugular Vein, Right* R **Vertebral Vein, Right** 　Deep cervical vein 　Suboccipital venous plexus S **Vertebral Vein, Left** 　*See R Vertebral Vein, Right* T **Face Vein, Right** 　Angular vein 　Anterior facial vein 　Common facial vein 　Deep facial vein 　Frontal vein 　Posterior facial 　　(retromandibular) vein 　Supraorbital vein V **Face Vein, Left** 　*See T Face Vein, Right* Y **Upper Vein**	Ø **Open** 3 **Percutaneous** 4 **Percutaneous Endoscopic**	Z **No Device**	X **Diagnostic** Z **No Qualifier**

Non-OR	Ø59[Ø,1,3,4,5,6,7,8,9,A,B,C,D,F,G,H,L,M,N,P,Q,R,S,T,V,Y][Ø,3,4]ØZ
Non-OR	Ø59[Ø,1,3,4,5,6,7,8,9,A,B,C,D,F,G,H,L,M,N,P,Q,R,S,T,V,Y]3ZX
Non-OR	Ø59[Ø,1,3,4,5,6,7,8,9,A,B,C,D,F,G,H,L,M,N,P,Q,R,S,T,V,Y][Ø,3,4]ZZ

Non-OR Procedure　　　　DRG Non-OR Procedure　　　　Valid OR Procedure　　　　HAC Associated Procedure　　　　Combination Only　　　　New/Revised GREEN

Ø	**Medical and Surgical**
5	**Upper Veins**
B	**Excision** Definition: Cutting out or off, without replacement, a portion of a body part
	Explanation: The qualifier DIAGNOSTIC is used to identify excision procedures that are biopsies

Body Part Character 4	Approach Character 5	Device Character 6	Qualifier Character 7
Ø Azygos Vein Right ascending lumbar vein Right subcostal vein **1 Hemiazygos Vein** Left ascending lumbar vein Left subcostal vein **3 Innominate Vein, Right** Brachiocephalic vein Inferior thyroid vein **4 Innominate Vein, Left** *See 3 Innominate Vein, Right* **5 Subclavian Vein, Right** **6 Subclavian Vein, Left** **7 Axillary Vein, Right** **8 Axillary Vein, Left** **9 Brachial Vein, Right** Radial vein Ulnar vein **A Brachial Vein, Left** *See 9 Brachial Vein, Right* **B Basilic Vein, Right** Median antebrachial vein Median cubital vein **C Basilic Vein, Left** *See B Basilic Vein, Right* **D Cephalic Vein, Right** Accessory cephalic vein **F Cephalic Vein, Left** *See D Cephalic Vein, Right* **G Hand Vein, Right** Dorsal metacarpal vein Palmar (volar) digital vein Palmar (volar) metacarpal vein Superficial palmar venous arch Volar (palmar) digital vein Volar (palmar) metacarpal vein **H Hand Vein, Left** *See G Hand Vein, Right* **L Intracranial Vein** Anterior cerebral vein Basal (internal) cerebral vein Dural venous sinus Great cerebral vein Inferior cerebellar vein Inferior cerebral vein Internal (basal) cerebral vein Middle cerebral vein Ophthalmic vein Superior cerebellar vein Superior cerebral vein **M Internal Jugular Vein, Right** **N Internal Jugular Vein, Left** **P External Jugular Vein, Right** Posterior auricular vein **Q External Jugular Vein, Left** *See P External Jugular Vein, Right* **R Vertebral Vein, Right** Deep cervical vein Suboccipital venous plexus **S Vertebral Vein, Left** *See R Vertebral Vein, Right* **T Face Vein, Right** Angular vein Anterior facial vein Common facial vein Deep facial vein Frontal vein Posterior facial (retromandibular) vein Supraorbital vein **V Face Vein, Left** *See T Face Vein, Right* **Y Upper Vein**	**Ø Open** **3 Percutaneous** **4 Percutaneous Endoscopic**	**Z No Device**	**X Diagnostic** **Z No Qualifier**

NC Noncovered Procedure   **LC** Limited Coverage   **QA** Questionable OB Admit   **NT** New Tech Add-on   ⊞ Combination Member   ♂ Male   ♀ Female

ICD-10-PCS 2022   **249**

Ø5B–Ø5B

0   Medical and Surgical
5   Upper Veins
C   Extirpation   Definition: Taking or cutting out solid matter from a body part

Explanation: The solid matter may be an abnormal byproduct of a biological function or a foreign body; it may be imbedded in a body part or in the lumen of a tubular body part. The solid matter may or may not have been previously broken into pieces.

Body Part Character 4	Approach Character 5	Device Character 6	Qualifier Character 7

0   **Azygos Vein**
   Right ascending lumbar vein
   Right subcostal vein
1   **Hemiazygos Vein**
   Left ascending lumbar vein
   Left subcostal vein
3   **Innominate Vein, Right**
   Brachiocephalic vein
   Inferior thyroid vein
4   **Innominate Vein, Left**
   See 3 Innominate Vein, Right
5   **Subclavian Vein, Right**
6   **Subclavian Vein, Left**
7   **Axillary Vein, Right**
8   **Axillary Vein, Left**
9   **Brachial Vein, Right**
   Radial vein
   Ulnar vein
A   **Brachial Vein, Left**
   See 9 Brachial Vein, Right
B   **Basilic Vein, Right**
   Median antebrachial vein
   Median cubital vein
C   **Basilic Vein, Left**
   See B Basilic Vein, Right
D   **Cephalic Vein, Right**
   Accessory cephalic vein
F   **Cephalic Vein, Left**
   See D Cephalic Vein, Right
G   **Hand Vein, Right**
   Dorsal metacarpal vein
   Palmar (volar) digital vein
   Palmar (volar) metacarpal vein
   Superficial palmar venous arch
   Volar (palmar) digital vein
   Volar (palmar) metacarpal vein
H   **Hand Vein, Left**
   See G Hand Vein, Right
L   **Intracranial Vein**
   Anterior cerebral vein
   Basal (internal) cerebral vein
   Dural venous sinus
   Great cerebral vein
   Inferior cerebellar vein
   Inferior cerebral vein
   Internal (basal) cerebral vein
   Middle cerebral vein
   Ophthalmic vein
   Superior cerebellar vein
   Superior cerebral vein
M   **Internal Jugular Vein, Right**
N   **Internal Jugular Vein, Left**
P   **External Jugular Vein, Right**
   Posterior auricular vein
Q   **External Jugular Vein, Left**
   See P External Jugular Vein, Right
R   **Vertebral Vein, Right**
   Deep cervical vein
   Suboccipital venous plexus
S   **Vertebral Vein, Left**
   See R Vertebral Vein, Right
T   **Face Vein, Right**
   Angular vein
   Anterior facial vein
   Common facial vein
   Deep facial vein
   Frontal vein
   Posterior facial (retromandibular) vein
   Supraorbital vein
V   **Face Vein, Left**
   See T Face Vein, Right
Y   **Upper Vein**
	0 Open
	3 Percutaneous
	4 Percutaneous Endoscopic
		Z No Device	**Z** No Qualifier

Ø   Medical and Surgical
5   Upper Veins
D   Extraction   Definition: Pulling or stripping out or off all or a portion of a body part by the use of force
                    Explanation: The qualifier DIAGNOSTIC is used to identify extraction procedures that are biopsies

Body Part Character 4	Approach Character 5	Device Character 6	Qualifier Character 7

9   **Brachial Vein, Right**
     Radial vein
     Ulnar vein
A   **Brachial Vein, Left**
     See 9 Brachial Vein, Right
B   **Basilic Vein, Right**
     Median antebrachial vein
     Median cubital vein
C   **Basilic Vein, Left**
     See B Basilic Vein, Right
D   **Cephalic Vein, Right**
     Accessory cephalic vein
F   **Cephalic Vein, Left**
     See D Cephalic Vein, Right
G   **Hand Vein, Right**
     Dorsal metacarpal vein
     Palmar (volar) digital vein
     Palmar (volar) metacarpal vein
     Superficial palmar venous arch
     Volar (palmar) digital vein
     Volar (palmar) metacarpal vein
H   **Hand Vein, Left**
     See G Hand Vein, Right
Y   **Upper Vein**
	Ø Open
	3 Percutaneous
		Z No Device	**Z** No Qualifier

Ø   Medical and Surgical
5   Upper Veins
F   Fragmentation   Definition: Breaking solid matter in a body part into pieces
                    Explanation: Physical force (e.g., manual, ultrasonic) applied directly or indirectly is used to break the solid matter into pieces. The solid matter may be an abnormal byproduct of a biological function or a foreign body. The pieces of solid matter are not taken out.

Body Part Character 4	Approach Character 5	Device Character 6	Qualifier Character 7

3   **Innominate Vein, Right**
     Brachiocephalic vein
     Inferior thyroid vein
4   **Innominate Vein, Left**
     See 3 Innominate Vein, Right
5   **Subclavian Vein, Right**
6   **Subclavian Vein, Left**
7   **Axillary Vein, Right**
8   **Axillary Vein, Left**
9   **Brachial Vein, Right**
     Radial vein
     Ulnar vein
A   **Brachial Vein, Left**
     See 9 Brachial Vein, Right
B   **Basilic Vein, Right**
     Median antebrachial vein
     Median cubital vein
C   **Basilic Vein, Left**
     See B Basilic Vein, Right
D   **Cephalic Vein, Right**
     Accessory cephalic vein
F   **Cephalic Vein, Left**
     See D Cephalic Vein, Right
Y   **Upper Vein**
	3 Percutaneous	**Z** No Device	**Ø** Ultrasonic
			Z No Qualifier

NC Noncovered Procedure   **LC** Limited Coverage   **QA** Questionable OB Admit   **NT** New Tech Add-on   ⊞ Combination Member   ♂Male   ♀Female

ICD-10-PCS 2022   **251**

Ø   **Medical and Surgical**
5   **Upper Veins**
H   **Insertion**   Definition: Putting in a nonbiological appliance that monitors, assists, performs, or prevents a physiological function but does not physically take the place of a body part
                  Explanation: None

Body Part Character 4		Approach Character 5	Device Character 6	Qualifier Character 7

Ø **Azygos Vein** ✚
    Right ascending lumbar vein
    Right subcostal vein
		Ø Open
		3 Percutaneous
		4 Percutaneous Endoscopic
			2 Monitoring Device
			3 Infusion Device
			D Intraluminal Device
			M Neurostimulator Lead
				Z No Qualifier

1 **Hemiazygos Vein**
    Left ascending lumbar vein
    Left subcostal vein
5 **Subclavian Vein, Right**
6 **Subclavian Vein, Left**
7 **Axillary Vein, Right**
8 **Axillary Vein, Left**
9 **Brachial Vein, Right**
    Radial vein
    Ulnar vein
A **Brachial Vein, Left**
    See 9 *Brachial Vein, Right*
B **Basilic Vein, Right**
    Median antebrachial vein
    Median cubital vein
C **Basilic Vein, Left**
    See B *Basilic Vein, Right*
D **Cephalic Vein, Right**
    Accessory cephalic vein
F **Cephalic Vein, Left**
    See D *Cephalic Vein, Right*
G **Hand Vein, Right**
    Dorsal metacarpal vein
    Palmar (volar) digital vein
    Palmar (volar) metacarpal vein
    Superficial palmar venous arch
    Volar (palmar) digital vein
    Volar (palmar) metacarpal vein
H **Hand Vein, Left**
    See G *Hand Vein, Right*
	L **Intracranial Vein**
	    Anterior cerebral vein
	    Basal (internal) cerebral vein
	    Dural venous sinus
	    Great cerebral vein
	    Inferior cerebellar vein
	    Inferior cerebral vein
	    Internal (basal) cerebral vein
	    Middle cerebral vein
	    Ophthalmic vein
	    Superior cerebellar vein
	    Superior cerebral vein
	M **Internal Jugular Vein, Right**
	N **Internal Jugular Vein, Left**
	P **External Jugular Vein, Right**
	    Posterior auricular vein
	Q **External Jugular Vein, Left**
	    See P *External Jugular Vein,*
	    Right
	R **Vertebral Vein, Right**
	    Deep cervical vein
	    Suboccipital venous plexus
	S **Vertebral Vein, Left**
	    See R *Vertebral Vein, Right*
	T **Face Vein, Right**
	    Angular vein
	    Anterior facial vein
	    Common facial vein
	    Deep facial vein
	    Frontal vein
	    Posterior facial
	       (retromandibular) vein
	    Supraorbital vein
	V **Face Vein, Left**
	    See T *Face Vein, Right*
		Ø Open
		3 Percutaneous
		4 Percutaneous Endoscopic
			3 Infusion Device
			D Intraluminal Device
				Z No Qualifier

3 **Innominate Vein, Right** ✚
    Brachiocephalic vein
    Inferior thyroid vein
4 **Innominate Vein, Left** ✚
    See 3 *Innominate Vein, Right*
		Ø Open
		3 Percutaneous
		4 Percutaneous Endoscopic
			3 Infusion Device
			D Intraluminal Device
			M Neurostimulator Lead
				Z No Qualifier

Y **Upper Vein**		**Ø** Open **3** Percutaneous **4** Percutaneous Endoscopic	**2** Monitoring Device **3** Infusion Device **D** Intraluminal Device **Y** Other Device	**Z** No Qualifier

Non-OR	Ø5HØ[Ø,3,4]3Z	
Non-OR	Ø5H[1,5,6,7,8,9,A,B,C,D,F,G,H,L,M,N,P,Q,R,S,T,V][Ø,3,4]3Z	
Non-OR	Ø5H[3,4][Ø,3,4]3Z	
Non-OR	Ø5HY[Ø,3,4]3Z	
Non-OR	Ø5HY32Z	
Non-OR	Ø5HY[3,4]YZ	
HAC	Ø5HØ[3,4]3Z when reported with SDx J95.811	
HAC	Ø5H[1,5,6][3,4]3Z when reported with SDx J95.811	
HAC	Ø5H[M,N,P,Q]33Z when reported with SDx J95.811	
HAC	Ø5H[3,4][3,4]3Z when reported with SDx J95.811	

See Appendix L for Procedure Combinations
✚   Ø5HØ[Ø,3,4]MZ
✚   Ø5H[3,4][Ø,3,4]MZ

Ø   **Medical and Surgical**
5   **Upper Veins**
J   **Inspection**   Definition: Visually and/or manually exploring a body part
                  Explanation: Visual exploration may be performed with or without optical instrumentation. Manual exploration may be performed directly or through intervening body layers.

Body Part Character 4	Approach Character 5	Device Character 6	Qualifier Character 7
Y **Upper Vein**	**Ø** Open **3** Percutaneous **4** Percutaneous Endoscopic **X** External	**Z** No Device	**Z** No Qualifier

Non-OR	Ø5JY[3,X]ZZ

Non-OR Procedure   DRG Non-OR Procedure   Valid OR Procedure   HAC Associated Procedure   Combination Only   New/Revised GREEN

Ø   Medical and Surgical
5   Upper Veins
L   Occlusion   Definition: Completely closing an orifice or the lumen of a tubular body part
                    Explanation: The orifice can be a natural orifice or an artificially created orifice

Body Part Character 4	Approach Character 5	Device Character 6	Qualifier Character 7

Ø **Azygos Vein**
    Right ascending lumbar vein
    Right subcostal vein
1 **Hemiazygos Vein**
    Left ascending lumbar vein
    Left subcostal vein
3 **Innominate Vein, Right**
    Brachiocephalic vein
    Inferior thyroid vein
4 **Innominate Vein, Left**
    See 3 Innominate Vein, Right
5 **Subclavian Vein, Right**
6 **Subclavian Vein, Left**
7 **Axillary Vein, Right**
8 **Axillary Vein, Left**
9 **Brachial Vein, Right**
    Radial vein
    Ulnar vein
A **Brachial Vein, Left**
    See 9 Brachial Vein, Right
B **Basilic Vein, Right**
    Median antebrachial vein
    Median cubital vein
C **Basilic Vein, Left**
    See B Basilic Vein, Right
D **Cephalic Vein, Right**
    Accessory cephalic vein
F **Cephalic Vein, Left**
    See D Cephalic Vein, Right
G **Hand Vein, Right**
    Dorsal metacarpal vein
    Palmar (volar) digital vein
    Palmar (volar) metacarpal vein
    Superficial palmar venous arch
    Volar (palmar) digital vein
    Volar (palmar) metacarpal vein
H **Hand Vein, Left**
    See G Hand Vein, Right
L **Intracranial Vein**
    Anterior cerebral vein
    Basal (internal) cerebral vein
    Dural venous sinus
    Great cerebral vein
    Inferior cerebellar vein
    Inferior cerebral vein
    Internal (basal) cerebral vein
    Middle cerebral vein
    Ophthalmic vein
    Superior cerebellar vein
    Superior cerebral vein
M **Internal Jugular Vein, Right**
N **Internal Jugular Vein, Left**
P **External Jugular Vein, Right**
    Posterior auricular vein
Q **External Jugular Vein, Left**
    See P External Jugular Vein, Right
R **Vertebral Vein, Right**
    Deep cervical vein
    Suboccipital venous plexus
S **Vertebral Vein, Left**
    See R Vertebral Vein, Right
T **Face Vein, Right**
    Angular vein
    Anterior facial vein
    Common facial vein
    Deep facial vein
    Frontal vein
    Posterior facial (retromandibular) vein
    Supraorbital vein
V **Face Vein, Left**
    See T Face Vein, Right
Y **Upper Vein**
	Ø Open
	3 Percutaneous
	4 Percutaneous Endoscopic
		C Extraluminal Device
		D Intraluminal Device
		Z No Device
			Z No Qualifier

NC Noncovered Procedure   **LC** Limited Coverage   **QA** Questionable OB Admit   **NT** New Tech Add-on   ⊞ Combination Member   ♂ Male   ♀ Female

ICD-10-PCS 2022   **253**

05L–05L

Ø   Medical and Surgical
5   Upper Veins
N   Release   Definition: Freeing a body part from an abnormal physical constraint by cutting or by the use of force
                   Explanation: Some of the restraining tissue may be taken out but none of the body part is taken out

Body Part Character 4	Approach Character 5	Device Character 6	Qualifier Character 7

Ø   Azygos Vein
     Right ascending lumbar vein
     Right subcostal vein
	Ø Open
	3 Percutaneous
	4 Percutaneous Endoscopic
		Z No Device	**Z No Qualifier**

1   Hemiazygos Vein
     Left ascending lumbar vein
     Left subcostal vein			

3   Innominate Vein, Right
     Brachiocephalic vein
     Inferior thyroid vein			

4 Innominate Vein, Left *See 3 Innominate Vein, Right*			
5 Subclavian Vein, Right			
6 Subclavian Vein, Left			
7 Axillary Vein, Right			
8 Axillary Vein, Left			

9   Brachial Vein, Right
     Radial vein
     Ulnar vein			

A Brachial Vein, Left *See 9 Brachial Vein, Right*			

B   Basilic Vein, Right
     Median antebrachial vein
     Median cubital vein			

C Basilic Vein, Left *See B Basilic Vein, Right*			
D Cephalic Vein, Right Accessory cephalic vein			
F Cephalic Vein, Left *See D Cephalic Vein, Right*			

G   Hand Vein, Right
     Dorsal metacarpal vein
     Palmar (volar) digital vein
     Palmar (volar) metacarpal vein
     Superficial palmar venous arch
     Volar (palmar) digital vein
     Volar (palmar) metacarpal vein			

H Hand Vein, Left *See G Hand Vein, Right*			

L   Intracranial Vein
     Anterior cerebral vein
     Basal (internal) cerebral vein
     Dural venous sinus
     Great cerebral vein
     Inferior cerebellar vein
     Inferior cerebral vein
     Internal (basal) cerebral vein
     Middle cerebral vein
     Ophthalmic vein
     Superior cerebellar vein
     Superior cerebral vein			

M Internal Jugular Vein, Right			
N Internal Jugular Vein, Left			
P External Jugular Vein, Right Posterior auricular vein			
Q External Jugular Vein, Left *See P External Jugular Vein, Right*			

R   Vertebral Vein, Right
     Deep cervical vein
     Suboccipital venous plexus			

S Vertebral Vein, Left *See R Vertebral Vein, Right*			

T   Face Vein, Right
     Angular vein
     Anterior facial vein
     Common facial vein
     Deep facial vein
     Frontal vein
     Posterior facial (retromandibular) vein
     Supraorbital vein			

V Face Vein, Left *See T Face Vein, Right*			
Y Upper Vein			

Non-OR Procedure   DRG Non-OR Procedure   Valid OR Procedure   HAC Associated Procedure   Combination Only   New/Revised GREEN

Ø   **Medical and Surgical**
5   **Upper Veins**
P   **Removal**   Definition: Taking out or off a device from a body part

Explanation: If a device is taken out and a similar device put in without cutting or puncturing the skin or mucous membrane, the procedure is coded to the root operation CHANGE. Otherwise, the procedure for taking out a device is coded to the root operation REMOVAL.

Body Part Character 4	Approach Character 5	Device Character 6	Qualifier Character 7

Ø   **Azygos Vein**
    Right ascending lumbar vein
    Right subcostal vein
	Ø Open
	3 Percutaneous
	4 Percutaneous Endoscopic
	X External
		2 Monitoring Device
		M Neurostimulator Lead
			Z No Qualifier

3   **Innominate Vein, Right**
    Brachiocephalic vein
    Inferior thyroid vein
4   **Innominate Vein, Left**
    See 3 Innominate Vein, Right
	Ø Open
	3 Percutaneous
	4 Percutaneous Endoscopic
	X External
		M Neurostimulator Lead	**Z** No Qualifier

Y **Upper Vein**	**Ø** Open **3** Percutaneous **4** Percutaneous Endoscopic	**Ø** Drainage Device **2** Monitoring Device **3** Infusion Device **7** Autologous Tissue Substitute **C** Extraluminal Device **D** Intraluminal Device **J** Synthetic Substitute **K** Nonautologous Tissue Substitute **Y** Other Device	**Z** No Qualifier
Y **Upper Vein**	**X** External	**Ø** Drainage Device **2** Monitoring Device **3** Infusion Device **D** Intraluminal Device	**Z** No Qualifier

Non-OR   05PØ[Ø,3,4,X]2Z
Non-OR   05PY3[Ø,2,3]Z
Non-OR   05PY[3,4]YZ
Non-OR   05PYX[Ø,2,3,D]Z

NC Noncovered Procedure   LC Limited Coverage   QA Questionable OB Admit   NT New Tech Add-on   ⊞ Combination Member   ♂ Male   ♀ Female

ICD-10-PCS 2022   255

05P–05P

Upper Veins *(left margin)*

Ø Medical and Surgical
5 Upper Veins
Q Repair   Definition: Restoring, to the extent possible, a body part to its normal anatomic structure and function

                   Explanation: Used only when the method to accomplish the repair is not one of the other root operations

Body Part Character 4	Approach Character 5	Device Character 6	Qualifier Character 7

Ø Azygos Vein
   Right ascending lumbar vein
   Right subcostal vein
1 Hemiazygos Vein
   Left ascending lumbar vein
   Left subcostal vein
3 Innominate Vein, Right
   Brachiocephalic vein
   Inferior thyroid vein
4 Innominate Vein, Left
   See 3 Innominate Vein, Right
5 Subclavian Vein, Right
6 Subclavian Vein, Left
7 Axillary Vein, Right
8 Axillary Vein, Left
9 Brachial Vein, Right
   Radial vein
   Ulnar vein
A Brachial Vein, Left
   See 9 Brachial Vein, Right
B Basilic Vein, Right
   Median antebrachial vein
   Median cubital vein
C Basilic Vein, Left
   See B Basilic Vein, Right
D Cephalic Vein, Right
   Accessory cephalic vein
F Cephalic Vein, Left
   See D Cephalic Vein, Right
G Hand Vein, Right
   Dorsal metacarpal vein
   Palmar (volar) digital vein
   Palmar (volar) metacarpal vein
   Superficial palmar venous arch
   Volar (palmar) digital vein
   Volar (palmar) metacarpal vein
H Hand Vein, Left
   See G Hand Vein, Right
L Intracranial Vein
   Anterior cerebral vein
   Basal (internal) cerebral vein
   Dural venous sinus
   Great cerebral vein
   Inferior cerebellar vein
   Inferior cerebral vein
   Internal (basal) cerebral vein
   Middle cerebral vein
   Ophthalmic vein
   Superior cerebellar vein
   Superior cerebral vein
M Internal Jugular Vein, Right
N Internal Jugular Vein, Left
P External Jugular Vein, Right
   Posterior auricular vein
Q External Jugular Vein, Left
   See P External Jugular Vein, Right
R Vertebral Vein, Right
   Deep cervical vein
   Suboccipital venous plexus
S Vertebral Vein, Left
   See R Vertebral Vein, Right
T Face Vein, Right
   Angular vein
   Anterior facial vein
   Common facial vein
   Deep facial vein
   Frontal vein
   Posterior facial (retromandibular) vein
   Supraorbital vein
V Face Vein, Left
   See T Face Vein, Right
Y Upper Vein
	Ø Open
	3 Percutaneous
	4 Percutaneous Endoscopic
		Z No Device	Z No Qualifier

Non-OR Procedure   DRG Non-OR Procedure   Valid OR Procedure   HAC Associated Procedure   Combination Only   New/Revised GREEN

Ø   Medical and Surgical
5   Upper Veins
R   Replacement   Definition: Putting in or on biological or synthetic material that physically takes the place and/or function of all or a portion of a body part

Explanation: The body part may have been taken out or replaced, or may be taken out, physically eradicated, or rendered nonfunctional during the REPLACEMENT procedure. A REMOVAL procedure is coded for taking out the device used in a previous replacement procedure.

Body Part Character 4	Approach Character 5	Device Character 6	Qualifier Character 7
Ø Azygos Vein Right ascending lumbar vein Right subcostal vein	**Ø Open** **4 Percutaneous Endoscopic**	**7 Autologous Tissue Substitute** **J Synthetic Substitute** **K Nonautologous Tissue Substitute**	**Z No Qualifier**
1 Hemiazygos Vein Left ascending lumbar vein Left subcostal vein			
3 Innominate Vein, Right Brachiocephalic vein Inferior thyroid vein			
4 Innominate Vein, Left *See 3 Innominate Vein, Right*			
5 Subclavian Vein, Right			
6 Subclavian Vein, Left			
7 Axillary Vein, Right			
8 Axillary Vein, Left			
9 Brachial Vein, Right Radial vein Ulnar vein			
A Brachial Vein, Left *See 9 Brachial Vein, Right*			
B Basilic Vein, Right Median antebrachial vein Median cubital vein			
C Basilic Vein, Left *See B Basilic Vein, Right*			
D Cephalic Vein, Right Accessory cephalic vein			
F Cephalic Vein, Left *See D Cephalic Vein, Right*			
G Hand Vein, Right Dorsal metacarpal vein Palmar (volar) digital vein Palmar (volar) metacarpal vein Superficial palmar venous arch Volar (palmar) digital vein Volar (palmar) metacarpal vein			
H Hand Vein, Left *See G Hand Vein, Right*			
L Intracranial Vein Anterior cerebral vein Basal (internal) cerebral vein Dural venous sinus Great cerebral vein Inferior cerebellar vein Inferior cerebral vein Internal (basal) cerebral vein Middle cerebral vein Ophthalmic vein Superior cerebellar vein Superior cerebral vein			
M Internal Jugular Vein, Right			
N Internal Jugular Vein, Left			
P External Jugular Vein, Right Posterior auricular vein			
Q External Jugular Vein, Left *See P External Jugular Vein, Right*			
R Vertebral Vein, Right Deep cervical vein Suboccipital venous plexus			
S Vertebral Vein, Left *See R Vertebral Vein, Right*			
T Face Vein, Right Angular vein Anterior facial vein Common facial vein Deep facial vein Frontal vein Posterior facial (retromandibular) vein Supraorbital vein			
V Face Vein, Left *See T Face Vein, Right*			
Y Upper Vein			

Ø   **Medical and Surgical**
5   **Upper Veins**
S   **Reposition**   Definition: Moving to its normal location, or other suitable location, all or a portion of a body part

                          Explanation: The body part is moved to a new location from an abnormal location, or from a normal location where it is not functioning correctly. The body part may or may not be cut out or off to be moved to the new location.

Body Part Character 4	Approach Character 5	Device Character 6	Qualifier Character 7

Ø **Azygos Vein**
    Right ascending lumbar vein
    Right subcostal vein
1 **Hemiazygos Vein**
    Left ascending lumbar vein
    Left subcostal vein
3 **Innominate Vein, Right**
    Brachiocephalic vein
    Inferior thyroid vein
4 **Innominate Vein, Left**
    See 3 Innominate Vein, Right
5 **Subclavian Vein, Right**
6 **Subclavian Vein, Left**
7 **Axillary Vein, Right**
8 **Axillary Vein, Left**
9 **Brachial Vein, Right**
    Radial vein
    Ulnar vein
A **Brachial Vein, Left**
    See 9 Brachial Vein, Right
B **Basilic Vein, Right**
    Median antebrachial vein
    Median cubital vein
C **Basilic Vein, Left**
    See B Basilic Vein, Right
D **Cephalic Vein, Right**
    Accessory cephalic vein
F **Cephalic Vein, Left**
    See D Cephalic Vein, Right
G **Hand Vein, Right**
    Dorsal metacarpal vein
    Palmar (volar) digital vein
    Palmar (volar) metacarpal vein
    Superficial palmar venous arch
    Volar (palmar) digital vein
    Volar (palmar) metacarpal vein
H **Hand Vein, Left**
    See G Hand Vein, Right
L **Intracranial Vein**
    Anterior cerebral vein
    Basal (internal) cerebral vein
    Dural venous sinus
    Great cerebral vein
    Inferior cerebellar vein
    Inferior cerebral vein
    Internal (basal) cerebral vein
    Middle cerebral vein
    Ophthalmic vein
    Superior cerebellar vein
    Superior cerebral vein
M **Internal Jugular Vein, Right**
N **Internal Jugular Vein, Left**
P **External Jugular Vein, Right**
    Posterior auricular vein
Q **External Jugular Vein, Left**
    See P External Jugular Vein, Right
R **Vertebral Vein, Right**
    Deep cervical vein
    Suboccipital venous plexus
S **Vertebral Vein, Left**
    See R Vertebral Vein, Right
T **Face Vein, Right**
    Angular vein
    Anterior facial vein
    Common facial vein
    Deep facial vein
    Frontal vein
    Posterior facial (retromandibular) vein
    Supraorbital vein
V **Face Vein, Left**
    See T Face Vein, Right
Y **Upper Vein**
	Ø Open
	3 Percutaneous
	4 Percutaneous Endoscopic
		Z No Device	**Z** No Qualifier

Ø   Medical and Surgical
5   Upper Veins
U   Supplement   Definition: Putting in or on biological or synthetic material that physically reinforces and/or augments the function of a portion of a body part

                      Explanation: The biological material is non-living, or is living and from the same individual. The body part may have been previously replaced, and the SUPPLEMENT procedure is performed to physically reinforce and/or augment the function of the replaced body part.

Body Part Character 4	Approach Character 5	Device Character 6	Qualifier Character 7

Ø   Azygos Vein
    Right ascending lumbar vein
    Right subcostal vein
1   Hemiazygos Vein
    Left ascending lumbar vein
    Left subcostal vein
3   Innominate Vein, Right
    Brachiocephalic vein
    Inferior thyroid vein
4   Innominate Vein, Left
    See 3 Innominate Vein, Right
5   Subclavian Vein, Right
6   Subclavian Vein, Left
7   Axillary Vein, Right
8   Axillary Vein, Left
9   Brachial Vein, Right
    Radial vein
    Ulnar vein
A   Brachial Vein, Left
    See 9 Brachial Vein, Right
B   Basilic Vein, Right
    Median antebrachial vein
    Median cubital vein
C   Basilic Vein, Left
    See B Basilic Vein, Right
D   Cephalic Vein, Right
    Accessory cephalic vein
F   Cephalic Vein, Left
    See D Cephalic Vein, Right
G   Hand Vein, Right
    Dorsal metacarpal vein
    Palmar (volar) digital vein
    Palmar (volar) metacarpal vein
    Superficial palmar venous arch
    Volar (palmar) digital vein
    Volar (palmar) metacarpal vein
H   Hand Vein, Left
    See G Hand Vein, Right
L   Intracranial Vein
    Anterior cerebral vein
    Basal (internal) cerebral vein
    Dural venous sinus
    Great cerebral vein
    Inferior cerebellar vein
    Inferior cerebral vein
    Internal (basal) cerebral vein
    Middle cerebral vein
    Ophthalmic vein
    Superior cerebellar vein
    Superior cerebral vein
M   Internal Jugular Vein, Right
N   Internal Jugular Vein, Left
P   External Jugular Vein, Right
    Posterior auricular vein
Q   External Jugular Vein, Left
    See P External Jugular Vein, Right
R   Vertebral Vein, Right
    Deep cervical vein
    Suboccipital venous plexus
S   Vertebral Vein, Left
    See R Vertebral Vein, Right
T   Face Vein, Right
    Angular vein
    Anterior facial vein
    Common facial vein
    Deep facial vein
    Frontal vein
    Posterior facial (retromandibular) vein
    Supraorbital vein
V   Face Vein, Left
    See T Face Vein, Right
Y   Upper Vein
	Ø Open
	3 Percutaneous
	4 Percutaneous Endoscopic
		7 Autologous Tissue Substitute
		J Synthetic Substitute
		K Nonautologous Tissue Substitute
			Z No Qualifier

NC Noncovered Procedure   **LC** Limited Coverage   **QA** Questionable OB Admit   **NT** New Tech Add-on   ⊞ Combination Member   ♂ Male   ♀ Female

ICD-10-PCS 2022   259

Ø   **Medical and Surgical**
5   **Upper Veins**
V   **Restriction**   Definition: Partially closing an orifice or the lumen of a tubular body part

                              Explanation: The orifice can be a natural orifice or an artificially created orifice

Body Part Character 4	Approach Character 5	Device Character 6	Qualifier Character 7

Ø **Azygos Vein**
   Right ascending lumbar vein
   Right subcostal vein
1 **Hemiazygos Vein**
   Left ascending lumbar vein
   Left subcostal vein
3 **Innominate Vein, Right**
   Brachiocephalic vein
   Inferior thyroid vein
4 **Innominate Vein, Left**
   See 3 Innominate Vein, Right
5 **Subclavian Vein, Right**
6 **Subclavian Vein, Left**
7 **Axillary Vein, Right**
8 **Axillary Vein, Left**
9 **Brachial Vein, Right**
   Radial vein
   Ulnar vein
A **Brachial Vein, Left**
   See 9 Brachial Vein, Right
B **Basilic Vein, Right**
   Median antebrachial vein
   Median cubital vein
C **Basilic Vein, Left**
   See B Basilic Vein, Right
D **Cephalic Vein, Right**
   Accessory cephalic vein
F **Cephalic Vein, Left**
   See D Cephalic Vein, Right
G **Hand Vein, Right**
   Dorsal metacarpal vein
   Palmar (volar) digital vein
   Palmar (volar) metacarpal vein
   Superficial palmar venous arch
   Volar (palmar) digital vein
   Volar (palmar) metacarpal vein
H **Hand Vein, Left**
   See G Hand Vein, Right
L **Intracranial Vein**
   Anterior cerebral vein
   Basal (internal) cerebral vein
   Dural venous sinus
   Great cerebral vein
   Inferior cerebellar vein
   Inferior cerebral vein
   Internal (basal) cerebral vein
   Middle cerebral vein
   Ophthalmic vein
   Superior cerebellar vein
   Superior cerebral vein
M **Internal Jugular Vein, Right**
N **Internal Jugular Vein, Left**
P **External Jugular Vein, Right**
   Posterior auricular vein
Q **External Jugular Vein, Left**
   See P External Jugular Vein, Right
R **Vertebral Vein, Right**
   Deep cervical vein
   Suboccipital venous plexus
S **Vertebral Vein, Left**
   See R Vertebral Vein, Right
T **Face Vein, Right**
   Angular vein
   Anterior facial vein
   Common facial vein
   Deep facial vein
   Frontal vein
   Posterior facial (retromandibular) vein
   Supraorbital vein
V **Face Vein, Left**
   See T Face Vein, Right
Y **Upper Vein**
	Ø Open
	3 Percutaneous
	4 Percutaneous Endoscopic
		C Extraluminal Device
		D Intraluminal Device
		Z No Device
			Z No Qualifier

Non-OR Procedure   DRG Non-OR Procedure   Valid OR Procedure   HAC Associated Procedure   Combination Only   New/Revised GREEN

Ø   Medical and Surgical
5   Upper Veins
W   Revision   Definition: Correcting, to the extent possible, a portion of a malfunctioning device or the position of a displaced device

Explanation: Revision can include correcting a malfunctioning or displaced device by taking out or putting in components of the device such as a screw or pin

Body Part Character 4	Approach Character 5	Device Character 6	Qualifier Character 7
Ø Azygos Vein Right ascending lumbar vein Right subcostal vein	**Ø Open** **3 Percutaneous** **4 Percutaneous Endoscopic** **X External**	**2 Monitoring Device** **M Neurostimulator Lead**	**Z No Qualifier**
3 Innominate Vein, Right Brachiocephalic vein Inferior thyroid vein **4 Innominate Vein, Left** *See 3 Innominate Vein, Right*	**Ø Open** **3 Percutaneous** **4 Percutaneous Endoscopic** **X External**	**M Neurostimulator Lead**	**Z No Qualifier**
Y Upper Vein	**Ø Open** **3 Percutaneous** **4 Percutaneous Endoscopic**	**Ø Drainage Device** **2 Monitoring Device** **3 Infusion Device** **7 Autologous Tissue Substitute** **C Extraluminal Device** **D Intraluminal Device** **J Synthetic Substitute** **K Nonautologous Tissue Substitute** **Y Other Device**	**Z No Qualifier**
Y Upper Vein	**X External**	**Ø Drainage Device** **2 Monitoring Device** **3 Infusion Device** **7 Autologous Tissue Substitute** **C Extraluminal Device** **D Intraluminal Device** **J Synthetic Substitute** **K Nonautologous Tissue Substitute**	**Z No Qualifier**

Non-OR	Ø5WØXMZ
Non-OR	Ø5W[3,4]XMZ
Non-OR	Ø5WY3[Ø,2,3,D]Z
Non-OR	Ø5WY[3,4]YZ
Non-OR	Ø5WYX[Ø,2,3,7,C,D,J,K]Z

NC Noncovered Procedure   **LC** Limited Coverage   **QA** Questionable OB Admit   **NT** New Tech Add-on   ⊞ Combination Member   ♂ Male   ♀ Female

ICD-10-PCS 2022   261

Lower Veins Ø61–Ø6W

Character Meanings

This Character Meaning table is provided as a guide to assist the user in the identification of character members that may be found in this section of code tables. It **SHOULD NOT** be used to build a PCS code.

Operation–Character 3	Body Part–Character 4	Approach–Character 5	Device–Character 6	Qualifier–Character 7
1 Bypass	Ø Inferior Vena Cava	Ø Open	Ø Drainage Device	Ø Ultrasonic
5 Destruction	1 Splenic Vein	3 Percutaneous	2 Monitoring Device	4 Hepatic Vein
7 Dilation	2 Gastric Vein	4 Percutaneous Endoscopic	3 Infusion Device	5 Superior Mesenteric Vein
9 Drainage	3 Esophageal Vein	7 Via Natural or Artificial Opening	7 Autologous Tissue Substitute	6 Inferior Mesenteric Vein
B Excision	4 Hepatic Vein	8 Via Natural or Artificial Opening Endoscopic	9 Autologous Venous Tissue	9 Renal Vein, Right
C Extirpation	5 Superior Mesenteric Vein	X External	A Autologous Arterial Tissue	B Renal Vein, Left
D Extraction	6 Inferior Mesenteric Vein		C Extraluminal Device	C Hemorrhoidal Plexus
F Fragmentation	7 Colic Vein		D Intraluminal Device	P Pulmonary Trunk
H Insertion	8 Portal Vein		J Synthetic Substitute	Q Pulmonary Artery, Right
J Inspection	9 Renal Vein, Right		K Nonautologous Tissue Substitute	R Pulmonary Artery, Left
L Occlusion	B Renal Vein, Left		Y Other Device	T Via Umbilical Vein
N Release	C Common Iliac Vein, Right		Z No Device	X Diagnostic
P Removal	D Common Iliac Vein, Left			Y Lower Vein
Q Repair	F External Iliac Vein, Right			Z No Qualifier
R Replacement	G External Iliac Vein, Left			
S Reposition	H Hypogastric Vein, Right			
U Supplement	J Hypogastric Vein, Left			
V Restriction	M Femoral Vein, Right			
W Revision	N Femoral Vein, Left			
	P Saphenous Vein, Right			
	Q Saphenous Vein, Left			
	T Foot Vein, Right			
	V Foot Vein, Left			
	Y Lower Vein			

AHA Coding Clinic for table Ø61
2017, 4Q, 36-38 Fontan completion procedure
2017, 4Q, 66-67 New qualifier values - Portal to hepatic shunt

AHA Coding Clinic for table Ø6B
2020, 1Q, 28 Free flap microvascular breast reconstruction
2017, 3Q, 5 Femoral artery to posterior tibial artery bypass using autologous and synthetic grafts
2017, 1Q, 31 Left to right common carotid artery bypass
2017, 1Q, 32 Peroneal artery to dorsalis pedis artery bypass using saphenous vein graft
2016, 3Q, 31 Femoral to peroneal artery bypass with in-situ saphenous vein graft and lysis of valves
2016, 2Q, 18 Femoral-tibial artery bypass and saphenous vein graft
2016, 1Q, 27 Aortocoronary bypass graft utilizing Y-graft
2014, 3Q, 8 Excision of saphenous vein for coronary artery bypass graft
2014, 3Q, 20 MAZE procedure performed with coronary artery bypass graft
2014, 1Q, 10 Repair of thoracic aortic aneurysm & coronary artery bypass graft

AHA Coding Clinic for table Ø6F
2020, 4Q, 45-49 New fragmentation tables
2020, 4Q, 49-50 Intravascular ultrasound assisted thrombolysis
2020, 4Q, 50 Intravascular lithotripsy

AHA Coding Clinic for table Ø6H
2017, 3Q, 11 Placement of peripherally inserted central catheter using 3CG ECG technology
2017, 1Q, 31 Umbilical vein catheterization
2017, 1Q, 31 Central catheter placement in femoral vein
2013, 3Q, 18 Heart transplant surgery

AHA Coding Clinic for table Ø6L
2020, 3Q, 44 Cardiophrenic vein embolization
2019, 4Q, 28 Transorifice occlusion of gastric varices
2018, 2Q, 18 Transverse rectus abdominis myocutaneous (TRAM) delay
2017, 4Q, 57-58 Added approach values - Transorifice esophageal vein banding
2013, 4Q, 112 Endoscopic banding of esophageal varices

AHA Coding Clinic for table Ø6V
2018, 3Q, 11 Transvenous transcatheter placement of valve in inferior vena cava
2018, 1Q, 10 Revision of transjugular intrahepatic portosystemic shunt

AHA Coding Clinic for table Ø6W
2019, 2Q, 39 Transjugular intrahepatic portosystemic shunt revision
2018, 1Q, 10 Revision of transjugular intrahepatic portosystemic shunt
2014, 3Q, 25 Revision of transjugular intrahepatic portosystemic shunt (TIPS)

Lower Veins

Inferior vena cava **Ø**

Common hepatic **4**

Portal **B**

Colic **7**

Internal pudendal **H, J**

Femoral **M, N**

Greater saphenous **P, Q**

Lesser saphenous **P, Q**

Anterior tibial **M, N**

Posterior tibial **M, N**

Digital **T, V**

Esophageal **3**

Gastric **2**

Splenic **1**

Renal **9, B**

Inferior mesenteric **6**

Superior mesenteric **5**

Common iliac **C, D**

Internal iliac (Hypogastric) **H, J**

External iliac **F, G**

Rectal venous plexus **H, J**

Popliteal **M, N**

Lesser saphenous **P, Q**

Greater saphenous **P, Q**

Dorsal venous arch **T, V**

Portal Venous Circulation

Inferior vena cava **Ø**

Portal **8**

Gastric **2**

Splenic **1**

Superior mesenteric **5**

Right colic **7**

Ileocolic **7**

Inferior mesenteric **6**

Left colic **7**

0 Medical and Surgical
6 Lower Veins
1 Bypass   Definition: Altering the route of passage of the contents of a tubular body part

Explanation: Rerouting contents of a body part to a downstream area of the normal route, to a similar route and body part, or to an abnormal route and dissimilar body part. Includes one or more anastomoses, with or without the use of a device.

Body Part Character 4		Approach Character 5	Device Character 6	Qualifier Character 7
0 Inferior Vena Cava Postcava Right inferior phrenic vein Right ovarian vein Right second lumbar vein Right suprarenal vein Right testicular vein		**0 Open** **4 Percutaneous Endoscopic**	**7 Autologous Tissue Substitute** **9 Autologous Venous Tissue** **A Autologous Arterial Tissue** **J Synthetic Substitute** **K Nonautologous Tissue Substitute** **Z No Device**	**5 Superior Mesenteric Vein** **6 Inferior Mesenteric Vein** **P Pulmonary Trunk** **Q Pulmonary Artery, Right** **R Pulmonary Artery, Left** **Y Lower Vein**
1 Splenic Vein Left gastroepiploic vein Pancreatic vein		**0 Open** **4 Percutaneous Endoscopic**	**7 Autologous Tissue Substitute** **9 Autologous Venous Tissue** **A Autologous Arterial Tissue** **J Synthetic Substitute** **K Nonautologous Tissue Substitute** **Z No Device**	**9 Renal Vein, Right** **B Renal Vein, Left** **Y Lower Vein**
2 Gastric Vein **3 Esophageal Vein** **4 Hepatic Vein** **5 Superior Mesenteric Vein** Right gastroepiploic vein **6 Inferior Mesenteric Vein** Sigmoid vein Superior rectal vein **7 Colic Vein** Ileocolic vein Left colic vein Middle colic vein Right colic vein **9 Renal Vein, Right** **B Renal Vein, Left** Left inferior phrenic vein Left ovarian vein Left second lumbar vein Left suprarenal vein Left testicular vein **C Common Iliac Vein, Right** **D Common Iliac Vein, Left** **F External Iliac Vein, Right** **G External Iliac Vein, Left** **H Hypogastric Vein, Right** Gluteal vein Internal iliac vein Internal pudendal vein Lateral sacral vein Middle hemorrhoidal vein Obturator vein Uterine vein Vaginal vein Vesical vein	**J Hypogastric Vein, Left** *See H Hypogastric Vein, Right* **M Femoral Vein, Right** Deep femoral (profunda femoris) vein Popliteal vein Profunda femoris (deep femoral) vein **N Femoral Vein, Left** *See M Femoral Vein, Right* **P Saphenous Vein, Right** External pudendal vein Great(er) saphenous vein Lesser saphenous vein Small saphenous vein Superficial circumflex iliac vein Superficial epigastric vein **Q Saphenous Vein, Left** *See P Saphenous Vein, Right* **T Foot Vein, Right** Common digital vein Dorsal metatarsal vein Dorsal venous arch Plantar digital vein Plantar metatarsal vein Plantar venous arch **V Foot Vein, Left** *See T Foot Vein, Right*	**0 Open** **4 Percutaneous Endoscopic**	**7 Autologous Tissue Substitute** **9 Autologous Venous Tissue** **A Autologous Arterial Tissue** **J Synthetic Substitute** **K Nonautologous Tissue Substitute** **Z No Device**	**Y Lower Vein**
8 Portal Vein Hepatic portal vein		**0 Open**	**7 Autologous Tissue Substitute** **9 Autologous Venous Tissue** **A Autologous Arterial Tissue** **J Synthetic Substitute** **K Nonautologous Tissue Substitute** **Z No Device**	**9 Renal Vein, Right** **B Renal Vein, Left** **Y Lower Vein**
8 Portal Vein Hepatic portal vein		**3 Percutaneous**	**J Synthetic Substitute**	**4 Hepatic Vein** **Y Lower Vein**
8 Portal Vein Hepatic portal vein		**4 Percutaneous Endoscopic**	**7 Autologous Tissue Substitute** **9 Autologous Venous Tissue** **A Autologous Arterial Tissue** **K Nonautologous Tissue Substitute** **Z No Device**	**9 Renal Vein, Right** **B Renal Vein, Left** **Y Lower Vein**
8 Portal Vein Hepatic portal vein		**4 Percutaneous Endoscopic**	**J Synthetic Substitute**	**4 Hepatic Vein** **9 Renal Vein, Right** **B Renal Vein, Left** **Y Lower Vein**

NC Noncovered Procedure   **LC** Limited Coverage   **QA** Questionable OB Admit   **NT** New Tech Add-on   ⊞ Combination Member   ♂ Male   ♀ Female

Ø   Medical and Surgical
6   Lower Veins
5   Destruction   Definition: Physical eradication of all or a portion of a body part by the direct use of energy, force, or a destructive agent

Explanation: None of the body part is physically taken out

Body Part Character 4	Approach Character 5	Device Character 6	Qualifier Character 7
Ø Inferior Vena Cava Postcava Right inferior phrenic vein Right ovarian vein Right second lumbar vein Right suprarenal vein Right testicular vein **1 Splenic Vein** Left gastroepiploic vein Pancreatic vein **2 Gastric Vein** **3 Esophageal Vein** **4 Hepatic Vein** **5 Superior Mesenteric Vein** Right gastroepiploic vein **6 Inferior Mesenteric Vein** Sigmoid vein Superior rectal vein **7 Colic Vein** Ileocolic vein Left colic vein Middle colic vein Right colic vein **8 Portal Vein** Hepatic portal vein **9 Renal Vein, Right** **B Renal Vein, Left** Left inferior phrenic vein Left ovarian vein Left second lumbar vein Left suprarenal vein Left testicular vein **C Common Iliac Vein, Right** **D Common Iliac Vein, Left** **F External Iliac Vein, Right** **G External Iliac Vein, Left** **H Hypogastric Vein, Right** Gluteal vein Internal iliac vein Internal pudendal vein Lateral sacral vein Middle hemorrhoidal vein Obturator vein Uterine vein Vaginal vein Vesical vein **J Hypogastric Vein, Left** *See H Hypogastric Vein, Right* **M Femoral Vein, Right** Deep femoral (profunda femoris) vein Popliteal vein Profunda femoris (deep femoral) vein **N Femoral Vein, Left** *See M Femoral Vein, Right* **P Saphenous Vein, Right** External pudendal vein Great(er) saphenous vein Lesser saphenous vein Small saphenous vein Superficial circumflex iliac vein Superficial epigastric vein **Q Saphenous Vein, Left** *See P Saphenous Vein, Right* **T Foot Vein, Right** Common digital vein Dorsal metatarsal vein Dorsal venous arch Plantar digital vein Plantar metatarsal vein Plantar venous arch **V Foot Vein, Left** *See T Foot Vein, Right*	**Ø Open** **3 Percutaneous** **4 Percutaneous Endoscopic**	**Z No Device**	**Z No Qualifier**
Y Lower Vein	**Ø Open** **3 Percutaneous** **4 Percutaneous Endoscopic**	**Z No Device**	**C Hemorrhoidal Plexus** **Z No Qualifier**

Ø   **Medical and Surgical**
6   **Lower Veins**
7   **Dilation**   Definition: Expanding an orifice or the lumen of a tubular body part

Explanation: The orifice can be a natural orifice or an artificially created orifice. Accomplished by stretching a tubular body part using intraluminal pressure or by cutting part of the orifice or wall of the tubular body part.

Body Part Character 4	Approach Character 5	Device Character 6	Qualifier Character 7

Ø   **Inferior Vena Cava**
     Postcava
     Right inferior phrenic vein
     Right ovarian vein
     Right second lumbar vein
     Right suprarenal vein
     Right testicular vein
1   **Splenic Vein**
     Left gastroepiploic vein
     Pancreatic vein
2   **Gastric Vein**
3   **Esophageal Vein**
4   **Hepatic Vein**
5   **Superior Mesenteric Vein**
     Right gastroepiploic vein
6   **Inferior Mesenteric Vein**
     Sigmoid vein
     Superior rectal vein
7   **Colic Vein**
     Ileocolic vein
     Left colic vein
     Middle colic vein
     Right colic vein
8   **Portal Vein**
     Hepatic portal vein
9   **Renal Vein, Right**
B   **Renal Vein, Left**
     Left inferior phrenic vein
     Left ovarian vein
     Left second lumbar vein
     Left suprarenal vein
     Left testicular vein
C   **Common Iliac Vein, Right**
D   **Common Iliac Vein, Left**
F   **External Iliac Vein, Right**
G   **External Iliac Vein, Left**
H   **Hypogastric Vein, Right**
     Gluteal vein
     Internal iliac vein
     Internal pudendal vein
     Lateral sacral vein
     Middle hemorrhoidal vein
     Obturator vein
     Uterine vein
     Vaginal vein
     Vesical vein
J   **Hypogastric Vein, Left**
     See H Hypogastric Vein, Right
M   **Femoral Vein, Right**
     Deep femoral (profunda femoris) vein
     Popliteal vein
     Profunda femoris (deep femoral) vein
N   **Femoral Vein, Left**
     See M Femoral Vein, Right
P   **Saphenous Vein, Right**
     External pudendal vein
     Great(er) saphenous vein
     Lesser saphenous vein
     Small saphenous vein
     Superficial circumflex iliac vein
     Superficial epigastric vein
Q   **Saphenous Vein, Left**
     See P Saphenous Vein, Right
T   **Foot Vein, Right**
     Common digital vein
     Dorsal metatarsal vein
     Dorsal venous arch
     Plantar digital vein
     Plantar metatarsal vein
     Plantar venous arch
V   **Foot Vein, Left**
     See T Foot Vein, Right
Y   **Lower Vein**
	Ø Open
	3 Percutaneous
	4 Percutaneous Endoscopic
		D Intraluminal Device
		Z No Device
			Z No Qualifier

NC Noncovered Procedure   LC Limited Coverage   OA Questionable OB Admit   NT New Tech Add-on   ⊞ Combination Member   ♂ Male   ♀ Female

Lower Veins

Ø **Medical and Surgical**
6 **Lower Veins**
9 **Drainage**　　　Definition: Taking or letting out fluids and/or gases from a body part
　　　　　　　　　　　Explanation: The qualifier DIAGNOSTIC is used to identify drainage procedures that are biopsies

Body Part Character 4	Approach Character 5	Device Character 6	Qualifier Character 7
Ø **Inferior Vena Cava** Postcava Right inferior phrenic vein Right ovarian vein Right second lumbar vein Right suprarenal vein Right testicular vein **1** **Splenic Vein** Left gastroepiploic vein Pancreatic vein **2** **Gastric Vein** **3** **Esophageal Vein** **4** **Hepatic Vein** **5** **Superior Mesenteric Vein** Right gastroepiploic vein **6** **Inferior Mesenteric Vein** Sigmoid vein Superior rectal vein **7** **Colic Vein** Ileocolic vein Left colic vein Middle colic vein Right colic vein **8** **Portal Vein** Hepatic portal vein **9** **Renal Vein, Right** **B** **Renal Vein, Left** Left inferior phrenic vein Left ovarian vein Left second lumbar vein Left suprarenal vein Left testicular vein **C** **Common Iliac Vein, Right** **D** **Common Iliac Vein, Left** **F** **External Iliac Vein, Right** **G** **External Iliac Vein, Left** **H** **Hypogastric Vein, Right** Gluteal vein Internal iliac vein Internal pudendal vein Lateral sacral vein Middle hemorrhoidal vein Obturator vein Uterine vein Vaginal vein Vesical vein **J** **Hypogastric Vein, Left** *See H Hypogastric Vein, Right* **M** **Femoral Vein, Right** Deep femoral (profunda femoris) vein Popliteal vein Profunda femoris (deep femoral) vein **N** **Femoral Vein, Left** *See M Femoral Vein, Right* **P** **Saphenous Vein, Right** External pudendal vein Great(er) saphenous vein Lesser saphenous vein Small saphenous vein Superficial circumflex iliac vein Superficial epigastric vein **Q** **Saphenous Vein, Left** *See P Saphenous Vein, Right* **T** **Foot Vein, Right** Common digital vein Dorsal metatarsal vein Dorsal venous arch Plantar digital vein Plantar metatarsal vein Plantar venous arch **V** **Foot Vein, Left** *See T Foot Vein, Right* **Y** **Lower Vein**	**Ø** Open **3** Percutaneous **4** Percutaneous Endoscopic	**Ø** Drainage Device	**Z** No Qualifier

Non-OR	Ø69[Ø,1,2,4,5,6,7,8,9,B,C,D,F,G,H,J,M,N,P,Q,T,V,Y][Ø,3,4]ØZ
Non-OR	Ø69330Z

Ø69 Continued on next page

Lower Veins *(side tab)*

Ø **Medical and Surgical**
6 **Lower Veins**
9 **Drainage**

069 Continued

Definition: Taking or letting out fluids and/or gases from a body part
Explanation: The qualifier DIAGNOSTIC is used to identify drainage procedures that are biopsies

Body Part Character 4	Approach Character 5	Device Character 6	Qualifier Character 7
Ø **Inferior Vena Cava** Postcava Right inferior phrenic vein Right ovarian vein Right second lumbar vein Right suprarenal vein Right testicular vein 1 **Splenic Vein** Left gastroepiploic vein Pancreatic vein 2 **Gastric Vein** 3 **Esophageal Vein** 4 **Hepatic Vein** 5 **Superior Mesenteric Vein** Right gastroepiploic vein 6 **Inferior Mesenteric Vein** Sigmoid vein Superior rectal vein 7 **Colic Vein** Ileocolic vein Left colic vein Middle colic vein Right colic vein 8 **Portal Vein** Hepatic portal vein 9 **Renal Vein, Right** B **Renal Vein, Left** Left inferior phrenic vein Left ovarian vein Left second lumbar vein Left suprarenal vein Left testicular vein C **Common Iliac Vein, Right** D **Common Iliac Vein, Left** F **External Iliac Vein, Right** G **External Iliac Vein, Left** H **Hypogastric Vein, Right** Gluteal vein Internal iliac vein Internal pudendal vein Lateral sacral vein Middle hemorrhoidal vein Obturator vein Uterine vein Vaginal vein Vesical vein J **Hypogastric Vein, Left** *See H Hypogastric Vein, Right* M **Femoral Vein, Right** Deep femoral (profunda femoris) vein Popliteal vein Profunda femoris (deep femoral) vein N **Femoral Vein, Left** *See M Femoral Vein, Right* P **Saphenous Vein, Right** External pudendal vein Great(er) saphenous vein Lesser saphenous vein Small saphenous vein Superficial circumflex iliac vein Superficial epigastric vein Q **Saphenous Vein, Left** *See P Saphenous Vein, Right* T **Foot Vein, Right** Common digital vein Dorsal metatarsal vein Dorsal venous arch Plantar digital vein Plantar metatarsal vein Plantar venous arch V **Foot Vein, Left** *See T Foot Vein, Right* Y **Lower Vein**	Ø **Open** 3 **Percutaneous** 4 **Percutaneous Endoscopic**	Z **No Device**	X **Diagnostic** Z **No Qualifier**

Non-OR   069[Ø,1,2,3,4,5,6,7,8,9,B,C,D,F,G,H,J,M,N,P,Q,T,V,Y]3ZX
Non-OR   069[Ø,1,2,4,5,6,7,8,9,B,C,D,F,G,H,J,M,N,P,Q,T,V,Y][Ø,3,4]ZZ
Non-OR   06933ZZ

 Noncovered Procedure   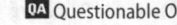 Limited Coverage   **UA** Questionable OB Admit   **NT** New Tech Add-on   ⊞ Combination Member   ♂ Male   ♀ Female

069–069 *(side tab)*

Lower Veins

Ø   **Medical and Surgical**
6   **Lower Veins**
B   **Excision**   Definition: Cutting out or off, without replacement, a portion of a body part
                     Explanation: The qualifier DIAGNOSTIC is used to identify excision procedures that are biopsies

Body Part Character 4	Approach Character 5	Device Character 6	Qualifier Character 7

Ø **Inferior Vena Cava**
   Postcava
   Right inferior phrenic vein
   Right ovarian vein
   Right second lumbar vein
   Right suprarenal vein
   Right testicular vein
1 **Splenic Vein**
   Left gastroepiploic vein
   Pancreatic vein
2 **Gastric Vein**
3 **Esophageal Vein**
4 **Hepatic Vein**
5 **Superior Mesenteric Vein**
   Right gastroepiploic vein
6 **Inferior Mesenteric Vein**
   Sigmoid vein
   Superior rectal vein
7 **Colic Vein**
   Ileocolic vein
   Left colic vein
   Middle colic vein
   Right colic vein
8 **Portal Vein**
   Hepatic portal vein
9 **Renal Vein, Right**
B **Renal Vein, Left**
   Left inferior phrenic vein
   Left ovarian vein
   Left second lumbar vein
   Left suprarenal vein
   Left testicular vein
C **Common Iliac Vein, Right**
D **Common Iliac Vein, Left**
F **External Iliac Vein, Right**
G **External Iliac Vein, Left**
H **Hypogastric Vein, Right**
   Gluteal vein
   Internal iliac vein
   Internal pudendal vein
   Lateral sacral vein
   Middle hemorrhoidal vein
   Obturator vein
   Uterine vein
   Vaginal vein
   Vesical vein
J **Hypogastric Vein, Left**
   See H Hypogastric Vein, Right
M **Femoral Vein, Right**
   Deep femoral (profunda femoris) vein
   Popliteal vein
   Profunda femoris (deep femoral) vein
N **Femoral Vein, Left**
   See M Femoral Vein, Right
P **Saphenous Vein, Right**
   External pudendal vein
   Great(er) saphenous vein
   Lesser saphenous vein
   Small saphenous vein
   Superficial circumflex iliac vein
   Superficial epigastric vein
Q **Saphenous Vein, Left**
   See P Saphenous Vein, Right
T **Foot Vein, Right**
   Common digital vein
   Dorsal metatarsal vein
   Dorsal venous arch
   Plantar digital vein
   Plantar metatarsal vein
   Plantar venous arch
V **Foot Vein, Left**
   See T Foot Vein, Right
	Ø Open
	3 Percutaneous
	4 Percutaneous Endoscopic
		Z No Device	**X** Diagnostic
			Z No Qualifier

Y Lower Vein	**Ø** Open **3** Percutaneous **4** Percutaneous Endoscopic	**Z** No Device	**C** Hemorrhoidal Plexus **X** Diagnostic **Z** No Qualifier

0　Medical and Surgical
6　Lower Veins
C　Extirpation　　Definition: Taking or cutting out solid matter from a body part

Explanation: The solid matter may be an abnormal byproduct of a biological function or a foreign body; it may be imbedded in a body part or in the lumen of a tubular body part. The solid matter may or may not have been previously broken into pieces.

Body Part Character 4	Approach Character 5	Device Character 6	Qualifier Character 7
0　Inferior Vena Cava Postcava Right inferior phrenic vein Right ovarian vein Right second lumbar vein Right suprarenal vein Right testicular vein **1　Splenic Vein** Left gastroepiploic vein Pancreatic vein **2　Gastric Vein** **3　Esophageal Vein** **4　Hepatic Vein** **5　Superior Mesenteric Vein** Right gastroepiploic vein **6　Inferior Mesenteric Vein** Sigmoid vein Superior rectal vein **7　Colic Vein** Ileocolic vein Left colic vein Middle colic vein Right colic vein **8　Portal Vein** Hepatic portal vein **9　Renal Vein, Right** **B　Renal Vein, Left** Left inferior phrenic vein Left ovarian vein Left second lumbar vein Left suprarenal vein Left testicular vein **C　Common Iliac Vein, Right** **D　Common Iliac Vein, Left** **F　External Iliac Vein, Right** **G　External Iliac Vein, Left** **H　Hypogastric Vein, Right** Gluteal vein Internal iliac vein Internal pudendal vein Lateral sacral vein Middle hemorrhoidal vein Obturator vein Uterine vein Vaginal vein Vesical vein **J　Hypogastric Vein, Left** *See* H Hypogastric Vein, Right **M　Femoral Vein, Right** Deep femoral (profunda femoris) vein Popliteal vein Profunda femoris (deep femoral) vein **N　Femoral Vein, Left** *See* M Femoral Vein, Right **P　Saphenous Vein, Right** External pudendal vein Great(er) saphenous vein Lesser saphenous vein Small saphenous vein Superficial circumflex iliac vein Superficial epigastric vein **Q　Saphenous Vein, Left** *See* P Saphenous Vein, Right **T　Foot Vein, Right** Common digital vein Dorsal metatarsal vein Dorsal venous arch Plantar digital vein Plantar metatarsal vein Plantar venous arch **V　Foot Vein, Left** *See* T Foot Vein, Right **Y　Lower Vein**	**0　Open** **3　Percutaneous** **4　Percutaneous Endoscopic**	**Z　No Device**	**Z　No Qualifier**

NC Noncovered Procedure　　LC Limited Coverage　　QA Questionable OB Admit　　NT New Tech Add-on　　⊞ Combination Member　　♂ Male　　♀ Female

Lower Veins

Ø   Medical and Surgical
6   Lower Veins
D   Extraction   Definition: Pulling or stripping out or off all or a portion of a body part by the use of force

Explanation: The qualifier DIAGNOSTIC is used to identify extraction procedures that are biopsies

Body Part Character 4	Approach Character 5	Device Character 6	Qualifier Character 7

M   Femoral Vein, Right
    Deep femoral (profunda femoris) vein
    Popliteal vein
    Profunda femoris (deep femoral) vein
N   Femoral Vein, Left
    See M Femoral Vein, Right
P   Saphenous Vein, Right
    External pudendal vein
    Great(er) saphenous vein
    Lesser saphenous vein
    Small saphenous vein
    Superficial circumflex iliac vein
    Superficial epigastric vein
Q   Saphenous Vein, Left
    See P Saphenous Vein, Right
T   Foot Vein, Right
    Common digital vein
    Dorsal metatarsal vein
    Dorsal venous arch
    Plantar digital vein
    Plantar metatarsal vein
    Plantar venous arch
V   Foot Vein, Left
    See T Foot Vein, Right
Y   Lower Vein
	Ø Open
	3 Percutaneous
	4 Percutaneous Endoscopic
		Z No Device	**Z** No Qualifier

Ø   Medical and Surgical
6   Lower Veins
F   Fragmentation   Definition: Breaking solid matter in a body part into pieces

Explanation: Physical force (e.g., manual, ultrasonic) applied directly or indirectly is used to break the solid matter into pieces. The solid matter may be an abnormal byproduct of a biological function or a foreign body. The pieces of solid matter are not taken out.

Body Part Character 4	Approach Character 5	Device Character 6	Qualifier Character 7

C   Common Iliac Vein, Right
D   Common Iliac Vein, Left
F   External Iliac Vein, Right
G   External Iliac Vein, Left
H   Hypogastric Vein, Right
    Gluteal vein
    Internal iliac vein
    Internal pudendal vein
    Lateral sacral vein
    Middle hemorrhoidal vein
    Obturator vein
    Uterine vein
    Vaginal vein
    Vesical vein
J   Hypogastric Vein, Left
    See H Hypogastric Vein, Right
M   Femoral Vein, Right
    Deep femoral (profunda femoris) vein
    Popliteal vein
    Profunda femoris (deep femoral) vein
N   Femoral Vein, Left
    See M Femoral Vein, Right
P   Saphenous Vein, Right
    External pudendal vein
    Great(er) saphenous vein
    Lesser saphenous vein
    Small saphenous vein
    Superficial circumflex iliac vein
    Superficial epigastric vein
Q   Saphenous Vein, Left
    See P Saphenous Vein, Right
Y   Lower Vein
	3 Percutaneous	**Z** No Device	**Ø** Ultrasonic
			Z No Qualifier

Ø　Medical and Surgical
6　Lower Veins
H　Insertion　　Definition: Putting in a nonbiological appliance that monitors, assists, performs, or prevents a physiological function but does not physically take the place of a body part
　　　　　　　　　Explanation: None

Body Part Character 4		Approach Character 5	Device Character 6	Qualifier Character 7
Ø Inferior Vena Cava Postcava Right inferior phrenic vein Right ovarian vein Right second lumbar vein Right suprarenal vein Right testicular vein		**Ø Open** **3 Percutaneous**	**3 Infusion Device**	**T Via Umbilical Vein** **Z No Qualifier**
Ø Inferior Vena Cava Postcava Right inferior phrenic vein Right ovarian vein Right second lumbar vein Right suprarenal vein Right testicular vein		**Ø Open** **3 Percutaneous**	**D Intraluminal Device**	**Z No Qualifier**
Ø Inferior Vena Cava Postcava Right inferior phrenic vein Right ovarian vein Right second lumbar vein Right suprarenal vein Right testicular vein		**4 Percutaneous Endoscopic**	**3 Infusion Device** **D Intraluminal Device**	**Z No Qualifier**
1 Splenic Vein Left gastroepiploic vein Pancreatic vein **2 Gastric Vein** **3 Esophageal Vein** **4 Hepatic Vein** **5 Superior Mesenteric Vein** Right gastroepiploic vein **6 Inferior Mesenteric Vein** Sigmoid vein Superior rectal vein **7 Colic Vein** Ileocolic vein Left colic vein Middle colic vein Right colic vein **8 Portal Vein** Hepatic portal vein **9 Renal Vein, Right** **B Renal Vein, Left** Left inferior phrenic vein Left ovarian vein Left second lumbar vein Left suprarenal vein Left testicular vein **C Common Iliac Vein, Right** **D Common Iliac Vein, Left** **F External Iliac Vein, Right** **G External Iliac Vein, Left**	**H Hypogastric Vein, Right** Gluteal vein Internal iliac vein Internal pudendal vein Lateral sacral vein Middle hemorrhoidal vein Obturator vein Uterine vein Vaginal vein Vesical vein **J Hypogastric Vein, Left** *See H Hypogastric Vein, Right* **M Femoral Vein, Right** Deep femoral (profunda 　femoris) vein Popliteal vein Profunda femoris (deep 　femoral) vein **N Femoral Vein, Left** *See M Femoral Vein, Right* **P Saphenous Vein, Right** External pudendal vein Great(er) saphenous vein Lesser saphenous vein Small saphenous vein Superficial circumflex iliac vein Superficial epigastric vein **Q Saphenous Vein, Left** *See P Saphenous Vein, Right* **T Foot Vein, Right** Common digital vein Dorsal metatarsal vein Dorsal venous arch Plantar digital vein Plantar metatarsal vein Plantar venous arch **V Foot Vein, Left** *See T Foot Vein, Right*	**Ø Open** **3 Percutaneous** **4 Percutaneous Endoscopic**	**3 Infusion Device** **D Intraluminal Device**	**Z No Qualifier**
Y Lower Vein		**Ø Open** **3 Percutaneous** **4 Percutaneous Endoscopic**	**2 Monitoring Device** **3 Infusion Device** **D Intraluminal Device** **Y Other Device**	**Z No Qualifier**

Non-OR	06HØ[Ø,3]3[T,Z]
Non-OR	06HØ3DZ
Non-OR	06HØ43Z
Non-OR	06H[1,2,3,4,5,6,7,8,9,B,C,D,F,G,H,J,M,N,P,Q,T,V][Ø,3,4]3Z
Non-OR	06HY[Ø,3,4]3Z
Non-OR	06HY32Z
Non-OR	06HY[3,4]YZ

NC Noncovered Procedure　　**LC** Limited Coverage　　**QA** Questionable OB Admit　　**NT** New Tech Add-on　　⊞ Combination Member　　♂ Male　　♀ Female

ICD-10-PCS 2022　　　　　　　　　　　　　　　　　　　　　　　　　　　　　　　　　273

06H–06H

Lower Veins

Ø **Medical and Surgical**
6 **Lower Veins**
J **Inspection**   Definition: Visually and/or manually exploring a body part

Explanation: Visual exploration may be performed with or without optical instrumentation. Manual exploration may be performed directly or through intervening body layers.

Body Part Character 4	Approach Character 5	Device Character 6	Qualifier Character 7
Y Lower Vein	Ø Open 3 Percutaneous 4 Percutaneous Endoscopic X External	Z No Device	Z No Qualifier

Non-OR Ø6JY[3,X]ZZ

Ø **Medical and Surgical**
6 **Lower Veins**
L **Occlusion**   Definition: Completely closing an orifice or the lumen of a tubular body part

Explanation: The orifice can be a natural orifice or an artificially created orifice

Body Part Character 4		Approach Character 5	Device Character 6	Qualifier Character 7

Ø Inferior Vena Cava
  Postcava
  Right inferior phrenic vein
  Right ovarian vein
  Right second lumbar vein
  Right suprarenal vein
  Right testicular vein
1 Splenic Vein
  Left gastroepiploic vein
  Pancreatic vein
4 Hepatic Vein
5 Superior Mesenteric Vein
  Right gastroepiploic vein
6 Inferior Mesenteric Vein
  Sigmoid vein
  Superior rectal vein
7 Colic Vein
  Ileocolic vein
  Left colic vein
  Middle colic vein
  Right colic vein
8 Portal Vein
  Hepatic portal vein
9 Renal Vein, Right
B Renal Vein, Left
  Left inferior phrenic vein
  Left ovarian vein
  Left second lumbar vein
  Left suprarenal vein
  Left testicular vein
C Common Iliac Vein, Right
D Common Iliac Vein, Left
F External Iliac Vein, Right
G External Iliac Vein, Left
	H Hypogastric Vein, Right
	  Gluteal vein
	  Internal iliac vein
	  Internal pudendal vein
	  Lateral sacral vein
	  Middle hemorrhoidal vein
	  Obturator vein
	  Uterine vein
	  Vaginal vein
	  Vesical vein
	J Hypogastric Vein, Left
	  See H Hypogastric Vein, Right
	M Femoral Vein, Right
	  Deep femoral (profunda
	    femoris) vein
	  Popliteal vein
	  Profunda femoris (deep
	    femoral) vein
	N Femoral Vein, Left
	  See M Femoral Vein, Right
	P Saphenous Vein, Right
	  External pudendal vein
	  Great(er) saphenous vein
	  Lesser saphenous vein
	  Small saphenous vein
	  Superficial circumflex iliac vein
	  Superficial epigastric vein
	Q Saphenous Vein, Left
	  See P Saphenous Vein, Right
	T Foot Vein, Right
	  Common digital vein
	  Dorsal metatarsal vein
	  Dorsal venous arch
	  Plantar digital vein
	  Plantar metatarsal vein
	  Plantar venous arch
	V Foot Vein, Left
	  See T Foot Vein, Right
		Ø Open
		3 Percutaneous
		4 Percutaneous Endoscopic
			C Extraluminal Device
			D Intraluminal Device
			Z No Device
				Z No Qualifier

2 Gastric Vein 3 Esophageal Vein		Ø Open 3 Percutaneous 4 Percutaneous Endoscopic 7 Via Natural or Artificial Opening 8 Via Natural or Artificial Opening Endoscopic	C Extraluminal Device D Intraluminal Device Z No Device	Z No Qualifier
Y Lower Vein		Ø Open 3 Percutaneous 4 Percutaneous Endoscopic 7 Via Natural or Artificial Opening 8 Via Natural or Artificial Opening Endoscopic	C Extraluminal Device D Intraluminal Device Z No Device	C Hemorrhoidal Plexus Z No Qualifier

Non-OR Ø6L2[7,8][C,D,Z]Z
Non-OR Ø6L3[3,4,7,8][C,D,Z]Z

Non-OR Procedure   DRG Non-OR Procedure   Valid OR Procedure   HAC Associated Procedure   Combination Only   New/Revised GREEN

Ø Medical and Surgical
6 Lower Veins
N Release
     Definition: Freeing a body part from an abnormal physical constraint by cutting or by the use of force
     Explanation: Some of the restraining tissue may be taken out but none of the body part is taken out

Body Part Character 4		Approach Character 5	Device Character 6	Qualifier Character 7

Ø Inferior Vena Cava
Postcava
Right inferior phrenic vein
Right ovarian vein
Right second lumbar vein
Right suprarenal vein
Right testicular vein
1 Splenic Vein
Left gastroepiploic vein
Pancreatic vein
2 Gastric Vein
3 Esophageal Vein
4 Hepatic Vein
5 Superior Mesenteric Vein
Right gastroepiploic vein
6 Inferior Mesenteric Vein
Sigmoid vein
Superior rectal vein
7 Colic Vein
Ileocolic vein
Left colic vein
Middle colic vein
Right colic vein
8 Portal Vein
Hepatic portal vein
9 Renal Vein, Right
B Renal Vein, Left
Left inferior phrenic vein
Left ovarian vein
Left second lumbar vein
Left suprarenal vein
Left testicular vein
C Common Iliac Vein, Right
D Common Iliac Vein, Left
F External Iliac Vein, Right
G External Iliac Vein, Left
	H Hypogastric Vein, Right
	Gluteal vein
	Internal iliac vein
	Internal pudendal vein
	Lateral sacral vein
	Middle hemorrhoidal vein
	Obturator vein
	Uterine vein
	Vaginal vein
	Vesical vein
	J Hypogastric Vein, Left
	 See *H Hypogastric Vein, Right*
	M Femoral Vein, Right
	Deep femoral (profunda
	   femoris) vein
	Popliteal vein
	Profunda femoris (deep
	   femoral) vein
	N Femoral Vein, Left
	 See *M Femoral Vein, Right*
	P Saphenous Vein, Right
	External pudendal vein
	Great(er) saphenous vein
	Lesser saphenous vein
	Small saphenous vein
	Superficial circumflex iliac vein
	Superficial epigastric vein
	Q Saphenous Vein, Left
	 See *P Saphenous Vein, Right*
	T Foot Vein, Right
	Common digital vein
	Dorsal metatarsal vein
	Dorsal venous arch
	Plantar digital vein
	Plantar metatarsal vein
	Plantar venous arch
	V Foot Vein, Left
	 See *T Foot Vein, Right*
	Y Lower Vein
		Ø Open
		3 Percutaneous
		4 Percutaneous Endoscopic
			Z No Device	**Z No Qualifier**

Ø Medical and Surgical
6 Lower Veins
P Removal
     Definition: Taking out or off a device from a body part
     Explanation: If a device is taken out and a similar device put in without cutting or puncturing the skin or mucous membrane, the procedure is coded to the root operation CHANGE. Otherwise, the procedure for taking out a device is coded to the root operation REMOVAL.

Body Part Character 4	Approach Character 5	Device Character 6	Qualifier Character 7

Y Lower Vein	**Ø Open**
	3 Percutaneous
	4 Percutaneous Endoscopic
		Ø Drainage Device
		2 Monitoring Device
		3 Infusion Device
		7 Autologous Tissue
		   Substitute
		C Extraluminal Device
		D Intraluminal Device
		J Synthetic Substitute
		K Nonautologous Tissue
		   Substitute
		Y Other Device
			Z No Qualifier

Y Lower Vein	**X External**	**Ø Drainage Device** **2 Monitoring Device** **3 Infusion Device** **D Intraluminal Device**	**Z No Qualifier**

Non-OR	06PY3[Ø,2,3]Z
Non-OR	06PY[3,4]YZ
Non-OR	06PYX[Ø,2,3,D]Z

NC Noncovered Procedure   **LC** Limited Coverage   **QA** Questionable OB Admit   **NT** New Tech Add-on   ⊞ Combination Member   ♂ Male   ♀ Female

ICD-10-PCS 2022   275

06N–06P

Ø   Medical and Surgical
6   Lower Veins
Q   Repair   Definition: Restoring, to the extent possible, a body part to its normal anatomic structure and function
                     Explanation: Used only when the method to accomplish the repair is not one of the other root operations

Body Part Character 4	Approach Character 5	Device Character 6	Qualifier Character 7
Ø **Inferior Vena Cava** Postcava Right inferior phrenic vein Right ovarian vein Right second lumbar vein Right suprarenal vein Right testicular vein	**Ø** Open **3** Percutaneous **4** Percutaneous Endoscopic	**Z** No Device	**Z** No Qualifier
1 **Splenic Vein** Left gastroepiploic vein Pancreatic vein			
2 **Gastric Vein**			
3 **Esophageal Vein**			
4 **Hepatic Vein**			
5 **Superior Mesenteric Vein** Right gastroepiploic vein			
6 **Inferior Mesenteric Vein** Sigmoid vein Superior rectal vein			
7 **Colic Vein** Ileocolic vein Left colic vein Middle colic vein Right colic vein			
8 **Portal Vein** Hepatic portal vein			
9 **Renal Vein, Right**			
B **Renal Vein, Left** Left inferior phrenic vein Left ovarian vein Left second lumbar vein Left suprarenal vein Left testicular vein			
C **Common Iliac Vein, Right**			
D **Common Iliac Vein, Left**			
F **External Iliac Vein, Right**			
G **External Iliac Vein, Left**			
H **Hypogastric Vein, Right** Gluteal vein Internal iliac vein Internal pudendal vein Lateral sacral vein Middle hemorrhoidal vein Obturator vein Uterine vein Vaginal vein Vesical vein			
J **Hypogastric Vein, Left** *See H Hypogastric Vein, Right*			
M **Femoral Vein, Right** Deep femoral (profunda femoris) vein Popliteal vein Profunda femoris (deep femoral) vein			
N **Femoral Vein, Left** *See M Femoral Vein, Right*			
P **Saphenous Vein, Right** External pudendal vein Great(er) saphenous vein Lesser saphenous vein Small saphenous vein Superficial circumflex iliac vein Superficial epigastric vein			
Q **Saphenous Vein, Left** *See P Saphenous Vein, Right*			
T **Foot Vein, Right** Common digital vein Dorsal metatarsal vein Dorsal venous arch Plantar digital vein Plantar metatarsal vein Plantar venous arch			
V **Foot Vein, Left** *See T Foot Vein, Right*			
Y **Lower Vein**			

Ø Medical and Surgical
6 Lower Veins
R Replacement Definition: Putting in or on biological or synthetic material that physically takes the place and/or function of all or a portion of a body part

      Explanation: The body part may have been taken out or replaced, or may be taken out, physically eradicated, or rendered nonfunctional during the REPLACEMENT procedure. A REMOVAL procedure is coded for taking out the device used in a previous replacement procedure.

Body Part Character 4	Approach Character 5	Device Character 6	Qualifier Character 7
Ø Inferior Vena Cava Postcava Right inferior phrenic vein Right ovarian vein Right second lumbar vein Right suprarenal vein Right testicular vein **1 Splenic Vein** Left gastroepiploic vein Pancreatic vein **2 Gastric Vein** **3 Esophageal Vein** **4 Hepatic Vein** **5 Superior Mesenteric Vein** Right gastroepiploic vein **6 Inferior Mesenteric Vein** Sigmoid vein Superior rectal vein **7 Colic Vein** Ileocolic vein Left colic vein Middle colic vein Right colic vein **8 Portal Vein** Hepatic portal vein **9 Renal Vein, Right** **B Renal Vein, Left** Left inferior phrenic vein Left ovarian vein Left second lumbar vein Left suprarenal vein Left testicular vein **C Common Iliac Vein, Right** **D Common Iliac Vein, Left** **F External Iliac Vein, Right** **G External Iliac Vein, Left** **H Hypogastric Vein, Right** Gluteal vein Internal iliac vein Internal pudendal vein Lateral sacral vein Middle hemorrhoidal vein Obturator vein Uterine vein Vaginal vein Vesical vein **J Hypogastric Vein, Left** *See H Hypogastric Vein, Right* **M Femoral Vein, Right** Deep femoral (profunda femoris) vein Popliteal vein Profunda femoris (deep femoral) vein **N Femoral Vein, Left** *See M Femoral Vein, Right* **P Saphenous Vein, Right** External pudendal vein Great(er) saphenous vein Lesser saphenous vein Small saphenous vein Superficial circumflex iliac vein Superficial epigastric vein **Q Saphenous Vein, Left** *See P Saphenous Vein, Right* **T Foot Vein, Right** Common digital vein Dorsal metatarsal vein Dorsal venous arch Plantar digital vein Plantar metatarsal vein Plantar venous arch **V Foot Vein, Left** *See T Foot Vein, Right* **Y Lower Vein**	**Ø Open** **4 Percutaneous Endoscopic**	**7 Autologous Tissue Substitute** **J Synthetic Substitute** **K Nonautologous Tissue Substitute**	**Z No Qualifier**

NC Noncovered Procedure LC Limited Coverage QA Questionable OB Admit NT New Tech Add-on ⊞ Combination Member ♂Male ♀Female

ICD-10-PCS 2022   277

06R–06R

Lower Veins

Ø   **Medical and Surgical**
6   **Lower Veins**
S   **Reposition**   Definition: Moving to its normal location, or other suitable location, all or a portion of a body part

Explanation: The body part is moved to a new location from an abnormal location, or from a normal location where it is not functioning correctly. The body part may or may not be cut out or off to be moved to the new location.

Body Part Character 4	Approach Character 5	Device Character 6	Qualifier Character 7
Ø Inferior Vena Cava Postcava Right inferior phrenic vein Right ovarian vein Right second lumbar vein Right suprarenal vein Right testicular vein **1 Splenic Vein** Left gastroepiploic vein Pancreatic vein **2 Gastric Vein** **3 Esophageal Vein** **4 Hepatic Vein** **5 Superior Mesenteric Vein** Right gastroepiploic vein **6 Inferior Mesenteric Vein** Sigmoid vein Superior rectal vein **7 Colic Vein** Ileocolic vein Left colic vein Middle colic vein Right colic vein **8 Portal Vein** Hepatic portal vein **9 Renal Vein, Right** **B Renal Vein, Left** Left inferior phrenic vein Left ovarian vein Left second lumbar vein Left suprarenal vein Left testicular vein **C Common Iliac Vein, Right** **D Common Iliac Vein, Left** **F External Iliac Vein, Right** **G External Iliac Vein, Left** **H Hypogastric Vein, Right** Gluteal vein Internal iliac vein Internal pudendal vein Lateral sacral vein Middle hemorrhoidal vein Obturator vein Uterine vein Vaginal vein Vesical vein **J Hypogastric Vein, Left** *See H Hypogastric Vein, Right* **M Femoral Vein, Right** Deep femoral (profunda femoris) vein Popliteal vein Profunda femoris (deep femoral) vein **N Femoral Vein, Left** *See M Femoral Vein, Right* **P Saphenous Vein, Right** External pudendal vein Great(er) saphenous vein Lesser saphenous vein Small saphenous vein Superficial circumflex iliac vein Superficial epigastric vein **Q Saphenous Vein, Left** *See P Saphenous Vein, Right* **T Foot Vein, Right** Common digital vein Dorsal metatarsal vein Dorsal venous arch Plantar digital vein Plantar metatarsal vein Plantar venous arch **V Foot Vein, Left** *See T Foot Vein, Right* **Y Lower Vein**	**Ø Open** **3 Percutaneous** **4 Percutaneous Endoscopic**	**Z No Device**	**Z No Qualifier**

0　**Medical and Surgical**
6　**Lower Veins**
U　**Supplement**　　Definition: Putting in or on biological or synthetic material that physically reinforces and/or augments the function of a portion of a body part

Explanation: The biological material is non-living, or is living and from the same individual. The body part may have been previously replaced, and the SUPPLEMENT procedure is performed to physically reinforce and/or augment the function of the replaced body part.

Body Part Character 4	Approach Character 5	Device Character 6	Qualifier Character 7
0 **Inferior Vena Cava** Postcava Right inferior phrenic vein Right ovarian vein Right second lumbar vein Right suprarenal vein Right testicular vein **1** **Splenic Vein** Left gastroepiploic vein Pancreatic vein **2** **Gastric Vein** **3** **Esophageal Vein** **4** **Hepatic Vein** **5** **Superior Mesenteric Vein** Right gastroepiploic vein **6** **Inferior Mesenteric Vein** Sigmoid vein Superior rectal vein **7** **Colic Vein** Ileocolic vein Left colic vein Middle colic vein Right colic vein **8** **Portal Vein** Hepatic portal vein **9** **Renal Vein, Right** **B** **Renal Vein, Left** Left inferior phrenic vein Left ovarian vein Left second lumbar vein Left suprarenal vein Left testicular vein **C** **Common Iliac Vein, Right** **D** **Common Iliac Vein, Left** **F** **External Iliac Vein, Right** **G** **External Iliac Vein, Left** **H** **Hypogastric Vein, Right** Gluteal vein Internal iliac vein Internal pudendal vein Lateral sacral vein Middle hemorrhoidal vein Obturator vein Uterine vein Vaginal vein Vesical vein **J** **Hypogastric Vein, Left** *See* H Hypogastric Vein, Right **M** **Femoral Vein, Right** Deep femoral (profunda femoris) vein Popliteal vein Profunda femoris (deep femoral) vein **N** **Femoral Vein, Left** *See* M Femoral Vein, Right **P** **Saphenous Vein, Right** External pudendal vein Great(er) saphenous vein Lesser saphenous vein Small saphenous vein Superficial circumflex iliac vein Superficial epigastric vein **Q** **Saphenous Vein, Left** *See* P Saphenous Vein, Right **T** **Foot Vein, Right** Common digital vein Dorsal metatarsal vein Dorsal venous arch Plantar digital vein Plantar metatarsal vein Plantar venous arch **V** **Foot Vein, Left** *See* T Foot Vein, Right **Y** **Lower Vein**	**0** Open **3** Percutaneous **4** Percutaneous Endoscopic	**7** Autologous Tissue Substitute **J** Synthetic Substitute **K** Nonautologous Tissue Substitute	**Z** No Qualifier

NC Noncovered Procedure　　**LC** Limited Coverage　　**QA** Questionable OB Admit　　**NT** New Tech Add-on　　✜ Combination Member　　♂ Male　　♀ Female

ICD-10-PCS 2022　　　　　　　　　　　　　　　　　　　　　　　　　　　　　　　　　　279

Lower Veins

Ø	**Medical and Surgical**
6	**Lower Veins**
V	**Restriction**

Definition: Partially closing an orifice or the lumen of a tubular body part

Explanation: The orifice can be a natural orifice or an artificially created orifice

Body Part Character 4	Approach Character 5	Device Character 6	Qualifier Character 7
Ø Inferior Vena Cava Postcava Right inferior phrenic vein Right ovarian vein Right second lumbar vein Right suprarenal vein Right testicular vein	**Ø** Open **3** Percutaneous **4** Percutaneous Endoscopic	**C** Extraluminal Device **D** Intraluminal Device **Z** No Device	**Z** No Qualifier
1 Splenic Vein Left gastroepiploic vein Pancreatic vein			
2 Gastric Vein			
3 Esophageal Vein			
4 Hepatic Vein			
5 Superior Mesenteric Vein Right gastroepiploic vein			
6 Inferior Mesenteric Vein Sigmoid vein Superior rectal vein			
7 Colic Vein Ileocolic vein Left colic vein Middle colic vein Right colic vein			
8 Portal Vein Hepatic portal vein			
9 Renal Vein, Right			
B Renal Vein, Left Left inferior phrenic vein Left ovarian vein Left second lumbar vein Left suprarenal vein Left testicular vein			
C Common Iliac Vein, Right			
D Common Iliac Vein, Left			
F External Iliac Vein, Right			
G External Iliac Vein, Left			
H Hypogastric Vein, Right Gluteal vein Internal iliac vein Internal pudendal vein Lateral sacral vein Middle hemorrhoidal vein Obturator vein Uterine vein Vaginal vein Vesical vein			
J Hypogastric Vein, Left *See H Hypogastric Vein, Right*			
M Femoral Vein, Right Deep femoral (profunda femoris) vein Popliteal vein Profunda femoris (deep femoral) vein			
N Femoral Vein, Left *See M Femoral Vein, Right*			
P Saphenous Vein, Right External pudendal vein Great(er) saphenous vein Lesser saphenous vein Small saphenous vein Superficial circumflex iliac vein Superficial epigastric vein			
Q Saphenous Vein, Left *See P Saphenous Vein, Right*			
T Foot Vein, Right Common digital vein Dorsal metatarsal vein Dorsal venous arch Plantar digital vein Plantar metatarsal vein Plantar venous arch			
V Foot Vein, Left *See T Foot Vein, Right*			
Y Lower Vein			

Ø   Medical and Surgical
6   Lower Veins
W   Revision   Definition: Correcting, to the extent possible, a portion of a malfunctioning device or the position of a displaced device

Explanation: Revision can include correcting a malfunctioning or displaced device by taking out or putting in components of the device such as a screw or pin

Body Part Character 4	Approach Character 5	Device Character 6	Qualifier Character 7
Y Lower Vein	Ø Open 3 Percutaneous 4 Percutaneous Endoscopic	Ø Drainage Device 2 Monitoring Device 3 Infusion Device 7 Autologous Tissue Substitute C Extraluminal Device D Intraluminal Device J Synthetic Substitute K Nonautologous Tissue Substitute Y Other Device	Z No Qualifier
Y Lower Vein	X External	Ø Drainage Device 2 Monitoring Device 3 Infusion Device 7 Autologous Tissue Substitute C Extraluminal Device D Intraluminal Device J Synthetic Substitute K Nonautologous Tissue Substitute	Z No Qualifier

Non-OR   Ø6WY3[Ø,2,3,D]Z
Non-OR   Ø6WY[3,4]YZ
Non-OR   Ø6WYX[Ø,2,3,7,C,D,J,K]Z

Lymphatic and Hemic Systems Ø72–Ø7Y

Character Meanings*

This Character Meaning table is provided as a guide to assist the user in the identification of character members that may be found in this section of code tables. It **SHOULD NOT** be used to build a PCS code.

Operation–Character 3	Body Part–Character 4	Approach–Character 5	Device–Character 6	Qualifier–Character 7
2 Change	Ø Lymphatic, Head	Ø Open	Ø Drainage Device	Ø Allogeneic
5 Destruction	1 Lymphatic, Right Neck	3 Percutaneous	1 Radioactive Element	1 Syngeneic
9 Drainage	2 Lymphatic, Left Neck	4 Percutaneous Endoscopic	3 Infusion Device	2 Zooplastic
B Excision	3 Lymphatic, Right Upper Extremity	8 Via Natural or Artificial Opening Endoscopic	7 Autologous Tissue Substitute	X Diagnostic
C Extirpation	4 Lymphatic, Left Upper Extremity	X External	C Extraluminal Device	Z No Qualifier
D Extraction	5 Lymphatic, Right Axillary		D Intraluminal Device	
H Insertion	6 Lymphatic, Left Axillary		J Synthetic Substitute	
J Inspection	7 Lymphatic, Thorax		K Nonautologous Tissue Substitute	
L Occlusion	8 Lymphatic, Internal Mammary, Right		Y Other Device	
N Release	9 Lymphatic, Internal Mammary, Left		Z No Device	
P Removal	B Lymphatic, Mesenteric			
Q Repair	C Lymphatic, Pelvis			
S Reposition	D Lymphatic, Aortic			
T Resection	F Lymphatic, Right Lower Extremity			
U Supplement	G Lymphatic, Left Lower Extremity			
V Restriction	H Lymphatic, Right Inguinal			
W Revision	J Lymphatic, Left Inguinal			
Y Transplantation	K Thoracic Duct			
	L Cisterna Chyli			
	M Thymus			
	N Lymphatic			
	P Spleen			
	Q Bone Marrow, Sternum			
	R Bone Marrow, Iliac			
	S Bone Marrow, Vertebral			
	T Bone Marrow			

* Includes lymph vessels and lymph nodes.

AHA Coding Clinic for table Ø79
2018, 4Q, 84	Fine needle aspiration biopsy of lymphatic tissue
2017, 1Q, 34	Lymphovenous bypass following mastectomy
2014, 1Q, 26	Transbronchial needle aspiration lymph node biopsy
2013, 4Q, 111	Transbronchial needle aspiration lymph node biopsy

AHA Coding Clinic for table Ø7B
2019, 1Q, 3-8	Whipple procedure
2018, 4Q, 84	Fine needle aspiration biopsy of lymphatic tissue
2018, 1Q, 22	Resection of lymph node chains
2016, 1Q, 30	Axillary lymph node resection with modified radical mastectomy
2014, 3Q, 10	Selective excision of paratracheal lymph nodes
2014, 1Q, 20	Fiducial marker placement
2014, 1Q, 26	Transbronchial endoscopic lymph node aspiration biopsy

AHA Coding Clinic for table Ø7D
2018, 4Q, 84	Fine needle aspiration biopsy of lymphatic tissue
2013, 4Q, 111	Root operation for bone marrow biopsy

AHA Coding Clinic for table Ø7H
2020, 4Q, 43-44	Insertion of radioactive element
2020, 4Q, 53	Bone marrow body part

AHA Coding Clinic for table Ø7Q
2017, 1Q, 34	Lymphovenous bypass following mastectomy

AHA Coding Clinic for table Ø7S
2019, 3Q, 29	Thymus transplant for T-Cell production

AHA Coding Clinic for table Ø7T
2018, 1Q, 22	Resection of lymph node chains
2016, 2Q, 12	Resection of malignant neoplasm of infratemporal fossa
2016, 1Q, 30	Axillary lymph node resection with modified radical mastectomy
2015, 4Q, 13	New Section X codes—New Technology procedures
2014, 3Q, 9	Radical resection of level I lymph nodes
2014, 3Q, 16	Repair of Tetralogy of Fallot

AHA Coding Clinic for table Ø7Y
2019, 3Q, 29	Thymus transplant for T-Cell production

Lymphatic System

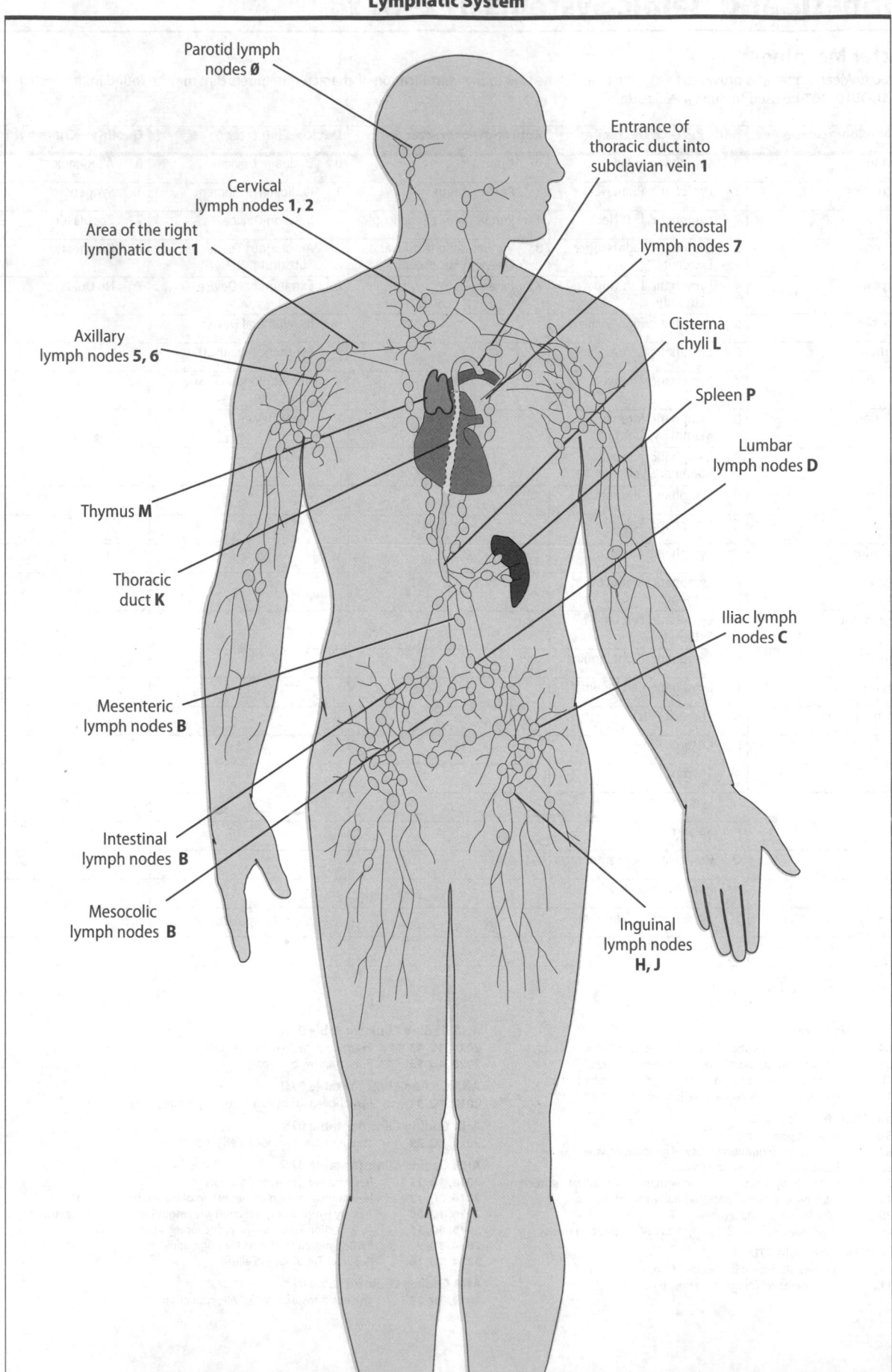

Parotid lymph nodes Ø

Entrance of thoracic duct into subclavian vein 1

Cervical lymph nodes 1, 2

Intercostal lymph nodes 7

Area of the right lymphatic duct 1

Cisterna chyli L

Axillary lymph nodes 5, 6

Spleen P

Lumbar lymph nodes D

Thymus M

Thoracic duct K

Mesenteric lymph nodes B

Iliac lymph nodes C

Intestinal lymph nodes B

Mesocolic lymph nodes B

Inguinal lymph nodes H, J

Lymphatic System

Ø   Medical and Surgical
7   Lymphatic and Hemic Systems
2   Change   Definition: Taking out or off a device from a body part and putting back an identical or similar device in or on the same body part without cutting or puncturing the skin or a mucous membrane

                    Explanation: All CHANGE procedures are coded using the approach EXTERNAL

Body Part Character 4		Approach Character 5	Device Character 6	Qualifier Character 7

K Thoracic Duct
    Left jugular trunk
    Left subclavian trunk
L Cisterna Chyli
    Intestinal lymphatic trunk
    Lumbar lymphatic trunk
	M Thymus
	    Thymus gland
	N Lymphatic
	P Spleen
	    Accessory spleen
	T Bone Marrow
		X External	**Ø** Drainage Device
			Y Other Device
				Z No Qualifier

Non-OR	All body part, approach, device, and qualifier values

Ø   Medical and Surgical
7   Lymphatic and Hemic Systems
5   Destruction   Definition: Physical eradication of all or a portion of a body part by the direct use of energy, force, or a destructive agent

                      Explanation: None of the body part is physically taken out

Body Part Character 4		Approach Character 5	Device Character 6	Qualifier Character 7

Ø Lymphatic, Head
    Buccinator lymph node
    Infraauricular lymph node
    Infraparotid lymph node
    Parotid lymph node
    Preauricular lymph node
    Submandibular lymph node
    Submaxillary lymph node
    Submental lymph node
    Subparotid lymph node
    Suprahyoid lymph node
1 Lymphatic, Right Neck
    Cervical lymph node
    Jugular lymph node
    Mastoid (postauricular) lymph node
    Occipital lymph node
    Postauricular (mastoid) lymph node
    Retropharyngeal lymph node
    Right jugular trunk
    Right lymphatic duct
    Right subclavian trunk
    Supraclavicular (Virchow's) lymph node
    Virchow's (supraclavicular) lymph node
2 Lymphatic, Left Neck
    Cervical lymph node
    Jugular lymph node
    Mastoid (postauricular) lymph node
    Occipital lymph node
    Postauricular (mastoid) lymph node
    Retropharyngeal lymph node
    Supraclavicular (Virchow's) lymph node
    Virchow's (supraclavicular) lymph node
3 Lymphatic, Right Upper Extremity
    Cubital lymph node
    Deltopectoral (infraclavicular) lymph
       node
    Epitrochlear lymph node
    Infraclavicular (deltopectoral) lymph
       node
    Supratrochlear lymph node
4 Lymphatic, Left Upper Extremity
    See 3 Lymphatic, Right Upper Extremity
5 Lymphatic, Right Axillary
    Anterior (pectoral) lymph node
    Apical (subclavicular) lymph node
    Brachial (lateral) lymph node
    Central axillary lymph node
    Lateral (brachial) lymph node
    Pectoral (anterior) lymph node
    Posterior (subscapular) lymph node
    Subclavicular (apical) lymph node
    Subscapular (posterior) lymph node
	6 Lymphatic, Left Axillary
	    See 5 Lymphatic, Right Axillary
	7 Lymphatic, Thorax
	    Intercostal lymph node
	    Mediastinal lymph node
	    Parasternal lymph node
	    Paratracheal lymph node
	    Tracheobronchial lymph node
	8 Lymphatic, Internal Mammary, Right
	9 Lymphatic, Internal Mammary, Left
	B Lymphatic, Mesenteric
	    Inferior mesenteric lymph node
	    Pararectal lymph node
	    Superior mesenteric lymph node
	C Lymphatic, Pelvis
	    Common iliac (subaortic) lymph node
	    Gluteal lymph node
	    Iliac lymph node
	    Inferior epigastric lymph node
	    Obturator lymph node
	    Sacral lymph node
	    Subaortic (common iliac) lymph node
	    Suprainguinal lymph node
	D Lymphatic, Aortic
	    Celiac lymph node
	    Gastric lymph node
	    Hepatic lymph node
	    Lumbar lymph node
	    Pancreaticosplenic lymph node
	    Paraaortic lymph node
	    Retroperitoneal lymph node
	F Lymphatic, Right Lower Extremity
	    Femoral lymph node
	    Popliteal lymph node
	G Lymphatic, Left Lower Extremity
	    See F Lymphatic, Right Lower Extremity
	H Lymphatic, Right Inguinal
	J Lymphatic, Left Inguinal
	K Thoracic Duct
	    Left jugular trunk
	    Left subclavian trunk
	L Cisterna Chyli
	    Intestinal lymphatic trunk
	    Lumbar lymphatic trunk
	M Thymus
	    Thymus gland
	P Spleen
	    Accessory spleen
		Ø Open
		3 Percutaneous
		4 Percutaneous Endoscopic
			Z No Device	**Z** No Qualifier

NC Noncovered Procedure   **LC** Limited Coverage   **QA** Questionable OB Admit   **NT** New Tech Add-on   ⊞ Combination Member   ♂ Male   ♀ Female

ICD-10-PCS 2022   285

Lymphatic and Hemic Systems

Ø   **Medical and Surgical**
7   **Lymphatic and Hemic Systems**
9   **Drainage**   Definition: Taking or letting out fluids and/or gases from a body part
                     Explanation: The qualifier DIAGNOSTIC is used to identify drainage procedures that are biopsies

Body Part Character 4		Approach Character 5	Device Character 6	Qualifier Character 7

Ø Lymphatic, Head
Buccinator lymph node
Infraauricular lymph node
Infraparotid lymph node
Parotid lymph node
Preauricular lymph node
Submandibular lymph node
Submaxillary lymph node
Submental lymph node
Subparotid lymph node
Suprahyoid lymph node
1 Lymphatic, Right Neck
Cervical lymph node
Jugular lymph node
Mastoid (postauricular) lymph node
Occipital lymph node
Postauricular (mastoid) lymph node
Retropharyngeal lymph node
Right jugular trunk
Right lymphatic duct
Right subclavian trunk
Supraclavicular (Virchow's) lymph
    node
Virchow's (supraclavicular) lymph
    node
2 Lymphatic, Left Neck
Cervical lymph node
Jugular lymph node
Mastoid (postauricular) lymph node
Occipital lymph node
Postauricular (mastoid) lymph node
Retropharyngeal lymph node
Supraclavicular (Virchow's) lymph
    node
Virchow's (supraclavicular) lymph
    node
3 Lymphatic, Right Upper Extremity
Cubital lymph node
Deltopectoral (infraclavicular) lymph
    node
Epitrochlear lymph node
Infraclavicular (deltopectoral) lymph
    node
Supratrochlear lymph node
4 Lymphatic, Left Upper Extremity
See 3 Lymphatic, Right Upper Extremity
5 Lymphatic, Right Axillary
Anterior (pectoral) lymph node
Apical (subclavicular) lymph node
Brachial (lateral) lymph node
Central axillary lymph node
Lateral (brachial) lymph node
Pectoral (anterior) lymph node
Posterior (subscapular) lymph node
Subclavicular (apical) lymph node
Subscapular (posterior) lymph node
	6 Lymphatic, Left Axillary
	See 5 Lymphatic, Right Axillary
	7 Lymphatic, Thorax
	Intercostal lymph node
	Mediastinal lymph node
	Parasternal lymph node
	Paratracheal lymph node
	Tracheobronchial lymph node
	8 Lymphatic, Internal Mammary, Right
	9 Lymphatic, Internal Mammary, Left
	B Lymphatic, Mesenteric
	Inferior mesenteric lymph node
	Pararectal lymph node
	Superior mesenteric lymph node
	C Lymphatic, Pelvis
	Common iliac (subaortic) lymph node
	Gluteal lymph node
	Iliac lymph node
	Inferior epigastric lymph node
	Obturator lymph node
	Sacral lymph node
	Subaortic (common iliac) lymph node
	Suprainguinal lymph node
	D Lymphatic, Aortic
	Celiac lymph node
	Gastric lymph node
	Hepatic lymph node
	Lumbar lymph node
	Pancreaticosplenic lymph node
	Paraaortic lymph node
	Retroperitoneal lymph node
	F Lymphatic, Right Lower Extremity
	Femoral lymph node
	Popliteal lymph node
	G Lymphatic, Left Lower Extremity
	See F Lymphatic, Right Lower Extremity
	H Lymphatic, Right Inguinal
	J Lymphatic, Left Inguinal
	K Thoracic Duct
	Left jugular trunk
	Left subclavian trunk
	L Cisterna Chyli
	Intestinal lymphatic trunk
	Lumbar lymphatic trunk
		Ø Open
		3 Percutaneous
		4 Percutaneous
		    Endoscopic
		8 Via Natural or
		    Artificial Opening
		    Endoscopic
			Ø Drainage Device	**Z No Qualifier**

Non-OR   Ø79[Ø,1,2,3,4,5,6,7,8,9,B,C,D,F,G,H,J,K,L][3,8]ØZ

Ø79 Continued on next page

Ø79 Continued

Ø   **Medical and Surgical**
7   **Lymphatic and Hemic Systems**
9   **Drainage**   Definition: Taking or letting out fluids and/or gases from a body part
                      Explanation: The qualifier DIAGNOSTIC is used to identify drainage procedures that are biopsies

Body Part Character 4		Approach Character 5	Device Character 6	Qualifier Character 7

Ø **Lymphatic, Head**
  Buccinator lymph node
  Infraauricular lymph node
  Infraparotid lymph node
  Parotid lymph node
  Preauricular lymph node
  Submandibular lymph node
  Submaxillary lymph node
  Submental lymph node
  Subparotid lymph node
  Suprahyoid lymph node
1 **Lymphatic, Right Neck**
  Cervical lymph node
  Jugular lymph node
  Mastoid (postauricular) lymph node
  Occipital lymph node
  Postauricular (mastoid) lymph node
  Retropharyngeal lymph node
  Right jugular trunk
  Right lymphatic duct
  Right subclavian trunk
  Supraclavicular (Virchow's) lymph
    node
  Virchow's (supraclavicular) lymph
    node
2 **Lymphatic, Left Neck**
  Cervical lymph node
  Jugular lymph node
  Mastoid (postauricular) lymph node
  Occipital lymph node
  Postauricular (mastoid) lymph node
  Retropharyngeal lymph node
  Supraclavicular (Virchow's) lymph
    node
  Virchow's (supraclavicular) lymph
    node
3 **Lymphatic, Right Upper Extremity**
  Cubital lymph node
  Deltopectoral (infraclavicular) lymph
    node
  Epitrochlear lymph node
  Infraclavicular (deltopectoral) lymph
    node
  Supratrochlear lymph node
4 **Lymphatic, Left Upper Extremity**
  See 3 Lymphatic, Right Upper Extremity
5 **Lymphatic, Right Axillary**
  Anterior (pectoral) lymph node
  Apical (subclavicular) lymph node
  Brachial (lateral) lymph node
  Central axillary lymph node
  Lateral (brachial) lymph node
  Pectoral (anterior) lymph node
  Posterior (subscapular) lymph node
  Subclavicular (apical) lymph node
  Subscapular (posterior) lymph node
	6 **Lymphatic, Left Axillary**
	  See 5 Lymphatic, Right Axillary
	7 **Lymphatic, Thorax**
	  Intercostal lymph node
	  Mediastinal lymph node
	  Parasternal lymph node
	  Paratracheal lymph node
	  Tracheobronchial lymph node
	8 **Lymphatic, Internal Mammary, Right**
	9 **Lymphatic, Internal Mammary, Left**
	B **Lymphatic, Mesenteric**
	  Inferior mesenteric lymph node
	  Pararectal lymph node
	  Superior mesenteric lymph node
	C **Lymphatic, Pelvis**
	  Common iliac (subaortic) lymph node
	  Gluteal lymph node
	  Iliac lymph node
	  Inferior epigastric lymph node
	  Obturator lymph node
	  Sacral lymph node
	  Subaortic (common iliac) lymph node
	  Suprainguinal lymph node
	D **Lymphatic, Aortic**
	  Celiac lymph node
	  Gastric lymph node
	  Hepatic lymph node
	  Lumbar lymph node
	  Pancreaticosplenic lymph node
	  Paraaortic lymph node
	  Retroperitoneal lymph node
	F **Lymphatic, Right Lower Extremity**
	  Femoral lymph node
	  Popliteal lymph node
	G **Lymphatic, Left Lower Extremity**
	  See F Lymphatic, Right Lower Extremity
	H **Lymphatic, Right Inguinal**
	J **Lymphatic, Left Inguinal**
	K **Thoracic Duct**
	  Left jugular trunk
	  Left subclavian trunk
	L **Cisterna Chyli**
	  Intestinal lymphatic trunk
	  Lumbar lymphatic trunk
		Ø Open
		3 Percutaneous
		4 Percutaneous
		  Endoscopic
		8 Via Natural or
		  Artificial Opening
		  Endoscopic
			Z No Device	X Diagnostic
				Z No Qualifier

M **Thymus**
  Thymus gland
P **Spleen**
  Accessory spleen
T **Bone Marrow**
		Ø Open
		3 Percutaneous
		4 Percutaneous
		  Endoscopic
			Ø Drainage Device	Z No Qualifier

M **Thymus**
  Thymus gland
P **Spleen**
  Accessory spleen
T **Bone Marrow**
		Ø Open
		3 Percutaneous
		4 Percutaneous
		  Endoscopic
			Z No Device	X Diagnostic
				Z No Qualifier

Non-OR	Ø79[Ø,1,2,3,4,5,6,7,8,9,B,C,D,F,G,H,J,K,L]8ZX
Non-OR	Ø79[Ø,1,2,3,4,5,6,7,8,9,B,C,D,F,G,H,J,K,L][3,8]ZZ
Non-OR	Ø79M3ØZ
Non-OR	Ø79P[3,4]ØZ
Non-OR	Ø79T[Ø,3,4]ØZ
Non-OR	Ø79M3ZZ
Non-OR	Ø79P[3,4]Z[X,Z]
Non-OR	Ø79T[Ø,3,4]Z[X,Z]

NC Noncovered Procedure   **LC** Limited Coverage   **QA** Questionable OB Admit   **NT** New Tech Add-on   ✛ Combination Member   ♂ Male   ♀ Female

ICD-10-PCS 2022   **287**

Ø   Medical and Surgical
7   Lymphatic and Hemic Systems
B   Excision   Definition: Cutting out or off, without replacement, a portion of a body part
                          Explanation: The qualifier DIAGNOSTIC is used to identify excision procedures that are biopsies

Body Part Character 4		Approach Character 5	Device Character 6	Qualifier Character 7

Ø   Lymphatic, Head
    Buccinator lymph node
    Infraauricular lymph node
    Infraparotid lymph node
    Parotid lymph node
    Preauricular lymph node
    Submandibular lymph node
    Submaxillary lymph node
    Submental lymph node
    Subparotid lymph node
    Suprahyoid lymph node
1   Lymphatic, Right Neck
    Cervical lymph node
    Jugular lymph node
    Mastoid (postauricular) lymph node
    Occipital lymph node
    Postauricular (mastoid) lymph node
    Retropharyngeal lymph node
    Right jugular trunk
    Right lymphatic duct
    Right subclavian trunk
    Supraclavicular (Virchow's) lymph
        node
    Virchow's (supraclavicular) lymph
        node
2   Lymphatic, Left Neck
    Cervical lymph node
    Jugular lymph node
    Mastoid (postauricular) lymph node
    Occipital lymph node
    Postauricular (mastoid) lymph node
    Retropharyngeal lymph node
    Supraclavicular (Virchow's) lymph
        node
    Virchow's (supraclavicular) lymph
        node
3   Lymphatic, Right Upper Extremity
    Cubital lymph node
    Deltopectoral (infraclavicular) lymph
        node
    Epitrochlear lymph node
    Infraclavicular (deltopectoral) lymph
        node
    Supratrochlear lymph node
4   Lymphatic, Left Upper Extremity
    See 3 Lymphatic, Right Upper Extremity
5   Lymphatic, Right Axillary
    Anterior (pectoral) lymph node
    Apical (subclavicular) lymph node
    Brachial (lateral) lymph node
    Central axillary lymph node
    Lateral (brachial) lymph node
    Pectoral (anterior) lymph node
    Posterior (subscapular) lymph node
    Subclavicular (apical) lymph node
    Subscapular (posterior) lymph node
	6 Lymphatic, Left Axillary
	    See 5 Lymphatic, Right Axillary
	7 Lymphatic, Thorax
	    Intercostal lymph node
	    Mediastinal lymph node
	    Parasternal lymph node
	    Paratracheal lymph node
	    Tracheobronchial lymph node
	8 Lymphatic, Internal Mammary, Right
	9 Lymphatic, Internal Mammary, Left
	B Lymphatic, Mesenteric
	    Inferior mesenteric lymph node
	    Pararectal lymph node
	    Superior mesenteric lymph node
	C Lymphatic, Pelvis
	    Common iliac (subaortic) lymph node
	    Gluteal lymph node
	    Iliac lymph node
	    Inferior epigastric lymph node
	    Obturator lymph node
	    Sacral lymph node
	    Subaortic (common iliac) lymph node
	    Suprainguinal lymph node
	D Lymphatic, Aortic
	    Celiac lymph node
	    Gastric lymph node
	    Hepatic lymph node
	    Lumbar lymph node
	    Pancreaticosplenic lymph node
	    Paraaortic lymph node
	    Retroperitoneal lymph node
	F Lymphatic, Right Lower Extremity
	    Femoral lymph node
	    Popliteal lymph node
	G Lymphatic, Left Lower Extremity
	    See F Lymphatic, Right Lower Extremity
	H Lymphatic, Right Inguinal ⊞
	J Lymphatic, Left Inguinal ⊞
	K Thoracic Duct
	    Left jugular trunk
	    Left subclavian trunk
	L Cisterna Chyli
	    Intestinal lymphatic trunk
	    Lumbar lymphatic trunk
	M Thymus
	    Thymus gland
	P Spleen
	    Accessory spleen
		Ø Open
		3 Percutaneous
		**4 Percutaneous
		    Endoscopic**
			Z No Device	**X Diagnostic**
				Z No Qualifier

Non-OR   Ø7BP[3,4]ZX

See Appendix L for Procedure Combinations
⊞   Ø7B[H,J][Ø,4]ZZ

Ø Medical and Surgical
7 Lymphatic and Hemic Systems
C Extirpation Definition: Taking or cutting out solid matter from a body part

Explanation: The solid matter may be an abnormal byproduct of a biological function or a foreign body; it may be imbedded in a body part or in the lumen of a tubular body part. The solid matter may or may not have been previously broken into pieces.

Body Part Character 4		Approach Character 5	Device Character 6	Qualifier Character 7
Ø Lymphatic, Head Buccinator lymph node Infraauricular lymph node Infraparotid lymph node Parotid lymph node Preauricular lymph node Submandibular lymph node Submaxillary lymph node Submental lymph node Subparotid lymph node Suprahyoid lymph node	**6 Lymphatic, Left Axillary** *See 5 Lymphatic, Right Axillary* **7 Lymphatic, Thorax** Intercostal lymph node Mediastinal lymph node Parasternal lymph node Paratracheal lymph node Tracheobronchial lymph node	**Ø Open** **3 Percutaneous** **4 Percutaneous Endoscopic**	**Z No Device**	**Z No Qualifier**
1 Lymphatic, Right Neck Cervical lymph node Jugular lymph node Mastoid (postauricular) lymph node Occipital lymph node Postauricular (mastoid) lymph node Retropharyngeal lymph node Right jugular trunk Right lymphatic duct Right subclavian trunk Supraclavicular (Virchow's) lymph node Virchow's (supraclavicular) lymph node	**8 Lymphatic, Internal Mammary, Right** **9 Lymphatic, Internal Mammary, Left** **B Lymphatic, Mesenteric** Inferior mesenteric lymph node Pararectal lymph node Superior mesenteric lymph node **C Lymphatic, Pelvis** Common iliac (subaortic) lymph node Gluteal lymph node Iliac lymph node Inferior epigastric lymph node Obturator lymph node Sacral lymph node Subaortic (common iliac) lymph node Suprainguinal lymph node			
2 Lymphatic, Left Neck Cervical lymph node Jugular lymph node Mastoid (postauricular) lymph node Occipital lymph node Postauricular (mastoid) lymph node Retropharyngeal lymph node Supraclavicular (Virchow's) lymph node Virchow's (supraclavicular) lymph node	**D Lymphatic, Aortic** Celiac lymph node Gastric lymph node Hepatic lymph node Lumbar lymph node Pancreaticosplenic lymph node Paraaortic lymph node Retroperitoneal lymph node			
3 Lymphatic, Right Upper Extremity Cubital lymph node Deltopectoral (infraclavicular) lymph node Epitrochlear lymph node Infraclavicular (deltopectoral) lymph node Supratrochlear lymph node	**F Lymphatic, Right Lower Extremity** Femoral lymph node Popliteal lymph node **G Lymphatic, Left Lower Extremity** *See F Lymphatic, Right Lower Extremity* **H Lymphatic, Right Inguinal** **J Lymphatic, Left Inguinal** **K Thoracic Duct** Left jugular trunk Left subclavian trunk **L Cisterna Chyli** Intestinal lymphatic trunk Lumbar lymphatic trunk			
4 Lymphatic, Left Upper Extremity *See 3 Lymphatic, Right Upper Extremity*	**M Thymus** Thymus gland			
5 Lymphatic, Right Axillary Anterior (pectoral) lymph node Apical (subclavicular) lymph node Brachial (lateral) lymph node Central axillary lymph node Lateral (brachial) lymph node Pectoral (anterior) lymph node Posterior (subscapular) lymph node Subclavicular (apical) lymph node Subscapular (posterior) lymph node	**P Spleen** Accessory spleen			

Non-OR 07CP[3,4]ZZ

NC Noncovered Procedure LC Limited Coverage QA Questionable OB Admit NT New Tech Add-on ⊞ Combination Member ♂ Male ♀ Female

ICD-10-PCS 2022 289

Lymphatic and Hemic Systems (side tab)

Ø Medical and Surgical
7 Lymphatic and Hemic Systems
D Extraction   Definition: Pulling or stripping out or off all or a portion of a body part by the use of force
         Explanation: The qualifier DIAGNOSTIC is used to identify extraction procedures that are biopsies

Body Part Character 4		Approach Character 5	Device Character 6	Qualifier Character 7
Ø Lymphatic, Head	**6 Lymphatic, Left Axillary**	**3** Percutaneous	**Z** No Device	**X** Diagnostic
Buccinator lymph node	*See 5 Lymphatic, Right Axillary*	**4** Percutaneous Endoscopic		
Infraauricular lymph node	**7 Lymphatic, Thorax**	**8** Via Natural or Artificial		
Infraparotid lymph node	Intercostal lymph node	Opening Endoscopic		
Parotid lymph node	Mediastinal lymph node			
Preauricular lymph node	Parasternal lymph node			
Submandibular lymph node	Paratracheal lymph node			
Submaxillary lymph node	Tracheobronchial lymph node			
Submental lymph node	**8 Lymphatic, Internal**			
Subparotid lymph node	**Mammary, Right**			
Suprahyoid lymph node	**9 Lymphatic, Internal**			
1 Lymphatic, Right Neck	**Mammary, Left**			
Cervical lymph node	**B Lymphatic, Mesenteric**			
Jugular lymph node	Inferior mesenteric lymph			
Mastoid (postauricular) lymph	node			
node	Pararectal lymph node			
Occipital lymph node	Superior mesenteric lymph			
Postauricular (mastoid) lymph	node			
node	**C Lymphatic, Pelvis**			
Retropharyngeal lymph node	Common iliac (subaortic)			
Right jugular trunk	lymph node			
Right lymphatic duct	Gluteal lymph node			
Right subclavian trunk	Iliac lymph node			
Supraclavicular (Virchow's)	Inferior epigastric lymph node			
lymph node	Obturator lymph node			
Virchow's (supraclavicular)	Sacral lymph node			
lymph node	Subaortic (common iliac)			
2 Lymphatic, Left Neck	lymph node			
Cervical lymph node	Suprainguinal lymph node			
Jugular lymph node	**D Lymphatic, Aortic**			
Mastoid (postauricular) lymph	Celiac lymph node			
node	Gastric lymph node			
Occipital lymph node	Hepatic lymph node			
Postauricular (mastoid) lymph	Lumbar lymph node			
node	Pancreaticosplenic lymph			
Retropharyngeal lymph node	node			
Supraclavicular (Virchow's)	Paraaortic lymph node			
lymph node	Retroperitoneal lymph node			
Virchow's (supraclavicular)	**F Lymphatic, Right Lower**			
lymph node	**Extremity**			
3 Lymphatic, Right Upper	Femoral lymph node			
Extremity	Popliteal lymph node			
Cubital lymph node	**G Lymphatic, Left Lower**			
Deltopectoral (infraclavicular)	**Extremity**			
lymph node	*See F Lymphatic, Right Lower*			
Epitrochlear lymph node	*Extremity*			
Infraclavicular (deltopectoral)	**H Lymphatic, Right Inguinal**			
lymph node	**J Lymphatic, Left Inguinal**			
Supratrochlear lymph node	**K Thoracic Duct**			
4 Lymphatic, Left Upper	Left jugular trunk			
Extremity	Left subclavian trunk			
See 3 Lymphatic, Right Upper	**L Cisterna Chyli**			
Extremity	Intestinal lymphatic trunk			
5 Lymphatic, Right Axillary	Lumbar lymphatic trunk			
Anterior (pectoral) lymph node				
Apical (subclavicular) lymph				
node				
Brachial (lateral) lymph node				
Central axillary lymph node				
Lateral (brachial) lymph node				
Pectoral (anterior) lymph node				
Posterior (subscapular) lymph				
node				
Subclavicular (apical) lymph				
node				
Subscapular (posterior) lymph				
node				
M Thymus		**3** Percutaneous	**Z** No Device	**X** Diagnostic
Thymus gland		**4** Percutaneous Endoscopic		
P Spleen				
Accessory spleen				
Q Bone Marrow, Sternum		**Ø** Open	**Z** No Device	**X** Diagnostic
R Bone Marrow, Iliac		**3** Percutaneous		**Z** No Qualifier
S Bone Marrow, Vertebral				
T Bone Marrow				

Non-OR   All body part, approach, device, and qualifier values

Ø   Medical and Surgical
7   Lymphatic and Hemic Systems
H   Insertion   Definition: Putting in a nonbiological appliance that monitors, assists, performs, or prevents a physiological function but does not physically take the place of a body part
                Explanation: None

Body Part Character 4	Approach Character 5	Device Character 6	Qualifier Character 7

K   Thoracic Duct
     Left jugular trunk
     Left subclavian trunk
L   Cisterna Chyli
     Intestinal lymphatic trunk
     Lumbar lymphatic trunk
M   Thymus
     Thymus gland
N   Lymphatic
P   Spleen
     Accessory spleen
T   Bone Marrow
	Ø Open
	3 Percutaneous
	4 Percutaneous Endoscopic
		1 Radioactive Element
		3 Infusion Device
		Y Other Device
			Z No Qualifier

Non-OR	Ø7H[K,L,M,N,P][Ø,4]3Z
Non-OR	Ø7H[K,L,M,N,P,T]3[1,3,Y]Z
Non-OR	Ø7H[N,P]4YZ
Non-OR	Ø7HT[Ø,4][1,3,Y]Z

Ø   Medical and Surgical
7   Lymphatic and Hemic Systems
J   Inspection   Definition: Visually and/or manually exploring a body part
                Explanation: Visual exploration may be performed with or without optical instrumentation. Manual exploration may be performed directly or through intervening body layers.

Body Part Character 4	Approach Character 5	Device Character 6	Qualifier Character 7

K   Thoracic Duct
     Left jugular trunk
     Left subclavian trunk
L   Cisterna Chyli
     Intestinal lymphatic trunk
     Lumbar lymphatic trunk
M   Thymus
     Thymus gland
T   Bone Marrow
	Ø Open
	3 Percutaneous
	4 Percutaneous Endoscopic
		Z No Device	Z No Qualifier

N Lymphatic	Ø Open 3 Percutaneous 4 Percutaneous Endoscopic 8 Via Natural or Artificial Opening Endoscopic X External	Z No Device	Z No Qualifier
P Spleen Accessory spleen	Ø Open 3 Percutaneous 4 Percutaneous Endoscopic X External	Z No Device	Z No Qualifier

Non-OR	Ø7J[K,L,M]3ZZ
Non-OR	Ø7JT[Ø,3,4]ZZ
Non-OR	Ø7JN[3,8,X]ZZ
Non-OR	Ø7JP[3,4,X]ZZ

NC Noncovered Procedure   **LC** Limited Coverage   **QA** Questionable OB Admit   **NT** New Tech Add-on   ⊞ Combination Member   ♂ Male   ♀ Female

ICD-10-PCS 2022   291

Ø   Medical and Surgical
7   Lymphatic and Hemic Systems
L   Occlusion   Definition: Completely closing an orifice or the lumen of a tubular body part
                Explanation: The orifice can be a natural orifice or an artificially created orifice

Body Part Character 4		Approach Character 5	Device Character 6	Qualifier Character 7

Ø Lymphatic, Head
  Buccinator lymph node
  Infraauricular lymph node
  Infraparotid lymph node
  Parotid lymph node
  Preauricular lymph node
  Submandibular lymph node
  Submaxillary lymph node
  Submental lymph node
  Subparotid lymph node
  Suprahyoid lymph node
1 Lymphatic, Right Neck
  Cervical lymph node
  Jugular lymph node
  Mastoid (postauricular) lymph node
  Occipital lymph node
  Postauricular (mastoid) lymph node
  Retropharyngeal lymph node
  Right jugular trunk
  Right lymphatic duct
  Right subclavian trunk
  Supraclavicular (Virchow's) lymph
    node
  Virchow's (supraclavicular) lymph
    node
2 Lymphatic, Left Neck
  Cervical lymph node
  Jugular lymph node
  Mastoid (postauricular) lymph node
  Occipital lymph node
  Postauricular (mastoid) lymph node
  Retropharyngeal lymph node
  Supraclavicular (Virchow's) lymph
    node
  Virchow's (supraclavicular) lymph
    node
3 Lymphatic, Right Upper Extremity
  Cubital lymph node
  Deltopectoral (infraclavicular) lymph
    node
  Epitrochlear lymph node
  Infraclavicular (deltopectoral) lymph
    node
  Supratrochlear lymph node
4 Lymphatic, Left Upper Extremity
  See 3 Lymphatic, Right Upper Extremity
5 Lymphatic, Right Axillary
  Anterior (pectoral) lymph node
  Apical (subclavicular) lymph node
  Brachial (lateral) lymph node
  Central axillary lymph node
  Lateral (brachial) lymph node
  Pectoral (anterior) lymph node
  Posterior (subscapular) lymph node
  Subclavicular (apical) lymph node
  Subscapular (posterior) lymph node
	6 Lymphatic, Left Axillary
	  See 5 Lymphatic, Right Axillary
	7 Lymphatic, Thorax
	  Intercostal lymph node
	  Mediastinal lymph node
	  Parasternal lymph node
	  Paratracheal lymph node
	  Tracheobronchial lymph node
	8 Lymphatic, Internal Mammary, Right
	9 Lymphatic, Internal Mammary, Left
	B Lymphatic, Mesenteric
	  Inferior mesenteric lymph node
	  Pararectal lymph node
	  Superior mesenteric lymph node
	C Lymphatic, Pelvis
	  Common iliac (subaortic) lymph node
	  Gluteal lymph node
	  Iliac lymph node
	  Inferior epigastric lymph node
	  Obturator lymph node
	  Sacral lymph node
	  Subaortic (common iliac) lymph node
	  Suprainguinal lymph node
	D Lymphatic, Aortic
	  Celiac lymph node
	  Gastric lymph node
	  Hepatic lymph node
	  Lumbar lymph node
	  Pancreaticosplenic lymph node
	  Paraaortic lymph node
	  Retroperitoneal lymph node
	F Lymphatic, Right Lower Extremity
	  Femoral lymph node
	  Popliteal lymph node
	G Lymphatic, Left Lower Extremity
	  See F Lymphatic, Right Lower Extremity
	H Lymphatic, Right Inguinal
	J Lymphatic, Left Inguinal
	K Thoracic Duct
	  Left jugular trunk
	  Left subclavian trunk
	L Cisterna Chyli
	  Intestinal lymphatic trunk
	  Lumbar lymphatic trunk
		Ø Open
		3 Percutaneous
		4 Percutaneous
		    Endoscopic
			C Extraluminal Device
			D Intraluminal Device
			Z No Device
				Z No Qualifier

Lymphatic and Hemic Systems

Ø   **Medical and Surgical**
7   **Lymphatic and Hemic Systems**
N   **Release**   Definition: Freeing a body part from an abnormal physical constraint by cutting or by the use of force
                     Explanation: Some of the restraining tissue may be taken out but none of the body part is taken out

Body Part Character 4		Approach Character 5	Device Character 6	Qualifier Character 7
Ø **Lymphatic, Head** Buccinator lymph node Infraauricular lymph node Infraparotid lymph node Parotid lymph node Preauricular lymph node Submandibular lymph node Submaxillary lymph node Submental lymph node Subparotid lymph node Suprahyoid lymph node **1** **Lymphatic, Right Neck** Cervical lymph node Jugular lymph node Mastoid (postauricular) lymph node Occipital lymph node Postauricular (mastoid) lymph node Retropharyngeal lymph node Right jugular trunk Right lymphatic duct Right subclavian trunk Supraclavicular (Virchow's) lymph node Virchow's (supraclavicular) lymph node **2** **Lymphatic, Left Neck** Cervical lymph node Jugular lymph node Mastoid (postauricular) lymph node Occipital lymph node Postauricular (mastoid) lymph node Retropharyngeal lymph node Supraclavicular (Virchow's) lymph node Virchow's (supraclavicular) lymph node **3** **Lymphatic, Right Upper Extremity** Cubital lymph node Deltopectoral (infraclavicular) lymph node Epitrochlear lymph node Infraclavicular (deltopectoral) lymph node Supratrochlear lymph node **4** **Lymphatic, Left Upper Extremity** *See 3 Lymphatic, Right Upper Extremity* **5** **Lymphatic, Right Axillary** Anterior (pectoral) lymph node Apical (subclavicular) lymph node Brachial (lateral) lymph node Central axillary lymph node Lateral (brachial) lymph node Pectoral (anterior) lymph node Posterior (subscapular) lymph node Subclavicular (apical) lymph node Subscapular (posterior) lymph node	**6** **Lymphatic, Left Axillary** *See 5 Lymphatic, Right Axillary* **7** **Lymphatic, Thorax** Intercostal lymph node Mediastinal lymph node Parasternal lymph node Paratracheal lymph node Tracheobronchial lymph node **8** **Lymphatic, Internal Mammary, Right** **9** **Lymphatic, Internal Mammary, Left** **B** **Lymphatic, Mesenteric** Inferior mesenteric lymph node Pararectal lymph node Superior mesenteric lymph node **C** **Lymphatic, Pelvis** Common iliac (subaortic) lymph node Gluteal lymph node Iliac lymph node Inferior epigastric lymph node Obturator lymph node Sacral lymph node Subaortic (common iliac) lymph node Suprainguinal lymph node **D** **Lymphatic, Aortic** Celiac lymph node Gastric lymph node Hepatic lymph node Lumbar lymph node Pancreaticosplenic lymph node Paraaortic lymph node Retroperitoneal lymph node **F** **Lymphatic, Right Lower Extremity** Femoral lymph node Popliteal lymph node **G** **Lymphatic, Left Lower Extremity** *See F Lymphatic, Right Lower Extremity* **H** **Lymphatic, Right Inguinal** **J** **Lymphatic, Left Inguinal** **K** **Thoracic Duct** Left jugular trunk Left subclavian trunk **L** **Cisterna Chyli** Intestinal lymphatic trunk Lumbar lymphatic trunk **M** **Thymus** Thymus gland **P** **Spleen** Accessory spleen	**Ø** Open **3** Percutaneous **4** Percutaneous Endoscopic	**Z** No Device	**Z** No Qualifier

0   Medical and Surgical
7   Lymphatic and Hemic Systems
P   Removal   Definition: Taking out or off a device from a body part

Explanation: If a device is taken out and a similar device put in without cutting or puncturing the skin or mucous membrane, the procedure is coded to the root operation CHANGE. Otherwise, the procedure for taking out a device is coded to the root operation REMOVAL.

Body Part Character 4	Approach Character 5	Device Character 6	Qualifier Character 7

K Thoracic Duct
  Left jugular trunk
  Left subclavian trunk
L Cisterna Chyli
  Intestinal lymphatic trunk
  Lumbar lymphatic trunk
N Lymphatic
	0 Open
	3 Percutaneous
	4 Percutaneous Endoscopic
		0 Drainage Device
		3 Infusion Device
		7 Autologous Tissue Substitute
		C Extraluminal Device
		D Intraluminal Device
		J Synthetic Substitute
		K Nonautologous Tissue Substitute
		Y Other Device
			Z No Qualifier

K Thoracic Duct
  Left jugular trunk
  Left subclavian trunk
L Cisterna Chyli
  Intestinal lymphatic trunk
  Lumbar lymphatic trunk
N Lymphatic
	X External	0 Drainage Device
		3 Infusion Device
		D Intraluminal Device
			Z No Qualifier

M Thymus
  Thymus gland
P Spleen
  Accessory spleen
	0 Open
	3 Percutaneous
	4 Percutaneous Endoscopic
		0 Drainage Device
		3 Infusion Device
		Y Other Device
			Z No Qualifier

M Thymus
  Thymus gland
P Spleen
  Accessory spleen
	X External	0 Drainage Device
		3 Infusion Device
			Z No Qualifier

T Bone Marrow	0 Open 3 Percutaneous 4 Percutaneous Endoscopic X External	0 Drainage Device	Z No Qualifier

Non-OR	07P[K,L,N][3,4]YZ
Non-OR	07P[K,L,N]X[0,3,D]Z
Non-OR	07P[M,P][3,4]YZ
Non-OR	07P[M,P]X[0,3]Z
Non-OR	07PT[0,3,4,X]0Z

Ø **Medical and Surgical**
7 **Lymphatic and Hemic Systems**
Q **Repair**　　　　Definition: Restoring, to the extent possible, a body part to its normal anatomic structure and function
　　　　　　　　　　Explanation: Used only when the method to accomplish the repair is not one of the other root operations

Body Part Character 4		Approach Character 5	Device Character 6	Qualifier Character 7
Ø **Lymphatic, Head** Buccinator lymph node Infraauricular lymph node Infraparotid lymph node Parotid lymph node Preauricular lymph node Submandibular lymph node Submaxillary lymph node Submental lymph node Subparotid lymph node Suprahyoid lymph node 1 **Lymphatic, Right Neck** Cervical lymph node Jugular lymph node Mastoid (postauricular) lymph node Occipital lymph node Postauricular (mastoid) lymph node Retropharyngeal lymph node Right jugular trunk Right lymphatic duct Right subclavian trunk Supraclavicular (Virchow's) lymph 　　node Virchow's (supraclavicular) lymph 　　node 2 **Lymphatic, Left Neck** Cervical lymph node Jugular lymph node Mastoid (postauricular) lymph node Occipital lymph node Postauricular (mastoid) lymph node Retropharyngeal lymph node Supraclavicular (Virchow's) lymph 　　node Virchow's (supraclavicular) lymph 　　node 3 **Lymphatic, Right Upper Extremity** Cubital lymph node Deltopectoral (infraclavicular) lymph 　　node Epitrochlear lymph node Infraclavicular (deltopectoral) lymph 　　node Supratrochlear lymph node 4 **Lymphatic, Left Upper Extremity** See 3 Lymphatic, Right Upper Extremity 5 **Lymphatic, Right Axillary** Anterior (pectoral) lymph node Apical (subclavicular) lymph node Brachial (lateral) lymph node Central axillary lymph node Lateral (brachial) lymph node Pectoral (anterior) lymph node Posterior (subscapular) lymph node Subclavicular (apical) lymph node Subscapular (posterior) lymph node	6 **Lymphatic, Left Axillary** See 5 Lymphatic, Right Axillary 7 **Lymphatic, Thorax** Intercostal lymph node Mediastinal lymph node Parasternal lymph node Paratracheal lymph node Tracheobronchial lymph node 8 **Lymphatic, Internal Mammary, Right** 9 **Lymphatic, Internal Mammary, Left** B **Lymphatic, Mesenteric** Inferior mesenteric lymph node Pararectal lymph node Superior mesenteric lymph node C **Lymphatic, Pelvis** Common iliac (subaortic) lymph node Gluteal lymph node Iliac lymph node Inferior epigastric lymph node Obturator lymph node Sacral lymph node Subaortic (common iliac) lymph node Suprainguinal lymph node D **Lymphatic, Aortic** Celiac lymph node Gastric lymph node Hepatic lymph node Lumbar lymph node Pancreaticosplenic lymph node Paraaortic lymph node Retroperitoneal lymph node F **Lymphatic, Right Lower Extremity** Femoral lymph node Popliteal lymph node G **Lymphatic, Left Lower Extremity** See F Lymphatic, Right Lower Extremity H **Lymphatic, Right Inguinal** J **Lymphatic, Left Inguinal** K **Thoracic Duct** Left jugular trunk Left subclavian trunk L **Cisterna Chyli** Intestinal lymphatic trunk Lumbar lymphatic trunk	Ø **Open** 3 **Percutaneous** 4 **Percutaneous Endoscopic** 8 **Via Natural or Artificial Opening Endoscopic**	Z **No Device**	Z **No Qualifier**
M **Thymus** Thymus gland P **Spleen** Accessory spleen		Ø **Open** 3 **Percutaneous** 4 **Percutaneous Endoscopic**	Z **No Device**	Z **No Qualifier**

NC Noncovered Procedure　　**LC** Limited Coverage　　**QA** Questionable OB Admit　　**NT** New Tech Add-on　　⊞ Combination Member　　♂ Male　　♀ Female

ICD-10-PCS 2022　　　　　　　　　　　　　　　　　　　　　　　　　　　　　　　　**295**

Lymphatic and Hemic Systems (side tab)

Ø Medical and Surgical
7 Lymphatic and Hemic Systems
S Reposition   Definition: Moving to its normal location, or other suitable location, all or a portion of a body part

Explanation: The body part is moved to a new location from an abnormal location, or from a normal location where it is not functioning correctly. The body part may or may not be cut out or off to be moved to the new location.

Body Part Character 4	Approach Character 5	Device Character 6	Qualifier Character 7

M Thymus
   Thymus gland
 P Spleen
   Accessory spleen
	Ø Open	Z No Device	Z No Qualifier

Ø Medical and Surgical
7 Lymphatic and Hemic Systems
T Resection   Definition: Cutting out or off, without replacement, all of a body part

Explanation: None

Body Part Character 4		Approach Character 5	Device Character 6	Qualifier Character 7

Ø Lymphatic, Head
 Buccinator lymph node
 Infraauricular lymph node
 Infraparotid lymph node
 Parotid lymph node
 Preauricular lymph node
 Submandibular lymph node
 Submaxillary lymph node
 Submental lymph node
 Subparotid lymph node
 Suprahyoid lymph node
 1 Lymphatic, Right Neck
 Cervical lymph node
 Jugular lymph node
 Mastoid (postauricular) lymph node
 Occipital lymph node
 Postauricular (mastoid) lymph node
 Retropharyngeal lymph node
 Right jugular trunk
 Right lymphatic duct
 Right subclavian trunk
 Supraclavicular (Virchow's) lymph
   node
 Virchow's (supraclavicular) lymph
   node
 2 Lymphatic, Left Neck
 Cervical lymph node
 Jugular lymph node
 Mastoid (postauricular) lymph node
 Occipital lymph node
 Postauricular (mastoid) lymph node
 Retropharyngeal lymph node
 Supraclavicular (Virchow's) lymph
   node
 Virchow's (supraclavicular) lymph
   node
 3 Lymphatic, Right Upper Extremity
 Cubital lymph node
 Deltopectoral (infraclavicular) lymph
   node
 Epitrochlear lymph node
 Infraclavicular (deltopectoral) lymph
   node
 Supratrochlear lymph node
 4 Lymphatic, Left Upper Extremity
 See 3 Lymphatic, Right Upper Extremity
 5 Lymphatic, Right Axillary ⊞
 Anterior (pectoral) lymph node
 Apical (subclavicular) lymph node
 Brachial (lateral) lymph node
 Central axillary lymph node
 Lateral (brachial) lymph node
 Pectoral (anterior) lymph node
 Posterior (subscapular) lymph node
 Subclavicular (apical) lymph node
 Subscapular (posterior) lymph node
	6 Lymphatic, Left Axillary ⊞
	 See 5 Lymphatic, Right Axillary
	 7 Lymphatic, Thorax ⊞
	 Intercostal lymph node
	 Mediastinal lymph node
	 Parasternal lymph node
	 Paratracheal lymph node
	 Tracheobronchial lymph node
	 8 Lymphatic, Internal ⊞
	 Mammary, Right
	 9 Lymphatic, Internal ⊞
	 Mammary, Left
	 B Lymphatic, Mesenteric
	 Inferior mesenteric lymph node
	 Pararectal lymph node
	 Superior mesenteric lymph node
	 C Lymphatic, Pelvis
	 Common iliac (subaortic) lymph node
	 Gluteal lymph node
	 Iliac lymph node
	 Inferior epigastric lymph node
	 Obturator lymph node
	 Sacral lymph node
	 Subaortic (common iliac) lymph node
	 Suprainguinal lymph node
	 D Lymphatic, Aortic
	 Celiac lymph node
	 Gastric lymph node
	 Hepatic lymph node
	 Lumbar lymph node
	 Pancreaticosplenic lymph node
	 Paraaortic lymph node
	 Retroperitoneal lymph node
	 F Lymphatic, Right Lower Extremity
	 Femoral lymph node
	 Popliteal lymph node
	 G Lymphatic, Left Lower Extremity
	 See F Lymphatic, Right Lower Extremity
	 H Lymphatic, Right Inguinal
	 J Lymphatic, Left Inguinal
	 K Thoracic Duct
	 Left jugular trunk
	 Left subclavian trunk
	 L Cisterna Chyli
	 Intestinal lymphatic trunk
	 Lumbar lymphatic trunk
	 M Thymus
	 Thymus gland
	 P Spleen
	 Accessory spleen
		Ø Open
		 4 Percutaneous Endoscopic
			Z No Device	**Z No Qualifier**

See Appendix L for Procedure Combinations
  ⊞   Ø7T[5,6,7,8,9]ØZZ

Ø   **Medical and Surgical**
7   **Lymphatic and Hemic Systems**
U   **Supplement**   Definition: Putting in or on biological or synthetic material that physically reinforces and/or augments the function of a portion of a body part

                       Explanation: The biological material is non-living, or is living and from the same individual. The body part may have been previously replaced, and the SUPPLEMENT procedure is performed to physically reinforce and/or augment the function of the replaced body part.

Body Part Character 4		Approach Character 5	Device Character 6	Qualifier Character 7

Ø Lymphatic, Head
  Buccinator lymph node
  Infraauricular lymph node
  Infraparotid lymph node
  Parotid lymph node
  Preauricular lymph node
  Submandibular lymph node
  Submaxillary lymph node
  Submental lymph node
  Subparotid lymph node
  Suprahyoid lymph node
1 Lymphatic, Right Neck
  Cervical lymph node
  Jugular lymph node
  Mastoid (postauricular) lymph node
  Occipital lymph node
  Postauricular (mastoid) lymph node
  Retropharyngeal lymph node
  Right jugular trunk
  Right lymphatic duct
  Right subclavian trunk
  Supraclavicular (Virchow's) lymph
    node
  Virchow's (supraclavicular) lymph
    node
2 Lymphatic, Left Neck
  Cervical lymph node
  Jugular lymph node
  Mastoid (postauricular) lymph node
  Occipital lymph node
  Postauricular (mastoid) lymph node
  Retropharyngeal lymph node
  Supraclavicular (Virchow's) lymph
    node
  Virchow's (supraclavicular) lymph
    node
3 Lymphatic, Right Upper Extremity
  Cubital lymph node
  Deltopectoral (infraclavicular) lymph
    node
  Epitrochlear lymph node
  Infraclavicular (deltopectoral) lymph
    node
  Supratrochlear lymph node
4 Lymphatic, Left Upper Extremity
  See 3 Lymphatic, Right Upper Extremity
5 Lymphatic, Right Axillary
  Anterior (pectoral) lymph node
  Apical (subclavicular) lymph node
  Brachial (lateral) lymph node
  Central axillary lymph node
  Lateral (brachial) lymph node
  Pectoral (anterior) lymph node
  Posterior (subscapular) lymph node
  Subclavicular (apical) lymph node
  Subscapular (posterior) lymph node
	6 Lymphatic, Left Axillary
	  See 5 Lymphatic, Right Axillary
	7 Lymphatic, Thorax
	  Intercostal lymph node
	  Mediastinal lymph node
	  Parasternal lymph node
	  Paratracheal lymph node
	  Tracheobronchial lymph node
	8 Lymphatic, Internal Mammary, Right
	9 Lymphatic, Internal Mammary, Left
	B Lymphatic, Mesenteric
	  Inferior mesenteric lymph node
	  Pararectal lymph node
	  Superior mesenteric lymph node
	C Lymphatic, Pelvis
	  Common iliac (subaortic) lymph node
	  Gluteal lymph node
	  Iliac lymph node
	  Inferior epigastric lymph node
	  Obturator lymph node
	  Sacral lymph node
	  Subaortic (common iliac) lymph node
	  Suprainguinal lymph node
	D Lymphatic, Aortic
	  Celiac lymph node
	  Gastric lymph node
	  Hepatic lymph node
	  Lumbar lymph node
	  Pancreaticosplenic lymph node
	  Paraaortic lymph node
	  Retroperitoneal lymph node
	F Lymphatic, Right Lower Extremity
	  Femoral lymph node
	  Popliteal lymph node
	G Lymphatic, Left Lower Extremity
	  See F Lymphatic, Right Lower Extremity
	H Lymphatic, Right Inguinal
	J Lymphatic, Left Inguinal
	K Thoracic Duct
	  Left jugular trunk
	  Left subclavian trunk
	L Cisterna Chyli
	  Intestinal lymphatic trunk
	  Lumbar lymphatic trunk
		Ø Open
		4 Percutaneous
		  Endoscopic
			7 Autologous Tissue
			  Substitute
			J Synthetic Substitute
			K Nonautologous
			  Tissue Substitute
				Z No Qualifier

Ø   Medical and Surgical
7   Lymphatic and Hemic Systems
V   Restriction   Definition: Partially closing an orifice or the lumen of a tubular body part
                              Explanation: The orifice can be a natural orifice or an artificially created orifice

Body Part Character 4		Approach Character 5	Device Character 6	Qualifier Character 7

Ø Lymphatic, Head
   Buccinator lymph node
   Infraauricular lymph node
   Infraparotid lymph node
   Parotid lymph node
   Preauricular lymph node
   Submandibular lymph node
   Submaxillary lymph node
   Submental lymph node
   Subparotid lymph node
   Suprahyoid lymph node
1 Lymphatic, Right Neck
   Cervical lymph node
   Jugular lymph node
   Mastoid (postauricular) lymph node
   Occipital lymph node
   Postauricular (mastoid) lymph node
   Retropharyngeal lymph node
   Right jugular trunk
   Right lymphatic duct
   Right subclavian trunk
   Supraclavicular (Virchow's) lymph
      node
   Virchow's (supraclavicular) lymph
      node
2 Lymphatic, Left Neck
   Cervical lymph node
   Jugular lymph node
   Mastoid (postauricular) lymph node
   Occipital lymph node
   Postauricular (mastoid) lymph node
   Retropharyngeal lymph node
   Supraclavicular (Virchow's) lymph
      node
   Virchow's (supraclavicular) lymph
      node
3 Lymphatic, Right Upper Extremity
   Cubital lymph node
   Deltopectoral (infraclavicular) lymph
      node
   Epitrochlear lymph node
   Infraclavicular (deltopectoral) lymph
      node
   Supratrochlear lymph node
4 Lymphatic, Left Upper Extremity
   See 3 Lymphatic, Right Upper Extremity
5 Lymphatic, Right Axillary
   Anterior (pectoral) lymph node
   Apical (subclavicular) lymph node
   Brachial (lateral) lymph node
   Central axillary lymph node
   Lateral (brachial) lymph node
   Pectoral (anterior) lymph node
   Posterior (subscapular) lymph node
   Subclavicular (apical) lymph node
   Subscapular (posterior) lymph node
	6 Lymphatic, Left Axillary
	   See 5 Lymphatic, Right Axillary
	7 Lymphatic, Thorax
	   Intercostal lymph node
	   Mediastinal lymph node
	   Parasternal lymph node
	   Paratracheal lymph node
	   Tracheobronchial lymph node
	8 Lymphatic, Internal Mammary, Right
	9 Lymphatic, Internal Mammary, Left
	B Lymphatic, Mesenteric
	   Inferior mesenteric lymph node
	   Pararectal lymph node
	   Superior mesenteric lymph node
	C Lymphatic, Pelvis
	   Common iliac (subaortic) lymph node
	   Gluteal lymph node
	   Iliac lymph node
	   Inferior epigastric lymph node
	   Obturator lymph node
	   Sacral lymph node
	   Subaortic (common iliac) lymph node
	   Suprainguinal lymph node
	D Lymphatic, Aortic
	   Celiac lymph node
	   Gastric lymph node
	   Hepatic lymph node
	   Lumbar lymph node
	   Pancreaticosplenic lymph node
	   Paraaortic lymph node
	   Retroperitoneal lymph node
	F Lymphatic, Right Lower Extremity
	   Femoral lymph node
	   Popliteal lymph node
	G Lymphatic, Left Lower Extremity
	   See F Lymphatic, Right Lower Extremity
	H Lymphatic, Right Inguinal
	J Lymphatic, Left Inguinal
	K Thoracic Duct
	   Left jugular trunk
	   Left subclavian trunk
	L Cisterna Chyli
	   Intestinal lymphatic trunk
	   Lumbar lymphatic trunk
		Ø Open
		3 Percutaneous
		4 Percutaneous
		   Endoscopic
			C Extraluminal Device
			D Intraluminal Device
			Z No Device
				Z No Qualifier

0   **Medical and Surgical**
7   **Lymphatic and Hemic Systems**
W   **Revision**   Definition: Correcting, to the extent possible, a portion of a malfunctioning device or the position of a displaced device

                 Explanation: Revision can include correcting a malfunctioning or displaced device by taking out or putting in components of the device such as a screw or pin

Body Part Character 4	Approach Character 5	Device Character 6	Qualifier Character 7

K Thoracic Duct
   Left jugular trunk
   Left subclavian trunk
L Cisterna Chyli
   Intestinal lymphatic trunk
   Lumbar lymphatic trunk
N Lymphatic
	0 Open
	3 Percutaneous
	4 Percutaneous Endoscopic
		0 Drainage Device
		3 Infusion Device
		7 Autologous Tissue
		   Substitute
		C Extraluminal Device
		D Intraluminal Device
		J Synthetic Substitute
		K Nonautologous Tissue
		   Substitute
		Y Other Device
			Z No Qualifier

K Thoracic Duct
   Left jugular trunk
   Left subclavian trunk
L Cisterna Chyli
   Intestinal lymphatic trunk
   Lumbar lymphatic trunk
N Lymphatic
	X External	**0** Drainage Device
		3 Infusion Device
		7 Autologous Tissue
		   Substitute
		C Extraluminal Device
		D Intraluminal Device
		J Synthetic Substitute
		K Nonautologous Tissue
		   Substitute
			Z No Qualifier

M Thymus
   Thymus gland
P Spleen
   Accessory spleen
	0 Open
	3 Percutaneous
	4 Percutaneous Endoscopic
		0 Drainage Device
		3 Infusion Device
		Y Other Device
			Z No Qualifier

M Thymus
   Thymus gland
P Spleen
   Accessory spleen
	X External	**0** Drainage Device
		3 Infusion Device
			Z No Qualifier

T Bone Marrow	**0** Open **3** Percutaneous **4** Percutaneous Endoscopic **X** External	**0** Drainage Device	**Z** No Qualifier

Non-OR	07W[K,L,N][3,4]YZ
Non-OR	07W[K,L,N]X[0,3,7,C,D,J,K]Z
Non-OR	07W[M,P][3,4]YZ
Non-OR	07W[M,P]X[0,3]Z
Non-OR	07WT[0,3,4,X]0Z

0   **Medical and Surgical**
7   **Lymphatic and Hemic Systems**
Y   **Transplantation**   Definition: Putting in or on all or a portion of a living body part taken from another individual or animal to physically take the place and/or function of all or a portion of a similar body part

                  Explanation: The native body part may or may not be taken out, and the transplanted body part may take over all or a portion of its function

Body Part Character 4	Approach Character 5	Device Character 6	Qualifier Character 7

M Thymus
   Thymus gland
P Spleen
   Accessory spleen
	0 Open	**Z** No Device	**0** Allogeneic
			1 Syngeneic
			2 Zooplastic

Eye Ø8Ø–Ø8X

Character Meanings

This Character Meaning table is provided as a guide to assist the user in the identification of character members that may be found in this section of code tables. It **SHOULD NOT** be used to build a PCS code.

Operation–Character 3		Body Part–Character 4		Approach–Character 5		Device–Character 6		Qualifier–Character 7	
Ø	Alteration	Ø	Eye, Right	Ø	Open	Ø	Drainage Device OR Synthetic Substitute, Intraocular Telescope	3	Nasal Cavity
1	Bypass	1	Eye, Left	3	Percutaneous	1	Radioactive Element	4	Sclera
2	Change	2	Anterior Chamber, Right	7	Via Natural or Artificial Opening	3	Infusion Device	X	Diagnostic
5	Destruction	3	Anterior Chamber, Left	8	Via Natural or Artificial Opening Endoscopic	5	Epiretinal Visual Prosthesis	Z	No Qualifier
7	Dilation	4	Vitreous, Right	X	External	7	Autologous Tissue Substitute		
9	Drainage	5	Vitreous, Left			C	Extraluminal Device		
B	Excision	6	Sclera, Right			D	Intraluminal Device		
C	Extirpation	7	Sclera, Left			J	Synthetic Substitute		
D	Extraction	8	Cornea, Right			K	Nonautologous Tissue Substitute		
F	Fragmentation	9	Cornea, Left			Y	Other Device		
H	Insertion	A	Choroid, Right			Z	No Device		
J	Inspection	B	Choroid, Left						
L	Occlusion	C	Iris, Right						
M	Reattachment	D	Iris, Left						
N	Release	E	Retina, Right						
P	Removal	F	Retina, Left						
Q	Repair	G	Retinal Vessel, Right						
R	Replacement	H	Retinal Vessel, Left						
S	Reposition	J	Lens, Right						
T	Resection	K	Lens, Left						
U	Supplement	L	Extraocular Muscle, Right						
V	Restriction	M	Extraocular Muscle, Left						
W	Revision	N	Upper Eyelid, Right						
X	Transfer	P	Upper Eyelid, Left						
		Q	Lower Eyelid, Right						
		R	Lower Eyelid, Left						
		S	Conjunctiva, Right						
		T	Conjunctiva, Left						
		V	Lacrimal Gland, Right						
		W	Lacrimal Gland, Left						
		X	Lacrimal Duct, Right						
		Y	Lacrimal Duct, Left						

AHA Coding Clinic for table Ø81
2019, 1Q, 27   Glaucoma tube shunt

AHA Coding Clinic for table Ø89
2016, 2Q, 21   Laser trabeculoplasty

AHA Coding Clinic for table Ø8B
2014, 4Q, 35   Vitrectomy with air/fluid exchange
2014, 4Q, 36   Pars plans vitrectomy without mention of instillation of oil, air or fluid

AHA Coding Clinic for table Ø8J
2015, 1Q, 35   Attempted removal of foreign body from cornea

AHA Coding Clinic for table Ø8N
2015, 2Q, 24   Penetrating keratoplasty and anterior segment reconstruction

AHA Coding Clinic for table Ø8Q
2018, 3Q, 13   Repair of ruptured globe

AHA Coding Clinic for table Ø8R
2015, 2Q, 24   Penetrating keratoplasty and anterior segment reconstruction
2015, 2Q, 25   Penetrating keratoplasty and placement of viscoelastic eye with paracentesis

AHA Coding Clinic for table Ø8T
2015, 2Q, 12   Orbital exenteration

AHA Coding Clinic for table Ø8U
2014, 3Q, 31   Corneal amniotic membrane transplantation

Eye

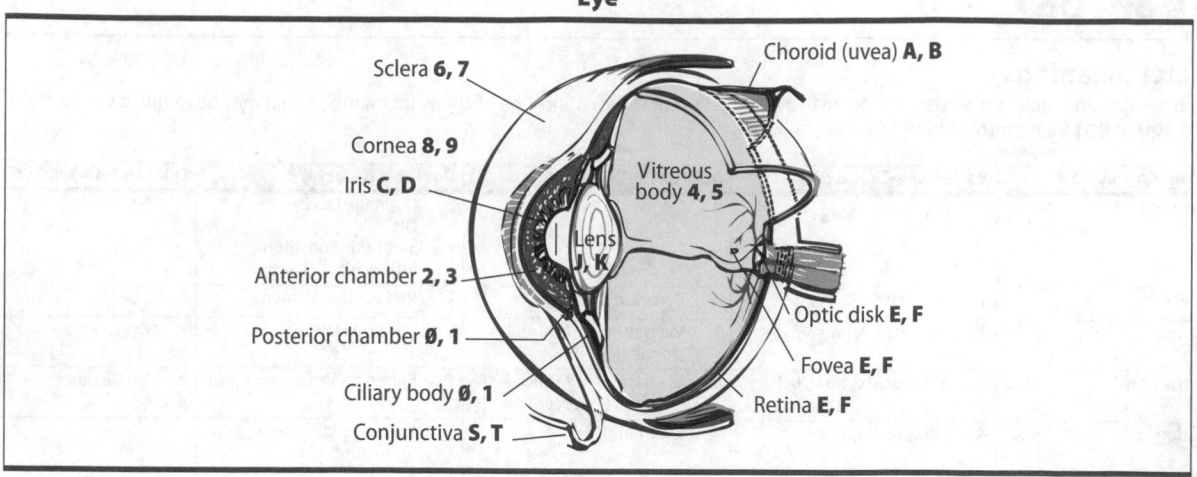

Sclera **6, 7**
Cornea **8, 9**
Iris **C, D**
Lens **J, K**
Anterior chamber **2, 3**
Posterior chamber **Ø, 1**
Ciliary body **Ø, 1**
Conjunctiva **S, T**
Choroid (uvea) **A, B**
Vitreous body **4, 5**
Optic disk **E, F**
Fovea **E, F**
Retina **E, F**

Eye Musculature

Superior rectus
Superior oblique
Lateral rectus
Medial rectus
Inferior oblique
Inferior rectus

Muscles and actions (right eye) **L, M**

Lacrimal System

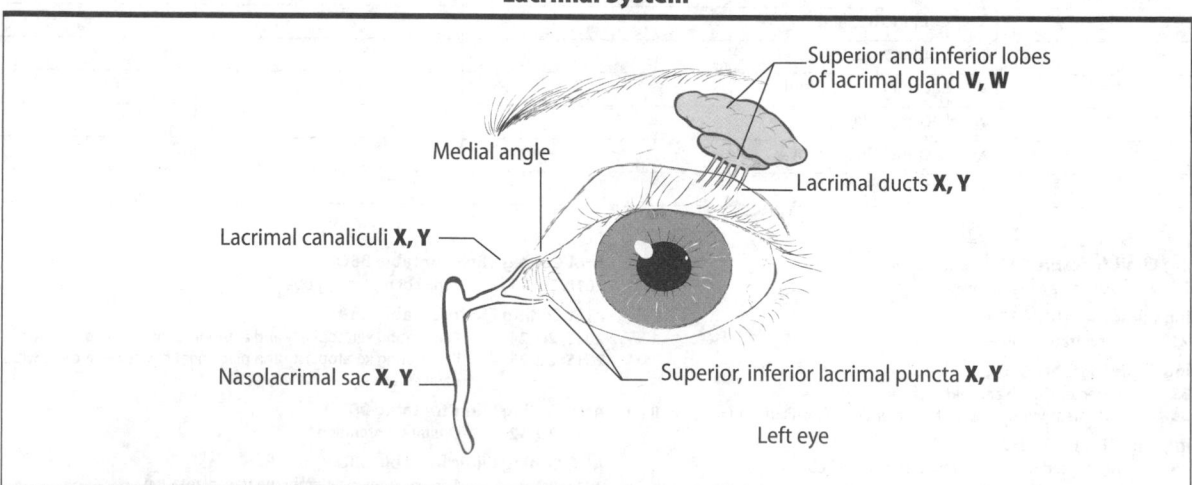

Superior and inferior lobes of lacrimal gland **V, W**
Medial angle
Lacrimal ducts **X, Y**
Lacrimal canaliculi **X, Y**
Nasolacrimal sac **X, Y**
Superior, inferior lacrimal puncta **X, Y**

Left eye

0 Medical and Surgical
8 Eye
0 Alteration

Definition: Modifying the anatomic structure of a body part without affecting the function of the body part

Explanation: Principal purpose is to improve appearance

Body Part Character 4	Approach Character 5	Device Character 6	Qualifier Character 7
N Upper Eyelid, Right Lateral canthus Levator palpebrae superioris muscle Orbicularis oculi muscle Superior tarsal plate P Upper Eyelid, Left *See N Upper Eyelid, Right* Q Lower Eyelid, Right Inferior tarsal plate Medial canthus R Lower Eyelid, Left *See Q Lower Eyelid, Right*	0 Open 3 Percutaneous X External	7 Autologous Tissue Substitute J Synthetic Substitute K Nonautologous Tissue Substitute Z No Device	Z No Qualifier

Non-OR All body part, approach, device, and qualifier values

0 Medical and Surgical
8 Eye
1 Bypass

Definition: Altering the route of passage of the contents of a tubular body part

Explanation: Rerouting contents of a body part to a downstream area of the normal route, to a similar route and body part, or to an abnormal route and dissimilar body part. Includes one or more anastomoses, with or without the use of a device.

Body Part Character 4	Approach Character 5	Device Character 6	Qualifier Character 7
2 Anterior Chamber, Right Aqueous humour 3 Anterior Chamber, Left *See 2 Anterior Chamber, Right*	3 Percutaneous	J Synthetic Substitute K Nonautologous Tissue Substitute Z No Device	4 Sclera
X Lacrimal Duct, Right Lacrimal canaliculus Lacrimal punctum Lacrimal sac Nasolacrimal duct Y Lacrimal Duct, Left *See X Lacrimal Duct, Right*	0 Open 3 Percutaneous	J Synthetic Substitute K Nonautologous Tissue Substitute Z No Device	3 Nasal Cavity

0 Medical and Surgical
8 Eye
2 Change

Definition: Taking out or off a device from a body part and putting back an identical or similar device in or on the same body part without cutting or puncturing the skin or a mucous membrane

Explanation: All CHANGE procedures are coded using the approach EXTERNAL

Body Part Character 4	Approach Character 5	Device Character 6	Qualifier Character 7
0 Eye, Right Ciliary body Posterior chamber 1 Eye, Left *See 0 Eye, Right*	X External	0 Drainage Device Y Other Device	Z No Qualifier

Non-OR All body part, approach, device, and qualifier values

Ø   Medical and Surgical
8   Eye
5   Destruction   Definition: Physical eradication of all or a portion of a body part by the direct use of energy, force, or a destructive agent
                             Explanation: None of the body part is physically taken out

Body Part Character 4		Approach Character 5	Device Character 6	Qualifier Character 7

Ø Eye, Right
    Ciliary body
    Posterior chamber
1 Eye, Left
    See Ø Eye, Right
6 Sclera, Right
7 Sclera, Left
	8 Cornea, Right
	9 Cornea, Left
	S Conjunctiva, Right
	    Plica semilunaris
	T Conjunctiva, Left
	    See S Conjunctiva, Right
		X External	Z No Device	Z No Qualifier

2 Anterior Chamber, Right
    Aqueous humour
3 Anterior Chamber, Left
    See 2 Anterior Chamber, Right
4 Vitreous, Right
    Vitreous body
5 Vitreous, Left
    See 4 Vitreous, Right
C Iris, Right
D Iris, Left
	E Retina, Right
	    Fovea
	    Macula
	    Optic disc
	F Retina, Left
	    See E Retina, Right
	G Retinal Vessel, Right
	H Retinal Vessel, Left
	J Lens, Right
	    Zonule of Zinn
	K Lens, Left
	    See J Lens, Right
		3 Percutaneous	Z No Device	Z No Qualifier

A Choroid, Right
B Choroid, Left
L Extraocular Muscle, Right
    Inferior oblique muscle
    Inferior rectus muscle
    Lateral rectus muscle
    Medial rectus muscle
    Superior oblique muscle
    Superior rectus muscle
	M Extraocular Muscle, Left
	    See L Extraocular Muscle, Right
	V Lacrimal Gland, Right
	W Lacrimal Gland, Left
		Ø Open
		3 Percutaneous
			Z No Device	Z No Qualifier

N Upper Eyelid, Right
    Lateral canthus
    Levator palpebrae superioris
        muscle
    Orbicularis oculi muscle
    Superior tarsal plate
P Upper Eyelid, Left
    See N Upper Eyelid, Right
	Q Lower Eyelid, Right
	    Inferior tarsal plate
	    Medial canthus
	R Lower Eyelid, Left
	    See Q Lower Eyelid, Right
		Ø Open
		3 Percutaneous
		X External
			Z No Device	Z No Qualifier

X Lacrimal Duct, Right
    Lacrimal canaliculus
    Lacrimal punctum
    Lacrimal sac
    Nasolacrimal duct
	Y Lacrimal Duct, Left
	    See X Lacrimal Duct, Right
		Ø Open
		3 Percutaneous
		7 Via Natural or Artificial
		    Opening
		8 Via Natural or Artificial
		    Opening Endoscopic
			Z No Device	Z No Qualifier

Non-OR   Ø85[E,F]3ZZ

Ø   Medical and Surgical
8   Eye
7   Dilation   Definition: Expanding an orifice or the lumen of a tubular body part
                          Explanation: The orifice can be a natural orifice or an artificially created orifice. Accomplished by stretching a tubular body part using intraluminal pressure or by cutting part of the orifice or wall of the tubular body part.

Body Part Character 4	Approach Character 5	Device Character 6	Qualifier Character 7

X Lacrimal Duct, Right
    Lacrimal canaliculus
    Lacrimal punctum
    Lacrimal sac
    Nasolacrimal duct
Y Lacrimal Duct, Left
    See X Lacrimal Duct, Right
	Ø Open
	3 Percutaneous
	7 Via Natural or Artificial
	    Opening
	8 Via Natural or Artificial
	    Opening Endoscopic
		D Intraluminal Device
		Z No Device
			Z No Qualifier

Non-OR Procedure   DRG Non-OR Procedure   Valid OR Procedure   HAC Associated Procedure   Combination Only   New/Revised GREEN

Ø   Medical and Surgical
8   Eye
9   Drainage   Definition: Taking or letting out fluids and/or gases from a body part
               Explanation: The qualifier DIAGNOSTIC is used to identify drainage procedures that are biopsies

Body Part Character 4		Approach Character 5	Device Character 6	Qualifier Character 7

Ø Eye, Right
   Ciliary body
   Posterior chamber
1 Eye, Left
   See Ø Eye, Right
6 Sclera, Right
7 Sclera, Left
	8 Cornea, Right
	9 Cornea, Left
	S Conjunctiva, Right
	   Plica semilunaris
	T Conjunctiva, Left
	   See S Conjunctiva, Right
		X External	Ø Drainage Device	Z No Qualifier

Ø Eye, Right
   Ciliary body
   Posterior chamber
1 Eye, Left
   See Ø Eye, Right
6 Sclera, Right
7 Sclera, Left
	8 Cornea, Right
	9 Cornea, Left
	S Conjunctiva, Right
	   Plica semilunaris
	T Conjunctiva, Left
	   See S Conjunctiva, Right
		X External	Z No Device	X Diagnostic
				Z No Qualifier

2 Anterior Chamber, Right
   Aqueous humour
3 Anterior Chamber, Left
   See 2 Anterior Chamber, Right
4 Vitreous, Right
   Vitreous body
5 Vitreous, Left
   See 4 Vitreous, Right
C Iris, Right
D Iris, Left
	E Retina, Right
	   Fovea
	   Macula
	   Optic disc
	F Retina, Left
	   See E Retina, Right
	G Retinal Vessel, Right
	H Retinal Vessel, Left
	J Lens, Right
	   Zonule of Zinn
	K Lens, Left
	   See J Lens, Right
		3 Percutaneous	Ø Drainage Device	Z No Qualifier

2 Anterior Chamber, Right
   Aqueous humour
3 Anterior Chamber, Left
   See 2 Anterior Chamber, Right
4 Vitreous, Right
   Vitreous body
5 Vitreous, Left
   See 4 Vitreous, Right
C Iris, Right
D Iris, Left
	E Retina, Right
	   Fovea
	   Macula
	   Optic disc
	F Retina, Left
	   See E Retina, Right
	G Retinal Vessel, Right
	H Retinal Vessel, Left
	J Lens, Right
	   Zonule of Zinn
	K Lens, Left
	   See J Lens, Right
		3 Percutaneous	Z No Device	X Diagnostic
				Z No Qualifier

A Choroid, Right
B Choroid, Left
L Extraocular Muscle, Right
   Inferior oblique muscle
   Inferior rectus muscle
   Lateral rectus muscle
   Medial rectus muscle
   Superior oblique muscle
   Superior rectus muscle
	M Extraocular Muscle, Left
	   See L Extraocular Muscle, Right
	V Lacrimal Gland, Right
	W Lacrimal Gland, Left
		Ø Open
		3 Percutaneous
			Ø Drainage Device	Z No Qualifier

A Choroid, Right
B Choroid, Left
L Extraocular Muscle, Right
   Inferior oblique muscle
   Inferior rectus muscle
   Lateral rectus muscle
   Medial rectus muscle
   Superior oblique muscle
   Superior rectus muscle
	M Extraocular Muscle, Left
	   See L Extraocular Muscle, Right
	V Lacrimal Gland, Right
	W Lacrimal Gland, Left
		Ø Open
		3 Percutaneous
			Z No Device	X Diagnostic
				Z No Qualifier

N Upper Eyelid, Right
   Lateral canthus
   Levator palpebrae superioris
     muscle
   Orbicularis oculi muscle
   Superior tarsal plate
P Upper Eyelid, Left
   See N Upper Eyelid, Right
	Q Lower Eyelid, Right
	   Inferior tarsal plate
	   Medial canthus
	R Lower Eyelid, Left
	   See Q Lower Eyelid, Right
		Ø Open
		3 Percutaneous
		X External
			Ø Drainage Device	Z No Qualifier

Non-OR   Ø89[Ø,1,6,7,8,9,S,T]XZ[X,Z]
Non-OR   Ø89[N,P,Q,R][Ø,3,X]ØZ

Ø89 Continued on next page

NC Noncovered Procedure   LC Limited Coverage   QA Questionable OB Admit   NT New Tech Add-on   ⊞ Combination Member   ♂ Male   ♀ Female

0   **Medical and Surgical**   *089 Continued*
8   **Eye**
9   **Drainage**   Definition: Taking or letting out fluids and/or gases from a body part

                           Explanation: The qualifier DIAGNOSTIC is used to identify drainage procedures that are biopsies

Body Part Character 4		Approach Character 5	Device Character 6	Qualifier Character 7

N Upper Eyelid, Right
   Lateral canthus
   Levator palpebrae superioris
      muscle
   Orbicularis oculi muscle
   Superior tarsal plate
P Upper Eyelid, Left
   See N Upper Eyelid, Right
	Q Lower Eyelid, Right
	   Inferior tarsal plate
	   Medial canthus
	R Lower Eyelid, Left
	   See Q Lower Eyelid, Right
		0 Open
		3 Percutaneous
		X External
			Z No Device	**X** Diagnostic
				Z No Qualifier

X Lacrimal Duct, Right
   Lacrimal canaliculus
   Lacrimal punctum
   Lacrimal sac
   Nasolacrimal duct
	Y Lacrimal Duct, Left
	   See X Lacrimal Duct, Right
		0 Open
		3 Percutaneous
		7 Via Natural or Artificial
		   Opening
		8 Via Natural or Artificial
		   Opening Endoscopic
			0 Drainage Device	**Z** No Qualifier

X Lacrimal Duct, Right
   Lacrimal canaliculus
   Lacrimal punctum
   Lacrimal sac
   Nasolacrimal duct
	Y Lacrimal Duct, Left
	   See X Lacrimal Duct, Right
		0 Open
		3 Percutaneous
		7 Via Natural or Artificial
		   Opening
		8 Via Natural or Artificial
		   Opening Endoscopic
			Z No Device	**X** Diagnostic
				Z No Qualifier

Non-OR	089[N,P,Q,R]0ZZ
Non-OR	089[N,P,Q,R][3,X]Z[X,Z]

0   **Medical and Surgical**
8   **Eye**
B   **Excision**   Definition: Cutting out or off, without replacement, a portion of a body part

                           Explanation: The qualifier DIAGNOSTIC is used to identify excision procedures that are biopsies

Body Part Character 4		Approach Character 5	Device Character 6	Qualifier Character 7

0 Eye, Right
   Ciliary body
   Posterior chamber
1 Eye, Left
   See 0 Eye, Right
N Upper Eyelid, Right
   Lateral canthus
   Levator palpebrae superioris
      muscle
   Orbicularis oculi muscle
   Superior tarsal plate
	P Upper Eyelid, Left
	   See N Upper Eyelid, Right
	Q Lower Eyelid, Right
	   Inferior tarsal plate
	   Medial canthus
	R Lower Eyelid, Left
	   See Q Lower Eyelid, Right
		0 Open
		3 Percutaneous
		X External
			Z No Device	**X** Diagnostic
				Z No Qualifier

4 Vitreous, Right
   Vitreous body
5 Vitreous, Left
   See 4 Vitreous, Right
C Iris, Right
D Iris, Left
E Retina, Right
   Fovea
   Macula
   Optic disc
	F Retina, Left
	   See E Retina, Right
	J Lens, Right
	   Zonule of Zinn
	K Lens, Left
	   See J Lens, Right
		3 Percutaneous	**Z** No Device	**X** Diagnostic
				Z No Qualifier

6 Sclera, Right
7 Sclera, Left
8 Cornea, Right
9 Cornea, Left
	S Conjunctiva, Right
	   Plica semilunaris
	T Conjunctiva, Left
	   See S Conjunctiva, Right
		X External	**Z** No Device	**X** Diagnostic
				Z No Qualifier

A Choroid, Right
B Choroid, Left
L Extraocular Muscle, Right
   Inferior oblique muscle
   Inferior rectus muscle
   Lateral rectus muscle
   Medial rectus muscle
   Superior oblique muscle
   Superior rectus muscle
	M Extraocular Muscle, Left
	   See L Extraocular Muscle, Right
	V Lacrimal Gland, Right
	W Lacrimal Gland, Left
		0 Open
		3 Percutaneous
			Z No Device	**X** Diagnostic
				Z No Qualifier

X Lacrimal Duct, Right
   Lacrimal canaliculus
   Lacrimal punctum
   Lacrimal sac
   Nasolacrimal duct
	Y Lacrimal Duct, Left
	   See X Lacrimal Duct, Right
		0 Open
		3 Percutaneous
		7 Via Natural or Artificial
		   Opening
		8 Via Natural or Artificial
		   Opening Endoscopic
			Z No Device	**X** Diagnostic
				Z No Qualifier

Ø   **Medical and Surgical**
8   **Eye**
C   **Extirpation**   Definition: Taking or cutting out solid matter from a body part

            Explanation: The solid matter may be an abnormal byproduct of a biological function or a foreign body; it may be imbedded in a body part or in the lumen of a tubular body part. The solid matter may or may not have been previously broken into pieces.

Body Part Character 4	Approach Character 5	Device Character 6	Qualifier Character 7

Ø Eye, Right
  Ciliary body
  Posterior chamber
1 Eye, Left
  See Ø Eye, Right
6 Sclera, Right
7 Sclera, Left
8 Cornea, Right
9 Cornea, Left
S Conjunctiva, Right
  Plica semilunaris
T Conjunctiva, Left
  See S Conjunctiva, Right
	X External	**Z** No Device	**Z** No Qualifier

2 Anterior Chamber, Right
  Aqueous humour
3 Anterior Chamber, Left
  See 2 Anterior Chamber, Right
4 Vitreous, Right
  Vitreous body
5 Vitreous, Left
  See 4 Vitreous, Right
C Iris, Right
D Iris, Left
E Retina, Right
  Fovea
  Macula
  Optic disc
F Retina, Left
  See E Retina, Right
G Retinal Vessel, Right
H Retinal Vessel, Left
J Lens, Right
  Zonule of Zinn
K Lens, Left
  See J Lens, Right
	3 Percutaneous
	X External
		Z No Device	**Z** No Qualifier

A Choroid, Right
B Choroid, Left
L Extraocular Muscle, Right
  Inferior oblique muscle
  Inferior rectus muscle
  Lateral rectus muscle
  Medial rectus muscle
  Superior oblique muscle
  Superior rectus muscle
M Extraocular Muscle, Left
  See L Extraocular Muscle, Right
N Upper Eyelid, Right
  Lateral canthus
  Levator palpebrae superioris muscle
  Orbicularis oculi muscle
  Superior tarsal plate
P Upper Eyelid, Left
  See N Upper Eyelid, Right
Q Lower Eyelid, Right
  Inferior tarsal plate
  Medial canthus
R Lower Eyelid, Left
  See Q Lower Eyelid, Right
V Lacrimal Gland, Right
W Lacrimal Gland, Left
	Ø Open
	3 Percutaneous
	X External
		Z No Device	**Z** No Qualifier

X Lacrimal Duct, Right
  Lacrimal canaliculus
  Lacrimal punctum
  Lacrimal sac
  Nasolacrimal duct
Y Lacrimal Duct, Left
  See X Lacrimal Duct, Right
	Ø Open
	3 Percutaneous
	7 Via Natural or Artificial Opening
	8 Via Natural or Artificial Opening
	    Endoscopic
		Z No Device	**Z** No Qualifier

Non-OR   Ø8C[Ø,1,6,7,S,T]XZZ
Non-OR   Ø8C[2,3]XZZ
Non-OR   Ø8C[N,P,Q,R][Ø,3,X]ZZ

NC Noncovered Procedure   **LC** Limited Coverage   **QA** Questionable OB Admit   **NT** New Tech Add-on   ⊞ Combination Member   ♂ Male   ♀ Female

ICD-10-PCS 2022   307

Ø8C–Ø8C

0 Medical and Surgical
8 Eye
D Extraction Definition: Pulling or stripping out or off all or a portion of a body part by the use of force

Explanation: The qualifier DIAGNOSTIC is used to identify extraction procedures that are biopsies

Body Part Character 4	Approach Character 5	Device Character 6	Qualifier Character 7
8 Cornea, Right 9 Cornea, Left	X External	Z No Device	X Diagnostic Z No Qualifier

J Lens, Right
   Zonule of Zinn
K Lens, Left
   See J Lens, Right
	3 Percutaneous	Z No Device	Z No Qualifier

0 Medical and Surgical
8 Eye
F Fragmentation Definition: Breaking solid matter in a body part into pieces

Explanation: Physical force (e.g., manual, ultrasonic) applied directly or indirectly is used to break the solid matter into pieces. The solid matter may be an abnormal byproduct of a biological function or a foreign body. The pieces of solid matter are not taken out.

Body Part Character 4	Approach Character 5	Device Character 6	Qualifier Character 7

4 Vitreous, Right   NC
   Vitreous body
5 Vitreous, Left   NC
   See 4 Vitreous, Right
	3 Percutaneous
	X External
		Z No Device	Z No Qualifier

Non-OR 08F[4,5]XZZ
NC 08F[4,5]XZZ

0 Medical and Surgical
8 Eye
H Insertion Definition: Putting in a nonbiological appliance that monitors, assists, performs, or prevents a physiological function but does not physically take the place of a body part

Explanation: None

Body Part Character 4	Approach Character 5	Device Character 6	Qualifier Character 7

0 Eye, Right
   Ciliary body
   Posterior chamber
1 Eye, Left
   See 0 Eye, Right
	0 Open	5 Epiretinal Visual Prosthesis
		Y Other Device
			Z No Qualifier

0 Eye, Right
   Ciliary body
   Posterior chamber
1 Eye, Left
   See 0 Eye, Right
	3 Percutaneous	1 Radioactive Element
		3 Infusion Device
		Y Other Device
			Z No Qualifier

0 Eye, Right
   Ciliary body
   Posterior chamber
1 Eye, Left
   See 0 Eye, Right
	7 Via Natural or Artificial Opening
	8 Via Natural or Artificial Opening Endoscopic
		Y Other Device	Z No Qualifier

0 Eye, Right
   Ciliary body
   Posterior chamber
1 Eye, Left
   See 0 Eye, Right
	X External	1 Radioactive Element
		3 Infusion Device
			Z No Qualifier

Non-OR 08H[0,1]3YZ
Non-OR 08H[0,1][7,8]YZ

Ø   Medical and Surgical
8   Eye
J   Inspection   Definition: Visually and/or manually exploring a body part

                     Explanation: Visual exploration may be performed with or without optical instrumentation. Manual exploration may be performed directly or through intervening body layers.

Body Part Character 4	Approach Character 5	Device Character 6	Qualifier Character 7

Ø   Eye, Right
   Ciliary body
   Posterior chamber
1   Eye, Left
   See Ø Eye, Right
J   Lens, Right
   Zonule of Zinn
K   Lens, Left
   See J Lens, Right
	X External	**Z No Device**	**Z No Qualifier**

L   Extraocular Muscle, Right
   Inferior oblique muscle
   Inferior rectus muscle
   Lateral rectus muscle
   Medial rectus muscle
   Superior oblique muscle
   Superior rectus muscle
M   Extraocular Muscle, Left
   See L Extraocular Muscle, Right
	Ø Open
	X External
		Z No Device	**Z No Qualifier**

Non-OR   Ø8J[Ø,1,J,K]XZZ
Non-OR   Ø8J[L,M]XZZ

Ø   Medical and Surgical
8   Eye
L   Occlusion   Definition: Completely closing an orifice or the lumen of a tubular body part

                 Explanation: The orifice can be a natural orifice or an artificially created orifice

Body Part Character 4	Approach Character 5	Device Character 6	Qualifier Character 7

X   Lacrimal Duct, Right
   Lacrimal canaliculus
   Lacrimal punctum
   Lacrimal sac
   Nasolacrimal duct
Y   Lacrimal Duct, Left
   See X Lacrimal Duct, Right
	Ø Open
	3 Percutaneous
		C Extraluminal Device
		D Intraluminal Device
		Z No Device
			Z No Qualifier

X   Lacrimal Duct, Right
   Lacrimal canaliculus
   Lacrimal punctum
   Lacrimal sac
   Nasolacrimal duct
Y   Lacrimal Duct, Left
   See X Lacrimal Duct, Right
	7 Via Natural or Artificial Opening
	8 Via Natural or Artificial Opening Endoscopic
		D Intraluminal Device
		Z No Device
			Z No Qualifier

Ø   Medical and Surgical
8   Eye
M   Reattachment   Definition: Putting back in or on all or a portion of a separated body part to its normal location or other suitable location

                    Explanation: Vascular circulation and nervous pathways may or may not be reestablished

Body Part Character 4	Approach Character 5	Device Character 6	Qualifier Character 7

N   Upper Eyelid, Right
   Lateral canthus
   Levator palpebrae superioris muscle
   Orbicularis oculi muscle
   Superior tarsal plate
P   Upper Eyelid, Left
   See N Upper Eyelid, Right
Q   Lower Eyelid, Right
   Inferior tarsal plate
   Medial canthus
R   Lower Eyelid, Left
   See Q Lower Eyelid, Right
	X External	**Z No Device**	**Z No Qualifier**

NC Noncovered Procedure   **LC** Limited Coverage   **QA** Questionable OB Admit   **NT** New Tech Add-on   ⊞ Combination Member   ♂ Male   ♀ Female

ICD-10-PCS 2022   309

Ø8J–Ø8M

Ø **Medical and Surgical**
8 **Eye**
N **Release**
Definition: Freeing a body part from an abnormal physical constraint by cutting or by the use of force
Explanation: Some of the restraining tissue may be taken out but none of the body part is taken out

Body Part Character 4	Approach Character 5	Device Character 6	Qualifier Character 7

Ø **Eye, Right**
  Ciliary body
  Posterior chamber
1 **Eye, Left**
  See Ø Eye, Right
6 **Sclera, Right**
7 **Sclera, Left**
8 **Cornea, Right**
9 **Cornea, Left**
S **Conjunctiva, Right**
  Plica semilunaris
T **Conjunctiva, Left**
  See S Conjunctiva, Right
	X External	Z No Device	Z No Qualifier

2 **Anterior Chamber, Right**
  Aqueous humour
3 **Anterior Chamber, Left**
  See 2 Anterior Chamber, Right
4 **Vitreous, Right**
  Vitreous body
5 **Vitreous, Left**
  See 4 Vitreous, Right
C **Iris, Right**
D **Iris, Left**
E **Retina, Right**
  Fovea
  Macula
  Optic disc
F **Retina, Left**
  See E Retina, Right
G **Retinal Vessel, Right**
H **Retinal Vessel, Left**
J **Lens, Right**
  Zonule of Zinn
K **Lens, Left**
  See J Lens, Right
	3 Percutaneous	Z No Device	Z No Qualifier

A **Choroid, Right**
B **Choroid, Left**
L **Extraocular Muscle, Right**
  Inferior oblique muscle
  Inferior rectus muscle
  Lateral rectus muscle
  Medial rectus muscle
  Superior oblique muscle
  Superior rectus muscle
M **Extraocular Muscle, Left**
  See L Extraocular Muscle, Right
V **Lacrimal Gland, Right**
W **Lacrimal Gland, Left**
	Ø Open
	3 Percutaneous
		Z No Device	Z No Qualifier

N **Upper Eyelid, Right**
  Lateral canthus
  Levator palpebrae superioris muscle
  Orbicularis oculi muscle
  Superior tarsal plate
P **Upper Eyelid, Left**
  See N Upper Eyelid, Right
Q **Lower Eyelid, Right**
  Inferior tarsal plate
  Medial canthus
R **Lower Eyelid, Left**
  See Q Lower Eyelid, Right
	Ø Open
	3 Percutaneous
	X External
		Z No Device	Z No Qualifier

X **Lacrimal Duct, Right**
  Lacrimal canaliculus
  Lacrimal punctum
  Lacrimal sac
  Nasolacrimal duct
Y **Lacrimal Duct, Left**
  See X Lacrimal Duct, Right
	Ø Open
	3 Percutaneous
	7 Via Natural or Artificial Opening
	8 Via Natural or Artificial Opening Endoscopic
		Z No Device	Z No Qualifier

0   **Medical and Surgical**
8   **Eye**
P   **Removal**   Definition: Taking out or off a device from a body part

Explanation: If a device is taken out and a similar device put in without cutting or puncturing the skin or mucous membrane, the procedure is coded to the root operation CHANGE. Otherwise, the procedure for taking out a device is coded to the root operation REMOVAL.

Body Part Character 4	Approach Character 5	Device Character 6	Qualifier Character 7

0 **Eye, Right**
   Ciliary body
   Posterior chamber
1 **Eye, Left**
   See 0 Eye, Right
	0 Open
	3 Percutaneous
	7 Via Natural or Artificial Opening
	8 Via Natural or Artificial Opening
	    Endoscopic
		0 Drainage Device
		1 Radioactive Element
		3 Infusion Device
		7 Autologous Tissue Substitute
		C Extraluminal Device
		D Intraluminal Device
		J Synthetic Substitute
		K Nonautologous Tissue Substitute
		Y Other Device
			Z No Qualifier

0 **Eye, Right**
   Ciliary body
   Posterior chamber
1 **Eye, Left**
   See 0 Eye, Right
	X External	**0** Drainage Device
		1 Radioactive Element
		3 Infusion Device
		7 Autologous Tissue Substitute
		C Extraluminal Device
		D Intraluminal Device
		J Synthetic Substitute
		K Nonautologous Tissue Substitute
			Z No Qualifier

J **Lens, Right**
   Zonule of Zinn
K **Lens, Left**
   See J Lens, Right
	3 Percutaneous	**J** Synthetic Substitute
		Y Other Device
			Z No Qualifier

L **Extraocular Muscle, Right**
   Inferior oblique muscle
   Inferior rectus muscle
   Lateral rectus muscle
   Medial rectus muscle
   Superior oblique muscle
   Superior rectus muscle
M **Extraocular Muscle, Left**
   See L Extraocular Muscle, Right
	0 Open
	3 Percutaneous
		0 Drainage Device
		7 Autologous Tissue Substitute
		J Synthetic Substitute
		K Nonautologous Tissue Substitute
		Y Other Device
			Z No Qualifier

Non-OR   08P[0,1]3YZ
Non-OR   08P[0,1][7,8][0,3,D,Y]Z
Non-OR   08P[0,1]X[0,1,3,C,D,J]Z
Non-OR   08P[J,K]3YZ
Non-OR   08P[L,M]3YZ

NC Noncovered Procedure   **LC** Limited Coverage   **QA** Questionable OB Admit   **NT** New Tech Add-on   ⊞ Combination Member   ♂ Male   ♀ Female

ICD-10-PCS 2022   311

Ø Medical and Surgical
8 Eye
Q Repair   Definition: Restoring, to the extent possible, a body part to its normal anatomic structure and function
                    Explanation: Used only when the method to accomplish the repair is not one of the other root operations

Body Part Character 4	Approach Character 5	Device Character 6	Qualifier Character 7

Ø Eye, Right
   Ciliary body
   Posterior chamber
1 Eye, Left
   See Ø Eye, Right
6 Sclera, Right
7 Sclera, Left
8 Cornea, Right   NC
9 Cornea, Left   NC
S Conjunctiva, Right
   Plica semilunaris
T Conjunctiva, Left
   See S Conjunctiva, Right
	X External	**Z No Device**	**Z No Qualifier**

2 Anterior Chamber, Right
   Aqueous humour
3 Anterior Chamber, Left
   See 2 Anterior Chamber, Right
4 Vitreous, Right
   Vitreous body
5 Vitreous, Left
   See 4 Vitreous, Right
C Iris, Right
D Iris, Left
E Retina, Right
   Fovea
   Macula
   Optic disc
F Retina, Left
   See E Retina, Right
G Retinal Vessel, Right
H Retinal Vessel, Left
J Lens, Right
   Zonule of Zinn
K Lens, Left
   See J Lens, Right
	3 Percutaneous	**Z No Device**	**Z No Qualifier**

A Choroid, Right
B Choroid, Left
L Extraocular Muscle, Right
   Inferior oblique muscle
   Inferior rectus muscle
   Lateral rectus muscle
   Medial rectus muscle
   Superior oblique muscle
   Superior rectus muscle
M Extraocular Muscle, Left
   See L Extraocular Muscle, Right
V Lacrimal Gland, Right
W Lacrimal Gland, Left
	Ø Open
	3 Percutaneous
		Z No Device	**Z No Qualifier**

N Upper Eyelid, Right
   Lateral canthus
   Levator palpebrae superioris muscle
   Orbicularis oculi muscle
   Superior tarsal plate
P Upper Eyelid, Left
   See N Upper Eyelid, Right
Q Lower Eyelid, Right
   Inferior tarsal plate
   Medial canthus
R Lower Eyelid, Left
   See Q Lower Eyelid, Right
	Ø Open
	3 Percutaneous
	X External
		Z No Device	**Z No Qualifier**

X Lacrimal Duct, Right
   Lacrimal canaliculus
   Lacrimal punctum
   Lacrimal sac
   Nasolacrimal duct
Y Lacrimal Duct, Left
   See X Lacrimal Duct, Right
	Ø Open
	3 Percutaneous
	7 Via Natural or Artificial Opening
	8 Via Natural or Artificial Opening Endoscopic
		Z No Device	**Z No Qualifier**

Non-OR	Ø8Q[N,P,Q,R][Ø,3,X]ZZ
NC	Ø8Q[8,9]XZZ

Ø   Medical and Surgical
8   Eye
R   Replacement   Definition: Putting in or on biological or synthetic material that physically takes the place and/or function of all or a portion of a body part

Explanation: The body part may have been taken out or replaced, or may be taken out, physically eradicated, or rendered nonfunctional during the REPLACEMENT procedure. A REMOVAL procedure is coded for taking out the device used in a previous replacement procedure.

Body Part Character 4	Approach Character 5	Device Character 6	Qualifier Character 7

Ø   Eye, Right
    Ciliary body
    Posterior chamber
1   Eye, Left
    See Ø Eye, Right
A   Choroid, Right
B   Choroid, Left
	Ø Open
	3 Percutaneous
		7 Autologous Tissue Substitute
		J Synthetic Substitute
		K Nonautologous Tissue Substitute
			Z No Qualifier

4   Vitreous, Right
    Vitreous body
5   Vitreous, Left
    See 4 Vitreous, Right
C   Iris, Right
D   Iris, Left
G   Retinal Vessel, Right
H   Retinal Vessel, Left
	3 Percutaneous	7 Autologous Tissue Substitute
		J Synthetic Substitute
		K Nonautologous Tissue Substitute
			Z No Qualifier

6   Sclera, Right
7   Sclera, Left
S   Conjunctiva, Right
    Plica semilunaris
T   Conjunctiva, Left
    See S Conjunctiva, Right
	X External	7 Autologous Tissue Substitute
		J Synthetic Substitute
		K Nonautologous Tissue Substitute
			Z No Qualifier

8 Cornea, Right 9 Cornea, Left	3 Percutaneous X External	7 Autologous Tissue Substitute J Synthetic Substitute K Nonautologous Tissue Substitute	Z No Qualifier

J   Lens, Right
    Zonule of Zinn
K   Lens, Left
    See J Lens, Right
	3 Percutaneous	Ø Synthetic Substitute, Intraocular
		    Telescope
		7 Autologous Tissue Substitute
		J Synthetic Substitute
		K Nonautologous Tissue Substitute
			Z No Qualifier

N   Upper Eyelid, Right
    Lateral canthus
    Levator palpebrae superioris muscle
    Orbicularis oculi muscle
    Superior tarsal plate
P   Upper Eyelid, Left
    See N Upper Eyelid, Right
Q   Lower Eyelid, Right
    Inferior tarsal plate
    Medial canthus
R   Lower Eyelid, Left
    See Q Lower Eyelid, Right
	Ø Open
	3 Percutaneous
	X External
		7 Autologous Tissue Substitute
		J Synthetic Substitute
		K Nonautologous Tissue Substitute
			Z No Qualifier

X   Lacrimal Duct, Right
    Lacrimal canaliculus
    Lacrimal punctum
    Lacrimal sac
    Nasolacrimal duct
Y   Lacrimal Duct, Left
    See X Lacrimal Duct, Right
	Ø Open
	3 Percutaneous
	7 Via Natural or Artificial Opening
	8 Via Natural or Artificial Opening
	    Endoscopic
		7 Autologous Tissue Substitute
		J Synthetic Substitute
		K Nonautologous Tissue Substitute
			Z No Qualifier

NC Noncovered Procedure   LC Limited Coverage   QA Questionable OB Admit   NT New Tech Add-on   ⊞ Combination Member   ♂ Male   ♀ Female

ICD-10-PCS 2022   313

Ø8R–Ø8R

Ø Medical and Surgical
8 Eye
S Reposition

Definition: Moving to its normal location, or other suitable location, all or a portion of a body part

Explanation: The body part is moved to a new location from an abnormal location, or from a normal location where it is not functioning correctly. The body part may or may not be cut out or off to be moved to the new location.

Body Part Character 4	Approach Character 5	Device Character 6	Qualifier Character 7

C Iris, Right
D Iris, Left
G Retinal Vessel, Right
H Retinal Vessel, Left
J Lens, Right
   Zonule of Zinn
K Lens, Left
   See J Lens, Right
	3 Percutaneous	Z No Device	Z No Qualifier

L Extraocular Muscle, Right
   Inferior oblique muscle
   Inferior rectus muscle
   Lateral rectus muscle
   Medial rectus muscle
   Superior oblique muscle
   Superior rectus muscle
M Extraocular Muscle, Left
   See L Extraocular Muscle, Right
V Lacrimal Gland, Right
W Lacrimal Gland, Left
	Ø Open
	3 Percutaneous
		Z No Device	Z No Qualifier

N Upper Eyelid, Right
   Lateral canthus
   Levator palpebrae superioris muscle
   Orbicularis oculi muscle
   Superior tarsal plate
P Upper Eyelid, Left
   See N Upper Eyelid, Right
Q Lower Eyelid, Right
   Inferior tarsal plate
   Medial canthus
R Lower Eyelid, Left
   See Q Lower Eyelid, Right
	Ø Open
	3 Percutaneous
	X External
		Z No Device	Z No Qualifier

X Lacrimal Duct, Right
   Lacrimal canaliculus
   Lacrimal punctum
   Lacrimal sac
   Nasolacrimal duct
Y Lacrimal Duct, Left
   See X Lacrimal Duct, Right
	Ø Open
	3 Percutaneous
	7 Via Natural or Artificial Opening
	8 Via Natural or Artificial Opening
	   Endoscopic
		Z No Device	Z No Qualifier

0   **Medical and Surgical**
8   **Eye**
T   **Resection**   Definition: Cutting out or off, without replacement, all of a body part
                   Explanation: None

Body Part Character 4	Approach Character 5	Device Character 6	Qualifier Character 7

0   **Eye, Right**
    Ciliary body
    Posterior chamber
1   **Eye, Left**
    See 0 Eye, Right
8   **Cornea, Right**
9   **Cornea, Left**
	X External	**Z** No Device	**Z** No Qualifier

4   **Vitreous, Right**
    Vitreous body
5   **Vitreous, Left**
    See 4 Vitreous, Right
C   **Iris, Right**
D   **Iris, Left**
J   **Lens, Right**
    Zonule of Zinn
K   **Lens, Left**
    See J Lens, Right
	3 Percutaneous	**Z** No Device	**Z** No Qualifier

L   **Extraocular Muscle, Right**
    Inferior oblique muscle
    Inferior rectus muscle
    Lateral rectus muscle
    Medial rectus muscle
    Superior oblique muscle
    Superior rectus muscle
M   **Extraocular Muscle, Left**
    See L Extraocular Muscle, Right
V   **Lacrimal Gland, Right**
W   **Lacrimal Gland, Left**
	0 Open
	3 Percutaneous
		Z No Device	**Z** No Qualifier

N   **Upper Eyelid, Right**
    Lateral canthus
    Levator palpebrae superioris muscle
    Orbicularis oculi muscle
    Superior tarsal plate
P   **Upper Eyelid, Left**
    See N Upper Eyelid, Right
Q   **Lower Eyelid, Right**
    Inferior tarsal plate
    Medial canthus
R   **Lower Eyelid, Left**
    See Q Lower Eyelid, Right
	0 Open
	X External
		Z No Device	**Z** No Qualifier

X   **Lacrimal Duct, Right**
    Lacrimal canaliculus
    Lacrimal punctum
    Lacrimal sac
    Nasolacrimal duct
Y   **Lacrimal Duct, Left**
    See X Lacrimal Duct, Right
	0 Open
	3 Percutaneous
	7 Via Natural or Artificial Opening
	8 Via Natural or Artificial Opening Endoscopic
		Z No Device	**Z** No Qualifier

NC Noncovered Procedure   **LC** Limited Coverage   **QA** Questionable OB Admit   **NT** New Tech Add-on   ⊞ Combination Member   ♂ Male   ♀ Female

ICD-10-PCS 2022

315

08T–08T

Ø   Medical and Surgical
8   Eye
U   Supplement

Definition: Putting in or on biological or synthetic material that physically reinforces and/or augments the function of a portion of a body part

Explanation: The biological material is non-living, or is living and from the same individual. The body part may have been previously replaced, and the SUPPLEMENT procedure is performed to physically reinforce and/or augment the function of the replaced body part.

Body Part Character 4	Approach Character 5	Device Character 6	Qualifier Character 7

Ø   **Eye, Right**
   Ciliary body
   Posterior chamber
1   **Eye, Left**
   See Ø Eye, Right
C   **Iris, Right**
D   **Iris, Left**
E   **Retina, Right**
   Fovea
   Macula
   Optic disc
F   **Retina, Left**
   See E Retina, Right
G   **Retinal Vessel, Right**
H   **Retinal Vessel, Left**
L   **Extraocular Muscle, Right**
   Inferior oblique muscle
   Inferior rectus muscle
   Lateral rectus muscle
   Medial rectus muscle
   Superior oblique muscle
   Superior rectus muscle
M   **Extraocular Muscle, Left**
   See L Extraocular Muscle, Right
	Ø Open
	3 Percutaneous
		7 Autologous Tissue Substitute
		J Synthetic Substitute
		K Nonautologous Tissue Substitute
			Z No Qualifier

8   **Cornea, Right**   `NC`
9   **Cornea, Left**   `NC`
N   **Upper Eyelid, Right**
   Lateral canthus
   Levator palpebrae superioris muscle
   Orbicularis oculi muscle
   Superior tarsal plate
P   **Upper Eyelid, Left**
   See N Upper Eyelid, Right
Q   **Lower Eyelid, Right**
   Inferior tarsal plate
   Medial canthus
R   **Lower Eyelid, Left**
   See Q Lower Eyelid, Right
	Ø Open
	3 Percutaneous
	X External
		7 Autologous Tissue Substitute
		J Synthetic Substitute
		K Nonautologous Tissue Substitute
			Z No Qualifier

X   **Lacrimal Duct, Right**
   Lacrimal canaliculus
   Lacrimal punctum
   Lacrimal sac
   Nasolacrimal duct
Y   **Lacrimal Duct, Left**
   See X Lacrimal Duct, Right
	Ø Open
	3 Percutaneous
	7 Via Natural or Artificial Opening
	8 Via Natural or Artificial Opening Endoscopic
		7 Autologous Tissue Substitute
		J Synthetic Substitute
		K Nonautologous Tissue Substitute
			Z No Qualifier

`NC` Ø8U[8,9][Ø,3,X]KZ

Ø   Medical and Surgical
8   Eye
V   Restriction

Definition: Partially closing an orifice or the lumen of a tubular body part

Explanation: The orifice can be a natural orifice or an artificially created orifice

Body Part Character 4	Approach Character 5	Device Character 6	Qualifier Character 7

X   **Lacrimal Duct, Right**
   Lacrimal canaliculus
   Lacrimal punctum
   Lacrimal sac
   Nasolacrimal duct
Y   **Lacrimal Duct, Left**
   See X Lacrimal Duct, Right
	Ø Open
	3 Percutaneous
		C Extraluminal Device
		D Intraluminal Device
		Z No Device
			Z No Qualifier

X   **Lacrimal Duct, Right**
   Lacrimal canaliculus
   Lacrimal punctum
   Lacrimal sac
   Nasolacrimal duct
Y   **Lacrimal Duct, Left**
   See X Lacrimal Duct, Right
	7 Via Natural or Artificial Opening
	8 Via Natural or Artificial Opening Endoscopic
		D Intraluminal Device
		Z No Device
			Z No Qualifier

Ø   Medical and Surgical
8   Eye
W   Revision   Definition: Correcting, to the extent possible, a portion of a malfunctioning device or the position of a displaced device

Explanation: Revision can include correcting a malfunctioning or displaced device by taking out or putting in components of the device such as a screw or pin

Body Part Character 4	Approach Character 5	Device Character 6	Qualifier Character 7

Ø Eye, Right
   Ciliary body
   Posterior chamber
1 Eye, Left
   See Ø Eye, Right
	Ø Open
	3 Percutaneous
	7 Via Natural or Artificial Opening
	8 Via Natural or Artificial Opening Endoscopic
		Ø Drainage Device
		3 Infusion Device
		7 Autologous Tissue Substitute
		C Extraluminal Device
		D Intraluminal Device
		J Synthetic Substitute
		K Nonautologous Tissue Substitute
		Y Other Device
			Z No Qualifier

Ø Eye, Right
   Ciliary body
   Posterior chamber
1 Eye, Left
   See Ø Eye, Right
	X External	**Ø** Drainage Device
		3 Infusion Device
		7 Autologous Tissue Substitute
		C Extraluminal Device
		D Intraluminal Device
		J Synthetic Substitute
		K Nonautologous Tissue Substitute
			Z No Qualifier

J Lens, Right
   Zonule of Zinn
K Lens, Left
   See J Lens, Right
	3 Percutaneous	**J** Synthetic Substitute
		Y Other Device
			Z No Qualifier

J Lens, Right
   Zonule of Zinn
K Lens, Left
   See J Lens, Right
	X External	**J** Synthetic Substitute	**Z** No Qualifier

L Extraocular Muscle, Right
   Inferior oblique muscle
   Inferior rectus muscle
   Lateral rectus muscle
   Medial rectus muscle
   Superior oblique muscle
   Superior rectus muscle
M Extraocular Muscle, Left
   See L Extraocular Muscle, Right
	Ø Open
	3 Percutaneous
		Ø Drainage Device
		7 Autologous Tissue Substitute
		J Synthetic Substitute
		K Nonautologous Tissue Substitute
		Y Other Device
			Z No Qualifier

Non-OR   Ø8W[Ø,1][3,7,8]YZ
Non-OR   Ø8W[Ø,1]X[Ø,3,7,C,D,J,K]Z
Non-OR   Ø8W[J,K]3YZ
Non-OR   Ø8W[J,K]XJZ
Non-OR   Ø8W[L,M]3YZ

Ø   Medical and Surgical
8   Eye
X   Transfer   Definition: Moving, without taking out, all or a portion of a body part to another location to take over the function of all or a portion of a body part

Explanation: The body part transferred remains connected to its vascular and nervous supply

Body Part Character 4	Approach Character 5	Device Character 6	Qualifier Character 7

L Extraocular Muscle, Right
   Inferior oblique muscle
   Inferior rectus muscle
   Lateral rectus muscle
   Medial rectus muscle
   Superior oblique muscle
   Superior rectus muscle
M Extraocular Muscle, Left
   See L Extraocular Muscle, Right
	Ø Open
	3 Percutaneous
		Z No Device	**Z** No Qualifier

NC Noncovered Procedure   **LC** Limited Coverage   **QA** Questionable OB Admit   **NT** New Tech Add-on   ⊞ Combination Member   ♂ Male   ♀ Female

ICD-10-PCS 2022   317

Ear, Nose, Sinus Ø9Ø–Ø9W

Character Meanings*

This Character Meaning table is provided as a guide to assist the user in the identification of character members that may be found in this section of code tables. It **SHOULD NOT** be used to build a PCS code.

Operation–Character 3	Body Part–Character 4	Approach–Character 5	Device–Character 6	Qualifier–Character 7
Ø Alteration	Ø External Ear, Right	Ø Open	Ø Drainage Device	Ø Endolymphatic
1 Bypass	1 External Ear, Left	3 Percutaneous	1 Radioactive Element	X Diagnostic
2 Change	2 External Ear, Bilateral	4 Percutaneous Endoscopic	4 Hearing Device, Bone Conduction	Z No Qualifier
3 Control	3 External Auditory Canal, Right	7 Via Natural or Artificial Opening	5 Hearing Device, Single Channel Cochlear Prosthesis	
5 Destruction	4 External Auditory Canal, Left	8 Via Natural or Artificial Opening Endoscopic	6 Hearing Device, Multiple Channel Cochlear Prosthesis	
7 Dilation	5 Middle Ear, Right	X External	7 Autologous Tissue Substitute	
8 Division	6 Middle Ear, Left		B Intraluminal Device, Airway	
9 Drainage	7 Tympanic Membrane, Right		D Intraluminal Device	
B Excision	8 Tympanic Membrane, Left		J Synthetic Substitute	
C Extirpation	9 Auditory Ossicle, Right		K Nonautologous Tissue Substitute	
D Extraction	A Auditory Ossicle, Left		S Hearing Device	
H Insertion	B Mastoid Sinus, Right		Y Other Device	
J Inspection	C Mastoid Sinus, Left		Z No Device	
M Reattachment	D Inner Ear, Right			
N Release	E Inner Ear, Left			
P Removal	F Eustachian Tube, Right			
Q Repair	G Eustachian Tube, Left			
R Replacement	H Ear, Right			
S Reposition	J Ear, Left			
T Resection	K Nasal Mucosa and Soft Tissue			
U Supplement	L Nasal Turbinate			
W Revision	M Nasal Septum			
	N Nasopharynx			
	P Accessory Sinus			
	Q Maxillary Sinus, Right			
	R Maxillary Sinus, Left			
	S Frontal Sinus, Right			
	T Frontal Sinus, Left			
	U Ethmoid Sinus, Right			
	V Ethmoid Sinus, Left			
	W Sphenoid Sinus, Right			
	X Sphenoid Sinus, Left			
	Y Sinus			

* Includes sinus ducts.

AHA Coding Clinic for table Ø93
2018, 4Q, 38   Control of epistaxis

AHA Coding Clinic for table Ø95
2018, 1Q, 19   Control of epistaxis via silver nitrate cauterization

AHA Coding Clinic for table Ø9H
2020, 4Q, 43-44   Insertion of radioactive element

AHA Coding Clinic for table Ø9Q
2018, 1Q, 19   Control of epistaxis via silver nitrate cauterization
2017, 4Q, 106   Control of bleeding of external naris using suture
2014, 4Q, 20   Control of epistaxis
2014, 3Q, 22   Transsphenoidal removal of pituitary tumor and fat graft placement
2013, 4Q, 114   Balloon sinuplasty

AHA Coding Clinic for table Ø9U
2019, 4Q, 28-29   Sinus supplement

Ear, Nose, Sinus

Ear Anatomy

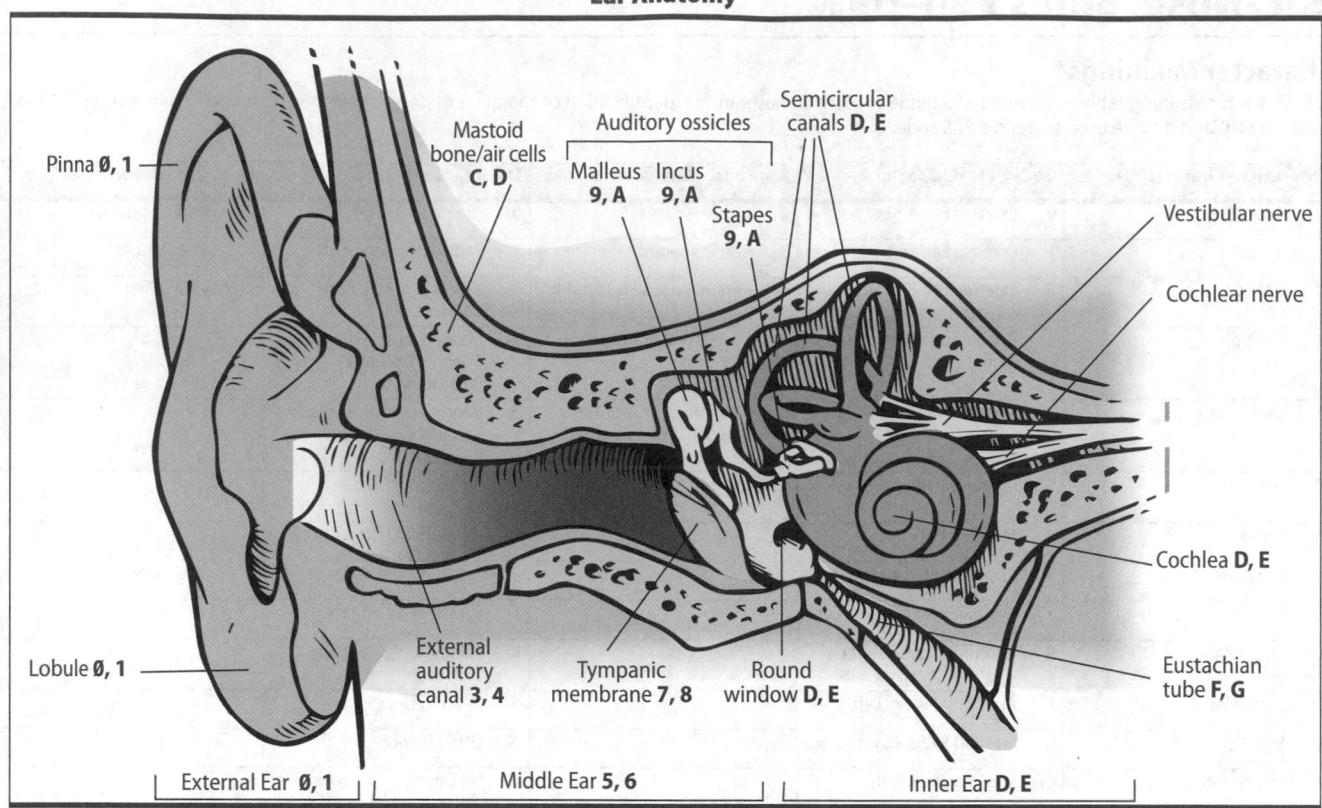

Pinna Ø, 1

Mastoid bone/air cells C, D

Auditory ossicles

Malleus 9, A

Incus 9, A

Stapes 9, A

Semicircular canals D, E

Vestibular nerve

Cochlear nerve

Cochlea D, E

Eustachian tube F, G

Round window D, E

Tympanic membrane 7, 8

External auditory canal 3, 4

Lobule Ø, 1

External Ear Ø, 1

Middle Ear 5, 6

Inner Ear D, E

Nasal Turbinates

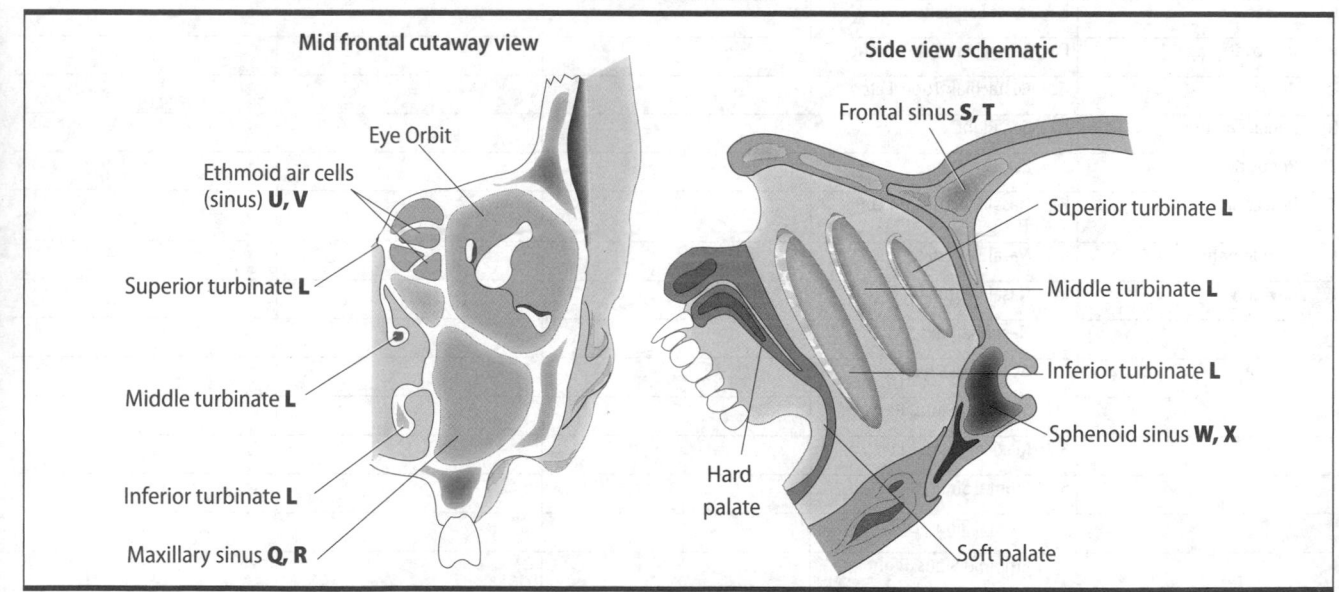

Mid frontal cutaway view

Eye Orbit

Ethmoid air cells (sinus) U, V

Superior turbinate L

Middle turbinate L

Inferior turbinate L

Maxillary sinus Q, R

Side view schematic

Frontal sinus S, T

Superior turbinate L

Middle turbinate L

Inferior turbinate L

Sphenoid sinus W, X

Hard palate

Soft palate

Paranasal Sinuses

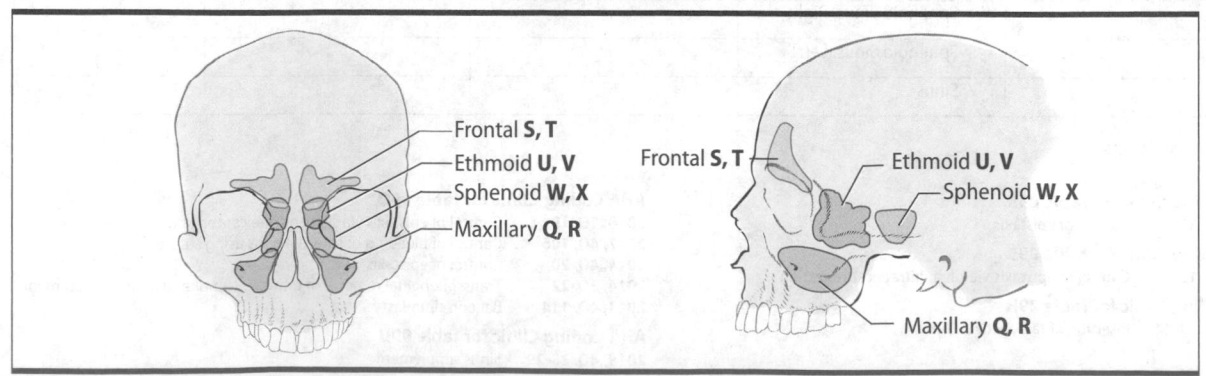

Frontal S, T
Ethmoid U, V
Sphenoid W, X
Maxillary Q, R

Frontal S, T
Ethmoid U, V
Sphenoid W, X
Maxillary Q, R

0 Medical and Surgical
9 Ear, Nose, Sinus
0 Alteration — Definition: Modifying the anatomic structure of a body part without affecting the function of the body part

Explanation: Principal purpose is to improve appearance

Body Part Character 4		Approach Character 5	Device Character 6	Qualifier Character 7

0 External Ear, Right
  Antihelix
  Antitragus
  Auricle
  Earlobe
  Helix
  Pinna
  Tragus
1 External Ear, Left
  See 0 External Ear, Right
	2 External Ear, Bilateral
	  See 0 External Ear, Right
	K Nasal Mucosa and Soft Tissue
	  Columella
	  External naris
	  Greater alar cartilage
	  Internal naris
	  Lateral nasal cartilage
	  Lesser alar cartilage
	  Nasal cavity
	  Nostril
		0 Open
		3 Percutaneous
		4 Percutaneous Endoscopic
		X External
			7 Autologous Tissue Substitute
			J Synthetic Substitute
			K Nonautologous Tissue Substitute
			Z No Device
				Z No Qualifier

0 Medical and Surgical
9 Ear, Nose, Sinus
1 Bypass — Definition: Altering the route of passage of the contents of a tubular body part

Explanation: Rerouting contents of a body part to a downstream area of the normal route, to a similar route and body part, or to an abnormal route and dissimilar body part. Includes one or more anastomoses, with or without the use of a device.

Body Part Character 4	Approach Character 5	Device Character 6	Qualifier Character 7

D Inner Ear, Right
  Bony labyrinth
  Bony vestibule
  Cochlea
  Round window
  Semicircular canal
E Inner Ear, Left
  See D Inner Ear, Right
	0 Open	7 Autologous Tissue Substitute
		J Synthetic Substitute
		K Nonautologous Tissue Substitute
		Z No Device
			0 Endolymphatic

0 Medical and Surgical
9 Ear, Nose, Sinus
2 Change — Definition: Taking out or off a device from a body part and putting back an identical or similar device in or on the same body part without cutting or puncturing the skin or a mucous membrane

Explanation: All CHANGE procedures are coded using the approach EXTERNAL

Body Part Character 4	Approach Character 5	Device Character 6	Qualifier Character 7

H Ear, Right
J Ear, Left
K Nasal Mucosa and Soft Tissue
  Columella
  External naris
  Greater alar cartilage
  Internal naris
  Lateral nasal cartilage
  Lesser alar cartilage
  Nasal cavity
  Nostril
Y Sinus
	X External	0 Drainage Device
		Y Other Device
			Z No Qualifier

Non-OR   All body part, approach, device, and qualifier values

0 Medical and Surgical
9 Ear, Nose, Sinus
3 Control — Definition: Stopping, or attempting to stop, postprocedural or other acute bleeding

Explanation: None

Body Part Character 4	Approach Character 5	Device Character 6	Qualifier Character 7

K Nasal Mucosa and Soft Tissue
  Columella
  External naris
  Greater alar cartilage
  Internal naris
  Lateral nasal cartilage
  Lesser alar cartilage
  Nasal cavity
  Nostril
	7 Via Natural or Artificial Opening
	8 Via Natural or Artificial Opening Endoscopic
		Z No Device	Z No Qualifier

Non-OR   093K[7,8]ZZ

NC Noncovered Procedure   LC Limited Coverage   QA Questionable OB Admit   NT New Tech Add-on   ⊞ Combination Member   ♂ Male   ♀ Female

Ø   Medical and Surgical
9   Ear, Nose, Sinus
5   Destruction   Definition: Physical eradication of all or a portion of a body part by the direct use of energy, force, or a destructive agent

Explanation: None of the body part is physically taken out

Body Part Character 4		Approach Character 5	Device Character 6	Qualifier Character 7
Ø External Ear, Right Antihelix Antitragus Auricle Earlobe Helix Pinna Tragus	**1 External Ear, Left** *See Ø External Ear, Right*	**Ø** Open **3** Percutaneous **4** Percutaneous Endoscopic **X** External	**Z** No Device	**Z** No Qualifier
3 External Auditory Canal, Right External auditory meatus	**4 External Auditory Canal, Left** *See 3 External Auditory Canal, Right*	**Ø** Open **3** Percutaneous **4** Percutaneous Endoscopic **7** Via Natural or Artificial Opening **8** Via Natural or Artificial Opening Endoscopic **X** External	**Z** No Device	**Z** No Qualifier
5 Middle Ear, Right Oval window Tympanic cavity **6 Middle Ear, Left** *See 5 Middle Ear, Right* **9 Auditory Ossicle, Right** Incus Malleus Stapes **A Auditory Ossicle, Left** *See 9 Auditory Ossicle, Right*	**D Inner Ear, Right** Bony labyrinth Bony vestibule Cochlea Round window Semicircular canal **E Inner Ear, Left** *See D Inner Ear, Right*	**Ø** Open **8** Via Natural or Artificial Opening Endoscopic	**Z** No Device	**Z** No Qualifier
7 Tympanic Membrane, Right Pars flaccida **8 Tympanic Membrane, Left** *See 7 Tympanic Membrane, Right* **F Eustachian Tube, Right** Auditory tube Pharyngotympanic tube **G Eustachian Tube, Left** *See F Eustachian Tube, Right*	**L Nasal Turbinate** Inferior turbinate Middle turbinate Nasal concha Superior turbinate **N Nasopharynx** Choana Fossa of Rosenmuller Pharyngeal recess Rhinopharynx	**Ø** Open **3** Percutaneous **4** Percutaneous Endoscopic **7** Via Natural or Artificial Opening **8** Via Natural or Artificial Opening Endoscopic	**Z** No Device	**Z** No Qualifier
B Mastoid Sinus, Right Mastoid air cells **C Mastoid Sinus, Left** *See B Mastoid Sinus, Right* **M Nasal Septum** Quadrangular cartilage Septal cartilage Vomer bone **P Accessory Sinus** **Q Maxillary Sinus, Right** Antrum of Highmore	**R Maxillary Sinus, Left** *See Q Maxillary Sinus, Right* **S Frontal Sinus, Right** **T Frontal Sinus, Left** **U Ethmoid Sinus, Right** Ethmoidal air cell **V Ethmoid Sinus, Left** *See U Ethmoid Sinus, Right* **W Sphenoid Sinus, Right** **X Sphenoid Sinus, Left**	**Ø** Open **3** Percutaneous **4** Percutaneous Endoscopic **8** Via Natural or Artificial Opening Endoscopic	**Z** No Device	**Z** No Qualifier
K Nasal Mucosa and Soft Tissue Columella External naris Greater alar cartilage Internal naris Lateral nasal cartilage Lesser alar cartilage Nasal cavity Nostril		**Ø** Open **3** Percutaneous **4** Percutaneous Endoscopic **8** Via Natural or Artificial Opening Endoscopic **X** External	**Z** No Device	**Z** No Qualifier

Non-OR	Ø95[Ø,1][Ø,3,4,X]ZZ	
Non-OR	Ø95[3,4][Ø,3,4,7,8,X]ZZ	
Non-OR	Ø95[F,G][Ø,3,4,7,8]ZZ	
Non-OR	Ø95M[Ø,3,4,8]ZZ	
Non-OR	Ø95K[Ø,3,4,8,X]ZZ	

Non-OR Procedure   DRG Non-OR Procedure   Valid OR Procedure   HAC Associated Procedure   Combination Only   New/Revised GREEN

Ø Medical and Surgical
9 Ear, Nose, Sinus
7 Dilation   Definition: Expanding an orifice or the lumen of a tubular body part

Explanation: The orifice can be a natural orifice or an artificially created orifice. Accomplished by stretching a tubular body part using intraluminal pressure or by cutting part of the orifice or wall of the tubular body part.

Body Part Character 4	Approach Character 5	Device Character 6	Qualifier Character 7

F Eustachian Tube, Right
    Auditory tube
    Pharyngotympanic tube
G Eustachian Tube, Left
    See F Eustachian Tube, Right
	Ø Open
	7 Via Natural or Artificial Opening
	8 Via Natural or Artificial Opening
	    Endoscopic
		D Intraluminal Device
		Z No Device
			Z No Qualifier

F Eustachian Tube, Right
    Auditory tube
    Pharyngotympanic tube
G Eustachian Tube, Left
    See F Eustachian Tube, Right
	3 Percutaneous
	4 Percutaneous Endoscopic
		Z No Device	Z No Qualifier

Non-OR   All body part, approach, device, and qualifier values

Ø Medical and Surgical
9 Ear, Nose, Sinus
8 Division   Definition: Cutting into a body part, without draining fluids and/or gases from the body part, in order to separate or transect a body part

Explanation: All or a portion of the body part is separated into two or more portions

Body Part Character 4	Approach Character 5	Device Character 6	Qualifier Character 7

L Nasal Turbinate
    Inferior turbinate
    Middle turbinate
    Nasal concha
    Superior turbinate
	Ø Open
	3 Percutaneous
	4 Percutaneous Endoscopic
	7 Via Natural or Artificial Opening
	8 Via Natural or Artificial Opening
	    Endoscopic
		Z No Device	Z No Qualifier

Ear, Nose, Sinus

Ø　**Medical and Surgical**
9　**Ear, Nose, Sinus**
9　**Drainage**　　　Definition: Taking or letting out fluids and/or gases from a body part

Explanation: The qualifier DIAGNOSTIC is used to identify drainage procedures that are biopsies

Body Part Character 4		Approach Character 5	Device Character 6	Qualifier Character 7
Ø **External Ear, Right** Antihelix Antitragus Auricle Earlobe Helix Pinna Tragus	1 **External Ear, Left** *See Ø External Ear, Right*	Ø Open 3 Percutaneous 4 Percutaneous Endoscopic X External	Ø Drainage Device	Z No Qualifier
Ø **External Ear, Right** Antihelix Antitragus Auricle Earlobe Helix Pinna Tragus	1 **External Ear, Left** *See Ø External Ear, Right*	Ø Open 3 Percutaneous 4 Percutaneous Endoscopic X External	Z No Device	X Diagnostic Z No Qualifier
3 **External Auditory Canal, Right** External auditory meatus 4 **External Auditory Canal, Left** *See 3 External Auditory Canal, Right*	K **Nasal Mucosa and Soft Tissue** Columella External naris Greater alar cartilage Internal naris Lateral nasal cartilage Lesser alar cartilage Nasal cavity Nostril	Ø Open 3 Percutaneous 4 Percutaneous Endoscopic 7 Via Natural or Artificial Opening 8 Via Natural or Artificial Opening Endoscopic X External	Ø Drainage Device	Z No Qualifier
3 **External Auditory Canal, Right** External auditory meatus 4 **External Auditory Canal, Left** *See 3 External Auditory Canal, Right*	K **Nasal Mucosa and Soft Tissue** Columella External naris Greater alar cartilage Internal naris Lateral nasal cartilage Lesser alar cartilage Nasal cavity Nostril	Ø Open 3 Percutaneous 4 Percutaneous Endoscopic 7 Via Natural or Artificial Opening 8 Via Natural or Artificial Opening Endoscopic X External	Z No Device	X Diagnostic Z No Qualifier
5 **Middle Ear, Right** Oval window Tympanic cavity 6 **Middle Ear, Left** *See 5 Middle Ear, Right* 9 **Auditory Ossicle, Right** Incus Malleus Stapes	A **Auditory Ossicle, Left** *See 9 Auditory Ossicle, Right* D **Inner Ear, Right** Bony labyrinth Bony vestibule Cochlea Round window Semicircular canal E **Inner Ear, Left** *See D Inner Ear, Right*	Ø Open 7 Via Natural or Artificial Opening 8 Via Natural or Artificial Opening Endoscopic	Ø Drainage Device	Z No Qualifier
5 **Middle Ear, Right** Oval window Tympanic cavity 6 **Middle Ear, Left** *See 5 Middle Ear, Right* 9 **Auditory Ossicle, Right** Incus Malleus Stapes	A **Auditory Ossicle, Left** *See 9 Auditory Ossicle, Right* D **Inner Ear, Right** Bony labyrinth Bony vestibule Cochlea Round window Semicircular canal E **Inner Ear, Left** *See D Inner Ear, Right*	Ø Open 7 Via Natural or Artificial Opening 8 Via Natural or Artificial Opening Endoscopic	Z No Device	X Diagnostic Z No Qualifier

Non-OR	Ø99[Ø,1][Ø,3,4,X]ØZ
Non-OR	Ø99[Ø,1][Ø,3,4,X]Z[X,Z]
Non-OR	Ø99[3,4,K][Ø,3,4,7,8,X]ØZ
Non-OR	Ø99[3,4,K][Ø,3,4,7,8,X]Z[X,Z]
Non-OR	Ø99[5,6]8ØZ
Non-OR	Ø99[9,A,D,E][7,8]ØZ
Non-OR	Ø99[5,6]ØZZ
Non-OR	Ø99[5,6,9,A,D,E][7,8]Z[X,Z]

Ø99 Continued on next page

Ø Medical and Surgical
9 Ear, Nose, Sinus
9 Drainage

Ø99 Continued

Definition: Taking or letting out fluids and/or gases from a body part
Explanation: The qualifier DIAGNOSTIC is used to identify drainage procedures that are biopsies

Body Part Character 4		Approach Character 5	Device Character 6	Qualifier Character 7
7 Tympanic Membrane, Right 　Pars flaccida 8 Tympanic Membrane, Left 　*See 7 Tympanic Membrane, Right* B Mastoid Sinus, Right 　Mastoid air cells C Mastoid Sinus, Left 　*See B Mastoid Sinus, Right* F Eustachian Tube, Right 　Auditory tube 　Pharyngotympanic tube G Eustachian Tube, Left 　*See F Eustachian Tube, Right* L Nasal Turbinate 　Inferior turbinate 　Middle turbinate 　Nasal concha 　Superior turbinate M Nasal Septum 　Quadrangular cartilage 　Septal cartilage 　Vomer bone	N Nasopharynx 　Choana 　Fossa of Rosenmuller 　Pharyngeal recess 　Rhinopharynx P Accessory Sinus Q Maxillary Sinus, Right 　Antrum of Highmore R Maxillary Sinus, Left 　*See Q Maxillary Sinus, Right* S Frontal Sinus, Right T Frontal Sinus, Left U Ethmoid Sinus, Right 　Ethmoidal air cell V Ethmoid Sinus, Left 　*See U Ethmoid Sinus, Right* W Sphenoid Sinus, Right X Sphenoid Sinus, Left	Ø Open 3 Percutaneous 4 Percutaneous Endoscopic 7 Via Natural or Artificial Opening 8 Via Natural or Artificial Opening Endoscopic	Ø Drainage Device	Z No Qualifier
7 Tympanic Membrane, Right 　Pars flaccida 8 Tympanic Membrane, Left 　*See 7 Tympanic Membrane, Right* B Mastoid Sinus, Right 　Mastoid air cells C Mastoid Sinus, Left 　*See B Mastoid Sinus, Right* F Eustachian Tube, Right 　Auditory tube 　Pharyngotympanic tube G Eustachian Tube, Left 　*See F Eustachian Tube, Right* L Nasal Turbinate 　Inferior turbinate 　Middle turbinate 　Nasal concha 　Superior turbinate M Nasal Septum 　Quadrangular cartilage 　Septal cartilage 　Vomer bone	N Nasopharynx 　Choana 　Fossa of Rosenmuller 　Pharyngeal recess 　Rhinopharynx P Accessory Sinus Q Maxillary Sinus, Right 　Antrum of Highmore R Maxillary Sinus, Left 　*See Q Maxillary Sinus, Right* S Frontal Sinus, Right T Frontal Sinus, Left U Ethmoid Sinus, Right 　Ethmoidal air cell V Ethmoid Sinus, Left 　*See U Ethmoid Sinus, Right* W Sphenoid Sinus, Right X Sphenoid Sinus, Left	Ø Open 3 Percutaneous 4 Percutaneous Endoscopic 7 Via Natural or Artificial Opening 8 Via Natural or Artificial Opening Endoscopic	Z No Device	X Diagnostic Z No Qualifier

Non-OR	Ø99[B,C][3,7,8]ØZ
Non-OR	Ø99[F,G,L,M][Ø,3,4,7,8]ØZ
Non-OR	Ø99N3ØZ
Non-OR	Ø99[P,Q,R,S,T,U,V,W,X][3,4,7,8]ØZ
Non-OR	Ø99[7,8][Ø,3,4,7,8]ZZ
Non-OR	Ø99[7,8][7,8]ZX
Non-OR	Ø99[B,C]3ZZ
Non-OR	Ø99[B,C][7,8]Z[X,Z]
Non-OR	Ø99[F,G][Ø,3,4,7,8]ZZ
Non-OR	Ø99[F,G][7,8]ZX
Non-OR	Ø99[L,M][Ø,3,4,7,8]Z[X,Z]
Non-OR	Ø99N[Ø,3,4,7,8]ZX
Non-OR	Ø99N3ZZ
Non-OR	Ø99[P,Q,R,S,T,U,V,W,X][3,4,7,8]Z[X,Z]

NC Noncovered Procedure　　LC Limited Coverage　　QA Questionable OB Admit　　NT New Tech Add-on　　⊞ Combination Member　　♂ Male　　♀ Female

Ear, Nose, Sinus

Ø   **Medical and Surgical**
9   **Ear, Nose, Sinus**
B   **Excision**   Definition: Cutting out or off, without replacement, a portion of a body part
                          Explanation: The qualifier DIAGNOSTIC is used to identify excision procedures that are biopsies

Body Part Character 4		Approach Character 5	Device Character 6	Qualifier Character 7
Ø **External Ear, Right** Antihelix Antitragus Auricle Earlobe Helix Pinna Tragus	1 **External Ear, Left** *See Ø External Ear, Right*	Ø Open 3 Percutaneous 4 Percutaneous Endoscopic X External	Z No Device	X Diagnostic Z No Qualifier

3 **External Auditory Canal,**
Right
External auditory meatus
	4 **External Auditory Canal, Left**
	*See 3 External Auditory Canal,
	Right*
		Ø Open
		3 Percutaneous
		4 Percutaneous Endoscopic
		7 Via Natural or Artificial
		  Opening
		8 Via Natural or Artificial
		  Opening Endoscopic
		X External
			Z No Device	X Diagnostic
				Z No Qualifier

5 **Middle Ear, Right** Oval window Tympanic cavity 6 **Middle Ear, Left** *See 5 Middle Ear, Right* 9 **Auditory Ossicle, Right** Incus Malleus Stapes	A **Auditory Ossicle, Left** *See 9 Auditory Ossicle, Right* D **Inner Ear, Right** Bony labyrinth Bony vestibule Cochlea Round window Semicircular canal E **Inner Ear, Left** *See D Inner Ear, Right*	Ø Open 8 Via Natural or Artificial Opening Endoscopic	Z No Device	X Diagnostic Z No Qualifier

7 **Tympanic Membrane, Right**
Pars flaccida
8 **Tympanic Membrane, Left**
*See 7 Tympanic Membrane,
Right*
F **Eustachian Tube, Right**
Auditory tube
Pharyngotympanic tube
G **Eustachian Tube, Left**
See F Eustachian Tube, Right
	L **Nasal Turbinate**
	Inferior turbinate
	Middle turbinate
	Nasal concha
	Superior turbinate
	N **Nasopharynx**
	Choana
	Fossa of Rosenmuller
	Pharyngeal recess
	Rhinopharynx
		Ø Open
		3 Percutaneous
		4 Percutaneous Endoscopic
		7 Via Natural or Artificial
		  Opening
		8 Via Natural or Artificial
		  Opening Endoscopic
			Z No Device	X Diagnostic
				Z No Qualifier

B **Mastoid Sinus, Right** Mastoid air cells C **Mastoid Sinus, Left** *See B Mastoid Sinus, Right* M **Nasal Septum** Quadrangular cartilage Septal cartilage Vomer bone P **Accessory Sinus** Q **Maxillary Sinus, Right** Antrum of Highmore	R **Maxillary Sinus, Left** *See Q Maxillary Sinus, Right* S **Frontal Sinus, Right** T **Frontal Sinus, Left** U **Ethmoid Sinus, Right** Ethmoidal air cell V **Ethmoid Sinus, Left** *See U Ethmoid Sinus, Right* W **Sphenoid Sinus, Right** X **Sphenoid Sinus, Left**	Ø Open 3 Percutaneous 4 Percutaneous Endoscopic 8 Via Natural or Artificial Opening Endoscopic	Z No Device	X Diagnostic Z No Qualifier
K **Nasal Mucosa and Soft Tissue** Columella External naris Greater alar cartilage Internal naris Lateral nasal cartilage Lesser alar cartilage Nasal cavity Nostril		Ø Open 3 Percutaneous 4 Percutaneous Endoscopic 8 Via Natural or Artificial Opening Endoscopic X External	Z No Device	X Diagnostic Z No Qualifier

Non-OR   Ø9B[Ø,1][Ø,3,4,X]Z[X,Z]
Non-OR   Ø9B[3,4][Ø,3,4,7,8,X]Z[X,Z]
Non-OR   Ø9B[F,G,L,N][Ø,3,4,7,8]Z[X,Z]
Non-OR   Ø9BM[Ø,3,4,8]ZX
Non-OR   Ø9B[P,Q,R,S,T,U,V,W,X][3,4,8]ZX
Non-OR   Ø9BK8Z[X,Z]

Non-OR Procedure   DRG Non-OR Procedure   Valid OR Procedure   HAC Associated Procedure   Combination Only   New/Revised GREEN

Ø   Medical and Surgical
9   Ear, Nose, Sinus
C   Extirpation   Definition: Taking or cutting out solid matter from a body part

Explanation: The solid matter may be an abnormal byproduct of a biological function or a foreign body; it may be imbedded in a body part or in the lumen of a tubular body part. The solid matter may or may not have been previously broken into pieces.

Body Part Character 4		Approach Character 5	Device Character 6	Qualifier Character 7
Ø External Ear, Right Antihelix Antitragus Auricle Earlobe Helix Pinna Tragus	**1 External Ear, Left** *See Ø External Ear, Right*	**Ø** Open **3** Percutaneous **4** Percutaneous Endoscopic **X** External	**Z** No Device	**Z** No Qualifier
3 External Auditory Canal, Right External auditory meatus	**4 External Auditory Canal, Left** *See 3 External Auditory Canal, Right*	**Ø** Open **3** Percutaneous **4** Percutaneous Endoscopic **7** Via Natural or Artificial Opening **8** Via Natural or Artificial Opening Endoscopic **X** External	**Z** No Device	**Z** No Qualifier
5 Middle Ear, Right Oval window Tympanic cavity **6 Middle Ear, Left** *See 5 Middle Ear, Right* **9 Auditory Ossicle, Right** Incus Malleus Stapes	**A Auditory Ossicle, Left** *See 9 Auditory Ossicle, Right* **D Inner Ear, Right** Bony labyrinth Bony vestibule Cochlea Round window Semicircular canal **E Inner Ear, Left** *See D Inner Ear, Right*	**Ø** Open **8** Via Natural or Artificial Opening Endoscopic	**Z** No Device	**Z** No Qualifier
7 Tympanic Membrane, Right Pars flaccida **8 Tympanic Membrane, Left** *See 7 Tympanic Membrane, Right* **F Eustachian Tube, Right** Auditory tube Pharyngotympanic tube **G Eustachian Tube, Left** *See F Eustachian Tube, Right*	**L Nasal Turbinate** Inferior turbinate Middle turbinate Nasal concha Superior turbinate **N Nasopharynx** Choana Fossa of Rosenmuller Pharyngeal recess Rhinopharynx	**Ø** Open **3** Percutaneous **4** Percutaneous Endoscopic **7** Via Natural or Artificial Opening **8** Via Natural or Artificial Opening Endoscopic	**Z** No Device	**Z** No Qualifier
B Mastoid Sinus, Right Mastoid air cells **C Mastoid Sinus, Left** *See B Mastoid Sinus, Right* **M Nasal Septum** Quadrangular cartilage Septal cartilage Vomer bone **P Accessory Sinus** **Q Maxillary Sinus, Right** Antrum of Highmore	**R Maxillary Sinus, Left** *See Q Maxillary Sinus, Right* **S Frontal Sinus, Right** **T Frontal Sinus, Left** **U Ethmoid Sinus, Right** Ethmoidal air cell **V Ethmoid Sinus, Left** *See U Ethmoid Sinus, Right* **W Sphenoid Sinus, Right** **X Sphenoid Sinus, Left**	**Ø** Open **3** Percutaneous **4** Percutaneous Endoscopic **8** Via Natural or Artificial Opening Endoscopic	**Z** No Device	**Z** No Qualifier
K Nasal Mucosa and Soft Tissue Columella External naris Greater alar cartilage Internal naris Lateral nasal cartilage Lesser alar cartilage Nasal cavity Nostril		**Ø** Open **3** Percutaneous **4** Percutaneous Endoscopic **8** Via Natural or Artificial Opening Endoscopic **X** External	**Z** No Device	**Z** No Qualifier

Non-OR	Ø9C[Ø,1][Ø,3,4,X]ZZ
Non-OR	Ø9C[3,4][Ø,3,4,7,8,X]ZZ
Non-OR	Ø9C[7,8,F,G,L][Ø,3,4,7,8]ZZ
Non-OR	Ø9CM[Ø,3,4,8]ZZ
Non-OR	Ø9CK8ZZ

NC Noncovered Procedure   **LC** Limited Coverage   **QA** Questionable OB Admit   **NT** New Tech Add-on   ⊞ Combination Member   ♂ Male   ♀ Female

ICD-10-PCS 2022   327

Ø   Medical and Surgical
9   Ear, Nose, Sinus
D   Extraction   Definition: Pulling or stripping out or off all or a portion of a body part by the use of force
                  Explanation: The qualifier DIAGNOSTIC is used to identify extraction procedures that are biopsies

Body Part Character 4	Approach Character 5	Device Character 6	Qualifier Character 7
7 Tympanic Membrane, Right Pars flaccida **8 Tympanic Membrane, Left** *See 7 Tympanic Membrane, Right* **L Nasal Turbinate** Inferior turbinate Middle turbinate Nasal concha Superior turbinate	**Ø** Open **3** Percutaneous **4** Percutaneous Endoscopic **7** Via Natural or Artificial Opening **8** Via Natural or Artificial Opening Endoscopic	**Z** No Device	**Z** No Qualifier
9 Auditory Ossicle, Right Incus Malleus Stapes **A Auditory Ossicle, Left** *See 9 Auditory Ossicle, Right*	**Ø** Open	**Z** No Device	**Z** No Qualifier
B Mastoid Sinus, Right Mastoid air cells **C Mastoid Sinus, Left** *See B Mastoid Sinus, Right* **M Nasal Septum** Quadrangular cartilage Septal cartilage Vomer bone **P Accessory Sinus** **Q Maxillary Sinus, Right** Antrum of Highmore **R Maxillary Sinus, Left** *See Q Maxillary Sinus, Right* **S Frontal Sinus, Right** **T Frontal Sinus, Left** **U Ethmoid Sinus, Right** Ethmoidal air cell **V Ethmoid Sinus, Left** *See U Ethmoid Sinus, Right* **W Sphenoid Sinus, Right** **X Sphenoid Sinus, Left**	**Ø** Open **3** Percutaneous **4** Percutaneous Endoscopic	**Z** No Device	**Z** No Qualifier

Ø   Medical and Surgical
9   Ear, Nose, Sinus
H   Insertion   Definition: Putting in a nonbiological appliance that monitors, assists, performs, or prevents a physiological function but does not physically
                take the place of a body part
                Explanation: None

Body Part Character 4	Approach Character 5	Device Character 6	Qualifier Character 7

D Inner Ear, Right
Bony labyrinth
Bony vestibule
Cochlea
Round window
Semicircular canal
E Inner Ear, Left
See D Inner Ear, Right
	Ø Open
	3 Percutaneous
	4 Percutaneous Endoscopic
		1 Radioactive Element
		4 Hearing Device, Bone Conduction
		5 Hearing Device, Single Channel
		    Cochlear Prosthesis
		6 Hearing Device, Multiple Channel
		    Cochlear Prosthesis
		S Hearing Device
			Z No Qualifier

H Ear, Right **J Ear, Left** **K Nasal Mucosa and Soft Tissue** Columella External naris Greater alar cartilage Internal naris Lateral nasal cartilage Lesser alar cartilage Nasal cavity Nostril **Y Sinus**	**Ø** Open **3** Percutaneous **4** Percutaneous Endoscopic **7** Via Natural or Artificial Opening **8** Via Natural or Artificial Opening Endoscopic	**1** Radioactive Element **Y** Other Device	**Z** No Qualifier
N Nasopharynx Choana Fossa of Rosenmuller Pharyngeal recess Rhinopharynx	**7** Via Natural or Artificial Opening **8** Via Natural or Artificial Opening Endoscopic	**1** Radioactive Element **B** Intraluminal Device, Airway	**Z** No Qualifier

Non-OR	Ø9H[H,J,K]Ø1Z	Non-OR	Ø9H[H,J,K,Y][3,4,7,8][1,Y]Z
Non-OR	Ø9HKØYZ	Non-OR	Ø9HN[7,8][1,B]Z

Non-OR Procedure   DRG Non-OR Procedure   Valid OR Procedure   HAC Associated Procedure   Combination Only   New/Revised GREEN

Ø   Medical and Surgical
9   Ear, Nose, Sinus
J   Inspection   Definition: Visually and/or manually exploring a body part

Explanation: Visual exploration may be performed with or without optical instrumentation. Manual exploration may be performed directly or through intervening body layers.

Body Part Character 4	Approach Character 5	Device Character 6	Qualifier Character 7
7 Tympanic Membrane, Right Pars flaccida **8** Tympanic Membrane, Left *See 7 Tympanic Membrane, Right* **H** Ear, Right **J** Ear, Left	**Ø** Open **3** Percutaneous **4** Percutaneous Endoscopic **7** Via Natural or Artificial Opening **8** Via Natural or Artificial Opening Endoscopic **X** External	**Z** No Device	**Z** No Qualifier
D Inner Ear, Right Bony labyrinth Bony vestibule Cochlea Round window Semicircular canal **E** Inner Ear, Left *See D Inner Ear, Right* **K** Nasal Mucosa and Soft Tissue Columella External naris Greater alar cartilage Internal naris Lateral nasal cartilage Lesser alar cartilage Nasal cavity Nostril **Y** Sinus	**Ø** Open **3** Percutaneous **4** Percutaneous Endoscopic **8** Via Natural or Artificial Opening Endoscopic **X** External	**Z** No Device	**Z** No Qualifier

Non-OR	Ø9J[7,8][3,7,8,X]ZZ
Non-OR	Ø9J[H,J][Ø,3,4,7,8,X]ZZ
Non-OR	Ø9J[D,E][3,8,X]ZZ
Non-OR	Ø9J[K,Y][Ø,3,4,8,X]ZZ

Ø   Medical and Surgical
9   Ear, Nose, Sinus
M   Reattachment   Definition: Putting back in or on all or a portion of a separated body part to its normal location or other suitable location

Explanation: Vascular circulation and nervous pathways may or may not be reestablished

Body Part Character 4	Approach Character 5	Device Character 6	Qualifier Character 7
Ø External Ear, Right Antihelix Antitragus Auricle Earlobe Helix Pinna Tragus **1** External Ear, Left *See Ø External Ear, Right* **K** Nasal Mucosa and Soft Tissue Columella External naris Greater alar cartilage Internal naris Lateral nasal cartilage Lesser alar cartilage Nasal cavity Nostril	**X** External	**Z** No Device	**Z** No Qualifier

Ear, Nose, Sinus (side margin)

Ø **Medical and Surgical**
9 **Ear, Nose, Sinus**
N **Release**   Definition: Freeing a body part from an abnormal physical constraint by cutting or by the use of force
            Explanation: Some of the restraining tissue may be taken out but none of the body part is taken out

Body Part Character 4		Approach Character 5	Device Character 6	Qualifier Character 7
Ø **External Ear, Right** Antihelix Antitragus Auricle Earlobe Helix Pinna Tragus	1 **External Ear, Left** *See Ø External Ear, Right*	Ø Open 3 Percutaneous 4 Percutaneous Endoscopic X External	Z No Device	Z No Qualifier
3 **External Auditory Canal, Right** External auditory meatus	4 **External Auditory Canal, Left** *See 3 External Auditory Canal, Right*	Ø Open 3 Percutaneous 4 Percutaneous Endoscopic 7 Via Natural or Artificial Opening 8 Via Natural or Artificial Opening Endoscopic X External	Z No Device	Z No Qualifier
5 **Middle Ear, Right** Oval window Tympanic cavity 6 **Middle Ear, Left** *See 5 Middle Ear, Right* 9 **Auditory Ossicle, Right** Incus Malleus Stapes	A **Auditory Ossicle, Left** *See 9 Auditory Ossicle, Right* D **Inner Ear, Right** Bony labyrinth Bony vestibule Cochlea Round window Semicircular canal E **Inner Ear, Left** *See D Inner Ear, Right*	Ø Open 8 Via Natural or Artificial Opening Endoscopic	Z No Device	Z No Qualifier
7 **Tympanic Membrane, Right** Pars flaccida 8 **Tympanic Membrane, Left** *See 7 Tympanic Membrane, Right* F **Eustachian Tube, Right** Auditory tube Pharyngotympanic tube G **Eustachian Tube, Left** *See F Eustachian Tube, Right*	L **Nasal Turbinate** Inferior turbinate Middle turbinate Nasal concha Superior turbinate N **Nasopharynx** Choana Fossa of Rosenmuller Pharyngeal recess Rhinopharynx	Ø Open 3 Percutaneous 4 Percutaneous Endoscopic 7 Via Natural or Artificial Opening 8 Via Natural or Artificial Opening Endoscopic	Z No Device	Z No Qualifier
B **Mastoid Sinus, Right** Mastoid air cells C **Mastoid Sinus, Left** *See B Mastoid Sinus, Right* M **Nasal Septum** Quadrangular cartilage Septal cartilage Vomer bone P **Accessory Sinus** Q **Maxillary Sinus, Right** Antrum of Highmore	R **Maxillary Sinus, Left** *See Q Maxillary Sinus, Right* S **Frontal Sinus, Right** T **Frontal Sinus, Left** U **Ethmoid Sinus, Right** Ethmoidal air cell V **Ethmoid Sinus, Left** *See U Ethmoid Sinus, Right* W **Sphenoid Sinus, Right** X **Sphenoid Sinus, Left**	Ø Open 3 Percutaneous 4 Percutaneous Endoscopic 8 Via Natural or Artificial Opening Endoscopic	Z No Device	Z No Qualifier
K **Nasal Mucosa and Soft Tissue** Columella External naris Greater alar cartilage Internal naris Lateral nasal cartilage Lesser alar cartilage Nasal cavity Nostril		Ø Open 3 Percutaneous 4 Percutaneous Endoscopic 8 Via Natural or Artificial Opening Endoscopic X External	Z No Device	Z No Qualifier

Non-OR Ø9N[Ø,1]XZZ
Non-OR Ø9N[3,4]XZZ
Non-OR Ø9N[F,G,L][Ø,3,4,7,8]ZZ
Non-OR Ø9NM[Ø,3,4,8]ZZ
Non-OR Ø9NK[Ø,3,4,8,X]ZZ

ICD-10-PCS 2022   Ear, Nose, Sinus   Ø9P–Ø9P

Ear, Nose, Sinus

Ø **Medical and Surgical**
9 **Ear, Nose, Sinus**
P **Removal** Definition: Taking out or off a device from a body part

Explanation: If a device is taken out and a similar device put in without cutting or puncturing the skin or mucous membrane, the procedure is coded to the root operation CHANGE. Otherwise, the procedure for taking out a device is coded to the root operation REMOVAL.

Body Part Character 4	Approach Character 5	Device Character 6	Qualifier Character 7
7 **Tympanic Membrane, Right** Pars flaccida 8 **Tympanic Membrane, Left** *See 7 Tympanic Membrane, Right*	Ø Open 7 Via Natural or Artificial Opening 8 Via Natural or Artificial Opening Endoscopic X External	Ø Drainage Device	Z No Qualifier
D **Inner Ear, Right** Bony labyrinth Bony vestibule Cochlea Round window Semicircular canal E **Inner Ear, Left** *See D Inner Ear, Right*	Ø Open 7 Via Natural or Artificial Opening 8 Via Natural or Artificial Opening Endoscopic	S Hearing Device	Z No Qualifier
H **Ear, Right** J **Ear, Left** K **Nasal Mucosa and Soft Tissue** Columella External naris Greater alar cartilage Internal naris Lateral nasal cartilage Lesser alar cartilage Nasal cavity Nostril	Ø Open 3 Percutaneous 4 Percutaneous Endoscopic 7 Via Natural or Artificial Opening 8 Via Natural or Artificial Opening Endoscopic	Ø Drainage Device 7 Autologous Tissue Substitute D Intraluminal Device J Synthetic Substitute K Nonautologous Tissue Substitute Y Other Device	Z No Qualifier
H **Ear, Right** J **Ear, Left** K **Nasal Mucosa and Soft Tissue** Columella External naris Greater alar cartilage Internal naris Lateral nasal cartilage Lesser alar cartilage Nasal cavity Nostril	X External	Ø Drainage Device 7 Autologous Tissue Substitute D Intraluminal Device J Synthetic Substitute K Nonautologous Tissue Substitute	Z No Qualifier
Y **Sinus**	Ø Open 3 Percutaneous 4 Percutaneous Endoscopic	Ø Drainage Device Y Other Device	Z No Qualifier
Y **Sinus**	7 Via Natural or Artificial Opening 8 Via Natural or Artificial Opening Endoscopic	Y Other Device	Z No Qualifier
Y **Sinus**	X External	Ø Drainage Device	Z No Qualifier

Non-OR	Ø9P[7,8][Ø,7,8,X]ØZ
Non-OR	Ø9P[H,J][3,4][Ø,J,K,Y]Z
Non-OR	Ø9P[H,J][7,8][Ø,D,Y]Z
Non-OR	Ø9PK[Ø,3,4,7,8][Ø,7,D,J,K,Y]Z
Non-OR	Ø9P[H,J]X[Ø,7,D,J,K]Z
Non-OR	Ø9PKX[Ø,7,D,J,K]Z
Non-OR	Ø9PY[3,4]YZ
Non-OR	Ø9PY[7,8]YZ
Non-OR	Ø9PYXØZ

NC Noncovered Procedure **LC** Limited Coverage **QA** Questionable OB Admit **NT** New Tech Add-on ⊞ Combination Member ♂ Male ♀ Female

ICD-10-PCS 2022   **331**

Ø9P–Ø9P

Ear, Nose, Sinus

Ø   **Medical and Surgical**
9   **Ear, Nose, Sinus**
Q   **Repair**

Definition: Restoring, to the extent possible, a body part to its normal anatomic structure and function

Explanation: Used only when the method to accomplish the repair is not one of the other root operations

Body Part Character 4		Approach Character 5	Device Character 6	Qualifier Character 7

Ø   **External Ear, Right**
Antihelix
Antitragus
Auricle
Earlobe
Helix
Pinna
Tragus
	1 **External Ear, Left**
	    See Ø External Ear, Right
	2 **External Ear, Bilateral**
	    See Ø External Ear, Right
		Ø Open
		3 Percutaneous
		4 Percutaneous Endoscopic
		X External
			Z No Device	**Z** No Qualifier

3   **External Auditory Canal, Right**
External auditory meatus
4   **External Auditory Canal, Left**
    See 3 External Auditory Canal, Right
	F **Eustachian Tube, Right**
	Auditory tube
	Pharyngotympanic tube
	G **Eustachian Tube, Left**
	    See F Eustachian Tube, Right
		Ø Open
		3 Percutaneous
		4 Percutaneous Endoscopic
		7 Via Natural or Artificial Opening
		8 Via Natural or Artificial Opening Endoscopic
		X External
			Z No Device	**Z** No Qualifier

5   **Middle Ear, Right**
Oval window
Tympanic cavity
6   **Middle Ear, Left**
    See 5 Middle Ear, Right
9   **Auditory Ossicle, Right**
Incus
Malleus
Stapes
	A **Auditory Ossicle, Left**
	    See 9 Auditory Ossicle, Right
	D **Inner Ear, Right**
	Bony labyrinth
	Bony vestibule
	Cochlea
	Round window
	Semicircular canal
	E **Inner Ear, Left**
	    See D Inner Ear, Right
		Ø Open
		8 Via Natural or Artificial Opening Endoscopic
			Z No Device	**Z** No Qualifier

7 **Tympanic Membrane, Right** Pars flaccida **8** **Tympanic Membrane, Left** *See 7 Tympanic Membrane, Right* **L** **Nasal Turbinate** Inferior turbinate Middle turbinate Nasal concha Superior turbinate	**N** **Nasopharynx** Choana Fossa of Rosenmuller Pharyngeal recess Rhinopharynx	**Ø** Open **3** Percutaneous **4** Percutaneous Endoscopic **7** Via Natural or Artificial Opening **8** Via Natural or Artificial Opening Endoscopic	**Z** No Device	**Z** No Qualifier

B   **Mastoid Sinus, Right**
Mastoid air cells
C   **Mastoid Sinus, Left**
    See B Mastoid Sinus, Right
M   **Nasal Septum**
Quadrangular cartilage
Septal cartilage
Vomer bone
P   **Accessory Sinus**
Q   **Maxillary Sinus, Right**
Antrum of Highmore
	R **Maxillary Sinus, Left**
	    See Q Maxillary Sinus, Right
	S **Frontal Sinus, Right**
	T **Frontal Sinus, Left**
	U **Ethmoid Sinus, Right**
	Ethmoidal air cell
	V **Ethmoid Sinus, Left**
	    See U Ethmoid Sinus, Right
	W **Sphenoid Sinus, Right**
	X **Sphenoid Sinus, Left**
		Ø Open
		3 Percutaneous
		4 Percutaneous Endoscopic
		8 Via Natural or Artificial Opening Endoscopic
			Z No Device	**Z** No Qualifier

K **Nasal Mucosa and Soft Tissue** Columella External naris Greater alar cartilage Internal naris Lateral nasal cartilage Lesser alar cartilage Nasal cavity Nostril		**Ø** Open **3** Percutaneous **4** Percutaneous Endoscopic **8** Via Natural or Artificial Opening Endoscopic **X** External	**Z** No Device	**Z** No Qualifier

Non-OR   Ø9Q[Ø,1,2]XZZ
Non-OR   Ø9Q[3,4]XZZ
Non-OR   Ø9Q[F,G][Ø,3,4,7,8,X]ZZ
Non-OR   Ø9QKXZZ

Ø   **Medical and Surgical**
9   **Ear, Nose, Sinus**
R   **Replacement**   Definition: Putting in or on biological or synthetic material that physically takes the place and/or function of all or a portion of a body part

Explanation: The body part may have been taken out or replaced, or may be taken out, physically eradicated, or rendered nonfunctional during the REPLACEMENT procedure. A REMOVAL procedure is coded for taking out the device used in a previous replacement procedure.

Body Part Character 4	Approach Character 5	Device Character 6	Qualifier Character 7

Ø   **External Ear, Right**
    Antihelix
    Antitragus
    Auricle
    Earlobe
    Helix
    Pinna
    Tragus
1   **External Ear, Left**
    See Ø External Ear, Right
2   **External Ear, Bilateral**
    See Ø External Ear, Right
K   **Nasal Mucosa and Soft Tissue**
    Columella
    External naris
    Greater alar cartilage
    Internal naris
    Lateral nasal cartilage
    Lesser alar cartilage
    Nasal cavity
    Nostril
	Ø Open
	X External
		7 Autologous Tissue Substitute
		J Synthetic Substitute
		K Nonautologous Tissue Substitute
			Z No Qualifier

5   **Middle Ear, Right**
    Oval window
    Tympanic cavity
6   **Middle Ear, Left**
    See 5 Middle Ear, Right
9   **Auditory Ossicle, Right**
    Incus
    Malleus
    Stapes
A   **Auditory Ossicle, Left**
    See 9 Auditory Ossicle, Right
D   **Inner Ear, Right**
    Bony labyrinth
    Bony vestibule
    Cochlea
    Round window
    Semicircular canal
E   **Inner Ear, Left**
    See D Inner Ear, Right
	Ø Open	**7** Autologous Tissue Substitute
		J Synthetic Substitute
		K Nonautologous Tissue Substitute
			Z No Qualifier

7   **Tympanic Membrane, Right**
    Pars flaccida
8   **Tympanic Membrane, Left**
    See 7 Tympanic Membrane, Right
N   **Nasopharynx**
    Choana
    Fossa of Rosenmuller
    Pharyngeal recess
    Rhinopharynx
	Ø Open
	7 Via Natural or Artificial Opening
	8 Via Natural or Artificial Opening Endoscopic
		7 Autologous Tissue Substitute
		J Synthetic Substitute
		K Nonautologous Tissue Substitute
			Z No Qualifier

L   **Nasal Turbinate**
    Inferior turbinate
    Middle turbinate
    Nasal concha
    Superior turbinate
	Ø Open
	3 Percutaneous
	4 Percutaneous Endoscopic
	7 Via Natural or Artificial Opening
	8 Via Natural or Artificial Opening Endoscopic
		7 Autologous Tissue Substitute
		J Synthetic Substitute
		K Nonautologous Tissue Substitute
			Z No Qualifier

M   **Nasal Septum**
    Quadrangular cartilage
    Septal cartilage
    Vomer bone
	Ø Open
	3 Percutaneous
	4 Percutaneous Endoscopic
		7 Autologous Tissue Substitute
		J Synthetic Substitute
		K Nonautologous Tissue Substitute
			Z No Qualifier

Ear, Nose, Sinus

Ø   **Medical and Surgical**
9   **Ear, Nose, Sinus**
S   **Reposition**

Definition: Moving to its normal location, or other suitable location, all or a portion of a body part

Explanation: The body part is moved to a new location from an abnormal location, or from a normal location where it is not functioning correctly. The body part may or may not be cut out or off to be moved to the new location.

Body Part Character 4	Approach Character 5	Device Character 6	Qualifier Character 7
Ø **External Ear, Right** Antihelix Antitragus Auricle Earlobe Helix Pinna Tragus 1 **External Ear, Left** *See Ø External Ear, Right* 2 **External Ear, Bilateral** *See Ø External Ear, Right* K **Nasal Mucosa and Soft Tissue** Columella External naris Greater alar cartilage Internal naris Lateral nasal cartilage Lesser alar cartilage Nasal cavity Nostril	Ø Open 4 Percutaneous Endoscopic X External	Z No Device	Z No Qualifier
7 **Tympanic Membrane, Right** Pars flaccida 8 **Tympanic Membrane, Left** *See 7 Tympanic Membrane, Right* F **Eustachian Tube, Right** Auditory tube Pharyngotympanic tube G **Eustachian Tube, Left** *See F Eustachian Tube, Right* L **Nasal Turbinate** Inferior turbinate Middle turbinate Nasal concha Superior turbinate	Ø Open 4 Percutaneous Endoscopic 7 Via Natural or Artificial Opening 8 Via Natural or Artificial Opening Endoscopic	Z No Device	Z No Qualifier
9 **Auditory Ossicle, Right** Incus Malleus Stapes A **Auditory Ossicle, Left** *See 9 Auditory Ossicle, Right* M **Nasal Septum** Quadrangular cartilage Septal cartilage Vomer bone	Ø Open 4 Percutaneous Endoscopic	Z No Device	Z No Qualifier

Non-OR   Ø9S[F,G][Ø,4,7,8]ZZ

Ø   **Medical and Surgical**
9   **Ear, Nose, Sinus**
T   **Resection**   Definition: Cutting out or off, without replacement, all of a body part
                  Explanation: None

Body Part Character 4		Approach Character 5	Device Character 6	Qualifier Character 7
Ø **External Ear, Right** Antihelix Antitragus Auricle Earlobe Helix Pinna Tragus	**1** **External Ear, Left** *See Ø External Ear, Right*	**Ø** Open **4** Percutaneous Endoscopic **X** External	**Z** No Device	**Z** No Qualifier
5 **Middle Ear, Right** Oval window Tympanic cavity **6** **Middle Ear, Left** *See 5 Middle Ear, Right* **9** **Auditory Ossicle, Right** Incus Malleus Stapes	**A** **Auditory Ossicle, Left** *See 9 Auditory Ossicle, Right* **D** **Inner Ear, Right** Bony labyrinth Bony vestibule Cochlea Round window Semicircular canal **E** **Inner Ear, Left** *See D Inner Ear, Right*	**Ø** Open **8** Via Natural or Artificial Opening Endoscopic	**Z** No Device	**Z** No Qualifier
7 **Tympanic Membrane, Right** Pars flaccida **8** **Tympanic Membrane, Left** *See 7 Tympanic Membrane, Right* **F** **Eustachian Tube, Right** Auditory tube Pharyngotympanic tube **G** **Eustachian Tube, Left** *See F Eustachian Tube, Right*	**L** **Nasal Turbinate** Inferior turbinate Middle turbinate Nasal concha Superior turbinate **N** **Nasopharynx** Choana Fossa of Rosenmuller Pharyngeal recess Rhinopharynx	**Ø** Open **4** Percutaneous Endoscopic **7** Via Natural or Artificial Opening **8** Via Natural or Artificial Opening Endoscopic	**Z** No Device	**Z** No Qualifier
B **Mastoid Sinus, Right** Mastoid air cells **C** **Mastoid Sinus, Left** *See B Mastoid Sinus, Right* **M** **Nasal Septum** Quadrangular cartilage Septal cartilage Vomer bone **P** **Accessory Sinus** **Q** **Maxillary Sinus, Right** Antrum of Highmore	**R** **Maxillary Sinus, Left** *See Q Maxillary Sinus, Right* **S** **Frontal Sinus, Right** **T** **Frontal Sinus, Left** **U** **Ethmoid Sinus, Right** Ethmoidal air cell **V** **Ethmoid Sinus, Left** *See U Ethmoid Sinus, Right* **W** **Sphenoid Sinus, Right** **X** **Sphenoid Sinus, Left**	**Ø** Open **4** Percutaneous Endoscopic **8** Via Natural or Artificial Opening Endoscopic	**Z** No Device	**Z** No Qualifier
K **Nasal Mucosa and Soft Tissue** Columella External naris Greater alar cartilage Internal naris Lateral nasal cartilage Lesser alar cartilage Nasal cavity Nostril		**Ø** Open **4** Percutaneous Endoscopic **8** Via Natural or Artificial Opening Endoscopic **X** External	**Z** No Device	**Z** No Qualifier

Non-OR   Ø9T[F,G][Ø,4,7,8]ZZ

NC Noncovered Procedure   **LC** Limited Coverage   **QA** Questionable OB Admit   **NT** New Tech Add-on   ⊞ Combination Member   ♂ Male   ♀ Female

ICD-10-PCS 2022   **335**

Ear, Nose, Sinus

Ø   **Medical and Surgical**
9   **Ear, Nose, Sinus**
U   **Supplement**

Definition: Putting in or on biological or synthetic material that physically reinforces and/or augments the function of a portion of a body part
Explanation: The biological material is non-living, or is living and from the same individual. The body part may have been previously replaced, and the SUPPLEMENT procedure is performed to physically reinforce and/or augment the function of the replaced body part.

Body Part Character 4		Approach Character 5	Device Character 6	Qualifier Character 7
Ø External Ear, Right Antihelix Antitragus Auricle Earlobe Helix Pinna Tragus	**1 External Ear, Left** *See Ø External Ear, Right* **2 External Ear, Bilateral** *See Ø External Ear, Right*	**Ø** Open **X** External	**7** Autologous Tissue Substitute **J** Synthetic Substitute **K** Nonautologous Tissue Substitute	**Z** No Qualifier
5 Middle Ear, Right Oval window Tympanic cavity **6 Middle Ear, Left** *See 5 Middle Ear, Right* **9 Auditory Ossicle, Right** Incus Malleus Stapes **A Auditory Ossicle, Left** *See 9 Auditory Ossicle, Right*	**D Inner Ear, Right** Bony labyrinth Bony vestibule Cochlea Round window Semicircular canal **E Inner Ear, Left** *See D Inner Ear, Right*	**Ø** Open **8** Via Natural or Artificial Opening Endoscopic	**7** Autologous Tissue Substitute **J** Synthetic Substitute **K** Nonautologous Tissue Substitute	**Z** No Qualifier
7 Tympanic Membrane, Right Pars flaccida **8 Tympanic Membrane, Left** *See 7 Tympanic Membrane, Right*	**N Nasopharynx** Choana Fossa of Rosenmuller Pharyngeal recess Rhinopharynx	**Ø** Open **7** Via Natural or Artificial Opening **8** Via Natural or Artificial Opening Endoscopic	**7** Autologous Tissue Substitute **J** Synthetic Substitute **K** Nonautologous Tissue Substitute	**Z** No Qualifier
B Mastoid Sinus, Right Mastoid air cells **C Mastoid Sinus, Left** *See B Mastoid Sinus, Right* **L Nasal Turbinate** Inferior turbinate Middle turbinate Nasal concha Superior turbinate **P Accessory Sinus** **Q Maxillary Sinus, Right** Antrum of Highmore	**R Maxillary Sinus, Left** *See Q Maxillary Sinus, Right* **S Frontal Sinus, Right** **T Frontal Sinus, Left** **U Ethmoid Sinus, Right** Ethmoidal air cell **V Ethmoid Sinus, Left** *See U Ethmoid Sinus, Right* **W Sphenoid Sinus, Right** **X Sphenoid Sinus, Left**	**Ø** Open **3** Percutaneous **4** Percutaneous Endoscopic **7** Via Natural or Artificial Opening **8** Via Natural or Artificial Opening Endoscopic	**7** Autologous Tissue Substitute **J** Synthetic Substitute **K** Nonautologous Tissue Substitute	**Z** No Qualifier
K Nasal Mucosa and Soft Tissue Columella External naris Greater alar cartilage Internal naris Lateral nasal cartilage Lesser alar cartilage Nasal cavity Nostril		**Ø** Open **8** Via Natural or Artificial Opening Endoscopic **X** External	**7** Autologous Tissue Substitute **J** Synthetic Substitute **K** Nonautologous Tissue Substitute	**Z** No Qualifier
M Nasal Septum Quadrangular cartilage Septal cartilage Vomer bone		**Ø** Open **3** Percutaneous **4** Percutaneous Endoscopic **8** Via Natural or Artificial Opening Endoscopic	**7** Autologous Tissue Substitute **J** Synthetic Substitute **K** Nonautologous Tissue Substitute	**Z** No Qualifier

Ø Medical and Surgical
9 Ear, Nose, Sinus
W Revision   Definition: Correcting, to the extent possible, a portion of a malfunctioning device or the position of a displaced device

Explanation: Revision can include correcting a malfunctioning or displaced device by taking out or putting in components of the device such as a screw or pin

Body Part Character 4	Approach Character 5	Device Character 6	Qualifier Character 7
7 **Tympanic Membrane, Right** Pars flaccida **8** **Tympanic Membrane, Left** *See 7 Tympanic Membrane, Right* **9** **Auditory Ossicle, Right** Incus Malleus Stapes **A** **Auditory Ossicle, Left** *See 9 Auditory Ossicle, Right*	**Ø** Open **7** Via Natural or Artificial Opening **8** Via Natural or Artificial Opening Endoscopic	**7** Autologous Tissue Substitute **J** Synthetic Substitute **K** Nonautologous Tissue Substitute	**Z** No Qualifier
D **Inner Ear, Right** Bony labyrinth Bony vestibule Cochlea Round window Semicircular canal **E** **Inner Ear, Left** *See D Inner Ear, Right*	**Ø** Open **7** Via Natural or Artificial Opening **8** Via Natural or Artificial Opening Endoscopic	**S** Hearing Device	**Z** No Qualifier
H **Ear, Right** **J** **Ear, Left** **K** **Nasal Mucosa and Soft Tissue** Columella External naris Greater alar cartilage Internal naris Lateral nasal cartilage Lesser alar cartilage Nasal cavity Nostril	**Ø** Open **3** Percutaneous **4** Percutaneous Endoscopic **7** Via Natural or Artificial Opening **8** Via Natural or Artificial Opening Endoscopic	**Ø** Drainage Device **7** Autologous Tissue Substitute **D** Intraluminal Device **J** Synthetic Substitute **K** Nonautologous Tissue Substitute **Y** Other Device	**Z** No Qualifier
H **Ear, Right** **J** **Ear, Left** **K** **Nasal Mucosa and Soft Tissue** Columella External naris Greater alar cartilage Internal naris Lateral nasal cartilage Lesser alar cartilage Nasal cavity Nostril	**X** External	**Ø** Drainage Device **7** Autologous Tissue Substitute **D** Intraluminal Device **J** Synthetic Substitute **K** Nonautologous Tissue Substitute	**Z** No Qualifier
Y **Sinus**	**Ø** Open **3** Percutaneous **4** Percutaneous Endoscopic	**Ø** Drainage Device **Y** Other Device	**Z** No Qualifier
Y **Sinus**	**7** Via Natural or Artificial Opening **8** Via Natural or Artificial Opening Endoscopic	**Y** Other Device	**Z** No Qualifier
Y **Sinus**	**X** External	**Ø** Drainage Device	**Z** No Qualifier

Non-OR	Ø9W[H,J][3,4][J,K,Y]Z
Non-OR	Ø9W[H,J][7,8][D,Y]Z
Non-OR	Ø9WK[Ø,3,4,7,8][Ø,7,D,J,K,Y]Z
Non-OR	Ø9W[H,J,K]X[Ø,7,D,J,K]Z
Non-OR	Ø9WY[3,4]YZ
Non-OR	Ø9WY[7,8]YZ
Non-OR	Ø9WYXØZ

Respiratory System 0B1–0BY

Character Meanings

This Character Meaning table is provided as a guide to assist the user in the identification of character members that may be found in this section of code tables. It **SHOULD NOT** be used to build a PCS code.

Operation–Character 3		Body Part–Character 4		Approach–Character 5		Device–Character 6		Qualifier–Character 7	
1	Bypass	0	Tracheobronchial Tree	0	Open	0	Drainage Device	0	Allogeneic
2	Change	1	Trachea	3	Percutaneous	1	Radioactive Element	1	Syngeneic
5	Destruction	2	Carina	4	Percutaneous Endoscopic	2	Monitoring Device	2	Zooplastic
7	Dilation	3	Main Bronchus, Right	7	Via Natural or Artificial Opening	3	Infusion Device	4	Cutaneous
9	Drainage	4	Upper Lobe Bronchus, Right	8	Via Natural or Artificial Opening Endoscopic	7	Autologous Tissue Substitute	6	Esophagus
B	Excision	5	Middle Lobe Bronchus, Right	X	External	C	Extraluminal Device	X	Diagnostic
C	Extirpation	6	Lower Lobe Bronchus, Right			D	Intraluminal Device	Z	No Qualifier
D	Extraction	7	Main Bronchus, Left			E	Intraluminal Device, Endotracheal Airway		
F	Fragmentation	8	Upper Lobe Bronchus, Left			F	Tracheostomy Device		
H	Insertion	9	Lingula Bronchus			G	Intraluminal Device, Endobronchial Valve		
J	Inspection	B	Lower Lobe Bronchus, Left			J	Synthetic Substitute		
L	Occlusion	C	Upper Lung Lobe, Right			K	Nonautologous Tissue Substitute		
M	Reattachment	D	Middle Lung Lobe, Right			M	Diaphragmatic Pacemaker Lead		
N	Release	F	Lower Lung Lobe, Right			Y	Other Device		
P	Removal	G	Upper Lung Lobe, Left			Z	No Device		
Q	Repair	H	Lung Lingula						
R	Replacement	J	Lower Lung Lobe, Left						
S	Reposition	K	Lung, Right						
T	Resection	L	Lung, Left						
U	Supplement	M	Lungs, Bilateral						
V	Restriction	N	Pleura, Right						
W	Revision	P	Pleura, Left						
Y	Transplantation	Q	Pleura						
		T	Diaphragm						

AHA Coding Clinic for table 0B5
2016, 2Q, 17   Photodynamic therapy for treatment of malignant mesothelioma
2015, 2Q, 31   Thoracoscopic talc pleurodesis

AHA Coding Clinic for table 0B7
2020, 3Q, 43   Tracheobronchomalacia with placement of tracheobronchial stent

AHA Coding Clinic for table 0B9
2017, 3Q, 15   Bronchoscopy with suctioning for removal of retained secretions
2017, 1Q, 51   Bronchoalveolar lavage
2016, 1Q, 26   Bronchoalveolar lavage, endobronchial biopsy and transbronchial biopsy
2016, 1Q, 27   Fiberoptic bronchoscopy with brushings and bronchoalveolar lavage

AHA Coding Clinic for table 0BB
2016, 1Q, 26   Bronchoalveolar lavage, endobronchial biopsy and transbronchial biopsy
2016, 1Q, 27   Fiberoptic bronchoscopy with brushings and bronchoalveolar lavage
2014, 1Q, 20   Fiducial marker placement

AHA Coding Clinic for table 0BC
2017, 3Q, 14   Bronchoscopy with suctioning and washings for removal of mucus plug

AHA Coding Clinic for table 0BD
2020, 3Q, 40   Transbronchial cryobiopsy of upper, middle and lower lobes of lung
2018, 3Q, 28   Lung decortication for empyema

AHA Coding Clinic for table 0BH
2019, 3Q, 33   Insertion of endobronchial valve
2014, 4Q, 3-10   Mechanical ventilation

AHA Coding Clinic for table 0BJ
2015, 2Q, 31   Thoracoscopic talc pleurodesis
2014, 1Q, 20   Fiducial marker placement

AHA Coding Clinic for table 0BL
2019, 3Q, 33   Insertion of endobronchial valve

AHA Coding Clinic for table 0BN
2019, 2Q, 20   Pericardiectomy for constrictive pericarditis
2018, 3Q, 28   Lung decortication
2018, 3Q, 28   Lung decortication for empyema
2015, 3Q, 15   Vascular ring surgery with release of esophagus and trachea

AHA Coding Clinic for table 0BQ
2020, 3Q, 41   Plication of diaphragm
2016, 2Q, 22   Esophageal lengthening Collis gastroplasty with Nissen fundoplication and hiatal hernia
2014, 3Q, 28   Laparoscopic Nissen fundoplication and diaphragmatic hernia repair

AHA Coding Clinic for table 0BU
2020, 3Q, 43   Tracheobronchomalacia with placement of tracheobronchial stent
2015, 1Q, 28   Repair of bronchopleural fistula using omental pedicle graft

AHA Coding Clinic for table 0BV
2020, 3Q, 41   Plication of diaphragm

Respiratory System

Trachea **1**

Right lung **K**

Right main/
primary
bronchus **3**

Diaphragm **T**

Pleura **N, P, Q**

Left lung **L**

Carina of trachea **2**

Left main/
primary
bronchus **7**

Right Lung Bronchi

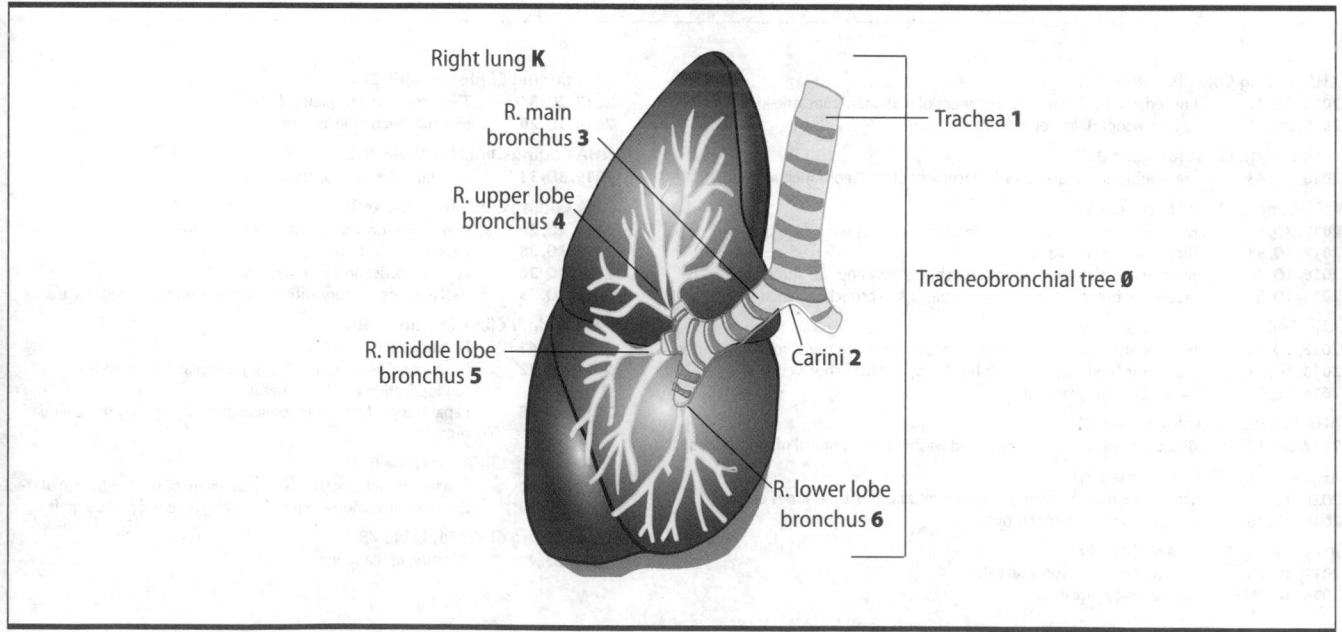

Right lung **K**

R. main
bronchus **3**

R. upper lobe
bronchus **4**

R. middle lobe
bronchus **5**

Trachea **1**

Tracheobronchial tree **Ø**

Carini **2**

R. lower lobe
bronchus **6**

0   **Medical and Surgical**
B   **Respiratory System**
1   **Bypass**   Definition: Altering the route of passage of the contents of a tubular body part

                   Explanation: Rerouting contents of a body part to a downstream area of the normal route, to a similar route and body part, or to an abnormal route and dissimilar body part. Includes one or more anastomoses, with or without the use of a device.

Body Part Character 4	Approach Character 5	Device Character 6	Qualifier Character 7
1 Trachea Cricoid cartilage	**0** Open	**D** Intraluminal Device	**6** Esophagus
1 Trachea Cricoid cartilage	**0** Open	**F** Tracheostomy Device **Z** No Device	**4** Cutaneous
1 Trachea Cricoid cartilage	**3** Percutaneous **4** Percutaneous Endoscopic	**F** Tracheostomy Device **Z** No Device	**4** Cutaneous

DRG Non-OR	0B113[F,Z]4
Non-OR	0B110D6

0   **Medical and Surgical**
B   **Respiratory System**
2   **Change**   Definition: Taking out or off a device from a body part and putting back an identical or similar device in or on the same body part without cutting or puncturing the skin or a mucous membrane

                   Explanation: All CHANGE procedures are coded using the approach EXTERNAL

Body Part Character 4	Approach Character 5	Device Character 6	Qualifier Character 7
0 Tracheobronchial Tree **K** Lung, Right **L** Lung, Left **Q** Pleura **T** Diaphragm	**X** External	**0** Drainage Device **Y** Other Device	**Z** No Qualifier
1 Trachea Cricoid cartilage	**X** External	**0** Drainage Device **E** Intraluminal Device, Endotracheal Airway **F** Tracheostomy Device **Y** Other Device	**Z** No Qualifier

Non-OR	All body part, approach, device, and qualifier values

0   **Medical and Surgical**
B   **Respiratory System**
5   **Destruction**   Definition: Physical eradication of all or a portion of a body part by the direct use of energy, force, or a destructive agent

                   Explanation: None of the body part is physically taken out

Body Part Character 4	Approach Character 5	Device Character 6	Qualifier Character 7

1 Trachea
    Cricoid cartilage
2 Carina
3 Main Bronchus, Right
    Bronchus intermedius
    Intermediate bronchus
4 Upper Lobe Bronchus, Right
5 Middle Lobe Bronchus, Right
6 Lower Lobe Bronchus, Right
7 Main Bronchus, Left
8 Upper Lobe Bronchus, Left
9 Lingula Bronchus
B Lower Lobe Bronchus, Left
C Upper Lung Lobe, Right
D Middle Lung Lobe, Right
F Lower Lung Lobe, Right
G Upper Lung Lobe, Left
H Lung Lingula
J Lower Lung Lobe, Left
K Lung, Right
L Lung, Left
M Lungs, Bilateral
	0 Open
	3 Percutaneous
	4 Percutaneous Endoscopic
	7 Via Natural or Artificial Opening
	8 Via Natural or Artificial Opening Endoscopic
		Z No Device	**Z** No Qualifier

N Pleura, Right **P** Pleura, Left **T** Diaphragm	**0** Open **3** Percutaneous **4** Percutaneous Endoscopic	**Z** No Device	**Z** No Qualifier

Non-OR	0B5[3,4,5,6,7,8,9,B][4,8]ZZ
Non-OR	0B5[C,D,F,G,H,J,K,L,M]8ZZ

0B1–0B5

NC Noncovered Procedure   **LC** Limited Coverage   **QA** Questionable OB Admit   **NT** New Tech Add-on   ⊞ Combination Member   ♂ Male   ♀ Female

ICD-10-PCS 2022   341

Respiratory System

Ø Medical and Surgical
B Respiratory System
7 Dilation   Definition: Expanding an orifice or the lumen of a tubular body part

Explanation: The orifice can be a natural orifice or an artificially created orifice. Accomplished by stretching a tubular body part using intraluminal pressure or by cutting part of the orifice or wall of the tubular body part.

Body Part — Character 4	Approach — Character 5	Device — Character 6	Qualifier — Character 7

1 Trachea
  Cricoid cartilage
2 Carina
3 Main Bronchus, Right
  Bronchus intermedius
  Intermediate bronchus
4 Upper Lobe Bronchus, Right
5 Middle Lobe Bronchus, Right
6 Lower Lobe Bronchus, Right
7 Main Bronchus, Left
8 Upper Lobe Bronchus, Left
9 Lingula Bronchus
B Lower Lobe Bronchus, Left
	Ø Open
	3 Percutaneous
	4 Percutaneous Endoscopic
	7 Via Natural or Artificial Opening
	8 Via Natural or Artificial Opening Endoscopic
		D Intraluminal Device
		Z No Device
			Z No Qualifier

Non-OR ØB7[3,4,5,6,7,8,9,B][Ø,3,4,7,8][D,Z]Z

Ø Medical and Surgical
B Respiratory System
9 Drainage   Definition: Taking or letting out fluids and/or gases from a body part

Explanation: The qualifier DIAGNOSTIC is used to identify drainage procedures that are biopsies

Body Part — Character 4	Approach — Character 5	Device — Character 6	Qualifier — Character 7
1 Trachea, Cricoid cartilage 2 Carina 3 Main Bronchus, Right, Bronchus intermedius, Intermediate bronchus 4 Upper Lobe Bronchus, Right 5 Middle Lobe Bronchus, Right 6 Lower Lobe Bronchus, Right 7 Main Bronchus, Left 8 Upper Lobe Bronchus, Left 9 Lingula Bronchus B Lower Lobe Bronchus, Left C Upper Lung Lobe, Right D Middle Lung Lobe, Right F Lower Lung Lobe, Right G Upper Lung Lobe, Left H Lung Lingula J Lower Lung Lobe, Left K Lung, Right L Lung, Left M Lungs, Bilateral	Ø Open 3 Percutaneous 4 Percutaneous Endoscopic 7 Via Natural or Artificial Opening 8 Via Natural or Artificial Opening Endoscopic	Ø Drainage Device	Z No Qualifier
1 Trachea, Cricoid cartilage 2 Carina 3 Main Bronchus, Right, Bronchus intermedius, Intermediate bronchus 4 Upper Lobe Bronchus, Right 5 Middle Lobe Bronchus, Right 6 Lower Lobe Bronchus, Right 7 Main Bronchus, Left 8 Upper Lobe Bronchus, Left 9 Lingula Bronchus B Lower Lobe Bronchus, Left C Upper Lung Lobe, Right D Middle Lung Lobe, Right F Lower Lung Lobe, Right G Upper Lung Lobe, Left H Lung Lingula J Lower Lung Lobe, Left K Lung, Right L Lung, Left M Lungs, Bilateral	Ø Open 3 Percutaneous 4 Percutaneous Endoscopic 7 Via Natural or Artificial Opening 8 Via Natural or Artificial Opening Endoscopic	Z No Device	X Diagnostic Z No Qualifier
N Pleura, Right P Pleura, Left	Ø Open 3 Percutaneous 4 Percutaneous Endoscopic 8 Via Natural or Artificial Opening Endoscopic	Ø Drainage Device	Z No Qualifier
N Pleura, Right P Pleura, Left	Ø Open 3 Percutaneous 4 Percutaneous Endoscopic 8 Via Natural or Artificial Opening Endoscopic	Z No Device	X Diagnostic Z No Qualifier
T Diaphragm	Ø Open 3 Percutaneous 4 Percutaneous Endoscopic	Ø Drainage Device	Z No Qualifier
T Diaphragm	Ø Open 3 Percutaneous 4 Percutaneous Endoscopic	Z No Device	X Diagnostic Z No Qualifier

Non-OR ØB9[1,2,3,4,5,6,7,8,9,B][7,8]ØZ
Non-OR ØB9[1,2,3,4,5,6,7,8,9,B][3,4]ZX
Non-OR ØB9[1,2,3,4,5,6,7,8,9,B][7,8]Z[X,Z]
Non-OR ØB9[C,D,F,G,H,J,K,L,M][3,4,7]ZX
Non-OR ØB9[C,D,F,G,H,J,K,L,M]8Z[X,Z]

Non-OR ØB9[N,P][Ø,3,8]ØZ
Non-OR ØB9[N,P][Ø,3,8]Z[X,Z]
Non-OR ØB9[N,P]4ZX
Non-OR ØB9T[3,4]ØZ
Non-OR ØB9T[3,4]Z[X,Z]

Ø **Medical and Surgical**
B **Respiratory System**
B **Excision**   Definition: Cutting out or off, without replacement, a portion of a body part

Explanation: The qualifier DIAGNOSTIC is used to identify excision procedures that are biopsies

Body Part Character 4	Approach Character 5	Device Character 6	Qualifier Character 7

1 Trachea
  Cricoid cartilage
2 Carina
3 Main Bronchus, Right
  Bronchus intermedius
  Intermediate bronchus
4 Upper Lobe Bronchus, Right
5 Middle Lobe Bronchus, Right
6 Lower Lobe Bronchus, Right
7 Main Bronchus, Left
8 Upper Lobe Bronchus, Left
9 Lingula Bronchus
B Lower Lobe Bronchus, Left
C Upper Lung Lobe, Right
D Middle Lung Lobe, Right
F Lower Lung Lobe, Right
G Upper Lung Lobe, Left
H Lung Lingula
J Lower Lung Lobe, Left
K Lung, Right
L Lung, Left
M Lungs, Bilateral
	Ø Open
	3 Percutaneous
	4 Percutaneous Endoscopic
	7 Via Natural or Artificial Opening
	8 Via Natural or Artificial Opening
	  Endoscopic
		Z No Device	X Diagnostic
			Z No Qualifier

N Pleura, Right P Pleura, Left	Ø Open 3 Percutaneous 4 Percutaneous Endoscopic 8 Via Natural or Artificial Opening Endoscopic	Z No Device	X Diagnostic Z No Qualifier
T Diaphragm	Ø Open 3 Percutaneous 4 Percutaneous Endoscopic	Z No Device	X Diagnostic Z No Qualifier

Non-OR ØBB[1,2,3,4,5,6,7,8,9,B][3,4,7,8]ZX
Non-OR ØBB[3,4,5,6,7,8,9,B,M][4,8]ZZ
Non-OR ØBB[C,D,F,G,H,J,K,L,M]3ZX

Non-OR ØBB[C,D,F,G,H,J,K,L]8ZZ
Non-OR ØBB[N,P][Ø,3]ZX

Ø **Medical and Surgical**
B **Respiratory System**
C **Extirpation**   Definition: Taking or cutting out solid matter from a body part

Explanation: The solid matter may be an abnormal byproduct of a biological function or a foreign body; it may be imbedded in a body part or in the lumen of a tubular body part. The solid matter may or may not have been previously broken into pieces.

Body Part Character 4	Approach Character 5	Device Character 6	Qualifier Character 7

1 Trachea
  Cricoid cartilage
2 Carina
3 Main Bronchus, Right
  Bronchus intermedius
  Intermediate bronchus
4 Upper Lobe Bronchus, Right
5 Middle Lobe Bronchus, Right
6 Lower Lobe Bronchus, Right
7 Main Bronchus, Left
8 Upper Lobe Bronchus, Left
9 Lingula Bronchus
B Lower Lobe Bronchus, Left
C Upper Lung Lobe, Right
D Middle Lung Lobe, Right
F Lower Lung Lobe, Right
G Upper Lung Lobe, Left
H Lung Lingula
J Lower Lung Lobe, Left
K Lung, Right
L Lung, Left
M Lungs, Bilateral
	Ø Open
	3 Percutaneous
	4 Percutaneous Endoscopic
	7 Via Natural or Artificial Opening
	8 Via Natural or Artificial Opening
	  Endoscopic
		Z No Device	Z No Qualifier

N Pleura, Right P Pleura, Left T Diaphragm	Ø Open 3 Percutaneous 4 Percutaneous Endoscopic	Z No Device	Z No Qualifier

Non-OR ØBC[1,2,3,4,5,6,7,8,9,B][7,8]ZZ
Non-OR ØBC[N,P]3ZZ

Respiratory System

Ø   **Medical and Surgical**
B   **Respiratory System**
D   **Extraction**   Definition: Pulling or stripping out or off all or a portion of a body part by the use of force
                       Explanation: The qualifier DIAGNOSTIC is used to identify extraction procedures that are biopsies

Body Part Character 4	Approach Character 5	Device Character 6	Qualifier Character 7

1 Trachea
   Cricoid cartilage
2 Carina
3 Main Bronchus, Right
   Bronchus intermedius
   Intermediate bronchus
4 Upper Lobe Bronchus, Right
5 Middle Lobe Bronchus, Right
6 Lower Lobe Bronchus, Right
7 Main Bronchus, Left
8 Upper Lobe Bronchus, Left
9 Lingula Bronchus
B Lower Lobe Bronchus, Left
C Upper Lung Lobe, Right
D Middle Lung Lobe, Right
F Lower Lung Lobe, Right
G Upper Lung Lobe, Left
H Lung Lingula
J Lower Lung Lobe, Left
K Lung, Right
L Lung, Left
M Lungs, Bilateral
	4 Percutaneous Endoscopic
	8 Via Natural or Artificial Opening
	   Endoscopic
		Z No Device	X Diagnostic

N Pleura, Right P Pleura, Left	Ø Open 3 Percutaneous 4 Percutaneous Endoscopic	Z No Device	X Diagnostic Z No Qualifier

Non-OR   ØBD[1,2,3,4,5,6,7,8,9,B,C,D,F,G,H,J,K,L,M][4,8]ZX

Ø   **Medical and Surgical**
B   **Respiratory System**
F   **Fragmentation**   Definition: Breaking solid matter in a body part into pieces
                       Explanation: Physical force (e.g., manual, ultrasonic) applied directly or indirectly is used to break the solid matter into pieces. The solid matter may be an abnormal byproduct of a biological function or a foreign body. The pieces of solid matter are not taken out.

Body Part Character 4	Approach Character 5	Device Character 6	Qualifier Character 7

1 Trachea   **NC**
   Cricoid cartilage
2 Carina   **NC**
3 Main Bronchus, Right   **NC**
   Bronchus intermedius
   Intermediate bronchus
4 Upper Lobe Bronchus, Right   **NC**
5 Middle Lobe Bronchus, Right   **NC**
6 Lower Lobe Bronchus, Right   **NC**
7 Main Bronchus, Left   **NC**
8 Upper Lobe Bronchus, Left   **NC**
9 Lingula Bronchus   **NC**
B Lower Lobe Bronchus, Left   **NC**
	Ø Open
	3 Percutaneous
	4 Percutaneous Endoscopic
	7 Via Natural or Artificial Opening
	8 Via Natural or Artificial Opening
	   Endoscopic
	X External
		Z No Device	Z No Qualifier

Non-OR   ØBF[1,2,3,4,5,6,7,8,9,B]XZZ
Non-OR   ØBF[3,4,5,6,7,8,9,B][7,8]ZZ
NC   ØBF[1,2,3,4,5,6,7,8,9,B]XZZ

Ø　Medical and Surgical
B　Respiratory System
H　Insertion　　　Definition: Putting in a nonbiological appliance that monitors, assists, performs, or prevents a physiological function but does not physically take the place of a body part
　　　　　　　　　　Explanation: None

Body Part Character 4	Approach Character 5	Device Character 6	Qualifier Character 7
Ø Tracheobronchial Tree	**Ø** Open **3** Percutaneous **4** Percutaneous Endoscopic **7** Via Natural or Artificial Opening **8** Via Natural or Artificial Opening Endoscopic	**1** Radioactive Element **2** Monitoring Device **3** Infusion Device **D** Intraluminal Device **Y** Other Device	**Z** No Qualifier
1 Trachea 　　Cricoid cartilage	**Ø** Open	**2** Monitoring Device **D** Intraluminal Device **Y** Other Device	**Z** No Qualifier
1 Trachea 　　Cricoid cartilage	**3** Percutaneous	**D** Intraluminal Device **E** Intraluminal Device, Endotracheal Airway **Y** Other Device	**Z** No Qualifier
1 Trachea 　　Cricoid cartilage	**4** Percutaneous Endoscopic	**D** Intraluminal Device **Y** Other Device	**Z** No Qualifier
1 Trachea 　　Cricoid cartilage	**7** Via Natural or Artificial Opening **8** Via Natural or Artificial Opening Endoscopic	**2** Monitoring Device **D** Intraluminal Device **E** Intraluminal Device, Endotracheal Airway **Y** Other Device	**Z** No Qualifier
3 Main Bronchus, Right 　　Bronchus intermedius 　　Intermediate bronchus **4** Upper Lobe Bronchus, Right **5** Middle Lobe Bronchus, Right **6** Lower Lobe Bronchus, Right **7** Main Bronchus, Left **8** Upper Lobe Bronchus, Left **9** Lingula Bronchus **B** Lower Lobe Bronchus, Left	**Ø** Open **3** Percutaneous **4** Percutaneous Endoscopic **7** Via Natural or Artificial Opening **8** Via Natural or Artificial Opening Endoscopic	**G** Intraluminal Device, Endobronchial Valve	**Z** No Qualifier
K Lung, Right **L** Lung, Left	**Ø** Open **3** Percutaneous **4** Percutaneous Endoscopic **7** Via Natural or Artificial Opening **8** Via Natural or Artificial Opening Endoscopic	**1** Radioactive Element **2** Monitoring Device **3** Infusion Device **Y** Other Device	**Z** No Qualifier
Q Pleura	**Ø** Open **3** Percutaneous **4** Percutaneous Endoscopic **7** Via Natural or Artificial Opening **8** Via Natural or Artificial Opening Endoscopic	**Y** Other Device	**Z** No Qualifier
T Diaphragm	**Ø** Open **3** Percutaneous **4** Percutaneous Endoscopic	**2** Monitoring Device **M** Diaphragmatic Pacemaker Lead **Y** Other Device	**Z** No Qualifier
T Diaphragm	**7** Via Natural or Artificial Opening **8** Via Natural or Artificial Opening Endoscopic	**Y** Other Device	**Z** No Qualifier

DRG Non-OR	ØBH[3,4,5,6,7,8,9,B]8GZ
Non-OR	ØBHØ3YZ
Non-OR	ØBHØ[7,8][2,3,D,Y]Z
Non-OR	ØBH13[E,Y]Z
Non-OR	ØBH1[7,8][2,D,E,Y]Z
Non-OR	ØBH[K,L]3YZ
Non-OR	ØBH[K,L]7[2,3,Y]Z
Non-OR	ØBH[K,L]8[2,3]Z
Non-OR	ØBHQ[3,7]YZ
Non-OR	ØBHT3YZ
Non-OR	ØBHT[7,8]YZ

NC Noncovered Procedure　　**LC** Limited Coverage　　**QA** Questionable OB Admit　　**NT** New Tech Add-on　　⊞ Combination Member　　♂ Male　　♀ Female

ICD-10-PCS 2022　　　　　　　　　　　　　　　　　　　　　　　　　　　　　　　　　　　　　　　345

ØBH–ØBH

Respiratory System

Ø Medical and Surgical
B Respiratory System
J Inspection   Definition: Visually and/or manually exploring a body part

Explanation: Visual exploration may be performed with or without optical instrumentation. Manual exploration may be performed directly or through intervening body layers.

Body Part Character 4	Approach Character 5	Device Character 6	Qualifier Character 7

Ø Tracheobronchial Tree
1 Trachea
   Cricoid cartilage
K Lung, Right
L Lung, Left
Q Pleura
T Diaphragm
	Ø Open
	3 Percutaneous
	4 Percutaneous Endoscopic
	7 Via Natural or Artificial Opening
	8 Via Natural or Artificial Opening
	   Endoscopic
	X External
		Z No Device	Z No Qualifier

Non-OR   ØBJ[Ø,K,L,Q,T][3,7,8,X]ZZ
Non-OR   ØBJ1[3,4,7,8,X]ZZ

Ø Medical and Surgical
B Respiratory System
L Occlusion   Definition: Completely closing an orifice or the lumen of a tubular body part

Explanation: The orifice can be a natural orifice or an artificially created orifice

Body Part Character 4	Approach Character 5	Device Character 6	Qualifier Character 7

1 Trachea
   Cricoid cartilage
2 Carina
3 Main Bronchus, Right
   Bronchus intermedius
   Intermediate bronchus
4 Upper Lobe Bronchus, Right
5 Middle Lobe Bronchus, Right
6 Lower Lobe Bronchus, Right
7 Main Bronchus, Left
8 Upper Lobe Bronchus, Left
9 Lingula Bronchus
B Lower Lobe Bronchus, Left
	Ø Open
	3 Percutaneous
	4 Percutaneous Endoscopic
		C Extraluminal Device
		D Intraluminal Device
		Z No Device
			Z No Qualifier

1 Trachea
   Cricoid cartilage
2 Carina
3 Main Bronchus, Right
   Bronchus intermedius
   Intermediate bronchus
4 Upper Lobe Bronchus, Right
5 Middle Lobe Bronchus, Right
6 Lower Lobe Bronchus, Right
7 Main Bronchus, Left
8 Upper Lobe Bronchus, Left
9 Lingula Bronchus
B Lower Lobe Bronchus, Left
	7 Via Natural or Artificial Opening
	8 Via Natural or Artificial Opening
	   Endoscopic
		D Intraluminal Device
		Z No Device
			Z No Qualifier

Ø　Medical and Surgical
B　Respiratory System
M　Reattachment　　Definition: Putting back in or on all or a portion of a separated body part to its normal location or other suitable location
　　　　　　　　　　　　Explanation: Vascular circulation and nervous pathways may or may not be reestablished

Body Part Character 4	Approach Character 5	Device Character 6	Qualifier Character 7
1　Trachea 　　Cricoid cartilage **2**　Carina **3**　Main Bronchus, Right 　　Bronchus intermedius 　　Intermediate bronchus **4**　Upper Lobe Bronchus, Right **5**　Middle Lobe Bronchus, Right **6**　Lower Lobe Bronchus, Right **7**　Main Bronchus, Left **8**　Upper Lobe Bronchus, Left **9**　Lingula Bronchus **B**　Lower Lobe Bronchus, Left **C**　Upper Lung Lobe, Right **D**　Middle Lung Lobe, Right **F**　Lower Lung Lobe, Right **G**　Upper Lung Lobe, Left **H**　Lung Lingula **J**　Lower Lung Lobe, Left **K**　Lung, Right **L**　Lung, Left **T**　Diaphragm	**Ø**　Open	**Z**　No Device	**Z**　No Qualifier

Ø　Medical and Surgical
B　Respiratory System
N　Release　　Definition: Freeing a body part from an abnormal physical constraint by cutting or by the use of force
　　　　　　　　　Explanation: Some of the restraining tissue may be taken out but none of the body part is taken out

Body Part Character 4	Approach Character 5	Device Character 6	Qualifier Character 7
1　Trachea 　　Cricoid cartilage **2**　Carina **3**　Main Bronchus, Right 　　Bronchus intermedius 　　Intermediate bronchus **4**　Upper Lobe Bronchus, Right **5**　Middle Lobe Bronchus, Right **6**　Lower Lobe Bronchus, Right **7**　Main Bronchus, Left **8**　Upper Lobe Bronchus, Left **9**　Lingula Bronchus **B**　Lower Lobe Bronchus, Left **C**　Upper Lung Lobe, Right **D**　Middle Lung Lobe, Right **F**　Lower Lung Lobe, Right **G**　Upper Lung Lobe, Left **H**　Lung Lingula **J**　Lower Lung Lobe, Left **K**　Lung, Right **L**　Lung, Left **M**　Lungs, Bilateral	**Ø**　Open **3**　Percutaneous **4**　Percutaneous Endoscopic **7**　Via Natural or Artificial Opening **8**　Via Natural or Artificial Opening 　　Endoscopic	**Z**　No Device	**Z**　No Qualifier
N　Pleura, Right **P**　Pleura, Left **T**　Diaphragm	**Ø**　Open **3**　Percutaneous **4**　Percutaneous Endoscopic	**Z**　No Device	**Z**　No Qualifier

Respiratory System

Ø   **Medical and Surgical**
B   **Respiratory System**
P   **Removal**   Definition: Taking out or off a device from a body part
                       Explanation: If a device is taken out and a similar device put in without cutting or puncturing the skin or mucous membrane, the procedure is coded to the root operation CHANGE. Otherwise, the procedure for taking out a device is coded to the root operation REMOVAL.

Body Part Character 4	Approach Character 5	Device Character 6	Qualifier Character 7
Ø Tracheobronchial Tree	Ø Open 3 Percutaneous 4 Percutaneous Endoscopic 7 Via Natural or Artificial Opening 8 Via Natural or Artificial Opening Endoscopic	Ø Drainage Device 1 Radioactive Element 2 Monitoring Device 3 Infusion Device 7 Autologous Tissue Substitute C Extraluminal Device D Intraluminal Device J Synthetic Substitute K Nonautologous Tissue Substitute Y Other Device	Z No Qualifier
Ø Tracheobronchial Tree	X External	Ø Drainage Device 1 Radioactive Element 2 Monitoring Device 3 Infusion Device D Intraluminal Device	Z No Qualifier
1 Trachea Cricoid cartilage	Ø Open 3 Percutaneous 4 Percutaneous Endoscopic 7 Via Natural or Artificial Opening 8 Via Natural or Artificial Opening Endoscopic	Ø Drainage Device 2 Monitoring Device 7 Autologous Tissue Substitute C Extraluminal Device D Intraluminal Device F Tracheostomy Device J Synthetic Substitute K Nonautologous Tissue Substitute	Z No Qualifier
1 Trachea Cricoid cartilage	X External	Ø Drainage Device 2 Monitoring Device D Intraluminal Device F Tracheostomy Device	Z No Qualifier
K Lung, Right L Lung, Left	Ø Open 3 Percutaneous 4 Percutaneous Endoscopic 7 Via Natural or Artificial Opening 8 Via Natural or Artificial Opening Endoscopic	Ø Drainage Device 1 Radioactive Element 2 Monitoring Device 3 Infusion Device Y Other Device	Z No Qualifier
K Lung, Right L Lung, Left	X External	Ø Drainage Device 1 Radioactive Element 2 Monitoring Device 3 Infusion Device	Z No Qualifier
Q Pleura	Ø Open 3 Percutaneous 4 Percutaneous Endoscopic 7 Via Natural or Artificial Opening 8 Via Natural or Artificial Opening Endoscopic	Ø Drainage Device 1 Radioactive Element 2 Monitoring Device Y Other Device	Z No Qualifier
Q Pleura	X External	Ø Drainage Device 1 Radioactive Element 2 Monitoring Device	Z No Qualifier
T Diaphragm	Ø Open 3 Percutaneous 4 Percutaneous Endoscopic 7 Via Natural or Artificial Opening 8 Via Natural or Artificial Opening Endoscopic	Ø Drainage Device 2 Monitoring Device 7 Autologous Tissue Substitute J Synthetic Substitute K Nonautologous Tissue Substitute M Diaphragmatic Pacemaker Lead Y Other Device	Z No Qualifier
T Diaphragm	X External	Ø Drainage Device 2 Monitoring Device M Diaphragmatic Pacemaker Lead	Z No Qualifier

Non-OR	ØBPØ[3,4]YZ		Non-OR	ØBPL7[Ø,2,3,Y]Z
Non-OR	ØBPØ[7,8][Ø,2,3,D,Y]Z		Non-OR	ØBPL8[Ø,2,3]Z
Non-OR	ØBPØX[Ø,1,2,3,D]Z		Non-OR	ØBP[K,L]X[Ø,1,2,3]Z
Non-OR	ØBP1[Ø,3,4]FZ		Non-OR	ØBPQ[Ø,3,4,7,8][Ø,1,2,]Z
Non-OR	ØBP1[7,8][Ø,2,D,F]Z		Non-OR	ØBPQ[3,7]YZ
Non-OR	ØBP1X[Ø,2,D,F]Z		Non-OR	ØBPQX[Ø,1,2]Z
Non-OR	ØBP[K,L]3YZ		Non-OR	ØBPT3YZ
Non-OR	ØBPK7[Ø,1,2,3,Y]Z		Non-OR	ØBPT[7,8][Ø,2,Y]Z
Non-OR	ØBPK8[Ø,1,2,3]Z		Non-OR	ØBPTX[Ø,2,M]Z

Non-OR Procedure   DRG Non-OR Procedure   Valid OR Procedure   HAC Associated Procedure   Combination Only   New/Revised GREEN

Respiratory System

Ø   **Medical and Surgical**
B   **Respiratory System**
Q   **Repair**   Definition: Restoring, to the extent possible, a body part to its normal anatomic structure and function
                 Explanation: Used only when the method to accomplish the repair is not one of the other root operations

Body Part Character 4	Approach Character 5	Device Character 6	Qualifier Character 7

1   Trachea
     Cricoid cartilage
2   Carina
3   Main Bronchus, Right
     Bronchus intermedius
     Intermediate bronchus
4   Upper Lobe Bronchus, Right
5   Middle Lobe Bronchus, Right
6   Lower Lobe Bronchus, Right
7   Main Bronchus, Left
8   Upper Lobe Bronchus, Left
9   Lingula Bronchus
B   Lower Lobe Bronchus, Left
C   Upper Lung Lobe, Right
D   Middle Lung Lobe, Right
F   Lower Lung Lobe, Right
G   Upper Lung Lobe, Left
H   Lung Lingula
J   Lower Lung Lobe, Left
K   Lung, Right
L   Lung, Left
M   Lungs, Bilateral
	Ø Open
	3 Percutaneous
	4 Percutaneous Endoscopic
	7 Via Natural or Artificial Opening
	8 Via Natural or Artificial Opening
	     Endoscopic
		Z No Device	Z No Qualifier

N Pleura, Right P Pleura, Left T Diaphragm	Ø Open 3 Percutaneous 4 Percutaneous Endoscopic	Z No Device	Z No Qualifier

NC Noncovered Procedure   **LC** Limited Coverage   **QA** Questionable OB Admit   **NT** New Tech Add-on   ⊞ Combination Member   ♂ Male   ♀ Female

ICD-10-PCS 2022   349

Respiratory System

Ø   **Medical and Surgical**
B   **Respiratory System**
R   **Replacement**   Definition: Putting in or on biological or synthetic material that physically takes the place and/or function of all or a portion of a body part

Explanation: The body part may have been taken out or replaced, or may be taken out, physically eradicated, or rendered nonfunctional during the REPLACEMENT procedure. A REMOVAL procedure is coded for taking out the device used in a previous replacement procedure.

Body Part Character 4	Approach Character 5	Device Character 6	Qualifier Character 7

1 Trachea
  Cricoid cartilage
2 Carina
3 Main Bronchus, Right
  Bronchus intermedius
  Intermediate bronchus
4 Upper Lobe Bronchus, Right
5 Middle Lobe Bronchus, Right
6 Lower Lobe Bronchus, Right
7 Main Bronchus, Left
8 Upper Lobe Bronchus, Left
9 Lingula Bronchus
B Lower Lobe Bronchus, Left
T Diaphragm
	Ø Open
	4 Percutaneous Endoscopic
		7 Autologous Tissue Substitute
		J Synthetic Substitute
		K Nonautologous Tissue Substitute
			Z No Qualifier

Ø   **Medical and Surgical**
B   **Respiratory System**
S   **Reposition**   Definition: Moving to its normal location, or other suitable location, all or a portion of a body part

Explanation: The body part is moved to a new location from an abnormal location, or from a normal location where it is not functioning correctly. The body part may or may not be cut out or off to be moved to the new location.

Body Part Character 4	Approach Character 5	Device Character 6	Qualifier Character 7

1 Trachea
  Cricoid cartilage
2 Carina
3 Main Bronchus, Right
  Bronchus intermedius
  Intermediate bronchus
4 Upper Lobe Bronchus, Right
5 Middle Lobe Bronchus, Right
6 Lower Lobe Bronchus, Right
7 Main Bronchus, Left
8 Upper Lobe Bronchus, Left
9 Lingula Bronchus
B Lower Lobe Bronchus, Left
C Upper Lung Lobe, Right
D Middle Lung Lobe, Right
F Lower Lung Lobe, Right
G Upper Lung Lobe, Left
H Lung Lingula
J Lower Lung Lobe, Left
K Lung, Right
L Lung, Left
T Diaphragm
	Ø Open	Z No Device	Z No Qualifier

Ø   Medical and Surgical
B   Respiratory System
T   Resection   Definition: Cutting out or off, without replacement, all of a body part
                Explanation: None

Body Part Character 4	Approach Character 5	Device Character 6	Qualifier Character 7

1   Trachea
      Cricoid cartilage
2   Carina
3   Main Bronchus, Right
      Bronchus intermedius
      Intermediate bronchus
4   Upper Lobe Bronchus, Right
5   Middle Lobe Bronchus, Right
6   Lower Lobe Bronchus, Right
7   Main Bronchus, Left
8   Upper Lobe Bronchus, Left
9   Lingula Bronchus
B   Lower Lobe Bronchus, Left
C   Upper Lung Lobe, Right
D   Middle Lung Lobe, Right
F   Lower Lung Lobe, Right
G   Upper Lung Lobe, Left
H   Lung Lingula
J   Lower Lung Lobe, Left
K   Lung, Right
L   Lung, Left
M   Lungs, Bilateral
T   Diaphragm
	Ø Open
	4 Percutaneous Endoscopic
		Z No Device	Z No Qualifier

Ø   Medical and Surgical
B   Respiratory System
U   Supplement   Definition: Putting in or on biological or synthetic material that physically reinforces and/or augments the function of a portion of a body part
                Explanation: The biological material is non-living, or is living and from the same individual. The body part may have been previously replaced, and the SUPPLEMENT procedure is performed to physically reinforce and/or augment the function of the replaced body part.

Body Part Character 4	Approach Character 5	Device Character 6	Qualifier Character 7

1   Trachea
      Cricoid cartilage
2   Carina
3   Main Bronchus, Right
      Bronchus intermedius
      Intermediate bronchus
4   Upper Lobe Bronchus, Right
5   Middle Lobe Bronchus, Right
6   Lower Lobe Bronchus, Right
7   Main Bronchus, Left
8   Upper Lobe Bronchus, Left
9   Lingula Bronchus
B   Lower Lobe Bronchus, Left
	Ø Open
	4 Percutaneous Endoscopic
	8 Via Natural or Artificial Opening
	      Endoscopic
		7 Autologous Tissue Substitute
		J Synthetic Substitute
		K Nonautologous Tissue Substitute
			Z No Qualifier

T Diaphragm	Ø Open 4 Percutaneous Endoscopic	7 Autologous Tissue Substitute J Synthetic Substitute K Nonautologous Tissue Substitute	Z No Qualifier

Ø   **Medical and Surgical**
B   **Respiratory System**
V   **Restriction**   Definition: Partially closing an orifice or the lumen of a tubular body part
                           Explanation: The orifice can be a natural orifice or an artificially created orifice

Body Part Character 4	Approach Character 5	Device Character 6	Qualifier Character 7

1 Trachea
   Cricoid cartilage
2 Carina
3 Main Bronchus, Right
   Bronchus intermedius
   Intermediate bronchus
4 Upper Lobe Bronchus, Right
5 Middle Lobe Bronchus, Right
6 Lower Lobe Bronchus, Right
7 Main Bronchus, Left
8 Upper Lobe Bronchus, Left
9 Lingula Bronchus
B Lower Lobe Bronchus, Left
	Ø Open
	3 Percutaneous
	4 Percutaneous Endoscopic
		C Extraluminal Device
		D Intraluminal Device
		Z No Device
			Z No Qualifier

1 Trachea
   Cricoid cartilage
2 Carina
3 Main Bronchus, Right
   Bronchus intermedius
   Intermediate bronchus
4 Upper Lobe Bronchus, Right
5 Middle Lobe Bronchus, Right
6 Lower Lobe Bronchus, Right
7 Main Bronchus, Left
8 Upper Lobe Bronchus, Left
9 Lingula Bronchus
B Lower Lobe Bronchus, Left
	7 Via Natural or Artificial Opening
	8 Via Natural or Artificial Opening
	   Endoscopic
		D Intraluminal Device
		Z No Device
			Z No Qualifier

Non-OR Procedure   DRG Non-OR Procedure   Valid OR Procedure   HAC Associated Procedure   Combination Only   New/Revised GREEN

Respiratory System

Ø   Medical and Surgical
B   Respiratory System
W   Revision   Definition: Correcting, to the extent possible, a portion of a malfunctioning device or the position of a displaced device

                     Explanation: Revision can include correcting a malfunctioning or displaced device by taking out or putting in components of the device such as a screw or pin

Body Part Character 4	Approach Character 5	Device Character 6	Qualifier Character 7
Ø Tracheobronchial Tree	Ø Open 3 Percutaneous 4 Percutaneous Endoscopic 7 Via Natural or Artificial Opening 8 Via Natural or Artificial Opening Endoscopic	Ø Drainage Device 2 Monitoring Device 3 Infusion Device 7 Autologous Tissue Substitute C Extraluminal Device D Intraluminal Device J Synthetic Substitute K Nonautologous Tissue Substitute Y Other Device	Z No Qualifier
Ø Tracheobronchial Tree	X External	Ø Drainage Device 2 Monitoring Device 3 Infusion Device 7 Autologous Tissue Substitute C Extraluminal Device D Intraluminal Device J Synthetic Substitute K Nonautologous Tissue Substitute	Z No Qualifier
1 Trachea Cricoid cartilage	Ø Open 3 Percutaneous 4 Percutaneous Endoscopic 7 Via Natural or Artificial Opening 8 Via Natural or Artificial Opening Endoscopic X External	Ø Drainage Device 2 Monitoring Device 7 Autologous Tissue Substitute C Extraluminal Device D Intraluminal Device F Tracheostomy Device J Synthetic Substitute K Nonautologous Tissue Substitute	Z No Qualifier
K Lung, Right L Lung, Left	Ø Open 3 Percutaneous 4 Percutaneous Endoscopic 7 Via Natural or Artificial Opening 8 Via Natural or Artificial Opening Endoscopic	Ø Drainage Device 2 Monitoring Device 3 Infusion Device Y Other Device	Z No Qualifier
K Lung, Right L Lung, Left	X External	Ø Drainage Device 2 Monitoring Device 3 Infusion Device	Z No Qualifier
Q Pleura	Ø Open 3 Percutaneous 4 Percutaneous Endoscopic 7 Via Natural or Artificial Opening 8 Via Natural or Artificial Opening Endoscopic	Ø Drainage Device 2 Monitoring Device Y Other Device	Z No Qualifier
Q Pleura	X External	Ø Drainage Device 2 Monitoring Device	Z No Qualifier
T Diaphragm	Ø Open 3 Percutaneous 4 Percutaneous Endoscopic 7 Via Natural or Artificial Opening 8 Via Natural or Artificial Opening Endoscopic	Ø Drainage Device 2 Monitoring Device 7 Autologous Tissue Substitute J Synthetic Substitute K Nonautologous Tissue Substitute M Diaphragmatic Pacemaker Lead Y Other Device	Z No Qualifier
T Diaphragm	X External	Ø Drainage Device 2 Monitoring Device 7 Autologous Tissue Substitute J Synthetic Substitute K Nonautologous Tissue Substitute M Diaphragmatic Pacemaker Lead	Z No Qualifier

Non-OR   ØBWØ[3,4]YZ
Non-OR   ØBWØ[7,8][2,3,D,Y]Z
Non-OR   ØBWØX[Ø,2,3,7,C,D,J,K]Z
Non-OR   ØBW1X[Ø,2,7,C,D,F,J,K]Z
Non-OR   ØBW[K,L]3YZ
Non-OR   ØBW[K,L]7[Ø,2,3,Y]Z
Non-OR   ØBW[K,L]8[Ø,2,3]Z
Non-OR   ØBW[K,L]X[Ø,2,3]Z
Non-OR   ØBWQ[Ø,3,4,7,8][Ø,2]Z
Non-OR   ØBWQ[Ø,3,7]YZ
Non-OR   ØBWQX[Ø,2]Z
Non-OR   ØBWT[3,7,8]YZ
Non-OR   ØBWTX[Ø,2,7,J,K,M]Z

NC Noncovered Procedure   LC Limited Coverage   QA Questionable OB Admit   NT New Tech Add-on   ⊞ Combination Member   ♂ Male   ♀ Female

Ø   Medical and Surgical
B   Respiratory System
Y   Transplantation   Definition: Putting in or on all or a portion of a living body part taken from another individual or animal to physically take the place and/or function of all or a portion of a similar body part

Explanation: The native body part may or may not be taken out, and the transplanted body part may take over all or a portion of its function

Body Part Character 4	Approach Character 5	Device Character 6	Qualifier Character 7
C Upper Lung Lobe, Right `LC` D Middle Lung Lobe, Right `LC` F Lower Lung Lobe, Right `LC` G Upper Lung Lobe, Left `LC` H Lung Lingula `LC` J Lower Lung Lobe, Left `LC` K Lung, Right `LC` L Lung, Left `LC` M Lungs, Bilateral `LC`	Ø Open	Z No Device	Ø Allogeneic 1 Syngeneic 2 Zooplastic

`LC`   ØBY[C,D,F,G,H,J,K,L,M]ØZ[Ø,1,2]

Mouth and Throat ØCØ–ØCX

Character Meanings

This Character Meaning table is provided as a guide to assist the user in the identification of character members that may be found in this section of code tables. It **SHOULD NOT** be used to build a PCS code.

Operation–Character 3		Body Part–Character 4		Approach–Character 5		Device–Character 6		Qualifier–Character 7	
Ø	Alteration	Ø	Upper Lip	Ø	Open	Ø	Drainage Device	Ø	Single
2	Change	1	Lower Lip	3	Percutaneous	1	Radioactive Element	1	Multiple
5	Destruction	2	Hard Palate	4	Percutaneous Endoscopic	5	External Fixation Device	2	All
7	Dilation	3	Soft Palate	7	Via Natural or Artificial Opening	7	Autologous Tissue Substitute	X	Diagnostic
9	Drainage	4	Buccal Mucosa	8	Via Natural or Artificial Opening Endoscopic	B	Intraluminal Device, Airway	Z	No Qualifier
B	Excision	5	Upper Gingiva	X	External	C	Extraluminal Device		
C	Extirpation	6	Lower Gingiva			D	Intraluminal Device		
D	Extraction	7	Tongue			J	Synthetic Substitute		
F	Fragmentation	8	Parotid Gland, Right			K	Nonautologous Tissue Substitute		
H	Insertion	9	Parotid Gland, Left			Y	Other Device		
J	Inspection	A	Salivary Gland			Z	No Device		
L	Occlusion	B	Parotid Duct, Right						
M	Reattachment	C	Parotid Duct, Left						
N	Release	D	Sublingual Gland, Right						
P	Removal	F	Sublingual Gland, Left						
Q	Repair	G	Submaxillary Gland, Right						
R	Replacement	H	Submaxillary Gland, Left						
S	Reposition	J	Minor Salivary Gland						
T	Resection	M	Pharynx						
U	Supplement	N	Uvula						
V	Restriction	P	Tonsils						
W	Revision	Q	Adenoids						
X	Transfer	R	Epiglottis						
		S	Larynx						
		T	Vocal Cord, Right						
		V	Vocal Cord, Left						
		W	Upper Tooth						
		X	Lower Tooth						
		Y	Mouth and Throat						

AHA Coding Clinic for table ØC9
2017, 2Q, 16   Incision and drainage of floor of mouth

AHA Coding Clinic for table ØCB
2017, 2Q, 16   Excision of floor of mouth
2016, 3Q, 28   Lingual tonsillectomy, tongue base excision and epiglottopexy
2016, 2Q, 19   Biopsy of the base of tongue
2014, 3Q, 21   Superficial parotidectomy

AHA Coding Clinic for table ØCC
2016, 2Q, 20   Sialendoscopy with stone removal

AHA Coding Clinic for table ØCH
2020, 4Q, 43-44   Insertion of radioactive element

AHA Coding Clinic for table ØCQ
2017, 1Q, 20   Preparatory nasal adhesion repair before definitive cleft palate repair

AHA Coding Clinic for table ØCR
2014, 3Q, 25   Excision of soft palate with placement of surgical obturator
2014, 2Q, 5   Oasis acellular matrix graft
2014, 2Q, 6   Composite grafting (synthetic versus nonautologous tissue substitute)

AHA Coding Clinic for table ØCS
2016, 3Q, 28   Lingual tonsillectomy, tongue base excision and epiglottopexy

AHA Coding Clinic for table ØCT
2016, 2Q, 12   Resection of malignant neoplasm of infratemporal fossa
2014, 3Q, 21   Superficial parotidectomy
2014, 3Q, 23   Le Fort I osteotomy

Salivary Glands

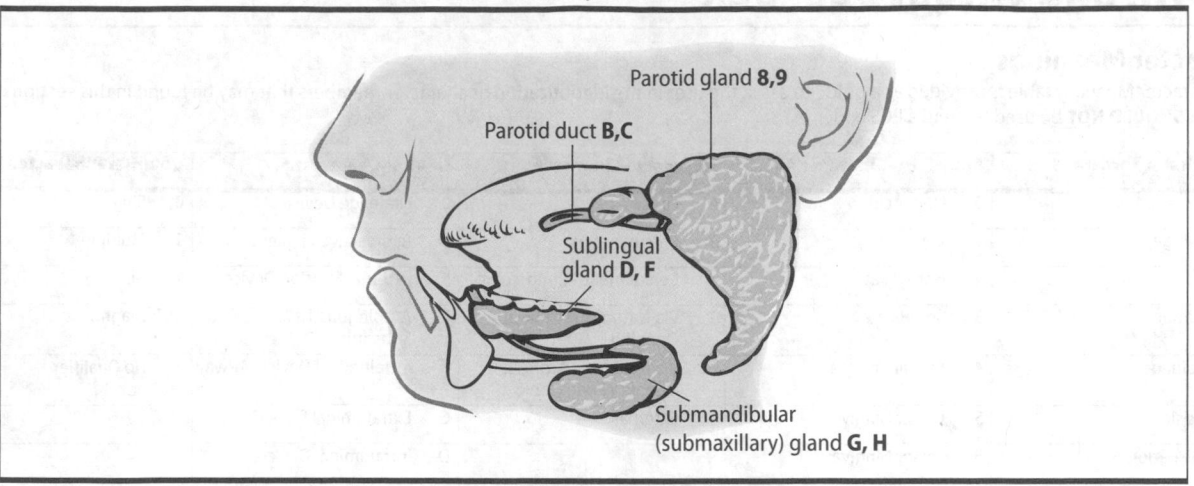

Parotid gland **8,9**

Parotid duct **B,C**

Sublingual gland **D, F**

Submandibular (submaxillary) gland **G, H**

Oral Anatomy

Nasal cavity

Hard palate **2**

Tongue **7**

Nasopharynx region **M**

Oropharynx region **M**

Hypopharynx region **M**

Vocal cords **T,V**

Soft palate **3**

Pharynx **M**

Epiglottis **R**

Larynx **S**

Mouth Frontal View (Upper)

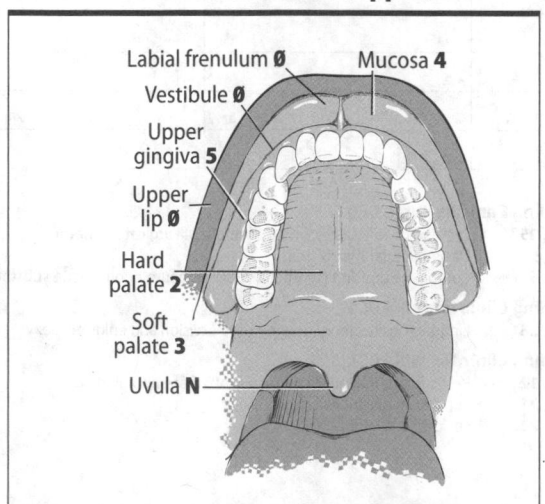

Labial frenulum **Ø**

Vestibule **Ø**

Upper gingiva **5**

Upper lip **Ø**

Hard palate **2**

Soft palate **3**

Uvula **N**

Mucosa **4**

Mouth Frontal View (Lower)

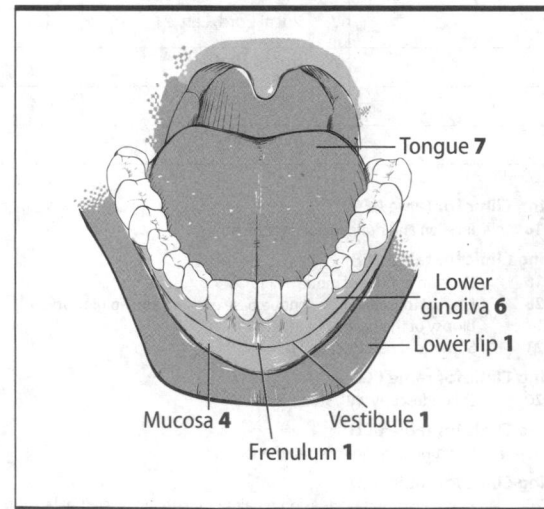

Tongue **7**

Lower gingiva **6**

Lower lip **1**

Vestibule **1**

Frenulum **1**

Mucosa **4**

0   **Medical and Surgical**
C   **Mouth and Throat**
0   **Alteration**   Definition: Modifying the anatomic structure of a body part without affecting the function of the body part
                     Explanation: Principal purpose is to improve appearance

Body Part Character 4	Approach Character 5	Device Character 6	Qualifier Character 7

0 Upper Lip
   Frenulum labii superioris
   Labial gland
   Vermilion border
1 Lower Lip
   Frenulum labii inferioris
   Labial gland
   Vermilion border
	X External	**7** Autologous Tissue Substitute
		J Synthetic Substitute
		K Nonautologous Tissue Substitute
		Z No Device
			Z No Qualifier

0   **Medical and Surgical**
C   **Mouth and Throat**
2   **Change**   Definition: Taking out or off a device from a body part and putting back an identical or similar device in or on the same body part without cutting or puncturing the skin or a mucous membrane
                     Explanation: All CHANGE procedures are coded using the approach EXTERNAL

Body Part Character 4	Approach Character 5	Device Character 6	Qualifier Character 7

A Salivary Gland
S Larynx
   Aryepiglottic fold
   Arytenoid cartilage
   Corniculate cartilage
   Cuneiform cartilage
   False vocal cord
   Glottis
   Rima glottidis
   Thyroid cartilage
   Ventricular fold
Y Mouth and Throat
	X External	**0** Drainage Device
		Y Other Device
			Z No Qualifier

Non-OR   All body part, approach, device, and qualifier values

Mouth and Throat

0   Medical and Surgical
C   Mouth and Throat
5   Destruction   Definition: Physical eradication of all or a portion of a body part by the direct use of energy, force, or a destructive agent
                        Explanation: None of the body part is physically taken out

Body Part Character 4		Approach Character 5	Device Character 6	Qualifier Character 7
0 Upper Lip Frenulum labii superioris Labial gland Vermilion border **1** Lower Lip Frenulum labii inferioris Labial gland Vermilion border **2** Hard Palate **3** Soft Palate **4** Buccal Mucosa Buccal gland Molar gland Palatine gland	**5** Upper Gingiva **6** Lower Gingiva **7** Tongue Frenulum linguae **N** Uvula Palatine uvula **P** Tonsils Palatine tonsil **Q** Adenoids Pharyngeal tonsil	**0** Open **3** Percutaneous **X** External	**Z** No Device	**Z** No Qualifier
8 Parotid Gland, Right **9** Parotid Gland, Left **B** Parotid Duct, Right Stensen's duct **C** Parotid Duct, Left *See B Parotid Duct, Right* **D** Sublingual Gland, Right	**F** Sublingual Gland, Left **G** Submaxillary Gland, Right Submandibular gland **H** Submaxillary Gland, Left *See G Submaxillary Gland, Right* **J** Minor Salivary Gland Anterior lingual gland	**0** Open **3** Percutaneous	**Z** No Device	**Z** No Qualifier
M Pharynx Base of tongue Hypopharynx Laryngopharynx Lingual tonsil Oropharynx Piriform recess (sinus) Tongue, base of **R** Epiglottis Glossoepiglottic fold	**S** Larynx Aryepiglottic fold Arytenoid cartilage Corniculate cartilage Cuneiform cartilage False vocal cord Glottis Rima glottidis Thyroid cartilage Ventricular fold **T** Vocal Cord, Right Vocal fold **V** Vocal Cord, Left *See T Vocal Cord, Right*	**0** Open **3** Percutaneous **4** Percutaneous Endoscopic **7** Via Natural or Artificial Opening **8** Via Natural or Artificial Opening Endoscopic	**Z** No Device	**Z** No Qualifier
W Upper Tooth **X** Lower Tooth		**0** Open **X** External	**Z** No Device	**0** Single **1** Multiple **2** All

Non-OR   0C5[5,6][0,3,X]ZZ
Non-OR   0C5[W,X][0,X]Z[0,1,2]

0   Medical and Surgical
C   Mouth and Throat
7   Dilation   Definition: Expanding an orifice or the lumen of a tubular body part
                     Explanation: The orifice can be a natural orifice or an artificially created orifice. Accomplished by stretching a tubular body part using intraluminal pressure or by cutting part of the orifice or wall of the tubular body part.

Body Part Character 4	Approach Character 5	Device Character 6	Qualifier Character 7
B Parotid Duct, Right Stensen's duct **C** Parotid Duct, Left *See B Parotid Duct, Right*	**0** Open **3** Percutaneous **7** Via Natural or Artificial Opening	**D** Intraluminal Device **Z** No Device	**Z** No Qualifier
M Pharynx Base of tongue Hypopharynx Laryngopharynx Lingual tonsil Oropharynx Piriform recess (sinus) Tongue, base of	**7** Via Natural or Artificial Opening **8** Via Natural or Artificial Opening Endoscopic	**D** Intraluminal Device **Z** No Device	**Z** No Qualifier
S Larynx Aryepiglottic fold Arytenoid cartilage Corniculate cartilage Cuneiform cartilage False vocal cord Glottis Rima glottidis Thyroid cartilage Ventricular fold	**0** Open **3** Percutaneous **4** Percutaneous Endoscopic **7** Via Natural or Artificial Opening **8** Via Natural or Artificial Opening Endoscopic	**D** Intraluminal Device **Z** No Device	**Z** No Qualifier

Non-OR   0C7[B,C][0,3,7][D,Z]Z
Non-OR   0C7M[7,8][D,Z]Z

Non-OR Procedure   DRG Non-OR Procedure   Valid OR Procedure   HAC Associated Procedure   Combination Only   New/Revised GREEN

0   **Medical and Surgical**
C   **Mouth and Throat**
9   **Drainage**   Definition: Taking or letting out fluids and/or gases from a body part

                 Explanation: The qualifier DIAGNOSTIC is used to identify drainage procedures that are biopsies

Body Part — Character 4		Approach — Character 5	Device — Character 6	Qualifier — Character 7
0 Upper Lip Frenulum labii superioris Labial gland Vermilion border **1** Lower Lip Frenulum labii inferioris Labial gland Vermilion border **2** Hard Palate **3** Soft Palate **4** Buccal Mucosa Buccal gland Molar gland Palatine gland	**5** Upper Gingiva **6** Lower Gingiva **7** Tongue Frenulum linguae **N** Uvula Palatine uvula **P** Tonsils Palatine tonsil **Q** Adenoids Pharyngeal tonsil	**0** Open **3** Percutaneous **X** External	**0** Drainage Device	**Z** No Qualifier
0 Upper Lip Frenulum labii superioris Labial gland Vermilion border **1** Lower Lip Frenulum labii inferioris Labial gland Vermilion border **2** Hard Palate **3** Soft Palate **4** Buccal Mucosa Buccal gland Molar gland Palatine gland	**5** Upper Gingiva **6** Lower Gingiva **7** Tongue Frenulum linguae **N** Uvula Palatine uvula **P** Tonsils Palatine tonsil **Q** Adenoids Pharyngeal tonsil	**0** Open **3** Percutaneous **X** External	**Z** No Device	**X** Diagnostic **Z** No Qualifier
8 Parotid Gland, Right **9** Parotid Gland, Left **B** Parotid Duct, Right Stensen's duct **C** Parotid Duct, Left *See B Parotid Duct, Right* **D** Sublingual Gland, Right	**F** Sublingual Gland, Left **G** Submaxillary Gland, Right Submandibular gland **H** Submaxillary Gland, Left *See G Submaxillary Gland, Right* **J** Minor Salivary Gland Anterior lingual gland	**0** Open **3** Percutaneous	**0** Drainage Device	**Z** No Qualifier
8 Parotid Gland, Right **9** Parotid Gland, Left **B** Parotid Duct, Right Stensen's duct **C** Parotid Duct, Left *See B Parotid Duct, Right*	**D** Sublingual Gland, Right **F** Sublingual Gland, Left **G** Submaxillary Gland, Right Submandibular gland **H** Submaxillary Gland, Left *See G Submaxillary Gland, Right* **J** Minor Salivary Gland Anterior lingual gland	**0** Open **3** Percutaneous	**Z** No Device	**X** Diagnostic **Z** No Qualifier
M Pharynx Base of tongue Hypopharynx Laryngopharynx Lingual tonsil Oropharynx Piriform recess (sinus) Tongue, base of **R** Epiglottis Glossoepiglottic fold	**S** Larynx Aryepiglottic fold Arytenoid cartilage Corniculate cartilage Cuneiform cartilage False vocal cord Glottis Rima glottidis Thyroid cartilage Ventricular fold **T** Vocal Cord, Right Vocal fold **V** Vocal Cord, Left *See T Vocal Cord, Right*	**0** Open **3** Percutaneous **4** Percutaneous Endoscopic **7** Via Natural or Artificial Opening **8** Via Natural or Artificial Opening Endoscopic	**0** Drainage Device	**Z** No Qualifier

Non-OR	0C9[0,1,2,3,4,7,N,P,Q]30Z
Non-OR	0C9[5,6][0,3,X]0Z
Non-OR	0C9[0,1,4][0,3,X]ZX
Non-OR	0C9[0,1,2,3,4,7,N,P,Q]3ZZ
Non-OR	0C9[5,6][0,3,X]Z[X,Z]
Non-OR	0C97[3,X]ZX
Non-OR	0C9[8,9,B,C,D,F,G,H,J][0,3]0Z
Non-OR	0C9[8,9,B,C,D,F,G,H,J]3ZX
Non-OR	0C9[8,9,G,H]3ZZ
Non-OR	0C9[B,C,D, F,J][0,3]ZZ
Non-OR	0C9[M,R,S,T,V]30Z

0C9 Continued on next page

NC Noncovered Procedure   **LC** Limited Coverage   **QA** Questionable OB Admit   **NT** New Tech Add-on   ⊞ Combination Member   ♂ Male   ♀ Female

Mouth and Throat

0	**Medical and Surgical**		*0C9 Continued*
C	**Mouth and Throat**		
9	**Drainage**	Definition: Taking or letting out fluids and/or gases from a body part	
		Explanation: The qualifier DIAGNOSTIC is used to identify drainage procedures that are biopsies	

Body Part Character 4		Approach Character 5	Device Character 6	Qualifier Character 7
M **Pharynx** Base of tongue Hypopharynx Laryngopharynx Lingual tonsil Oropharynx Piriform recess (sinus) Tongue, base of **R** **Epiglottis** Glossoepiglottic fold	**S** **Larynx** Aryepiglottic fold Arytenoid cartilage Corniculate cartilage Cuneiform cartilage False vocal cord Glottis Rima glottidis Thyroid cartilage Ventricular fold **T** **Vocal Cord, Right** Vocal fold **V** **Vocal Cord, Left** *See T Vocal Cord, Right*	**0** Open **3** Percutaneous **4** Percutaneous Endoscopic **7** Via Natural or Artificial Opening **8** Via Natural or Artificial Opening Endoscopic	**Z** No Device	**X** Diagnostic **Z** No Qualifier
W **Upper Tooth** **X** **Lower Tooth**		**0** Open **X** External	**0** Drainage Device **Z** No Device	**0** Single **1** Multiple **2** All

Non-OR	0C9M[0,3,4,7,8]ZX
Non-OR	0C9[M,R,S,T,V]3ZZ
Non-OR	0C9[R,S,T,V][3,4,7,8]ZX
Non-OR	0C9[W,X][0,X][0,Z][0,1,2]

0	**Medical and Surgical**
C	**Mouth and Throat**
B	**Excision**

Definition: Cutting out or off, without replacement, a portion of a body part

Explanation: The qualifier DIAGNOSTIC is used to identify excision procedures that are biopsies

Body Part Character 4		Approach Character 5	Device Character 6	Qualifier Character 7
0 **Upper Lip** Frenulum labii superioris Labial gland Vermilion border **1** **Lower Lip** Frenulum labii inferioris Labial gland Vermilion border **2** **Hard Palate** **3** **Soft Palate** **4** **Buccal Mucosa** Buccal gland Molar gland Palatine gland	**5** **Upper Gingiva** **6** **Lower Gingiva** **7** **Tongue** Frenulum linguae **N** **Uvula** Palatine uvula **P** **Tonsils** Palatine tonsil **Q** **Adenoids** Pharyngeal tonsil	**0** Open **3** Percutaneous **X** External	**Z** No Device	**X** Diagnostic **Z** No Qualifier
8 **Parotid Gland, Right** **9** **Parotid Gland, Left** **B** **Parotid Duct, Right** Stensen's duct **C** **Parotid Duct, Left** *See B Parotid Duct, Right* **D** **Sublingual Gland, Right**	**F** **Sublingual Gland, Left** **G** **Submaxillary Gland, Right** Submandibular gland **H** **Submaxillary Gland, Left** *See G Submaxillary Gland, Right* **J** **Minor Salivary Gland** Anterior lingual gland	**0** Open **3** Percutaneous	**Z** No Device	**X** Diagnostic **Z** No Qualifier
M **Pharynx** Base of tongue Hypopharynx Laryngopharynx Lingual tonsil Oropharynx Piriform recess (sinus) Tongue, base of **R** **Epiglottis** Glossoepiglottic fold	**S** **Larynx** Aryepiglottic fold Arytenoid cartilage Corniculate cartilage Cuneiform cartilage False vocal cord Glottis Rima glottidis Thyroid cartilage Ventricular fold **T** **Vocal Cord, Right** Vocal fold **V** **Vocal Cord, Left** *See T Vocal Cord, Right*	**0** Open **3** Percutaneous **4** Percutaneous Endoscopic **7** Via Natural or Artificial Opening **8** Via Natural or Artificial Opening Endoscopic	**Z** No Device	**X** Diagnostic **Z** No Qualifier
W **Upper Tooth** **X** **Lower Tooth**		**0** Open **X** External	**Z** No Device	**0** Single **1** Multiple **2** All

Non-OR	0CB[0,1,4][0,3,X]ZX		Non-OR	0CBM[0,3,4,7,8]ZX
Non-OR	0CB[5,6][0,3,X]Z[X,Z]		Non-OR	0CB[R,S,T,V][3,4,7,8]ZX
Non-OR	0CB7[3,X]ZX		Non-OR	0CB[W,X][0,X]Z[0,1,2]
Non-OR	0CB[8,9,B,C,D,F,G,H,J]3ZX			

Non-OR Procedure   DRG Non-OR Procedure   Valid OR Procedure   HAC Associated Procedure   Combination Only   New/Revised GREEN

Ø Medical and Surgical
C Mouth and Throat
C Extirpation Definition: Taking or cutting out solid matter from a body part

Explanation: The solid matter may be an abnormal byproduct of a biological function or a foreign body; it may be imbedded in a body part or in the lumen of a tubular body part. The solid matter may or may not have been previously broken into pieces.

Body Part Character 4		Approach Character 5	Device Character 6	Qualifier Character 7
Ø Upper Lip Frenulum labii superioris Labial gland Vermilion border **1 Lower Lip** Frenulum labii inferioris Labial gland Vermilion border **2 Hard Palate** **3 Soft Palate** **4 Buccal Mucosa** Buccal gland Molar gland Palatine gland	**5 Upper Gingiva** **6 Lower Gingiva** **7 Tongue** Frenulum linguae **N Uvula** Palatine uvula **P Tonsils** Palatine tonsil **Q Adenoids** Pharyngeal tonsil	**Ø** Open **3** Percutaneous **X** External	**Z** No Device	**Z** No Qualifier
8 Parotid Gland, Right **9 Parotid Gland, Left** **B Parotid Duct, Right** Stensen's duct **C Parotid Duct, Left** See B Parotid Duct, Right **D Sublingual Gland, Right**	**F Sublingual Gland, Left** **G Submaxillary Gland, Right** Submandibular gland **H Submaxillary Gland, Left** See G Submaxillary Gland, Right **J Minor Salivary Gland** Anterior lingual gland	**Ø** Open **3** Percutaneous	**Z** No Device	**Z** No Qualifier
M Pharynx Base of tongue Hypopharynx Laryngopharynx Lingual tonsil Oropharynx Piriform recess (sinus) Tongue, base of **R Epiglottis** Glossoepiglottic fold	**S Larynx** Aryepiglottic fold Arytenoid cartilage Corniculate cartilage Cuneiform cartilage False vocal cord Glottis Rima glottidis Thyroid cartilage Ventricular fold **T Vocal Cord, Right** Vocal fold **V Vocal Cord, Left** See T Vocal Cord, Right	**Ø** Open **3** Percutaneous **4** Percutaneous Endoscopic **7** Via Natural or Artificial Opening **8** Via Natural or Artificial Opening Endoscopic	**Z** No Device	**Z** No Qualifier
W Upper Tooth **X Lower Tooth**		**Ø** Open **X** External	**Z** No Device	**Ø** Single **1** Multiple **2** All

Non-OR	ØCC[Ø,1,2,3,4,7,N,P,Q]XZZ
Non-OR	ØCC[5,6][Ø,3,X]ZZ
Non-OR	ØCC[8,9,G,H]3ZZ
Non-OR	ØCC[B,C,D, F,J][Ø,3]ZZ
Non-OR	ØCC[M,S][7,8]ZZ
Non-OR	ØCC[W,X][Ø,X]Z[Ø,1,2]

Ø Medical and Surgical
C Mouth and Throat
D Extraction Definition: Pulling or stripping out or off all or a portion of a body part by the use of force

Explanation: The qualifier DIAGNOSTIC is used to identify extraction procedures that are biopsies

Body Part Character 4	Approach Character 5	Device Character 6	Qualifier Character 7
T Vocal Cord, Right Vocal fold **V Vocal Cord, Left** See T Vocal Cord, Right	**Ø** Open **3** Percutaneous **4** Percutaneous Endoscopic **7** Via Natural or Artificial Opening **8** Via Natural or Artificial Opening Endoscopic	**Z** No Device	**Z** No Qualifier
W Upper Tooth **X Lower Tooth**	**X** External	**Z** No Device	**Ø** Single **1** Multiple **2** All

Non-OR	ØCD[W,X]XZ[Ø,1,2]

NC Noncovered Procedure   **LC** Limited Coverage   **QA** Questionable OB Admit   **NT** New Tech Add-on   ✚ Combination Member   ♂ Male   ♀ Female

ICD-10-PCS 2022   361

Ø Medical and Surgical
C Mouth and Throat
F Fragmentation   Definition: Breaking solid matter in a body part into pieces

Explanation: Physical force (e.g., manual, ultrasonic) applied directly or indirectly is used to break the solid matter into pieces. The solid matter may be an abnormal byproduct of a biological function or a foreign body. The pieces of solid matter are not taken out.

Body Part Character 4		Approach Character 5	Device Character 6	Qualifier Character 7
B Parotid Duct, Right `NC` Stensen's duct **C** Parotid Duct, Left `NC` *See B Parotid Duct, Right*	**Ø** Open **3** Percutaneous **7** Via Natural or Artificial Opening **X** External		**Z** No Device	**Z** No Qualifier

Non-OR All body part, approach, device, and qualifier values
`NC` ØCF[B,C]XZZ

Ø Medical and Surgical
C Mouth and Throat
H Insertion   Definition: Putting in a nonbiological appliance that monitors, assists, performs, or prevents a physiological function but does not physically take the place of a body part

Explanation: None

Body Part Character 4	Approach Character 5	Device Character 6	Qualifier Character 7
7 Tongue Frenulum linguae	**Ø** Open **3** Percutaneous **X** External	**1** Radioactive Element	**Z** No Qualifier
A Salivary Gland **S** Larynx Aryepiglottic fold Arytenoid cartilage Corniculate cartilage Cuneiform cartilage False vocal cord Glottis Rima glottidis Thyroid cartilage Ventricular fold	**Ø** Open **3** Percutaneous **7** Via Natural or Artificial Opening **8** Via Natural or Artificial Opening Endoscopic	**1** Radioactive Element **Y** Other Device	**Z** No Qualifier
Y Mouth and Throat	**Ø** Open **3** Percutaneous	**1** Radioactive Element **Y** Other Device	**Z** No Qualifier
Y Mouth and Throat	**7** Via Natural or Artificial Opening **8** Via Natural or Artificial Opening Endoscopic	**1** Radioactive Element **B** Intraluminal Device, Airway **Y** Other Device	**Z** No Qualifier

Non-OR ØCH[A,S]Ø1Z
Non-OR ØCHSØYZ
Non-OR ØCH[A,S][3,7,8][1,Y]Z
Non-OR ØCHY[Ø,3][1,Y]Z
Non-OR ØCHY[7,8][1,B,Y]Z

Ø Medical and Surgical
C Mouth and Throat
J Inspection   Definition: Visually and/or manually exploring a body part

Explanation: Visual exploration may be performed with or without optical instrumentation. Manual exploration may be performed directly or through intervening body layers.

Body Part Character 4	Approach Character 5	Device Character 6	Qualifier Character 7
A Salivary Gland	**Ø** Open **3** Percutaneous **X** External	**Z** No Device	**Z** No Qualifier
S Larynx Aryepiglottic fold Arytenoid cartilage Corniculate cartilage Cuneiform cartilage False vocal cord Glottis Rima glottidis Thyroid cartilage Ventricular fold **Y** Mouth and Throat	**Ø** Open **3** Percutaneous **4** Percutaneous Endoscopic **7** Via Natural or Artificial Opening **8** Via Natural or Artificial Opening Endoscopic **X** External	**Z** No Device	**Z** No Qualifier

Non-OR All body part, approach, device, and qualifier values

0   **Medical and Surgical**
C   **Mouth and Throat**
L   **Occlusion**   Definition: Completely closing an orifice or the lumen of a tubular body part
                Explanation: The orifice can be a natural orifice or an artificially created orifice

Body Part Character 4	Approach Character 5	Device Character 6	Qualifier Character 7

B   Parotid Duct, Right
    Stensen's duct
C   Parotid Duct, Left
    See B Parotid Duct, Right
	0 Open
	3 Percutaneous
	4 Percutaneous Endoscopic
		C Extraluminal Device
		D Intraluminal Device
		Z No Device
			Z No Qualifier

B   Parotid Duct, Right
    Stensen's duct
C   Parotid Duct, Left
    See B Parotid Duct, Right
	7 Via Natural or Artificial Opening
	8 Via Natural or Artificial Opening
	     Endoscopic
		D Intraluminal Device
		Z No Device
			Z No Qualifier

0   **Medical and Surgical**
C   **Mouth and Throat**
M   **Reattachment**   Definition: Putting back in or on all or a portion of a separated body part to its normal location or other suitable location
                        Explanation: Vascular circulation and nervous pathways may or may not be reestablished

Body Part Character 4	Approach Character 5	Device Character 6	Qualifier Character 7

0   Upper Lip
    Frenulum labii superioris
    Labial gland
    Vermilion border
1   Lower Lip
    Frenulum labii inferioris
    Labial gland
    Vermilion border
3   Soft Palate
7   Tongue
    Frenulum linguae
N   Uvula
    Palatine uvula
	0 Open	**Z** No Device	**Z** No Qualifier

W Upper Tooth **X** Lower Tooth	**0** Open **X** External	**Z** No Device	**0** Single **1** Multiple **2** All

Non-OR   0CM[W,X][0,X]Z[0,1,2]

Mouth and Throat

Ø   **Medical and Surgical**
C   **Mouth and Throat**
N   **Release**   Definition: Freeing a body part from an abnormal physical constraint by cutting or by the use of force
                        Explanation: Some of the restraining tissue may be taken out but none of the body part is taken out

Body Part Character 4	Approach Character 5	Device Character 6	Qualifier Character 7

Ø **Upper Lip**
    Frenulum labii superioris
    Labial gland
    Vermilion border
1 **Lower Lip**
    Frenulum labii inferioris
    Labial gland
    Vermilion border
2 **Hard Palate**
3 **Soft Palate**
4 **Buccal Mucosa**
    Buccal gland
    Molar gland
    Palatine gland
5 **Upper Gingiva**
6 **Lower Gingiva**
7 **Tongue**
    Frenulum linguae
N **Uvula**
    Palatine uvula
P **Tonsils**
    Palatine tonsil
Q **Adenoids**
    Pharyngeal tonsil
	Ø Open
	3 Percutaneous
	X External
		Z No Device	**Z** No Qualifier

8 **Parotid Gland, Right**
9 **Parotid Gland, Left**
B **Parotid Duct, Right**
    Stensen's duct
C **Parotid Duct, Left**
    See B Parotid Duct, Right
D **Sublingual Gland, Right**
F **Sublingual Gland, Left**
G **Submaxillary Gland, Right**
    Submandibular gland
H **Submaxillary Gland, Left**
    See G Submaxillary Gland, Right
J **Minor Salivary Gland**
    Anterior lingual gland
	Ø Open
	3 Percutaneous
		Z No Device	**Z** No Qualifier

M **Pharynx**
    Base of tongue
    Hypopharynx
    Laryngopharynx
    Lingual tonsil
    Oropharynx
    Piriform recess (sinus)
    Tongue, base of
R **Epiglottis**
    Glossoepiglottic fold
S **Larynx**
    Aryepiglottic fold
    Arytenoid cartilage
    Corniculate cartilage
    Cuneiform cartilage
    False vocal cord
    Glottis
    Rima glottidis
    Thyroid cartilage
    Ventricular fold
T **Vocal Cord, Right**
    Vocal fold
V **Vocal Cord, Left**
    See T Vocal Cord, Right
	Ø Open
	3 Percutaneous
	4 Percutaneous Endoscopic
	7 Via Natural or Artificial Opening
	8 Via Natural or Artificial Opening Endoscopic
		Z No Device	**Z** No Qualifier

W **Upper Tooth** **X** **Lower Tooth**	**Ø** Open **X** External	**Z** No Device	**Ø** Single **1** Multiple **2** All

Non-OR   ØCN[Ø,1,5,6,7][Ø,3,X]ZZ
Non-OR   ØCN[W,X][Ø,X]Z[Ø,1,2]

Non-OR Procedure   DRG Non-OR Procedure   Valid OR Procedure   HAC Associated Procedure   Combination Only   New/Revised GREEN

0   **Medical and Surgical**
C   **Mouth and Throat**
P   **Removal**   Definition: Taking out or off a device from a body part

                        Explanation: If a device is taken out and a similar device put in without cutting or puncturing the skin or mucous membrane, the procedure is coded to the root operation CHANGE. Otherwise, the procedure for taking out a device is coded to the root operation REMOVAL.

Body Part Character 4	Approach Character 5	Device Character 6	Qualifier Character 7
A Salivary Gland	**0** Open **3** Percutaneous	**0** Drainage Device **C** Extraluminal Device **Y** Other Device	**Z** No Qualifier
A Salivary Gland	**7** Via Natural or Artificial Opening **8** Via Natural or Artificial Opening Endoscopic	**Y** Other Device	**Z** No Qualifier

S   Larynx
     Aryepiglottic fold
     Arytenoid cartilage
     Corniculate cartilage
     Cuneiform cartilage
     False vocal cord
     Glottis
     Rima glottidis
     Thyroid cartilage
     Ventricular fold
	0 Open
	3 Percutaneous
	7 Via Natural or Artificial Opening
	8 Via Natural or Artificial Opening Endoscopic
		0 Drainage Device
		7 Autologous Tissue Substitute
		D Intraluminal Device
		J Synthetic Substitute
		K Nonautologous Tissue Substitute
		Y Other Device
			Z No Qualifier

S   Larynx
     Aryepiglottic fold
     Arytenoid cartilage
     Corniculate cartilage
     Cuneiform cartilage
     False vocal cord
     Glottis
     Rima glottidis
     Thyroid cartilage
     Ventricular fold
	X External	**0** Drainage Device
		7 Autologous Tissue Substitute
		D Intraluminal Device
		J Synthetic Substitute
		K Nonautologous Tissue Substitute
			Z No Qualifier

Y Mouth and Throat	**0** Open **3** Percutaneous **7** Via Natural or Artificial Opening **8** Via Natural or Artificial Opening Endoscopic	**0** Drainage Device **1** Radioactive Element **7** Autologous Tissue Substitute **D** Intraluminal Device **J** Synthetic Substitute **K** Nonautologous Tissue Substitute **Y** Other Device	**Z** No Qualifier
Y Mouth and Throat	**X** External	**0** Drainage Device **1** Radioactive Element **7** Autologous Tissue Substitute **D** Intraluminal Device **J** Synthetic Substitute **K** Nonautologous Tissue Substitute	**Z** No Qualifier

Non-OR	0CPA[0,3][0,C,Y]Z
Non-OR	0CPA[7,8]YZ
Non-OR	0CPS3YZ
Non-OR	0CPS[7,8][0,D,Y]Z
Non-OR	0CPSX[0,7,D,J,K]Z
Non-OR	0CPY3YZ
Non-OR	0CPY[7,8][0,D,Y]Z
Non-OR	0CPYX[0,1,7,D,J,K]Z

NC Noncovered Procedure   **LC** Limited Coverage   **QA** Questionable OB Admit   **NT** New Tech Add-on   ⊞ Combination Member   ♂ Male   ♀ Female

ICD-10-PCS 2022   **365**

Mouth and Throat

Ø   **Medical and Surgical**
C   **Mouth and Throat**
Q   **Repair**   Definition: Restoring, to the extent possible, a body part to its normal anatomic structure and function
                   Explanation: Used only when the method to accomplish the repair is not one of the other root operations

Body Part Character 4	Approach Character 5	Device Character 6	Qualifier Character 7

Ø   **Upper Lip**
     Frenulum labii superioris
     Labial gland
     Vermilion border
1   **Lower Lip**
     Frenulum labii inferioris
     Labial gland
     Vermilion border
2   **Hard Palate**
3   **Soft Palate**
4   **Buccal Mucosa**
     Buccal gland
     Molar gland
     Palatine gland
5   **Upper Gingiva**
6   **Lower Gingiva**
7   **Tongue**
     Frenulum linguae
N   **Uvula**
     Palatine uvula
P   **Tonsils**
     Palatine tonsil
Q   **Adenoids**
     Pharyngeal tonsil
	Ø Open
	3 Percutaneous
	X External
		Z No Device	**Z** No Qualifier

8   **Parotid Gland, Right**
9   **Parotid Gland, Left**
B   **Parotid Duct, Right**
     Stensen's duct
C   **Parotid Duct, Left**
     See B Parotid Duct, Right
D   **Sublingual Gland, Right**
F   **Sublingual Gland, Left**
G   **Submaxillary Gland, Right**
     Submandibular gland
H   **Submaxillary Gland, Left**
     See G Submaxillary Gland, Right
J   **Minor Salivary Gland**
     Anterior lingual gland
	Ø Open
	3 Percutaneous
		Z No Device	**Z** No Qualifier

M   **Pharynx**
     Base of tongue
     Hypopharynx
     Laryngopharynx
     Lingual tonsil
     Oropharynx
     Piriform recess (sinus)
     Tongue, base of
R   **Epiglottis**
     Glossoepiglottic fold
S   **Larynx**
     Aryepiglottic fold
     Arytenoid cartilage
     Corniculate cartilage
     Cuneiform cartilage
     False vocal cord
     Glottis
     Rima glottidis
     Thyroid cartilage
     Ventricular fold
T   **Vocal Cord, Right**
     Vocal fold
V   **Vocal Cord, Left**
     See T Vocal Cord, Right
	Ø Open
	3 Percutaneous
	4 Percutaneous Endoscopic
	7 Via Natural or Artificial Opening
	8 Via Natural or Artificial Opening Endoscopic
		Z No Device	**Z** No Qualifier

W **Upper Tooth** **X** **Lower Tooth**	**Ø** Open **X** External	**Z** No Device	**Ø** Single **1** Multiple **2** All

Non-OR   ØCQ[Ø,1,4,7]XZZ
Non-OR   ØCQ[5,6][Ø,3,X]ZZ
Non-OR   ØCQ[W,X][Ø,X]Z[Ø,1,2]

Ø   Medical and Surgical
C   Mouth and Throat
R   Replacement   Definition: Putting in or on biological or synthetic material that physically takes the place and/or function of all or a portion of a body part

Explanation: The body part may have been taken out or replaced, or may be taken out, physically eradicated, or rendered nonfunctional during the REPLACEMENT procedure. A REMOVAL procedure is coded for taking out the device used in a previous replacement procedure.

Body Part Character 4	Approach Character 5	Device Character 6	Qualifier Character 7

Ø   **Upper Lip**
    Frenulum labii superioris
    Labial gland
    Vermilion border
1   **Lower Lip**
    Frenulum labii inferioris
    Labial gland
    Vermilion border
2   **Hard Palate**
3   **Soft Palate**
4   **Buccal Mucosa**
    Buccal gland
    Molar gland
    Palatine gland
5   **Upper Gingiva**
6   **Lower Gingiva**
7   **Tongue**
    Frenulum linguae
N   **Uvula**
    Palatine uvula
	Ø Open
	3 Percutaneous
	X External
		7 Autologous Tissue Substitute
		J Synthetic Substitute
		K Nonautologous Tissue Substitute
			Z No Qualifier

B   **Parotid Duct, Right**
    Stensen's duct
C   **Parotid Duct, Left**
    See B Parotid Duct, Right
	Ø Open
	3 Percutaneous
		7 Autologous Tissue Substitute
		J Synthetic Substitute
		K Nonautologous Tissue Substitute
			Z No Qualifier

M   **Pharynx**
    Base of tongue
    Hypopharynx
    Laryngopharynx
    Lingual tonsil
    Oropharynx
    Piriform recess (sinus)
    Tongue, base of
R   **Epiglottis**
    Glossoepiglottic fold
S   **Larynx**
    Aryepiglottic fold
    Arytenoid cartilage
    Corniculate cartilage
    Cuneiform cartilage
    False vocal cord
    Glottis
    Rima glottidis
    Thyroid cartilage
    Ventricular fold
T   **Vocal Cord, Right**
    Vocal fold
V   **Vocal Cord, Left**
    See T Vocal Cord, Right
	Ø Open
	7 Via Natural or Artificial Opening
	8 Via Natural or Artificial Opening
	    Endoscopic
		7 Autologous Tissue Substitute
		J Synthetic Substitute
		K Nonautologous Tissue Substitute
			Z No Qualifier

W **Upper Tooth** X **Lower Tooth**	Ø Open X External	7 Autologous Tissue Substitute J Synthetic Substitute K Nonautologous Tissue Substitute	Ø Single 1 Multiple 2 All

Non-OR   ØCR[W,X][Ø,X][7,J,K][Ø,1,2]

Mouth and Throat

Ø   **Medical and Surgical**
C   **Mouth and Throat**
S   **Reposition**   Definition: Moving to its normal location, or other suitable location, all or a portion of a body part

Explanation: The body part is moved to a new location from an abnormal location, or from a normal location where it is not functioning correctly. The body part may or may not be cut out or off to be moved to the new location.

Body Part Character 4	Approach Character 5	Device Character 6	Qualifier Character 7

Ø   **Upper Lip**
    Frenulum labii superioris
    Labial gland
    Vermilion border
1   **Lower Lip**
    Frenulum labii inferioris
    Labial gland
    Vermilion border
2   **Hard Palate**
3   **Soft Palate**
7   **Tongue**
    Frenulum linguae
N   **Uvula**
    Palatine uvula
	Ø Open
	X External
		Z No Device	Z No Qualifier

B   **Parotid Duct, Right**
    Stensen's duct
C   **Parotid Duct, Left**
    See B Parotid Duct, Right
	Ø Open
	3 Percutaneous
		Z No Device	Z No Qualifier

R   **Epiglottis**
    Glossoepiglottic fold
T   **Vocal Cord, Right**
    Vocal fold
V   **Vocal Cord, Left**
    See T Vocal Cord, Right
	Ø Open
	7 Via Natural or Artificial Opening
	8 Via Natural or Artificial Opening
	    Endoscopic
		Z No Device	Z No Qualifier

W **Upper Tooth** X **Lower Tooth**	Ø Open X External	5 External Fixation Device Z No Device	Ø Single 1 Multiple 2 All

Non-OR   ØCS[W,X][Ø,X][5,Z][Ø,1,2]

Ø   Medical and Surgical
C   Mouth and Throat
T   Resection   Definition: Cutting out or off, without replacement, all of a body part
                Explanation: None

Body Part Character 4	Approach Character 5	Device Character 6	Qualifier Character 7

Ø Upper Lip
  Frenulum labii superioris
  Labial gland
  Vermilion border
1 Lower Lip
  Frenulum labii inferioris
  Labial gland
  Vermilion border
2 Hard Palate
3 Soft Palate
7 Tongue
  Frenulum linguae
N Uvula
  Palatine uvula
P Tonsils
  Palatine tonsil
Q Adenoids
  Pharyngeal tonsil
	Ø Open
	X External
		Z No Device	Z No Qualifier

8 Parotid Gland, Right
9 Parotid Gland, Left
B Parotid Duct, Right
  Stensen's duct
C Parotid Duct, Left
  See B Parotid Duct, Right
D Sublingual Gland, Right
F Sublingual Gland, Left
G Submaxillary Gland, Right
  Submandibular gland
H Submaxillary Gland, Left
  See G Submaxillary Gland, Right
J Minor Salivary Gland
  Anterior lingual gland
	Ø Open	Z No Device	Z No Qualifier

M Pharynx
  Base of tongue
  Hypopharynx
  Laryngopharynx
  Lingual tonsil
  Oropharynx
  Piriform recess (sinus)
  Tongue, base of
R Epiglottis
  Glossoepiglottic fold
S Larynx
  Aryepiglottic fold
  Arytenoid cartilage
  Corniculate cartilage
  Cuneiform cartilage
  False vocal cord
  Glottis
  Rima glottidis
  Thyroid cartilage
  Ventricular fold
T Vocal Cord, Right
  Vocal fold
V Vocal Cord, Left
  See T Vocal Cord, Right
	Ø Open
	4 Percutaneous Endoscopic
	7 Via Natural or Artificial Opening
	8 Via Natural or Artificial Opening
	  Endoscopic
		Z No Device	Z No Qualifier

W Upper Tooth X Lower Tooth	Ø Open	Z No Device	Ø Single 1 Multiple 2 All

Non-OR   ØCT[W,X]ØZ[Ø,1,2]

NC Noncovered Procedure   LC Limited Coverage   QA Questionable OB Admit   NT New Tech Add-on   ⊞ Combination Member   ♂ Male   ♀ Female

ICD-10-PCS 2022   369

Mouth and Throat

Ø   **Medical and Surgical**
C   **Mouth and Throat**
U   **Supplement**   Definition: Putting in or on biological or synthetic material that physically reinforces and/or augments the function of a portion of a body part

            Explanation: The biological material is non-living, or is living and from the same individual. The body part may have been previously replaced, and the SUPPLEMENT procedure is performed to physically reinforce and/or augment the function of the replaced body part.

Body Part Character 4	Approach Character 5	Device Character 6	Qualifier Character 7

Ø **Upper Lip**
    Frenulum labii superioris
    Labial gland
    Vermilion border
1 **Lower Lip**
    Frenulum labii inferioris
    Labial gland
    Vermilion border
2 **Hard Palate**
3 **Soft Palate**
4 **Buccal Mucosa**
    Buccal gland
    Molar gland
    Palatine gland
5 **Upper Gingiva**
6 **Lower Gingiva**
7 **Tongue**
    Frenulum linguae
N **Uvula**
    Palatine uvula
	Ø Open
	3 Percutaneous
	X External
		7 Autologous Tissue Substitute
		J Synthetic Substitute
		K Nonautologous Tissue Substitute
			Z No Qualifier

M **Pharynx**
    Base of tongue
    Hypopharynx
    Laryngopharynx
    Lingual tonsil
    Oropharynx
    Piriform recess (sinus)
    Tongue, base of
R **Epiglottis**
    Glossoepiglottic fold
S **Larynx**
    Aryepiglottic fold
    Arytenoid cartilage
    Corniculate cartilage
    Cuneiform cartilage
    False vocal cord
    Glottis
    Rima glottidis
    Thyroid cartilage
    Ventricular fold
T **Vocal Cord, Right**
    Vocal fold
V **Vocal Cord, Left**
    See T Vocal Cord, Right
	Ø Open
	7 Via Natural or Artificial Opening
	8 Via Natural or Artificial Opening Endoscopic
		7 Autologous Tissue Substitute
		J Synthetic Substitute
		K Nonautologous Tissue Substitute
			Z No Qualifier

Non-OR   ØCU2[Ø,3]JZ

Ø   **Medical and Surgical**
C   **Mouth and Throat**
V   **Restriction**   Definition: Partially closing an orifice or the lumen of a tubular body part

            Explanation: The orifice can be a natural orifice or an artificially created orifice

Body Part Character 4	Approach Character 5	Device Character 6	Qualifier Character 7

B **Parotid Duct, Right**
    Stensen's duct
C **Parotid Duct, Left**
    See B Parotid Duct, Right
	Ø Open
	3 Percutaneous
		C Extraluminal Device
		D Intraluminal Device
		Z No Device
			Z No Qualifier

B **Parotid Duct, Right**
    Stensen's duct
C **Parotid Duct, Left**
    See B Parotid Duct, Right
	7 Via Natural or Artificial Opening
	8 Via Natural or Artificial Opening Endoscopic
		D Intraluminal Device
		Z No Device
			Z No Qualifier

Ø   Medical and Surgical
C   Mouth and Throat
W   Revision   Definition: Correcting, to the extent possible, a portion of a malfunctioning device or the position of a displaced device

                 Explanation: Revision can include correcting a malfunctioning or displaced device by taking out or putting in components of the device such as a screw or pin

Body Part Character 4	Approach Character 5	Device Character 6	Qualifier Character 7
A Salivary Gland	**Ø** Open **3** Percutaneous	**Ø** Drainage Device **C** Extraluminal Device **Y** Other Device	**Z** No Qualifier
A Salivary Gland	**7** Via Natural or Artificial Opening **8** Via Natural or Artificial Opening Endoscopic	**Y** Other Device	**Z** No Qualifier
A Salivary Gland	**X** External	**Ø** Drainage Device **C** Extraluminal Device	**Z** No Qualifier

S   Larynx
    Aryepiglottic fold
    Arytenoid cartilage
    Corniculate cartilage
    Cuneiform cartilage
    False vocal cord
    Glottis
    Rima glottidis
    Thyroid cartilage
    Ventricular fold
	Ø Open
	3 Percutaneous
	7 Via Natural or Artificial Opening
	8 Via Natural or Artificial Opening Endoscopic
		Ø Drainage Device
		7 Autologous Tissue Substitute
		D Intraluminal Device
		J Synthetic Substitute
		K Nonautologous Tissue Substitute
		Y Other Device
			Z No Qualifier

S   Larynx
    Aryepiglottic fold
    Arytenoid cartilage
    Corniculate cartilage
    Cuneiform cartilage
    False vocal cord
    Glottis
    Rima glottidis
    Thyroid cartilage
    Ventricular fold
	X External	**Ø** Drainage Device
		7 Autologous Tissue Substitute
		D Intraluminal Device
		J Synthetic Substitute
		K Nonautologous Tissue Substitute
			Z No Qualifier

Y Mouth and Throat	**Ø** Open **3** Percutaneous **7** Via Natural or Artificial Opening **8** Via Natural or Artificial Opening Endoscopic	**Ø** Drainage Device **1** Radioactive Element **7** Autologous Tissue Substitute **D** Intraluminal Device **J** Synthetic Substitute **K** Nonautologous Tissue Substitute **Y** Other Device	**Z** No Qualifier
Y Mouth and Throat	**X** External	**Ø** Drainage Device **1** Radioactive Element **7** Autologous Tissue Substitute **D** Intraluminal Device **J** Synthetic Substitute **K** Nonautologous Tissue Substitute	**Z** No Qualifier

Non-OR	ØCWA[Ø,3][Ø,C,Y]Z
Non-OR	ØCWA[7,8]YZ
Non-OR	ØCWAX[Ø,C]Z
Non-OR	ØCWS[3,7,8]YZ
Non-OR	ØCWSX[Ø,7,D,J,K]Z
Non-OR	ØCWYØ7Z
Non-OR	ØCWY[3,7,8]YZ
Non-OR	ØCWYX[Ø,1,7,D,J,K]Z

NC Noncovered Procedure   LC Limited Coverage   QA Questionable OB Admit   NT New Tech Add-on   ⊞ Combination Member   ♂ Male   ♀ Female

ICD-10-PCS 2022   371

Ø **Medical and Surgical**
C **Mouth and Throat**
X **Transfer**   Definition: Moving, without taking out, all or a portion of a body part to another location to take over the function of all or a portion of a body part
Explanation: The body part transferred remains connected to its vascular and nervous supply

Body Part Character 4	Approach Character 5	Device Character 6	Qualifier Character 7
Ø **Upper Lip** Frenulum labii superioris Labial gland Vermilion border **1** **Lower Lip** Frenulum labii inferioris Labial gland Vermilion border **3** **Soft Palate** **4** **Buccal Mucosa** Buccal gland Molar gland Palatine gland **5** **Upper Gingiva** **6** **Lower Gingiva** **7** **Tongue** Frenulum linguae	**Ø** Open **X** External	**Z** No Device	**Z** No Qualifier

Gastrointestinal System ØD1–ØDY

Character Meanings

This Character Meaning table is provided as a guide to assist the user in the identification of character members that may be found in this section of code tables. It **SHOULD NOT** be used to build a PCS code.

Operation–Character 3		Body Part–Character 4		Approach–Character 5		Device–Character 6		Qualifier–Character 7	
1	Bypass	Ø	Upper Intestinal Tract	Ø	Open	Ø	Drainage Device	Ø	Allogeneic
2	Change	1	Esophagus, Upper	3	Percutaneous	1	Radioactive Element	1	Syngeneic
5	Destruction	2	Esophagus, Middle	4	Percutaneous Endoscopic	2	Monitoring Device	2	Zooplastic
7	Dilation	3	Esophagus, Lower	7	Via Natural or Artificial Opening	3	Infusion Device	3	Vertical
8	Division	4	Esophagogastric Junction	8	Via Natural or Artificial Opening Endoscopic	7	Autologous Tissue Substitute	4	Cutaneous
9	Drainage	5	Esophagus	F	Via Natural or Artificial Opening with Percutaneous Endoscopic Assistance	B	Intraluminal Device, Airway	5	Esophagus
B	Excision	6	Stomach	X	External	C	Extraluminal Device	6	Stomach
C	Extirpation	7	Stomach, Pylorus			D	Intraluminal Device	7	Vagina
D	Extraction	8	Small Intestine			J	Synthetic Substitute	8	Small Intestine
F	Fragmentation	9	Duodenum			K	Nonautologous Tissue Substitute	9	Duodenum
H	Insertion	A	Jejunum			L	Artificial Sphincter	A	Jejunum
J	Inspection	B	Ileum			M	Stimulator Lead	B	Ileum
L	Occlusion	C	Ileocecal Valve			U	Feeding Device	E	Large Intestine
M	Reattachment	D	Lower Intestinal Tract			Y	Other Device	H	Cecum
N	Release	E	Large Intestine			Z	No Device	K	Ascending Colon
P	Removal	F	Large Intestine, Right					L	Transverse Colon
Q	Repair	G	Large Intestine, Left					M	Descending Colon
R	Replacement	H	Cecum					N	Sigmoid Colon
S	Reposition	J	Appendix					P	Rectum
T	Resection	K	Ascending Colon					Q	Anus
U	Supplement	L	Transverse Colon					X	Diagnostic
V	Restriction	M	Descending Colon					Z	No Qualifier
W	Revision	N	Sigmoid Colon						
X	Transfer	P	Rectum						
Y	Transplantation	Q	Anus						
		R	Anal Sphincter						
		U	Omentum						
		V	Mesentery						
		W	Peritoneum						

Gastrointestinal System

AHA Coding Clinic for table ØD1
2021, 1Q, 19	Kock pouch revision surgery
2019, 4Q, 29	Intestinal bypass
2017, 2Q, 17	Billroth II (distal gastrectomy and gastrojejunostomy)
2016, 2Q, 31	Laparoscopic biliopancreatic diversion with duodenal switch
2014, 4Q, 41	Abdominoperineal resection (APR) with flap closure of perineum and colostomy

AHA Coding Clinic for table ØD2
2019, 1Q, 26	Exchange of clogged gastrojejunostomy tube

AHA Coding Clinic for table ØD5
2017, 1Q, 34	Debulking of tumor and peritoneum ablation

AHA Coding Clinic for table ØD7
2020, 3Q, 45	Dilation versus drainage of perirectal cyst
2017, 3Q, 23	Laparoscopic pyloromyotomy
2014, 4Q, 40	Dilation of gastrojejunostomy anastomosis stricture

AHA Coding Clinic for table ØD8
2019, 2Q, 15	Reversal of Roux-en-Y bypass
2017, 3Q, 22	Laparoscopic esophagomyotomy (Heller type) and Toupet fundoplication
2017, 3Q, 23	Laparoscopic pyloromyotomy

AHA Coding Clinic for table ØD9
2020, 3Q, 45	Dilation versus drainage of perirectal cyst
2015, 2Q, 29	Insertion of nasogastric tube for drainage and feeding

AHA Coding Clinic for table ØDB
2021, 2Q, 11	Serosal injury with excision of small intestine
2021, 1Q, 20	Rectal suction biopsy
2021, 1Q, 22	Total proctocolectomy with creation of J-pouch
2019, 2Q, 15	Reversal of Roux-en-Y bypass
2019, 1Q, 3-8	Whipple procedure
2019, 1Q, 27	Excision of pelvic sidewall mass
2017, 2Q, 17	Billroth II (distal gastrectomy and gastrojejunostomy)
2017, 1Q, 16	Hepatic flexure versus transverse colon
2016, 3Q, 3-7	Stoma creation & takedown procedures
2016, 2Q, 31	Laparoscopic biliopancreatic diversion with duodenal switch
2016, 1Q, 22	Perineal proctectomy
2016, 1Q, 24	Endoscopic brush biopsy of esophagus
2014, 4Q, 40	Abdominoperineal resection (APR) with flap closure of perineum and colostomy
2014, 3Q, 28	Ileostomy takedown and parastomal hernia repair
2014, 3Q, 32	Pyloric-sparing Whipple procedure

AHA Coding Clinic for table ØDD
2021, 1Q, 20	Rectal suction biopsy
2017, 4Q, 41-42	Extraction procedures

AHA Coding Clinic for table ØDH
2020, 4Q, 43-44	Insertion of radioactive element
2020, 3Q, 43	Staged laparoscopic gastric conduit and placement of feeding tube
2019, 2Q, 18	Endoscopic wound VAC placement
2016, 3Q, 26	Insertion of gastrostomy tube
2013, 4Q, 117	Percutaneous endoscopic placement of gastrostomy tube

AHA Coding Clinic for table ØDJ
2019, 1Q, 25	Laparoscopic appendectomy converted to open procedure
2019, 1Q, 25	Milking of inspissated material from ileum to colon
2017, 2Q, 15	Low anterior resection with sigmoidoscopy
2016, 2Q, 20	Capsule endoscopy of small intestine
2015, 3Q, 24	Esophagogastroduodenoscopy with epinephrine injection for control of bleeding

AHA Coding Clinic for table ØDL
2013, 4Q, 112	Endoscopic banding of esophageal varices

AHA Coding Clinic for table ØDN
2017, 4Q, 49-50	New and revised body part values - Repositioning of the intestine
2017, 1Q, 35	Lysis of omental and peritoneal adhesions
2015, 3Q, 15	Vascular ring surgery with release of esophagus and trachea
2015, 3Q, 16	Vascular ring surgery and double aortic arch

AHA Coding Clinic for table ØDP
2019, 2Q, 18	Removal of wound VAC

AHA Coding Clinic for table ØDQ
2019, 2Q, 15	Reversal of Roux-en-Y bypass
2018, 2Q, 25	Third and fourth degree obstetric lacerations
2018, 1Q, 11	Repair of internal hernia at Petersen space
2017, 3Q, 17	Posterior sagittal anorectoplasty
2016, 3Q, 3-7	Stoma creation & takedown procedures
2016, 3Q, 26	Insertion of gastrostomy tube
2016, 1Q, 7	Obstetrical perineal laceration repair
2016, 1Q, 8	Obstetrical perineal laceration repair
2014, 4Q, 20	Control of bleeding duodenal ulcer

AHA Coding Clinic for table ØDS
2019, 1Q, 30	Laparoscopic-assisted rectopexy with manual reduction of prolapse
2017, 4Q, 49-50	New and revised body part values - Repositioning of the intestine
2017, 3Q, 9	Ileocolic intussusception reduction via air enema
2017, 3Q, 17	Posterior sagittal anorectoplasty
2016, 3Q, 3-5	Stoma creation & takedown procedures

AHA Coding Clinic for table ØDT
2021, 1Q, 22	Total proctocolectomy with creation of J-pouch
2020, 4Q, 100	Robotic-assisted sigmoid colectomy with extension of incision for specimen removal
2019, 1Q, 3-8	Whipple procedure
2019, 1Q, 14	Esophagectomy with colon interposition
2017, 4Q, 49-50	New and revised body part values - Repositioning of the intestine
2014, 4Q, 40	Abdominoperineal resection (APR) with flap closure of perineum and colostomy
2014, 4Q, 42	Right colectomy with side-to-side functional end-to-end anastomosis
2014, 3Q, 6	Ileocecectomy including cecum, terminal ileum and appendix
2014, 3Q, 6	Right colectomy

AHA Coding Clinic for table ØDU
2021, 2Q, 20	Malone antegrade continence enema procedure
2021, 1Q, 22	Total proctocolectomy with creation of J-pouch
2019, 1Q, 30	Laparoscopic-assisted rectopexy with manual reduction of prolapse

AHA Coding Clinic for table ØDV
2017, 3Q, 22	Laparoscopic esophagomyotomy (Heller type) and Toupet fundoplication
2016, 2Q, 22	Esophageal lengthening Collis gastroplasty with Nissen fundoplication and hiatal hernia
2014, 3Q, 28	Laparoscopic Nissen fundoplication and diaphragmatic hernia repair

AHA Coding Clinic for table ØDW
2021, 1Q, 19	Kock pouch revision surgery
2018, 1Q, 20	Adjustment of gastric band

AHA Coding Clinic for table ØDX
2019, 4Q, 29-30	Transfer large intestine to vagina
2019, 1Q, 14	Esophagectomy with colon interposition
2017, 2Q, 18	Esophagectomy and esophagogastrectomy with cervical esophagogastrostomy
2016, 2Q, 22	Esophageal lengthening Collis gastroplasty with Nissen fundoplication and hiatal hernia
2015, 1Q, 28	Repair of bronchopleural fistula using omental pedicle graft

Upper Intestinal Tract (Ø) and Lower Intestinal Tract (D)

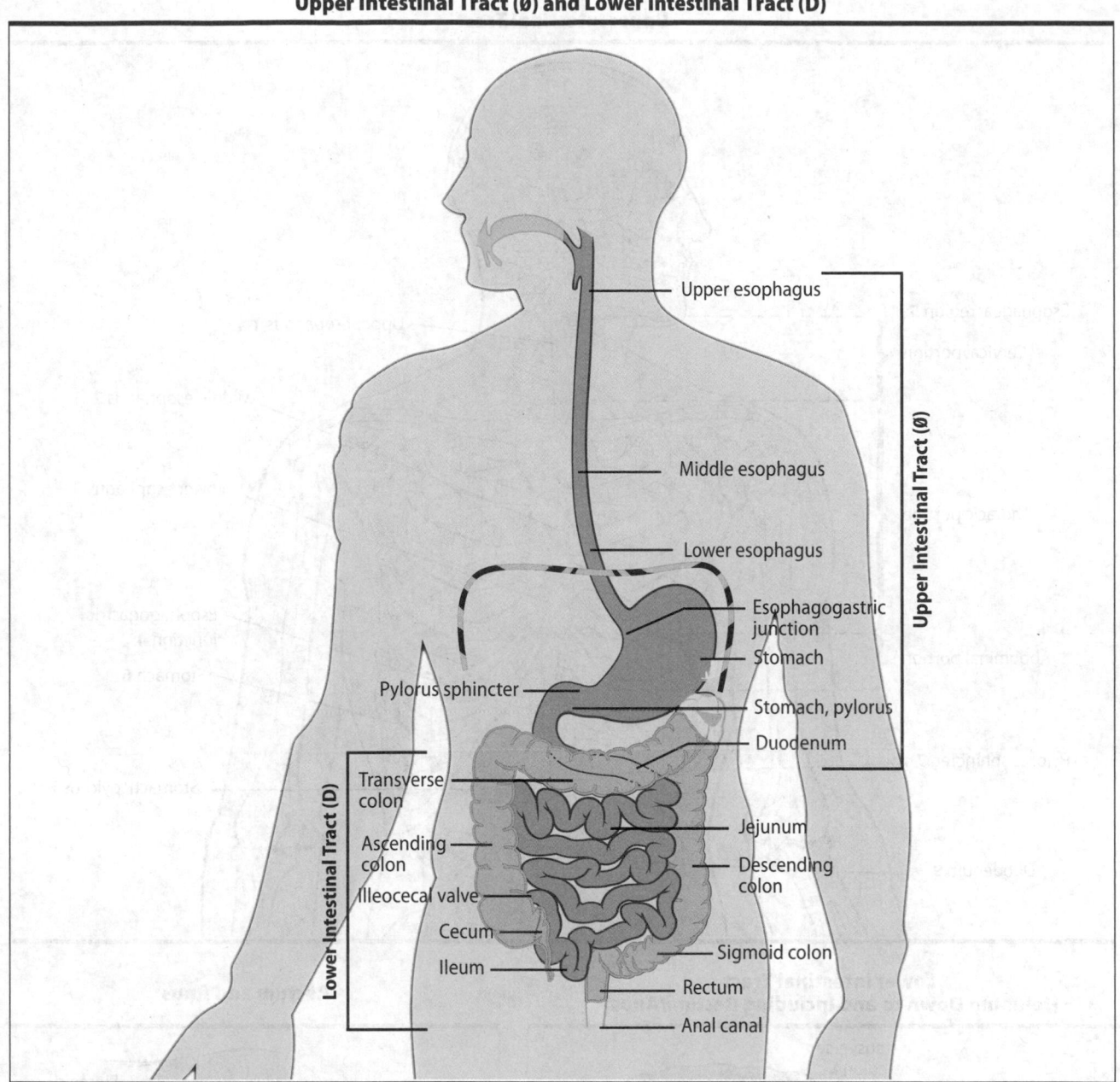

Upper Intestinal Tract

Esophageal region **5**:

Cervical portion

Thoracic portion

Abdominal portion

Pylorus sphincter **7**

Duodenum **9**

Upper esophagus **1**

Middle esophagus **2**

Lower esophagus **3**

Esophagogastric junction **4**

Stomach **6**

Stomach, pylorus **7**

Lower Intestinal Tract
(Jejunum Down to and Including Rectum/Anus)

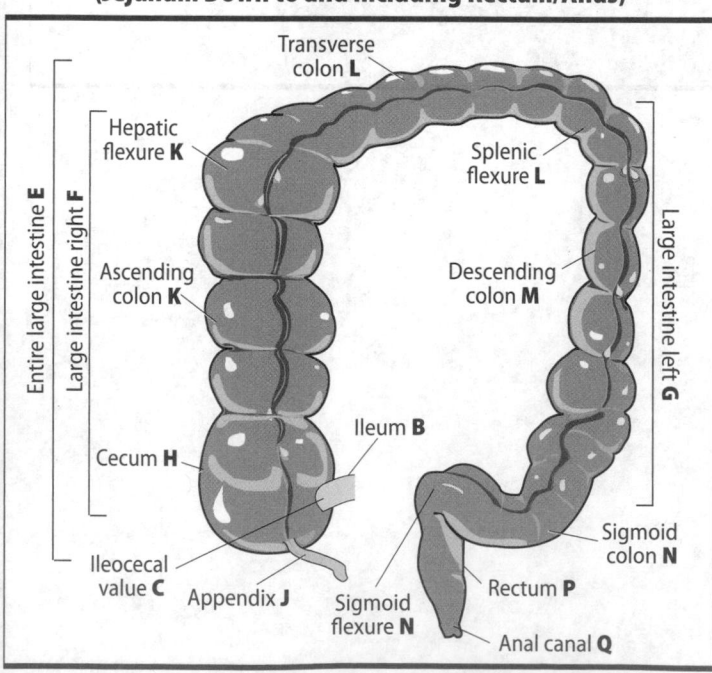

Transverse colon **L**

Hepatic flexure **K**

Splenic flexure **L**

Entire large intestine **E**

Large intestine right **F**

Ascending colon **K**

Descending colon **M**

Large intestine left **G**

Cecum **H**

Ileum **B**

Ileocecal value **C**

Appendix **J**

Sigmoid flexure **N**

Rectum **P**

Sigmoid colon **N**

Anal canal **Q**

Rectum and Anus

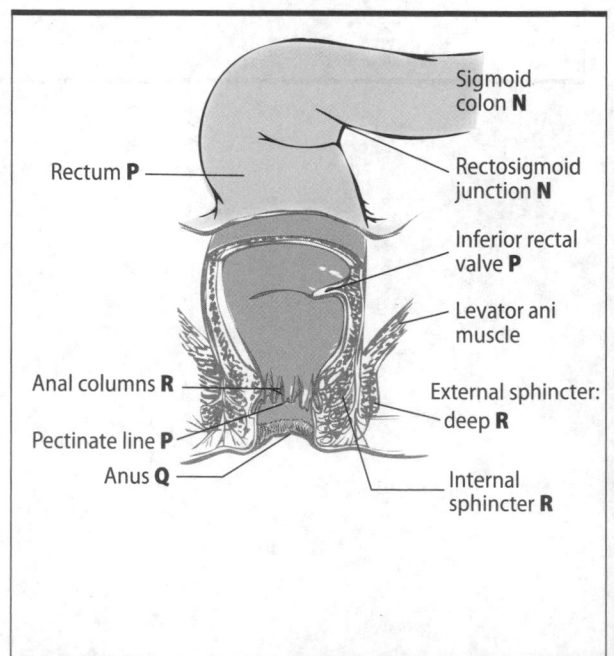

Rectum **P**

Anal columns **R**

Pectinate line **P**

Anus **Q**

Sigmoid colon **N**

Rectosigmoid junction **N**

Inferior rectal valve **P**

Levator ani muscle

External sphincter: deep **R**

Internal sphincter **R**

Ø　Medical and Surgical
D　Gastrointestinal System
1　Bypass　　Definition: Altering the route of passage of the contents of a tubular body part
　　　　　　　　Explanation: Rerouting contents of a body part to a downstream area of the normal route, to a similar route and body part, or to an abnormal route and dissimilar body part. Includes one or more anastomoses, with or without the use of a device.

Body Part Character 4	Approach Character 5	Device Character 6	Qualifier Character 7
1 Esophagus, Upper 　Cervical esophagus **2** Esophagus, Middle 　Thoracic esophagus **3** Esophagus, Lower 　Abdominal esophagus **5** Esophagus	**Ø** Open **4** Percutaneous Endoscopic **8** Via Natural or Artificial Opening Endoscopic	**7** Autologous Tissue Substitute **J** Synthetic Substitute **K** Nonautologous Tissue Substitute **Z** No Device	**4** Cutaneous **6** Stomach **9** Duodenum **A** Jejunum **B** Ileum
1 Esophagus, Upper 　Cervical esophagus **2** Esophagus, Middle 　Thoracic esophagus **3** Esophagus, Lower 　Abdominal esophagus **5** Esophagus	**3** Percutaneous	**J** Synthetic Substitute	**4** Cutaneous
6 Stomach **9** Duodenum	**Ø** Open **4** Percutaneous Endoscopic **8** Via Natural or Artificial Opening Endoscopic	**7** Autologous Tissue Substitute **J** Synthetic Substitute **K** Nonautologous Tissue Substitute **Z** No Device	**4** Cutaneous **9** Duodenum **A** Jejunum **B** Ileum **L** Transverse Colon
6 Stomach **9** Duodenum	**3** Percutaneous	**J** Synthetic Substitute	**4** Cutaneous
8 Small Intestine	**Ø** Open **4** Percutaneous Endoscopic **8** Via Natural or Artificial Opening Endoscopic	**7** Autologous Tissue Substitute **J** Synthetic Substitute **K** Nonautologous Tissue Substitute **Z** No Device	**4** Cutaneous **8** Small Intestine **H** Cecum **K** Ascending Colon **L** Transverse Colon **M** Descending Colon **N** Sigmoid Colon **P** Rectum **Q** Anus
A Jejunum 　Duodenojejunal flexure	**Ø** Open **4** Percutaneous Endoscopic **8** Via Natural or Artificial Opening Endoscopic	**7** Autologous Tissue Substitute **J** Synthetic Substitute **K** Nonautologous Tissue Substitute **Z** No Device	**4** Cutaneous **A** Jejunum **B** Ileum **H** Cecum **K** Ascending Colon **L** Transverse Colon **M** Descending Colon **N** Sigmoid Colon **P** Rectum **Q** Anus
A Jejunum 　Duodenojejunal flexure	**3** Percutaneous	**J** Synthetic Substitute	**4** Cutaneous
B Ileum	**Ø** Open **4** Percutaneous Endoscopic **8** Via Natural or Artificial Opening Endoscopic	**7** Autologous Tissue Substitute **J** Synthetic Substitute **K** Nonautologous Tissue Substitute **Z** No Device	**4** Cutaneous **B** Ileum **H** Cecum **K** Ascending Colon **L** Transverse Colon **M** Descending Colon **N** Sigmoid Colon **P** Rectum **Q** Anus
B Ileum	**3** Percutaneous	**J** Synthetic Substitute	**4** Cutaneous
E Large Intestine	**Ø** Open **4** Percutaneous Endoscopic **8** Via Natural or Artificial Opening Endoscopic	**7** Autologous Tissue Substitute **J** Synthetic Substitute **K** Nonautologous Tissue Substitute **Z** No Device	**4** Cutaneous **E** Large Intestine **P** Rectum
H Cecum	**Ø** Open **4** Percutaneous Endoscopic **8** Via Natural or Artificial Opening Endoscopic	**7** Autologous Tissue Substitute **J** Synthetic Substitute **K** Nonautologous Tissue Substitute **Z** No Device	**4** Cutaneous **H** Cecum **K** Ascending Colon **L** Transverse Colon **M** Descending Colon **N** Sigmoid Colon **P** Rectum
H Cecum	**3** Percutaneous	**J** Synthetic Substitute	**4** Cutaneous

Non-OR　ØD16[Ø,4,8][7,J,K,Z]4
Non-OR　ØD163J4
HAC　ØD16[Ø,4,8][7,J,K,Z][9,A,B,L] when reported with PDx E66.Ø1 and SDx K68.11, K95.Ø1, K95.81 or T81.4Ø–T81.49 with 7th character A

ØD1 Continued on next page

ØD1 Continued

Ø **Medical and Surgical**
D **Gastrointestinal System**
1 **Bypass**　　　Definition: Altering the route of passage of the contents of a tubular body part

Explanation: Rerouting contents of a body part to a downstream area of the normal route, to a similar route and body part, or to an abnormal route and dissimilar body part. Includes one or more anastomoses, with or without the use of a device.

Body Part Character 4	Approach Character 5	Device Character 6	Qualifier Character 7
K　Ascending Colon	Ø　Open 4　Percutaneous Endoscopic 8　Via Natural or Artificial Opening 　　Endoscopic	7　Autologous Tissue Substitute J　Synthetic Substitute K　Nonautologous Tissue Substitute Z　No Device	4　Cutaneous K　Ascending Colon L　Transverse Colon M　Descending Colon N　Sigmoid Colon P　Rectum
K　Ascending Colon	3　Percutaneous	J　Synthetic Substitute	4　Cutaneous
L　Transverse Colon 　　Hepatic flexure 　　Splenic flexure	Ø　Open 4　Percutaneous Endoscopic 8　Via Natural or Artificial Opening 　　Endoscopic	7　Autologous Tissue Substitute J　Synthetic Substitute K　Nonautologous Tissue Substitute Z　No Device	4　Cutaneous L　Transverse Colon M　Descending Colon N　Sigmoid Colon P　Rectum
L　Transverse Colon 　　Hepatic flexure 　　Splenic flexure	3　Percutaneous	J　Synthetic Substitute	4　Cutaneous
M　Descending Colon	Ø　Open 4　Percutaneous Endoscopic 8　Via Natural or Artificial Opening 　　Endoscopic	7　Autologous Tissue Substitute J　Synthetic Substitute K　Nonautologous Tissue Substitute Z　No Device	4　Cutaneous M　Descending Colon N　Sigmoid Colon P　Rectum
M　Descending Colon	3　Percutaneous	J　Synthetic Substitute	4　Cutaneous
N　Sigmoid Colon 　　Rectosigmoid junction 　　Sigmoid flexure	Ø　Open 4　Percutaneous Endoscopic 8　Via Natural or Artificial Opening 　　Endoscopic	7　Autologous Tissue Substitute J　Synthetic Substitute K　Nonautologous Tissue Substitute Z　No Device	4　Cutaneous N　Sigmoid Colon P　Rectum
N　Sigmoid Colon 　　Rectosigmoid junction 　　Sigmoid flexure	3　Percutaneous	J　Synthetic Substitute	4　Cutaneous

Ø **Medical and Surgical**
D **Gastrointestinal System**
2 **Change**　　　Definition: Taking out or off a device from a body part and putting back an identical or similar device in or on the same body part without cutting or puncturing the skin or a mucous membrane

Explanation: All CHANGE procedures are coded using the approach EXTERNAL

Body Part Character 4	Approach Character 5	Device Character 6	Qualifier Character 7
Ø　Upper Intestinal Tract D　Lower Intestinal Tract	X　External	Ø　Drainage Device U　Feeding Device Y　Other Device	Z　No Qualifier
U　Omentum 　　Gastrocolic ligament 　　Gastrocolic omentum 　　Gastrohepatic omentum 　　Gastrophrenic ligament 　　Gastrosplenic ligament 　　Greater Omentum 　　Hepatogastric ligament 　　Lesser Omentum V　Mesentery 　　Mesoappendix 　　Mesocolon W　Peritoneum 　　Epiploic foramen	X　External	Ø　Drainage Device Y　Other Device	Z　No Qualifier

Non-OR　All body part, approach, device, and qualifier values

Ø	**Medical and Surgical**
D	**Gastrointestinal System**
5	**Destruction** Definition: Physical eradication of all or a portion of a body part by the direct use of energy, force, or a destructive agent
	Explanation: None of the body part is physically taken out

Body Part Character 4	Approach Character 5	Device Character 6	Qualifier Character 7
1 Esophagus, Upper Cervical esophagus **2 Esophagus, Middle** Thoracic esophagus **3 Esophagus, Lower** Abdominal esophagus **4 Esophagogastric Junction** Cardia Cardioesophageal junction Gastroesophageal (GE) junction **5 Esophagus** **6 Stomach** **7 Stomach, Pylorus** Pyloric antrum Pyloric canal Pyloric sphincter **8 Small Intestine** **9 Duodenum** **A Jejunum** Duodenojejunal flexure **B Ileum** **C Ileocecal Valve** **E Large Intestine** **F Large Intestine, Right** **G Large Intestine, Left** **H Cecum** **J Appendix** Vermiform appendix **K Ascending Colon** **L Transverse Colon** Hepatic flexure Splenic flexure **M Descending Colon** **N Sigmoid Colon** Rectosigmoid junction Sigmoid flexure **P Rectum** Anorectal junction	**Ø Open** **3 Percutaneous** **4 Percutaneous Endoscopic** **7 Via Natural or Artificial Opening** **8 Via Natural or Artificial Opening Endoscopic**	**Z No Device**	**Z No Qualifier**
Q Anus Anal orifice	**Ø Open** **3 Percutaneous** **4 Percutaneous Endoscopic** **7 Via Natural or Artificial Opening** **8 Via Natural or Artificial Opening Endoscopic** **X External**	**Z No Device**	**Z No Qualifier**
R Anal Sphincter External anal sphincter Internal anal sphincter **U Omentum** Gastrocolic ligament Gastrocolic omentum Gastrohepatic omentum Gastrophrenic ligament Gastrosplenic ligament Greater Omentum Hepatogastric ligament Lesser Omentum **V Mesentery** Mesoappendix Mesocolon **W Peritoneum** Epiploic foramen	**Ø Open** **3 Percutaneous** **4 Percutaneous Endoscopic**	**Z No Device**	**Z No Qualifier**

Non-OR   0D5[1,2,3,4,5,6,7,9,E,F,G,H,K,L,M,N][4,8]ZZ
Non-OR   0D5[8,A,B,C]8ZZ
Non-OR   0D5P[0,3,4,7,8]ZZ
Non-OR   0D5Q[4,8]ZZ
Non-OR   0D5R4ZZ

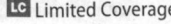 Noncovered Procedure   **LC** Limited Coverage   **QA** Questionable OB Admit   **NT** New Tech Add-on   ⊞ Combination Member   ♂ Male   ♀ Female

ICD-10-PCS 2022   379

0D5–0D5

Ø   Medical and Surgical
D   Gastrointestinal System
7   Dilation   Definition: Expanding an orifice or the lumen of a tubular body part

Explanation: The orifice can be a natural orifice or an artificially created orifice. Accomplished by stretching a tubular body part using intraluminal pressure or by cutting part of the orifice or wall of the tubular body part.

Body Part Character 4	Approach Character 5	Device Character 6	Qualifier Character 7

1 Esophagus, Upper
   Cervical esophagus
2 Esophagus, Middle
   Thoracic esophagus
3 Esophagus, Lower
   Abdominal esophagus
4 Esophagogastric Junction
   Cardia
   Cardioesophageal junction
   Gastroesophageal (GE) junction
5 Esophagus
6 Stomach
7 Stomach, Pylorus
   Pyloric antrum
   Pyloric canal
   Pyloric sphincter
8 Small Intestine
9 Duodenum
A Jejunum
   Duodenojejunal flexure
B Ileum
C Ileocecal Valve
E Large Intestine
F Large Intestine, Right
G Large Intestine, Left
H Cecum
K Ascending Colon
L Transverse Colon
   Hepatic flexure
   Splenic flexure
M Descending Colon
N Sigmoid Colon
   Rectosigmoid junction
   Sigmoid flexure
P Rectum
   Anorectal junction
Q Anus
   Anal orifice
	Ø Open
	3 Percutaneous
	4 Percutaneous Endoscopic
	7 Via Natural or Artificial Opening
	8 Via Natural or Artificial Opening
	   Endoscopic
		D Intraluminal Device
		Z No Device
			Z No Qualifier

Non-OR	ØD7[1,2,3,4,5,6,8,9,A,B,C,E,F,G,H,K,L,M,N,P,Q][7,8][D,Z]Z
Non-OR	ØD77[4,8]DZ
Non-OR	ØD777[D,Z]Z
Non-OR	ØD7[8,9,A,B,C,E,F,G,H,K,L,M,N][Ø,3,4]DZ

Ø   Medical and Surgical
D   Gastrointestinal System
8   Division   Definition: Cutting into a body part, without draining fluids and/or gases from the body part, in order to separate or transect a body part

Explanation: All or a portion of the body part is separated into two or more portions

Body Part Character 4	Approach Character 5	Device Character 6	Qualifier Character 7

4 Esophagogastric Junction
   Cardia
   Cardioesophageal junction
   Gastroesophageal (GE) junction
7 Stomach, Pylorus
   Pyloric antrum
   Pyloric canal
   Pyloric sphincter
	Ø Open
	3 Percutaneous
	4 Percutaneous Endoscopic
	7 Via Natural or Artificial Opening
	8 Via Natural or Artificial Opening
	   Endoscopic
		Z No Device	Z No Qualifier

R Anal Sphincter
   External anal sphincter
   Internal anal sphincter
	Ø Open
	3 Percutaneous
		Z No Device	Z No Qualifier

Ø Medical and Surgical
D Gastrointestinal System
9 Drainage   Definition: Taking or letting out fluids and/or gases from a body part
         Explanation: The qualifier DIAGNOSTIC is used to identify drainage procedures that are biopsies

Body Part Character 4		Approach Character 5	Device Character 6	Qualifier Character 7

1 Esophagus, Upper
  Cervical esophagus
2 Esophagus, Middle
  Thoracic esophagus
3 Esophagus, Lower
  Abdominal esophagus
4 Esophagogastric Junction
  Cardia
  Cardioesophageal junction
  Gastroesophageal (GE) junction
5 Esophagus
6 Stomach
7 Stomach, Pylorus
  Pyloric antrum
  Pyloric canal
  Pyloric sphincter
8 Small Intestine
9 Duodenum
	A Jejunum
	  Duodenojejunal flexure
	B Ileum
	C Ileocecal Valve
	E Large Intestine
	F Large Intestine, Right
	G Large Intestine, Left
	H Cecum
	J Appendix
	  Vermiform appendix
	K Ascending Colon
	L Transverse Colon
	  Hepatic flexure
	  Splenic flexure
	M Descending Colon
	N Sigmoid Colon
	  Rectosigmoid junction
	  Sigmoid flexure
	P Rectum
	  Anorectal junction
		Ø Open
		3 Percutaneous
		4 Percutaneous Endoscopic
		7 Via Natural or Artificial Opening
		8 Via Natural or Artificial Opening Endoscopic
			Ø Drainage Device	Z No Qualifier

1 Esophagus, Upper
  Cervical esophagus
2 Esophagus, Middle
  Thoracic esophagus
3 Esophagus, Lower
  Abdominal esophagus
4 Esophagogastric Junction
  Cardia
  Cardioesophageal junction
  Gastroesophageal (GE) junction
5 Esophagus
6 Stomach
7 Stomach, Pylorus
  Pyloric antrum
  Pyloric canal
  Pyloric sphincter
8 Small Intestine
9 Duodenum
	A Jejunum
	  Duodenojejunal flexure
	B Ileum
	C Ileocecal Valve
	E Large Intestine
	F Large Intestine, Right
	G Large Intestine, Left
	H Cecum
	J Appendix
	  Vermiform appendix
	K Ascending Colon
	L Transverse Colon
	  Hepatic flexure
	  Splenic flexure
	M Descending Colon
	N Sigmoid Colon
	  Rectosigmoid junction
	  Sigmoid flexure
	P Rectum
	  Anorectal junction
		Ø Open
		3 Percutaneous
		4 Percutaneous Endoscopic
		7 Via Natural or Artificial Opening
		8 Via Natural or Artificial Opening Endoscopic
			Z No Device	X Diagnostic
				Z No Qualifier

Q Anus Anal orifice		Ø Open 3 Percutaneous 4 Percutaneous Endoscopic 7 Via Natural or Artificial Opening 8 Via Natural or Artificial Opening Endoscopic X External	Ø Drainage Device	Z No Qualifier
Q Anus Anal orifice		Ø Open 3 Percutaneous 4 Percutaneous Endoscopic 7 Via Natural or Artificial Opening 8 Via Natural or Artificial Opening Endoscopic X External	Z No Device	X Diagnostic Z No Qualifier

Non-OR	ØD9[1,2,3,4,5,C,J]3ØZ
Non-OR	ØD9[6,7,8,9,A,B,E,F,G,H,K,L,M,N,P][3,7,8]ØZ
Non-OR	ØD9[1,2,3,4,5,6,7,8,9,A,B,C,E,F,G,H,K,L,M,N,P][3,4,7,8]ZX
Non-OR	ØD9[1,2,3,4,5,6,7,8,9,A,B,C,E,F,G,H,J,K,L,M,N,P]3ZZ
Non-OR	ØD9Q3ØZ
Non-OR	ØD9Q[Ø,3,4,7,8,X]ZX
Non-OR	ØD9Q3ZZ

ØD9 Continued on next page

ØD9 Continued

Ø   **Medical and Surgical**
D   **Gastrointestinal System**
9   **Drainage**   Definition: Taking or letting out fluids and/or gases from a body part
                       Explanation: The qualifier DIAGNOSTIC is used to identify drainage procedures that are biopsies

Body Part Character 4	Approach Character 5	Device Character 6	Qualifier Character 7
R Anal Sphincter External anal sphincter Internal anal sphincter **U Omentum** Gastrocolic ligament Gastrocolic omentum Gastrohepatic omentum Gastrophrenic ligament Gastrosplenic ligament Greater Omentum Hepatogastric ligament Lesser Omentum **V Mesentery** Mesoappendix Mesocolon **W Peritoneum** Epiploic foramen	**Ø** Open **3** Percutaneous **4** Percutaneous Endoscopic	**Ø** Drainage Device	**Z** No Qualifier
R Anal Sphincter External anal sphincter Internal anal sphincter **U Omentum** Gastrocolic ligament Gastrocolic omentum Gastrohepatic omentum Gastrophrenic ligament Gastrosplenic ligament Greater Omentum Hepatogastric ligament Lesser Omentum **V Mesentery** Mesoappendix Mesocolon **W Peritoneum** Epiploic foramen	**Ø** Open **3** Percutaneous **4** Percutaneous Endoscopic	**Z** No Device	**X** Diagnostic **Z** No Qualifier

Non-OR	ØD9[R,W]3ØZ
Non-OR	ØD9[U,V][3,4]ØZ
Non-OR	ØD9[R,U,V,W]3Z[X,Z]
Non-OR	ØD9R[Ø,4]ZX
Non-OR	ØD9[U,V]4ZZ

Gastrointestinal System

Ø   **Medical and Surgical**
D   **Gastrointestinal System**
B   **Excision**   Definition: Cutting out or off, without replacement, a portion of a body part

                       Explanation: The qualifier DIAGNOSTIC is used to identify excision procedures that are biopsies

Body Part Character 4		Approach Character 5	Device Character 6	Qualifier Character 7

1   **Esophagus, Upper**
     Cervical esophagus
2   **Esophagus, Middle**
     Thoracic esophagus
3   **Esophagus, Lower**
     Abdominal esophagus
4   **Esophagogastric**
     Junction
     Cardia
     Cardioesophageal
       junction
     Gastroesophageal (GE)
       junction
5   **Esophagus**
7   **Stomach, Pylorus**
     Pyloric antrum
     Pyloric canal
     Pyloric sphincter
	8 **Small Intestine**
	9 **Duodenum**
	A **Jejunum**
	     Duodenojejunal flexure
	B **Ileum**
	C **Ileocecal Valve**
	E **Large Intestine**
	F **Large Intestine, Right**
	H **Cecum**
	J **Appendix**
	     Vermiform appendix
	K **Ascending Colon**
	P **Rectum**
	     Anorectal junction
		Ø Open
		3 Percutaneous
		4 Percutaneous Endoscopic
		7 Via Natural or Artificial
		     Opening
		8 Via Natural or Artificial
		     Opening Endoscopic
			Z No Device	**X** Diagnostic
				Z No Qualifier

6 **Stomach**		**Ø** Open
		3 Percutaneous
		4 Percutaneous Endoscopic
		7 Via Natural or Artificial
		     Opening
		8 Via Natural or Artificial
		     Opening Endoscopic
			Z No Device	**3** Vertical
				X Diagnostic
				Z No Qualifier

G   **Large Intestine, Left**
L   **Transverse Colon**
     Hepatic flexure
     Splenic flexure
M   **Descending Colon**
N   **Sigmoid Colon**
     Rectosigmoid junction
     Sigmoid flexure
		Ø Open
		3 Percutaneous
		4 Percutaneous Endoscopic
		7 Via Natural or Artificial
		     Opening
		8 Via Natural or Artificial
		     Opening Endoscopic
			Z No Device	**X** Diagnostic
				Z No Qualifier

G   **Large Intestine, Left**
L   **Transverse Colon**
     Hepatic flexure
     Splenic flexure
M   **Descending Colon**
N   **Sigmoid Colon**
     Rectosigmoid junction
     Sigmoid flexure
		F Via Natural or Artificial
		     Opening with Percutaneous
		     Endoscopic Assistance
			Z No Device	**Z** No Qualifier

Q   **Anus**
     Anal orifi
		Ø Open
		3 Percutaneous
		4 Percutaneous Endoscopic
		7 Via Natural or Artificial
		     Opening
		8 Via Natural or Artificial
		     Opening Endoscopic
		X External
			Z No Device	**X** Diagnostic
				Z No Qualifier

R   **Anal Sphincter**
     External anal sphincter
     Internal anal sphincter
U   **Omentum**
     Gastrocolic ligament
     Gastrocolic omentum
     Gastrohepatic omentum
     Gastrophrenic ligament
     Gastrosplenic ligament
     Greater Omentum
     Hepatogastric ligament
     Lesser Omentum
V   **Mesentery**
     Mesoappendix
     Mesocolon
W   **Peritoneum**
     Epiploic foramen
		Ø Open
		3 Percutaneous
		4 Percutaneous Endoscopic
			Z No Device	**X** Diagnostic
				Z No Qualifier

Non-OR	ØDB[1,2,3,4,5,7,8,9,A,B,C,E,F,H,K,P][3,4,7,8]ZX	**Non-OR**	ØDB[G,L,M,N]8ZZ
Non-OR	ØDB[1,2,3,5,7,9][4,8]ZZ	**Non-OR**	ØDBQ[Ø,3,4,7,8,X]ZX
Non-OR	ØDB[4,E,F,H,K,P]8ZZ	**Non-OR**	ØDBQ8ZZ
Non-OR	ØDB6[3,7]ZX	**Non-OR**	ØDBR[Ø,3,4]ZX
Non-OR	ØDB68Z[X,Z]	**Non-OR**	ØDB[U,V,W][3,4]ZX
Non-OR	ØDB[G,L,M,N][3,4,7,8]ZX		

NC Noncovered Procedure   **LC** Limited Coverage   **QA** Questionable OB Admit   **NT** New Tech Add-on   ⊞ Combination Member   ♂ Male   ♀ Female

ICD-10-PCS 2022   383

ØDB–ØDB

Gastrointestinal System

Ø   **Medical and Surgical**
D   **Gastrointestinal System**
C   **Extirpation**   Definition: Taking or cutting out solid matter from a body part

Explanation: The solid matter may be an abnormal byproduct of a biological function or a foreign body; it may be imbedded in a body part or in the lumen of a tubular body part. The solid matter may or may not have been previously broken into pieces.

Body Part Character 4	Approach Character 5	Device Character 6	Qualifier Character 7

1   **Esophagus, Upper**
    Cervical esophagus
2   **Esophagus, Middle**
    Thoracic esophagus
3   **Esophagus, Lower**
    Abdominal esophagus
4   **Esophagogastric Junction**
    Cardia
    Cardioesophageal junction
    Gastroesophageal (GE) junction
5   **Esophagus**
6   **Stomach**
7   **Stomach, Pylorus**
    Pyloric antrum
    Pyloric canal
    Pyloric sphincter
8   **Small Intestine**
9   **Duodenum**
A   **Jejunum**
    Duodenojejunal flexure
B   **Ileum**
C   **Ileocecal Valve**
E   **Large Intestine**
F   **Large Intestine, Right**
G   **Large Intestine, Left**
H   **Cecum**
J   **Appendix**
    Vermiform appendix
K   **Ascending Colon**
L   **Transverse Colon**
    Hepatic flexure
    Splenic flexure
M   **Descending Colon**
N   **Sigmoid Colon**
    Rectosigmoid junction
    Sigmoid flexure
P   **Rectum**
    Anorectal junction
	Ø **Open**
	3 **Percutaneous**
	4 **Percutaneous Endoscopic**
	7 **Via Natural or Artificial Opening**
	8 **Via Natural or Artificial Opening Endoscopic**
		Z **No Device**	**Z** **No Qualifier**

Q **Anus** Anal orifice	Ø **Open** 3 **Percutaneous** 4 **Percutaneous Endoscopic** 7 **Via Natural or Artificial Opening** 8 **Via Natural or Artificial Opening Endoscopic** X **External**	**Z** **No Device**	**Z** **No Qualifier**

R   **Anal Sphincter**
    External anal sphincter
    Internal anal sphincter
U   **Omentum**
    Gastrocolic ligament
    Gastrocolic omentum
    Gastrohepatic omentum
    Gastrophrenic ligament
    Gastrosplenic ligament
    Greater Omentum
    Hepatogastric ligament
    Lesser Omentum
V   **Mesentery**
    Mesoappendix
    Mesocolon
W   **Peritoneum**
    Epiploic foramen
	Ø **Open**
	3 **Percutaneous**
	4 **Percutaneous Endoscopic**
		Z **No Device**	**Z** **No Qualifier**

Non-OR   ØDC[1,2,3,4,5,6,7,8,9,A,B,C,E,F,G,H,K,L,M,N,P][7,8]ZZ
Non-OR   ØDCQ[7,8,X]ZZ

Ø   **Medical and Surgical**
D   **Gastrointestinal System**
D   **Extraction**   Definition: Pulling or stripping out or off all or a portion of a body part by the use of force
                             Explanation: The qualifier DIAGNOSTIC is used to identify extraction procedures that are biopsies

Body Part Character 4	Approach Character 5	Device Character 6	Qualifier Character 7

1 **Esophagus, Upper**
    Cervical esophagus
2 **Esophagus, Middle**
    Thoracic esophagus
3 **Esophagus, Lower**
    Abdominal esophagus
4 **Esophagogastric Junction**
    Cardia
    Cardioesophageal junction
    Gastroesophageal (GE) junction
5 **Esophagus**
6 **Stomach**
7 **Stomach, Pylorus**
    Pyloric antrum
    Pyloric canal
    Pyloric sphincter
8 **Small Intestine**
9 **Duodenum**
A **Jejunum**
    Duodenojejunal flexure
B **Ileum**
C **Ileocecal Valve**
E **Large Intestine**
F **Large Intestine, Right**
G **Large Intestine, Left**
H **Cecum**
J **Appendix**
    Vermiform appendix
K **Ascending Colon**
L **Transverse Colon**
    Hepatic flexure
    Splenic flexure
M **Descending Colon**
N **Sigmoid Colon**
    Rectosigmoid junction
    Sigmoid flexure
P **Rectum**
    Anorectal junction
	3 Percutaneous
	4 Percutaneous Endoscopic
	8 Via Natural or Artificial Opening
	    Endoscopic
		Z No Device	**X** Diagnostic

Q **Anus**
    Anal orifice
	3 Percutaneous
	4 Percutaneous Endoscopic
	8 Via Natural or Artificial Opening
	    Endoscopic
	X External
		Z No Device	**X** Diagnostic

Non-OR   ØDD[1,2,3,4,5,6,7,8,9,A,B,C,E,F,G,H,K,L,M,N,P][3,4,8]ZX
Non-OR   ØDDQ[3,4,8,X]ZX

Ø Medical and Surgical
D Gastrointestinal System
F Fragmentation   Definition: Breaking solid matter in a body part into pieces

Explanation: Physical force (e.g., manual, ultrasonic) applied directly or indirectly is used to break the solid matter into pieces. The solid matter may be an abnormal byproduct of a biological function or a foreign body. The pieces of solid matter are not taken out.

Body Part Character 4	Approach Character 5	Device Character 6	Qualifier Character 7

5 Esophagus `NC`
6 Stomach `NC`
8 Small Intestine `NC`
9 Duodenum `NC`
A Jejunum `NC`
  Duodenojejunal flexure
B Ileum `NC`
E Large Intestine `NC`
F Large Intestine, Right `NC`
G Large Intestine, Left `NC`
H Cecum `NC`
J Appendix `NC`
  Vermiform appendix
K Ascending Colon `NC`
L Transverse Colon `NC`
  Hepatic flexure
  Splenic flexure
M Descending Colon `NC`
N Sigmoid Colon `NC`
  Rectosigmoid junction
  Sigmoid flexure
P Rectum `NC`
  Anorectal junction
Q Anus `NC`
  Anal orifice
	Ø Open
	3 Percutaneous
	4 Percutaneous Endoscopic
	7 Via Natural or Artificial Opening
	8 Via Natural or Artificial Opening
	  Endoscopic
	X External
		Z No Device	Z No Qualifier

Non-OR   ØDF[5,6,8,9,A,B,E,F,G,H,J,K,L,M,N,P,Q]XZZ
`NC`   ØDF[5,6,8,9,A,B,E,F,G,H,J,K,L,M,N,P,Q]XZZ

Ø　Medical and Surgical
D　Gastrointestinal System
H　Insertion　　　Definition: Putting in a nonbiological appliance that monitors, assists, performs, or prevents a physiological function but does not physically take the place of a body part
　　　　　　　　　　Explanation: None

Body Part Character 4	Approach Character 5	Device Character 6	Qualifier Character 7
Ø　Upper Intestinal Tract D　Lower Intestinal Tract	Ø　Open 3　Percutaneous 4　Percutaneous Endoscopic 7　Via Natural or Artificial Opening 8　Via Natural or Artificial Opening Endoscopic	Y　Other Device	Z　No Qualifier
5　Esophagus	Ø　Open 3　Percutaneous 4　Percutaneous Endoscopic	1　Radioactive Element 2　Monitoring Device 3　Infusion Device D　Intraluminal Device U　Feeding Device Y　Other Device	Z　No Qualifier
5　Esophagus	7　Via Natural or Artificial Opening 8　Via Natural or Artificial Opening Endoscopic	1　Radioactive Element 2　Monitoring Device 3　Infusion Device B　Intraluminal Device, Airway D　Intraluminal Device U　Feeding Device Y　Other Device	Z　No Qualifier
6　Stomach　⊞	Ø　Open 3　Percutaneous 4　Percutaneous Endoscopic	1　Radioactive Element 2　Monitoring Device 3　Infusion Device D　Intraluminal Device M　Stimulator Lead U　Feeding Device Y　Other Device	Z　No Qualifier
6　Stomach	7　Via Natural or Artificial Opening 8　Via Natural or Artificial Opening Endoscopic	1　Radioactive Element 2　Monitoring Device 3　Infusion Device D　Intraluminal Device U　Feeding Device Y　Other Device	Z　No Qualifier
8　Small Intestine 9　Duodenum A　Jejunum 　　Duodenojejunal flexure B　Ileum	Ø　Open 3　Percutaneous 4　Percutaneous Endoscopic 7　Via Natural or Artificial Opening 8　Via Natural or Artificial Opening Endoscopic	1　Radioactive Element 2　Monitoring Device 3　Infusion Device D　Intraluminal Device U　Feeding Device	Z　No Qualifier
E　Large Intestine P　Rectum 　　Anorectal junction	Ø　Open 3　Percutaneous 4　Percutaneous Endoscopic 7　Via Natural or Artificial Opening 8　Via Natural or Artificial Opening Endoscopic	1　Radioactive Element D　Intraluminal Device	Z　No Qualifier
Q　Anus 　　Anal orifice	Ø　Open 3　Percutaneous 4　Percutaneous Endoscopic	D　Intraluminal Device L　Artificial Sphincter	Z　No Qualifier
Q　Anus 　　Anal orifice	7　Via Natural or Artificial Opening 8　Via Natural or Artificial Opening Endoscopic	D　Intraluminal Device	Z　No Qualifier
R　Anal Sphincter 　　External anal sphincter 　　Internal anal sphincter	Ø　Open 3　Percutaneous 4　Percutaneous Endoscopic	M　Stimulator Lead	Z　No Qualifier

Non-OR	ØDH[Ø,D][Ø,3,4,7,8]YZ
Non-OR	ØDH5[Ø,3,4][D,U]Z
Non-OR	ØDH5[3,4]YZ
Non-OR	ØDH5[7,8][2,3,B,D,U,Y]Z
Non-OR	ØDH631Z
Non-OR	ØDH6[3,4][U,Y]Z
Non-OR	ØDH6[7,8][1,2,3,D,U,Y]Z
Non-OR	ØDH[8,9,A,B][Ø,3,4,7,8][1,D,U]Z
Non-OR	ØDH[8,9,A,B][7,8][2,3]Z
Non-OR	ØDHE[Ø,3,4,7,8][1,D]Z
Non-OR	ØDHP[Ø,3,4,7,8]DZ

See Appendix L for Procedure Combinations
⊞　　ØDH6[Ø,3,4]MZ

NC Noncovered Procedure　　LC Limited Coverage　　QA Questionable OB Admit　　NT New Tech Add-on　　⊞ Combination Member　　♂ Male　　♀ Female

ICD-10-PCS 2022　　　　　　　　　　　　　　　　　　　　　　　　　　　　　　　　　387

ØDH–ØDH

Ø   Medical and Surgical
D   Gastrointestinal System
J   Inspection   Definition: Visually and/or manually exploring a body part

Explanation: Visual exploration may be performed with or without optical instrumentation. Manual exploration may be performed directly or through intervening body layers.

Body Part Character 4	Approach Character 5	Device Character 6	Qualifier Character 7
Ø Upper Intestinal Tract **6 Stomach** **D Lower Intestinal Tract**	**Ø** Open **3** Percutaneous **4** Percutaneous Endoscopic **7** Via Natural or Artificial Opening **8** Via Natural or Artificial Opening Endoscopic **X** External	**Z** No Device	**Z** No Qualifier

U Omentum
   Gastrocolic ligament
   Gastrocolic omentum
   Gastrohepatic omentum
   Gastrophrenic ligament
   Gastrosplenic ligament
   Greater Omentum
   Hepatogastric ligament
   Lesser Omentum
V Mesentery
   Mesoappendix
   Mesocolon
W Peritoneum
   Epiploic foramen
	Ø Open
	3 Percutaneous
	4 Percutaneous Endoscopic
	X External
		Z No Device	**Z** No Qualifier

Non-OR	ØDJ[Ø,6,D][3,7,8,X]ZZ
Non-OR	ØDJ[U,V,W][3,X]ZZ

Ø   Medical and Surgical
D   Gastrointestinal System
L   Occlusion   Definition: Completely closing an orifice or the lumen of a tubular body part
                            Explanation: The orifice can be a natural orifice or an artificially created orifice

Body Part Character 4		Approach Character 5	Device Character 6	Qualifier Character 7

1 Esophagus, Upper
  Cervical esophagus
2 Esophagus, Middle .
  Thoracic esophagus
3 Esophagus, Lower
  Abdominal esophagus
4 Esophagogastric
  Junction
  Cardia
  Cardioesophageal
    junction
  Gastroesophageal (GE)
    junction
5 Esophagus
6 Stomach
7 Stomach, Pylorus
  Pyloric antrum
  Pyloric canal
  Pyloric sphincter
8 Small Intestine
	9 Duodenum
	A Jejunum
	  Duodenojejunal flexure
	B Ileum
	C Ileocecal Valve
	E Large Intestine
	F Large Intestine, Right
	G Large Intestine, Left
	H Cecum
	K Ascending Colon
	L Transverse Colon
	  Hepatic flexure
	  Splenic flexure
	M Descending Colon
	N Sigmoid Colon
	  Rectosigmoid junction
	  Sigmoid flexure
	P Rectum
	  Anorectal junction
		Ø Open
		3 Percutaneous
		4 Percutaneous Endoscopic
			C Extraluminal Device
			D Intraluminal Device
			Z No Device
				Z No Qualifier

1 Esophagus, Upper
  Cervical esophagus
2 Esophagus, Middle
  Thoracic esophagus
3 Esophagus, Lower
  Abdominal esophagus
4 Esophagogastric
  Junction
  Cardia
  Cardioesophageal
    junction
  Gastroesophageal (GE)
    junction
5 Esophagus
6 Stomach
7 Stomach, Pylorus
  Pyloric antrum
  Pyloric canal
  Pyloric sphincter
8 Small Intestine
	9 Duodenum
	A Jejunum
	  Duodenojejunal flexure
	B Ileum
	C Ileocecal Valve
	E Large Intestine
	F Large Intestine, Right
	G Large Intestine, Left
	H Cecum
	K Ascending Colon
	L Transverse Colon
	  Hepatic flexure
	  Splenic flexure
	M Descending Colon
	N Sigmoid Colon
	  Rectosigmoid junction
	  Sigmoid flexure
	P Rectum
	  Anorectal junction
		7 Via Natural or Artificial
		   Opening
		8 Via Natural or Artificial
		   Opening Endoscopic
			D Intraluminal Device
			Z No Device
				Z No Qualifier

Q Anus Anal orifice		Ø Open 3 Percutaneous 4 Percutaneous Endoscopic X External	C Extraluminal Device D Intraluminal Device Z No Device	Z No Qualifier

Q Anus
  Anal orifice
		7 Via Natural or Artificial
		   Opening
		8 Via Natural or Artificial
		   Opening Endoscopic
			D Intraluminal Device
			Z No Device
				Z No Qualifier

Non-OR ØDL[1,2,3,4,5][Ø,3,4][C,D,Z]Z
Non-OR ØDL[1,2,3,4,5][7,8][D,Z]Z

NC Noncovered Procedure   LC Limited Coverage   QA Questionable OB Admit   NT New Tech Add-on   ⊞ Combination Member   ♂ Male   ♀ Female
ICD-10-PCS 2022   389

ØDL–ØDL

Gastrointestinal System

Ø   **Medical and Surgical**
D   **Gastrointestinal System**
M   **Reattachment**   Definition: Putting back in or on all or a portion of a separated body part to its normal location or other suitable location
         Explanation: Vascular circulation and nervous pathways may or may not be reestablished

Body Part Character 4	Approach Character 5	Device Character 6	Qualifier Character 7

5   Esophagus
6   Stomach
8   Small Intestine
9   Duodenum
A   Jejunum
     Duodenojejunal flexure
B   Ileum
E   Large Intestine
F   Large Intestine, Right
G   Large Intestine, Left
H   Cecum
K   Ascending Colon
L   Transverse Colon
     Hepatic flexure
     Splenic flexure
M   Descending Colon
N   Sigmoid Colon
     Rectosigmoid junction
     Sigmoid flexure
P   Rectum
     Anorectal junction
	Ø Open
	4 Percutaneous Endoscopic
		Z No Device	Z No Qualifier

Ø   **Medical and Surgical**
D   **Gastrointestinal System**
N   **Release**   Definition: Freeing a body part from an abnormal physical constraint by cutting or by the use of force
         Explanation: Some of the restraining tissue may be taken out but none of the body part is taken out

Body Part Character 4	Approach Character 5	Device Character 6	Qualifier Character 7

1   Esophagus, Upper
     Cervical esophagus
2   Esophagus, Middle
     Thoracic esophagus
3   Esophagus, Lower
     Abdominal esophagus
4   Esophagogastric
     Junction
     Cardia
     Cardioesophageal
       junction
     Gastroesophageal (GE)
       junction
5   Esophagus
6   Stomach
7   Stomach, Pylorus
     Pyloric antrum
     Pyloric canal
     Pyloric sphincter
8   Small Intestine
9   Duodenum
 	
A   Jejunum
     Duodenojejunal flexure
B   Ileum
C   Ileocecal Valve
E   Large Intestine
F   Large Intestine, Right
G   Large Intestine, Left
H   Cecum
J   Appendix
     Vermiform appendix
K   Ascending Colon
L   Transverse Colon
     Hepatic flexure
     Splenic flexure
M   Descending Colon
N   Sigmoid Colon
     Rectosigmoid junction
     Sigmoid flexure
P   Rectum
     Anorectal junction
	Ø Open
	3 Percutaneous
	4 Percutaneous Endoscopic
	7 Via Natural or Artificial
	     Opening
	8 Via Natural or Artificial
	     Opening Endoscopic
		Z No Device	Z No Qualifier

Q   Anus
     Anal orifice
	Ø Open
	3 Percutaneous
	4 Percutaneous Endoscopic
	7 Via Natural or Artificial
	     Opening
	8 Via Natural or Artificial
	     Opening Endoscopic
	X External
		Z No Device	Z No Qualifier

R   Anal Sphincter
     External anal sphincter
     Internal anal sphincter
U   Omentum
     Gastrocolic ligament
     Gastrocolic omentum
     Gastrohepatic omentum
     Gastrophrenic ligament
     Gastrosplenic ligament
     Greater Omentum
     Hepatogastric ligament
     Lesser Omentum
V   Mesentery
     Mesoappendix
     Mesocolon
W   Peritoneum
     Epiploic foramen
	Ø Open
	3 Percutaneous
	4 Percutaneous Endoscopic
		Z No Device	Z No Qualifier

Non-OR   ØDN[8,9,A,B,E,F,G,H,K,L,M,N][7,8]ZZ

Ø   Medical and Surgical
D   Gastrointestinal System
P   Removal   Definition: Taking out or off a device from a body part

Explanation: If a device is taken out and a similar device put in without cutting or puncturing the skin or mucous membrane, the procedure is coded to the root operation CHANGE. Otherwise, the procedure for taking out a device is coded to the root operation REMOVAL.

Body Part Character 4	Approach Character 5	Device Character 6	Qualifier Character 7
Ø Upper Intestinal Tract D Lower Intestinal Tract	Ø Open 3 Percutaneous 4 Percutaneous Endoscopic 7 Via Natural or Artificial Opening 8 Via Natural or Artificial Opening Endoscopic	Ø Drainage Device 2 Monitoring Device 3 Infusion Device 7 Autologous Tissue Substitute C Extraluminal Device D Intraluminal Device J Synthetic Substitute K Nonautologous Tissue Substitute U Feeding Device Y Other Device	Z No Qualifier
Ø Upper Intestinal Tract D Lower Intestinal Tract	X External	Ø Drainage Device 2 Monitoring Device 3 Infusion Device D Intraluminal Device U Feeding Device	Z No Qualifier
5 Esophagus	Ø Open 3 Percutaneous 4 Percutaneous Endoscopic	1 Radioactive Element 2 Monitoring Device 3 Infusion Device U Feeding Device Y Other Device	Z No Qualifier
5 Esophagus	7 Via Natural or Artificial Opening 8 Via Natural or Artificial Opening Endoscopic	1 Radioactive Element D Intraluminal Device Y Other Device	Z No Qualifier
5 Esophagus	X External	1 Radioactive Element 2 Monitoring Device 3 Infusion Device D Intraluminal Device U Feeding Device	Z No Qualifier
6 Stomach	Ø Open 3 Percutaneous 4 Percutaneous Endoscopic	Ø Drainage Device 2 Monitoring Device 3 Infusion Device 7 Autologous Tissue Substitute C Extraluminal Device D Intraluminal Device J Synthetic Substitute K Nonautologous Tissue Substitute M Stimulator Lead U Feeding Device Y Other Device	Z No Qualifier
6 Stomach	7 Via Natural or Artificial Opening 8 Via Natural or Artificial Opening Endoscopic	Ø Drainage Device 2 Monitoring Device 3 Infusion Device 7 Autologous Tissue Substitute C Extraluminal Device D Intraluminal Device J Synthetic Substitute K Nonautologous Tissue Substitute U Feeding Device Y Other Device	Z No Qualifier
6 Stomach	X External	Ø Drainage Device 2 Monitoring Device 3 Infusion Device D Intraluminal Device U Feeding Device	Z No Qualifier

Non-OR   ØDP[Ø,D][3,4]YZ
Non-OR   ØDP[Ø,D][7,8][Ø,2,3,D,U,Y]Z
Non-OR   ØDP[Ø,D]X[Ø,2,3,D,U]Z
Non-OR   ØDP5[3,4]YZ
Non-OR   ØDP5[7,8][1,D,Y]Z
Non-OR   ØDP5X[1,2,3,D,U]Z
Non-OR   ØDP6[3,4]YZ
Non-OR   ØDP6[7,8][Ø,2,3,D,U,Y]Z
Non-OR   ØDP6X[Ø,2,3,D,U]Z

ØDP Continued on next page

NC Noncovered Procedure   LC Limited Coverage   QA Questionable OB Admit   NT New Tech Add-on   ⊞ Combination Member   ♂ Male   ♀ Female

ICD-10-PCS 2022   391

Ø   Medical and Surgical
D   Gastrointestinal System
P   Removal   Definition: Taking out or off a device from a body part

Explanation: If a device is taken out and a similar device put in without cutting or puncturing the skin or mucous membrane, the procedure is coded to the root operation CHANGE. Otherwise, the procedure for taking out a device is coded to the root operation REMOVAL.

Body Part Character 4	Approach Character 5	Device Character 6	Qualifier Character 7
P Rectum Anorectal junction	**Ø** Open **3** Percutaneous **4** Percutaneous Endoscopic **7** Via Natural or Artificial Opening **8** Via Natural or Artificial Opening Endoscopic **X** External	**1** Radioactive Element	**Z** No Qualifier
Q Anus Anal orifice	**Ø** Open **3** Percutaneous **4** Percutaneous Endoscopic **7** Via Natural or Artificial Opening **8** Via Natural or Artificial Opening Endoscopic	**L** Artificial Sphincter	**Z** No Qualifier
R Anal Sphincter External anal sphincter Internal anal sphincter	**Ø** Open **3** Percutaneous **4** Percutaneous Endoscopic	**M** Stimulator Lead	**Z** No Qualifier
U Omentum Gastrocolic ligament Gastrocolic omentum Gastrohepatic omentum Gastrophrenic ligament Gastrosplenic ligament Greater Omentum Hepatogastric ligament Lesser Omentum **V Mesentery** Mesoappendix Mesocolon **W Peritoneum** Epiploic foramen	**Ø** Open **3** Percutaneous **4** Percutaneous Endoscopic	**Ø** Drainage Device **1** Radioactive Element **7** Autologous Tissue Substitute **J** Synthetic Substitute **K** Nonautologous Tissue Substitute	**Z** No Qualifier

Non-OR   ØDPP[7,8,X]1Z

Ø   **Medical and Surgical**
D   **Gastrointestinal System**
Q   **Repair**   Definition: Restoring, to the extent possible, a body part to its normal anatomic structure and function

                     Explanation: Used only when the method to accomplish the repair is not one of the other root operations

Body Part Character 4	Approach Character 5	Device Character 6	Qualifier Character 7

1 **Esophagus, Upper**
  Cervical esophagus
2 **Esophagus, Middle**
  Thoracic esophagus
3 **Esophagus, Lower**
  Abdominal esophagus
4 **Esophagogastric Junction**
  Cardia
  Cardioesophageal junction
  Gastroesophageal (GE) junction
5 **Esophagus**
6 **Stomach**
7 **Stomach, Pylorus**
  Pyloric antrum
  Pyloric canal
  Pyloric sphincter
8 **Small Intestine** ⊞
9 **Duodenum** ⊞
A **Jejunum** ⊞
  Duodenojejunal flexure
B **Ileum** ⊞
C **Ileocecal Valve**
E **Large Intestine** ⊞
F **Large Intestine, Right** ⊞
G **Large Intestine, Left** ⊞
H **Cecum** ⊞
J **Appendix**
  Vermiform appendix
K **Ascending Colon** ⊞
L **Transverse Colon** ⊞
  Hepatic flexure
  Splenic flexure
M **Descending Colon** ⊞
N **Sigmoid Colon** ⊞
  Rectosigmoid junction
  Sigmoid flexure
P **Rectum**
  Anorectal junction
	Ø **Open**
	3 **Percutaneous**
	4 **Percutaneous Endoscopic**
	7 **Via Natural or Artificial Opening**
	8 **Via Natural or Artificial Opening**
	  Endoscopic
		Z **No Device**	Z **No Qualifier**

Q **Anus**
  Anal orifice
	Ø **Open**
	3 **Percutaneous**
	4 **Percutaneous Endoscopic**
	7 **Via Natural or Artificial Opening**
	8 **Via Natural or Artificial Opening**
	  Endoscopic
	X **External**
		Z **No Device**	Z **No Qualifier**

R **Anal Sphincter**
  External anal sphincter
  Internal anal sphincter
U **Omentum**
  Gastrocolic ligament
  Gastrocolic omentum
  Gastrohepatic omentum
  Gastrophrenic ligament
  Gastrosplenic ligament
  Greater Omentum
  Hepatogastric ligament
  Lesser Omentum
V **Mesentery**
  Mesoappendix
  Mesocolon
W **Peritoneum**
  Epiploic foramen
	Ø **Open**
	3 **Percutaneous**
	4 **Percutaneous Endoscopic**
		Z **No Device**	Z **No Qualifier**

Non-OR   ØDQU[Ø,3,4]ZZ

See Appendix L for Procedure Combinations
⊞   ØDQ[8,9,A,B,E,F,G,H,K,L,M,N]ØZZ

NC Noncovered Procedure   LC Limited Coverage   QA Questionable OB Admit   NT New Tech Add-on   ⊞ Combination Member   ♂ Male   ♀ Female

Gastrointestinal System

Ø   **Medical and Surgical**
D   **Gastrointestinal System**
R   **Replacement**   Definition: Putting in or on biological or synthetic material that physically takes the place and/or function of all or a portion of a body part
                     Explanation: The body part may have been taken out or replaced, or may be taken out, physically eradicated, or rendered nonfunctional during the REPLACEMENT procedure. A REMOVAL procedure is coded for taking out the device used in a previous replacement procedure.

Body Part Character 4	Approach Character 5	Device Character 6	Qualifier Character 7
5 Esophagus	**Ø** Open **4** Percutaneous Endoscopic **7** Via Natural or Artificial Opening **8** Via Natural or Artificial Opening Endoscopic	**7** Autologous Tissue Substitute **J** Synthetic Substitute **K** Nonautologous Tissue Substitute	**Z** No Qualifier

R   Anal Sphincter
     External anal sphincter
     Internal anal sphincter
U   Omentum
     Gastrocolic ligament
     Gastrocolic omentum
     Gastrohepatic omentum
     Gastrophrenic ligament
     Gastrosplenic ligament
     Greater Omentum
     Hepatogastric ligament
     Lesser Omentum
V   Mesentery
     Mesoappendix
     Mesocolon
W   Peritoneum
     Epiploic foramen
	Ø Open
	4 Percutaneous Endoscopic
		7 Autologous Tissue Substitute
		J Synthetic Substitute
		K Nonautologous Tissue Substitute
			Z No Qualifier

Ø   **Medical and Surgical**
D   **Gastrointestinal System**
S   **Reposition**   Definition: Moving to its normal location, or other suitable location, all or a portion of a body part
                  Explanation: The body part is moved to a new location from an abnormal location, or from a normal location where it is not functioning correctly. The body part may or may not be cut out or off to be moved to the new location.

Body Part Character 4	Approach Character 5	Device Character 6	Qualifier Character 7

5   Esophagus
6   Stomach
9   Duodenum
A   Jejunum
     Duodenojejunal flexure
B   Ileum
H   Cecum
K   Ascending Colon
L   Transverse Colon
     Hepatic flexure
     Splenic flexure
M   Descending Colon
N   Sigmoid Colon
     Rectosigmoid junction
     Sigmoid flexure
P   Rectum
     Anorectal junction
Q   Anus
     Anal orifice
	Ø Open
	4 Percutaneous Endoscopic
	7 Via Natural or Artificial Opening
	8 Via Natural or Artificial Opening Endoscopic
	X External
		Z No Device	**Z** No Qualifier

8 Small Intestine **E** Large Intestine	**Ø** Open **4** Percutaneous Endoscopic **7** Via Natural or Artificial Opening **8** Via Natural or Artificial Opening Endoscopic	**Z** No Device	**Z** No Qualifier

Non-OR   ØDS[5,6,9,A,B,H,K,L,M,N,P,Q]XZZ

Ø Medical and Surgical
D Gastrointestinal System
T Resection Definition: Cutting out or off, without replacement, all of a body part
Explanation: None

Body Part Character 4	Approach Character 5	Device Character 6	Qualifier Character 7
1 Esophagus, Upper Cervical esophagus **2 Esophagus, Middle** Thoracic esophagus **3 Esophagus, Lower** Abdominal esophagus **4 Esophagogastric Junction** Cardia Cardioesophageal junction Gastroesophageal (GE) junction **5 Esophagus** **6 Stomach** **7 Stomach, Pylorus** Pyloric antrum Pyloric canal Pyloric sphincter **8 Small Intestine** **9 Duodenum** ⊞ **A Jejunum** Duodenojejunal flexure **B Ileum** **C Ileocecal Valve** **E Large Intestine** **F Large Intestine, Right** **H Cecum** **J Appendix** Vermiform appendix **K Ascending Colon** **P Rectum** Anorectal junction **Q Anus** Anal orifice	**Ø Open** **4 Percutaneous Endoscopic** **7 Via Natural or Artificial Opening** **8 Via Natural or Artificial Opening Endoscopic**	**Z No Device**	**Z No Qualifier**
G Large Intestine, Left **L Transverse Colon** Hepatic flexure Splenic flexure **M Descending Colon** **N Sigmoid Colon** Rectosigmoid junction Sigmoid flexure	**Ø Open** **4 Percutaneous Endoscopic** **7 Via Natural or Artificial Opening** **8 Via Natural or Artificial Opening Endoscopic** **F Via Natural or Artificial Opening with Percutaneous Endoscopic Assistance**	**Z No Device**	**Z No Qualifier**
R Anal Sphincter External anal sphincter Internal anal sphincter **U Omentum** Gastrocolic ligament Gastrocolic omentum Gastrohepatic omentum Gastrophrenic ligament Gastrosplenic ligament Greater Omentum Hepatogastric ligament Lesser Omentum	**Ø Open** **4 Percutaneous Endoscopic**	**Z No Device**	**Z No Qualifier**

See Appendix L for Procedure Combinations
⊞ ØDT9ØZZ

Ø   Medical and Surgical
D   Gastrointestinal System
U   Supplement   Definition: Putting in or on biological or synthetic material that physically reinforces and/or augments the function of a portion of a body part

Explanation: The biological material is non-living, or is living and from the same individual. The body part may have been previously replaced, and the SUPPLEMENT procedure is performed to physically reinforce and/or augment the function of the replaced body part.

Body Part Character 4	Approach Character 5	Device Character 6	Qualifier Character 7

1 Esophagus, Upper
    Cervical esophagus
2 Esophagus, Middle
    Thoracic esophagus
3 Esophagus, Lower
    Abdominal esophagus
4 Esophagogastric Junction
    Cardia
    Cardioesophageal junction
    Gastroesophageal (GE) junction
5 Esophagus
6 Stomach
7 Stomach, Pylorus
    Pyloric antrum
    Pyloric canal
    Pyloric sphincter
8 Small Intestine
9 Duodenum
A Jejunum
    Duodenojejunal flexure
B Ileum
C Ileocecal Valve
E Large Intestine
F Large Intestine, Right
G Large Intestine, Left
H Cecum
K Ascending Colon
L Transverse Colon
    Hepatic flexure
    Splenic flexure
M Descending Colon
N Sigmoid Colon
    Rectosigmoid junction
    Sigmoid flexure
P Rectum
    Anorectal junction
	Ø Open
	4 Percutaneous Endoscopic
	7 Via Natural or Artificial Opening
	**8 Via Natural or Artificial Opening
	    Endoscopic**
		7 Autologous Tissue Substitute
		J Synthetic Substitute
		K Nonautologous Tissue Substitute
			Z No Qualifier

Q Anus
    Anal orifice
	Ø Open
	4 Percutaneous Endoscopic
	7 Via Natural or Artificial Opening
	**8 Via Natural or Artificial Opening
	    Endoscopic**
	X External
		7 Autologous Tissue Substitute
		J Synthetic Substitute
		K Nonautologous Tissue Substitute
			Z No Qualifier

R Anal Sphincter
    External anal sphincter
    Internal anal sphincter
U Omentum
    Gastrocolic ligament
    Gastrocolic omentum
    Gastrohepatic omentum
    Gastrophrenic ligament
    Gastrosplenic ligament
    Greater Omentum
    Hepatogastric ligament
    Lesser Omentum
V Mesentery
    Mesoappendix
    Mesocolon
W Peritoneum
    Epiploic foramen
	Ø Open
	4 Percutaneous Endoscopic
		7 Autologous Tissue Substitute
		J Synthetic Substitute
		K Nonautologous Tissue Substitute
			Z No Qualifier

Ø   **Medical and Surgical**
D   **Gastrointestinal System**
V   **Restriction**   Definition: Partially closing an orifice or the lumen of a tubular body part
                  Explanation: The orifice can be a natural orifice or an artificially created orifice

Body Part Character 4		Approach Character 5	Device Character 6	Qualifier Character 7
1 Esophagus, Upper Cervical esophagus 2 Esophagus, Middle Thoracic esophagus 3 Esophagus, Lower Abdominal esophagus 4 Esophagogastric Junction Cardia Cardioesophageal junction Gastroesophageal (GE) junction 5 Esophagus 6 Stomach 7 Stomach, Pylorus Pyloric antrum Pyloric canal Pyloric sphincter 8 Small Intestine	9 Duodenum A Jejunum Duodenojejunal flexure B Ileum C Ileocecal Valve E Large Intestine F Large Intestine, Right G Large Intestine, Left H Cecum K Ascending Colon L Transverse Colon Hepatic flexure Splenic flexure M Descending Colon N Sigmoid Colon Rectosigmoid junction Sigmoid flexure P Rectum Anorectal junction	Ø Open 3 Percutaneous 4 Percutaneous Endoscopic	C Extraluminal Device D Intraluminal Device Z No Device	Z No Qualifier
1 Esophagus, Upper Cervical esophagus 2 Esophagus, Middle Thoracic esophagus 3 Esophagus, Lower Abdominal esophagus 4 Esophagogastric Junction Cardia Cardioesophageal junction Gastroesophageal (GE) junction 5 Esophagus 6 Stomach **NC** 7 Stomach, Pylorus Pyloric antrum Pyloric canal Pyloric sphincter 8 Small Intestine	9 Duodenum A Jejunum Duodenojejunal flexure B Ileum C Ileocecal Valve E Large Intestine F Large Intestine, Right G Large Intestine, Left H Cecum K Ascending Colon L Transverse Colon Hepatic flexure Splenic flexure M Descending Colon N Sigmoid Colon Rectosigmoid junction Sigmoid flexure P Rectum Anorectal junction	7 Via Natural or Artificial Opening 8 Via Natural or Artificial Opening Endoscopic	D Intraluminal Device Z No Device	Z No Qualifier
Q Anus Anal orifice		Ø Open 3 Percutaneous 4 Percutaneous Endoscopic X External	C Extraluminal Device D Intraluminal Device Z No Device	Z No Qualifier
Q Anus Anal orifice		7 Via Natural or Artificial Opening 8 Via Natural or Artificial Opening Endoscopic	D Intraluminal Device Z No Device	Z No Qualifier

Non-OR   ØDV6[7,8]DZ
HAC   ØDV64CZ when reported with PDx E66.Ø1 and SDx K68.11, K95.Ø1, K95.81, or T81.4Ø–T81.49 with 7th character A
NC   ØDV6[7,8]DZ

NC Noncovered Procedure   **LC** Limited Coverage   **QA** Questionable OB Admit   **NT** New Tech Add-on   ⊞ Combination Member   ♂ Male   ♀ Female

ICD-10-PCS 2022   397

ØDV–ØDV

Gastrointestinal System

Ø   **Medical and Surgical**
D   **Gastrointestinal System**
W   **Revision**   Definition: Correcting, to the extent possible, a portion of a malfunctioning device or the position of a displaced device
                     Explanation: Revision can include correcting a malfunctioning or displaced device by taking out or putting in components of the device such as a screw or pin

Body Part Character 4	Approach Character 5	Device Character 6	Qualifier Character 7
Ø Upper Intestinal Tract **D** Lower Intestinal Tract	**Ø** Open **3** Percutaneous **4** Percutaneous Endoscopic **7** Via Natural or Artificial Opening **8** Via Natural or Artificial Opening Endoscopic	**Ø** Drainage Device **2** Monitoring Device **3** Infusion Device **7** Autologous Tissue Substitute **C** Extraluminal Device **D** Intraluminal Device **J** Synthetic Substitute **K** Nonautologous Tissue Substitute **U** Feeding Device **Y** Other Device	**Z** No Qualifier
Ø Upper Intestinal Tract **D** Lower Intestinal Tract	**X** External	**Ø** Drainage Device **2** Monitoring Device **3** Infusion Device **7** Autologous Tissue Substitute **C** Extraluminal Device **D** Intraluminal Device **J** Synthetic Substitute **K** Nonautologous Tissue Substitute **U** Feeding Device	**Z** No Qualifier
5 Esophagus	**Ø** Open **3** Percutaneous **4** Percutaneous Endoscopic	**Y** Other Device	**Z** No Qualifier
5 Esophagus	**7** Via Natural or Artificial Opening **8** Via Natural or Artificial Opening Endoscopic	**D** Intraluminal Device **Y** Other Device	**Z** No Qualifier
5 Esophagus	**X** External	**D** Intraluminal Device	**Z** No Qualifier
6 Stomach	**Ø** Open **3** Percutaneous **4** Percutaneous Endoscopic	**Ø** Drainage Device **2** Monitoring Device **3** Infusion Device **7** Autologous Tissue Substitute **C** Extraluminal Device **D** Intraluminal Device **J** Synthetic Substitute **K** Nonautologous Tissue Substitute **M** Stimulator Lead **U** Feeding Device **Y** Other Device	**Z** No Qualifier
6 Stomach	**7** Via Natural or Artificial Opening **8** Via Natural or Artificial Opening Endoscopic	**Ø** Drainage Device **2** Monitoring Device **3** Infusion Device **7** Autologous Tissue Substitute **C** Extraluminal Device **D** Intraluminal Device **J** Synthetic Substitute **K** Nonautologous Tissue Substitute **U** Feeding Device **Y** Other Device	**Z** No Qualifier
6 Stomach	**X** External	**Ø** Drainage Device **2** Monitoring Device **3** Infusion Device **7** Autologous Tissue Substitute **C** Extraluminal Device **D** Intraluminal Device **J** Synthetic Substitute **K** Nonautologous Tissue Substitute **U** Feeding Device	**Z** No Qualifier

Non-OR	ØDW[Ø,D][3,4,7,8]YZ
Non-OR	ØDW[Ø,D]8UZ
Non-OR	ØDW[Ø,D]X[Ø,2,3,7,C,D,J,K,U]Z
Non-OR	ØDW5[Ø,3,4]YZ
Non-OR	ØDW5[7,8]YZ
Non-OR	ØDW5XDZ
Non-OR	ØDW6[3,4]YZ
Non-OR	ØDW68UZ
Non-OR	ØDW6[7,8]YZ
Non-OR	ØDW6X[Ø,2,3,7,C,D,J,K,U]Z

ØDW Continued on next page

Non-OR Procedure   DRG Non-OR Procedure   Valid OR Procedure   HAC Associated Procedure   Combination Only   New/Revised GREEN

Ø Medical and Surgical
D Gastrointestinal System
W Revision

ØDW Continued

Definition: Correcting, to the extent possible, a portion of a malfunctioning device or the position of a displaced device

Explanation: Revision can include correcting a malfunctioning or displaced device by taking out or putting in components of the device such as a screw or pin

Body Part Character 4	Approach Character 5	Device Character 6	Qualifier Character 7
8 Small Intestine E Large Intestine	Ø Open 4 Percutaneous Endoscopic 7 Via Natural or Artificial Opening 8 Via Natural or Artificial Opening Endoscopic	7 Autologous Tissue Substitute J Synthetic Substitute K Nonautologous Tissue Substitute	Z No Qualifier

Q Anus
   Anal orifice
	Ø Open
	3 Percutaneous
	4 Percutaneous Endoscopic
	7 Via Natural or Artificial Opening
	8 Via Natural or Artificial Opening
	   Endoscopic
		L Artificial Sphincter	Z No Qualifier

R Anal Sphincter
   External anal sphincter
   Internal anal sphincter
	Ø Open
	3 Percutaneous
	4 Percutaneous Endoscopic
		M Stimulator Lead	Z No Qualifier

U Omentum
   Gastrocolic ligament
   Gastrocolic omentum
   Gastrohepatic omentum
   Gastrophrenic ligament
   Gastrosplenic ligament
   Greater Omentum
   Hepatogastric ligament
   Lesser Omentum
V Mesentery
   Mesoappendix
   Mesocolon
W Peritoneum
   Epiploic foramen
	Ø Open
	3 Percutaneous
	4 Percutaneous Endoscopic
		Ø Drainage Device
		7 Autologous Tissue Substitute
		J Synthetic Substitute
		K Nonautologous Tissue Substitute
			Z No Qualifier

Non-OR ØDW[U,V,W][Ø,3,4]ØZ

Ø Medical and Surgical
D Gastrointestinal System
X Transfer

Definition: Moving, without taking out, all or a portion of a body part to another location to take over the function of all or a portion of a body part

Explanation: The body part transferred remains connected to its vascular and nervous supply

Body Part Character 4	Approach Character 5	Device Character 6	Qualifier Character 7
6 Stomach 8 Small Intestine	Ø Open 4 Percutaneous Endoscopic	Z No Device	5 Esophagus
E Large Intestine	Ø Open 4 Percutaneous Endoscopic	Z No Device	5 Esophagus 7 Vagina ♀

♀ ØDXE[Ø,4]Z7

Ø Medical and Surgical
D Gastrointestinal System
Y Transplantation

Definition: Putting in or on all or a portion of a living body part taken from another individual or animal to physically take the place and/or function of all or a portion of a similar body part

Explanation: The native body part may or may not be taken out, and the transplanted body part may take over all or a portion of its function

Body Part Character 4	Approach Character 5	Device Character 6	Qualifier Character 7
5 Esophagus 6 Stomach 8 Small Intestine LC E Large Intestine LC	Ø Open	Z No Device	Ø Allogeneic 1 Syngeneic 2 Zooplastic

Non-OR ØDY5ØZ[Ø,1,2]
LC ØDY[8,E]ØZ[Ø,1,2]

Hepatobiliary System and Pancreas ØF1–ØFY

Character Meanings

This Character Meaning table is provided as a guide to assist the user in the identification of character members that may be found in this section of code tables. It **SHOULD NOT** be used to build a PCS code.

Operation–Character 3	Body Part–Character 4	Approach–Character 5	Device–Character 6	Qualifier–Character 7
1 Bypass	Ø Liver	Ø Open	Ø Drainage Device	Ø Allogeneic
2 Change	1 Liver, Right Lobe	3 Percutaneous	1 Radioactive Element	1 Syngeneic
5 Destruction	2 Liver, Left Lobe	4 Percutaneous Endoscopic	2 Monitoring Device	2 Zooplastic
7 Dilation	4 Gallbladder	7 Via Natural or Artificial Opening	3 Infusion Device	3 Duodenum
8 Division	5 Hepatic Duct, Right	8 Via Natural or Artificial Opening Endoscopic	7 Autologous Tissue Substitute	4 Stomach
9 Drainage	6 Hepatic Duct, Left	X External	C Extraluminal Device	5 Hepatic Duct, Right
B Excision	7 Hepatic Duct, Common		D Intraluminal Device	6 Hepatic Duct, Left
C Extirpation	8 Cystic Duct		J Synthetic Substitute	7 Hepatic Duct, Caudate
D Extraction	9 Common Bile Duct		K Nonautologous Tissue Substitute	8 Cystic Duct
F Fragmentation	B Hepatobiliary Duct		Y Other Device	9 Common Bile Duct
H Insertion	C Ampulla of Vater		Z No Device	B Small Intestine
J Inspection	D Pancreatic Duct			C Large Intestine
L Occlusion	F Pancreatic Duct, Accessory			F Irreversible Electroporation
M Reattachment	G Pancreas			X Diagnostic
N Release				Z No Qualifier
P Removal				
Q Repair				
R Replacement				
S Reposition				
T Resection				
U Supplement				
V Restriction				
W Revision				
Y Transplantation				

AHA Coding Clinic for table ØF1
2020, 4Q, 53   Bypass pancreatic duct to stomach

AHA Coding Clinic for table ØF5
2018, 4Q, 39   Irreversible electroporation

AHA Coding Clinic for table ØF7
2016, 3Q, 27   Endoscopic retrograde cholangiopancreatography with sphincterotomy and insertion of pancreatic stent
2016, 1Q, 25   Endoscopic retrograde cholangiopancreatography with brush biopsy of pancreatic and common bile ducts
2015, 1Q, 32   Percutaneous transhepatic biliary drainage catheter placement
2014, 3Q, 15   Drainage of pancreatic pseudocyst

AHA Coding Clinic for table ØF9
2020, 3Q, 34   Cystogastrostomy with stent insertion
2015, 1Q, 32   Percutaneous transhepatic biliary drainage catheter placement
2014, 3Q, 15   Drainage of pancreatic pseudocyst

AHA Coding Clinic for table ØFB
2019, 1Q, 3-8   Whipple procedure
2016, 3Q, 41   Open cholecystectomy with needle biopsy of liver
2016, 1Q, 23   Endoscopic ultrasound with aspiration biopsy of common hepatic duct
2016, 1Q, 25   Endoscopic retrograde cholangiopancreatography with brush biopsy of pancreatic and common bile ducts
2014, 3Q, 32   Pyloric-sparing Whipple procedure

AHA Coding Clinic for table ØFC
2016, 3Q, 27   Endoscopic retrograde cholangiopancreatography with sphincterotomy and insertion of pancreatic stent

AHA Coding Clinic for table ØFH
2020, 4Q, 43-44   Insertion of radioactive element

AHA Coding Clinic for table ØFQ
2016, 3Q, 27   Revision of common bile duct anastomosis
2013, 4Q, 109   Separating conjoined twins

AHA Coding Clinic for table ØFT
2019, 1Q, 3-8   Whipple Procedure
2012, 4Q, 99   Domino liver transplant

AHA Coding Clinic for table ØFY
2014, 3Q, 13   Orthotopic liver transplant with end to side cavoplasty
2012, 4Q, 99   Domino liver transplant

Liver

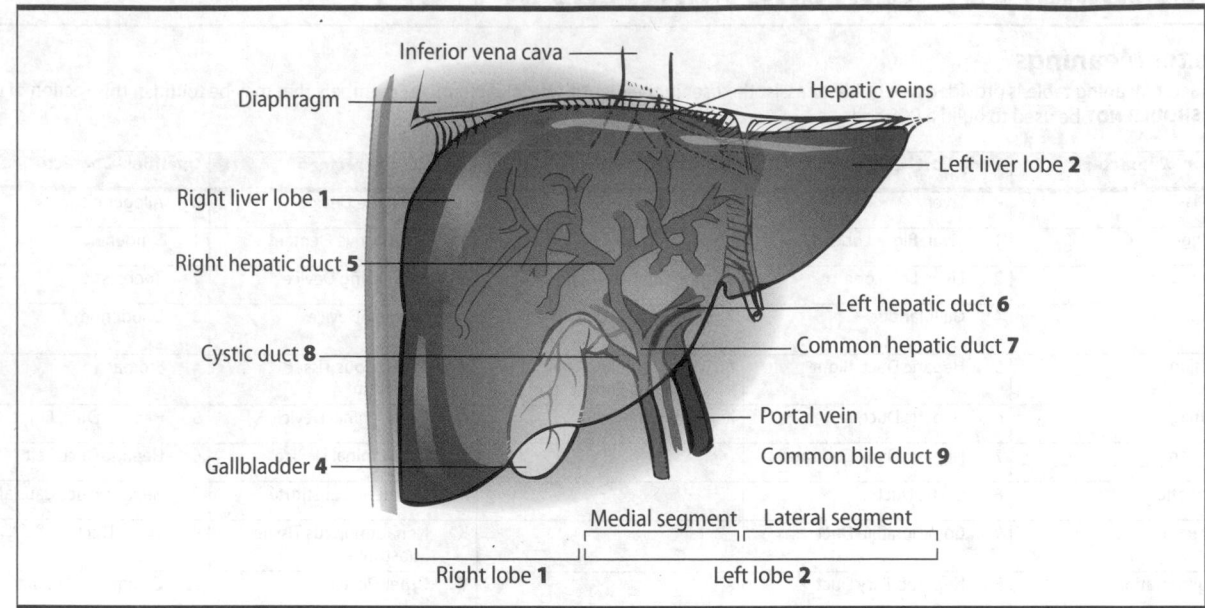

Inferior vena cava

Diaphragm

Hepatic veins

Left liver lobe **2**

Right liver lobe **1**

Right hepatic duct **5**

Left hepatic duct **6**

Cystic duct **8**

Common hepatic duct **7**

Portal vein

Gallbladder **4**

Common bile duct **9**

Medial segment Lateral segment

Right lobe **1** Left lobe **2**

Pancreas

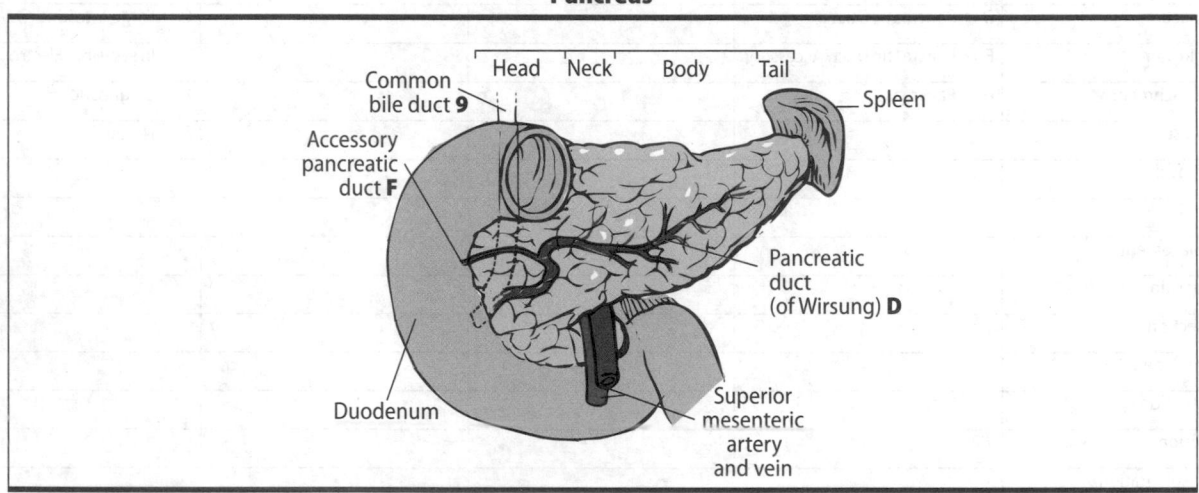

Head Neck Body Tail

Common bile duct **9**

Spleen

Accessory pancreatic duct **F**

Pancreatic duct (of Wirsung) **D**

Duodenum

Superior mesenteric artery and vein

Gallbladder and Ducts

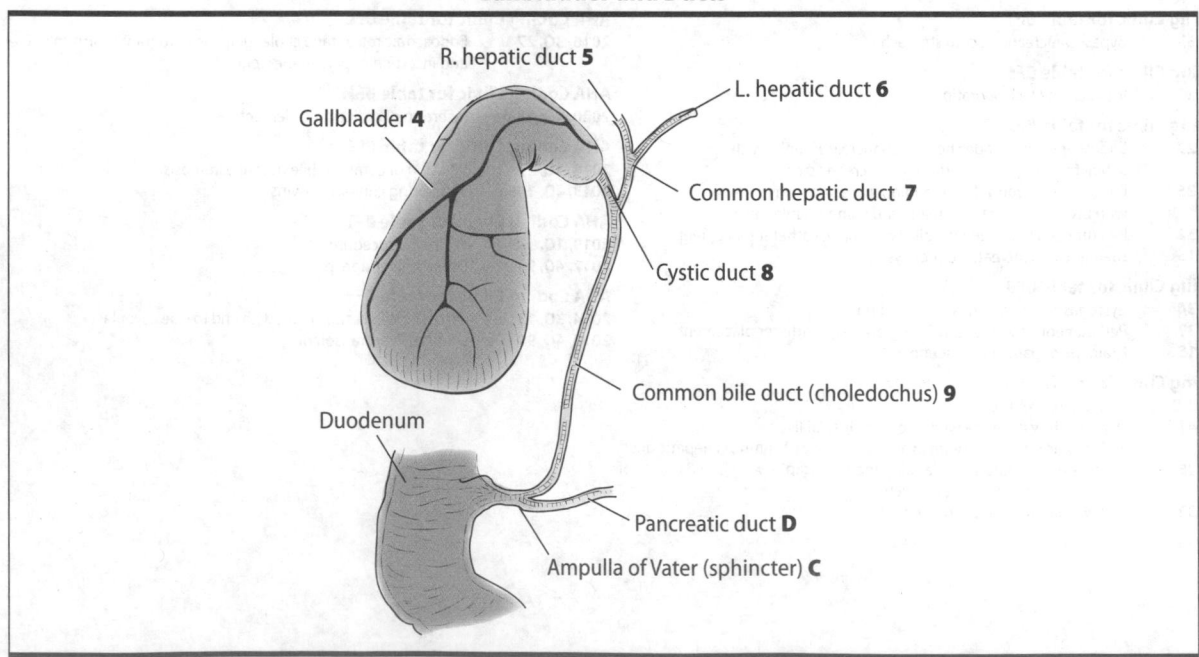

R. hepatic duct **5**

L. hepatic duct **6**

Gallbladder **4**

Common hepatic duct **7**

Cystic duct **8**

Common bile duct (choledochus) **9**

Duodenum

Pancreatic duct **D**

Ampulla of Vater (sphincter) **C**

Ø **Medical and Surgical**
F **Hepatobiliary System and Pancreas**
1 **Bypass**   Definition: Altering the route of passage of the contents of a tubular body part

Explanation: Rerouting contents of a body part to a downstream area of the normal route, to a similar route and body part, or to an abnormal route and dissimilar body part. Includes one or more anastomoses, with or without the use of a device.

Body Part Character 4	Approach Character 5	Device Character 6	Qualifier Character 7
4 Gallbladder 5 Hepatic Duct, Right 6 Hepatic Duct, Left 7 Hepatic Duct, Common 8 Cystic Duct 9 Common Bile Duct	Ø Open 4 Percutaneous Endoscopic	D Intraluminal Device Z No Device	3 Duodenum 4 Stomach 5 Hepatic Duct, Right 6 Hepatic Duct, Left 7 Hepatic Duct, Caudate 8 Cystic Duct 9 Common Bile Duct B Small Intestine
D Pancreatic Duct Duct of Wirsung	Ø Open 4 Percutaneous Endoscopic	D Intraluminal Device Z No Device	3 Duodenum 4 Stomach B Small Intestine C Large Intestine
F Pancreatic Duct, Accessory Duct of Santorini G Pancreas	Ø Open 4 Percutaneous Endoscopic	D Intraluminal Device Z No Device	3 Duodenum B Small Intestine C Large Intestine

Ø **Medical and Surgical**
F **Hepatobiliary System and Pancreas**
2 **Change**   Definition: Taking out or off a device from a body part and putting back an identical or similar device in or on the same body part without cutting or puncturing the skin or a mucous membrane

Explanation: All CHANGE procedures are coded using the approach EXTERNAL

Body Part Character 4	Approach Character 5	Device Character 6	Qualifier Character 7

Ø Liver
   Quadrate lobe
4 Gallbladder
B Hepatobiliary Duct
D Pancreatic Duct
   Duct of Wirsung
G Pancreas
	X External	Ø Drainage Device
		Y Other Device
			Z No Qualifier

Non-OR All body part, approach, device, and qualifier values

Ø **Medical and Surgical**
F **Hepatobiliary System and Pancreas**
5 **Destruction**   Definition: Physical eradication of all or a portion of a body part by the direct use of energy, force, or a destructive agent

Explanation: None of the body part is physically taken out

Body Part Character 4	Approach Character 5	Device Character 6	Qualifier Character 7
Ø Liver Quadrate lobe 1 Liver, Right Lobe 2 Liver, Left Lobe	Ø Open 3 Percutaneous 4 Percutaneous Endoscopic	Z No Device	F Irreversible Electroporation Z No Qualifier
4 Gallbladder	Ø Open 3 Percutaneous 4 Percutaneous Endoscopic 8 Via Natural or Artificial Opening Endoscopic	Z No Device	Z No Qualifier

5 Hepatic Duct, Right
6 Hepatic Duct, Left
7 Hepatic Duct, Common
8 Cystic Duct
9 Common Bile Duct
C Ampulla of Vater
   Duodenal ampulla
   Hepatopancreatic ampulla
D Pancreatic Duct
   Duct of Wirsung
F Pancreatic Duct, Accessory
   Duct of Santorini
	Ø Open
	3 Percutaneous
	4 Percutaneous Endoscopic
	7 Via Natural or Artificial Opening
	8 Via Natural or Artificial Opening Endoscopic
		Z No Device	Z No Qualifier

G Pancreas	Ø Open 3 Percutaneous 4 Percutaneous Endoscopic	Z No Device	F Irreversible Electroporation Z No Qualifier
G Pancreas	8 Via Natural or Artificial Opening Endoscopic	Z No Device	Z No Qualifier

Non-OR ØF5[5,6,7,8,9,C,D,F][4,8]ZZ   **Non-OR** ØF5G8ZZ
Non-OR ØF5G4Z[F,Z]

NC Noncovered Procedure   **LC** Limited Coverage   **QA** Questionable OB Admit   **NT** New Tech Add-on   ⊞ Combination Member   ♂ Male   ♀ Female

ICD-10-PCS 2022   403

ØF1–ØF5

Ø   **Medical and Surgical**
F   **Hepatobiliary System and Pancreas**
7   **Dilation**   Definition: Expanding an orifice or the lumen of a tubular body part

Explanation: The orifice can be a natural orifice or an artificially created orifice. Accomplished by stretching a tubular body part using intraluminal pressure or by cutting part of the orifice or wall of the tubular body part.

Body Part Character 4	Approach Character 5	Device Character 6	Qualifier Character 7

5   Hepatic Duct, Right
6   Hepatic Duct, Left
7   Hepatic Duct, Common
8   Cystic Duct
9   Common Bile Duct
C   Ampulla of Vater
     Duodenal ampulla
     Hepatopancreatic ampulla
D   Pancreatic Duct
     Duct of Wirsung
F   Pancreatic Duct, Accessory
     Duct of Santorini
	Ø Open
	3 Percutaneous
	4 Percutaneous Endoscopic
	7 Via Natural or Artificial Opening
	8 Via Natural or Artificial Opening
	     Endoscopic
		D Intraluminal Device
		Z No Device
			Z No Qualifier

Non-OR	ØF7[5,6,7,8,9][3,4,8][D,Z]Z
Non-OR	ØF7[5,6,7,8,9,D]]7DZ
Non-OR	ØF7C8[D,Z]Z
Non-OR	ØF7[D,F][4,8][D,Z]Z

Ø   **Medical and Surgical**
F   **Hepatobiliary System and Pancreas**
8   **Division**   Definition: Cutting into a body part, without draining fluids and/or gases from the body part, in order to separate or transect a body part

Explanation: All or a portion of the body part is separated into two or more portions

Body Part Character 4	Approach Character 5	Device Character 6	Qualifier Character 7
Ø Liver **1** Liver, Right Lobe **2** Liver, Left Lobe **G** Pancreas	**Ø** Open **3** Percutaneous **4** Percutaneous Endoscopic	**Z** No Device	**Z** No Qualifier

Non-OR	ØF8[Ø,1,2]3ZZ

0   Medical and Surgical
F   Hepatobiliary System and Pancreas
9   Drainage   Definition: Taking or letting out fluids and/or gases from a body part
                       Explanation: The qualifier DIAGNOSTIC is used to identify drainage procedures that are biopsies

Body Part Character 4	Approach Character 5	Device Character 6	Qualifier Character 7
0 Liver Quadrate lobe **1 Liver, Right Lobe** **2 Liver, Left Lobe**	**0** Open **3** Percutaneous **4** Percutaneous Endoscopic	**0** Drainage Device	**Z** No Qualifier
0 Liver Quadrate lobe **1 Liver, Right Lobe** **2 Liver, Left Lobe**	**0** Open **3** Percutaneous **4** Percutaneous Endoscopic	**Z** No Device	**X** Diagnostic **Z** No Qualifier
4 Gallbladder **G Pancreas**	**0** Open **3** Percutaneous **4** Percutaneous Endoscopic **8** Via Natural or Artificial Opening Endoscopic	**0** Drainage Device	**Z** No Qualifier
4 Gallbladder **G Pancreas**	**0** Open **3** Percutaneous **4** Percutaneous Endoscopic **8** Via Natural or Artificial Opening Endoscopic	**Z** No Device	**X** Diagnostic **Z** No Qualifier
5 Hepatic Duct, Right **6 Hepatic Duct, Left** **7 Hepatic Duct, Common** **8 Cystic Duct** **9 Common Bile Duct** **C Ampulla of Vater** Duodenal ampulla Hepatopancreatic ampulla **D Pancreatic Duct** Duct of Wirsung **F Pancreatic Duct, Accessory** Duct of Santorini	**0** Open **3** Percutaneous **4** Percutaneous Endoscopic **7** Via Natural or Artificial Opening **8** Via Natural or Artificial Opening Endoscopic	**0** Drainage Device	**Z** No Qualifier
5 Hepatic Duct, Right **6 Hepatic Duct, Left** **7 Hepatic Duct, Common** **8 Cystic Duct** **9 Common Bile Duct** **C Ampulla of Vater** Duodenal ampulla Hepatopancreatic ampulla **D Pancreatic Duct** Duct of Wirsung **F Pancreatic Duct, Accessory** Duct of Santorini	**0** Open **3** Percutaneous **4** Percutaneous Endoscopic **7** Via Natural or Artificial Opening **8** Via Natural or Artificial Opening Endoscopic	**Z** No Device	**X** Diagnostic **Z** No Qualifier

Non-OR 0F9[0,1,2][3,4]0Z	**Non-OR** 0F99[3,8]0Z
Non-OR 0F9[0,1,2][3,4]Z[X,Z]	**Non-OR** 0F9C[3,4,8]0Z
Non-OR 0F9[4,G]80Z	**Non-OR** 0F9[D,F][3,8]0Z
Non-OR 0F9G30Z	**Non-OR** 0F9[5,6,8,9,C,D,F]3Z[X,Z]
Non-OR 0F9[4,G]8Z[X,Z]	**Non-OR** 0F9[5,6,8,9,C,D,F][4,7,8]ZX
Non-OR 0F9G3Z[XZ]	**Non-OR** 0F9[5,6,8,D,F]8ZZ
Non-OR 0F9G4ZX	**Non-OR** 0F97[3,4,7,8]Z[X,Z]
Non-OR 0F9[5,6,8][3,8]0Z	**Non-OR** 0F99[4,7,8]ZZ
Non-OR 0F97[3,4,7,8]0Z	**Non-OR** 0F9C[4,8]ZZ

NC Noncovered Procedure   **LC** Limited Coverage   **QA** Questionable OB Admit   **NT** New Tech Add-on   ⊞ Combination Member   ♂ Male   ♀ Female

ICD-10-PCS 2022   405

0F9–0F9

Ø **Medical and Surgical**
F **Hepatobiliary System and Pancreas**
B **Excision**　　　Definition: Cutting out or off, without replacement, a portion of a body part
　　　　　　　　　Explanation: The qualifier DIAGNOSTIC is used to identify excision procedures that are biopsies

Body Part Character 4	Approach Character 5	Device Character 6	Qualifier Character 7
Ø Liver 　　Quadrate lobe **1** Liver, Right Lobe **2** Liver, Left Lobe	**Ø** Open **3** Percutaneous **4** Percutaneous Endoscopic	**Z** No Device	**X** Diagnostic **Z** No Qualifier
4 Gallbladder **G** Pancreas	**Ø** Open **3** Percutaneous **4** Percutaneous Endoscopic **8** Via Natural or Artificial Opening 　　Endoscopic	**Z** No Device	**X** Diagnostic **Z** No Qualifier
5 Hepatic Duct, Right **6** Hepatic Duct, Left **7** Hepatic Duct, Common **8** Cystic Duct **9** Common Bile Duct **C** Ampulla of Vater 　　Duodenal ampulla 　　Hepatopancreatic ampulla **D** Pancreatic Duct 　　Duct of Wirsung **F** Pancreatic Duct, Accessory 　　Duct of Santorini	**Ø** Open **3** Percutaneous **4** Percutaneous Endoscopic **7** Via Natural or Artificial Opening **8** Via Natural or Artificial Opening 　　Endoscopic	**Z** No Device	**X** Diagnostic **Z** No Qualifier

Non-OR	ØFB[Ø,1,2]3ZX
Non-OR	ØFB[4,G][3,4,8]ZX
Non-OR	ØFB[5,6,7,8,9,C,D,F][3,4,7,8]ZX
Non-OR	ØFB[5,6,7,8,9,C,D,F][4,8]ZZ

Ø **Medical and Surgical**
F **Hepatobiliary System and Pancreas**
C **Extirpation**　　　Definition: Taking or cutting out solid matter from a body part
　　　　　　　　　Explanation: The solid matter may be an abnormal byproduct of a biological function or a foreign body; it may be imbedded in a body part or in the lumen of a tubular body part. The solid matter may or may not have been previously broken into pieces.

Body Part Character 4	Approach Character 5	Device Character 6	Qualifier Character 7
Ø Liver 　　Quadrate lobe **1** Liver, Right Lobe **2** Liver, Left Lobe	**Ø** Open **3** Percutaneous **4** Percutaneous Endoscopic	**Z** No Device	**Z** No Qualifier
4 Gallbladder **G** Pancreas	**Ø** Open **3** Percutaneous **4** Percutaneous Endoscopic **8** Via Natural or Artificial Opening 　　Endoscopic	**Z** No Device	**Z** No Qualifier
5 Hepatic Duct, Right **6** Hepatic Duct, Left **7** Hepatic Duct, Common **8** Cystic Duct **9** Common Bile Duct **C** Ampulla of Vater 　　Duodenal ampulla 　　Hepatopancreatic ampulla **D** Pancreatic Duct 　　Duct of Wirsung **F** Pancreatic Duct, Accessory 　　Duct of Santorini	**Ø** Open **3** Percutaneous **4** Percutaneous Endoscopic **7** Via Natural or Artificial Opening **8** Via Natural or Artificial Opening 　　Endoscopic	**Z** No Device	**Z** No Qualifier

Non-OR	ØFC[5,6,7,8,9][3,4,7,8]ZZ
Non-OR	ØFCC[4,8]ZZ
Non-OR	ØFC[D,F][3,4,8]ZZ

Ø　**Medical and Surgical**
F　**Hepatobiliary System and Pancreas**
D　**Extraction**　　Definition: Pulling or stripping out or off all or a portion of a body part by the use of force
　　　　　　　　　　Explanation: The qualifier DIAGNOSTIC is used to identify extraction procedures that are biopsies

Body Part Character 4	Approach Character 5	Device Character 6	Qualifier Character 7
Ø　Liver 　　Quadrate lobe 1　Liver, Right Lobe 2　Liver, Left Lobe	3　Percutaneous 4　Percutaneous Endoscopic	Z　No Device	X　Diagnostic
4　Gallbladder 5　Hepatic Duct, Right 6　Hepatic Duct, Left 7　Hepatic Duct, Common 8　Cystic Duct 9　Common Bile Duct C　Ampulla of Vater 　　Duodenal ampulla 　　Hepatopancreatic ampulla D　Pancreatic Duct 　　Duct of Wirsung F　Pancreatic Duct, Accessory 　　Duct of Santorini G　Pancreas	3　Percutaneous 4　Percutaneous Endoscopic 8　Via Natural or Artificial Opening 　　Endoscopic	Z　No Device	X　Diagnostic

Non-OR　ØFD[Ø,1,2]3ZX
Non-OR　ØFD[4,5,6,7,8,9,C,D,F,G][3,4,8]ZX

Ø　**Medical and Surgical**
F　**Hepatobiliary System and Pancreas**
F　**Fragmentation**　　Definition: Breaking solid matter in a body part into pieces
　　　　　　　　　　Explanation: Physical force (e.g., manual, ultrasonic) applied directly or indirectly is used to break the solid matter into pieces. The solid matter may be an abnormal byproduct of a biological function or a foreign body. The pieces of solid matter are not taken out.

Body Part Character 4	Approach Character 5	Device Character 6	Qualifier Character 7
4　Gallbladder　　**NC** 5　Hepatic Duct, Right　　**NC** 6　Hepatic Duct, Left　　**NC** 7　Hepatic Duct, Common 8　Cystic Duct　　**NC** 9　Common Bile Duct　　**NC** C　Ampulla of Vater　　**NC** 　　Duodenal ampulla 　　Hepatopancreatic ampulla D　Pancreatic Duct　　**NC** 　　Duct of Wirsung F　Pancreatic Duct, Accessory　　**NC** 　　Duct of Santorini	Ø　Open 3　Percutaneous 4　Percutaneous Endoscopic 7　Via Natural or Artificial Opening 8　Via Natural or Artificial Opening 　　Endoscopic X　External	Z　No Device	Z　No Qualifier

Non-OR　ØFF[4,5,6,7,8,9,C,D,F][8,X]ZZ
NC　　ØFF[4,5,6,8,9,C,D,F]XZZ

Ø　**Medical and Surgical**
F　**Hepatobiliary System and Pancreas**
H　**Insertion**　　Definition: Putting in a nonbiological appliance that monitors, assists, performs, or prevents a physiological function but does not physically take the place of a body part
　　　　　　　　　　Explanation: None

Body Part Character 4	Approach Character 5	Device Character 6	Qualifier Character 7
Ø　Liver 　　Quadrate lobe 4　Gallbladder G　Pancreas	Ø　Open 3　Percutaneous 4　Percutaneous Endoscopic	1　Radioactive Element 2　Monitoring Device 3　Infusion Device Y　Other Device	Z　No Qualifier
1　Liver, Right Lobe 2　Liver, Left Lobe	Ø　Open 3　Percutaneous 4　Percutaneous Endoscopic	2　Monitoring Device 3　Infusion Device	Z　No Qualifier
B　Hepatobiliary Duct　　⊞ D　Pancreatic Duct 　　Duct of Wirsung	Ø　Open 3　Percutaneous 4　Percutaneous Endoscopic 7　Via Natural or Artificial Opening 8　Via Natural or Artificial Opening 　　Endoscopic	1　Radioactive Element 2　Monitoring Device 3　Infusion Device D　Intraluminal Device Y　Other Device	Z　No Qualifier

Non-OR　ØFH[Ø,4,G]31Z	**Non-OR**　ØFH[B,D][Ø,3,4]3Z	See Appendix L for Procedure Combinations
Non-OR　ØFH[Ø,4,G][Ø,3,4]3Z	**Non-OR**　ØFH[B,D][4,8]DZ	⊞　　ØFHB7DZ
Non-OR　ØFH[Ø,4,G][3,4]YZ	**Non-OR**　ØFH[B,D][7,8][2,3]Z	
Non-OR　ØFH[1,2][Ø,3,4]3Z	**Non-OR**　ØFH[B,D][3,4,7,8]YZ	

NC Noncovered Procedure　　**LC** Limited Coverage　　**QA** Questionable OB Admit　　**NT** New Tech Add-on　　⊞ Combination Member　　♂ Male　　♀ Female

Ø **Medical and Surgical**
F **Hepatobiliary System and Pancreas**
J **Inspection**   Definition: Visually and/or manually exploring a body part

Explanation: Visual exploration may be performed with or without optical instrumentation. Manual exploration may be performed directly or through intervening body layers.

Body Part Character 4	Approach Character 5	Device Character 6	Qualifier Character 7
Ø Liver Quadrate lobe	Ø Open 3 Percutaneous 4 Percutaneous Endoscopic X External	Z No Device	Z No Qualifier
4 Gallbladder G Pancreas	Ø Open 3 Percutaneous 4 Percutaneous Endoscopic 8 Via Natural or Artificial Opening Endoscopic X External	Z No Device	Z No Qualifier
B Hepatobiliary Duct D Pancreatic Duct Duct of Wirsung	Ø Open 3 Percutaneous 4 Percutaneous Endoscopic 7 Via Natural or Artificial Opening 8 Via Natural or Artificial Opening Endoscopic	Z No Device	Z No Qualifier

Non-OR   ØFJØ[3,X]ZZ
Non-OR   ØFJ[4,G][3,8,X]ZZ
Non-OR   ØFJ[B,D][3,7,8]ZZ

Ø **Medical and Surgical**
F **Hepatobiliary System and Pancreas**
L **Occlusion**   Definition: Completely closing an orifice or the lumen of a tubular body part

Explanation: The orifice can be a natural orifice or an artificially created orifice

Body Part Character 4	Approach Character 5	Device Character 6	Qualifier Character 7

5 Hepatic Duct, Right
6 Hepatic Duct, Left
7 Hepatic Duct, Common
8 Cystic Duct
9 Common Bile Duct
C Ampulla of Vater
   Duodenal ampulla
   Hepatopancreatic ampulla
D Pancreatic Duct
   Duct of Wirsung
F Pancreatic Duct, Accessory
   Duct of Santorini
	Ø Open
	3 Percutaneous
	4 Percutaneous Endoscopic
		C Extraluminal Device
		D Intraluminal Device
		Z No Device
			Z No Qualifier

5 Hepatic Duct, Right
6 Hepatic Duct, Left
7 Hepatic Duct, Common
8 Cystic Duct
9 Common Bile Duct
C Ampulla of Vater
   Duodenal ampulla
   Hepatopancreatic ampulla
D Pancreatic Duct
   Duct of Wirsung
F Pancreatic Duct, Accessory
   Duct of Santorini
	7 Via Natural or Artificial Opening
	8 Via Natural or Artificial Opening Endoscopic
		D Intraluminal Device
		Z No Device
			Z No Qualifier

Non-OR   ØFL[5,6,7,8,9][3,4][C,D,Z]Z
Non-OR   ØFL[5,6,7,8,9][7,8][D,Z]Z

Ø   Medical and Surgical
F   Hepatobiliary System and Pancreas
M   Reattachment   Definition: Putting back in or on all or a portion of a separated body part to its normal location or other suitable location
                      Explanation: Vascular circulation and nervous pathways may or may not be reestablished

Body Part Character 4	Approach Character 5	Device Character 6	Qualifier Character 7

Ø   Liver
     Quadrate lobe
1   Liver, Right Lobe
2   Liver, Left Lobe
4   Gallbladder
5   Hepatic Duct, Right
6   Hepatic Duct, Left
7   Hepatic Duct, Common
8   Cystic Duct
9   Common Bile Duct
C   Ampulla of Vater
     Duodenal ampulla
     Hepatopancreatic ampulla
D   Pancreatic Duct
     Duct of Wirsung
F   Pancreatic Duct, Accessory
     Duct of Santorini
G   Pancreas
	Ø Open
	4 Percutaneous Endoscopic
		Z No Device	**Z** No Qualifier

Non-OR   ØFM[4,5,6,7,8,9]4ZZ

Ø   Medical and Surgical
F   Hepatobiliary System and Pancreas
N   Release   Definition: Freeing a body part from an abnormal physical constraint by cutting or by the use of force
              Explanation: Some of the restraining tissue may be taken out but none of the body part is taken out

Body Part Character 4	Approach Character 5	Device Character 6	Qualifier Character 7
Ø Liver Quadrate lobe **1** Liver, Right Lobe **2** Liver, Left Lobe	**Ø** Open **3** Percutaneous **4** Percutaneous Endoscopic	**Z** No Device	**Z** No Qualifier
4 Gallbladder **G** Pancreas	**Ø** Open **3** Percutaneous **4** Percutaneous Endoscopic **8** Via Natural or Artificial Opening Endoscopic	**Z** No Device	**Z** No Qualifier

5   Hepatic Duct, Right
6   Hepatic Duct, Left
7   Hepatic Duct, Common
8   Cystic Duct
9   Common Bile Duct
C   Ampulla of Vater
     Duodenal ampulla
     Hepatopancreatic ampulla
D   Pancreatic Duct
     Duct of Wirsung
F   Pancreatic Duct, Accessory
     Duct of Santorini
	Ø Open
	3 Percutaneous
	4 Percutaneous Endoscopic
	7 Via Natural or Artificial Opening
	8 Via Natural or Artificial Opening Endoscopic
		Z No Device	**Z** No Qualifier

Ø **Medical and Surgical**
F **Hepatobiliary System and Pancreas**
P **Removal**   Definition: Taking out or off a device from a body part

Explanation: If a device is taken out and a similar device put in without cutting or puncturing the skin or mucous membrane, the procedure is coded to the root operation CHANGE. Otherwise, the procedure for taking out a device is coded to the root operation REMOVAL.

Body Part Character 4	Approach Character 5	Device Character 6	Qualifier Character 7
Ø Liver Quadrate lobe	**Ø** Open **3** Percutaneous **4** Percutaneous Endoscopic	**Ø** Drainage Device **2** Monitoring Device **3** Infusion Device **Y** Other Device	**Z** No Qualifier
Ø Liver Quadrate lobe	**X** External	**Ø** Drainage Device **2** Monitoring Device **3** Infusion Device	**Z** No Qualifier
4 Gallbladder **G** Pancreas	**Ø** Open **3** Percutaneous **4** Percutaneous Endoscopic	**Ø** Drainage Device **2** Monitoring Device **3** Infusion Device **D** Intraluminal Device **Y** Other Device	**Z** No Qualifier
4 Gallbladder **G** Pancreas	**X** External	**Ø** Drainage Device **2** Monitoring Device **3** Infusion Device **D** Intraluminal Device	**Z** No Qualifier
B Hepatobiliary Duct **D** Pancreatic Duct Duct of Wirsung	**Ø** Open **3** Percutaneous **4** Percutaneous Endoscopic **7** Via Natural or Artificial Opening **8** Via Natural or Artificial Opening Endoscopic	**Ø** Drainage Device **1** Radioactive Element **2** Monitoring Device **3** Infusion Device **7** Autologous Tissue Substitute **C** Extraluminal Device **D** Intraluminal Device **J** Synthetic Substitute **K** Nonautologous Tissue Substitute **Y** Other Device	**Z** No Qualifier
B Hepatobiliary Duct **D** Pancreatic Duct Duct of Wirsung	**X** External	**Ø** Drainage Device **1** Radioactive Element **2** Monitoring Device **3** Infusion Device **D** Intraluminal Device	**Z** No Qualifier

Non-OR	ØFPØ[3,4]YZ	
Non-OR	ØFPØX[Ø,2,3]Z	
Non-OR	ØFPG3ØZ	
Non-OR	ØFP[4,G][3,4]YZ	
Non-OR	ØFP4X[Ø,2,3,D]Z	
Non-OR	ØFPGX[Ø,2,3]Z	
Non-OR	ØFP[B,D][3,4]YZ	
Non-OR	ØFP[B,D][7,8][Ø,2,3,D,Y]Z	
Non-OR	ØFP[B,D]X[Ø,1,2,3,D]Z	

See Appendix L for Procedure Combinations

Combo-only	ØFP[B,D][7,8]DZ
Combo-only	ØFP[B,D]XDZ

Ø **Medical and Surgical**
F **Hepatobiliary System and Pancreas**
Q **Repair**　　　Definition: Restoring, to the extent possible, a body part to its normal anatomic structure and function

Explanation: Used only when the method to accomplish the repair is not one of the other root operations

Body Part Character 4	Approach Character 5	Device Character 6	Qualifier Character 7
Ø Liver Quadrate lobe **1** Liver, Right Lobe **2** Liver, Left Lobe	**Ø** Open **3** Percutaneous **4** Percutaneous Endoscopic	**Z** No Device	**Z** No Qualifier
4 Gallbladder **G** Pancreas	**Ø** Open **3** Percutaneous **4** Percutaneous Endoscopic **8** Via Natural or Artificial Opening Endoscopic	**Z** No Device	**Z** No Qualifier

5 Hepatic Duct, Right
6 Hepatic Duct, Left
7 Hepatic Duct, Common
8 Cystic Duct
9 Common Bile Duct
C Ampulla of Vater
  Duodenal ampulla
  Hepatopancreatic ampulla
D Pancreatic Duct
  Duct of Wirsung
F Pancreatic Duct, Accessory
  Duct of Santorini
	Ø Open
	3 Percutaneous
	4 Percutaneous Endoscopic
	7 Via Natural or Artificial Opening
	8 Via Natural or Artificial Opening
	  Endoscopic
		Z No Device	**Z** No Qualifier

Ø **Medical and Surgical**
F **Hepatobiliary System and Pancreas**
R **Replacement**　　　Definition: Putting in or on biological or synthetic material that physically takes the place and/or function of all or a portion of a body part

Explanation: The body part may have been taken out or replaced, or may be taken out, physically eradicated, or rendered nonfunctional during the REPLACEMENT procedure. A REMOVAL procedure is coded for taking out the device used in a previous replacement procedure.

Body Part Character 4	Approach Character 5	Device Character 6	Qualifier Character 7

5 Hepatic Duct, Right
6 Hepatic Duct, Left
7 Hepatic Duct, Common
8 Cystic Duct
9 Common Bile Duct
C Ampulla of Vater
  Duodenal ampulla
  Hepatopancreatic ampulla
D Pancreatic Duct
  Duct of Wirsung
F Pancreatic Duct, Accessory
  Duct of Santorini
	Ø Open
	4 Percutaneous Endoscopic
	8 Via Natural or Artificial Opening
	  Endoscopic
		7 Autologous Tissue Substitute
		J Synthetic Substitute
		K Nonautologous Tissue Substitute
			Z No Qualifier

Ø **Medical and Surgical**
F **Hepatobiliary System and Pancreas**
S **Reposition**　　　Definition: Moving to its normal location, or other suitable location, all or a portion of a body part

Explanation: The body part is moved to a new location from an abnormal location, or from a normal location where it is not functioning correctly. The body part may or may not be cut out or off to be moved to the new location.

Body Part Character 4	Approach Character 5	Device Character 6	Qualifier Character 7

Ø Liver
  Quadrate lobe
4 Gallbladder
5 Hepatic Duct, Right
6 Hepatic Duct, Left
7 Hepatic Duct, Common
8 Cystic Duct
9 Common Bile Duct
C Ampulla of Vater
  Duodenal ampulla
  Hepatopancreatic ampulla
D Pancreatic Duct
  Duct of Wirsung
F Pancreatic Duct, Accessory
  Duct of Santorini
G Pancreas
	Ø Open
	4 Percutaneous Endoscopic
		Z No Device	**Z** No Qualifier

NC Noncovered Procedure　　**LC** Limited Coverage　　**QA** Questionable OB Admit　　**NT** New Tech Add-on　　⊞ Combination Member　　♂ Male　　♀ Female

Ø   Medical and Surgical
F   Hepatobiliary System and Pancreas
T   Resection   Definition: Cutting out or off, without replacement, all of a body part
Explanation: None

Body Part Character 4	Approach Character 5	Device Character 6	Qualifier Character 7
Ø Liver Quadrate lobe **1** Liver, Right Lobe **2** Liver, Left Lobe **4** Gallbladder **G** Pancreas ⊞	**Ø** Open **4** Percutaneous Endoscopic	**Z** No Device	**Z** No Qualifier

5 Hepatic Duct, Right
6 Hepatic Duct, Left
7 Hepatic Duct, Common
8 Cystic Duct
9 Common Bile Duct
C Ampulla of Vater
   Duodenal ampulla
   Hepatopancreatic ampulla
D Pancreatic Duct
   Duct of Wirsung
F Pancreatic Duct, Accessory
   Duct of Santorini
	Ø Open
	4 Percutaneous Endoscopic
	7 Via Natural or Artificial Opening
	8 Via Natural or Artificial Opening
	   Endoscopic
		Z No Device	**Z** No Qualifier

Non-OR   ØFT[D,F][4,8]ZZ

See Appendix L for Procedure Combinations
⊞   ØFTGØZZ

Ø   Medical and Surgical
F   Hepatobiliary System and Pancreas
U   Supplement   Definition: Putting in or on biological or synthetic material that physically reinforces and/or augments the function of a portion of a body part
Explanation: The biological material is non-living, or is living and from the same individual. The body part may have been previously replaced, and the SUPPLEMENT procedure is performed to physically reinforce and/or augment the function of the replaced body part.

Body Part Character 4	Approach Character 5	Device Character 6	Qualifier Character 7

5 Hepatic Duct, Right
6 Hepatic Duct, Left
7 Hepatic Duct, Common
8 Cystic Duct
9 Common Bile Duct
C Ampulla of Vater
   Duodenal ampulla
   Hepatopancreatic ampulla
D Pancreatic Duct
   Duct of Wirsung
F Pancreatic Duct, Accessory
   Duct of Santorini
	Ø Open
	3 Percutaneous
	4 Percutaneous Endoscopic
	8 Via Natural or Artificial Opening
	   Endoscopic
		7 Autologous Tissue Substitute
		J Synthetic Substitute
		K Nonautologous Tissue Substitute
			Z No Qualifier

Non-OR Procedure   DRG Non-OR Procedure   Valid OR Procedure   HAC Associated Procedure   Combination Only   New/Revised GREEN

Ø   Medical and Surgical
F   Hepatobiliary System and Pancreas
V   Restriction   Definition: Partially closing an orifice or the lumen of a tubular body part

                      Explanation: The orifice can be a natural orifice or an artificially created orifice

Body Part Character 4	Approach Character 5	Device Character 6	Qualifier Character 7

5   Hepatic Duct, Right
6   Hepatic Duct, Left
7   Hepatic Duct, Common
8   Cystic Duct
9   Common Bile Duct
C   Ampulla of Vater
     Duodenal ampulla
     Hepatopancreatic ampulla
D   Pancreatic Duct
     Duct of Wirsung
F   Pancreatic Duct, Accessory
     Duct of Santorini
	Ø Open
	3 Percutaneous
	4 Percutaneous Endoscopic
		C Extraluminal Device
		D Intraluminal Device
		Z No Device
			Z No Qualifier

5   Hepatic Duct, Right
6   Hepatic Duct, Left
7   Hepatic Duct, Common
8   Cystic Duct
9   Common Bile Duct
C   Ampulla of Vater
     Duodenal ampulla
     Hepatopancreatic ampulla
D   Pancreatic Duct
     Duct of Wirsung
F   Pancreatic Duct, Accessory
     Duct of Santorini
	7 Via Natural or Artificial Opening
	8 Via Natural or Artificial Opening
	     Endoscopic
		D Intraluminal Device
		Z No Device
			Z No Qualifier

Non-OR   ØFV[5,6,7,8,9][3,4][C,D,Z]Z
Non-OR   ØFV[5,6,7,8,9][7,8][D,Z]Z

NC Noncovered Procedure   LC Limited Coverage   QA Questionable OB Admit   NT New Tech Add-on   ⊞ Combination Member   ♂ Male   ♀ Female

ICD-10-PCS 2022   413

Hepatobiliary System and Pancreas

Ø   Medical and Surgical
F   Hepatobiliary System and Pancreas
W   Revision   Definition: Correcting, to the extent possible, a portion of a malfunctioning device or the position of a displaced device

Explanation: Revision can include correcting a malfunctioning or displaced device by taking out or putting in components of the device such as a screw or pin

Body Part Character 4	Approach Character 5	Device Character 6	Qualifier Character 7
Ø Liver Quadrate lobe	Ø Open 3 Percutaneous 4 Percutaneous Endoscopic	Ø Drainage Device 2 Monitoring Device 3 Infusion Device Y Other Device	Z No Qualifier
Ø Liver Quadrate lobe	X External	Ø Drainage Device 2 Monitoring Device 3 Infusion Device	Z No Qualifier
4 Gallbladder G Pancreas	Ø Open 3 Percutaneous 4 Percutaneous Endoscopic	Ø Drainage Device 2 Monitoring Device 3 Infusion Device D Intraluminal Device Y Other Device	Z No Qualifier
4 Gallbladder G Pancreas	X External	Ø Drainage Device 2 Monitoring Device 3 Infusion Device D Intraluminal Device	Z No Qualifier
B Hepatobiliary Duct D Pancreatic Duct Duct of Wirsung	Ø Open 3 Percutaneous 4 Percutaneous Endoscopic 7 Via Natural or Artificial Opening 8 Via Natural or Artificial Opening Endoscopic	Ø Drainage Device 2 Monitoring Device 3 Infusion Device 7 Autologous Tissue Substitute C Extraluminal Device D Intraluminal Device J Synthetic Substitute K Nonautologous Tissue Substitute Y Other Device	Z No Qualifier
B Hepatobiliary Duct D Pancreatic Duct Duct of Wirsung	X External	Ø Drainage Device 2 Monitoring Device 3 Infusion Device 7 Autologous Tissue Substitute C Extraluminal Device D Intraluminal Device J Synthetic Substitute K Nonautologous Tissue Substitute	Z No Qualifier

Non-OR   ØFWØ[3,4]YZ
Non-OR   ØFWØX[Ø,2,3]Z
Non-OR   ØFW[4,G][3,4]YZ
Non-OR   ØFW[4,G]X[Ø,2,3,D]Z
Non-OR   ØFW[B,D][3,4,7,8]YZ
Non-OR   ØFW[B,D]X[Ø,2,3,7,C,D,J,K]Z

Ø   Medical and Surgical
F   Hepatobiliary System and Pancreas
Y   Transplantation   Definition: Putting in or on all or a portion of a living body part taken from another individual or animal to physically take the place and/or function of all or a portion of a similar body part

Explanation: The native body part may or may not be taken out, and the transplanted body part may take over all or a portion of its function

Body Part Character 4	Approach Character 5	Device Character 6	Qualifier Character 7
Ø Liver `LC` Quadrate lobe G Pancreas `LC` `NC` ⊞	Ø Open	Z No Device	Ø Allogeneic 1 Syngeneic 2 Zooplastic

`LC`   ØFYØØZ[Ø,1,2]
`LC`   ØFYGØZ[Ø,1]
`NC`   ØFYGØZ2
`NC`   ØFYGØZ[Ø,1] If reported alone without one of the following procedures
      ØTYØØZ[Ø,1,2], ØTY1ØZ[Ø,1,2] and without one of the following
      diagnoses E1Ø.1Ø-E1Ø.9, E89.1

See Appendix L for Procedure Combinations
⊞   ØFYGØZ[Ø,1,2]

Endocrine System ØG2–ØGW

Character Meanings

This Character Meaning table is provided as a guide to assist the user in the identification of character members that may be found in this section of code tables. It **SHOULD NOT** be used to build a PCS code.

Operation–Character 3	Body Part–Character 4	Approach–Character 5	Device–Character 6	Qualifier–Character 7
2 Change	Ø Pituitary Gland	Ø Open	Ø Drainage Device	X Diagnostic
5 Destruction	1 Pineal Body	3 Percutaneous	1 Radioactive Element	Z No Qualifier
8 Division	2 Adrenal Gland, Left	4 Percutaneous Endoscopic	2 Monitoring Device	
9 Drainage	3 Adrenal Gland, Right	X External	3 Infusion Device	
B Excision	4 Adrenal Glands, Bilateral		Y Other Device	
C Extirpation	5 Adrenal Gland		Z No Device	
H Insertion	6 Carotid Body, Left			
J Inspection	7 Carotid Body, Right			
M Reattachment	8 Carotid Bodies, Bilateral			
N Release	9 Para-aortic Body			
P Removal	B Coccygeal Glomus			
Q Repair	C Glomus Jugulare			
S Reposition	D Aortic Body			
T Resection	F Paraganglion Extremity			
W Revision	G Thyroid Gland Lobe, Left			
	H Thyroid Gland Lobe, Right			
	J Thyroid Gland Isthmus			
	K Thyroid Gland			
	L Superior Parathyroid Gland, Right			
	M Superior Parathyroid Gland, Left			
	N Inferior Parathyroid Gland, Right			
	P Inferior Parathyroid Gland, Left			
	Q Parathyroid Glands, Multiple			
	R Parathyroid Gland			
	S Endocrine Gland			

AHA Coding Clinic for table ØGB

2021, 2Q, 7	Infrarenal para-aortic paraganglioma with excision
2017, 2Q, 20	Near total thyroidectomy
2014, 3Q, 22	Transsphenoidal removal of pituitary tumor and fat graft placement

AHA Coding Clinic for table ØGH

2020, 4Q, 43-44	Insertion of radioactive element

AHA Coding Clinic for table ØGT

2017, 2Q, 20	Near total thyroidectomy

Endocrine System

Pineal gland **1**

Pituitary **Ø**

Parathyroid glands **L, M, N, P, Q, R**

Thyroid gland **G, H, J, K**

Thymus gland

Thoracic duct

Adrenals (suprarenal) gland **2, 3, 4, 5**

Pancreas

Left Adrenal Gland

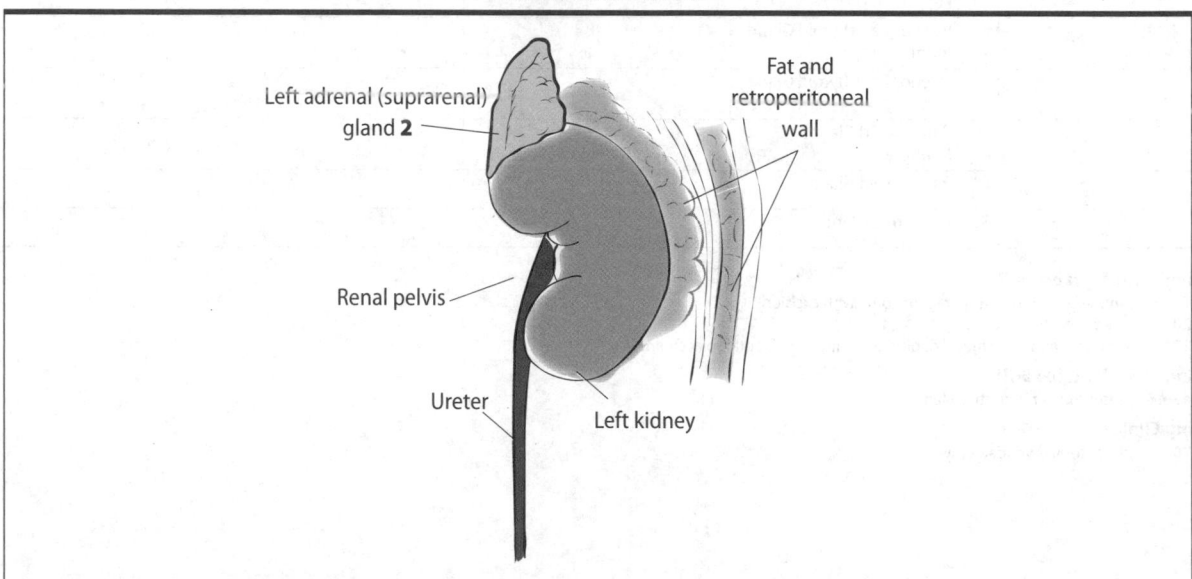

Left adrenal (suprarenal) gland **2**

Fat and retroperitoneal wall

Renal pelvis

Ureter

Left kidney

Thyroid

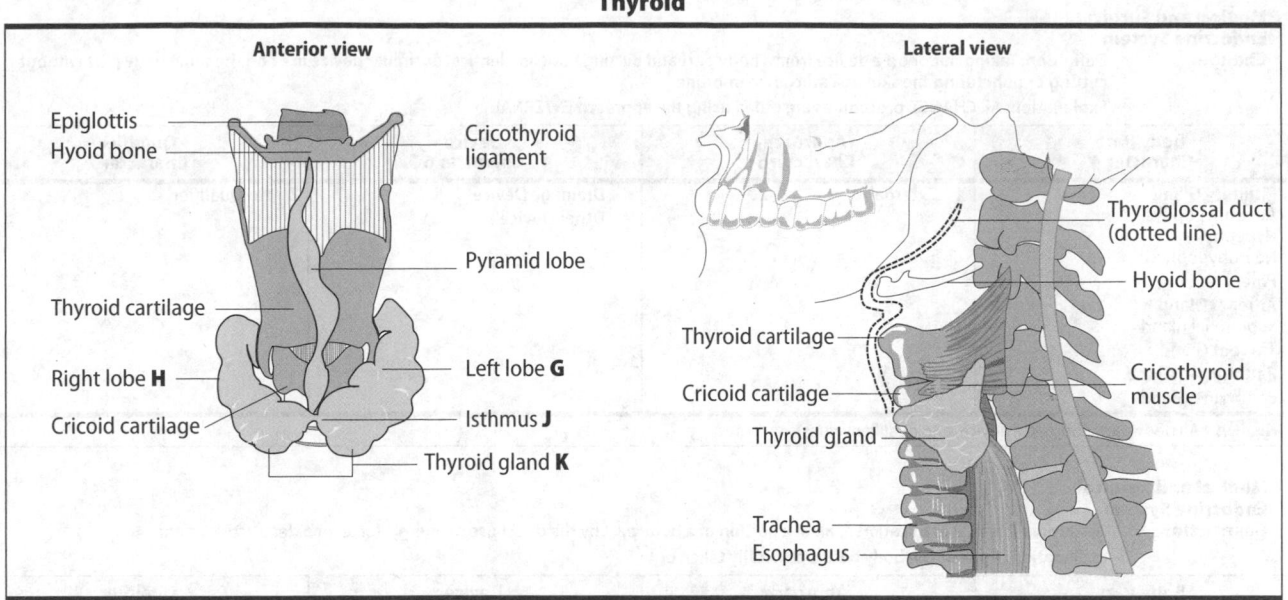

Anterior view

- Epiglottis
- Hyoid bone
- Cricothyroid ligament
- Pyramid lobe
- Thyroid cartilage
- Right lobe **H**
- Left lobe **G**
- Cricoid cartilage
- Isthmus **J**
- Thyroid gland **K**

Lateral view

- Thyroglossal duct (dotted line)
- Hyoid bone
- Thyroid cartilage
- Cricothyroid muscle
- Cricoid cartilage
- Thyroid gland
- Trachea
- Esophagus

Thyroid and Parathyroid Glands

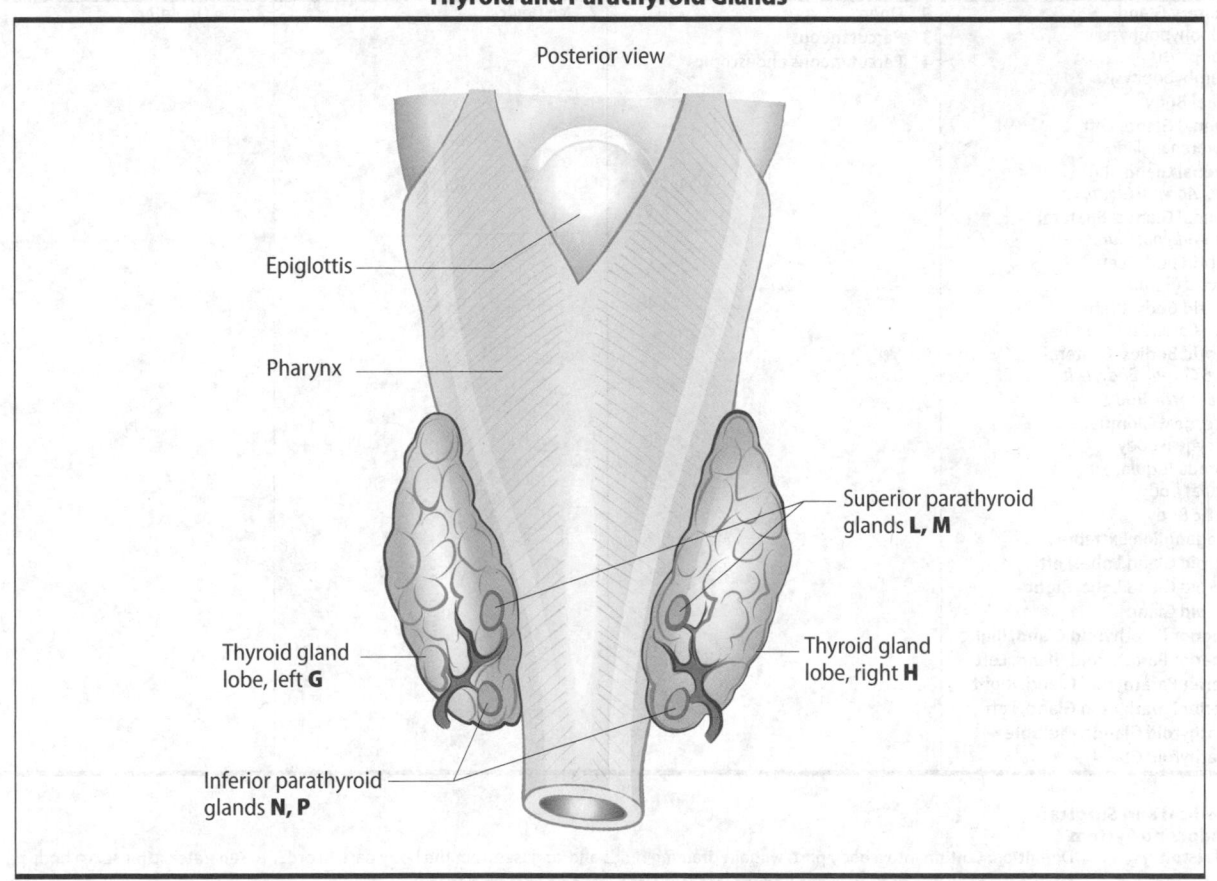

Posterior view

- Epiglottis
- Pharynx
- Superior parathyroid glands **L, M**
- Thyroid gland lobe, left **G**
- Thyroid gland lobe, right **H**
- Inferior parathyroid glands **N, P**

Ø	**Medical and Surgical**
G	**Endocrine System**
2	**Change**

Definition: Taking out or off a device from a body part and putting back an identical or similar device in or on the same body part without cutting or puncturing the skin or a mucous membrane

Explanation: All CHANGE procedures are coded using the approach EXTERNAL

Body Part Character 4	Approach Character 5	Device Character 6	Qualifier Character 7

Ø **Pituitary Gland**
  Adenohypophysis
  Hypophysis
  Neurohypophysis
1 **Pineal Body**
5 **Adrenal Gland**
  Suprarenal gland
K **Thyroid Gland**
R **Parathyroid Gland**
S **Endocrine Gland**
	X External	Ø Drainage Device
		Y Other Device
			Z No Qualifier

Non-OR   All body part, approach, device, and qualifier values

Ø	**Medical and Surgical**
G	**Endocrine System**
5	**Destruction**

Definition: Physical eradication of all or a portion of a body part by the direct use of energy, force, or a destructive agent

Explanation: None of the body part is physically taken out

Body Part Character 4	Approach Character 5	Device Character 6	Qualifier Character 7

Ø **Pituitary Gland**
  Adenohypophysis
  Hypophysis
  Neurohypophysis
1 **Pineal Body**
2 **Adrenal Gland, Left**
  Suprarenal gland
3 **Adrenal Gland, Right**
  See 2 Adrenal Gland, Left
4 **Adrenal Glands, Bilateral**
  See 2 Adrenal Gland, Left
6 **Carotid Body, Left**
  Carotid glomus
7 **Carotid Body, Right**
  See 6 Carotid Body, Left
8 **Carotid Bodies, Bilateral**
  See 6 Carotid Body, Left
9 **Para-aortic Body**
B **Coccygeal Glomus**
  Coccygeal body
C **Glomus Jugulare**
  Jugular body
D **Aortic Body**
F **Paraganglion Extremity**
G **Thyroid Gland Lobe, Left**
H **Thyroid Gland Lobe, Right**
K **Thyroid Gland**
L **Superior Parathyroid Gland, Right**
M **Superior Parathyroid Gland, Left**
N **Inferior Parathyroid Gland, Right**
P **Inferior Parathyroid Gland, Left**
Q **Parathyroid Glands, Multiple**
R **Parathyroid Gland**
	Ø Open
	3 Percutaneous
	4 Percutaneous Endoscopic
		Z No Device	Z No Qualifier

Ø	**Medical and Surgical**
G	**Endocrine System**
8	**Division**

Definition: Cutting into a body part, without draining fluids and/or gases from the body part, in order to separate or transect a body part

Explanation: All or a portion of the body part is separated into two or more portions

Body Part Character 4	Approach Character 5	Device Character 6	Qualifier Character 7

Ø **Pituitary Gland**
  Adenohypophysis
  Hypophysis
  Neurohypophysis
J **Thyroid Gland Isthmus**
	Ø Open
	3 Percutaneous
	4 Percutaneous Endoscopic
		Z No Device	Z No Qualifier

Ø   **Medical and Surgical**
G   **Endocrine System**
9   **Drainage**   Definition: Taking or letting out fluids and/or gases from a body part
                    Explanation: The qualifier DIAGNOSTIC is used to identify drainage procedures that are biopsies

Body Part Character 4	Approach Character 5	Device Character 6	Qualifier Character 7

Ø Pituitary Gland
    Adenohypophysis
    Hypophysis
    Neurohypophysis
1 Pineal Body
2 Adrenal Gland, Left
    Suprarenal gland
3 Adrenal Gland, Right
    See 2 Adrenal Gland, Left
4 Adrenal Glands, Bilateral
    See 2 Adrenal Gland, Left
6 Carotid Body, Left
    Carotid glomus
7 Carotid Body, Right
    See 6 Carotid Body, Left
8 Carotid Bodies, Bilateral
    See 6 Carotid Body, Left
9 Para-aortic Body
B Coccygeal Glomus
    Coccygeal body
C Glomus Jugulare
    Jugular body
D Aortic Body
F Paraganglion Extremity
G Thyroid Gland Lobe, Left
H Thyroid Gland Lobe, Right
K Thyroid Gland
L Superior Parathyroid Gland, Right
M Superior Parathyroid Gland, Left
N Inferior Parathyroid Gland, Right
P Inferior Parathyroid Gland, Left
Q Parathyroid Glands, Multiple
R Parathyroid Gland
	Ø Open
	3 Percutaneous
	4 Percutaneous Endoscopic
		Ø Drainage Device	**Z** No Qualifier

Ø Pituitary Gland
    Adenohypophysis
    Hypophysis
    Neurohypophysis
1 Pineal Body
2 Adrenal Gland, Left
    Suprarenal gland
3 Adrenal Gland, Right
    See 2 Adrenal Gland, Left
4 Adrenal Glands, Bilateral
    See 2 Adrenal Gland, Left
6 Carotid Body, Left
    Carotid glomus
7 Carotid Body, Right
    See 6 Carotid Body, Left
8 Carotid Bodies, Bilateral
    See 6 Carotid Body, Left
9 Para-aortic Body
B Coccygeal Glomus
    Coccygeal body
C Glomus Jugulare
    Jugular body
D Aortic Body
F Paraganglion Extremity
G Thyroid Gland Lobe, Left
H Thyroid Gland Lobe, Right
K Thyroid Gland
L Superior Parathyroid Gland, Right
M Superior Parathyroid Gland, Left
N Inferior Parathyroid Gland, Right
P Inferior Parathyroid Gland, Left
Q Parathyroid Glands, Multiple
R Parathyroid Gland
	Ø Open
	3 Percutaneous
	4 Percutaneous Endoscopic
		Z No Device	**X** Diagnostic
			Z No Qualifier

Non-OR	0G9[0,1,2,3,4,6,7,8,9,B,C,D,F,G,H,K,L,M,N,P,Q,R]30Z
Non-OR	0G9[G,H,K,L,M,N,P,Q,R]40Z
Non-OR	0G9[2,3,4,G,H,K][3,4]ZX
Non-OR	0G9[0,1,2,3,4,6,7,8,9,B,C,D,F,G,H,K,L,M,N,P,Q,R]3ZZ
Non-OR	0G9[G,H,K,L,M,N,P,Q,R]4ZZ

Ø   **Medical and Surgical**
G   **Endocrine System**
B   **Excision**   Definition: Cutting out or off, without replacement, a portion of a body part

Explanation: The qualifier DIAGNOSTIC is used to identify excision procedures that are biopsies

Body Part Character 4	Approach Character 5	Device Character 6	Qualifier Character 7
Ø **Pituitary Gland** Adenohypophysis Hypophysis Neurohypophysis **1** **Pineal Body** **2** **Adrenal Gland, Left** Suprarenal gland **3** **Adrenal Gland, Right** *See 2 Adrenal Gland, Left* **4** **Adrenal Glands, Bilateral** *See 2 Adrenal Gland, Left* **6** **Carotid Body, Left** Carotid glomus **7** **Carotid Body, Right** *See 6 Carotid Body, Left* **8** **Carotid Bodies, Bilateral** *See 6 Carotid Body, Left* **9** **Para-aortic Body** **B** **Coccygeal Glomus** Coccygeal body **C** **Glomus Jugulare** Jugular body **D** **Aortic Body** **F** **Paraganglion Extremity** **G** **Thyroid Gland Lobe, Left** **H** **Thyroid Gland Lobe, Right** **J** **Thyroid Gland Isthmus** **L** **Superior Parathyroid Gland, Right** **M** **Superior Parathyroid Gland, Left** **N** **Inferior Parathyroid Gland, Right** **P** **Inferior Parathyroid Gland, Left** **Q** **Parathyroid Glands, Multiple** **R** **Parathyroid Gland**	**Ø** Open **3** Percutaneous **4** Percutaneous Endoscopic	**Z** No Device	**X** Diagnostic **Z** No Qualifier

Non-OR   ØGB[2,3,4,G,H,J][3,4]ZX

Ø   **Medical and Surgical**
G   **Endocrine System**
C   **Extirpation**   Definition: Taking or cutting out solid matter from a body part

Explanation: The solid matter may be an abnormal byproduct of a biological function or a foreign body; it may be imbedded in a body part or in the lumen of a tubular body part. The solid matter may or may not have been previously broken into pieces.

Body Part Character 4	Approach Character 5	Device Character 6	Qualifier Character 7
Ø **Pituitary Gland** Adenohypophysis Hypophysis Neurohypophysis **1** **Pineal Body** **2** **Adrenal Gland, Left** Suprarenal gland **3** **Adrenal Gland, Right** *See 2 Adrenal Gland, Left* **4** **Adrenal Glands, Bilateral** *See 2 Adrenal Gland, Left* **6** **Carotid Body, Left** Carotid glomus **7** **Carotid Body, Right** *See 6 Carotid Body, Left* **8** **Carotid Bodies, Bilateral** *See 6 Carotid Body, Left* **9** **Para-aortic Body** **B** **Coccygeal Glomus** Coccygeal body **C** **Glomus Jugulare** Jugular body **D** **Aortic Body** **F** **Paraganglion Extremity** **G** **Thyroid Gland Lobe, Left** **H** **Thyroid Gland Lobe, Right** **K** **Thyroid Gland** **L** **Superior Parathyroid Gland, Right** **M** **Superior Parathyroid Gland, Left** **N** **Inferior Parathyroid Gland, Right** **P** **Inferior Parathyroid Gland, Left** **Q** **Parathyroid Glands, Multiple** **R** **Parathyroid Gland**	**Ø** Open **3** Percutaneous **4** Percutaneous Endoscopic	**Z** No Device	**Z** No Qualifier

Ø   Medical and Surgical
G   Endocrine System
H   Insertion   Definition: Putting in a nonbiological appliance that monitors, assists, performs, or prevents a physiological function but does not physically take the place of a body part
                     Explanation: None

Body Part Character 4	Approach Character 5	Device Character 6	Qualifier Character 7
S Endocrine Gland	**Ø** Open **3** Percutaneous **4** Percutaneous Endoscopic	**1** Radioactive Element **2** Monitoring Device **3** Infusion Device **Y** Other Device	**Z** No Qualifier

Non-OR   ØGHS31Z
Non-OR   ØGHS[3,4]YZ

Ø   Medical and Surgical
G   Endocrine System
J   Inspection   Definition: Visually and/or manually exploring a body part
                     Explanation: Visual exploration may be performed with or without optical instrumentation. Manual exploration may be performed directly or through intervening body layers.

Body Part Character 4	Approach Character 5	Device Character 6	Qualifier Character 7

Ø   Pituitary Gland
     Adenohypophysis
     Hypophysis
     Neurohypophysis
1   Pineal Body
5   Adrenal Gland
     Suprarenal gland
K   Thyroid Gland
R   Parathyroid Gland
S   Endocrine Gland
	Ø Open
	3 Percutaneous
	4 Percutaneous Endoscopic
		Z No Device	**Z** No Qualifier

Non-OR   ØGJ[Ø,1,5,K,R,S]3ZZ

Ø   Medical and Surgical
G   Endocrine System
M   Reattachment   Definition: Putting back in or on all or a portion of a separated body part to its normal location or other suitable location
                     Explanation: Vascular circulation and nervous pathways may or may not be reestablished

Body Part Character 4	Approach Character 5	Device Character 6	Qualifier Character 7

2   Adrenal Gland, Left
     Suprarenal gland
3   Adrenal Gland, Right
     See 2 Adrenal Gland, Left
G   Thyroid Gland Lobe, Left
H   Thyroid Gland Lobe, Right
L   Superior Parathyroid Gland, Right
M   Superior Parathyroid Gland, Left
N   Inferior Parathyroid Gland, Right
P   Inferior Parathyroid Gland, Left
Q   Parathyroid Glands, Multiple
R   Parathyroid Gland
	Ø Open
	4 Percutaneous Endoscopic
		Z No Device	**Z** No Qualifier

Endocrine System

Ø   **Medical and Surgical**
G   **Endocrine System**
N   **Release**   Definition: Freeing a body part from an abnormal physical constraint by cutting or by the use of force
                  Explanation: Some of the restraining tissue may be taken out but none of the body part is taken out

Body Part Character 4	Approach Character 5	Device Character 6	Qualifier Character 7

Ø   Pituitary Gland
    Adenohypophysis
    Hypophysis
    Neurohypophysis
1   Pineal Body
2   Adrenal Gland, Left
    Suprarenal gland
3   Adrenal Gland, Right
    See 2 Adrenal Gland, Left
4   Adrenal Glands, Bilateral
    See 2 Adrenal Gland, Left
6   Carotid Body, Left
    Carotid glomus
7   Carotid Body, Right
    See 6 Carotid Body, Left
8   Carotid Bodies, Bilateral
    See 6 Carotid Body, Left
9   Para-aortic Body
B   Coccygeal Glomus
    Coccygeal body
C   Glomus Jugulare
    Jugular body
D   Aortic Body
F   Paraganglion Extremity
G   Thyroid Gland Lobe, Left
H   Thyroid Gland Lobe, Right
K   Thyroid Gland
L   Superior Parathyroid Gland, Right
M   Superior Parathyroid Gland, Left
N   Inferior Parathyroid Gland, Right
P   Inferior Parathyroid Gland, Left
Q   Parathyroid Glands, Multiple
R   Parathyroid Gland
	Ø Open
	3 Percutaneous
	4 Percutaneous Endoscopic
		Z No Device	Z No Qualifier

Non-OR   ØGN[6,7,8,9,B,C,D,F][Ø,3,4]ZZ

Ø   **Medical and Surgical**
G   **Endocrine System**
P   **Removal**   Definition: Taking out or off a device from a body part
                   Explanation: If a device is taken out and a similar device put in without cutting or puncturing the skin or mucous membrane, the procedure is coded to the root operation CHANGE. Otherwise, the procedure for taking out a device is coded to the root operation REMOVAL.

Body Part Character 4	Approach Character 5	Device Character 6	Qualifier Character 7

Ø   Pituitary Gland
    Adenohypophysis
    Hypophysis
    Neurohypophysis
1   Pineal Body
5   Adrenal Gland
    Suprarenal gland
K   Thyroid Gland
R   Parathyroid Gland
	Ø Open
	3 Percutaneous
	4 Percutaneous Endoscopic
	X External
		Ø Drainage Device	Z No Qualifier

S Endocrine Gland	Ø Open 3 Percutaneous 4 Percutaneous Endoscopic	Ø Drainage Device 2 Monitoring Device 3 Infusion Device Y Other Device	Z No Qualifier
S Endocrine Gland	X External	Ø Drainage Device 2 Monitoring Device 3 Infusion Device	Z No Qualifier

Non-OR   ØGP[Ø,1,5,K,R]XØZ
Non-OR   ØGPS[3,4]YZ
Non-OR   ØGPSX[Ø,2,3]Z

Ø   **Medical and Surgical**
G   **Endocrine System**
Q   **Repair**   Definition: Restoring, to the extent possible, a body part to its normal anatomic structure and function

                     Explanation: Used only when the method to accomplish the repair is not one of the other root operations

Body Part Character 4	Approach Character 5	Device Character 6	Qualifier Character 7

Ø   **Pituitary Gland**
     Adenohypophysis
     Hypophysis
     Neurohypophysis
1   **Pineal Body**
2   **Adrenal Gland, Left**
     Suprarenal gland
3   **Adrenal Gland, Right**
     See 2 Adrenal Gland, Left
4   **Adrenal Glands, Bilateral**
     See 2 Adrenal Gland, Left
6   **Carotid Body, Left**
     Carotid glomus
7   **Carotid Body, Right**
     See 6 Carotid Body, Left
8   **Carotid Bodies, Bilateral**
     See 6 Carotid Body, Left
9   **Para-aortic Body**
B   **Coccygeal Glomus**
     Coccygeal body
C   **Glomus Jugulare**
     Jugular body
D   **Aortic Body**
F   **Paraganglion Extremity**
G   **Thyroid Gland Lobe, Left**
H   **Thyroid Gland Lobe, Right**
J   **Thyroid Gland Isthmus**
K   **Thyroid Gland**
L   **Superior Parathyroid Gland, Right**
M   **Superior Parathyroid Gland, Left**
N   **Inferior Parathyroid Gland, Right**
P   **Inferior Parathyroid Gland, Left**
Q   **Parathyroid Glands, Multiple**
R   **Parathyroid Gland**
	Ø Open
	3 Percutaneous
	4 Percutaneous Endoscopic
		Z No Device	**Z** No Qualifier

Ø   **Medical and Surgical**
G   **Endocrine System**
S   **Reposition**   Definition: Moving to its normal location, or other suitable location, all or a portion of a body part

                     Explanation: The body part is moved to a new location from an abnormal location, or from a normal location where it is not functioning correctly. The body part may or may not be cut out or off to be moved to the new location.

Body Part Character 4	Approach Character 5	Device Character 6	Qualifier Character 7

2   **Adrenal Gland, Left**
     Suprarenal gland
3   **Adrenal Gland, Right**
     See 2 Adrenal Gland, Left
G   **Thyroid Gland Lobe, Left**
H   **Thyroid Gland Lobe, Right**
L   **Superior Parathyroid Gland, Right**
M   **Superior Parathyroid Gland, Left**
N   **Inferior Parathyroid Gland, Right**
P   **Inferior Parathyroid Gland, Left**
Q   **Parathyroid Glands, Multiple**
R   **Parathyroid Gland**
	Ø Open
	4 Percutaneous Endoscopic
		Z No Device	**Z** No Qualifier

Endocrine System

Ø **Medical and Surgical**
G **Endocrine System**
T **Resection**   Definition: Cutting out or off, without replacement, all of a body part
                   Explanation: None

Body Part Character 4	Approach Character 5	Device Character 6	Qualifier Character 7

Ø   Pituitary Gland
     Adenohypophysis
     Hypophysis
     Neurohypophysis
1   Pineal Body
2   Adrenal Gland, Left
     Suprarenal gland
3   Adrenal Gland, Right
     See 2 Adrenal Gland, Left
4   Adrenal Glands, Bilateral
     See 2 Adrenal Gland, Left
6   Carotid Body, Left
     Carotid glomus
7   Carotid Body, Right
     See 6 Carotid Body, Left
8   Carotid Bodies, Bilateral
     See 6 Carotid Body, Left
9   Para-aortic Body
B   Coccygeal Glomus
     Coccygeal body
C   Glomus Jugulare
     Jugular body
D   Aortic Body
F   Paraganglion Extremity
G   Thyroid Gland Lobe, Left
H   Thyroid Gland Lobe, Right
J   Thyroid Gland Isthmus
K   Thyroid Gland
L   Superior Parathyroid Gland, Right
M   Superior Parathyroid Gland, Left
N   Inferior Parathyroid Gland, Right
P   Inferior Parathyroid Gland, Left
Q   Parathyroid Glands, Multiple
R   Parathyroid Gland
	Ø Open
	4 Percutaneous Endoscopic
		Z No Device	Z No Qualifier

Non-OR   ØGT[6,7,8,9,B,C,D,F][Ø,4]ZZ

Ø **Medical and Surgical**
G **Endocrine System**
W **Revision**   Definition: Correcting, to the extent possible, a portion of a malfunctioning device or the position of a displaced device
                   Explanation: Revision can include correcting a malfunctioning or displaced device by taking out or putting in components of the device such as a screw or pin

Body Part Character 4	Approach Character 5	Device Character 6	Qualifier Character 7

Ø   Pituitary Gland
     Adenohypophysis
     Hypophysis
     Neurohypophysis
1   Pineal Body
5   Adrenal Gland
     Suprarenal gland
K   Thyroid Gland
R   Parathyroid Gland
	Ø Open
	3 Percutaneous
	4 Percutaneous Endoscopic
	X External
		Ø Drainage Device	Z No Qualifier

S Endocrine Gland	Ø Open 3 Percutaneous 4 Percutaneous Endoscopic	Ø Drainage Device 2 Monitoring Device 3 Infusion Device Y Other Device	Z No Qualifier
S Endocrine Gland	X External	Ø Drainage Device 2 Monitoring Device 3 Infusion Device	Z No Qualifier

Non-OR   ØGW[Ø,1,5,K,R]XØZ
Non-OR   ØGWS[3,4]YZ
Non-OR   ØGWSX[Ø,2,3]Z

Skin and Breast ØHØ–ØHX

Character Meanings*

This Character Meaning table is provided as a guide to assist the user in the identification of character members that may be found in this section of code tables. It **SHOULD NOT** be used to build a PCS code.

Operation–Character 3		Body Part–Character 4		Approach–Character 5		Device–Character 6		Qualifier–Character 7	
Ø	Alteration	Ø	Skin, Scalp	Ø	Open	Ø	Drainage Device	2	Cell Suspension Technique
2	Change	1	Skin, Face	3	Percutaneous	1	Radioactive Element	3	Full Thickness
5	Destruction	2	Skin, Right Ear	7	Via Natural or Artificial Opening	7	Autologous Tissue Substitute	4	Partial Thickness
8	Division	3	Skin, Left Ear	8	Via Natural or Artificial Opening Endoscopic	J	Synthetic Substitute	5	Latissimus Dorsi Myocutaneous Flap
9	Drainage	4	Skin, Neck	X	External	K	Nonautologous Tissue Substitute	6	Transverse Rectus Abdominis Myocutaneous Flap
B	Excision	5	Skin, Chest			N	Tissue Expander	7	Deep Inferior Epigastric Artery Perforator Flap
C	Extirpation	6	Skin, Back			Y	Other Device	8	Superficial Inferior Epigastric Artery Flap
D	Extraction	7	Skin, Abdomen			Z	No Device	9	Gluteal Artery Perforator Flap
H	Insertion	8	Skin, Buttock					D	Multiple
J	Inspection	9	Skin, Perineum					X	Diagnostic
M	Reattachment	A	Skin, Inguinal					Z	No Qualifier
N	Release	B	Skin, Right Upper Arm						
P	Removal	C	Skin, Left Upper Arm						
Q	Repair	D	Skin, Right Lower Arm						
R	Replacement	E	Skin, Left Lower Arm						
S	Reposition	F	Skin, Right Hand						
T	Resection	G	Skin, Left Hand						
U	Supplement	H	Skin, Right Upper Leg						
W	Revision	J	Skin, Left Upper Leg						
X	Transfer	K	Skin, Right Lower Leg						
		L	Skin, Left Lower Leg						
		M	Skin, Right Foot						
		N	Skin, Left Foot						
		P	Skin						
		Q	Finger Nail						
		R	Toe Nail						
		S	Hair						
		T	Breast, Right						
		U	Breast, Left						
		V	Breast, Bilateral						
		W	Nipple, Right						
		X	Nipple, Left						
		Y	Supernumerary Breast						

* Includes skin and breast glands and ducts.

AHA Coding Clinic for table ØHØ

2019, 4Q, 30-31	Breast procedures

AHA Coding Clinic for table ØH5

2019, 4Q, 30-31	Breast procedures

AHA Coding Clinic for table ØH9

2019, 4Q, 30-31	Breast procedures

AHA Coding Clinic for table ØHB

2020, 1Q, 31	Repair of buried penis
2019, 4Q, 30-31	Breast procedures
2018, 1Q, 14	Excisional debridement of breast tissue and skin
2016, 3Q, 29	Closure of bilateral alveolar clefts
2015, 3Q, 3-8	Excisional and nonexcisional debridement

AHA Coding Clinic for table ØHC

2019, 4Q, 30-31	Breast procedures

AHA Coding Clinic for table ØHD

2019, 4Q, 30-31	Breast procedures
2016, 1Q, 40	Nonexcisional debridement of skin and subcutaneous tissue
2015, 3Q, 3-8	Excisional and nonexcisional debridement

AHA Coding Clinic for table ØHH

2019, 4Q, 30-31	Breast procedures
2017, 4Q, 67	New qualifier values - Pedicle flap procedures
2014, 2Q, 12	Pedicle latissimus myocutaneous flap with placement of breast tissue expanders
2013, 4Q, 107	Breast tissue expander placement using acellular dermal matrix

AHA Coding Clinic for table ØHJ

2019, 4Q, 30-31	Breast procedures

AHA Coding Clinic for table ØHN

2019, 4Q, 30-31	Breast procedures

AHA Coding Clinic for table ØHP

2019, 4Q, 30-31	Breast procedures
2018, 3Q, 13	Deep inferior epigastric artery perforator flap breast reconstruction
2016, 2Q, 27	Removal of nonviable transverse rectus abdominis myocutaneous (TRAM) flaps

AHA Coding Clinic for table ØHQ

2019, 4Q, 30-31	Breast procedures
2018, 2Q, 25	Third and fourth degree obstetric lacerations
2016, 1Q, 7	Obstetrical perineal laceration repair
2014, 4Q, 31	Delayed wound closure following fracture treatment

AHA Coding Clinic for table ØHR

2020, 1Q, 27	Delayed reconstruction following mastectomy using gracilis musculocutaneous free flap
2020, 1Q, 28	Free flap microvascular breast reconstruction
2020, 1Q, 30	Polarity Skin TE™ application
2019, 4Q, 30-31	Breast procedures
2019, 4Q, 32	Cell suspension epithelial autograft
2019, 3Q, 32	Breast reconstruction with neurotization
2018, 3Q, 13	Deep inferior epigastric artery perforator flap breast reconstruction
2017, 1Q, 35	Epifix® allograft
2014, 3Q, 14	Application of TheraSkin® and excisional debridement

AHA Coding Clinic for table ØHT

2021, 2Q, 16	Goldilocks breast reconstruction
2018, 3Q, 13	Deep inferior epigastric artery perforator flap breast reconstruction
2014, 4Q, 34	Skin-sparing mastectomy

AHA Coding Clinic for table ØHU

2019, 4Q, 30-31	Breast procedures

AHA Coding Clinic for table ØHW

2019, 4Q, 30-31	Breast procedures

Integumentary Anatomy

Hair follicle **S**
Hair **S**
Sebaceous gland **Ø-9, A-P**
Arrector pili muscle
Epidermis
Thick-skin epidermis
Dermis
Hair shaft **S**
Pacinian corpuscle
Hair matrix **S**
Hypodermis (subcutaneous layer)
Sweat (eccrine gland) **Ø-9, A-P**
Sensory nerve
Bulb
Blood vessels

Nail Anatomy

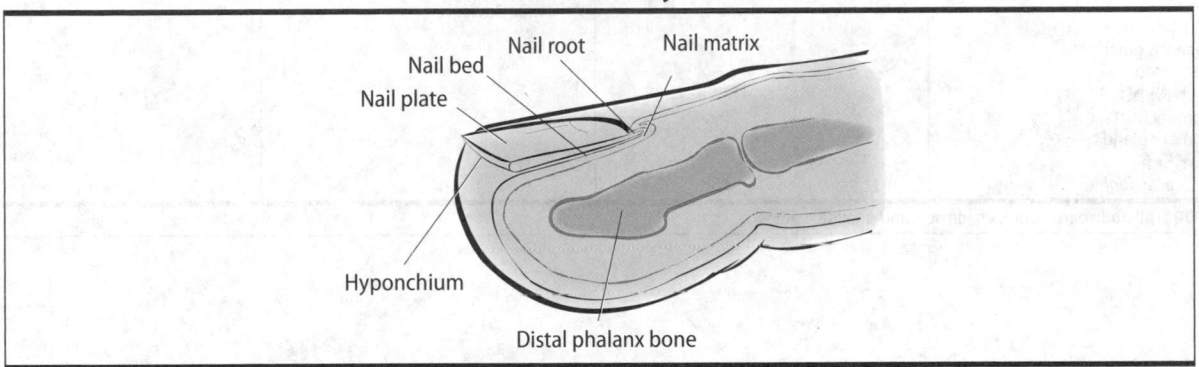

Nail bed
Nail root
Nail matrix
Nail plate
Hyponchium
Distal phalanx bone

Breast

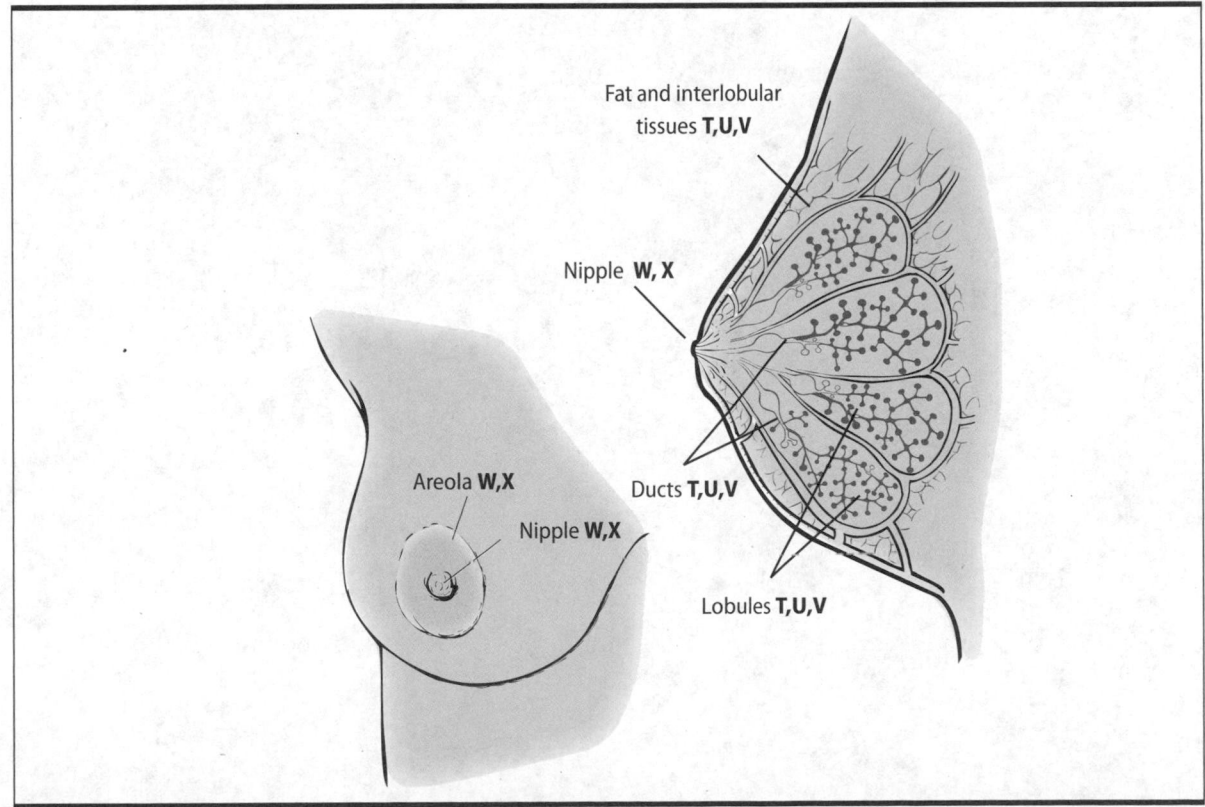

Fat and interlobular tissues **T,U,V**
Nipple **W, X**
Areola **W,X**
Nipple **W,X**
Ducts **T,U,V**
Lobules **T,U,V**

Skin and Breast (side tab)

Ø   **Medical and Surgical**
H   **Skin and Breast**
Ø   **Alteration**   Definition: Modifying the anatomic structure of a body part without affecting the function of the body part

Explanation: Principal purpose is to improve appearance

Body Part Character 4	Approach Character 5	Device Character 6	Qualifier Character 7

T **Breast, Right**
   Mammary duct
   Mammary gland
 U **Breast, Left**
   See T Breast, Right
 V **Breast, Bilateral**
   See T Breast, Right
	Ø Open
	 3 Percutaneous
		7 Autologous Tissue Substitute
		 J Synthetic Substitute
		 K Nonautologous Tissue Substitute
		 Z No Device
			Z No Qualifier

Non-OR   ØHØ[T,U,V]3JZ

Ø   **Medical and Surgical**
H   **Skin and Breast**
2   **Change**   Definition: Taking out or off a device from a body part and putting back an identical or similar device in or on the same body part without cutting or puncturing the skin or a mucous membrane

Explanation: All CHANGE procedures are coded using the approach EXTERNAL

Body Part Character 4	Approach Character 5	Device Character 6	Qualifier Character 7

P **Skin**
   Dermis
   Epidermis
   Sebaceous gland
   Sweat gland
 T **Breast, Right**
   Mammary duct
   Mammary gland
 U **Breast, Left**
   See T Breast, Right
	X External	**Ø** Drainage Device
		 Y Other Device
			Z No Qualifier

Non-OR   All body part, approach, device, and qualifier values

Ø Medical and Surgical
H Skin and Breast
5 Destruction

Definition: Physical eradication of all or a portion of a body part by the direct use of energy, force, or a destructive agent

Explanation: None of the body part is physically taken out

Body Part Character 4	Approach Character 5	Device Character 6	Qualifier Character 7
Ø Skin, Scalp 1 Skin, Face 2 Skin, Right Ear 3 Skin, Left Ear 4 Skin, Neck 5 Skin, Chest Breast procedures, skin only 6 Skin, Back 7 Skin, Abdomen 8 Skin, Buttock 9 Skin, Perineum A Skin, Inguinal B Skin, Right Upper Arm C Skin, Left Upper Arm D Skin, Right Lower Arm E Skin, Left Lower Arm F Skin, Right Hand G Skin, Left Hand H Skin, Right Upper Leg J Skin, Left Upper Leg K Skin, Right Lower Leg L Skin, Left Lower Leg M Skin, Right Foot N Skin, Left Foot	X External	Z No Device	D Multiple Z No Qualifier

Q Finger Nail
   Nail bed
   Nail plate
R Toe Nail
   See Q Finger Nail
	X External	Z No Device	Z No Qualifier

T Breast, Right
   Mammary duct
   Mammary gland
U Breast, Left
   See T Breast, Right
V Breast, Bilateral
   See T Breast, Right
	Ø Open
	3 Percutaneous
	7 Via Natural or Artificial Opening
	8 Via Natural or Artificial Opening Endoscopic
		Z No Device	Z No Qualifier

W Nipple, Right
   Areola
X Nipple, Left
   See W Nipple, Right
	Ø Open
	3 Percutaneous
	7 Via Natural or Artificial Opening
	8 Via Natural or Artificial Opening Endoscopic
	X External
		Z No Device	Z No Qualifier

DRG Non-OR	ØH5[Ø,1,4,5,6,7,8,9,A,B,C,D,E,F,G,H,J,K,L,M,N]XZ[D,Z]
DRG Non-OR	ØH5[Q,R]XZZ
Non-OR	ØH5[2,3]XZ[D,Z]

NC Noncovered Procedure   LC Limited Coverage   QA Questionable OB Admit   NT New Tech Add-on   ⊞ Combination Member   ♂ Male   ♀ Female

ICD-10-PCS 2022   429

ØH5–ØH5

Ø Medical and Surgical
H Skin and Breast
8 Division

Definition: Cutting into a body part, without draining fluids and/or gases from the body part, in order to separate or transect a body part

Explanation: All or a portion of the body part is separated into two or more portions

Body Part Character 4	Approach Character 5	Device Character 6	Qualifier Character 7
Ø Skin, Scalp	X External	Z No Device	Z No Qualifier
1 Skin, Face			
2 Skin, Right Ear			
3 Skin, Left Ear			
4 Skin, Neck			
5 Skin, Chest Breast procedures, skin only			
6 Skin, Back			
7 Skin, Abdomen			
8 Skin, Buttock			
9 Skin, Perineum			
A Skin, Inguinal			
B Skin, Right Upper Arm			
C Skin, Left Upper Arm			
D Skin, Right Lower Arm			
E Skin, Left Lower Arm			
F Skin, Right Hand			
G Skin, Left Hand			
H Skin, Right Upper Leg			
J Skin, Left Upper Leg			
K Skin, Right Lower Leg			
L Skin, Left Lower Leg			
M Skin, Right Foot			
N Skin, Left Foot			

Non-OR   All body part, approach, device, and qualifier values

Skin and Breast

Ø   **Medical and Surgical**
H   **Skin and Breast**
9   **Drainage**   Definition: Taking or letting out fluids and/or gases from a body part
                     Explanation: The qualifier DIAGNOSTIC is used to identify drainage procedures that are biopsies

Body Part Character 4		Approach Character 5	Device Character 6	Qualifier Character 7

Ø Skin, Scalp
1 Skin, Face
2 Skin, Right Ear
3 Skin, Left Ear
4 Skin, Neck
5 Skin, Chest
   Breast procedures, skin
     only
6 Skin, Back
7 Skin, Abdomen
8 Skin, Buttock
9 Skin, Perineum
A Skin, Inguinal
B Skin, Right Upper Arm
C Skin, Left Upper Arm
D Skin, Right Lower Arm
	E Skin, Left Lower Arm
	F Skin, Right Hand
	G Skin, Left Hand
	H Skin, Right Upper Leg
	J Skin, Left Upper Leg
	K Skin, Right Lower Leg
	L Skin, Left Lower Leg
	M Skin, Right Foot
	N Skin, Left Foot
	Q Finger Nail
	   Nail bed
	   Nail plate
	R Toe Nail
	   See Q Finger Nail
		X External	Ø Drainage Device	Z No Qualifier

Ø Skin, Scalp
1 Skin, Face
2 Skin, Right Ear
3 Skin, Left Ear
4 Skin, Neck
5 Skin, Chest
   Breast procedures, skin
     only
6 Skin, Back
7 Skin, Abdomen
8 Skin, Buttock
9 Skin, Perineum
A Skin, Inguinal
B Skin, Right Upper Arm
C Skin, Left Upper Arm
D Skin, Right Lower Arm
	E Skin, Left Lower Arm
	F Skin, Right Hand
	G Skin, Left Hand
	H Skin, Right Upper Leg
	J Skin, Left Upper Leg
	K Skin, Right Lower Leg
	L Skin, Left Lower Leg
	M Skin, Right Foot
	N Skin, Left Foot
	Q Finger Nail
	   Nail bed
	   Nail plate
	R Toe Nail
	   See Q Finger Nail
		X External	Z No Device	X Diagnostic
				Z No Qualifier

T Breast, Right
   Mammary duct
   Mammary gland
U Breast, Left
   See T Breast, Right
V Breast, Bilateral
   See T Breast, Right
		Ø Open
		3 Percutaneous
		7 Via Natural or Artificial
		   Opening
		8 Via Natural or Artificial
		   Opening Endoscopic
			Ø Drainage Device	Z No Qualifier

T Breast, Right
   Mammary duct
   Mammary gland
U Breast, Left
   See T Breast, Right
V Breast, Bilateral
   See T Breast, Right
		Ø Open
		3 Percutaneous
		7 Via Natural or Artificial
		   Opening
		8 Via Natural or Artificial
		   Opening Endoscopic
			Z No Device	X Diagnostic
				Z No Qualifier

W Nipple, Right
   Areola
X Nipple, Left
   See W Nipple, Right
		Ø Open
		3 Percutaneous
		7 Via Natural or Artificial
		   Opening
		8 Via Natural or Artificial
		   Opening Endoscopic
		X External
			Ø Drainage Device	Z No Qualifier

W Nipple, Right
   Areola
X Nipple, Left
   See W Nipple, Right
		Ø Open
		3 Percutaneous
		7 Via Natural or Artificial
		   Opening
		8 Via Natural or Artificial
		   Opening Endoscopic
		X External
			Z No Device	X Diagnostic
				Z No Qualifier

Non-OR   ØH9[Ø,1,2,3,4,5,6,7,8,A,B,C,D,E,F,G,H,J,K,L,M,N,Q,R]XØZ
Non-OR   ØH9[Ø,1,2,3,4,5,6,7,8,A,B,C,D,E,F,G,H,J,K,L,M,N,Q,R]XZ[X,Z]
Non-OR   ØH99XZX
Non-OR   ØH9[T,U,V][Ø,3,7,8]ØZ
Non-OR   ØH9[T,U,V][3,7,8]Z[X,Z]
Non-OR   ØH9[W,X][Ø,3,7,8,X]ØZ
Non-OR   ØH9[W,X][3,7,8,X]Z[X,Z]

NC Noncovered Procedure   LC Limited Coverage   QA Questionable OB Admit   NT New Tech Add-on   ⊞ Combination Member   ♂ Male   ♀ Female

ICD-10-PCS 2022   **431**

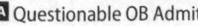

Skin and Breast

Ø   **Medical and Surgical**
H   **Skin and Breast**
B   **Excision**   Definition: Cutting out or off, without replacement, a portion of a body part
                      Explanation: The qualifier DIAGNOSTIC is used to identify excision procedures that are biopsies

Body Part Character 4	Approach Character 5	Device Character 6	Qualifier Character 7

Ø Skin, Scalp
1 Skin, Face
2 Skin, Right Ear
3 Skin, Left Ear
4 Skin, Neck
5 Skin, Chest
     Breast procedures, skin only
6 Skin, Back
7 Skin, Abdomen
8 Skin, Buttock
9 Skin, Perineum
A Skin, Inguinal
B Skin, Right Upper Arm
C Skin, Left Upper Arm
D Skin, Right Lower Arm
E Skin, Left Lower Arm
F Skin, Right Hand
G Skin, Left Hand
H Skin, Right Upper Leg
J Skin, Left Upper Leg
K Skin, Right Lower Leg
L Skin, Left Lower Leg
M Skin, Right Foot
N Skin, Left Foot
Q Finger Nail
     Nail bed
     Nail plate
R Toe Nail
     See Q Finger Nail
	X External	**Z** No Device	**X** Diagnostic
			Z No Qualifier

T Breast, Right
     Mammary duct
     Mammary gland
U Breast, Left
     See T Breast, Right
V Breast, Bilateral
     See T Breast, Right
Y Supernumerary Breast
	Ø Open
	3 Percutaneous
	7 Via Natural or Artificial Opening
	8 Via Natural or Artificial Opening
	     Endoscopic
		Z No Device	**X** Diagnostic
			Z No Qualifier

W Nipple, Right
     Areola
X Nipple, Left
     See W Nipple, Right
	Ø Open
	3 Percutaneous
	7 Via Natural or Artificial Opening
	8 Via Natural or Artificial Opening
	     Endoscopic
	X External
		Z No Device	**X** Diagnostic
			Z No Qualifier

DRG Non-OR	ØHB9XZZ
Non-OR	ØHB[Ø,1,2,3,4,5,6,7,8,A,B,C,D,E,F,G,H,J,K,L,M,N,Q,R]XZ[X,Z]
Non-OR	ØHB9XZX
Non-OR	ØHB[T,U,V,Y][3,7,8]ZX
Non-OR	ØHB[W,X][3,7,8,X]ZX

Ø Medical and Surgical
H Skin and Breast
C Extirpation

Definition: Taking or cutting out solid matter from a body part

Explanation: The solid matter may be an abnormal byproduct of a biological function or a foreign body; it may be imbedded in a body part or in the lumen of a tubular body part. The solid matter may or may not have been previously broken into pieces.

Body Part Character 4	Approach Character 5	Device Character 6	Qualifier Character 7
Ø Skin, Scalp	X External	Z No Device	Z No Qualifier
1 Skin, Face			
2 Skin, Right Ear			
3 Skin, Left Ear			
4 Skin, Neck			
5 Skin, Chest Breast procedures, skin only			
6 Skin, Back			
7 Skin, Abdomen			
8 Skin, Buttock			
9 Skin, Perineum			
A Skin, Inguinal			
B Skin, Right Upper Arm			
C Skin, Left Upper Arm			
D Skin, Right Lower Arm			
E Skin, Left Lower Arm			
F Skin, Right Hand			
G Skin, Left Hand			
H Skin, Right Upper Leg			
J Skin, Left Upper Leg			
K Skin, Right Lower Leg			
L Skin, Left Lower Leg			
M Skin, Right Foot			
N Skin, Left Foot			
Q Finger Nail Nail bed Nail plate			
R Toe Nail *See Q Finger Nail*			
T Breast, Right Mammary duct Mammary gland	Ø Open	Z No Device	Z No Qualifier
U Breast, Left *See T Breast, Right*	3 Percutaneous		
V Breast, Bilateral *See T Breast, Right*	7 Via Natural or Artificial Opening		
	8 Via Natural or Artificial Opening Endoscopic		
W Nipple, Right Areola	Ø Open	Z No Device	Z No Qualifier
X Nipple, Left *See W Nipple, Right*	3 Percutaneous		
	7 Via Natural or Artificial Opening		
	8 Via Natural or Artificial Opening Endoscopic		
	X External		

Non-OR   ØHC[Ø,1,2,3,4,5,6,7,8,9,A,B,C,D,E,F,G,H,J,K,L,M,N,Q,R]XZZ
Non-OR   ØHC[T,U,V][3,7,8]ZZ
Non-OR   ØHC[W,X][3,7,8,X]ZZ

Skin and Breast

Ø   Medical and Surgical
H   Skin and Breast
D   Extraction   Definition: Pulling or stripping out or off all or a portion of a body part by the use of force
                             Explanation: The qualifier DIAGNOSTIC is used to identify extraction procedures that are biopsies

Body Part Character 4	Approach Character 5	Device Character 6	Qualifier Character 7
Ø Skin, Scalp	**X** External	**Z** No Device	**Z** No Qualifier
1 Skin, Face			
2 Skin, Right Ear			
3 Skin, Left Ear			
4 Skin, Neck			
5 Skin, Chest Breast procedures, skin only			
6 Skin, Back			
7 Skin, Abdomen			
8 Skin, Buttock			
9 Skin, Perineum			
A Skin, Inguinal			
B Skin, Right Upper Arm			
C Skin, Left Upper Arm			
D Skin, Right Lower Arm			
E Skin, Left Lower Arm			
F Skin, Right Hand			
G Skin, Left Hand			
H Skin, Right Upper Leg			
J Skin, Left Upper Leg			
K Skin, Right Lower Leg			
L Skin, Left Lower Leg			
M Skin, Right Foot			
N Skin, Left Foot			

Q Finger Nail
      Nail bed
      Nail plate			

R Toe Nail *See* Q *Finger Nail*			
S Hair			

T Breast, Right
      Mammary duct
      Mammary gland
	Ø Open	**Z** No Device	**Z** No Qualifier

U Breast, Left *See* T *Breast, Right*			
V Breast, Bilateral *See* T *Breast, Right*			
Y Supernumerary Breast			

Non-OR   All body part, approach, device, and qualifier values

Ø   Medical and Surgical
H   Skin and Breast
H   Insertion

Definition: Putting in a nonbiological appliance that monitors, assists, performs, or prevents a physiological function but does not physically take the place of a body part

Explanation: None

Body Part Character 4	Approach Character 5	Device Character 6	Qualifier Character 7
P Skin	**X** External	**Y** Other Device	**Z** No Qualifier
T Breast, Right Mammary duct Mammary gland **U** Breast, Left *See T Breast, Right*	**Ø** Open **3** Percutaneous **7** Via Natural or Artificial Opening **8** Via Natural or Artificial Opening Endoscopic	**1** Radioactive Element **N** Tissue Expander **Y** Other Device	**Z** No Qualifier
V Breast, Bilateral Mammary duct Mammary gland	**Ø** Open **3** Percutaneous **7** Via Natural or Artificial Opening **8** Via Natural or Artificial Opening Endoscopic	**1** Radioactive Element **N** Tissue Expander	**Z** No Qualifier
W Nipple, Right Areola **X** Nipple, Left *See W Nipple, Right*	**Ø** Open **3** Percutaneous **7** Via Natural or Artificial Opening **8** Via Natural or Artificial Opening Endoscopic	**1** Radioactive Element **N** Tissue Expander	**Z** No Qualifier
W Nipple, Right Areola **X** Nipple, Left *See W Nipple, Right*	**X** External	**1** Radioactive Element	**Z** No Qualifier

Non-OR   ØHHPXYZ
Non-OR   ØHH[T,U][3,7,8]YZ

Ø   Medical and Surgical
H   Skin and Breast
J   Inspection

Definition: Visually and/or manually exploring a body part

Explanation: Visual exploration may be performed with or without optical instrumentation. Manual exploration may be performed directly or through intervening body layers.

Body Part Character 4	Approach Character 5	Device Character 6	Qualifier Character 7
P Skin Dermis Epidermis Sebaceous gland Sweat gland **Q** Finger Nail Nail bed Nail plate **R** Toe Nail *See Q Finger Nail*	**X** External	**Z** No Device	**Z** No Qualifier
T Breast, Right Mammary duct Mammary gland **U** Breast, Left *See T Breast, Right*	**Ø** Open **3** Percutaneous **7** Via Natural or Artificial Opening **8** Via Natural or Artificial Opening Endoscopic	**Z** No Device	**Z** No Qualifier

Non-OR   All body part, approach, device and qualifier values

NC Noncovered Procedure   **LC** Limited Coverage   **QA** Questionable OB Admit   **NT** New Tech Add-on   ⊞ Combination Member   ♂ Male   ♀ Female

ICD-10-PCS 2022   435

ØHH–ØHJ

Skin and Breast

Ø　**Medical and Surgical**
H　**Skin and Breast**
M　**Reattachment**　Definition: Putting back in or on all or a portion of a separated body part to its normal location or other suitable location
　　　　　　　　　　　　Explanation: Vascular circulation and nervous pathways may or may not be reestablished

Body Part Character 4	Approach Character 5	Device Character 6	Qualifier Character 7
Ø　Skin, Scalp	X　External	Z　No Device	Z　No Qualifier
1　Skin, Face			
2　Skin, Right Ear			
3　Skin, Left Ear			
4　Skin, Neck			
5　Skin, Chest 　　Breast procedures, skin only			
6　Skin, Back			
7　Skin, Abdomen			
8　Skin, Buttock			
9　Skin, Perineum			
A　Skin, Inguinal			
B　Skin, Right Upper Arm			
C　Skin, Left Upper Arm			
D　Skin, Right Lower Arm			
E　Skin, Left Lower Arm			
F　Skin, Right Hand			
G　Skin, Left Hand			
H　Skin, Right Upper Leg			
J　Skin, Left Upper Leg			
K　Skin, Right Lower Leg			
L　Skin, Left Lower Leg			
M　Skin, Right Foot			
N　Skin, Left Foot			
T　Breast, Right 　　Mammary duct 　　Mammary gland			
U　Breast, Left 　　See T Breast, Right			
V　Breast, Bilateral 　　See T Breast, Right			
W　Nipple, Right 　　Areola			
X　Nipple, Left 　　See W Nipple, Right			

Non-OR　ØHMØXZZ

Ø   Medical and Surgical
H   Skin and Breast
N   Release   Definition: Freeing a body part from an abnormal physical constraint by cutting or by the use of force
                      Explanation: Some of the restraining tissue may be taken out but none of the body part is taken out

Body Part Character 4	Approach Character 5	Device Character 6	Qualifier Character 7

Ø Skin, Scalp
1 Skin, Face
2 Skin, Right Ear
3 Skin, Left Ear
4 Skin, Neck
5 Skin, Chest
   Breast procedures, skin only
6 Skin, Back
7 Skin, Abdomen
8 Skin, Buttock
9 Skin, Perineum
A Skin, Inguinal
B Skin, Right Upper Arm
C Skin, Left Upper Arm
D Skin, Right Lower Arm
E Skin, Left Lower Arm
F Skin, Right Hand
G Skin, Left Hand
H Skin, Right Upper Leg
J Skin, Left Upper Leg
K Skin, Right Lower Leg
L Skin, Left Lower Leg
M Skin, Right Foot
N Skin, Left Foot
Q Finger Nail
   Nail bed
   Nail plate
R Toe Nail
   See Q Finger Nail
	X External	**Z** No Device	**Z** No Qualifier

T Breast, Right
   Mammary duct
   Mammary gland
U Breast, Left
   See T Breast, Right
V Breast, Bilateral
   See T Breast, Right
	Ø Open
	3 Percutaneous
	7 Via Natural or Artificial Opening
	8 Via Natural or Artificial Opening
	   Endoscopic
		Z No Device	**Z** No Qualifier

W Nipple, Right
   Areola
X Nipple, Left
   See W Nipple, Right
	Ø Open
	3 Percutaneous
	7 Via Natural or Artificial Opening
	8 Via Natural or Artificial Opening
	   Endoscopic
	X External
		Z No Device	**Z** No Qualifier

🆖 Noncovered Procedure   🆑 Limited Coverage   🆀🅰 Questionable OB Admit   🆕🆃 New Tech Add-on   ⊞ Combination Member   ♂Male   ♀Female

ICD-10-PCS 2022   **437**

Ø   Medical and Surgical
H   Skin and Breast
P   Removal   Definition: Taking out or off a device from a body part

Explanation: If a device is taken out and a similar device put in without cutting or puncturing the skin or mucous membrane, the procedure is coded to the root operation CHANGE. Otherwise, the procedure for taking out a device is coded to the root operation REMOVAL.

Body Part Character 4	Approach Character 5	Device Character 6	Qualifier Character 7
P Skin Dermis Epidermis Sebaceous gland Sweat gland	**X External**	**Ø Drainage Device** **7 Autologous Tissue Substitute** **J Synthetic Substitute** **K Nonautologous Tissue Substitute** **Y Other Device**	**Z No Qualifier**
Q Finger Nail Nail bed Nail plate **R Toe Nail** *See Q Finger Nail*	**X External**	**Ø Drainage Device** **7 Autologous Tissue Substitute** **J Synthetic Substitute** **K Nonautologous Tissue Substitute**	**Z No Qualifier**
S Hair	**X External**	**7 Autologous Tissue Substitute** **J Synthetic Substitute** **K Nonautologous Tissue Substitute**	**Z No Qualifier**
T Breast, Right Mammary duct Mammary gland **U Breast, Left** *See T Breast, Right*	**Ø Open** **3 Percutaneous** **7 Via Natural or Artificial Opening** **8 Via Natural or Artificial Opening Endoscopic**	**Ø Drainage Device** **1 Radioactive Element** **7 Autologous Tissue Substitute** **J Synthetic Substitute** **K Nonautologous Tissue Substitute** **N Tissue Expander** **Y Other Device**	**Z No Qualifier**

Non-OR	ØHPPX[Ø,7,J,K,Y]Z
Non-OR	ØHP[Q,R]X[Ø,7,J,K]Z
Non-OR	ØHPSX[7,J,K]Z
Non-OR	ØHP[T,U]Ø[Ø,1,7,K]Z
Non-OR	ØHP[T,U]3[Ø,1,7,K,Y]Z
Non-OR	ØHP[T,U][7,8][Ø,1,7,J,K,N,Y]Z

Ø   Medical and Surgical
H   Skin and Breast
Q   Repair   Definition: Restoring, to the extent possible, a body part to its normal anatomic structure and function

                        Explanation: Used only when the method to accomplish the repair is not one of the other root operations

Body Part Character 4	Approach Character 5	Device Character 6	Qualifier Character 7
Ø Skin, Scalp	**X** External	**Z** No Device	**Z** No Qualifier
1 Skin, Face			
2 Skin, Right Ear			
3 Skin, Left Ear			
4 Skin, Neck			
5 Skin, Chest Breast procedures, skin only			
6 Skin, Back			
7 Skin, Abdomen			
8 Skin, Buttock			
9 Skin, Perineum			
A Skin, Inguinal			
B Skin, Right Upper Arm			
C Skin, Left Upper Arm			
D Skin, Right Lower Arm			
E Skin, Left Lower Arm			
F Skin, Right Hand			
G Skin, Left Hand			
H Skin, Right Upper Leg			
J Skin, Left Upper Leg			
K Skin, Right Lower Leg			
L Skin, Left Lower Leg			
M Skin, Right Foot			
N Skin, Left Foot			

Q   Finger Nail
     Nail bed
     Nail plate			

R Toe Nail *See Q Finger Nail*			

T   Breast, Right
     Mammary duct
     Mammary gland
	Ø Open
	3 Percutaneous
	7 Via Natural or Artificial Opening
	8 Via Natural or Artificial Opening
	     Endoscopic
		Z No Device	**Z** No Qualifier

U Breast, Left *See T Breast, Right*			
V Breast, Bilateral *See T Breast, Right*			
Y Supernumerary Breast			

W   Nipple, Right
     Areola
	Ø Open
	3 Percutaneous
	7 Via Natural or Artificial Opening
	8 Via Natural or Artificial Opening
	     Endoscopic
	X External
		Z No Device	**Z** No Qualifier

X Nipple, Left *See W Nipple, Right*			

DRG Non-OR	ØHQ9XZZ
Non-OR	ØHQ[Ø,1,2,3,4,5,6,7,8,A,B,C,D,E,F,G,H,J,K,L,M,N]XZZ

NC Noncovered Procedure   LC Limited Coverage   QA Questionable OB Admit   NT New Tech Add-on   ⊞ Combination Member   ♂ Male   ♀ Female

ICD-10-PCS 2022   **439**

Skin and Breast

Ø   **Medical and Surgical**
H   **Skin and Breast**
R   **Replacement**   Definition: Putting in or on biological or synthetic material that physically takes the place and/or function of all or a portion of a body part
               Explanation: The body part may have been taken out or replaced, or may be taken out, physically eradicated, or rendered nonfunctional during
               the REPLACEMENT procedure. A REMOVAL procedure is coded for taking out the device used in a previous replacement procedure.

Body Part Character 4		Approach Character 5	Device Character 6	Qualifier Character 7
Ø Skin, Scalp 1 Skin, Face 2 Skin, Right Ear 3 Skin, Left Ear 4 Skin, Neck 5 Skin, Chest Breast procedures, skin only 6 Skin, Back 7 Skin, Abdomen 8 Skin, Buttock 9 Skin, Perineum A Skin, Inguinal	B Skin, Right Upper Arm C Skin, Left Upper Arm D Skin, Right Lower Arm E Skin, Left Lower Arm F Skin, Right Hand G Skin, Left Hand H Skin, Right Upper Leg J Skin, Left Upper Leg K Skin, Right Lower Leg L Skin, Left Lower Leg M Skin, Right Foot N Skin, Left Foot	X External	7 Autologous Tissue Substitute	2 Cell Suspension Technique 3 Full Thickness 4 Partial Thickness
Ø Skin, Scalp 1 Skin, Face 2 Skin, Right Ear 3 Skin, Left Ear 4 Skin, Neck 5 Skin, Chest Breast procedures, skin only 6 Skin, Back 7 Skin, Abdomen 8 Skin, Buttock 9 Skin, Perineum A Skin, Inguinal	B Skin, Right Upper Arm C Skin, Left Upper Arm D Skin, Right Lower Arm E Skin, Left Lower Arm F Skin, Right Hand G Skin, Left Hand H Skin, Right Upper Leg J Skin, Left Upper Leg K Skin, Right Lower Leg L Skin, Left Lower Leg M Skin, Right Foot N Skin, Left Foot	X External	J Synthetic Substitute	3 Full Thickness 4 Partial Thickness Z No Qualifier
Ø Skin, Scalp 1 Skin, Face 2 Skin, Right Ear 3 Skin, Left Ear 4 Skin, Neck 5 Skin, Chest Breast procedures, skin only 6 Skin, Back 7 Skin, Abdomen 8 Skin Buttock 9 Skin, Perineum A Skin, Inguinal	B Skin, Right Upper Arm C Skin, Left Upper Arm D Skin, Right Lower Arm E Skin, Left Lower Arm F Skin, Right Hand G Skin, Left Hand H Skin, Right Upper Leg J Skin, Left Upper Leg K Skin, Right Lower Leg L Skin, Left Lower Leg M Skin, Right Foot N Skin, Left Foot	X External	K Nonautologous Tissue Substitute	3 Full Thickness 4 Partial Thickness

Q Finger Nail
  Nail bed
  Nail plate
	R Toe Nail
	  See Q Finger Nail
	S Hair
		X External	7 Autologous Tissue Substitute
			J Synthetic Substitute
			K Nonautologous Tissue Substitute
				Z No Qualifier

T Breast, Right
  Mammary duct
  Mammary gland
	U Breast, Left
	  See T Breast, Right
	V Breast, Bilateral
	  See T Breast, Right
		Ø Open	7 Autologous Tissue Substitute	5 Latissimus Dorsi Myocutaneous Flap
				6 Transverse Rectus Abdominis Myocutaneous Flap
				7 Deep Inferior Epigastric Artery Perforator Flap
				8 Superficial Inferior Epigastric Artery Flap
				9 Gluteal Artery Perforator Flap
				Z No Qualifier

T Breast, Right
  Mammary duct
  Mammary gland
	U Breast, Left
	  See T Breast, Right
	V Breast, Bilateral
	  See T Breast, Right
		Ø Open	J Synthetic Substitute
			K Nonautologous Tissue Substitute
				Z No Qualifier

T Breast, Right ⊞
  Mammary duct
  Mammary gland
U Breast, Left ⊞
  See T Breast, Right
	V Breast, Bilateral ⊞
	  See T Breast, Right
		3 Percutaneous	7 Autologous Tissue Substitute
			J Synthetic Substitute
			K Nonautologous Tissue Substitute
				Z No Qualifier

W Nipple, Right
  Areola
	X Nipple, Left
	  See W Nipple, Right
		Ø Open
		3 Percutaneous
		X External
			7 Autologous Tissue Substitute
			J Synthetic Substitute
			K Nonautologous Tissue Substitute
				Z No Qualifier

Non-OR   ØHRSX7Z

See Appendix L for Procedure Combinations
     ⊞   ØHR[T,U,V]37Z

Non-OR Procedure   DRG Non-OR Procedure   Valid OR Procedure   HAC Associated Procedure   Combination Only   New/Revised GREEN

Ø   Medical and Surgical
H   Skin and Breast
S   Reposition   Definition: Moving to its normal location, or other suitable location, all or a portion of a body part

                 Explanation: The body part is moved to a new location from an abnormal location, or from a normal location where it is not functioning correctly. The body part may or may not be cut out or off to be moved to the new location.

Body Part Character 4	Approach Character 5	Device Character 6	Qualifier Character 7

S Hair
W Nipple, Right
   Areola
X Nipple, Left
   See W Nipple, Right
	X External	**Z** No Device	**Z** No Qualifier

T Breast, Right
   Mammary duct
   Mammary gland
U Breast, Left
   See T Breast, Right
V Breast, Bilateral
   See T Breast, Right
	Ø Open	**Z** No Device	**Z** No Qualifier

Non-OR   ØHSSXZZ

Ø   Medical and Surgical
H   Skin and Breast
T   Resection   Definition: Cutting out or off, without replacement, all of a body part

                 Explanation: None

Body Part Character 4	Approach Character 5	Device Character 6	Qualifier Character 7

Q Finger Nail
   Nail bed
   Nail plate
R Toe Nail
   See Q Finger Nail
W Nipple, Right
   Areola
X Nipple, Left
   See W Nipple, Right
	X External	**Z** No Device	**Z** No Qualifier

T Breast, Right ⊞
   Mammary duct
   Mammary gland
U Breast, Left ⊞
   See T Breast, Right
V Breast, Bilateral ⊞
   See T Breast, Right
Y Supernumerary Breast
	Ø Open	**Z** No Device	**Z** No Qualifier

Non-OR   ØHT[Q,R]XZZ   **See Appendix L for Procedure Combinations**
                                     ⊞   ØHT[T,U,V]ØZZ

Ø   Medical and Surgical
H   Skin and Breast
U   Supplement   Definition: Putting in or on biological or synthetic material that physically reinforces and/or augments the function of a portion of a body part

                 Explanation: The biological material is non-living, or is living and from the same individual. The body part may have been previously replaced, and the SUPPLEMENT procedure is performed to physically reinforce and/or augment the function of the replaced body part.

Body Part Character 4	Approach Character 5	Device Character 6	Qualifier Character 7

T Breast, Right
   Mammary duct
   Mammary gland
U Breast, Left
   See T Breast, Right
V Breast, Bilateral
   See T Breast, Right
	Ø Open
	3 Percutaneous
	7 Via Natural or Artificial Opening
	8 Via Natural or Artificial Opening
	   Endoscopic
		7 Autologous Tissue Substitute
		J Synthetic Substitute
		K Nonautologous Tissue Substitute
			Z No Qualifier

W Nipple, Right
   Areola
X Nipple, Left
   See W Nipple, Right
	Ø Open
	3 Percutaneous
	7 Via Natural or Artificial Opening
	8 Via Natural or Artificial Opening
	   Endoscopic
	X External
		7 Autologous Tissue Substitute
		J Synthetic Substitute
		K Nonautologous Tissue Substitute
			Z No Qualifier

Non-OR   ØHU[T,U,V]3JZ

Skin and Breast

Ø   **Medical and Surgical**
H   **Skin and Breast**
W   **Revision**   Definition: Correcting, to the extent possible, a portion of a malfunctioning device or the position of a displaced device

Explanation: Revision can include correcting a malfunctioning or displaced device by taking out or putting in components of the device such as a screw or pin

Body Part Character 4	Approach Character 5	Device Character 6	Qualifier Character 7

P Skin
   Dermis
   Epidermis
   Sebaceous gland
   Sweat gland
	X External	**Ø** Drainage Device
		7 Autologous Tissue Substitute
		J Synthetic Substitute
		K Nonautologous Tissue Substitute
		Y Other Device
			Z No Qualifier

Q Finger Nail
   Nail bed
   Nail plate
R Toe Nail
   See Q Finger Nail
	X External	**Ø** Drainage Device
		7 Autologous Tissue Substitute
		J Synthetic Substitute
		K Nonautologous Tissue Substitute
			Z No Qualifier

S Hair	**X** External	**7** Autologous Tissue Substitute **J** Synthetic Substitute **K** Nonautologous Tissue Substitute	**Z** No Qualifier

T Breast, Right
   Mammary duct
   Mammary gland
U Breast, Left
   See T Breast, Right
	Ø Open
	3 Percutaneous
	7 Via Natural or Artificial Opening
	8 Via Natural or Artificial Opening Endoscopic
		Ø Drainage Device
		7 Autologous Tissue Substitute
		J Synthetic Substitute
		K Nonautologous Tissue Substitute
		N Tissue Expander
		Y Other Device
			Z No Qualifier

Non-OR	ØHWPX[Ø,7,J,K,Y]Z
Non-OR	ØHW[Q,R]X[Ø,7,J,K]Z
Non-OR	ØHWSX[7,J,K]Z
Non-OR	ØHW[T,U]Ø[Ø,7,K,N]Z
Non-OR	ØHW[T,U]3[Ø,7,K,N,Y]Z
Non-OR	ØHW[T,U][7,8][Ø,7,J,K,N,Y]Z

Ø   **Medical and Surgical**
H   **Skin and Breast**
X   **Transfer**   Definition: Moving, without taking out, all or a portion of a body part to another location to take over the function of all or a portion of a body part

Explanation: The body part transferred remains connected to its vascular and nervous supply

Body Part Character 4	Approach Character 5	Device Character 6	Qualifier Character 7
Ø Skin, Scalp **1** Skin, Face **2** Skin, Right Ear **3** Skin, Left Ear **4** Skin, Neck **5** Skin, Chest Breast procedures, skin only **6** Skin, Back **7** Skin, Abdomen **8** Skin, Buttock **9** Skin, Perineum **A** Skin, Inguinal **B** Skin, Right Upper Arm **C** Skin, Left Upper Arm **D** Skin, Right Lower Arm **E** Skin, Left Lower Arm **F** Skin, Right Hand **G** Skin, Left Hand **H** Skin, Right Upper Leg **J** Skin, Left Upper Leg **K** Skin, Right Lower Leg **L** Skin, Left Lower Leg **M** Skin, Right Foot **N** Skin, Left Foot	**X** External	**Z** No Device	**Z** No Qualifier

Subcutaneous Tissue and Fascia ØJØ–ØJX

Character Meanings

This Character Meaning table is provided as a guide to assist the user in the identification of character members that may be found in this section of code tables. It **SHOULD NOT** be used to build a PCS code.

Operation–Character 3		Body Part–Character 4		Approach–Character 5		Device–Character 6		Qualifier–Character 7	
Ø	Alteration	Ø	Subcutaneous Tissue and Fascia, Scalp	Ø	Open	Ø	Drainage Device OR Monitoring Device, Hemodynamic	B	Skin and Subcutaneous Tissue
2	Change	1	Subcutaneous Tissue and Fascia, Face	3	Percutaneous	1	Radioactive Element	C	Skin, Subcutaneous Tissue and Fascia
5	Destruction	4	Subcutaneous Tissue and Fascia, Right Neck	X	External	2	Monitoring Device	X	Diagnostic
8	Division	5	Subcutaneous Tissue and Fascia, Left Neck			3	Infusion Device	Z	No Qualifier
9	Drainage	6	Subcutaneous Tissue and Fascia, Chest			4	Pacemaker, Single Chamber		
B	Excision	7	Subcutaneous Tissue and Fascia, Back			5	Pacemaker, Single Chamber Rate Responsive		
C	Extirpation	8	Subcutaneous Tissue and Fascia, Abdomen			6	Pacemaker, Dual Chamber		
D	Extraction	9	Subcutaneous Tissue and Fascia, Buttock			7	Autologous Tissue Substitute OR Cardiac Resynchronization Pacemaker Pulse Generator		
H	Insertion	B	Subcutaneous Tissue and Fascia, Perineum			8	Defibrillator Generator		
J	Inspection	C	Subcutaneous Tissue and Fascia, Pelvic Region			9	Cardiac Resynchronization Defibrillator Pulse Generator		
N	Release	D	Subcutaneous Tissue and Fascia, Right Upper Arm			A	Contractility Modulation Device		
P	Removal	F	Subcutaneous Tissue and Fascia, Left Upper Arm			B	Stimulator Generator, Single Array		
Q	Repair	G	Subcutaneous Tissue and Fascia, Right Lower Arm			C	Stimulator Generator, Single Array Rechargeable		
R	Replacement	H	Subcutaneous Tissue and Fascia, Left Lower Arm			D	Stimulator Generator, Multiple Array		
U	Supplement	J	Subcutaneous Tissue and Fascia, Right Hand			E	Stimulator Generator, Multiple Array Rechargeable		
W	Revision	K	Subcutaneous Tissue and Fascia, Left Hand			F	Subcutaneous Defibrillator Lead		
X	Transfer	L	Subcutaneous Tissue and Fascia, Right Upper Leg			H	Contraceptive Device		
		M	Subcutaneous Tissue and Fascia, Left Upper Leg			J	Synthetic Substitute		
		N	Subcutaneous Tissue and Fascia, Right Lower Leg			K	Nonautologous Tissue Substitute		
		P	Subcutaneous Tissue and Fascia, Left Lower Leg			M	Stimulator Generator		
		Q	Subcutaneous Tissue and Fascia, Right Foot			N	Tissue Expander		
		R	Subcutaneous Tissue and Fascia, Left Foot			P	Cardiac Rhythm Related Device		
		S	Subcutaneous Tissue and Fascia, Head and Neck			V	Infusion Device, Pump		
		T	Subcutaneous Tissue and Fascia, Trunk			W	Vascular Access Device, Totally Implantable		
		V	Subcutaneous Tissue and Fascia, Upper Extremity			X	Vascular Access Device, Tunneled		
		W	Subcutaneous Tissue and Fascia, Lower Extremity			Y	Other Device		
						Z	No Device		

AHA Coding Clinic for table ØJ2

2018, 3Q, 10	Disruption of perma-catheter fibrin sheath via angioplasty of superior vena cava
2017, 2Q, 26	Exchange of tunneled catheter

AHA Coding Clinic for table ØJ5

2019, 3Q, 25	Endoscopic removal of pilonidal sinus and cyst

AHA Coding Clinic for table ØJ8

2017, 3Q, 11	Bilateral escharotomy of leg, thigh and foot

AHA Coding Clinic for table ØJ9

2018, 3Q, 16	Incision and drainage of submandibular space
2018, 3Q, 16	Incision and drainage of neck abscess
2015, 3Q, 23	Incision and drainage of multiple abscess cavities using vessel loop

AHA Coding Clinic for table ØJB

2020, 1Q, 31	Repair of buried penis
2019, 3Q, 25	Endoscopic removal of pilonidal sinus and cyst
2018, 3Q, 17	Excisional debridement of periosteum
2018, 1Q, 7	Placement of fat graft following lumbar decompression surgery
2015, 3Q, 3-8	Excisional and nonexcisional debridement
2015, 2Q, 13	Transfer of free flap to reconstruct orbital defect
2015, 1Q, 29	Fistulectomy with placement of seton
2014, 4Q, 38	Abdominoplasty and abdominal wall plication for hernia repair
2014, 3Q, 22	Transsphenoidal removal of pituitary tumor and fat graft placement

AHA Coding Clinic for table ØJC

2017, 3Q, 22	Replacement of native skull bone flap

AHA Coding Clinic for table ØJD

2016, 3Q, 20	VersaJet™ nonexcisional debridement of leg muscle
2016, 3Q, 21	Nonexcisional debridement of infected lumbar wound
2016, 3Q, 21	Nonexcisional pulsed lavage debridement
2016, 3Q, 22	Debridement of bone and tendon using Tenex ultrasound device
2016, 1Q, 40	Nonexcisional debridement of skin and subcutaneous tissue
2015, 3Q, 3-8	Excisional and nonexcisional debridement
2015, 1Q, 23	Non-Excisional debridement with lavage of wound

AHA Coding Clinic for table ØJH

2020, 4Q, 54	Insertion of other device into subcutaneous tissue and fascia
2020, 4Q, 55	Insertion of subcutaneous pump system for ascites drainage
2020, 2Q, 15	Ommaya Reservoir with Ventricular Catheter Placement
2020, 2Q, 16	Ommaya Reservoir Placement for Cerebrospinal Fluid Infusion Therapy
2019, 4Q, 33	Subcutaneous implantable cardioverter defibrillator lead
2017, 4Q, 63-64	Added and revised device values - Vascular access reservoir
2017, 2Q, 24	Tunneled catheter versus totally implantable catheter
2017, 2Q, 26	Exchange of tunneled catheter
2016, 4Q, 97-98	Phrenic neurostimulator
2016, 2Q, 14	Insertion of peritoneal totally implantable venous access device
2016, 2Q, 15	Removal and replacement of tunneled internal jugular catheter
2015, 4Q, 14	New Section X codes—New Technology procedures
2015, 4Q, 30-31	Vascular access devices
2015, 2Q, 33	Totally implantable central venous access device (Port-a-Cath)
2014, 3Q, 19	End of life replacement of Baclofen pump
2013, 4Q, 116	Device character for Port-A-Cath placement
2012, 4Q, 104	Placement of subcutaneous implantable cardioverter defibrillator

AHA Coding Clinic for table ØJN

2017, 3Q, 11	Bilateral escharotomy of leg, thigh and foot

AHA Coding Clinic for table ØJP

2019, 4Q, 33	Subcutaneous implantable cardioverter defibrillator lead
2018, 4Q, 86	Placement of lumboatrial shunt
2018, 3Q, 29	Decommissioning of left ventricular assist device with exploration of mediastinum
2016, 2Q, 15	Removal and replacement of tunneled internal jugular catheter
2015, 4Q, 31	Vascular access devices
2014, 3Q, 19	End of life replacement of Baclofen pump
2013, 4Q, 109	Separating conjoined twins
2012, 4Q, 104	Placement of subcutaneous implantable cardioverter defibrillator

AHA Coding Clinic for table ØJQ

2017, 3Q, 19	Anterior repair of cystocele
2014, 4Q, 44	Posterior colporrhaphy/rectocele repair

AHA Coding Clinic for table ØJR

2015, 2Q, 13	Transfer of free flap to reconstruct orbital defect

AHA Coding Clinic for table ØJU

2018, 2Q, 20	Prelaminated free flap graft using Alloderm™
2018, 1Q, 7	Placement of fat graft following lumbar decompression surgery

AHA Coding Clinic for table ØJW

2019, 4Q, 33	Subcutaneous implantable cardioverter defibrillator lead
2018, 1Q, 8	Ventricular peritoneal shunt ligation
2015, 4Q, 33	Externalization of peritoneal dialysis catheter
2015, 2Q, 9	Revision of ventriculoperitoneal (VP) shunt
2012, 4Q, 104	Placement of subcutaneous implantable cardioverter defibrillator

AHA Coding Clinic for table ØJX

2021, 2Q, 16	Goldilocks breast reconstruction
2018, 1Q, 10	Complex wound closure using pericranial flap
2014, 3Q, 18	Placement of reverse sural fasciocutaneous pedicle flap
2013, 4Q, 109	Separating conjoined twins

Ø   **Medical and Surgical**
J   **Subcutaneous Tissue and Fascia**
Ø   **Alteration**   Definition: Modifying the anatomic structure of a body part without affecting the function of the body part
                       Explanation: Principal purpose is to improve appearance

Body Part Character 4		Approach Character 5	Device Character 6	Qualifier Character 7
1 Subcutaneous Tissue and Fascia, Face Masseteric fascia Orbital fascia Submandibular space **4 Subcutaneous Tissue and Fascia, Right Neck** Deep cervical fascia Pretracheal fascia Prevertebral fascia **5 Subcutaneous Tissue and Fascia, Left Neck** *See 4 Subcutaneous Tissue and Fascia, Right Neck* **6 Subcutaneous Tissue and Fascia, Chest** Pectoral fascia **7 Subcutaneous Tissue and Fascia, Back** **8 Subcutaneous Tissue and Fascia, Abdomen** **9 Subcutaneous Tissue and Fascia, Buttock** **D Subcutaneous Tissue and Fascia, Right Upper Arm** Axillary fascia Deltoid fascia Infraspinatus fascia Subscapular aponeurosis Supraspinatus fascia	**F Subcutaneous Tissue and Fascia, Left Upper Arm** *See D Subcutaneous Tissue and Fascia, Right Upper Arm* **G Subcutaneous Tissue and Fascia, Right Lower Arm** Antebrachial fascia Bicipital aponeurosis **H Subcutaneous Tissue and Fascia, Left Lower Arm** *See G Subcutaneous Tissue and Fascia, Right Lower Arm* **L Subcutaneous Tissue and Fascia, Right Upper Leg** Crural fascia Fascia lata Iliac fascia Iliotibial tract (band) **M Subcutaneous Tissue and Fascia, Left Upper Leg** *See L Subcutaneous Tissue and Fascia, Right Upper Leg* **N Subcutaneous Tissue and Fascia, Right Lower Leg** **P Subcutaneous Tissue and Fascia, Left Lower Leg**	**Ø Open** **3 Percutaneous**	**Z No Device**	**Z No Qualifier**

Ø   **Medical and Surgical**
J   **Subcutaneous Tissue and Fascia**
2   **Change**   Definition: Taking out or off a device from a body part and putting back an identical or similar device in or on the same body part without cutting or puncturing the skin or a mucous membrane
                     Explanation: All CHANGE procedures are coded using the approach EXTERNAL

Body Part Character 4	Approach Character 5	Device Character 6	Qualifier Character 7
S Subcutaneous Tissue and Fascia, Head and Neck **T Subcutaneous Tissue and Fascia, Trunk** External oblique aponeurosis Transversalis fascia **V Subcutaneous Tissue and Fascia, Upper Extremity** **W Subcutaneous Tissue and Fascia, Lower Extremity**	**X External**	**Ø Drainage Device** **Y Other Device**	**Z No Qualifier**

Non-OR	All body part, approach, device, and qualifier values

Ø   **Medical and Surgical**
J   **Subcutaneous Tissue and Fascia**
5   **Destruction**   Definition: Physical eradication of all or a portion of a body part by the direct use of energy, force, or a destructive agent
                           Explanation: None of the body part is physically taken out

Body Part Character 4		Approach Character 5	Device Character 6	Qualifier Character 7
Ø Subcutaneous Tissue and Fascia, Scalp Galea aponeurotica **1 Subcutaneous Tissue and Fascia, Face** Masseteric fascia Orbital fascia Submandibular space **4 Subcutaneous Tissue and Fascia, Right Neck** Deep cervical fascia Pretracheal fascia Prevertebral fascia **5 Subcutaneous Tissue and Fascia, Left Neck** *See 4 Subcutaneous Tissue and Fascia, Right Neck* **6 Subcutaneous Tissue and Fascia, Chest** Pectoral fascia **7 Subcutaneous Tissue and Fascia, Back** **8 Subcutaneous Tissue and Fascia, Abdomen** **9 Subcutaneous Tissue and Fascia, Buttock** **B Subcutaneous Tissue and Fascia, Perineum** **C Subcutaneous Tissue and Fascia, Pelvic Region** **D Subcutaneous Tissue and Fascia, Right Upper Arm** Axillary fascia Deltoid fascia Infraspinatus fascia Subscapular aponeurosis Supraspinatus fascia **F Subcutaneous Tissue and Fascia, Left Upper Arm** *See D Subcutaneous Tissue and Fascia, Right Upper Arm*	**G Subcutaneous Tissue and Fascia, Right Lower Arm** Antebrachial fascia Bicipital aponeurosis **H Subcutaneous Tissue and Fascia, Left Lower Arm** *See G Subcutaneous Tissue and Fascia, Right Lower Arm* **J Subcutaneous Tissue and Fascia, Right Hand** Palmar fascia (aponeurosis) **K Subcutaneous Tissue and Fascia, Left Hand** *See J Subcutaneous Tissue and Fascia, Right Hand* **L Subcutaneous Tissue and Fascia, Right Upper Leg** Crural fascia Fascia lata Iliac fascia Iliotibial tract (band) **M Subcutaneous Tissue and Fascia, Left Upper Leg** *See L Subcutaneous Tissue and Fascia, Right Upper Leg* **N Subcutaneous Tissue and Fascia, Right Lower Leg** **P Subcutaneous Tissue and Fascia, Left Lower Leg** **Q Subcutaneous Tissue and Fascia, Right Foot** Plantar fascia (aponeurosis) **R Subcutaneous Tissue and Fascia, Left Foot** *See Q Subcutaneous Tissue and Fascia, Right Foot*	**Ø Open** **3 Percutaneous**	**Z No Device**	**Z No Qualifier**

DRG Non-OR   All body part, approach, device, and qualifier values

Ø   **Medical and Surgical**
J   **Subcutaneous Tissue and Fascia**
8   **Division**   Definition: Cutting into a body part, without draining fluids and/or gases from the body part, in order to separate or transect a body part
                      Explanation: All or a portion of the body part is separated into two or more portions

Body Part Character 4		Approach Character 5	Device Character 6	Qualifier Character 7

Ø   **Subcutaneous Tissue and Fascia, Scalp**
    Galea aponeurotica
1   **Subcutaneous Tissue and Fascia, Face**
    Masseteric fascia
    Orbital fascia
    Submandibular space
4   **Subcutaneous Tissue and Fascia, Right Neck**
    Deep cervical fascia
    Pretracheal fascia
    Prevertebral fascia
5   **Subcutaneous Tissue and Fascia, Left Neck**
    See 4 Subcutaneous Tissue and Fascia, Right Neck
6   **Subcutaneous Tissue and Fascia, Chest**
    Pectoral fascia
7   **Subcutaneous Tissue and Fascia, Back**
8   **Subcutaneous Tissue and Fascia, Abdomen**
9   **Subcutaneous Tissue and Fascia, Buttock**
B   **Subcutaneous Tissue and Fascia, Perineum**
C   **Subcutaneous Tissue and Fascia, Pelvic Region**
D   **Subcutaneous Tissue and Fascia, Right Upper Arm**
    Axillary fascia
    Deltoid fascia
    Infraspinatus fascia
    Subscapular aponeurosis
    Supraspinatus fascia
F   **Subcutaneous Tissue and Fascia, Left Upper Arm**
    See D Subcutaneous Tissue and Fascia, Right Upper Arm
G   **Subcutaneous Tissue and Fascia, Right Lower Arm**
    Antebrachial fascia
    Bicipital aponeurosis
	H **Subcutaneous Tissue and Fascia, Left Lower Arm**
	    See G Subcutaneous Tissue and Fascia, Right Lower Arm
	J **Subcutaneous Tissue and Fascia, Right Hand**
	    Palmar fascia (aponeurosis)
	K **Subcutaneous Tissue and Fascia, Left Hand**
	    See J Subcutaneous Tissue and Fascia, Right Hand
	L **Subcutaneous Tissue and Fascia, Right Upper Leg**
	    Crural fascia
	    Fascia lata
	    Iliac fascia
	    Iliotibial tract (band)
	M **Subcutaneous Tissue and Fascia, Left Upper Leg**
	    See L Subcutaneous Tissue and Fascia, Right Upper Leg
	N **Subcutaneous Tissue and Fascia, Right Lower Leg**
	P **Subcutaneous Tissue and Fascia, Left Lower Leg**
	Q **Subcutaneous Tissue and Fascia, Right Foot**
	    Plantar fascia (aponeurosis)
	R **Subcutaneous Tissue and Fascia, Left Foot**
	    See Q Subcutaneous Tissue and Fascia, Right Foot
	S **Subcutaneous Tissue and Fascia, Head and Neck**
	T **Subcutaneous Tissue and Fascia, Trunk**
	    External oblique aponeurosis
	    Transversalis fascia
	V **Subcutaneous Tissue and Fascia, Upper Extremity**
	W **Subcutaneous Tissue and Fascia, Lower Extremity**
		Ø Open
		3 Percutaneous
			Z No Device	**Z** No Qualifier

Subcutaneous Tissue and Fascia

Ø   **Medical and Surgical**
J   **Subcutaneous Tissue and Fascia**
9   **Drainage**   Definition: Taking or letting out fluids and/or gases from a body part
                       Explanation: The qualifier DIAGNOSTIC is used to identify drainage procedures that are biopsies

Body Part Character 4		Approach Character 5	Device Character 6	Qualifier Character 7
Ø **Subcutaneous Tissue and Fascia, Scalp** Galea aponeurotica 1 **Subcutaneous Tissue and Fascia, Face** Masseteric fascia Orbital fascia Submandibular space 4 **Subcutaneous Tissue and Fascia, Right Neck** Deep cervical fascia Pretracheal fascia Prevertebral fascia 5 **Subcutaneous Tissue and Fascia, Left Neck** *See 4 Subcutaneous Tissue and Fascia, Right Neck* 6 **Subcutaneous Tissue and Fascia, Chest** Pectoral fascia 7 **Subcutaneous Tissue and Fascia, Back** 8 **Subcutaneous Tissue and Fascia, Abdomen** 9 **Subcutaneous Tissue and Fascia, Buttock** B **Subcutaneous Tissue and Fascia, Perineum** C **Subcutaneous Tissue and Fascia, Pelvic Region** D **Subcutaneous Tissue and Fascia, Right Upper Arm** Axillary fascia Deltoid fascia Infraspinatus fascia Subscapular aponeurosis Supraspinatus fascia F **Subcutaneous Tissue and Fascia, Left Upper Arm** *See D Subcutaneous Tissue and Fascia, Right Upper Arm*	G **Subcutaneous Tissue and Fascia, Right Lower Arm** Antebrachial fascia Bicipital aponeurosis H **Subcutaneous Tissue and Fascia, Left Lower Arm** *See G Subcutaneous Tissue and Fascia, Right Lower Arm* J **Subcutaneous Tissue and Fascia, Right Hand** Palmar fascia (aponeurosis) K **Subcutaneous Tissue and Fascia, Left Hand** *See J Subcutaneous Tissue and Fascia, Right Hand* L **Subcutaneous Tissue and Fascia, Right Upper Leg** Crural fascia Fascia lata Iliac fascia Iliotibial tract (band) M **Subcutaneous Tissue and Fascia, Left Upper Leg** *See L Subcutaneous Tissue and Fascia, Right Upper Leg* N **Subcutaneous Tissue and Fascia, Right Lower Leg** P **Subcutaneous Tissue and Fascia, Left Lower Leg** Q **Subcutaneous Tissue and Fascia, Right Foot** Plantar fascia (aponeurosis) R **Subcutaneous Tissue and Fascia, Left Foot** *See Q Subcutaneous Tissue and Fascia, Right Foot*	Ø Open 3 Percutaneous	Ø Drainage Device	Z No Qualifier

Non-OR   ØJ9[Ø,1,4,5,6,7,8,9,B,C,D,F,G,H,J,K,L,M,N,P,Q,R][Ø,3]ØZ

ØJ9 Continued on next page

Subcutaneous Tissue and Fascia

Ø   **Medical and Surgical**
J   **Subcutaneous Tissue and Fascia**
9   **Drainage**   Definition: Taking or letting out fluids and/or gases from a body part

                       Explanation: The qualifier DIAGNOSTIC is used to identify drainage procedures that are biopsies

Body Part Character 4		Approach Character 5	Device Character 6	Qualifier Character 7
Ø Subcutaneous Tissue and Fascia, Scalp Galea aponeurotica **1 Subcutaneous Tissue and Fascia, Face** Masseteric fascia Orbital fascia Submandibular space **4 Subcutaneous Tissue and Fascia, Right Neck** Deep cervical fascia Pretracheal fascia Prevertebral fascia **5 Subcutaneous Tissue and Fascia, Left Neck** *See 4 Subcutaneous Tissue and Fascia, Right Neck* **6 Subcutaneous Tissue and Fascia, Chest** Pectoral fascia **7 Subcutaneous Tissue and Fascia, Back** **8 Subcutaneous Tissue and Fascia, Abdomen** **9 Subcutaneous Tissue and Fascia, Buttock** **B Subcutaneous Tissue and Fascia, Perineum** **C Subcutaneous Tissue and Fascia, Pelvic Region** **D Subcutaneous Tissue and Fascia, Right Upper Arm** Axillary fascia Deltoid fascia Infraspinatus fascia Subscapular aponeurosis Supraspinatus fascia **F Subcutaneous Tissue and Fascia, Left Upper Arm** *See D Subcutaneous Tissue and Fascia, Right Upper Arm*	**G Subcutaneous Tissue and Fascia, Right Lower Arm** Antebrachial fascia Bicipital aponeurosis **H Subcutaneous Tissue and Fascia, Left Lower Arm** *See G Subcutaneous Tissue and Fascia, Right Lower Arm* **J Subcutaneous Tissue and Fascia, Right Hand** Palmar fascia (aponeurosis) **K Subcutaenous Tissue and Fascia, Left Hand** *See J Subcutaneous Tissue and Fascia, Right Hand* **L Subcutaneous Tissue and Fascia, Right Upper Leg** Crural fascia Fascia lata Iliac fascia Iliotibial tract (band) **M Subcutaneous Tissue and Fascia, Left Upper Leg** *See L Subcutaneous Tissue and Fascia, Right Upper Leg* **N Subcutaneous Tissue and Fascia, Right Lower Leg** **P Subcutaneous Tissue and Fascia, Left Lower Leg** **Q Subcutaneous Tissue and Fascia, Right Foot** Plantar fascia (aponeurosis) **R Subcutaneous Tissue and Fascia, Left Foot** *See Q Subcutaneous Tissue and Fascia, Right Foot*	**Ø Open** **3 Percutaneous**	**Z No Device**	**X Diagnostic** **Z No Qualifier**

Non-OR   ØJ9[Ø,1,4,5,6,7,8,9,B,C,D,F,G,H,J,K,L,M,N,P,Q,R][Ø,3]ZX
Non-OR   ØJ9[Ø,1,4,5,6,7,8,9,B,C,D,F,G,H,J,K,L,M,N,P,Q,R]3ZZ

Ø Medical and Surgical
J Subcutaneous Tissue and Fascia
B Excision　　　Definition: Cutting out or off, without replacement, a portion of a body part
　　　　　　　　　　Explanation: The qualifier DIAGNOSTIC is used to identify excision procedures that are biopsies

Body Part Character 4		Approach Character 5	Device Character 6	Qualifier Character 7
Ø Subcutaneous Tissue and Fascia, Scalp Galea aponeurotica	**G Subcutaneous Tissue and Fascia, Right Lower Arm** Antebrachial fascia Bicipital aponeurosis	**Ø Open** **3 Percutaneous**	**Z No Device**	**X Diagnostic** **Z No Qualifier**
1 Subcutaneous Tissue and Fascia, Face Masseteric fascia Orbital fascia Submandibular space	**H Subcutaneous Tissue and Fascia, Left Lower Arm** *See G Subcutaneous Tissue and Fascia, Right Lower Arm*			
4 Subcutaneous Tissue and Fascia, Right Neck Deep cervical fascia Pretracheal fascia Prevertebral fascia	**J Subcutaneous Tissue and Fascia, Right Hand** Palmar fascia (aponeurosis)			
5 Subcutaneous Tissue and Fascia, Left Neck *See 4 Subcutaneous Tissue and Fascia, Right Neck*	**K Subcutaneous Tissue and Fascia, Left Hand** *See J Subcutaneous Tissue and Fascia, Right Hand*			
6 Subcutaneous Tissue and Fascia, Chest Pectoral fascia	**L Subcutaneous Tissue and Fascia, Right Upper Leg** Crural fascia Fascia lata Iliac fascia Iliotibial tract (band)			
7 Subcutaneous Tissue and Fascia, Back	**M Subcutaneous Tissue and Fascia, Left Upper Leg** *See L Subcutaneous Tissue and Fascia, Right Upper Leg*			
8 Subcutaneous Tissue and Fascia, Abdomen	**N Subcutaneous Tissue and Fascia, Right Lower Leg**			
9 Subcutaneous Tissue and Fascia, Buttock	**P Subcutaneous Tissue and Fascia, Left Lower Leg**			
B Subcutaneous Tissue and Fascia, Perineum	**Q Subcutaneous Tissue and Fascia, Right Foot** Plantar fascia (aponeurosis)			
C Subcutaneous Tissue and Fascia, Pelvic Region	**R Subcutaneous Tissue and Fascia, Left Foot** *See Q Subcutaneous Tissue and Fascia, Right Foot*			
D Subcutaneous Tissue and Fascia, Right Upper Arm Axillary fascia Deltoid fascia Infraspinatus fascia Subscapular aponeurosis Supraspinatus fascia				
F Subcutaneous Tissue and Fascia, Left Upper Arm *See D Subcutaneous Tissue and Fascia, Right Upper Arm*				

DRG Non-OR　ØJB[Ø,4,5,6,7,8,9,B,C,D,F,G,H,L,M,N,P,Q,R]3ZZ
Non-OR　　　ØJB[Ø,1,4,5,6,7,8,9,B,C,D,F,G,H,J,K,L,M,N,P,Q,R][Ø,3]ZX

Ø   Medical and Surgical
J   Subcutaneous Tissue and Fascia
C   Extirpation   Definition: Taking or cutting out solid matter from a body part

Explanation: The solid matter may be an abnormal byproduct of a biological function or a foreign body; it may be imbedded in a body part or in the lumen of a tubular body part. The solid matter may or may not have been previously broken into pieces.

Body Part Character 4		Approach Character 5	Device Character 6	Qualifier Character 7
Ø **Subcutaneous Tissue and Fascia, Scalp** Galea aponeurotica **1** **Subcutaneous Tissue and Fascia, Face** Masseteric fascia Orbital fascia Submandibular space **4** **Subcutaneous Tissue and Fascia, Right Neck** Deep cervical fascia Pretracheal fascia Prevertebral fascia **5** **Subcutaneous Tissue and Fascia, Left Neck** *See 4 Subcutaneous Tissue and Fascia, Right Neck* **6** **Subcutaneous Tissue and Fascia, Chest** Pectoral fascia **7** **Subcutaneous Tissue and Fascia, Back** **8** **Subcutaneous Tissue and Fascia, Abdomen** **9** **Subcutaneous Tissue and Fascia, Buttock** **B** **Subcutaneous Tissue and Fascia, Perineum** **C** **Subcutaneous Tissue and Fascia, Pelvic Region** **D** **Subcutaneous Tissue and Fascia, Right Upper Arm** Axillary fascia Deltoid fascia Infraspinatus fascia Subscapular aponeurosis Supraspinatus fascia **F** **Subcutaneous Tissue and Fascia, Left Upper Arm** *See D Subcutaneous Tissue and Fascia, Right Upper Arm*	**G** **Subcutaneous Tissue and Fascia, Right Lower Arm** Antebrachial fascia Bicipital aponeurosis **H** **Subcutaneous Tissue and Fascia, Left Lower Arm** *See G Subcutaneous Tissue and Fascia, Right Lower Arm* **J** **Subcutaneous Tissue and Fascia, Right Hand** Palmar fascia (aponeurosis) **K** **Subcutaneous Tissue and Fascia, Left Hand** *See J Subcutaneous Tissue and Fascia, Right Hand* **L** **Subcutaneous Tissue and Fascia, Right Upper Leg** Crural fascia Fascia lata Iliac fascia Iliotibial tract (band) **M** **Subcutaneous Tissue and Fascia, Left Upper Leg** *See L Subcutaneous Tissue and Fascia, Right Upper Leg* **N** **Subcutaneous Tissue and Fascia, Right Lower Leg** **P** **Subcutaneous Tissue and Fascia, Left Lower Leg** **Q** **Subcutaneous Tissue and Fascia, Right Foot** Plantar fascia (aponeurosis) **R** **Subcutaneous Tissue and Fascia, Left Foot** *See Q Subcutaneous Tissue and Fascia, Right Foot*	**Ø** Open **3** Percutaneous	**Z** No Device	**Z** No Qualifier

Non-OR   All body part, approach, device, and qualifier values

Ø   **Medical and Surgical**
J   **Subcutaneous Tissue and Fascia**
D   **Extraction**   Definition: Pulling or stripping out or off all or a portion of a body part by the use of force
                    Explanation: The qualifier DIAGNOSTIC is used to identify extraction procedures that are biopsies

Body Part Character 4		Approach Character 5	Device Character 6	Qualifier Character 7
Ø **Subcutaneous Tissue and Fascia, Scalp**	G **Subcutaneous Tissue and Fascia, Right Lower Arm**	Ø Open	Z No Device	Z No Qualifier
Galea aponeurotica	Antebrachial fascia	3 Percutaneous		
1 **Subcutaneous Tissue and Fascia, Face**	Bicipital aponeurosis			
Masseteric fascia	H **Subcutaneous Tissue and Fascia, Left Lower Arm**			
Orbital fascia	*See G Subcutaneous Tissue and Fascia, Right Lower Arm*			
Submandibular space				
4 **Subcutaneous Tissue and Fascia, Right Neck**	J **Subcutaneous Tissue and Fascia, Right Hand**			
Deep cervical fascia	Palmar fascia (aponeurosis)			
Pretracheal fascia	K **Subcutaneous Tissue and Fascia, Left Hand**			
Prevertebral fascia	*See J Subcutaneous Tissue and Fascia, Right Hand*			
5 **Subcutaneous Tissue and Fascia, Left Neck**				
See 4 Subcutaneous Tissue and Fascia, Right Neck	L **Subcutaneous Tissue and Fascia, Right Upper Leg**			
6 **Subcutaneous Tissue and Fascia, Chest**	Crural fascia			
Pectoral fascia	Fascia lata			
7 **Subcutaneous Tissue and Fascia, Back**	Iliac fascia			
8 **Subcutaneous Tissue and Fascia, Abdomen**	Iliotibial tract (band)			
9 **Subcutaneous Tissue and Fascia, Buttock**	M **Subcutaneous Tissue and Fascia, Left Upper Leg**			
B **Subcutaneous Tissue and Fascia, Perineum**	*See L Subcutaneous Tissue and Fascia, Right Upper Leg*			
C **Subcutaneous Tissue and Fascia, Pelvic Region**	N **Subcutaneous Tissue and Fascia, Right Lower Leg**			
D **Subcutaneous Tissue and Fascia, Right Upper Arm**	P **Subcutaneous Tissue and Fascia, Left Lower Leg**			
Axillary fascia	Q **Subcutaneous Tissue and Fascia, Right Foot**			
Deltoid fascia	Plantar fascia (aponeurosis)			
Infraspinatus fascia	R **Subcutaneous Tissue and Fascia, Left Foot**			
Subscapular aponeurosis	*See Q Subcutaneous Tissue and Fascia, Right Foot*			
Supraspinatus fascia				
F **Subcutaneous Tissue and Fascia, Left Upper Arm**				
See D Subcutaneous Tissue and Fascia, Right Upper Arm				

Non-OR   ØJD[Ø,1,4,5,B,C,D,F,G,H,J,K,N,P,Q,R]3ZZ

See Appendix L for Procedure Combinations
Combo-only   ØJD[6,7,8,9,L,M]3ZZ

Ø   **Medical and Surgical**
J   **Subcutaneous Tissue and Fascia**
H   **Insertion**   Definition: Putting in a nonbiological appliance that monitors, assists, performs, or prevents a physiological function but does not physically take the place of a body part
                   Explanation: None

Body Part Character 4		Approach Character 5	Device Character 6	Qualifier Character 7
Ø Subcutaneous Tissue and Fascia, Scalp Galea aponeurotica **1** Subcutaneous Tissue and Fascia, Face Masseteric fascia Orbital fascia Submandibular space **4** Subcutaneous Tissue and Fascia, Right Neck Deep cervical fascia Pretracheal fascia Prevertebral fascia **5** Subcutaneous Tissue and Fascia, Left Neck *See 4 Subcutaneous Tissue and Fascia, Right Neck* **9** Subcutaneous Tissue and Fascia, Buttock **B** Subcutaneous Tissue and Fascia, Perineum	**C** Subcutaneous Tissue and Fascia, Pelvic Region **J** Subcutaneous Tissue and Fascia, Right Hand Palmar fascia (aponeurosis) **K** Subcutaneous Tissue and Fascia, Left Hand *See J Subcutaneous Tissue and Fascia, Right Hand* **Q** Subcutaneous Tissue and Fascia, Right Foot Plantar fascia (aponeurosis) **R** Subcutaneous Tissue and Fascia, Left Foot *See Q Subcutaneous Tissue and Fascia, Right Foot*	**Ø** Open **3** Percutaneous	**N** Tissue Expander	**Z** No Qualifier
6 Subcutaneous Tissue and Fascia, Chest ⊞ Pectoral fascia		**Ø** Open **3** Percutaneous	**Ø** Monitoring Device, Hemodynamic **2** Monitoring Device **4** Pacemaker, Single Chamber **5** Pacemaker, Single Chamber Rate Responsive **6** Pacemaker, Dual Chamber **7** Cardiac Resynchronization Pacemaker Pulse Generator **8** Defibrillator Generator **9** Cardiac Resynchronization Defibrillator Pulse Generator **A** Contractility Modulation Device NT **B** Stimulator Generator, Single Array **C** Stimulator Generator, Single Array Rechargeable **D** Stimulator Generator, Multiple Array **E** Stimulator Generator, Multiple Array Rechargeable **F** Subcutaneous Defibrillator Lead **H** Contraceptive Device **M** Stimulator Generator NT **N** Tissue Expander **P** Cardiac Rhythm Related Device **V** Infusion Device, Pump **W** Vascular Access Device, Totally Implantable **X** Vascular Access Device, Tunneled **Y** Other Device	**Z** No Qualifier
7 Subcutaneous Tissue and Fascia, Back NC ⊞		**Ø** Open **3** Percutaneous	**B** Stimulator Generator, Single Array **C** Stimulator Generator, Single Array Rechargeable **D** Stimulator Generator, Multiple Array **E** Stimulator Generator, Multiple Array Rechargeable **M** Stimulator Generator **N** Tissue Expander **V** Infusion Device, Pump **Y** Other Device	**Z** No Qualifier

DRG Non-OR	ØJH6[Ø,3][4,5,6,7,H,P,X]Z	NC	ØJH7[Ø,3]MZ
DRG Non-OR	ØJH63WX	NT	ØJH6[Ø,3]AZ
Non-OR	ØJH63YZ		*See* Appendix H for applicable device trade name
Non-OR	ØJH73YZ	NT	ØJH6ØMZ in combination with Ø3HK3MZ or Ø3HL3MZ
HAC	ØJH6[Ø,3][4,5,6,7,8,9,P]Z when reported with SDx K68.11 or T81.4Ø-T81.49, T82.6-T82.7 with 7th character A		*See* Appendix H for applicable device trade name
HAC	ØJH63XZ when reported with SDx J95.811		**See Appendix L for Procedure Combinations**
		⊞	ØJH6[Ø,3][4,5,6,7,8,9,A,B,C,D,E,F,P]Z
		⊞	ØJH7[Ø,3][B,C,D,E]Z

ØJH Continued on next page

NC Noncovered Procedure   LC Limited Coverage   QA Questionable OB Admit   NT New Tech Add-on   ⊞ Combination Member   ♂ Male   ♀ Female

ICD-10-PCS 2022   453

ØJH Continued

Ø **Medical and Surgical**
J **Subcutaneous Tissue and Fascia**
H **Insertion**   Definition: Putting in a nonbiological appliance that monitors, assists, performs, or prevents a physiological function but does not physically take the place of a body part
Explanation: None

Body Part Character 4	Approach Character 5	Device Character 6	Qualifier Character 7
8 Subcutaneous Tissue and Fascia, Abdomen **NC ⊞**	Ø Open 3 Percutaneous	Ø Monitoring Device, Hemodynamic 2 Monitoring Device 4 Pacemaker, Single Chamber 5 Pacemaker, Single Chamber Rate Responsive 6 Pacemaker, Dual Chamber 7 Cardiac Resynchronization Pacemaker Pulse Generator 8 Defibrillator Generator 9 Cardiac Resynchronization Defibrillator Pulse Generator A Contractility Modulation Device **NT** B Stimulator Generator, Single Array C Stimulator Generator, Single Array Rechargeable D Stimulator Generator, Multiple Array E Stimulator Generator, Multiple Array Rechargeable H Contraceptive Device M Stimulator Generator N Tissue Expander P Cardiac Rhythm Related Device V Infusion Device, Pump W Vascular Access Device, Totally Implantable X Vascular Access Device, Tunneled Y Other Device	Z No Qualifier

D Subcutaneous Tissue and Fascia, Right Upper Arm
  Axillary fascia
  Deltoid fascia
  Infraspinatus fascia
  Subscapular aponeurosis
  Supraspinatus fascia
F Subcutaneous Tissue and Fascia, Left Upper Arm
  See D Subcutaneous Tissue and Fascia, Right Upper Arm
G Subcutaneous Tissue and Fascia, Right Lower Arm
  Antebrachial fascia
  Bicipital aponeurosis
H Subcutaneous Tissue and Fascia, Left Lower Arm
  See G Subcutaneous Tissue and Fascia, Right Lower Arm
L Subcutaneous Tissue and Fascia, Right Upper Leg
  Crural fascia
  Fascia lata
  Iliac fascia
  Iliotibial tract (band)
M Subcutaneous Tissue and Fascia, Left Upper Leg
  See L Subcutaneous Tissue and Fascia, Right Upper Leg
N Subcutaneous Tissue and Fascia, Right Lower Leg
P Subcutaneous Tissue and Fascia, Left Lower Leg
	Ø Open
	3 Percutaneous
		H Contraceptive Device
		N Tissue Expander
		V Infusion Device, Pump
		W Vascular Access Device, Totally Implantable
		X Vascular Access Device, Tunneled
			Z No Qualifier

S Subcutaneous Tissue and Fascia, Head and Neck V Subcutaneous Tissue and Fascia, Upper Extremity W Subcutaneous Tissue and Fascia, Lower Extremity	Ø Open 3 Percutaneous	1 Radioactive Element 3 Infusion Device Y Other Device	Z No Qualifier

T Subcutaneous Tissue and Fascia, Trunk
  External oblique aponeurosis
  Transversalis fascia
	Ø Open
	3 Percutaneous
		1 Radioactive Element
		3 Infusion Device
		V Infusion Device, Pump
		Y Other Device
			Z No Qualifier

DRG Non-OR	ØJH8[Ø,3][2,4,5,6,7,H,P,X]Z	Non-OR ØJH83YZ	HAC ØJH8[Ø,3][4,5,6,7,8,9,P]Z when reported with SDx K68.11 or T81.4Ø-T81.49, T82.6-T82.7 with 7th character A
DRG Non-OR	ØJH83WX	Non-OR ØJH[D,F,G,H,L,M][Ø,3]HZ	
DRG Non-OR	ØJH[D,F,G,H,L,M,N,P]ØXZ	Non-OR ØJHNØHZ	**NC** ØJH8[Ø,3]MZ
DRG Non-OR	ØJH[D,F,G,H,L,M,N,P]3[W,X]Z	Non-OR ØJH[S,V,W]Ø3Z	**NT** ØJHB[Ø,3]AZ *See* Appendix H for applicable device trade name
DRG Non-OR	ØJHN3HZ	Non-OR ØJH[S,V,W]3[3,Y]Z	**See Appendix L for Procedure Combinations**
DRG Non-OR	ØJHP[Ø,3]HZ	Non-OR ØJHTØ3Z	⊞ ØJH8[Ø,3][4,5,6,7,8,9,A,B,C,D,E,P]Z
		Non-OR ØJHT3[3,Y]Z	

Non-OR Procedure | DRG Non-OR Procedure | Valid OR Procedure | HAC Associated Procedure | Combination Only | New/Revised GREEN

Ø   Medical and Surgical
J   Subcutaneous Tissue and Fascia
J   Inspection   Definition: Visually and/or manually exploring a body part

Explanation: Visual exploration may be performed with or without optical instrumentation. Manual exploration may be performed directly or through intervening body layers.

Body Part Character 4	Approach Character 5	Device Character 6	Qualifier Character 7

S Subcutaneous Tissue and Fascia, Head and Neck
 T Subcutaneous Tissue and Fascia, Trunk
     External oblique aponeurosis
     Transversalis fascia
 V Subcutaneous Tissue and Fascia, Upper Extremity
 W Subcutaneous Tissue and Fascia, Lower Extremity
	Ø Open
	 3 Percutaneous
	 X External
		Z No Device	**Z** No Qualifier

Non-OR   All body part, approach, device, and qualifier values

---

Ø   Medical and Surgical
J   Subcutaneous Tissue and Fascia
N   Release   Definition: Freeing a body part from an abnormal physical constraint by cutting or by the use of force

Explanation: Some of the restraining tissue may be taken out but none of the body part is taken out

Body Part Character 4	Approach Character 5	Device Character 6	Qualifier Character 7

Ø Subcutaneous Tissue and Fascia, Scalp
     Galea aponeurotica
 1 Subcutaneous Tissue and Fascia, Face
     Masseteric fascia
     Orbital fascia
     Submandibular space
 4 Subcutaneous Tissue and Fascia, Right Neck
     Deep cervical fascia
     Pretracheal fascia
     Prevertebral fascia
 5 Subcutaneous Tissue and Fascia, Left Neck
     See 4 Subcutaneous Tissue and Fascia, Right Neck
 6 Subcutaneous Tissue and Fascia, Chest
     Pectoral fascia
 7 Subcutaneous Tissue and Fascia, Back
 8 Subcutaneous Tissue and Fascia, Abdomen
 9 Subcutaneous Tissue and Fascia, Buttock
 B Subcutaneous Tissue and Fascia, Perineum
 C Subcutaneous Tissue and Fascia, Pelvic Region
 D Subcutaneous Tissue and Fascia, Right Upper Arm
     Axillary fascia
     Deltoid fascia
     Infraspinatus fascia
     Subscapular aponeurosis
     Supraspinatus fascia
 F Subcutaneous Tissue and Fascia, Left Upper Arm
     See D Subcutaneous Tissue and Fascia, Right Upper Arm
 	
 G Subcutaneous Tissue and Fascia, Right Lower Arm
     Antebrachial fascia
     Bicipital aponeurosis
 H Subcutaneous Tissue and Fascia, Left Lower Arm
     See G Subcutaneous Tissue and Fascia, Right Lower Arm
 J Subcutaneous Tissue and Fascia, Right Hand
     Palmar fascia (aponeurosis)
 K Subcutaneous Tissue and Fascia, Left Hand
     See J Subcutaneous Tissue and Fascia, Right Hand
 L Subcutaneous Tissue and Fascia, Right Upper Leg
     Crural fascia
     Fascia lata
     Iliac fascia
     Iliotibial tract (band)
 M Subcutaneous Tissue and Fascia, Left Upper Leg
     See L Subcutaneous Tissue and Fascia, Right Upper Leg
 N Subcutaneous Tissue and Fascia, Right Lower Leg
 P Subcutaneous Tissue and Fascia, Left Lower Leg
 Q Subcutaneous Tissue and Fascia, Right Foot
     Plantar fascia (aponeurosis)
 R Subcutaneous Tissue and Fascia, Left Foot
     See Q Subcutaneous Tissue and Fascia, Right Foot
	Ø Open
	 3 Percutaneous
	 X External
		Z No Device	**Z** No Qualifier

Non-OR   ØJN[Ø,1,4,5,6,7,8,9,B,C,D,F,G,H,J,K,L,M,N,P,Q,R]XZZ

NC Noncovered Procedure   **LC** Limited Coverage   **QA** Questionable OB Admit   **NT** New Tech Add-on   ⊞ Combination Member   ♂ Male   ♀ Female

ICD-10-PCS 2022   455

Subcutaneous Tissue and Fascia *(side tab)*

Ø   Medical and Surgical
J   Subcutaneous Tissue and Fascia
P   Removal   Definition: Taking out or off a device from a body part

Explanation: If a device is taken out and a similar device put in without cutting or puncturing the skin or mucous membrane, the procedure is coded to the root operation CHANGE. Otherwise, the procedure for taking out a device is coded to the root operation REMOVAL.

Body Part Character 4	Approach Character 5	Device Character 6	Qualifier Character 7
S Subcutaneous Tissue and Fascia, Head and Neck	**Ø** Open **3** Percutaneous	**Ø** Drainage Device **1** Radioactive Element **3** Infusion Device **7** Autologous Tissue Substitute **J** Synthetic Substitute **K** Nonautologous Tissue Substitute **N** Tissue Expander **Y** Other Device	**Z** No Qualifier
S Subcutaneous Tissue and Fascia, Head and Neck	**X** External	**Ø** Drainage Device **1** Radioactive Element **3** Infusion Device	**Z** No Qualifier
T Subcutaneous Tissue and Fascia, Trunk External oblique aponeurosis Transversalis fascia	**Ø** Open **3** Percutaneous	**Ø** Drainage Device **1** Radioactive Element **2** Monitoring Device **3** Infusion Device **7** Autologous Tissue Substitute **F** Subcutaneous Defibrillator Lead **H** Contraceptive Device **J** Synthetic Substitute **K** Nonautologous Tissue Substitute **M** Stimulator Generator **N** Tissue Expander **P** Cardiac Rhythm Related Device **V** Infusion Device, Pump **W** Vascular Access Device, Totally Implantable **X** Vascular Access Device, Tunneled **Y** Other Device	**Z** No Qualifier
T Subcutaneous Tissue and Fascia, Trunk External oblique aponeurosis Transversalis fascia	**X** External	**Ø** Drainage Device **1** Radioactive Element **2** Monitoring Device **3** Infusion Device **H** Contraceptive Device **V** Infusion Device, Pump **X** Vascular Access Device, Tunneled	**Z** No Qualifier
V Subcutaneous Tissue and Fascia, Upper Extremity **W** Subcutaneous Tissue and Fascia, Lower Extremity	**Ø** Open **3** Percutaneous	**Ø** Drainage Device **1** Radioactive Element **3** Infusion Device **7** Autologous Tissue Substitute **H** Contraceptive Device **J** Synthetic Substitute **K** Nonautologous Tissue Substitute **N** Tissue Expander **V** Infusion Device, Pump **W** Vascular Access Device, Totally Implantable **X** Vascular Access Device, Tunneled **Y** Other Device	**Z** No Qualifier
V Subcutaneous Tissue and Fascia, Upper Extremity **W** Subcutaneous Tissue and Fascia, Lower Extremity	**X** External	**Ø** Drainage Device **1** Radioactive Element **3** Infusion Device **H** Contraceptive Device **V** Infusion Device, Pump **X** Vascular Access Device, Tunneled	**Z** No Qualifier

Non-OR	ØJPS[Ø,3][Ø,1,3,7,J,K,N,Y]Z
Non-OR	ØJPSX[Ø,1,3]Z
Non-OR	ØJPT[Ø,3][Ø,1,2,3,7,H,J,K,M,N,V,W,X,Y]Z
Non-OR	ØJPTX[Ø,1,2,3,H,V,X]Z
Non-OR	ØJP[V,W][Ø,3][Ø,1,3,7,H,J,K,N,V,W,X,Y]Z
Non-OR	ØJP[V,W]X[Ø,1,3,H,V,X]Z
HAC	ØJPT[Ø,3][F,P]Z when reported with SDx K68.11 or T81.4Ø-T81.49, T82.6-T82.7 with 7th character A

Non-OR Procedure   DRG Non-OR Procedure   Valid OR Procedure   HAC Associated Procedure   Combination Only   New/Revised GREEN
456   ICD-10-PCS 2022

ØJP–ØJP *(side tab)*

Ø   **Medical and Surgical**
J   **Subcutaneous Tissue and Fascia**
Q   **Repair**   Definition: Restoring, to the extent possible, a body part to its normal anatomic structure and function
                     Explanation: Used only when the method to accomplish the repair is not one of the other root operations

Body Part Character 4		Approach Character 5	Device Character 6	Qualifier Character 7
Ø Subcutaneous Tissue and Fascia, Scalp Galea aponeurotica **1** Subcutaneous Tissue and Fascia, Face Masseteric fascia Orbital fascia Submandibular space **4** Subcutaneous Tissue and Fascia, Right Neck Deep cervical fascia Pretracheal fascia Prevertebral fascia **5** Subcutaneous Tissue and Fascia, Left Neck *See 4 Subcutaneous Tissue and Fascia, Right Neck* **6** Subcutaneous Tissue and Fascia, Chest Pectoral fascia **7** Subcutaneous Tissue and Fascia, Back **8** Subcutaneous Tissue and Fascia, Abdomen **9** Subcutaneous Tissue and Fascia, Buttock **B** Subcutaneous Tissue and Fascia, Perineum **C** Subcutaneous Tissue and Fascia, Pelvic Region **D** Subcutaneous Tissue and Fascia, Right Upper Arm Axillary fascia Deltoid fascia Infraspinatus fascia Subscapular aponeurosis Supraspinatus fascia **F** Subcutaneous Tissue and Fascia, Left Upper Arm *See D Subcutaneous Tissue and Fascia, Right Upper Arm*	**G** Subcutaneous Tissue and Fascia, Right Lower Arm Antebrachial fascia Bicipital aponeurosis **H** Subcutaneous Tissue and Fascia, Left Lower Arm *See G Subcutaneous Tissue and Fascia, Right Lower Arm* **J** Subcutaneous Tissue and Fascia, Right Hand Palmar fascia (aponeurosis) **K** Subcutaneous Tissue and Fascia, Left Hand *See J Subcutaneous Tissue and Fascia, Right Hand* **L** Subcutaneous Tissue and Fascia, Right Upper Leg Crural fascia Fascia lata Iliac fascia Iliotibial tract (band) **M** Subcutaneous Tissue and Fascia, Left Upper Leg *See L Subcutaneous Tissue and Fascia, Right Upper Leg* **N** Subcutaneous Tissue and Fascia, Right Lower Leg **P** Subcutaneous Tissue and Fascia, Left Lower Leg **Q** Subcutaneous Tissue and Fascia, Right Foot Plantar fascia (aponeurosis) **R** Subcutaneous Tissue and Fascia, Left Foot *See Q Subcutaneous Tissue and Fascia, Right Foot*	**Ø** Open **3** Percutaneous	**Z** No Device	**Z** No Qualifier

Non-OR   ØJQ[Ø,1,4,5,6,7,8,9,B,C,D,F,G,H,J,K,L,M,N,P,Q,R]3ZZ

Ø   **Medical and Surgical**
J   **Subcutaneous Tissue and Fascia**
R   **Replacement**   Definition: Putting in or on biological or synthetic material that physically takes the place and/or function of all or a portion of a body part
                        Explanation: The body part may have been taken out or replaced, or may be taken out, physically eradicated, or rendered nonfunctional during
                        the REPLACEMENT procedure. A REMOVAL procedure is coded for taking out the device used in a previous replacement procedure.

Body Part Character 4		Approach Character 5	Device Character 6	Qualifier Character 7
Ø **Subcutaneous Tissue and Fascia, Scalp** Galea aponeurotica **1** **Subcutaneous Tissue and Fascia, Face** Masseteric fascia Orbital fascia Submandibular space **4** **Subcutaneous Tissue and Fascia, Right Neck** Deep cervical fascia Pretracheal fascia Prevertebral fascia **5** **Subcutaneous Tissue and Fascia, Left Neck** *See* 4 *Subcutaneous Tissue and Fascia, Right Neck* **6** **Subcutaneous Tissue and Fascia, Chest** Pectoral fascia **7** **Subcutaneous Tissue and Fascia, Back** **8** **Subcutaneous Tissue and Fascia, Abdomen** **9** **Subcutaneous Tissue and Fascia, Buttock** **B** **Subcutaneous Tissue and Fascia, Perineum** **C** **Subcutaneous Tissue and Fascia, Pelvic Region** **D** **Subcutaneous Tissue and Fascia, Right Upper Arm** Axillary fascia Deltoid fascia Infraspinatus fascia Subscapular aponeurosis Supraspinatus fascia **F** **Subcutaneous Tissue and Fascia, Left Upper Arm** *See* D *Subcutaneous Tissue and Fascia, Right Upper Arm*	**G** **Subcutaneous Tissue and Fascia, Right Lower Arm** Antebrachial fascia Bicipital aponeurosis **H** **Subcutaneous Tissue and Fascia, Left Lower Arm** *See* G *Subcutaneous Tissue and Fascia, Right Lower Arm* **J** **Subcutaneous Tissue and Fascia, Right Hand** Palmar fascia (aponeurosis) **K** **Subcutaneous Tissue and Fascia, Left Hand** *See* J *Subcutaneous Tissue and Fascia, Right Hand* **L** **Subcutaneous Tissue and Fascia, Right Upper Leg** Crural fascia Fascia lata Iliac fascia Iliotibial tract (band) **M** **Subcutaneous Tissue and Fascia, Left Upper Leg** *See* L *Subcutaneous Tissue and Fascia, Right Upper Leg* **N** **Subcutaneous Tissue and Fascia, Right Lower Leg** **P** **Subcutaneous Tissue and Fascia, Left Lower Leg** **Q** **Subcutaneous Tissue and Fascia, Right Foot** Plantar fascia (aponeurosis) **R** **Subcutaneous Tissue and Fascia, Left Foot** *See* Q *Subcutaneous Tissue and Fascia, Right Foot*	**Ø** Open **3** Percutaneous	**7** Autologous Tissue Substitute **J** Synthetic Substitute **K** Nonautologous Tissue Substitute	**Z** No Qualifier

Ø   Medical and Surgical
J   Subcutaneous Tissue and Fascia
U   Supplement: Definition: Putting in or on biological or synthetic material that physically reinforces and/or augments the function of a portion of a body part

Explanation: The biological material is non-living, or is living and from the same individual. The body part may have been previously replaced, and the SUPPLEMENT procedure is performed to physically reinforce and/or augment the function of the replaced body part.

Body Part Character 4		Approach Character 5	Device Character 6	Qualifier Character 7
Ø **Subcutaneous Tissue and Fascia, Scalp** Galea aponeurotica **1** **Subcutaneous Tissue and Fascia, Face** Masseteric fascia Orbital fascia Submandibular space **4** **Subcutaneous Tissue and Fascia, Right Neck** Deep cervical fascia Pretracheal fascia Prevertebral fascia **5** **Subcutaneous Tissue and Fascia, Left Neck** *See* 4 Subcutaneous Tissue and *Fascia, Right Neck* **6** **Subcutaneous Tissue and Fascia, Chest** Pectoral fascia **7** **Subcutaneous Tissue and Fascia, Back** **8** **Subcutaneous Tissue and Fascia, Abdomen** **9** **Subcutaneous Tissue and Fascia, Buttock** **B** **Subcutaneous Tissue and Fascia, Perineum** **C** **Subcutaneous Tissue and Fascia, Pelvic Region** **D** **Subcutaneous Tissue and Fascia, Right Upper Arm** Axillary fascia Deltoid fascia Infraspinatus fascia Subscapular aponeurosis Supraspinatus fascia **F** **Subcutaneous Tissue and Fascia, Left Upper Arm** *See* D Subcutaneous Tissue and *Fascia, Right Upper Arm*	**G** **Subcutaneous Tissue and Fascia, Right Lower Arm** Antebrachial fascia Bicipital aponeurosis **H** **Subcutaneous Tissue and Fascia, Left Lower Arm** *See* G Subcutaneous Tissue and *Fascia, Right Lower Arm* **J** **Subcutaneous Tissue and Fascia, Right Hand** Palmar fascia (aponeurosis) **K** **Subcutaneous Tissue and Fascia, Left Hand** *See* J Subcutaneous Tissue and *Fascia, Right Hand* **L** **Subcutaneous Tissue and Fascia, Right Upper Leg** Crural fascia Fascia lata Iliac fascia Iliotibial tract (band) **M** **Subcutaneous Tissue and Fascia, Left Upper Leg** *See* L Subcutaneous Tissue and *Fascia, Right Upper Leg* **N** **Subcutaneous Tissue and Fascia, Right Lower Leg** **P** **Subcutaneous Tissue and Fascia, Left Lower Leg** **Q** **Subcutaneous Tissue and Fascia, Right Foot** Plantar fascia (aponeurosis) **R** **Subcutaneous Tissue and Fascia, Left Foot** *See* Q Subcutaneous Tissue and *Fascia, Right Foot*	**Ø** Open **3** Percutaneous	**7** Autologous Tissue Substitute **J** Synthetic Substitute **K** Nonautologous Tissue Substitute	**Z** No Qualifier

NC Noncovered Procedure   **LC** Limited Coverage   **QA** Questionable OB Admit   **NT** New Tech Add-on   ⊞ Combination Member   ♂ Male   ♀ Female

ICD-10-PCS 2022   459

Subcutaneous Tissue and Fascia *(side tab)*

Ø **Medical and Surgical**
J **Subcutaneous Tissue and Fascia**
W **Revision**

Definition: Correcting, to the extent possible, a portion of a malfunctioning device or the position of a displaced device

Explanation: Revision can include correcting a malfunctioning or displaced device by taking out or putting in components of the device such as a screw or pin

Body Part Character 4	Approach Character 5	Device Character 6	Qualifier Character 7
S Subcutaneous Tissue and Fascia, Head and Neck	**Ø** Open **3** Percutaneous	**Ø** Drainage Device **3** Infusion Device **7** Autologous Tissue Substitute **J** Synthetic Substitute **K** Nonautologous Tissue Substitute **N** Tissue Expander **Y** Other Device	**Z** No Qualifier
S Subcutaneous Tissue and Fascia, Head and Neck	**X** External	**Ø** Drainage Device **3** Infusion Device **7** Autologous Tissue Substitute **J** Synthetic Substitute **K** Nonautologous Tissue Substitute **N** Tissue Expander	**Z** No Qualifier
T Subcutaneous Tissue and Fascia, Trunk External oblique aponeurosis Transversalis fascia	**Ø** Open **3** Percutaneous	**Ø** Drainage Device **2** Monitoring Device **3** Infusion Device **7** Autologous Tissue Substitute **F** Subcutaneous Defibrillator Lead **H** Contraceptive Device **J** Synthetic Substitute **K** Nonautologous Tissue Substitute **M** Stimulator Generator **N** Tissue Expander **P** Cardiac Rhythm Related Device **V** Infusion Device, Pump **W** Vascular Access Device, Totally Implantable **X** Vascular Access Device, Tunneled **Y** Other Device	**Z** No Qualifier
T Subcutaneous Tissue and Fascia, Trunk External oblique aponeurosis Transversalis fascia	**X** External	**Ø** Drainage Device **2** Monitoring Device **3** Infusion Device **7** Autologous Tissue Substitute **F** Subcutaneous Defibrillator Lead **H** Contraceptive Device **J** Synthetic Substitute **K** Nonautologous Tissue Substitute **M** Stimulator Generator **N** Tissue Expander **P** Cardiac Rhythm Related Device **V** Infusion Device, Pump **W** Vascular Access Device, Totally Implantable **X** Vascular Access Device, Tunneled	**Z** No Qualifier
V Subcutaneous Tissue and Fascia, Upper Extremity **W** Subcutaneous Tissue and Fascia, Lower Extremity	**Ø** Open **3** Percutaneous	**Ø** Drainage Device **3** Infusion Device **7** Autologous Tissue Substitute **H** Contraceptive Device **J** Synthetic Substitute **K** Nonautologous Tissue Substitute **N** Tissue Expander **V** Infusion Device, Pump **W** Vascular Access Device, Totally Implantable **X** Vascular Access Device, Tunneled **Y** Other Device	**Z** No Qualifier
V Subcutaneous Tissue and Fascia, Upper Extremity **W** Subcutaneous Tissue and Fascia, Lower Extremity	**X** External	**Ø** Drainage Device **3** Infusion Device **7** Autologous Tissue Substitute **H** Contraceptive Device **J** Synthetic Substitute **K** Nonautologous Tissue Substitute **N** Tissue Expander **V** Infusion Device, Pump **W** Vascular Access Device, Totally Implantable **X** Vascular Access Device, Tunneled	**Z** No Qualifier

DRG Non-OR ØJWS[Ø,3][Ø,3,7,J,K,N,Y]Z
DRG Non-OR ØJWT[Ø,3][Ø,3,7,H,J,K,M,N,V,W,X]Z
DRG Non-OR ØJWTXMZ
DRG Non-OR ØJW[V,W][Ø,3][Ø,3,7,H,J,K,N,V,W,X,Y]Z
Non-OR ØJWSX[Ø,3,7,J,K,N]Z
Non-OR ØJWT3YZ
Non-OR ØJWTX[Ø,2,3,7,F,H,J,K,N,P,V,W,X]Z
Non-OR ØJW[V,W]X[Ø,3,7,H,J,K,N,V,W,X]Z

HAC ØJWT[Ø,3][F,P]Z when reported with SDx K68.11 or T81.40-T81.49, T82.6-T82.7 with 7th character A

Ø   Medical and Surgical
J   Subcutaneous Tissue and Fascia
X   Transfer   Definition: Moving, without taking out, all or a portion of a body part to another location to take over the function of all or a portion of a body part
                   Explanation: The body part transferred remains connected to its vascular and nervous supply

Body Part Character 4		Approach Character 5	Device Character 6	Qualifier Character 7

Ø **Subcutaneous Tissue and Fascia, Scalp**
  Galea aponeurotica
1 **Subcutaneous Tissue and Fascia, Face**
  Masseteric fascia
  Orbital fascia
  Submandibular space
4 **Subcutaneous Tissue and Fascia, Right Neck**
  Deep cervical fascia
  Pretracheal fascia
  Prevertebral fascia
5 **Subcutaneous Tissue and Fascia, Left Neck**
  See 4 *Subcutaneous Tissue and Fascia, Right Neck*
6 **Subcutaneous Tissue and Fascia, Chest**
  Pectoral fascia
7 **Subcutaneous Tissue and Fascia, Back**
8 **Subcutaneous Tissue and Fascia, Abdomen**
9 **Subcutaneous Tissue and Fascia, Buttock**
B **Subcutaneous Tissue and Fascia, Perineum**
C **Subcutaneous Tissue and Fascia, Pelvic Region**
D **Subcutaneous Tissue and Fascia, Right Upper Arm**
  Axillary fascia
  Deltoid fascia
  Infraspinatus fascia
  Subscapular aponeurosis
  Supraspinatus fascia
F **Subcutaneous Tissue and Fascia, Left Upper Arm**
  See D *Subcutaneous Tissue and Fascia, Right Upper Arm*
	G **Subcutaneous Tissue and Fascia, Right Lower Arm**
	  Antebrachial fascia
	  Bicipital aponeurosis
	H **Subcutaneous Tissue and Fascia, Left Lower Arm**
	  See G *Subcutaneous Tissue and Fascia, Right Lower Arm*
	J **Subcutaneous Tissue and Fascia, Right Hand**
	  Palmar fascia (aponeurosis)
	K **Subcutaneous Tissue and Fascia, Left Hand**
	  See J *Subcutaneous Tissue and Fascia, Right Hand*
	L **Subcutaneous Tissue and Fascia, Right Upper Leg**
	  Crural fascia
	  Fascia lata
	  Iliac fascia
	  Iliotibial tract (band)
	M **Subcutaneous Tissue and Fascia, Left Upper Leg**
	  See L *Subcutaneous Tissue and Fascia, Right Upper Leg*
	N **Subcutaneous Tissue and Fascia, Right Lower Leg**
	P **Subcutaneous Tissue and Fascia, Left Lower Leg**
	Q **Subcutaneous Tissue and Fascia, Right Foot**
	  Plantar fascia (aponeurosis)
	R **Subcutaneous Tissue and Fascia, Left Foot**
	  See Q *Subcutaneous Tissue and Fascia, Right Foot*
		Ø Open
		3 Percutaneous
			Z No Device	**B** Skin and Subcutaneous Tissue
				C Skin, Subcutaneous Tissue and Fascia
				Z No Qualifier

NC Noncovered Procedure   **LC** Limited Coverage   **QA** Questionable OB Admit   **NT** New Tech Add-on   ⊞ Combination Member   ♂ Male   ♀ Female

ICD-10-PCS 2022   461

Muscles ØK2–ØKX

Character Meanings

This Character Meaning table is provided as a guide to assist the user in the identification of character members that may be found in this section of code tables. It **SHOULD NOT** be used to build a PCS code.

Operation–Character 3	Body Part–Character 4	Approach–Character 5	Device–Character 6	Qualifier–Character 7
2 Change	Ø Head Muscle	Ø Open	Ø Drainage Device	Ø Skin
5 Destruction	1 Facial Muscle	3 Percutaneous	7 Autologous Tissue Substitute	1 Subcutaneous Tissue
8 Division	2 Neck Muscle, Right	4 Percutaneous Endoscopic	J Synthetic Substitute	2 Skin and Subcutaneous Tissue
9 Drainage	3 Neck Muscle, Left	7 Via Natural or Artificial Opening	K Nonautologous Tissue Substitute	5 Latissimus Dorsi Myocutaneous Flap
B Excision	4 Tongue, Palate, Pharynx Muscle	8 Via Natural or Artificial Opening Endoscopic	M Stimulator Lead	6 Transverse Rectus Abdominis Myocutaneous Flap
C Extirpation	5 Shoulder Muscle, Right	X External	Y Other Device	7 Deep Inferior Epigastric Artery Perforator Flap
D Extraction	6 Shoulder Muscle, Left		Z No Device	8 Superficial Inferior Epigastric Artery Flap
H Insertion	7 Upper Arm Muscle, Right			9 Gluteal Artery Perforator Flap
J Inspection	8 Upper Arm Muscle, Left			X Diagnostic
M Reattachment	9 Lower Arm and Wrist Muscle, Right			Z No Qualifier
N Release	B Lower Arm and Wrist Muscle, Left			
P Removal	C Hand Muscle, Right			
Q Repair	D Hand Muscle, Left			
R Replacement	F Trunk Muscle, Right			
S Reposition	G Trunk Muscle, Left			
T Resection	H Thorax Muscle, Right			
U Supplement	J Thorax Muscle, Left			
W Revision	K Abdomen Muscle, Right			
X Transfer	L Abdomen Muscle, Left			
	M Perineum Muscle			
	N Hip Muscle, Right			
	P Hip Muscle, Left			
	Q Upper Leg Muscle, Right			
	R Upper Leg Muscle, Left			
	S Lower Leg Muscle, Right			
	T Lower Leg Muscle, Left			
	V Foot Muscle, Right			
	W Foot Muscle, Left			
	X Upper Muscle			
	Y Lower Muscle			

AHA Coding Clinic for table ØK8
2020, 2Q, 25   Endoscopic Stapling of Zenker's Diverticulum

AHA Coding Clinic for table ØKB
2020, 1Q, 27   Delayed reconstruction following mastectomy using gracilis musculocutaneous free flap
2016, 3Q, 20   Excisional debridement of sacrum
2015, 3Q, 3-8   Excisional and nonexcisional debridement

AHA Coding Clinic for table ØKD
2017, 4Q, 41-42   Extraction procedures

AHA Coding Clinic for table ØKH
2020, 4Q, 63   Intercompartmental pressure measurement

AHA Coding Clinic for table ØKN
2017, 2Q, 12   Compartment syndrome and fasciotomy of foot
2017, 2Q, 13   Compartment syndrome and fasciotomy of leg
2015, 2Q, 22   Arthroscopic subacromial decompression
2014, 4Q, 39   Abdominal component release with placement of mesh for hernia repair

AHA Coding Clinic for table ØKQ
2018, 2Q, 25   Third and fourth degree obstetric lacerations
2016, 2Q, 34   Assisted vaginal delivery
2016, 1Q, 7   Obstetrical perineal laceration repair
2014, 4Q, 43   Second degree obstetric perineal laceration
2013, 4Q, 120   Repair of second degree perineum obstetric laceration

AHA Coding Clinic for table ØKS
2017, 1Q, 41   Manual reduction of hernia

AHA Coding Clinic for table ØKT
2016, 2Q, 12   Resection of malignant neoplasm of infratemporal fossa
2015, 1Q, 38   Abdominoperineal resection with flap closure of the perineum and colostomy

AHA Coding Clinic for table ØKX
2018, 2Q, 18   Transverse rectus abdominis myocutaneous (TRAM) delay
2017, 4Q, 67   New qualifier values - Pedicle flap procedures
2016, 3Q, 30   Resection of femur with interposition arthroplasty
2015, 3Q, 33   Cleft lip repair using Millard rotation advancement
2015, 2Q, 26   Pharyngeal flap to soft palate
2014, 4Q, 41   Abdominoperineal resection (APR) with flap closure of perineum and colostomy
2014, 2Q, 10   Transverse abdominomyocutaneous (TRAM) breast reconstruction
2014, 2Q, 12   Pedicle latissimus myocutaneous flap with placement of breast tissue expanders

Muscles

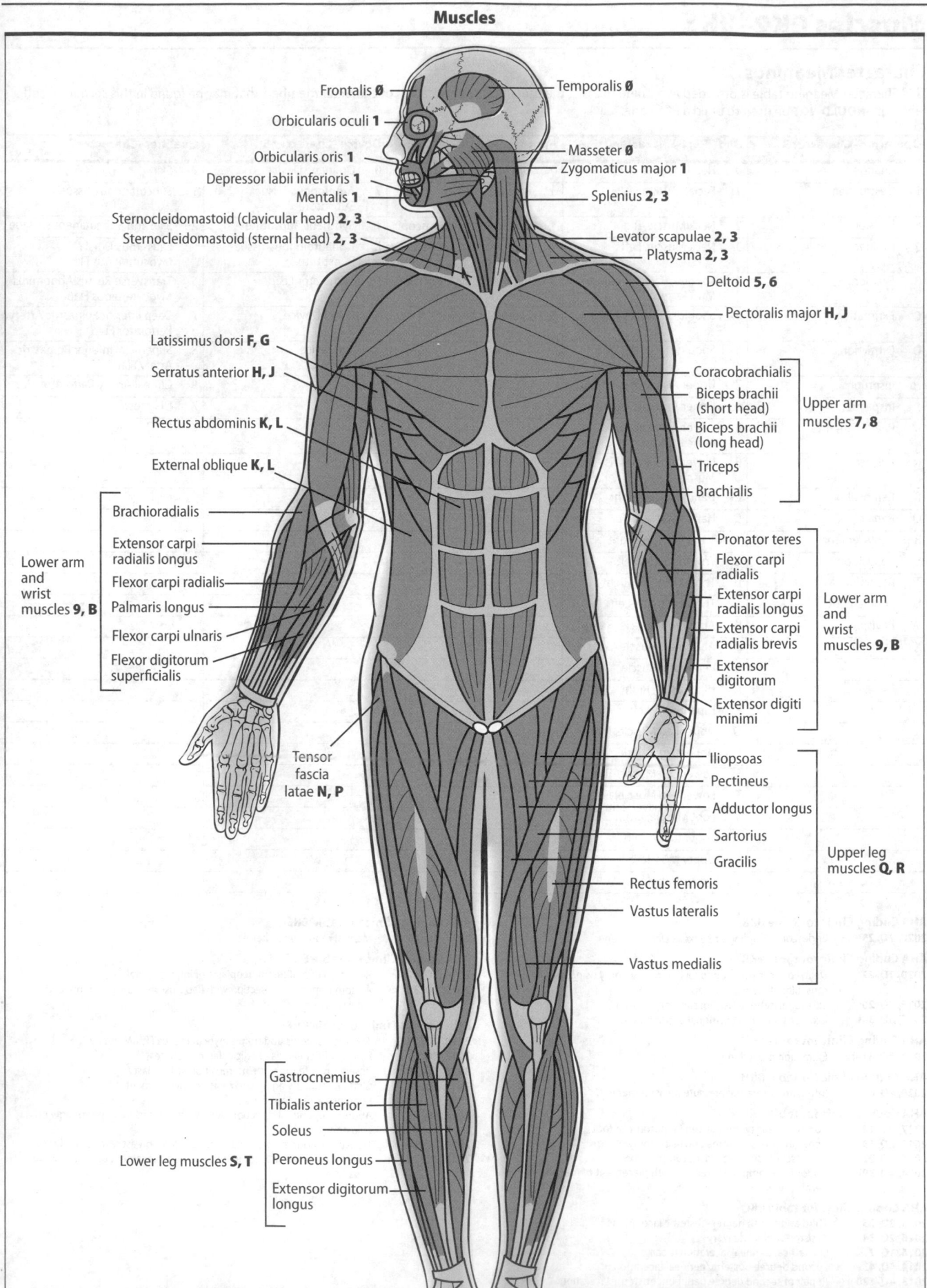

Frontalis **Ø**
Temporalis **Ø**
Orbicularis oculi **1**
Orbicularis oris **1**
Masseter **Ø**
Zygomaticus major **1**
Depressor labii inferioris **1**
Mentalis **1**
Splenius **2, 3**
Sternocleidomastoid (clavicular head) **2, 3**
Sternocleidomastoid (sternal head) **2, 3**
Levator scapulae **2, 3**
Platysma **2, 3**
Deltoid **5, 6**
Pectoralis major **H, J**
Latissimus dorsi **F, G**
Serratus anterior **H, J**
Coracobrachialis
Biceps brachii (short head)
Biceps brachii (long head)
Rectus abdominis **K, L**
External oblique **K, L**
Triceps
Brachialis
Upper arm muscles **7, 8**
Brachioradialis
Extensor carpi radialis longus
Flexor carpi radialis
Palmaris longus
Flexor carpi ulnaris
Flexor digitorum superficialis
Lower arm and wrist muscles **9, B**
Pronator teres
Flexor carpi radialis
Extensor carpi radialis longus
Extensor carpi radialis brevis
Extensor digitorum
Extensor digiti minimi
Lower arm and wrist muscles **9, B**
Tensor fascia latae **N, P**
Iliopsoas
Pectineus
Adductor longus
Sartorius
Gracilis
Rectus femoris
Vastus lateralis
Vastus medialis
Upper leg muscles **Q, R**
Gastrocnemius
Tibialis anterior
Soleus
Peroneus longus
Extensor digitorum longus
Lower leg muscles **S, T**

Ø   **Medical and Surgical**
K   **Muscles**
2   **Change**   Definition: Taking out or off a device from a body part and putting back an identical or similar device in or on the same body part without cutting or puncturing the skin or a mucous membrane
                Explanation: All CHANGE procedures are coded using the approach EXTERNAL

Body Part Character 4	Approach Character 5	Device Character 6	Qualifier Character 7
X Upper Muscle Y Lower Muscle	X External	Ø Drainage Device Y Other Device	Z No Qualifier

Non-OR   All body part, approach, device, and qualifier values

Ø   **Medical and Surgical**
K   **Muscles**
5   **Destruction**   Definition: Physical eradication of all or a portion of a body part by the direct use of energy, force, or a destructive agent
                      Explanation: None of the body part is physically taken out

Body Part Character 4			Approach Character 5	Device Character 6	Qualifier Character 7

Ø Head Muscle
   Auricularis muscle
   Masseter muscle
   Pterygoid muscle
   Splenius capitis muscle
   Temporalis muscle
   Temporoparietalis muscle
1 Facial Muscle
   Buccinator muscle
   Corrugator supercilii muscle
   Depressor anguli oris muscle
   Depressor labii inferioris muscle
   Depressor septi nasi muscle
   Depressor supercilii muscle
   Levator anguli oris muscle
   Levator labii superioris alaeque
      nasi muscle
   Levator labii superioris muscle
   Mentalis muscle
   Nasalis muscle
   Occipitofrontalis muscle
   Orbicularis oris muscle
   Procerus muscle
   Risorius muscle
   Zygomaticus muscle
2 Neck Muscle, Right
   Anterior vertebral muscle
   Arytenoid muscle
   Cricothyroid muscle
   Infrahyoid muscle
   Levator scapulae muscle
   Platysma muscle
   Scalene muscle
   Splenius cervicis muscle
   Sternocleidomastoid muscle
   Suprahyoid muscle
   Thyroarytenoid muscle
3 Neck Muscle, Left
   See 2 Neck Muscle, Right
4 Tongue, Palate, Pharynx
   Muscle
   Chondroglossus muscle
   Genioglossus muscle
   Hyoglossus muscle
   Inferior longitudinal muscle
   Levator veli palatini muscle
   Palatoglossal muscle
   Palatopharyngeal muscle
   Pharyngeal constrictor muscle
   Salpingopharyngeus muscle
   Styloglossus muscle
   Stylopharyngeus muscle
   Superior longitudinal muscle
   Tensor veli palatini muscle
5 Shoulder Muscle, Right
   Deltoid muscle
   Infraspinatus muscle
   Subscapularis muscle
   Supraspinatus muscle
   Teres major muscle
   Teres minor muscle
6 Shoulder Muscle, Left
   See 5 Shoulder Muscle, Right
	7 Upper Arm Muscle, Right
	   Biceps brachii muscle
	   Brachialis muscle
	   Coracobrachialis muscle
	   Triceps brachii muscle
	8 Upper Arm Muscle, Left
	   See 7 Upper Arm Muscle, Right
	9 Lower Arm and Wrist Muscle,
	   Right
	   Anatomical snuffbox
	   Brachioradialis muscle
	   Extensor carpi radialis muscle
	   Extensor carpi ulnaris muscle
	   Flexor carpi radialis muscle
	   Flexor carpi ulnaris muscle
	   Flexor pollicis longus muscle
	   Palmaris longus muscle
	   Pronator quadratus muscle
	   Pronator teres muscle
	B Lower Arm and Wrist Muscle,
	   Left
	   See 9 Lower Arm and Wrist
	      Muscle, Right
	C Hand Muscle, Right
	   Hypothenar muscle
	   Palmar interosseous muscle
	   Thenar muscle
	D Hand Muscle, Left
	   See C Hand Muscle, Right
	F Trunk Muscle, Right
	   Coccygeus muscle
	   Erector spinae muscle
	   Interspinalis muscle
	   Intertransversarius muscle
	   Latissimus dorsi muscle
	   Quadratus lumborum muscle
	   Rhomboid major muscle
	   Rhomboid minor muscle
	   Serratus posterior muscle
	   Transversospinalis muscle
	   Trapezius muscle
	G Trunk Muscle, Left
	   See F Trunk Muscle, Right
	H Thorax Muscle, Right
	   Intercostal muscle
	   Levatores costarum muscle
	   Pectoralis major muscle
	   Pectoralis minor muscle
	   Serratus anterior muscle
	   Subclavius muscle
	   Subcostal muscle
	   Transverse thoracis muscle
	J Thorax Muscle, Left
	   See H Thorax Muscle, Right
	K Abdomen Muscle, Right
	   External oblique muscle
	   Internal oblique muscle
	   Pyramidalis muscle
	   Rectus abdominis muscle
	   Transversus abdominis muscle
	L Abdomen Muscle, Left
	   See K Abdomen Muscle, Right
		M Perineum Muscle
		   Bulbospongiosus muscle
		   Cremaster muscle
		   Deep transverse perineal muscle
		   Ischiocavernosus muscle
		   Levator ani muscle
		   Superficial transverse perineal
		      muscle
		N Hip Muscle, Right
		   Gemellus muscle
		   Gluteus maximus muscle
		   Gluteus medius muscle
		   Gluteus minimus muscle
		   Iliacus muscle
		   Obturator muscle
		   Piriformis muscle
		   Psoas muscle
		   Quadratus femoris muscle
		   Tensor fasciae latae muscle
		P Hip Muscle, Left
		   See N Hip Muscle, Right
		Q Upper Leg Muscle, Right
		   Adductor brevis muscle
		   Adductor longus muscle
		   Adductor magnus muscle
		   Biceps femoris muscle
		   Gracilis muscle
		   Pectineus muscle
		   Quadriceps (femoris)
		   Rectus femoris muscle
		   Sartorius muscle
		   Semimembranosus muscle
		   Semitendinosus muscle
		   Vastus intermedius muscle
		   Vastus lateralis muscle
		   Vastus medialis muscle
		R Upper Leg Muscle, Left
		   See Q Upper Leg Muscle, Right
		S Lower Leg Muscle, Right
		   Extensor digitorum longus muscle
		   Extensor hallucis longus muscle
		   Fibularis brevis muscle
		   Fibularis longus muscle
		   Flexor digitorum longus muscle
		   Flexor hallucis longus muscle
		   Gastrocnemius muscle
		   Peroneus brevis muscle
		   Peroneus longus muscle
		   Popliteus muscle
		   Soleus muscle
		   Tibialis anterior muscle
		   Tibialis posterior muscle
		T Lower Leg Muscle, Left
		   See S Lower Leg Muscle, Right
		V Foot Muscle, Right
		   Abductor hallucis muscle
		   Adductor hallucis muscle
		   Extensor digitorum brevis muscle
		   Extensor hallucis brevis muscle
		   Flexor digitorum brevis muscle
		   Flexor hallucis brevis muscle
		   Quadratus plantae muscle
		W Foot Muscle, Left
		   See V Foot Muscle, Right
			Ø Open
			3 Percutaneous
			4 Percutaneous
			    Endoscopic
				Z No Device	Z No Qualifier

NC Noncovered Procedure   **LC** Limited Coverage   **QA** Questionable OB Admit   **NT** New Tech Add-on   ⊞ Combination Member   ♂ Male   ♀ Female

ICD-10-PCS 2022   465

ØK2–ØK5

Ø   Medical and Surgical
K   Muscles
8   Division

Definition: Cutting into a body part, without draining fluids and/or gases from the body part, in order to separate or transect a body part

Explanation: All or a portion of the body part is separated into two or more portions

Body Part Character 4			Approach Character 5	Device Character 6	Qualifier Character 7

Ø Head Muscle
Auricularis muscle
Masseter muscle
Pterygoid muscle
Splenius capitis muscle
Temporalis muscle
Temporoparietalis muscle
1 Facial Muscle
Buccinator muscle
Corrugator supercilii
  muscle
Depressor anguli oris
  muscle
Depressor labii inferioris
  muscle
Depressor septi nasi muscle
Depressor supercilii muscle
Levator anguli oris muscle
Levator labii superioris
  alaeque nasi muscle
Levator labii superioris
  muscle
Mentalis muscle
Nasalis muscle
Occipitofrontalis muscle
Orbicularis oris muscle
Procerus muscle
Risorius muscle
Zygomaticus muscle
2 Neck Muscle, Right
Anterior vertebral muscle
Arytenoid muscle
Cricothyroid muscle
Infrahyoid muscle
Levator scapulae muscle
Platysma muscle
Scalene muscle
Splenius cervicis muscle
Sternocleidomastoid
  muscle
Suprahyoid muscle
Thyroarytenoid muscle
3 Neck Muscle, Left
See 2 Neck Muscle, Right
Tensor veli palatini muscle
5 Shoulder Muscle, Right
Deltoid muscle
Infraspinatus muscle
Subscapularis muscle
Supraspinatus muscle
Teres major muscle
Teres minor muscle
6 Shoulder Muscle, Left
See 5 Shoulder Muscle, Right
7 Upper Arm Muscle, Right
Biceps brachii muscle
Brachialis muscle
Coracobrachialis muscle
Triceps brachii muscle
8 Upper Arm Muscle, Left
*See 7 Upper Arm Muscle,
  Right*
	**9 Lower Arm and Wrist Muscle,
	Right**
	Anatomical snuffbox
	Brachioradialis muscle
	Extensor carpi radialis muscle
	Extensor carpi ulnaris muscle
	Flexor carpi radialis muscle
	Flexor carpi ulnaris muscle
	Flexor pollicis longus muscle
	Palmaris longus muscle
	Pronator quadratus muscle
	Pronator teres muscle
	**B Lower Arm and Wrist Muscle,
	Left**
	*See 9 Lower Arm and Wrist
	  Muscle, Right*
	C Hand Muscle, Right
	Hypothenar muscle
	Palmar interosseous muscle
	Thenar muscle
	D Hand Muscle, Left
	See C Hand Muscle, Right
	F Trunk Muscle, Right
	Coccygeus muscle
	Erector spinae muscle
	Interspinalis muscle
	Intertransversarius muscle
	Latissimus dorsi muscle
	Quadratus lumborum muscle
	Rhomboid major muscle
	Rhomboid minor muscle
	Serratus posterior muscle
	Transversospinalis muscle
	Trapezius muscle
	G Trunk Muscle, Left
	See F Trunk Muscle, Right
	H Thorax Muscle, Right
	Intercostal muscle
	Levatores costarum muscle
	Pectoralis major muscle
	Pectoralis minor muscle
	Serratus anterior muscle
	Subclavius muscle
	Subcostal muscle
	Transverse thoracis muscle
	J Thorax Muscle, Left
	See H Thorax Muscle, Right
	K Abdomen Muscle, Right
	External oblique muscle
	Internal oblique muscle
	Pyramidalis muscle
	Rectus abdominis muscle
	Transversus abdominis muscle
	L Abdomen Muscle, Left
	See K Abdomen Muscle, Right
	M Perineum Muscle
	Bulbospongiosus muscle
	Cremaster muscle
	Deep transverse perineal muscle
	Ischiocavernosus muscle
	Levator ani muscle
	Superficial transverse perineal
	  muscle
		N Hip Muscle, Right
		Gemellus muscle
		Gluteus maximus muscle
		Gluteus medius muscle
		Gluteus minimus muscle
		Iliacus muscle
		Obturator muscle
		Piriformis muscle
		Psoas muscle
		Quadratus femoris muscle
		Tensor fasciae latae muscle
		P Hip Muscle, Left
		See N Hip Muscle, Right
		Q Upper Leg Muscle, Right
		Adductor brevis muscle
		Adductor longus muscle
		Adductor magnus muscle
		Biceps femoris muscle
		Gracilis muscle
		Pectineus muscle
		Quadriceps (femoris)
		Rectus femoris muscle
		Sartorius muscle
		Semimembranosus muscle
		Semitendinosus muscle
		Vastus intermedius muscle
		Vastus lateralis muscle
		Vastus medialis muscle
		R Upper Leg Muscle, Left
		See Q Upper Leg Muscle, Right
		S Lower Leg Muscle, Right
		Extensor digitorum longus
		  muscle
		Extensor hallucis longus
		  muscle
		Fibularis brevis muscle
		Fibularis longus muscle
		Flexor digitorum longus
		  muscle
		Flexor hallucis longus muscle
		Gastrocnemius muscle
		Peroneus brevis muscle
		Peroneus longus muscle
		Popliteus muscle
		Soleus muscle
		Tibialis anterior muscle
		Tibialis posterior muscle
		T Lower Leg Muscle, Left
		See S Lower Leg Muscle, Right
		V Foot Muscle, Right
		Abductor hallucis muscle
		Adductor hallucis muscle
		Extensor digitorum brevis
		  muscle
		Extensor hallucis brevis
		  muscle
		Flexor digitorum brevis
		  muscle
		Flexor hallucis brevis muscle
		Quadratus plantae muscle
		W Foot Muscle, Left
		See V Foot Muscle, Right
			Ø Open
			3 Percutaneous
			4 Percutaneous
			  Endoscopic
				Z No Device	**Z** No Qualifier

4 Tongue, Palate, Pharynx Muscle
Chondroglossus muscle
Genioglossus muscle
Hyoglossus muscle
Inferior longitudinal muscle
Levator veli palatini muscle
Palatoglossal muscle
Palatopharyngeal muscle
Pharyngeal constrictor muscle
Salpingopharyngeus muscle
Styloglossus muscle
Stylopharyngeus muscle
Superior longitudinal muscle
Tensor veli palatini muscle
			Ø Open
			3 Percutaneous
			4 Percutaneous
			  Endoscopic
			7 Via Natural or
			  Artificial Opening
			8 Via Natural or
			  Artificial Opening
			  Endoscopic
				Z No Device	**Z** No Qualifier

Ø **Medical and Surgical**
K **Muscles**
9 **Drainage** 　　Definition: Taking or letting out fluids and/or gases from a body part
　　　　　　　　　　　Explanation: The qualifier DIAGNOSTIC is used to identify drainage procedures that are biopsies

Body Part Character 4		Approach Character 5	Device Character 6	Qualifier Character 7
Ø **Head Muscle** Auricularis muscle Masseter muscle Pterygoid muscle Splenius capitis muscle Temporalis muscle Temporoparietalis muscle **1** **Facial Muscle** Buccinator muscle Corrugator supercilii muscle Depressor anguli oris muscle Depressor labii inferioris muscle Depressor septi nasi muscle Depressor supercilii muscle Levator anguli oris muscle Levator labii superioris alaeque nasi muscle Levator labii superioris muscle Mentalis muscle Nasalis muscle Occipitofrontalis muscle Orbicularis oris muscle Procerus muscle Risorius muscle Zygomaticus muscle **2** **Neck Muscle, Right** Anterior vertebral muscle Arytenoid muscle Cricothyroid muscle Infrahyoid muscle Levator scapulae muscle Platysma muscle Scalene muscle Splenius cervicis muscle Sternocleidomastoid muscle Suprahyoid muscle Thyroarytenoid muscle **3** **Neck Muscle, Left** *See 2 Neck Muscle, Right* **4** **Tongue, Palate, Pharynx Muscle** Chondroglossus muscle Genioglossus muscle Hyoglossus muscle Inferior longitudinal muscle Levator veli palatini muscle Palatoglossal muscle Palatopharyngeal muscle Pharyngeal constrictor muscle Salpingopharyngeus muscle Styloglossus muscle Stylopharyngeus muscle Superior longitudinal muscle Tensor veli palatini muscle **5** **Shoulder Muscle, Right** Deltoid muscle Infraspinatus muscle Subscapularis muscle Supraspinatus muscle Teres major muscle Teres minor muscle **6** **Shoulder Muscle, Left** *See 5 Shoulder Muscle, Right*	**7** **Upper Arm Muscle, Right** Biceps brachii muscle Brachialis muscle Coracobrachialis muscle Triceps brachii muscle **8** **Upper Arm Muscle, Left** *See 7 Upper Arm Muscle, Right* **9** **Lower Arm and Wrist Muscle, Right** Anatomical snuffbox Brachioradialis muscle Extensor carpi radialis muscle Extensor carpi ulnaris muscle Flexor carpi radialis muscle Flexor carpi ulnaris muscle Flexor pollicis longus muscle Palmaris longus muscle Pronator quadratus muscle Pronator teres muscle **B** **Lower Arm and Wrist Muscle, Left** *See 9 Lower Arm and Wrist Muscle, Right* **C** **Hand Muscle, Right** Hypothenar muscle Palmar interosseous muscle Thenar muscle **D** **Hand Muscle, Left** *See C Hand Muscle, Right* **F** **Trunk Muscle, Right** Coccygeus muscle Erector spinae muscle Interspinalis muscle Intertransversarius muscle Latissimus dorsi muscle Quadratus lumborum muscle Rhomboid major muscle Rhomboid minor muscle Serratus posterior muscle Transversospinalis muscle Trapezius muscle **G** **Trunk Muscle, Left** *See F Trunk Muscle, Right* **H** **Thorax Muscle, Right** Intercostal muscle Levatores costarum muscle Pectoralis major muscle Pectoralis minor muscle Serratus anterior muscle Subclavius muscle Subcostal muscle Transverse thoracis muscle **J** **Thorax Muscle, Left** *See H Thorax Muscle, Right* **K** **Abdomen Muscle, Right** External oblique muscle Internal oblique muscle Pyramidalis muscle Rectus abdominis muscle Transversus abdominis muscle **L** **Abdomen Muscle, Left** *See K Abdomen Muscle, Right*	**M** **Perineum Muscle** Bulbospongiosus muscle Cremaster muscle Deep transverse perineal muscle Ischiocavernosus muscle Levator ani muscle Superficial transverse perineal muscle **N** **Hip Muscle, Right** Gemellus muscle Gluteus maximus muscle Gluteus medius muscle Gluteus minimus muscle Iliacus muscle Obturator muscle Piriformis muscle Psoas muscle Quadratus femoris muscle Tensor fasciae latae muscle **P** **Hip Muscle, Left** *See N Hip Muscle, Right* **Q** **Upper Leg Muscle, Right** Adductor brevis muscle Adductor longus muscle Adductor magnus muscle Biceps femoris muscle Gracilis muscle Pectineus muscle Quadriceps (femoris) Rectus femoris muscle Sartorius muscle Semimembranosus muscle Semitendinosus muscle Vastus intermedius muscle Vastus lateralis muscle Vastus medialis muscle **R** **Upper Leg Muscle, Left** *See Q Upper Leg Muscle, Right* **S** **Lower Leg Muscle, Right** Extensor digitorum longus muscle Extensor hallucis longus muscle Fibularis brevis muscle Fibularis longus muscle Flexor digitorum longus muscle Flexor hallucis longus muscle Gastrocnemius muscle Peroneus brevis muscle Peroneus longus muscle Popliteus muscle Soleus muscle Tibialis anterior muscle Tibialis posterior muscle **T** **Lower Leg Muscle, Left** *See S Lower Leg Muscle, Right* **V** **Foot Muscle, Right** Abductor hallucis muscle Adductor hallucis muscle Extensor digitorum brevis muscle Extensor hallucis brevis muscle Flexor digitorum brevis muscle Flexor hallucis brevis muscle Quadratus plantae muscle **W** **Foot Muscle, Left** *See V Foot Muscle, Right*	**Ø** Open **3** Percutaneous **4** Percutaneous Endoscopic	**Ø** Drainage Device	**Z** No Qualifier

Non-OR　ØK9[Ø,1,2,3,4,5,6,7,8,9,B,C,D,F,G,H,J,K,L,M,N,P,Q,R,S,T,V,W]3ØZ

ØK9 Continued on next page

NC Noncovered Procedure　　**LC** Limited Coverage　　**QA** Questionable OB Admit　　**NT** New Tech Add-on　　✚ Combination Member　　♂ Male　　♀ Female

Ø	**Medical and Surgical**
K	**Muscles**
9	**Drainage**

ØK9 Continued

Definition: Taking or letting out fluids and/or gases from a body part
Explanation: The qualifier DIAGNOSTIC is used to identify drainage procedures that are biopsies

Body Part Character 4	Approach Character 5	Device Character 6	Qualifier Character 7
Ø Head Muscle Auricularis muscle Masseter muscle Pterygoid muscle Splenius capitis muscle Temporalis muscle Temporoparietalis muscle **1 Facial Muscle** Buccinator muscle Corrugator supercilii muscle Depressor anguli oris muscle Depressor labii inferioris muscle Depressor septi nasi muscle Depressor supercilii muscle Levator anguli oris muscle Levator labii superioris alaeque nasi muscle Levator labii superioris muscle Mentalis muscle Nasalis muscle Occipitofrontalis muscle Orbicularis oris muscle Procerus muscle Risorius muscle Zygomaticus muscle **2 Neck Muscle, Right** Anterior vertebral muscle Arytenoid muscle Cricothyroid muscle Infrahyoid muscle Levator scapulae muscle Platysma muscle Scalene muscle Splenius cervicis muscle Sternocleidomastoid muscle Suprahyoid muscle Thyroarytenoid muscle **3 Neck Muscle, Left** *See 2 Neck Muscle, Right* **4 Tongue, Palate, Pharynx Muscle** Chondroglossus muscle Genioglossus muscle Hyoglossus muscle Inferior longitudinal muscle Levator veli palatini muscle Palatoglossal muscle Palatopharyngeal muscle Pharyngeal constrictor muscle Salpingopharyngeus muscle Styloglossus muscle Stylopharyngeus muscle Superior longitudinal muscle Tensor veli palatini muscle **5 Shoulder Muscle, Right** Deltoid muscle Infraspinatus muscle Subscapularis muscle Supraspinatus muscle Teres major muscle Teres minor muscle **6 Shoulder Muscle, Left** *See 5 Shoulder Muscle, Right* **7 Upper Arm Muscle, Right** Biceps brachii muscle Brachialis muscle Coracobrachialis muscle Triceps brachii muscle **8 Upper Arm Muscle, Left** *See 7 Upper Arm Muscle, Right* **9 Lower Arm and Wrist Muscle, Right** Anatomical snuffbox Brachioradialis muscle Extensor carpi radialis muscle Extensor carpi ulnaris muscle Flexor carpi radialis muscle Flexor carpi ulnaris muscle Flexor pollicis longus muscle Palmaris longus muscle Pronator quadratus muscle Pronator teres muscle **B Lower Arm and Wrist Muscle, Left** *See 9 Lower Arm and Wrist Muscle, Right* **C Hand Muscle, Right** Hypothenar muscle Palmar interosseous muscle Thenar muscle **D Hand Muscle, Left** *See C Hand Muscle, Right* **F Trunk Muscle, Right** Coccygeus muscle Erector spinae muscle Interspinalis muscle Intertransversarius muscle Latissimus dorsi muscle Quadratus lumborum muscle Rhomboid major muscle Rhomboid minor muscle Serratus posterior muscle Transversospinalis muscle Trapezius muscle **G Trunk Muscle, Left** *See F Trunk Muscle, Right* **H Thorax Muscle, Right** Intercostal muscle Levatores costarum muscle Pectoralis major muscle Pectoralis minor muscle Serratus anterior muscle Subclavius muscle Subcostal muscle Transverse thoracis muscle **J Thorax Muscle, Left** *See H Thorax Muscle, Right* **K Abdomen Muscle, Right** External oblique muscle Internal oblique muscle Pyramidalis muscle Rectus abdominis muscle Transversus abdominis muscle **L Abdomen Muscle, Left** *See K Abdomen Muscle, Right* **M Perineum Muscle** Bulbospongiosus muscle Cremaster muscle Deep transverse perineal muscle Ischiocavernosus muscle Levator ani muscle Superficial transverse perineal muscle **N Hip Muscle, Right** Gemellus muscle Gluteus maximus muscle Gluteus medius muscle Gluteus minimus muscle Iliacus muscle Obturator muscle Piriformis muscle Psoas muscle Quadratus femoris muscle Tensor fasciae latae muscle **P Hip Muscle, Left** *See N Hip Muscle, Right* **Q Upper Leg Muscle, Right** Adductor brevis muscle Adductor longus muscle Adductor magnus muscle Biceps femoris muscle Gracilis muscle Pectineus muscle Quadriceps (femoris) Rectus femoris muscle Sartorius muscle Semimembranosus muscle Semitendinosus muscle Vastus intermedius muscle Vastus lateralis muscle Vastus medialis muscle **R Upper Leg Muscle, Left** *See Q Upper Leg Muscle, Right* **S Lower Leg Muscle, Right** Extensor digitorum longus muscle Extensor hallucis longus muscle Fibularis brevis muscle Fibularis longus muscle Flexor digitorum longus muscle Flexor hallucis longus muscle Gastrocnemius muscle Peroneus brevis muscle Peroneus longus muscle Popliteus muscle Soleus muscle Tibialis anterior muscle Tibialis posterior muscle **T Lower Leg Muscle, Left** *See S Lower Leg Muscle, Right* **V Foot Muscle, Right** Abductor hallucis muscle Adductor hallucis muscle Extensor digitorum brevis muscle Extensor hallucis brevis muscle Flexor digitorum brevis muscle Flexor hallucis brevis muscle Quadratus plantae muscle **W Foot Muscle, Left** *See V Foot Muscle, Right*	**Ø** Open **3** Percutaneous **4** Percutaneous Endoscopic	**Z** No Device	**X** Diagnostic **Z** No Qualifier

Non-OR ØK9[Ø,1,2,3,4,5,6,7,8,9,B,F,G,H,J,K,L,M,N,P,Q,R,S,T,V,W]3ZZ
Non-OR ØK9[C,D][3,4]ZZ

Ø Medical and Surgical
K Muscles
B Excision   Definition: Cutting out or off, without replacement, a portion of a body part
                    Explanation: The qualifier DIAGNOSTIC is used to identify excision procedures that are biopsies

Body Part Character 4		Approach Character 5	Device Character 6	Qualifier Character 7
Ø Head Muscle	**7 Upper Arm Muscle, Right**	**Ø Open**	**Z No Device**	**X Diagnostic**
Auricularis muscle	Biceps brachii muscle	**3 Percutaneous**		**Z No Qualifier**
Masseter muscle	Brachialis muscle	**4 Percutaneous Endoscopic**		
Pterygoid muscle	Coracobrachialis muscle			
Splenius capitis muscle	Triceps brachii muscle			
Temporalis muscle	**8 Upper Arm Muscle, Left**			
Temporoparietalis muscle	*See 7 Upper Arm Muscle, Right*			
1 Facial Muscle	**9 Lower Arm and Wrist Muscle, Right**			
Buccinator muscle	Anatomical snuffbox			
Corrugator supercilii muscle	Brachioradialis muscle			
Depressor anguli oris muscle	Extensor carpi radialis muscle			
Depressor labii inferioris muscle	Extensor carpi ulnaris muscle			
Depressor septi nasi muscle	Flexor carpi radialis muscle			
Depressor supercilii muscle	Flexor carpi ulnaris muscle			
Levator anguli oris muscle	Flexor pollicis longus muscle			
Levator labii superioris alaeque nasi muscle	Palmaris longus muscle			
Levator labii superioris muscle	Pronator quadratus muscle			
Mentalis muscle	Pronator teres muscle			
Nasalis muscle	**B Lower Arm and Wrist Muscle, Left**			
Occipitofrontalis muscle	*See 9 Lower Arm and Wrist Muscle, Right*			
Orbicularis oris muscle	**C Hand Muscle, Right**			
Procerus muscle	Hypothenar muscle			
Risorius muscle	Palmar interosseous muscle			
Zygomaticus muscle	Thenar muscle			
2 Neck Muscle, Right	**D Hand Muscle, Left**			
Anterior vertebral muscle	*See C Hand Muscle, Right*			
Arytenoid muscle	**F Trunk Muscle, Right**			
Cricothyroid muscle	Coccygeus muscle			
Infrahyoid muscle	Erector spinae muscle			
Levator scapulae muscle	Interspinalis muscle			
Platysma muscle	Intertransversarius muscle			
Scalene muscle	Latissimus dorsi muscle			
Splenius cervicis muscle	Quadratus lumborum muscle			
Sternocleidomastoid muscle	Rhomboid major muscle			
Suprahyoid muscle	Rhomboid minor muscle			
Thyroarytenoid muscle	Serratus posterior muscle			
3 Neck Muscle, Left	Transversospinalis muscle			
See 2 Neck Muscle, Right	Trapezius muscle			
4 Tongue, Palate, Pharynx Muscle	**G Trunk Muscle, Left**			
Chondroglossus muscle	*See F Trunk Muscle, Right*			
Genioglossus muscle	**H Thorax Muscle, Right**			
Hyoglossus muscle	Intercostal muscle			
Inferior longitudinal muscle	Levatores costarum muscle			
Levator veli palatini muscle	Pectoralis major muscle			
Palatoglossal muscle	Pectoralis minor muscle			
Palatopharyngeal muscle	Serratus anterior muscle			
Pharyngeal constrictor muscle	Subclavius muscle			
Salpingopharyngeus muscle	Subcostal muscle			
Styloglossus muscle	Transverse thoracis muscle			
Stylopharyngeus muscle	**J Thorax Muscle, Left**			
Superior longitudinal muscle	*See H Thorax Muscle, Right*			
Tensor veli palatini muscle	**K Abdomen Muscle, Right**			
5 Shoulder Muscle, Right	External oblique muscle			
Deltoid muscle	Internal oblique muscle			
Infraspinatus muscle	Pyramidalis muscle			
Subscapularis muscle	Rectus abdominis muscle			
Supraspinatus muscle	Transversus abdominis muscle			
Teres major muscle	**L Abdomen Muscle, Left**			
Teres minor muscle	*See K Abdomen Muscle, Right*			
6 Shoulder Muscle, Left				
See 5 Shoulder Muscle, Right				

M Perineum Muscle
Bulbospongiosus muscle
Cremaster muscle
Deep transverse perineal muscle
Ischiocavernosus muscle
Levator ani muscle
Superficial transverse perineal muscle

N Hip Muscle, Right
Gemellus muscle
Gluteus maximus muscle
Gluteus medius muscle
Gluteus minimus muscle
Iliacus muscle
Obturator muscle
Piriformis muscle
Psoas muscle
Quadratus femoris muscle
Tensor fasciae latae muscle

P Hip Muscle, Left
See N Hip Muscle, Right

Q Upper Leg Muscle, Right
Adductor brevis muscle
Adductor longus muscle
Adductor magnus muscle
Biceps femoris muscle
Gracilis muscle
Pectineus muscle
Quadriceps (femoris)
Rectus femoris muscle
Sartorius muscle
Semimembranosus muscle
Semitendinosus muscle
Vastus intermedius muscle
Vastus lateralis muscle
Vastus medialis muscle

R Upper Leg Muscle, Left
See Q Upper Leg Muscle, Right

S Lower Leg Muscle, Right
Extensor digitorum longus muscle
Extensor hallucis longus muscle
Fibularis brevis muscle
Fibularis longus muscle
Flexor digitorum longus muscle
Flexor hallucis longus muscle
Gastrocnemius muscle
Peroneus brevis muscle
Peroneus longus muscle
Popliteus muscle
Soleus muscle
Tibialis anterior muscle
Tibialis posterior muscle

T Lower Leg Muscle, Left
See S Lower Leg Muscle, Right

V Foot Muscle, Right
Abductor hallucis muscle
Adductor hallucis muscle
Extensor digitorum brevis muscle
Extensor hallucis brevis muscle
Flexor digitorum brevis muscle
Flexor hallucis brevis muscle
Quadratus plantae muscle

W Foot Muscle, Left
See V Foot Muscle, Right

Ø   **Medical and Surgical**
K   **Muscles**
C   **Extirpation**   Definition: Taking or cutting out solid matter from a body part

Explanation: The solid matter may be an abnormal byproduct of a biological function or a foreign body; it may be imbedded in a body part or in the lumen of a tubular body part. The solid matter may or may not have been previously broken into pieces.

Body Part Character 4			Approach Character 5	Device Character 6	Qualifier Character 7

Ø **Head Muscle**
 Auricularis muscle
 Masseter muscle
 Pterygoid muscle
 Splenius capitis muscle
 Temporalis muscle
 Temporoparietalis muscle
1 **Facial Muscle**
 Buccinator muscle
 Corrugator supercilii
  muscle
 Depressor anguli oris
  muscle
 Depressor labii inferioris
  muscle
 Depressor septi nasi
  muscle
 Depressor supercilii
  muscle
 Levator anguli oris muscle
 Levator labii superioris
  alaeque nasi muscle
 Levator labii superioris
  muscle
 Mentalis muscle
 Nasalis muscle
 Occipitofrontalis muscle
 Orbicularis oris muscle
 Procerus muscle
 Risorius muscle
 Zygomaticus muscle
2 **Neck Muscle, Right**
 Anterior vertebral muscle
 Arytenoid muscle
 Cricothyroid muscle
 Infrahyoid muscle
 Levator scapulae muscle
 Platysma muscle
 Scalene muscle
 Splenius cervicis muscle
 Sternocleidomastoid
  muscle
 Suprahyoid muscle
 Thyroarytenoid muscle
3 **Neck Muscle, Left**
 See 2 Neck Muscle, Right
4 **Tongue, Palate, Pharynx**
 Muscle
 Chondroglossus muscle
 Genioglossus muscle
 Hyoglossus muscle
 Inferior longitudinal
  muscle
 Levator veli palatini
  muscle
 Palatoglossal muscle
 Palatopharyngeal muscle
 Pharyngeal constrictor
  muscle
 Salpingopharyngeus
  muscle
 Styloglossus muscle
 Stylopharyngeus muscle
 Superior longitudinal
  muscle
 Tensor veli palatini muscle
5 **Shoulder Muscle, Right**
 Deltoid muscle
 Infraspinatus muscle
 Subscapularis muscle
 Supraspinatus muscle
 Teres major muscle
 Teres minor muscle
6 **Shoulder Muscle, Left**
 See 5 Shoulder Muscle,
  Right
	7 **Upper Arm Muscle, Right**
	 Biceps brachii muscle
	 Brachialis muscle
	 Coracobrachialis muscle
	 Triceps brachii muscle
	8 **Upper Arm Muscle, Left**
	 See 7 Upper Arm Muscle,
	  Right
	9 **Lower Arm and Wrist**
	 Muscle, Right
	 Anatomical snuffbox
	 Brachioradialis muscle
	 Extensor carpi radialis
	  muscle
	 Extensor carpi ulnaris
	  muscle
	 Flexor carpi radialis
	  muscle
	 Flexor carpi ulnaris muscle
	 Flexor pollicis longus
	  muscle
	 Palmaris longus muscle
	 Pronator quadratus
	  muscle
	 Pronator teres muscle
	B **Lower Arm and Wrist**
	 Muscle, Left
	 See 9 Lower Arm and Wrist
	  Muscle, Right
	C **Hand Muscle, Right**
	 Hypothenar muscle
	 Palmar interosseous
	  muscle
	 Thenar muscle
	D **Hand Muscle, Left**
	 See C Hand Muscle, Right
	F **Trunk Muscle, Right**
	 Coccygeus muscle
	 Erector spinae muscle
	 Interspinalis muscle
	 Intertransversarius muscle
	 Latissimus dorsi muscle
	 Quadratus lumborum
	  muscle
	 Rhomboid major muscle
	 Rhomboid minor muscle
	 Serratus posterior muscle
	 Transversospinalis muscle
	 Trapezius muscle
	G **Trunk Muscle, Left**
	 See F Trunk Muscle, Right
	H **Thorax Muscle, Right**
	 Intercostal muscle
	 Levatores costarum
	  muscle
	 Pectoralis major muscle
	 Pectoralis minor muscle
	 Serratus anterior muscle
	 Subclavius muscle
	 Subcostal muscle
	 Transverse thoracis
	  muscle
	J **Thorax Muscle, Left**
	 See H Thorax Muscle, Right
	K **Abdomen Muscle, Right**
	 External oblique muscle
	 Internal oblique muscle
	 Pyramidalis muscle
	 Rectus abdominis muscle
	 Transversus abdominis
	  muscle
	L **Abdomen Muscle, Left**
	 See K Abdomen Muscle,
	  Right
		M **Perineum Muscle**
		 Bulbospongiosus muscle
		 Cremaster muscle
		 Deep transverse perineal
		  muscle
		 Ischiocavernosus muscle
		 Levator ani muscle
		 Superficial transverse
		  perineal muscle
		N **Hip Muscle, Right**
		 Gemellus muscle
		 Gluteus maximus muscle
		 Gluteus medius muscle
		 Gluteus minimus muscle
		 Iliacus muscle
		 Obturator muscle
		 Piriformis muscle
		 Psoas muscle
		 Quadratus femoris muscle
		 Tensor fasciae latae
		  muscle
		P **Hip Muscle, Left**
		 See N Hip Muscle, Right
		Q **Upper Leg Muscle, Right**
		 Adductor brevis muscle
		 Adductor longus muscle
		 Adductor magnus muscle
		 Biceps femoris muscle
		 Gracilis muscle
		 Pectineus muscle
		 Quadriceps (femoris)
		 Rectus femoris muscle
		 Sartorius muscle
		 Semimembranosus
		  muscle
		 Semitendinosus muscle
		 Vastus intermedius muscle
		 Vastus lateralis muscle
		 Vastus medialis muscle
		R **Upper Leg Muscle, Left**
		 See Q Upper Leg Muscle,
		  Right
		S **Lower Leg Muscle, Right**
		 Extensor digitorum longus
		  muscle
		 Extensor hallucis longus
		  muscle
		 Fibularis brevis muscle
		 Fibularis longus muscle
		 Flexor digitorum longus
		  muscle
		 Flexor hallucis longus
		  muscle
		 Gastrocnemius muscle
		 Peroneus brevis muscle
		 Peroneus longus muscle
		 Popliteus muscle
		 Soleus muscle
		 Tibialis anterior muscle
		 Tibialis posterior muscle
		T **Lower Leg Muscle, Left**
		 See S Lower Leg Muscle,
		  Right
		V **Foot Muscle, Right**
		 Abductor hallucis muscle
		 Adductor hallucis muscle
		 Extensor digitorum brevis
		  muscle
		 Extensor hallucis brevis
		  muscle
		 Flexor digitorum brevis
		  muscle
		 Flexor hallucis brevis
		  muscle
		 Quadratus plantae muscle
		W **Foot Muscle, Left**
		 See V Foot Muscle, Right
			Ø **Open**
			3 **Percutaneous**
			4 **Percutaneous**
			 Endoscopic
				Z **No Device**	Z **No Qualifier**

Ø　Medical and Surgical
K　Muscles
D　Extraction　　Definition: Pulling or stripping out or off all or a portion of a body part by the use of force
　　　　　　　　　　Explanation: The qualifier DIAGNOSTIC is used to identify extraction procedures that are biopsies

Body Part Character 4			Approach Character 5	Device Character 6	Qualifier Character 7
Ø Head Muscle Auricularis muscle Masseter muscle Pterygoid muscle Splenius capitis muscle Temporalis muscle Temporoparietalis muscle **1 Facial Muscle** Buccinator muscle Corrugator supercilii muscle Depressor anguli oris muscle Depressor labii inferioris muscle Depressor septi nasi muscle Depressor supercilii muscle Levator anguli oris muscle Levator labii superioris alaeque nasi muscle Levator labii superioris muscle Mentalis muscle Nasalis muscle Occipitofrontalis muscle Orbicularis oris muscle Procerus muscle Risorius muscle Zygomaticus muscle **2 Neck Muscle, Right** Anterior vertebral muscle Arytenoid muscle Cricothyroid muscle Infrahyoid muscle Levator scapulae muscle Platysma muscle Scalene muscle Splenius cervicis muscle Sternocleidomastoid muscle Suprahyoid muscle Thyroarytenoid muscle **3 Neck Muscle, Left** *See 2 Neck Muscle, Right* **4 Tongue, Palate, Pharynx Muscle** Chondroglossus muscle Genioglossus muscle Hyoglossus muscle Inferior longitudinal muscle Levator veli palatini muscle Palatoglossal muscle Palatopharyngeal muscle Pharyngeal constrictor muscle Salpingopharyngeus muscle Styloglossus muscle Stylopharyngeus muscle Superior longitudinal muscle Tensor veli palatini muscle **5 Shoulder Muscle, Right** Deltoid muscle Infraspinatus muscle Subscapularis muscle Supraspinatus muscle Teres major muscle Teres minor muscle **6 Shoulder Muscle, Left** *See 5 Shoulder Muscle, Right*	**7 Upper Arm Muscle, Right** Biceps brachii muscle Brachialis muscle Coracobrachialis muscle Triceps brachii muscle **8 Upper Arm Muscle, Left** *See 7 Upper Arm Muscle, Right* **9 Lower Arm and Wrist Muscle, Right** Anatomical snuffbox Brachioradialis muscle Extensor carpi radialis muscle Extensor carpi ulnaris muscle Flexor carpi radialis muscle Flexor carpi ulnaris muscle Flexor pollicis longus muscle Palmaris longus muscle Pronator quadratus muscle Pronator teres muscle **B Lower Arm and Wrist Muscle, Left** *See 9 Lower Arm and Wrist Muscle, Right* **C Hand Muscle, Right** Hypothenar muscle Palmar interosseous muscle Thenar muscle **D Hand Muscle, Left** *See C Hand Muscle, Right* **F Trunk Muscle, Right** Coccygeus muscle Erector spinae muscle Interspinalis muscle Intertransversarius muscle Latissimus dorsi muscle Quadratus lumborum muscle Rhomboid major muscle Rhomboid minor muscle Serratus posterior muscle Transversospinalis muscle Trapezius muscle **G Trunk Muscle, Left** *See F Trunk Muscle, Right* **H Thorax Muscle, Right** Intercostal muscle Levatores costarum muscle Pectoralis major muscle Pectoralis minor muscle Serratus anterior muscle Subclavius muscle Subcostal muscle Transverse thoracis muscle **J Thorax Muscle, Left** *See H Thorax Muscle, Right* **K Abdomen Muscle, Right** External oblique muscle Internal oblique muscle Pyramidalis muscle Rectus abdominis muscle Transversus abdominis muscle **L Abdomen Muscle, Left** *See K Abdomen Muscle, Right*	**M Perineum Muscle** Bulbospongiosus muscle Cremaster muscle Deep transverse perineal muscle Ischiocavernosus muscle Levator ani muscle Superficial transverse perineal muscle **N Hip Muscle, Right** Gemellus muscle Gluteus maximus muscle Gluteus medius muscle Gluteus minimus muscle Iliacus muscle Obturator muscle Piriformis muscle Psoas muscle Quadratus femoris muscle Tensor fasciae latae muscle **P Hip Muscle, Left** *See N Hip Muscle, Right* **Q Upper Leg Muscle, Right** Adductor brevis muscle Adductor longus muscle Adductor magnus muscle Biceps femoris muscle Gracilis muscle Pectineus muscle Quadriceps (femoris) Rectus femoris muscle Sartorius muscle Semimembranosus muscle Semitendinosus muscle Vastus intermedius muscle Vastus lateralis muscle Vastus medialis muscle **R Upper Leg Muscle, Left** *See Q Upper Leg Muscle, Right* **S Lower Leg Muscle, Right** Extensor digitorum longus muscle Extensor hallucis longus muscle Fibularis brevis muscle Fibularis longus muscle Flexor digitorum longus muscle Flexor hallucis longus muscle Gastrocnemius muscle Peroneus brevis muscle Peroneus longus muscle Popliteus muscle Soleus muscle Tibialis anterior muscle Tibialis posterior muscle **T Lower Leg Muscle, Left** *See S Lower Leg Muscle, Right* **V Foot Muscle, Right** Abductor hallucis muscle Adductor hallucis muscle Extensor digitorum brevis muscle Extensor hallucis brevis muscle Flexor digitorum brevis muscle Flexor hallucis brevis muscle Quadratus plantae muscle **W Foot Muscle, Left** *See V Foot Muscle, Right*	**Ø Open**	**Z No Device**	**Z No Qualifier**

NC Noncovered Procedure　　LC Limited Coverage　　OA Questionable OB Admit　　NT New Tech Add-on　　✚ Combination Member　　♂ Male　　♀ Female

Ø Medical and Surgical
K Muscles
H Insertion
Definition: Putting in a nonbiological appliance that monitors, assists, performs, or prevents a physiological function but does not physically take the place of a body part
Explanation: None

Body Part Character 4	Approach Character 5	Device Character 6	Qualifier Character 7
X Upper Muscle Y Lower Muscle	Ø Open 3 Percutaneous 4 Percutaneous Endoscopic	M Stimulator Lead Y Other Device	Z No Qualifier

Non-OR   ØKH[X,Y][3,4]YZ

Ø Medical and Surgical
K Muscles
J Inspection
Definition: Visually and/or manually exploring a body part
Explanation: Visual exploration may be performed with or without optical instrumentation. Manual exploration may be performed directly or through intervening body layers.

Body Part Character 4	Approach Character 5	Device Character 6	Qualifier Character 7
X Upper Muscle Y Lower Muscle	Ø Open 3 Percutaneous 4 Percutaneous Endoscopic X External	Z No Device	Z No Qualifier

Non-OR   ØKJ[X,Y][3,X]ZZ

Ø   **Medical and Surgical**
K   **Muscles**
M   **Reattachment**   Definition: Putting back in or on all or a portion of a separated body part to its normal location or other suitable location

Explanation: Vascular circulation and nervous pathways may or may not be reestablished

Body Part Character 4		Approach Character 5	Device Character 6	Qualifier Character 7
Ø **Head Muscle** Auricularis muscle Masseter muscle Pterygoid muscle Splenius capitis muscle Temporalis muscle Temporoparietalis muscle **1** **Facial Muscle** Buccinator muscle Corrugator supercilii muscle Depressor anguli oris muscle Depressor labii inferioris muscle Depressor septi nasi muscle Depressor supercilii muscle Levator anguli oris muscle Levator labii superioris alaeque nasi muscle Levator labii superioris muscle Mentalis muscle Nasalis muscle Occipitofrontalis muscle Orbicularis oris muscle Procerus muscle Risorius muscle Zygomaticus muscle **2** **Neck Muscle, Right** Anterior vertebral muscle Arytenoid muscle Cricothyroid muscle Infrahyoid muscle Levator scapulae muscle Platysma muscle Scalene muscle Splenius cervicis muscle Sternocleidomastoid muscle Suprahyoid muscle Thyroarytenoid muscle **3** **Neck Muscle, Left** *See 2 Neck Muscle, Right* **4** **Tongue, Palate, Pharynx Muscle** Chondroglossus muscle Genioglossus muscle Hyoglossus muscle Inferior longitudinal muscle Levator veli palatini muscle Palatoglossal muscle Palatopharyngeal muscle Pharyngeal constrictor muscle Salpingopharyngeus muscle Styloglossus muscle Stylopharyngeus muscle Superior longitudinal muscle Tensor veli palatini muscle **5** **Shoulder Muscle, Right** Deltoid muscle Infraspinatus muscle Subscapularis muscle Supraspinatus muscle Teres major muscle Teres minor muscle **6** **Shoulder Muscle, Left** *See 5 Shoulder Muscle, Right*	**7** **Upper Arm Muscle, Right** Biceps brachii muscle Brachialis muscle Coracobrachialis muscle Triceps brachii muscle **8** **Upper Arm Muscle, Left** *See 7 Upper Arm Muscle, Right* **9** **Lower Arm and Wrist Muscle, Right** Anatomical snuffbox Brachioradialis muscle Extensor carpi radialis muscle Extensor carpi ulnaris muscle Flexor carpi radialis muscle Flexor carpi ulnaris muscle Flexor pollicis longus muscle Palmaris longus muscle Pronator quadratus muscle Pronator teres muscle **B** **Lower Arm and Wrist Muscle, Left** *See 9 Lower Arm and Wrist Muscle, Right* **C** **Hand Muscle, Right** Hypothenar muscle Palmar interosseous muscle Thenar muscle **D** **Hand Muscle, Left** *See C Hand Muscle, Right* **F** **Trunk Muscle, Right** Coccygeus muscle Erector spinae muscle Interspinalis muscle Intertransversarius muscle Latissimus dorsi muscle Quadratus lumborum muscle Rhomboid major muscle Rhomboid minor muscle Serratus posterior muscle Transversospinalis muscle Trapezius muscle **G** **Trunk Muscle, Left** *See F Trunk Muscle, Right* **H** **Thorax Muscle, Right** Intercostal muscle Levatores costarum muscle Pectoralis major muscle Pectoralis minor muscle Serratus anterior muscle Subclavius muscle Subcostal muscle Transverse thoracis muscle **J** **Thorax Muscle, Left** *See H Thorax Muscle, Right* **K** **Abdomen Muscle, Right** External oblique muscle Internal oblique muscle Pyramidalis muscle Rectus abdominis muscle Transversus abdominis muscle **L** **Abdomen Muscle, Left** *See K Abdomen Muscle, Right*	**M** **Perineum Muscle** Bulbospongiosus muscle Cremaster muscle Deep transverse perineal muscle Ischiocavernosus muscle Levator ani muscle Superficial transverse perineal muscle **N** **Hip Muscle, Right** Gemellus muscle Gluteus maximus muscle Gluteus medius muscle Gluteus minimus muscle Iliacus muscle Obturator muscle Piriformis muscle Psoas muscle Quadratus femoris muscle Tensor fasciae latae muscle **P** **Hip Muscle, Left** *See N Hip Muscle, Right* **Q** **Upper Leg Muscle, Right** Adductor brevis muscle Adductor longus muscle Adductor magnus muscle Biceps femoris muscle Gracilis muscle Pectineus muscle Quadriceps (femoris) Rectus femoris muscle Sartorius muscle Semimembranosus muscle Semitendinosus muscle Vastus intermedius muscle Vastus lateralis muscle Vastus medialis muscle **R** **Upper Leg Muscle, Left** *See Q Upper Leg Muscle, Right* **S** **Lower Leg Muscle, Right** Extensor digitorum longus muscle Extensor hallucis longus muscle Fibularis brevis muscle Fibularis longus muscle Flexor digitorum longus muscle Flexor hallucis longus muscle Gastrocnemius muscle Peroneus brevis muscle Peroneus longus muscle Popliteus muscle Soleus muscle Tibialis anterior muscle Tibialis posterior muscle **T** **Lower Leg Muscle, Left** *See S Lower Leg Muscle, Right* **V** **Foot Muscle, Right** Abductor hallucis muscle Adductor hallucis muscle Extensor digitorum brevis muscle Extensor hallucis brevis muscle Flexor digitorum brevis muscle Flexor hallucis brevis muscle Quadratus plantae muscle **W** **Foot Muscle, Left** *See V Foot Muscle, Right*	**Ø** Open **4** Percutaneous Endoscopic	**Z** No Device	**Z** No Qualifier

NC Noncovered Procedure   **LC** Limited Coverage   **QA** Questionable OB Admit   **NT** New Tech Add-on   ⊞ Combination Member   ♂ Male   ♀ Female

ICD-10-PCS 2022   473

Muscles

Ø　Medical and Surgical
K　Muscles
N　Release　Definition: Freeing a body part from an abnormal physical constraint by cutting or by the use of force
　　　　　Explanation: Some of the restraining tissue may be taken out but none of the body part is taken out

Body Part Character 4			Approach Character 5	Device Character 6	Qualifier Character 7
Ø Head Muscle 　Auricularis muscle 　Masseter muscle 　Pterygoid muscle 　Splenius capitis muscle 　Temporalis muscle 　Temporoparietalis muscle **1 Facial Muscle** 　Buccinator muscle 　Corrugator supercilii 　　muscle 　Depressor anguli oris 　　muscle 　Depressor labii inferioris 　　muscle 　Depressor septi nasi 　　muscle 　Depressor supercilii 　　muscle 　Levator anguli oris muscle 　Levator labii superioris 　　alaeque nasi muscle 　Levator labii superioris 　　muscle 　Mentalis muscle 　Nasalis muscle 　Occipitofrontalis muscle 　Orbicularis oris muscle 　Procerus muscle 　Risorius muscle 　Zygomaticus muscle **2 Neck Muscle, Right** 　Anterior vertebral muscle 　Arytenoid muscle 　Cricothyroid muscle 　Infrahyoid muscle 　Levator scapulae muscle 　Platysma muscle 　Scalene muscle 　Splenius cervicis muscle 　Sternocleidomastoid 　　muscle 　Suprahyoid muscle 　Thyroarytenoid muscle **3 Neck Muscle, Left** 　*See 2 Neck Muscle, Right* **4 Tongue, Palate, Pharynx** 　**Muscle** 　Chondroglossus muscle 　Genioglossus muscle 　Hyoglossus muscle 　Inferior longitudinal 　　muscle 　Levator veli palatini 　　muscle 　Palatoglossal muscle 　Palatopharyngeal muscle 　Pharyngeal constrictor 　　muscle 　Salpingopharyngeus 　　muscle 　Styloglossus muscle 　Stylopharyngeus muscle 　Superior longitudinal 　　muscle 　Tensor veli palatini muscle **5 Shoulder Muscle, Right** 　Deltoid muscle 　Infraspinatus muscle 　Subscapularis muscle 　Supraspinatus muscle 　Teres major muscle 　Teres minor muscle **6 Shoulder Muscle, Left** 　*See 5 Shoulder Muscle,* 　　*Right*	**7 Upper Arm Muscle, Right** 　Biceps brachii muscle 　Brachialis muscle 　Coracobrachialis muscle 　Triceps brachii muscle **8 Upper Arm Muscle, Left** 　*See 7 Upper Arm Muscle,* 　　*Right* **9 Lower Arm and Wrist** 　**Muscle, Right** 　Anatomical snuffbox 　Brachioradialis muscle 　Extensor carpi radialis 　　muscle 　Extensor carpi ulnaris 　　muscle 　Flexor carpi radialis 　　muscle 　Flexor carpi ulnaris muscle 　Flexor pollicis longus 　　muscle 　Palmaris longus muscle 　Pronator quadratus 　　muscle 　Pronator teres muscle **B Lower Arm and Wrist** 　**Muscle, Left** 　*See 9 Lower Arm and Wrist* 　　*Muscle, Right* **C Hand Muscle, Right** 　Hypothenar muscle 　Palmar interosseous 　　muscle 　Thenar muscle **D Hand Muscle, Left** 　*See C Hand Muscle, Right* **F Trunk Muscle, Right** 　Coccygeus muscle 　Erector spinae muscle 　Interspinalis muscle 　Intertransversarius muscle 　Latissimus dorsi muscle 　Quadratus lumborum 　　muscle 　Rhomboid major muscle 　Rhomboid minor muscle 　Serratus posterior muscle 　Transversospinalis muscle 　Trapezius muscle **G Trunk Muscle, Left** 　*See F Trunk Muscle, Right* **H Thorax Muscle, Right** 　Intercostal muscle 　Levatores costarum 　　muscle 　Pectoralis major muscle 　Pectoralis minor muscle 　Serratus anterior muscle 　Subclavius muscle 　Subcostal muscle 　Transverse thoracis 　　muscle **J Thorax Muscle, Left** 　*See H Thorax Muscle, Right* **K Abdomen Muscle, Right** 　External oblique muscle 　Internal oblique muscle 　Pyramidalis muscle 　Rectus abdominis muscle 　Transversus abdominis 　　muscle **L Abdomen Muscle, Left** 　*See K Abdomen Muscle,* 　　*Right*	**M Perineum Muscle** 　Bulbospongiosus muscle 　Cremaster muscle 　Deep transverse perineal 　　muscle 　Ischiocavernosus muscle 　Levator ani muscle 　Superficial transverse 　　perineal muscle **N Hip Muscle, Right** 　Gemellus muscle 　Gluteus maximus muscle 　Gluteus medius muscle 　Gluteus minimus muscle 　Iliacus muscle 　Obturator muscle 　Piriformis muscle 　Psoas muscle 　Quadratus femoris muscle 　Tensor fasciae latae 　　muscle **P Hip Muscle, Left** 　*See N Hip Muscle, Right* **Q Upper Leg Muscle, Right** 　Adductor brevis muscle 　Adductor longus muscle 　Adductor magnus muscle 　Biceps femoris muscle 　Gracilis muscle 　Pectineus muscle 　Quadriceps (femoris) 　Rectus femoris muscle 　Sartorius muscle 　Semimembranosus 　　muscle 　Semitendinosus muscle 　Vastus intermedius muscle 　Vastus lateralis muscle 　Vastus medialis muscle **R Upper Leg Muscle, Left** 　*See Q Upper Leg Muscle,* 　　*Right* **S Lower Leg Muscle, Right** 　Extensor digitorum longus 　　muscle 　Extensor hallucis longus 　　muscle 　Fibularis brevis muscle 　Fibularis longus muscle 　Flexor digitorum longus 　　muscle 　Flexor hallucis longus 　　muscle 　Gastrocnemius muscle 　Peroneus brevis muscle 　Peroneus longus muscle 　Popliteus muscle 　Soleus muscle 　Tibialis anterior muscle 　Tibialis posterior muscle **T Lower Leg Muscle, Left** 　*See S Lower Leg Muscle,* 　　*Right* **V Foot Muscle, Right** 　Abductor hallucis muscle 　Adductor hallucis muscle 　Extensor digitorum brevis 　　muscle 　Extensor hallucis brevis 　　muscle 　Flexor digitorum brevis 　　muscle 　Flexor hallucis brevis 　　muscle 　Quadratus plantae muscle **W Foot Muscle, Left** 　*See V Foot Muscle, Right*	**Ø Open** **3 Percutaneous** **4 Percutaneous** 　**Endoscopic** **X External**	**Z No Device**	**Z No Qualifier**

Non-OR　ØKN[Ø,1,2,3,4,5,6,7,8,9,B,C,D,F,G,H,J,K,L,M,N,P,Q,R,S,T,V,W]XZZ

Ø   **Medical and Surgical**
K   **Muscles**
P   **Removal**   Definition: Taking out or off a device from a body part

Explanation: If a device is taken out and a similar device put in without cutting or puncturing the skin or mucous membrane, the procedure is coded to the root operation CHANGE. Otherwise, the procedure for taking out a device is coded to the root operation REMOVAL.

Body Part Character 4	Approach Character 5	Device Character 6	Qualifier Character 7
X Upper Muscle **Y** Lower Muscle	**Ø** Open **3** Percutaneous **4** Percutaneous Endoscopic	**Ø** Drainage Device **7** Autologous Tissue Substitute **J** Synthetic Substitute **K** Nonautologous Tissue Substitute **M** Stimulator Lead **Y** Other Device	**Z** No Qualifier
X Upper Muscle **Y** Lower Muscle	**X** External	**Ø** Drainage Device **M** Stimulator Lead	**Z** No Qualifier

Non-OR   ØKP[X,Y][3,4]YZ
Non-OR   ØKP[X,Y]X[Ø,M]Z

NC Noncovered Procedure   LC Limited Coverage   QA Questionable OB Admit   NT New Tech Add-on   ⊞ Combination Member   ♂ Male   ♀ Female

ICD-10-PCS 2022   475

Muscles

Ø Medical and Surgical
K Muscles
Q Repair

Definition: Restoring, to the extent possible, a body part to its normal anatomic structure and function
Explanation: Used only when the method to accomplish the repair is not one of the other root operations

Body Part Character 4		Approach Character 5	Device Character 6	Qualifier Character 7
Ø Head Muscle Auricularis muscle Masseter muscle Pterygoid muscle Splenius capitis muscle Temporalis muscle Temporoparietalis muscle **1 Facial Muscle** Buccinator muscle Corrugator supercilii muscle Depressor anguli oris muscle Depressor labii inferioris muscle Depressor septi nasi muscle Depressor supercilii muscle Levator anguli oris muscle Levator labii superioris alaeque nasi muscle Levator labii superioris muscle Mentalis muscle Nasalis muscle Occipitofrontalis muscle Orbicularis oris muscle Procerus muscle Risorius muscle Zygomaticus muscle **2 Neck Muscle, Right** Anterior vertebral muscle Arytenoid muscle Cricothyroid muscle Infrahyoid muscle Levator scapulae muscle Platysma muscle Scalene muscle Splenius cervicis muscle Sternocleidomastoid muscle Suprahyoid muscle Thyroarytenoid muscle **3 Neck Muscle, Left** *See 2 Neck Muscle, Right* **4 Tongue, Palate, Pharynx Muscle** Chondroglossus muscle Genioglossus muscle Hyoglossus muscle Inferior longitudinal muscle Levator veli palatini muscle Palatoglossal muscle Palatopharyngeal muscle Pharyngeal constrictor muscle Salpingopharyngeus muscle Styloglossus muscle Stylopharyngeus muscle Superior longitudinal muscle Tensor veli palatini muscle **5 Shoulder Muscle, Right** Deltoid muscle Infraspinatus muscle Subscapularis muscle Supraspinatus muscle Teres major muscle Teres minor muscle **6 Shoulder Muscle, Left** *See 5 Shoulder Muscle, Right*	**7 Upper Arm Muscle, Right** Biceps brachii muscle Brachialis muscle Coracobrachialis muscle Triceps brachii muscle **8 Upper Arm Muscle, Left** *See 7 Upper Arm Muscle, Right* **9 Lower Arm and Wrist Muscle, Right** Anatomical snuffbox Brachioradialis muscle Extensor carpi radialis muscle Extensor carpi ulnaris muscle Flexor carpi radialis muscle Flexor carpi ulnaris muscle Flexor pollicis longus muscle Palmaris longus muscle Pronator quadratus muscle Pronator teres muscle **B Lower Arm and Wrist Muscle, Left** *See 9 Lower Arm and Wrist Muscle, Right* **C Hand Muscle, Right** Hypothenar muscle Palmar interosseous muscle Thenar muscle **D Hand Muscle, Left** *See C Hand Muscle, Right* **F Trunk Muscle, Right** Coccygeus muscle Erector spinae muscle Interspinalis muscle Intertransversarius muscle Latissimus dorsi muscle Quadratus lumborum muscle Rhomboid major muscle Rhomboid minor muscle Serratus posterior muscle Transversospinalis muscle Trapezius muscle **G Trunk Muscle, Left** *See F Trunk Muscle, Right* **H Thorax Muscle, Right** Intercostal muscle Levatores costarum muscle Pectoralis major muscle Pectoralis minor muscle Serratus anterior muscle Subclavius muscle Subcostal muscle Transverse thoracis muscle **J Thorax Muscle, Left** *See H Thorax Muscle, Right* **K Abdomen Muscle, Right** External oblique muscle Internal oblique muscle Pyramidalis muscle Rectus abdominis muscle Transversus abdominis muscle **L Abdomen Muscle, Left** *See K Abdomen Muscle, Right*	**M Perineum Muscle** Bulbospongiosus muscle Cremaster muscle Deep transverse perineal muscle Ischiocavernosus muscle Levator ani muscle Superficial transverse perineal muscle **N Hip Muscle, Right** Gemellus muscle Gluteus maximus muscle Gluteus medius muscle Gluteus minimus muscle Iliacus muscle Obturator muscle Piriformis muscle Psoas muscle Quadratus femoris muscle Tensor fasciae latae muscle **P Hip Muscle, Left** *See N Hip Muscle, Right* **Q Upper Leg Muscle, Right** Adductor brevis muscle Adductor longus muscle Adductor magnus muscle Biceps femoris muscle Gracilis muscle Pectineus muscle Quadriceps (femoris) Rectus femoris muscle Sartorius muscle Semimembranosus muscle Semitendinosus muscle Vastus intermedius muscle Vastus lateralis muscle Vastus medialis muscle **R Upper Leg Muscle, Left** *See Q Upper Leg Muscle, Right* **S Lower Leg Muscle, Right** Extensor digitorum longus muscle Extensor hallucis longus muscle Fibularis brevis muscle Fibularis longus muscle Flexor digitorum longus muscle Flexor hallucis longus muscle Gastrocnemius muscle Peroneus brevis muscle Peroneus longus muscle Popliteus muscle Soleus muscle Tibialis anterior muscle Tibialis posterior muscle **T Lower Leg Muscle, Left** *See S Lower Leg Muscle, Right* **V Foot Muscle, Right** Abductor hallucis muscle Adductor hallucis muscle Extensor digitorum brevis muscle Extensor hallucis brevis muscle Flexor digitorum brevis muscle Flexor hallucis brevis muscle Quadratus plantae muscle **W Foot Muscle, Left** *See V Foot Muscle, Right*	**Ø** Open **3** Percutaneous **4** Percutaneous Endoscopic	**Z** No Device	**Z** No Qualifier

Ø   **Medical and Surgical**
K   **Muscles**
R   **Replacement**   Definition: Putting in or on biological or synthetic material that physically takes the place and/or function of all or a portion of a body part
                 Explanation: The body part may have been taken out or replaced, or may be taken out, physically eradicated, or rendered nonfunctional during the REPLACEMENT procedure. A REMOVAL procedure is coded for taking out the device used in a previous replacement procedure.

Body Part Character 4			Approach Character 5	Device Character 6	Qualifier Character 7

Ø Head Muscle
Auricularis muscle
Masseter muscle
Pterygoid muscle
Splenius capitis muscle
Temporalis muscle
Temporoparietalis muscle
1 Facial Muscle
Buccinator muscle
Corrugator supercilii
  muscle
Depressor anguli oris
  muscle
Depressor labii inferioris
  muscle
Depressor septi nasi
  muscle
Depressor supercilii
  muscle
Levator anguli oris muscle
Levator labii superioris
  alaeque nasi muscle
Levator labii superioris
  muscle
Mentalis muscle
Nasalis muscle
Occipitofrontalis muscle
Orbicularis oris muscle
Procerus muscle
Risorius muscle
Zygomaticus muscle
2 Neck Muscle, Right
Anterior vertebral muscle
Arytenoid muscle
Cricothyroid muscle
Infrahyoid muscle
Levator scapulae muscle
Platysma muscle
Scalene muscle
Splenius cervicis muscle
Sternocleidomastoid
  muscle
Suprahyoid muscle
Thyroarytenoid muscle
3 Neck Muscle, Left
See 2 Neck Muscle, Right
4 Tongue, Palate, Pharynx
Muscle
Chondroglossus muscle
Genioglossus muscle
Hyoglossus muscle
Inferior longitudinal
  muscle
Levator veli palatini
  muscle
Palatoglossal muscle
Palatopharyngeal muscle
Pharyngeal constrictor
  muscle
Salpingopharyngeus
  muscle
Styloglossus muscle
Stylopharyngeus muscle
Superior longitudinal
  muscle
Tensor veli palatini muscle
5 Shoulder Muscle, Right
Deltoid muscle
Infraspinatus muscle
Subscapularis muscle
Supraspinatus muscle
Teres major muscle
Teres minor muscle
6 Shoulder Muscle, Left
See 5 Shoulder Muscle,
Right
	7 Upper Arm Muscle, Right
	Biceps brachii muscle
	Brachialis muscle
	Coracobrachialis muscle
	Triceps brachii muscle
	8 Upper Arm Muscle, Left
	See 7 Upper Arm Muscle,
	Right
	9 Lower Arm and Wrist
	Muscle, Right
	Anatomical snuffbox
	Brachioradialis muscle
	Extensor carpi radialis
	  muscle
	Extensor carpi ulnaris
	  muscle
	Flexor carpi radialis
	  muscle
	Flexor carpi ulnaris muscle
	Flexor pollicis longus
	  muscle
	Palmaris longus muscle
	Pronator quadratus
	  muscle
	Pronator teres muscle
	B Lower Arm and Wrist
	Muscle, Left
	See 9 Lower Arm and Wrist
	Muscle, Right
	C Hand Muscle, Right
	Hypothenar muscle
	Palmar interosseous
	  muscle
	Thenar muscle
	D Hand Muscle, Left
	See C Hand Muscle, Right
	F Trunk Muscle, Right
	Coccygeus muscle
	Erector spinae muscle
	Interspinalis muscle
	Intertransversarius muscle
	Latissimus dorsi muscle
	Quadratus lumborum
	  muscle
	Rhomboid major muscle
	Rhomboid minor muscle
	Serratus posterior muscle
	Transversospinalis muscle
	Trapezius muscle
	G Trunk Muscle, Left
	See F Trunk Muscle, Right
	H Thorax Muscle, Right
	Intercostal muscle
	Levatores costarum
	  muscle
	Pectoralis major muscle
	Pectoralis minor muscle
	Serratus anterior muscle
	Subclavius muscle
	Subcostal muscle
	Transverse thoracis
	  muscle
	J Thorax Muscle, Left
	See H Thorax Muscle, Right
	K Abdomen Muscle, Right
	External oblique muscle
	Internal oblique muscle
	Pyramidalis muscle
	Rectus abdominis muscle
	Transversus abdominis
	  muscle
	L Abdomen Muscle, Left
	See K Abdomen Muscle,
	Right
		M Perineum Muscle
		Bulbospongiosus muscle
		Cremaster muscle
		Deep transverse perineal
		  muscle
		Ischiocavernosus muscle
		Levator ani muscle
		Superficial transverse
		  perineal muscle
		N Hip Muscle, Right
		Gemellus muscle
		Gluteus maximus muscle
		Gluteus medius muscle
		Gluteus minimus muscle
		Iliacus muscle
		Obturator muscle
		Piriformis muscle
		Psoas muscle
		Quadratus femoris muscle
		Tensor fasciae latae
		  muscle
		P Hip Muscle, Left
		See N Hip Muscle, Right
		Q Upper Leg Muscle, Right
		Adductor brevis muscle
		Adductor longus muscle
		Adductor magnus muscle
		Biceps femoris muscle
		Gracilis muscle
		Pectineus muscle
		Quadriceps (femoris)
		Rectus femoris muscle
		Sartorius muscle
		Semimembranosus
		  muscle
		Semitendinosus muscle
		Vastus intermedius muscle
		Vastus lateralis muscle
		Vastus medialis muscle
		R Upper Leg Muscle, Left
		See Q Upper Leg Muscle,
		Right
		S Lower Leg Muscle, Right
		Extensor digitorum longus
		  muscle
		Extensor hallucis longus
		  muscle
		Fibularis brevis muscle
		Fibularis longus muscle
		Flexor digitorum longus
		  muscle
		Flexor hallucis longus
		  muscle
		Gastrocnemius muscle
		Peroneus brevis muscle
		Peroneus longus muscle
		Popliteus muscle
		Soleus muscle
		Tibialis anterior muscle
		Tibialis posterior muscle
		T Lower Leg Muscle, Left
		See S Lower Leg Muscle,
		Right
		V Foot Muscle, Right
		Abductor hallucis muscle
		Adductor hallucis muscle
		Extensor digitorum brevis
		  muscle
		Extensor hallucis brevis
		  muscle
		Flexor digitorum brevis
		  muscle
		Flexor hallucis brevis
		  muscle
		Quadratus plantae muscle
		W Foot Muscle, Left
		See V Foot Muscle, Right
			Ø Open
			4 Percutaneous
			  Endoscopic
				7 Autologous Tissue
				  Substitute
				J Synthetic
				  Substitute
				K Nonautologous
				  Tissue Substitute
					Z No Qualifier

🄽🄲 Noncovered Procedure   🄻🄲 Limited Coverage   🄾🄰 Questionable OB Admit   🄽🅃 New Tech Add-on   ⊞ Combination Member   ♂ Male   ♀ Female

ICD-10-PCS 2022   **477**

Ø   **Medical and Surgical**
K   **Muscles**
S   **Reposition**   Definition: Moving to its normal location, or other suitable location, all or a portion of a body part

Explanation: The body part is moved to a new location from an abnormal location, or from a normal location where it is not functioning correctly. The body part may or may not be cut out or off to be moved to the new location.

Body Part Character 4			Approach Character 5	Device Character 6	Qualifier Character 7
Ø Head Muscle Auricularis muscle Masseter muscle Pterygoid muscle Splenius capitis muscle Temporalis muscle Temporoparietalis muscle **1 Facial Muscle** Buccinator muscle Corrugator supercilii muscle Depressor anguli oris muscle Depressor labii inferioris muscle Depressor septi nasi muscle Depressor supercilii muscle Levator anguli oris muscle Levator labii superioris alaeque nasi muscle Levator labii superioris muscle Mentalis muscle Nasalis muscle Occipitofrontalis muscle Orbicularis oris muscle Procerus muscle Risorius muscle Zygomaticus muscle **2 Neck Muscle, Right** Anterior vertebral muscle Arytenoid muscle Cricothyroid muscle Infrahyoid muscle Levator scapulae muscle Platysma muscle Scalene muscle Splenius cervicis muscle Sternocleidomastoid muscle Suprahyoid muscle Thyroarytenoid muscle **3 Neck Muscle, Left** *See 2 Neck Muscle, Right* **4 Tongue, Palate, Pharynx Muscle** Chondroglossus muscle Genioglossus muscle Hyoglossus muscle Inferior longitudinal muscle Levator veli palatini muscle Palatoglossal muscle Palatopharyngeal muscle Pharyngeal constrictor muscle Salpingopharyngeus muscle Styloglossus muscle Stylopharyngeus muscle Superior longitudinal muscle Tensor veli palatini muscle **5 Shoulder Muscle, Right** Deltoid muscle Infraspinatus muscle Subscapularis muscle Supraspinatus muscle Teres major muscle Teres minor muscle **6 Shoulder Muscle, Left** *See 5 Shoulder Muscle, Right*	**7 Upper Arm Muscle, Right** Biceps brachii muscle Brachialis muscle Coracobrachialis muscle Triceps brachii muscle **8 Upper Arm Muscle, Left** *See 7 Upper Arm Muscle, Right* **9 Lower Arm and Wrist Muscle, Right** Anatomical snuffbox Brachioradialis muscle Extensor carpi radialis muscle Extensor carpi ulnaris muscle Flexor carpi radialis muscle Flexor carpi ulnaris muscle Flexor pollicis longus muscle Palmaris longus muscle Pronator quadratus muscle Pronator teres muscle **B Lower Arm and Wrist Muscle, Left** *See 9 Lower Arm and Wrist Muscle, Right* **C Hand Muscle, Right** Hypothenar muscle Palmar interosseous muscle Thenar muscle **D Hand Muscle, Left** *See C Hand Muscle, Right* **F Trunk Muscle, Right** Coccygeus muscle Erector spinae muscle Interspinalis muscle Intertransversarius muscle Latissimus dorsi muscle Quadratus lumborum muscle Rhomboid major muscle Rhomboid minor muscle Serratus posterior muscle Transversospinalis muscle Trapezius muscle **G Trunk Muscle, Left** *See F Trunk Muscle, Right* **H Thorax Muscle, Right** Intercostal muscle Levatores costarum muscle Pectoralis major muscle Pectoralis minor muscle Serratus anterior muscle Subclavius muscle Subcostal muscle Transverse thoracis muscle **J Thorax Muscle, Left** *See H Thorax Muscle, Right* **K Abdomen Muscle, Right** External oblique muscle Internal oblique muscle Pyramidalis muscle Rectus abdominis muscle Transversus abdominis muscle **L Abdomen Muscle, Left** *See K Abdomen Muscle, Right*	**M Perineum Muscle** Bulbospongiosus muscle Cremaster muscle Deep transverse perineal muscle Ischiocavernosus muscle Levator ani muscle Superficial transverse perineal muscle **N Hip Muscle, Right** Gemellus muscle Gluteus maximus muscle Gluteus medius muscle Gluteus minimus muscle Iliacus muscle Obturator muscle Piriformis muscle Psoas muscle Quadratus femoris muscle Tensor fasciae latae muscle **P Hip Muscle, Left** *See N Hip Muscle, Right* **Q Upper Leg Muscle, Right** Adductor brevis muscle Adductor longus muscle Adductor magnus muscle Biceps femoris muscle Gracilis muscle Pectineus muscle Quadriceps (femoris) Rectus femoris muscle Sartorius muscle Semimembranosus muscle Semitendinosus muscle Vastus intermedius muscle Vastus lateralis muscle Vastus medialis muscle **R Upper Leg Muscle, Left** *See Q Upper Leg Muscle, Right* **S Lower Leg Muscle, Right** Extensor digitorum longus muscle Extensor hallucis longus muscle Fibularis brevis muscle Fibularis longus muscle Flexor digitorum longus muscle Flexor hallucis longus muscle Gastrocnemius muscle Peroneus brevis muscle Peroneus longus muscle Popliteus muscle Soleus muscle Tibialis anterior muscle Tibialis posterior muscle **T Lower Leg Muscle, Left** *See S Lower Leg Muscle, Right* **V Foot Muscle, Right** Abductor hallucis muscle Adductor hallucis muscle Extensor digitorum brevis muscle Extensor hallucis brevis muscle Flexor digitorum brevis muscle Flexor hallucis brevis muscle Quadratus plantae muscle **W Foot Muscle, Left** *See V Foot Muscle, Right*	**Ø Open** **4 Percutaneous Endoscopic**	**Z No Device**	**Z No Qualifier**

Ø　**Medical and Surgical**
K　**Muscles**
T　**Resection**　　Definition: Cutting out or off, without replacement, all of a body part
　　　　　　　　　　　　Explanation: None

Body Part Character 4			Approach Character 5	Device Character 6	Qualifier Character 7
Ø Head Muscle 　Auricularis muscle 　Masseter muscle 　Pterygoid muscle 　Splenius capitis muscle 　Temporalis muscle 　Temporoparietalis muscle **1 Facial Muscle** 　Buccinator muscle 　Corrugator supercilii 　　muscle 　Depressor anguli oris 　　muscle 　Depressor labii inferioris 　　muscle 　Depressor septi nasi 　　muscle 　Depressor supercilii 　　muscle 　Levator anguli oris muscle 　Levator labii superioris 　　alaeque nasi muscle 　Levator labii superioris 　　muscle 　Mentalis muscle 　Nasalis muscle 　Occipitofrontalis muscle 　Orbicularis oris muscle 　Procerus muscle 　Risorius muscle 　Zygomaticus muscle **2 Neck Muscle, Right** 　Anterior vertebral muscle 　Arytenoid muscle 　Cricothyroid muscle 　Infrahyoid muscle 　Levator scapulae muscle 　Platysma muscle 　Scalene muscle 　Splenius cervicis muscle 　Sternocleidomastoid 　　muscle 　Suprahyoid muscle 　Thyroarytenoid muscle **3 Neck Muscle, Left** 　*See 2 Neck Muscle, Right* **4 Tongue, Palate, Pharynx** 　**Muscle** 　Chondroglossus muscle 　Genioglossus muscle 　Hyoglossus muscle 　Inferior longitudinal 　　muscle 　Levator veli palatini muscle 　Palatoglossal muscle 　Palatopharyngeal muscle 　Pharyngeal constrictor 　　muscle 　Salpingopharyngeus 　　muscle 　Styloglossus muscle 　Stylopharyngeus muscle 　Superior longitudinal 　　muscle 　Tensor veli palatini muscle **5 Shoulder Muscle, Right** 　Deltoid muscle 　Infraspinatus muscle 　Subscapularis muscle 　Supraspinatus muscle 　Teres major muscle 　Teres minor muscle **6 Shoulder Muscle, Left** 　*See 5 Shoulder Muscle,* 　　*Right*	**7 Upper Arm Muscle, Right** 　Biceps brachii muscle 　Brachialis muscle 　Coracobrachialis muscle 　Triceps brachii muscle **8 Upper Arm Muscle, Left** 　*See 7 Upper Arm Muscle,* 　　*Right* **9 Lower Arm and Wrist** 　**Muscle, Right** 　Anatomical snuffbox 　Brachioradialis muscle 　Extensor carpi radialis 　　muscle 　Extensor carpi ulnaris 　　muscle 　Flexor carpi radialis 　　muscle 　Flexor carpi ulnaris muscle 　Flexor pollicis longus 　　muscle 　Palmaris longus muscle 　Pronator quadratus 　　muscle 　Pronator teres muscle **B Lower Arm and Wrist** 　**Muscle, Left** 　*See 9 Lower Arm and Wrist* 　　*Muscle, Right* **C Hand Muscle, Right** 　Hypothenar muscle 　Palmar interosseous 　　muscle 　Thenar muscle **D Hand Muscle, Left** 　*See C Hand Muscle, Right* **F Trunk Muscle, Right** 　Coccygeus muscle 　Erector spinae muscle 　Interspinalis muscle 　Intertransversarius muscle 　Latissimus dorsi muscle 　Quadratus lumborum 　　muscle 　Rhomboid major muscle 　Rhomboid minor muscle 　Serratus posterior muscle 　Transversospinalis muscle 　Trapezius muscle **G Trunk Muscle, Left** 　*See F Trunk Muscle, Right* **H Thorax Muscle, Right** ⊞ 　Intercostal muscle 　Levatores costarum 　　muscle 　Pectoralis major muscle 　Pectoralis minor muscle 　Serratus anterior muscle 　Subclavius muscle 　Subcostal muscle 　Transverse thoracis 　　muscle **J Thorax Muscle, Left** ⊞ 　*See H Thorax Muscle, Right* **K Abdomen Muscle, Right** 　External oblique muscle 　Internal oblique muscle 　Pyramidalis muscle 　Rectus abdominis muscle 　Transversus abdominis 　　muscle **L Abdomen Muscle, Left** 　*See K Abdomen Muscle,* 　　*Right*	**M Perineum Muscle** 　Bulbospongiosus muscle 　Cremaster muscle 　Deep transverse perineal 　　muscle 　Ischiocavernosus muscle 　Levator ani muscle 　Superficial transverse 　　perineal muscle **N Hip Muscle, Right** 　Gemellus muscle 　Gluteus maximus muscle 　Gluteus medius muscle 　Gluteus minimus muscle 　Iliacus muscle 　Obturator muscle 　Piriformis muscle 　Psoas muscle 　Quadratus femoris muscle 　Tensor fasciae latae 　　muscle **P Hip Muscle, Left** 　*See N Hip Muscle, Right* **Q Upper Leg Muscle, Right** 　Adductor brevis muscle 　Adductor longus muscle 　Adductor magnus muscle 　Biceps femoris muscle 　Gracilis muscle 　Pectineus muscle 　Quadriceps (femoris) 　Rectus femoris muscle 　Sartorius muscle 　Semimembranosus muscle 　Semitendinosus muscle 　Vastus intermedius muscle 　Vastus lateralis muscle 　Vastus medialis muscle **R Upper Leg Muscle, Left** 　*See Q Upper Leg Muscle,* 　　*Right* **S Lower Leg Muscle, Right** 　Extensor digitorum longus 　　muscle 　Extensor hallucis longus 　　muscle 　Fibularis brevis muscle 　Fibularis longus muscle 　Flexor digitorum longus 　　muscle 　Flexor hallucis longus 　　muscle 　Gastrocnemius muscle 　Peroneus brevis muscle 　Peroneus longus muscle 　Popliteus muscle 　Soleus muscle 　Tibialis anterior muscle 　Tibialis posterior muscle **T Lower Leg Muscle, Left** 　*See S Lower Leg Muscle,* 　　*Right* **V Foot Muscle, Right** 　Abductor hallucis muscle 　Adductor hallucis muscle 　Extensor digitorum brevis 　　muscle 　Extensor hallucis brevis 　　muscle 　Flexor digitorum brevis 　　muscle 　Flexor hallucis brevis 　　muscle 　Quadratus plantae muscle **W Foot Muscle, Left** 　*See V Foot Muscle, Right*	**Ø Open** **4 Percutaneous** 　**Endoscopic**	**Z No Device**	**Z No Qualifier**

See Appendix L for Procedure Combinations
　⊞　　ØKT[H,J]ØZZ

NC Noncovered Procedure　　**LC** Limited Coverage　　**QA** Questionable OB Admit　　**NT** New Tech Add-on　　⊞ Combination Member　　♂ Male　　♀ Female

ICD-10-PCS 2022　　　　　　　　　　　　　　　　　　　　　　　　　　　　　　　　　　479

Muscles

Ø Medical and Surgical
K Muscles
U Supplement

Definition: Putting in or on biological or synthetic material that physically reinforces and/or augments the function of a portion of a body part

Explanation: The biological material is non-living, or is living and from the same individual. The body part may have been previously replaced, and the SUPPLEMENT procedure is performed to physically reinforce and/or augment the function of the replaced body part.

Body Part Character 4			Approach Character 5	Device Character 6	Qualifier Character 7
Ø Head Muscle Auricularis muscle Masseter muscle Pterygoid muscle Splenius capitis muscle Temporalis muscle Temporoparietalis muscle **1 Facial Muscle** Buccinator muscle Corrugator supercilii muscle Depressor anguli oris muscle Depressor labii inferioris muscle Depressor septi nasi muscle Depressor supercilii muscle Levator anguli oris muscle Levator labii superioris alaeque nasi muscle Levator labii superioris muscle Mentalis muscle Nasalis muscle Occipitofrontalis muscle Orbicularis oris muscle Procerus muscle Risorius muscle Zygomaticus muscle **2 Neck Muscle, Right** Anterior vertebral muscle Arytenoid muscle Cricothyroid muscle Infrahyoid muscle Levator scapulae muscle Platysma muscle Scalene muscle Splenius cervicis muscle Sternocleidomastoid muscle Suprahyoid muscle Thyroarytenoid muscle **3 Neck Muscle, Left** *See 2 Neck Muscle, Right* **4 Tongue, Palate, Pharynx Muscle** Chondroglossus muscle Genioglossus muscle Hyoglossus muscle Inferior longitudinal muscle Levator veli palatini muscle Palatoglossal muscle Palatopharyngeal muscle Pharyngeal constrictor muscle Salpingopharyngeus muscle Styloglossus muscle Stylopharyngeus muscle Superior longitudinal muscle Tensor veli palatini muscle **5 Shoulder Muscle, Right** Deltoid muscle Infraspinatus muscle Subscapularis muscle Supraspinatus muscle Teres major muscle Teres minor muscle **6 Shoulder Muscle, Left** *See 5 Shoulder Muscle, Right*	**7 Upper Arm Muscle, Right** Biceps brachii muscle Brachialis muscle Coracobrachialis muscle Triceps brachii muscle **8 Upper Arm Muscle, Left** *See 7 Upper Arm Muscle, Right* **9 Lower Arm and Wrist Muscle, Right** Anatomical snuffbox Brachioradialis muscle Extensor carpi radialis muscle Extensor carpi ulnaris muscle Flexor carpi radialis muscle Flexor carpi ulnaris muscle Flexor pollicis longus muscle Palmaris longus muscle Pronator quadratus muscle Pronator teres muscle **B Lower Arm and Wrist Muscle, Left** *See 9 Lower Arm and Wrist Muscle, Right* **C Hand Muscle, Right** Hypothenar muscle Palmar interosseous muscle Thenar muscle **D Hand Muscle, Left** *See C Hand Muscle, Right* **F Trunk Muscle, Right** Coccygeus muscle Erector spinae muscle Interspinalis muscle Intertransversarius muscle Latissimus dorsi muscle Quadratus lumborum muscle Rhomboid major muscle Rhomboid minor muscle Serratus posterior muscle Transversospinalis muscle Trapezius muscle **G Trunk Muscle, Left** *See F Trunk Muscle, Right* **H Thorax Muscle, Right** Intercostal muscle Levatores costarum muscle Pectoralis major muscle Pectoralis minor muscle Serratus anterior muscle Subclavius muscle Subcostal muscle Transverse thoracis muscle **J Thorax Muscle, Left** *See H Thorax Muscle, Right* **K Abdomen Muscle, Right** External oblique muscle Internal oblique muscle Pyramidalis muscle Rectus abdominis muscle Transversus abdominis muscle **L Abdomen Muscle, Left** *See K Abdomen Muscle, Right*	**M Perineum Muscle** Bulbospongiosus muscle Cremaster muscle Deep transverse perineal muscle Ischiocavernosus muscle Levator ani muscle Superficial transverse perineal muscle **N Hip Muscle, Right** Gemellus muscle Gluteus maximus muscle Gluteus medius muscle Gluteus minimus muscle Iliacus muscle Obturator muscle Piriformis muscle Psoas muscle Quadratus femoris muscle Tensor fasciae latae muscle **P Hip Muscle, Left** *See N Hip Muscle, Right* **Q Upper Leg Muscle, Right** Adductor brevis muscle Adductor longus muscle Adductor magnus muscle Biceps femoris muscle Gracilis muscle Pectineus muscle Quadriceps (femoris) Rectus femoris muscle Sartorius muscle Semimembranosus muscle Semitendinosus muscle Vastus intermedius muscle Vastus lateralis muscle Vastus medialis muscle **R Upper Leg Muscle, Left** *See Q Upper Leg Muscle, Right* **S Lower Leg Muscle, Right** Extensor digitorum longus muscle Extensor hallucis longus muscle Fibularis brevis muscle Fibularis longus muscle Flexor digitorum longus muscle Flexor hallucis longus muscle Gastrocnemius muscle Peroneus brevis muscle Peroneus longus muscle Popliteus muscle Soleus muscle Tibialis anterior muscle Tibialis posterior muscle **T Lower Leg Muscle, Left** *See S Lower Leg Muscle, Right* **V Foot Muscle, Right** Abductor hallucis muscle Adductor hallucis muscle Extensor digitorum brevis muscle Extensor hallucis brevis muscle Flexor digitorum brevis muscle Flexor hallucis brevis muscle Quadratus plantae muscle **W Foot Muscle, Left** *See V Foot Muscle, Right*	**Ø Open** **4 Percutaneous Endoscopic**	**7 Autologous Tissue Substitute** **J Synthetic Substitute** **K Nonautologous Tissue Substitute**	**Z No Qualifier**

Ø   Medical and Surgical
K   Muscles
W   Revision   Definition: Correcting, to the extent possible, a portion of a malfunctioning device or the position of a displaced device

Explanation: Revision can include correcting a malfunctioning or displaced device by taking out or putting in components of the device such as a screw or pin

Body Part Character 4	Approach Character 5	Device Character 6	Qualifier Character 7
X Upper Muscle **Y** Lower Muscle	**Ø** Open **3** Percutaneous **4** Percutaneous Endoscopic	**Ø** Drainage Device **7** Autologous Tissue Substitute **J** Synthetic Substitute **K** Nonautologous Tissue Substitute **M** Stimulator Lead **Y** Other Device	**Z** No Qualifier
X Upper Muscle **Y** Lower Muscle	**X** External	**Ø** Drainage Device **7** Autologous Tissue Substitute **J** Synthetic Substitute **K** Nonautologous Tissue Substitute **M** Stimulator Lead	**Z** No Qualifier

Non-OR   ØKW[X,Y][3,4]YZ
Non-OR   ØKW[X,Y]X[Ø,7,J,K,M]Z

Muscles

Ø   **Medical and Surgical**
K   **Muscles**
X   **Transfer**   Definition: Moving, without taking out, all or a portion of a body part to another location to take over the function of all or a portion of a body part
                          Explanation: The body part transferred remains connected to its vascular and nervous supply

Body Part Character 4			Approach Character 5	Device Character 6	Qualifier Character 7
Ø **Head Muscle**	6 **Shoulder Muscle, Left**	P **Hip Muscle, Left**	Ø Open	Z No Device	Ø Skin
Auricularis muscle	*See 5 Shoulder Muscle,*	*See N Hip Muscle, Right*	4 Percutaneous		1 Subcutaneous
Masseter muscle	*Right*	Q **Upper Leg Muscle, Right**	Endoscopic		Tissue
Pterygoid muscle	7 **Upper Arm Muscle, Right**	Adductor brevis muscle			2 Skin and
Splenius capitis muscle	Biceps brachii muscle	Adductor longus muscle			Subcutaneous
Temporalis muscle	Brachialis muscle	Adductor magnus muscle			Tissue
Temporoparietalis muscle	Coracobrachialis muscle	Biceps femoris muscle			Z No Qualifier
1 **Facial Muscle**	Triceps brachii muscle	Gracilis muscle			
Buccinator muscle	8 **Upper Arm Muscle, Left**	Pectineus muscle			
Corrugator supercilii muscle	*See 7 Upper Arm Muscle,*	Quadriceps (femoris)			
Depressor anguli oris	*Right*	Rectus femoris muscle			
muscle	9 **Lower Arm and Wrist**	Sartorius muscle			
Depressor labii inferioris	**Muscle, Right**	Semimembranosus muscle			
muscle	Anatomical snuffbox	Semitendinosus muscle			
Depressor septi nasi	Brachioradialis muscle	Vastus intermedius muscle			
muscle	Extensor carpi radialis	Vastus lateralis muscle			
Depressor supercilii	muscle	Vastus medialis muscle			
muscle	Extensor carpi ulnaris	R **Upper Leg Muscle, Left**			
Levator anguli oris muscle	muscle	*See Q Upper Leg Muscle,*			
Levator labii superioris	Flexor carpi radialis	*Right*			
alaeque nasi muscle	muscle	S **Lower Leg Muscle,**			
Levator labii superioris	Flexor carpi ulnaris muscle	**Right**			
muscle	Flexor pollicis longus	Extensor digitorum longus			
Mentalis muscle	muscle	muscle			
Nasalis muscle	Palmaris longus muscle	Extensor hallucis longus			
Occipitofrontalis muscle	Pronator quadratus	muscle			
Orbicularis oris muscle	muscle	Fibularis brevis muscle			
Procerus muscle	Pronator teres muscle	Fibularis longus muscle			
Risorius muscle	B **Lower Arm and Wrist**	Flexor digitorum longus			
Zygomaticus muscle	**Muscle, Left**	muscle			
2 **Neck Muscle, Right**	*See 9 Lower Arm and Wrist*	Flexor hallucis longus			
Anterior vertebral muscle	*Muscle, Right*	muscle			
Arytenoid muscle	C **Hand Muscle, Right**	Gastrocnemius muscle			
Cricothyroid muscle	Hypothenar muscle	Peroneus brevis muscle			
Infrahyoid muscle	Palmar interosseous	Peroneus longus muscle			
Levator scapulae muscle	muscle	Popliteus muscle			
Platysma muscle	Thenar muscle	Soleus muscle			
Scalene muscle	D **Hand Muscle, Left**	Tibialis anterior muscle			
Splenius cervicis muscle	*See C Hand Muscle, Right*	Tibialis posterior muscle			
Sternocleidomastoid	H **Thorax Muscle, Right**	T **Lower Leg Muscle, Left**			
muscle	Intercostal muscle	*See S Lower Leg Muscle,*			
Suprahyoid muscle	Levatores costarum	*Right*			
Thyroarytenoid muscle	muscle	V **Foot Muscle, Right**			
3 **Neck Muscle, Left**	Pectoralis major muscle	Abductor hallucis muscle			
See 2 Neck Muscle, Right	Pectoralis minor muscle	Adductor hallucis muscle			
4 **Tongue, Palate, Pharynx**	Serratus anterior muscle	Extensor digitorum brevis			
Muscle	Subclavius muscle	muscle			
Chondroglossus muscle	Subcostal muscle	Extensor hallucis brevis			
Genioglossus muscle	Transverse thoracis	muscle			
Hyoglossus muscle	muscle	Flexor digitorum brevis			
Inferior longitudinal muscle	J **Thorax Muscle, Left**	muscle			
Levator veli palatini muscle	*See H Thorax Muscle, Right*	Flexor hallucis brevis			
Palatoglossal muscle	M **Perineum Muscle**	muscle			
Palatopharyngeal muscle	Bulbospongiosus muscle	Quadratus plantae muscle			
Pharyngeal constrictor	Cremaster muscle	W **Foot Muscle, Left**			
muscle	Deep transverse perineal	*See V Foot Muscle, Right*			
Salpingopharyngeus	muscle				
muscle	Ischiocavernosus muscle				
Styloglossus muscle	Levator ani muscle				
Stylopharyngeus muscle	Superficial transverse				
Superior longitudinal	perineal muscle				
muscle	N **Hip Muscle, Right**				
Tensor veli palatini muscle	Gemellus muscle				
5 **Shoulder Muscle, Right**	Gluteus maximus muscle				
Deltoid muscle	Gluteus medius muscle				
Infraspinatus muscle	Gluteus minimus muscle				
Subscapularis muscle	Iliacus muscle				
Supraspinatus muscle	Obturator muscle				
Teres major muscle	Piriformis muscle				
Teres minor muscle	Psoas muscle				
	Quadratus femoris muscle				
	Tensor fasciae latae muscle				

ØKX Continued on next page

Non-OR Procedure   DRG Non-OR Procedure   Valid OR Procedure   HAC Associated Procedure   Combination Only   New/Revised GREEN

Ø   Medical and Surgical   *ØKX Continued*
K   Muscles
X   Transfer   Definition: Moving, without taking out, all or a portion of a body part to another location to take over the function of all or a portion of a body part
                      Explanation: The body part transferred remains connected to its vascular and nervous supply

Body Part Character 4	Approach Character 5	Device Character 6	Qualifier Character 7
F Trunk Muscle, Right Coccygeus muscle Erector spinae muscle Interspinalis muscle Intertransversarius muscle Latissimus dorsi muscle Quadratus lumborum muscle Rhomboid major muscle Rhomboid minor muscle Serratus posterior muscle Transversospinalis muscle Trapezius muscle **G Trunk Muscle, Left** *See F Trunk Muscle, Right*	**Ø Open** **4 Percutaneous Endoscopic**	**Z No Device**	**Ø Skin** **1 Subcutaneous Tissue** **2 Skin and Subcutaneous Tissue** **5 Latissimus Dorsi Myocutaneous Flap** **7 Deep Inferior Epigastric Artery Perforator Flap** **8 Superficial Inferior Epigastric Artery Flap** **9 Gluteal Artery Perforator Flap** **Z No Qualifier**
K Abdomen Muscle, Right External oblique muscle Internal oblique muscle Pyramidalis muscle Rectus abdominis muscle Transversus abdominis muscle **L Abdomen Muscle, Left** *See K Abdomen Muscle, Right*	**Ø Open** **4 Percutaneous Endoscopic**	**Z No Device**	**Ø Skin** **1 Subcutaneous Tissue** **2 Skin and Subcutaneous Tissue** **6 Transverse Rectus Abdominis Myocutaneous Flap** **Z No Qualifier**

Tendons ØL2–ØLX

Character Meanings*

This Character Meaning table is provided as a guide to assist the user in the identification of character members that may be found in this section of code tables. It **SHOULD NOT** be used to build a PCS code.

Operation–Character 3	Body Part–Character 4	Approach–Character 5	Device–Character 6	Qualifier–Character 7
2 Change	Ø Head and Neck Tendon	Ø Open	Ø Drainage Device	X Diagnostic
5 Destruction	1 Shoulder Tendon, Right	3 Percutaneous	7 Autologous Tissue Substitute	Z No Qualifier
8 Division	2 Shoulder Tendon, Left	4 Percutaneous Endoscopic	J Synthetic Substitute	
9 Drainage	3 Upper Arm Tendon, Right	X External	K Nonautologous Tissue Substitute	
B Excision	4 Upper Arm Tendon, Left		Y Other Device	
C Extirpation	5 Lower Arm and Wrist Tendon, Right		Z No Device	
D Extraction	6 Lower Arm and Wrist Tendon, Left			
H Insertion	7 Hand Tendon, Right			
J Inspection	8 Hand Tendon, Left			
M Reattachment	9 Trunk Tendon, Right			
N Release	B Trunk Tendon, Left			
P Removal	C Thorax Tendon, Right			
Q Repair	D Thorax Tendon, Left			
R Replacement	F Abdomen Tendon, Right			
S Reposition	G Abdomen Tendon, Left			
T Resection	H Perineum Tendon			
U Supplement	J Hip Tendon, Right			
W Revision	K Hip Tendon, Left			
X Transfer	L Upper Leg Tendon, Right			
	M Upper Leg Tendon, Left			
	N Lower Leg Tendon, Right			
	P Lower Leg Tendon, Left			
	Q Knee Tendon, Right			
	R Knee Tendon, Left			
	S Ankle Tendon, Right			
	T Ankle Tendon, Left			
	V Foot Tendon, Right			
	W Foot Tendon, Left			
	X Upper Tendon			
	Y Lower Tendon			

* Includes synovial membrane.

AHA Coding Clinic for table ØL8
2016, 3Q, 30   Resection of femur with interposition arthroplasty

AHA Coding Clinic for table ØLB
2017, 2Q, 21   Arthroscopic anterior cruciate ligament revision using autograft with anterolateral ligament reconstruction
2015, 3Q, 26   Thumb arthroplasty with resection of trapezium
2014, 3Q, 14   Application of TheraSkin® and excisional debridement
2014, 3Q, 18   Placement of reverse sural fasciocutaneous pedicle flap

AHA Coding Clinic for table ØLD
2017, 4Q, 41   Extraction procedures

AHA Coding Clinic for table ØLQ
2016, 3Q, 32   Rotator cuff repair, tenodesis, decompression, acromioplasty and coracoplasty
2015, 2Q, 11   Repair of patellar and quadriceps tendons with allograft
2013, 3Q, 20   Superior labrum anterior posterior (SLAP) repair and subacromial decompression

AHA Coding Clinic for table ØLS
2016, 3Q, 32   Rotator cuff repair, tenodesis, decompression, acromioplasty and coracoplasty
2015, 3Q, 14   Endoprosthetic replacement of humerus and tendon reattachment

AHA Coding Clinic for table ØLU
2015, 2Q, 11   Repair of patellar and quadriceps tendons with allograft

Foot Tendons

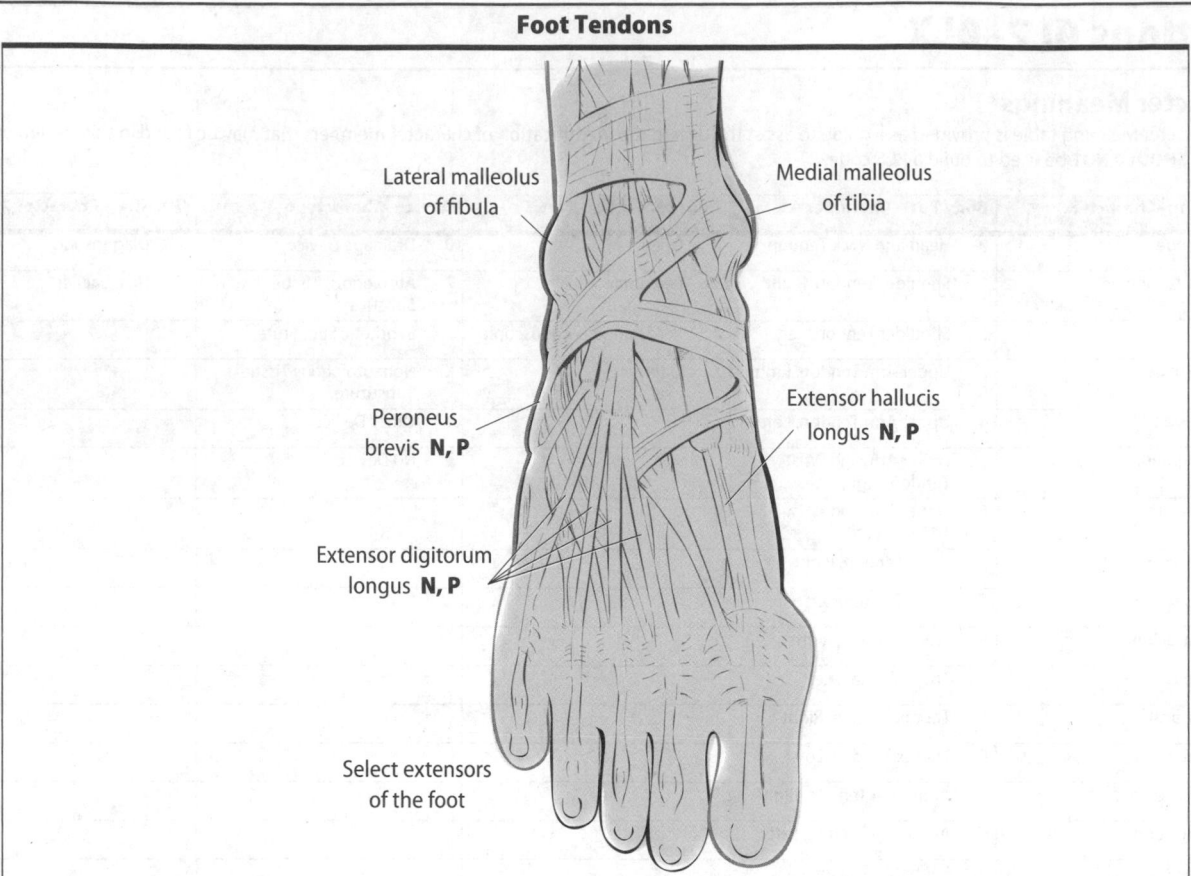

Lateral malleolus
of fibula

Medial malleolus
of tibia

Peroneus
brevis **N, P**

Extensor hallucis
longus **N, P**

Extensor digitorum
longus **N, P**

Select extensors
of the foot

Shoulder Tendons

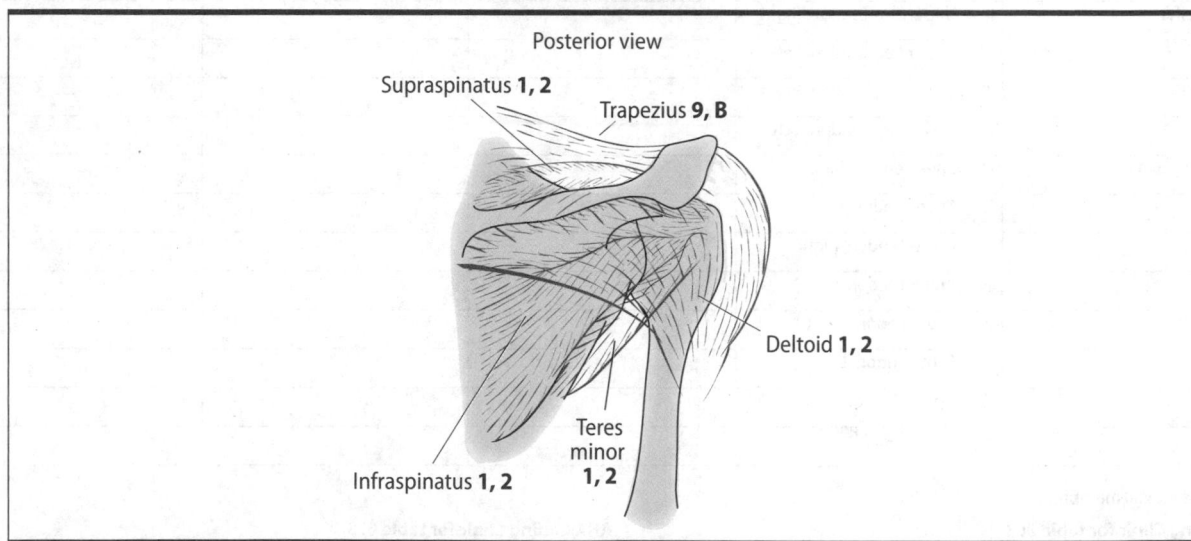

Posterior view

Supraspinatus **1, 2**

Trapezius **9, B**

Deltoid **1, 2**

Teres
minor
1, 2

Infraspinatus **1, 2**

Tendons of Wrist and Hand

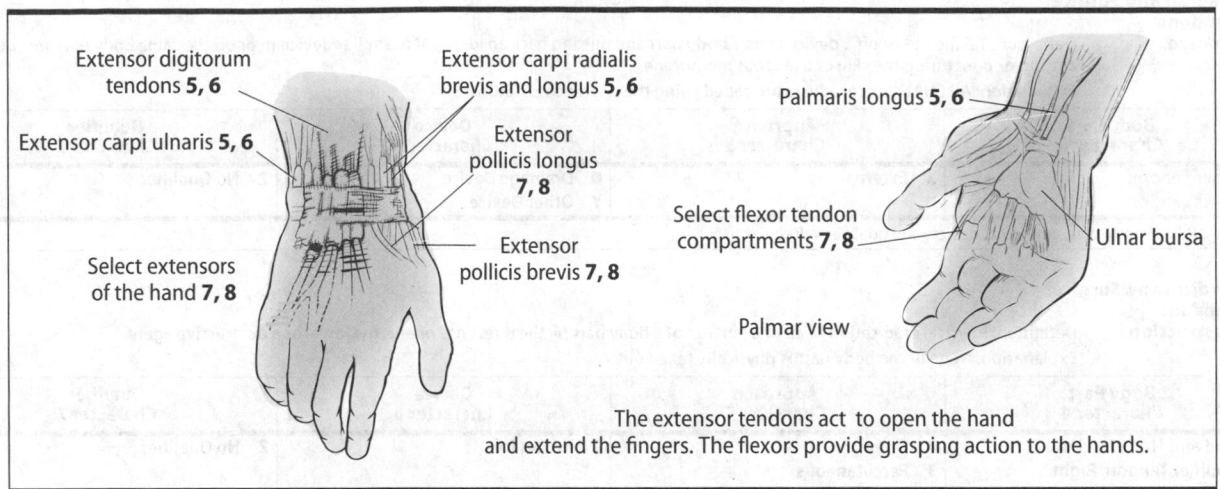

Extensor digitorum tendons **5, 6**

Extensor carpi ulnaris **5, 6**

Select extensors of the hand **7, 8**

Extensor carpi radialis brevis and longus **5, 6**

Extensor pollicis longus **7, 8**

Extensor pollicis brevis **7, 8**

Palmaris longus **5, 6**

Select flexor tendon compartments **7, 8**

Ulnar bursa

Palmar view

The extensor tendons act to open the hand and extend the fingers. The flexors provide grasping action to the hands.

Leg Muscles and Tendons

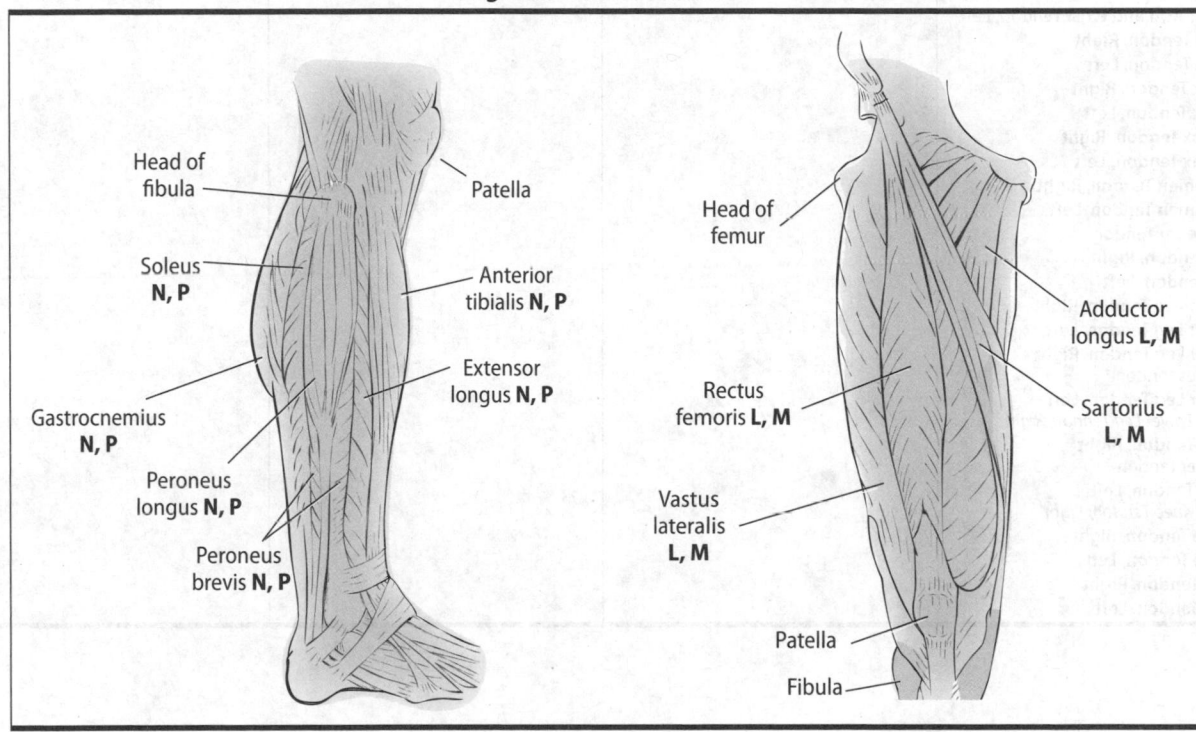

Head of fibula

Patella

Soleus **N, P**

Anterior tibialis **N, P**

Extensor longus **N, P**

Gastrocnemius **N, P**

Peroneus longus **N, P**

Peroneus brevis **N, P**

Head of femur

Adductor longus **L, M**

Rectus femoris **L, M**

Sartorius **L, M**

Vastus lateralis **L, M**

Patella

Fibula

Tendons

Ø   **Medical and Surgical**
L   **Tendons**
2   **Change**   Definition: Taking out or off a device from a body part and putting back an identical or similar device in or on the same body part without cutting or puncturing the skin or a mucous membrane
                       Explanation: All CHANGE procedures are coded using the approach EXTERNAL

Body Part Character 4	Approach Character 5	Device Character 6	Qualifier Character 7
X Upper Tendon Y Lower Tendon	X External	Ø Drainage Device Y Other Device	Z No Qualifier

Non-OR	All body part, approach, device, and qualifier values

Ø   **Medical and Surgical**
L   **Tendons**
5   **Destruction**   Definition: Physical eradication of all or a portion of a body part by the direct use of energy, force, or a destructive agent
                          Explanation: None of the body part is physically taken out

Body Part Character 4	Approach Character 5	Device Character 6	Qualifier Character 7

Ø   Head and Neck Tendon
1   Shoulder Tendon, Right
2   Shoulder Tendon, Left
3   Upper Arm Tendon, Right
4   Upper Arm Tendon, Left
5   Lower Arm and Wrist Tendon, Right
6   Lower Arm and Wrist Tendon, Left
7   Hand Tendon, Right
8   Hand Tendon, Left
9   Trunk Tendon, Right
B   Trunk Tendon, Left
C   Thorax Tendon, Right
D   Thorax Tendon, Left
F   Abdomen Tendon, Right
G   Abdomen Tendon, Left
H   Perineum Tendon
J   Hip Tendon, Right
K   Hip Tendon, Left
L   Upper Leg Tendon, Right
M   Upper Leg Tendon, Left
N   Lower Leg Tendon, Right
     Achilles tendon
P   Lower Leg Tendon, Left
     See N Lower Leg Tendon, Right
Q   Knee Tendon, Right
     Patellar tendon
R   Knee Tendon, Left
     See Q Knee Tendon, Right
S   Ankle Tendon, Right
T   Ankle Tendon, Left
V   Foot Tendon, Right
W   Foot Tendon, Left
	Ø Open
	3 Percutaneous
	4 Percutaneous Endoscopic
		Z No Device	Z No Qualifier

Ø   **Medical and Surgical**
L   **Tendons**
8   **Division**   Definition: Cutting into a body part, without draining fluids and/or gases from the body part, in order to separate or transect a body part
                      Explanation: All or a portion of the body part is separated into two or more portions

Body Part Character 4	Approach Character 5	Device Character 6	Qualifier Character 7

Ø   Head and Neck Tendon
1   Shoulder Tendon, Right
2   Shoulder Tendon, Left
3   Upper Arm Tendon, Right
4   Upper Arm Tendon, Left
5   Lower Arm and Wrist Tendon, Right
6   Lower Arm and Wrist Tendon, Left
7   Hand Tendon, Right
8   Hand Tendon, Left
9   Trunk Tendon, Right
B   Trunk Tendon, Left
C   Thorax Tendon, Right
D   Thorax Tendon, Left
F   Abdomen Tendon, Right
G   Abdomen Tendon, Left
H   Perineum Tendon
J   Hip Tendon, Right
K   Hip Tendon, Left
L   Upper Leg Tendon, Right
M   Upper Leg Tendon, Left
N   Lower Leg Tendon, Right
      Achilles tendon
P   Lower Leg Tendon, Left
      See N Lower Leg Tendon, Right
Q   Knee Tendon, Right
      Patellar tendon
R   Knee Tendon, Left
      See Q Knee Tendon, Right
S   Ankle Tendon, Right
T   Ankle Tendon, Left
V   Foot Tendon, Right
W   Foot Tendon, Left
	Ø Open
	3 Percutaneous
	4 Percutaneous Endoscopic
		Z No Device	Z No Qualifier

Ø   **Medical and Surgical**
L   **Tendons**
9   **Drainage**   Definition: Taking or letting out fluids and/or gases from a body part
                     Explanation: The qualifier DIAGNOSTIC is used to identify drainage procedures that are biopsies

Body Part Character 4	Approach Character 5	Device Character 6	Qualifier Character 7

Ø Head and Neck Tendon
1 Shoulder Tendon, Right
2 Shoulder Tendon, Left
3 Upper Arm Tendon, Right
4 Upper Arm Tendon, Left
5 Lower Arm and Wrist Tendon, Right
6 Lower Arm and Wrist Tendon, Left
7 Hand Tendon, Right
8 Hand Tendon, Left
9 Trunk Tendon, Right
B Trunk Tendon, Left
C Thorax Tendon, Right
D Thorax Tendon, Left
F Abdomen Tendon, Right
G Abdomen Tendon, Left
H Perineum Tendon
J Hip Tendon, Right
K Hip Tendon, Left
L Upper Leg Tendon, Right
M Upper Leg Tendon, Left
N Lower Leg Tendon, Right
    Achilles tendon
P Lower Leg Tendon, Left
    See N Lower Leg Tendon, Right
Q Knee Tendon, Right
    Patellar tendon
R Knee Tendon, Left
    See Q Knee Tendon, Right
S Ankle Tendon, Right
T Ankle Tendon, Left
V Foot Tendon, Right
W Foot Tendon, Left
	Ø Open
	3 Percutaneous
	4 Percutaneous Endoscopic
		Ø Drainage Device	**Z** No Qualifier

Ø Head and Neck Tendon
1 Shoulder Tendon, Right
2 Shoulder Tendon, Left
3 Upper Arm Tendon, Right
4 Upper Arm Tendon, Left
5 Lower Arm and Wrist Tendon, Right
6 Lower Arm and Wrist Tendon, Left
7 Hand Tendon, Right
8 Hand Tendon, Left
9 Trunk Tendon, Right
B Trunk Tendon, Left
C Thorax Tendon, Right
D Thorax Tendon, Left
F Abdomen Tendon, Right
G Abdomen Tendon, Left
H Perineum Tendon
J Hip Tendon, Right
K Hip Tendon, Left
L Upper Leg Tendon, Right
M Upper Leg Tendon, Left
N Lower Leg Tendon, Right
    Achilles tendon
P Lower Leg Tendon, Left
    See N Lower Leg Tendon, Right
Q Knee Tendon, Right
    Patellar tendon
R Knee Tendon, Left
    See Q Knee Tendon, Right
S Ankle Tendon, Right
T Ankle Tendon, Left
V Foot Tendon, Right
W Foot Tendon, Left
	Ø Open
	3 Percutaneous
	4 Percutaneous Endoscopic
		Z No Device	**X** Diagnostic
			Z No Qualifier

Non-OR   ØL9[Ø,1,2,3,4,5,6,7,8,9,B,C,D,F,G,H,J,K,L,M,N,P,Q,R,S,T,V,W]3ØZ
Non-OR   ØL9[Ø,1,2,3,4,5,6,7,8,9,B,C,D,F,G,H,J,K,L,M,N,P,Q,R,S,T,V,W]3ZZ

Non-OR   ØL9[7,8]4ZZ

Non-OR Procedure   DRG Non-OR Procedure   Valid OR Procedure   HAC Associated Procedure   Combination Only   New/Revised GREEN

Ø   Medical and Surgical
L   Tendons
B   Excision   Definition: Cutting out or off, without replacement, a portion of a body part
                Explanation: The qualifier DIAGNOSTIC is used to identify excision procedures that are biopsies

Body Part Character 4	Approach Character 5	Device Character 6	Qualifier Character 7

Ø Head and Neck Tendon
1 Shoulder Tendon, Right
2 Shoulder Tendon, Left
3 Upper Arm Tendon, Right
4 Upper Arm Tendon, Left
5 Lower Arm and Wrist Tendon, Right
6 Lower Arm and Wrist Tendon, Left
7 Hand Tendon, Right
8 Hand Tendon, Left
9 Trunk Tendon, Right
B Trunk Tendon, Left
C Thorax Tendon, Right
D Thorax Tendon, Left
F Abdomen Tendon, Right
G Abdomen Tendon, Left
H Perineum Tendon
J Hip Tendon, Right
K Hip Tendon, Left
L Upper Leg Tendon, Right
M Upper Leg Tendon, Left
N Lower Leg Tendon, Right
    Achilles tendon
P Lower Leg Tendon, Left
    See N Lower Leg Tendon, Right
Q Knee Tendon, Right
    Patellar tendon
R Knee Tendon, Left
    See Q Knee Tendon, Right
S Ankle Tendon, Right
T Ankle Tendon, Left
V Foot Tendon, Right
W Foot Tendon, Left
	Ø Open
	3 Percutaneous
	4 Percutaneous Endoscopic
		Z No Device	X Diagnostic
			Z No Qualifier

NC Noncovered Procedure   LC Limited Coverage   QA Questionable OB Admit   NT New Tech Add-on   ⊞ Combination Member   ♂ Male   ♀ Female

ICD-10-PCS 2022   491

Ø **Medical and Surgical**
L **Tendons**
C **Extirpation** Definition: Taking or cutting out solid matter from a body part

Explanation: The solid matter may be an abnormal byproduct of a biological function or a foreign body; it may be imbedded in a body part or in the lumen of a tubular body part. The solid matter may or may not have been previously broken into pieces.

Body Part Character 4	Approach Character 5	Device Character 6	Qualifier Character 7
Ø Head and Neck Tendon	**Ø** Open	**Z** No Device	**Z** No Qualifier
1 Shoulder Tendon, Right	**3** Percutaneous		
2 Shoulder Tendon, Left	**4** Percutaneous Endoscopic		
3 Upper Arm Tendon, Right			
4 Upper Arm Tendon, Left			
5 Lower Arm and Wrist Tendon, Right			
6 Lower Arm and Wrist Tendon, Left			
7 Hand Tendon, Right			
8 Hand Tendon, Left			
9 Trunk Tendon, Right			
B Trunk Tendon, Left			
C Thorax Tendon, Right			
D Thorax Tendon, Left			
F Abdomen Tendon, Right			
G Abdomen Tendon, Left			
H Perineum Tendon			
J Hip Tendon, Right			
K Hip Tendon, Left			
L Upper Leg Tendon, Right			
M Upper Leg Tendon, Left			
N Lower Leg Tendon, Right Achilles tendon			
P Lower Leg Tendon, Left See N Lower Leg Tendon, Right			
Q Knee Tendon, Right Patellar tendon			
R Knee Tendon, Left See Q Knee Tendon, Right			
S Ankle Tendon, Right			
T Ankle Tendon, Left			
V Foot Tendon, Right			
W Foot Tendon, Left			

Ø   **Medical and Surgical**
L   **Tendons**
D   **Extraction**   Definition: Pulling or stripping out or off all or a portion of a body part by the use of force

                           Explanation: The qualifier DIAGNOSTIC is used to identify extraction procedures that are biopsies

Body Part Character 4	Approach Character 5	Device Character 6	Qualifier Character 7

Ø Head and Neck Tendon
1 Shoulder Tendon, Right
2 Shoulder Tendon, Left
3 Upper Arm Tendon, Right
4 Upper Arm Tendon, Left
5 Lower Arm and Wrist Tendon, Right
6 Lower Arm and Wrist Tendon, Left
7 Hand Tendon, Right
8 Hand Tendon, Left
9 Trunk Tendon, Right
B Trunk Tendon, Left
C Thorax Tendon, Right
D Thorax Tendon, Left
F Abdomen Tendon, Right
G Abdomen Tendon, Left
H Perineum Tendon
J Hip Tendon, Right
K Hip Tendon, Left
L Upper Leg Tendon, Right
M Upper Leg Tendon, Left
N Lower Leg Tendon, Right
    Achilles tendon
P Lower Leg Tendon, Left
    See N Lower Leg Tendon, Right
Q Knee Tendon, Right
    Patellar tendon
R Knee Tendon, Left
    See Q Knee Tendon, Right
S Ankle Tendon, Right
T Ankle Tendon, Left
V Foot Tendon, Right
W Foot Tendon, Left
	Ø Open	**Z** No Device	**Z** No Qualifier

Ø   **Medical and Surgical**
L   **Tendons**
H   **Insertion**   Definition: Putting in a nonbiological appliance that monitors, assists, performs, or prevents a physiological function but does not physically take the place of a body part

                           Explanation: None

Body Part Character 4	Approach Character 5	Device Character 6	Qualifier Character 7
X Upper Tendon **Y** Lower Tendon	**Ø** Open **3** Percutaneous **4** Percutaneous Endoscopic	**Y** Other Device	**Z** No Qualifier

Non-OR   ØLH[X,Y][3,4]YZ

Ø   **Medical and Surgical**
L   **Tendons**
J   **Inspection**   Definition: Visually and/or manually exploring a body part

                           Explanation: Visual exploration may be performed with or without optical instrumentation. Manual exploration may be performed directly or through intervening body layers.

Body Part Character 4	Approach Character 5	Device Character 6	Qualifier Character 7
X Upper Tendon **Y** Lower Tendon	**Ø** Open **3** Percutaneous **4** Percutaneous Endoscopic **X** External	**Z** No Device	**Z** No Qualifier

Non-OR   ØLJ[X,Y][3,X]ZZ

NC Noncovered Procedure   **LC** Limited Coverage   **QA** Questionable OB Admit   **NT** New Tech Add-on   ⊞ Combination Member   ♂ Male   ♀ Female

ICD-10-PCS 2022   493

ØLD–ØLJ

Ø Medical and Surgical
L Tendons
M Reattachment Definition: Putting back in or on all or a portion of a separated body part to its normal location or other suitable location

Explanation: Vascular circulation and nervous pathways may or may not be reestablished

Body Part Character 4	Approach Character 5	Device Character 6	Qualifier Character 7
Ø Head and Neck Tendon	Ø Open	Z No Device	Z No Qualifier
1 Shoulder Tendon, Right	4 Percutaneous Endoscopic		
2 Shoulder Tendon, Left			
3 Upper Arm Tendon, Right			
4 Upper Arm Tendon, Left			
5 Lower Arm and Wrist Tendon, Right			
6 Lower Arm and Wrist Tendon, Left			
7 Hand Tendon, Right			
8 Hand Tendon, Left			
9 Trunk Tendon, Right			
B Trunk Tendon, Left			
C Thorax Tendon, Right			
D Thorax Tendon, Left			
F Abdomen Tendon, Right			
G Abdomen Tendon, Left			
H Perineum Tendon			
J Hip Tendon, Right			
K Hip Tendon, Left			
L Upper Leg Tendon, Right			
M Upper Leg Tendon, Left			
N Lower Leg Tendon, Right Achilles tendon			
P Lower Leg Tendon, Left See N Lower Leg Tendon, Right			
Q Knee Tendon, Right Patellar tendon			
R Knee Tendon, Left See Q Knee Tendon, Right			
S Ankle Tendon, Right			
T Ankle Tendon, Left			
V Foot Tendon, Right			
W Foot Tendon, Left			

Ø Medical and Surgical
L Tendons
N Release Definition: Freeing a body part from an abnormal physical constraint by cutting or by the use of force

Explanation: Some of the restraining tissue may be taken out but none of the body part is taken out

Body Part Character 4	Approach Character 5	Device Character 6	Qualifier Character 7
Ø Head and Neck Tendon	Ø Open	Z No Device	Z No Qualifier
1 Shoulder Tendon, Right	3 Percutaneous		
2 Shoulder Tendon, Left	4 Percutaneous Endoscopic		
3 Upper Arm Tendon, Right	X External		
4 Upper Arm Tendon, Left			
5 Lower Arm and Wrist Tendon, Right			
6 Lower Arm and Wrist Tendon, Left			
7 Hand Tendon, Right			
8 Hand Tendon, Left			
9 Trunk Tendon, Right			
B Trunk Tendon, Left			
C Thorax Tendon, Right			
D Thorax Tendon, Left			
F Abdomen Tendon, Right			
G Abdomen Tendon, Left			
H Perineum Tendon			
J Hip Tendon, Right			
K Hip Tendon, Left			
L Upper Leg Tendon, Right			
M Upper Leg Tendon, Left			
N Lower Leg Tendon, Right Achilles tendon			
P Lower Leg Tendon, Left See N Lower Leg Tendon, Right			
Q Knee Tendon, Right Patellar tendon			
R Knee Tendon, Left See Q Knee Tendon, Right			
S Ankle Tendon, Right			
T Ankle Tendon, Left			
V Foot Tendon, Right			
W Foot Tendon, Left			

Non-OR ØLN[Ø,1,2,3,4,5,6,7,8,9,B,C,D,F,G,H,J,K,L,M,N,P,Q,R,S,T,V,W]XZZ

Ø   Medical and Surgical
L   Tendons
P   Removal   Definition: Taking out or off a device from a body part

Explanation: If a device is taken out and a similar device put in without cutting or puncturing the skin or mucous membrane, the procedure is coded to the root operation CHANGE. Otherwise, the procedure for taking out a device is coded to the root operation REMOVAL.

Body Part Character 4	Approach Character 5	Device Character 6	Qualifier Character 7
X Upper Tendon Y Lower Tendon	Ø Open 3 Percutaneous 4 Percutaneous Endoscopic	Ø Drainage Device 7 Autologous Tissue Substitute J Synthetic Substitute K Nonautologous Tissue Substitute Y Other Device	Z No Qualifier
X Upper Tendon Y Lower Tendon	X External	Ø Drainage Device	Z No Qualifier

Non-OR   ØLP[X,Y]3ØZ
Non-OR   ØLP[X,Y][3,4]YZ
Non-OR   ØLP[X,Y]XØZ

Ø   Medical and Surgical
L   Tendons
Q   Repair   Definition: Restoring, to the extent possible, a body part to its normal anatomic structure and function

Explanation: Used only when the method to accomplish the repair is not one of the other root operations

Body Part Character 4	Approach Character 5	Device Character 6	Qualifier Character 7

Ø   Head and Neck Tendon
1   Shoulder Tendon, Right
2   Shoulder Tendon, Left
3   Upper Arm Tendon, Right
4   Upper Arm Tendon, Left
5   Lower Arm and Wrist Tendon, Right
6   Lower Arm and Wrist Tendon, Left
7   Hand Tendon, Right
8   Hand Tendon, Left
9   Trunk Tendon, Right
B   Trunk Tendon, Left
C   Thorax Tendon, Right
D   Thorax Tendon, Left
F   Abdomen Tendon, Right
G   Abdomen Tendon, Left
H   Perineum Tendon
J   Hip Tendon, Right
K   Hip Tendon, Left
L   Upper Leg Tendon, Right
M   Upper Leg Tendon, Left
N   Lower Leg Tendon, Right
     Achilles tendon
P   Lower Leg Tendon, Left
     See N Lower Leg Tendon, Right
Q   Knee Tendon, Right
     Patellar tendon
R   Knee Tendon, Left
     See Q Knee Tendon, Right
S   Ankle Tendon, Right
T   Ankle Tendon, Left
V   Foot Tendon, Right
W   Foot Tendon, Left
	Ø Open
	3 Percutaneous
	4 Percutaneous Endoscopic
		Z No Device	Z No Qualifier

NC Noncovered Procedure   LC Limited Coverage   QA Questionable OB Admit   NT New Tech Add-on   ⊞ Combination Member   ♂ Male   ♀ Female

ICD-10-PCS 2022   495

ØLP–ØLQ

Ø **Medical and Surgical**
L **Tendons**
R **Replacement**   Definition: Putting in or on biological or synthetic material that physically takes the place and/or function of all or a portion of a body part
Explanation: The body part may have been taken out or replaced, or may be taken out, physically eradicated, or rendered nonfunctional during the REPLACEMENT procedure. A REMOVAL procedure is coded for taking out the device used in a previous replacement procedure.

Body Part Character 4	Approach Character 5	Device Character 6	Qualifier Character 7

Ø Head and Neck Tendon
1 Shoulder Tendon, Right
2 Shoulder Tendon, Left
3 Upper Arm Tendon, Right
4 Upper Arm Tendon, Left
5 Lower Arm and Wrist Tendon, Right
6 Lower Arm and Wrist Tendon, Left
7 Hand Tendon, Right
8 Hand Tendon, Left
9 Trunk Tendon, Right
B Trunk Tendon, Left
C Thorax Tendon, Right
D Thorax Tendon, Left
F Abdomen Tendon, Right
G Abdomen Tendon, Left
H Perineum Tendon
J Hip Tendon, Right
K Hip Tendon, Left
L Upper Leg Tendon, Right
M Upper Leg Tendon, Left
N Lower Leg Tendon, Right
    Achilles tendon
P Lower Leg Tendon, Left
    See N Lower Leg Tendon, Right
Q Knee Tendon, Right
    Patellar tendon
R Knee Tendon, Left
    See Q Knee Tendon, Right
S Ankle Tendon, Right
T Ankle Tendon, Left
V Foot Tendon, Right
W Foot Tendon, Left
	Ø Open
	4 Percutaneous Endoscopic
		7 Autologous Tissue Substitute
		J Synthetic Substitute
		K Nonautologous Tissue Substitute
			Z No Qualifier

Ø **Medical and Surgical**
L **Tendons**
S **Reposition**   Definition: Moving to its normal location, or other suitable location, all or a portion of a body part
Explanation: The body part is moved to a new location from an abnormal location, or from a normal location where it is not functioning correctly. The body part may or may not be cut out or off to be moved to the new location.

Body Part Character 4	Approach Character 5	Device Character 6	Qualifier Character 7

Ø Head and Neck Tendon
1 Shoulder Tendon, Right
2 Shoulder Tendon, Left
3 Upper Arm Tendon, Right
4 Upper Arm Tendon, Left
5 Lower Arm and Wrist Tendon, Right
6 Lower Arm and Wrist Tendon, Left
7 Hand Tendon, Right
8 Hand Tendon, Left
9 Trunk Tendon, Right
B Trunk Tendon, Left
C Thorax Tendon, Right
D Thorax Tendon, Left
F Abdomen Tendon, Right
G Abdomen Tendon, Left
H Perineum Tendon
J Hip Tendon, Right
K Hip Tendon, Left
L Upper Leg Tendon, Right
M Upper Leg Tendon, Left
N Lower Leg Tendon, Right
    Achilles tendon
P Lower Leg Tendon, Left
    See N Lower Leg Tendon, Right
Q Knee Tendon, Right
    Patellar tendon
R Knee Tendon, Left
    See Q Knee Tendon, Right
S Ankle Tendon, Right
T Ankle Tendon, Left
V Foot Tendon, Right
W Foot Tendon, Left
	Ø Open
	4 Percutaneous Endoscopic
		Z No Device	**Z** No Qualifier

Non-OR Procedure   DRG Non-OR Procedure   Valid OR Procedure   HAC Associated Procedure   Combination Only   New/Revised GREEN

Tendons

Ø   **Medical and Surgical**
L   **Tendons**
T   **Resection**   Definition: Cutting out or off, without replacement, all of a body part
               Explanation: None

Body Part Character 4	Approach Character 5	Device Character 6	Qualifier Character 7

Ø Head and Neck Tendon
1 Shoulder Tendon, Right
2 Shoulder Tendon, Left
3 Upper Arm Tendon, Right
4 Upper Arm Tendon, Left
5 Lower Arm and Wrist Tendon, Right
6 Lower Arm and Wrist Tendon, Left
7 Hand Tendon, Right
8 Hand Tendon, Left
9 Trunk Tendon, Right
B Trunk Tendon, Left
C Thorax Tendon, Right
D Thorax Tendon, Left
F Abdomen Tendon, Right
G Abdomen Tendon, Left
H Perineum Tendon
J Hip Tendon, Right
K Hip Tendon, Left
L Upper Leg Tendon, Right
M Upper Leg Tendon, Left
N Lower Leg Tendon, Right
    Achilles tendon
P Lower Leg Tendon, Left
    See N Lower Leg Tendon, Right
Q Knee Tendon, Right
    Patellar tendon
R Knee Tendon, Left
    See Q Knee Tendon, Right
S Ankle Tendon, Right
T Ankle Tendon, Left
V Foot Tendon, Right
W Foot Tendon, Left
	Ø Open
	4 Percutaneous Endoscopic
		Z No Device	Z No Qualifier

Ø   **Medical and Surgical**
L   **Tendons**
U   **Supplement**   Definition: Putting in or on biological or synthetic material that physically reinforces and/or augments the function of a portion of a body part
               Explanation: The biological material is non-living, or is living and from the same individual. The body part may have been previously replaced, and the SUPPLEMENT procedure is performed to physically reinforce and/or augment the function of the replaced body part.

Body Part Character 4	Approach Character 5	Device Character 6	Qualifier Character 7

Ø Head and Neck Tendon
1 Shoulder Tendon, Right
2 Shoulder Tendon, Left
3 Upper Arm Tendon, Right
4 Upper Arm Tendon, Left
5 Lower Arm and Wrist Tendon, Right
6 Lower Arm and Wrist Tendon, Left
7 Hand Tendon, Right
8 Hand Tendon, Left
9 Trunk Tendon, Right
B Trunk Tendon, Left
C Thorax Tendon, Right
D Thorax Tendon, Left
F Abdomen Tendon, Right
G Abdomen Tendon, Left
H Perineum Tendon
J Hip Tendon, Right
K Hip Tendon, Left
L Upper Leg Tendon, Right
M Upper Leg Tendon, Left
N Lower Leg Tendon, Right
    Achilles tendon
P Lower Leg Tendon, Left
    See N Lower Leg Tendon, Right
Q Knee Tendon, Right
    Patellar tendon
R Knee Tendon, Left
    See Q Knee Tendon, Right
S Ankle Tendon, Right
T Ankle Tendon, Left
V Foot Tendon, Right
W Foot Tendon, Left
	Ø Open
	4 Percutaneous Endoscopic
		7 Autologous Tissue Substitute
		J Synthetic Substitute
		K Nonautologous Tissue Substitute
			Z No Qualifier

NC Noncovered Procedure   **LC** Limited Coverage   **QA** Questionable OB Admit   **NT** New Tech Add-on   ✚ Combination Member   ♂ Male   ♀ Female

Ø　Medical and Surgical
L　Tendons
W　Revision　　　Definition: Correcting, to the extent possible, a portion of a malfunctioning device or the position of a displaced device

　　　Explanation: Revision can include correcting a malfunctioning or displaced device by taking out or putting in components of the device such as a screw or pin

Body Part Character 4	Approach Character 5	Device Character 6	Qualifier Character 7
X　Upper Tendon Y　Lower Tendon	Ø　Open 3　Percutaneous 4　Percutaneous Endoscopic	Ø　Drainage Device 7　Autologous Tissue Substitute J　Synthetic Substitute K　Nonautologous Tissue Substitute Y　Other Device	Z　No Qualifier
X　Upper Tendon Y　Lower Tendon	X　External	Ø　Drainage Device 7　Autologous Tissue Substitute J　Synthetic Substitute K　Nonautologous Tissue Substitute	Z　No Qualifier

Non-OR　ØLW[X,Y][3,4]YZ
Non-OR　ØLW[X,Y]X[Ø,7,J,K]Z

Ø　Medical and Surgical
L　Tendons
X　Transfer　　　Definition: Moving, without taking out, all or a portion of a body part to another location to take over the function of all or a portion of a body part

　　　Explanation: The body part transferred remains connected to its vascular and nervous supply

Body Part Character 4	Approach Character 5	Device Character 6	Qualifier Character 7
Ø　Head and Neck Tendon 1　Shoulder Tendon, Right 2　Shoulder Tendon, Left 3　Upper Arm Tendon, Right 4　Upper Arm Tendon, Left 5　Lower Arm and Wrist Tendon, Right 6　Lower Arm and Wrist Tendon, Left 7　Hand Tendon, Right 8　Hand Tendon, Left 9　Trunk Tendon, Right B　Trunk Tendon, Left C　Thorax Tendon, Right D　Thorax Tendon, Left F　Abdomen Tendon, Right G　Abdomen Tendon, Left H　Perineum Tendon J　Hip Tendon, Right K　Hip Tendon, Left L　Upper Leg Tendon, Right M　Upper Leg Tendon, Left N　Lower Leg Tendon, Right 　　Achilles tendon P　Lower Leg Tendon, Left 　　*See N Lower Leg Tendon, Right* Q　Knee Tendon, Right 　　Patellar tendon R　Knee Tendon, Left 　　*See Q Knee Tendon, Right* S　Ankle Tendon, Right T　Ankle Tendon, Left V　Foot Tendon, Right W　Foot Tendon, Left	Ø　Open 4　Percutaneous Endoscopic	Z　No Device	Z　No Qualifier

Non-OR Procedure　　　DRG Non-OR Procedure　　　Valid OR Procedure　　　HAC Associated Procedure　　　Combination Only　　　New/Revised GREEN

Bursae and Ligaments ØM2–ØMX

Character Meanings*

This Character Meaning table is provided as a guide to assist the user in the identification of character members that may be found in this section of code tables. It **SHOULD NOT** be used to build a PCS code.

Operation–Character 3		Body Part–Character 4		Approach–Character 5		Device–Character 6		Qualifier–Character 7	
2	Change	Ø	Head and Neck Bursa and Ligament	Ø	Open	Ø	Drainage Device	X	Diagnostic
5	Destruction	1	Shoulder Bursa and Ligament, Right	3	Percutaneous	7	Autologous Tissue Substitute	Z	No Qualifier
8	Division	2	Shoulder Bursa and Ligament, Left	4	Percutaneous Endoscopic	J	Synthetic Substitute		
9	Drainage	3	Elbow Bursa and Ligament, Right	X	External	K	Nonautologous Tissue Substitute		
B	Excision	4	Elbow Bursa and Ligament, Left			Y	Other Device		
C	Extirpation	5	Wrist Bursa and Ligament, Right			Z	No Device		
D	Extraction	6	Wrist Bursa and Ligament, Left						
H	Insertion	7	Hand Bursa and Ligament, Right						
J	Inspection	8	Hand Bursa and Ligament, Left						
M	Reattachment	9	Upper Extremity Bursa and Ligament, Right						
N	Release	B	Upper Extremity Bursa and Ligament, Left						
P	Removal	C	Upper Spine Bursa and Ligament						
Q	Repair	D	Lower Spine Bursa and Ligament						
R	Replacement	F	Sternum Bursa and Ligament						
S	Reposition	G	Rib(s) Bursa and Ligament						
T	Resection	H	Abdomen Bursa and Ligament, Right						
U	Supplement	J	Abdomen Bursa and Ligament, Left						
W	Revision	K	Perineum Bursa and Ligament						
X	Transfer	L	Hip Bursa and Ligament, Right						
		M	Hip Bursa and Ligament, Left						
		N	Knee Bursa and Ligament, Right						
		P	Knee Bursa and Ligament, Left						
		Q	Ankle Bursa and Ligament, Right						
		R	Ankle Bursa and Ligament, Left						
		S	Foot Bursa and Ligament, Right						
		T	Foot Bursa and Ligament, Left						
		V	Lower Extremity Bursa and Ligament, Right						
		W	Lower Extremity Bursa and Ligament, Left						
		X	Upper Bursa and Ligament						
		Y	Lower Bursa and Ligament						

* Includes synovial membrane.

AHA Coding Clinic for table ØMB
2018, 3Q, 17   Excisional debridement of periosteum

AHA Coding Clinic for table ØMM
2013, 3Q, 20   Superior labrum anterior posterior (SLAP) repair and subacromial decompression

AHA Coding Clinic for table ØMQ
2014, 3Q, 9   Interspinous ligamentoplasty

AHA Coding Clinic for table ØMT
2017, 2Q, 21   Arthroscopic anterior cruciate ligament revision using autograft with anterolateral ligament reconstruction

AHA Coding Clinic for table ØMU
2017, 2Q, 21   Arthroscopic anterior cruciate ligament revision using autograft with anterolateral ligament reconstruction

Shoulder Ligaments

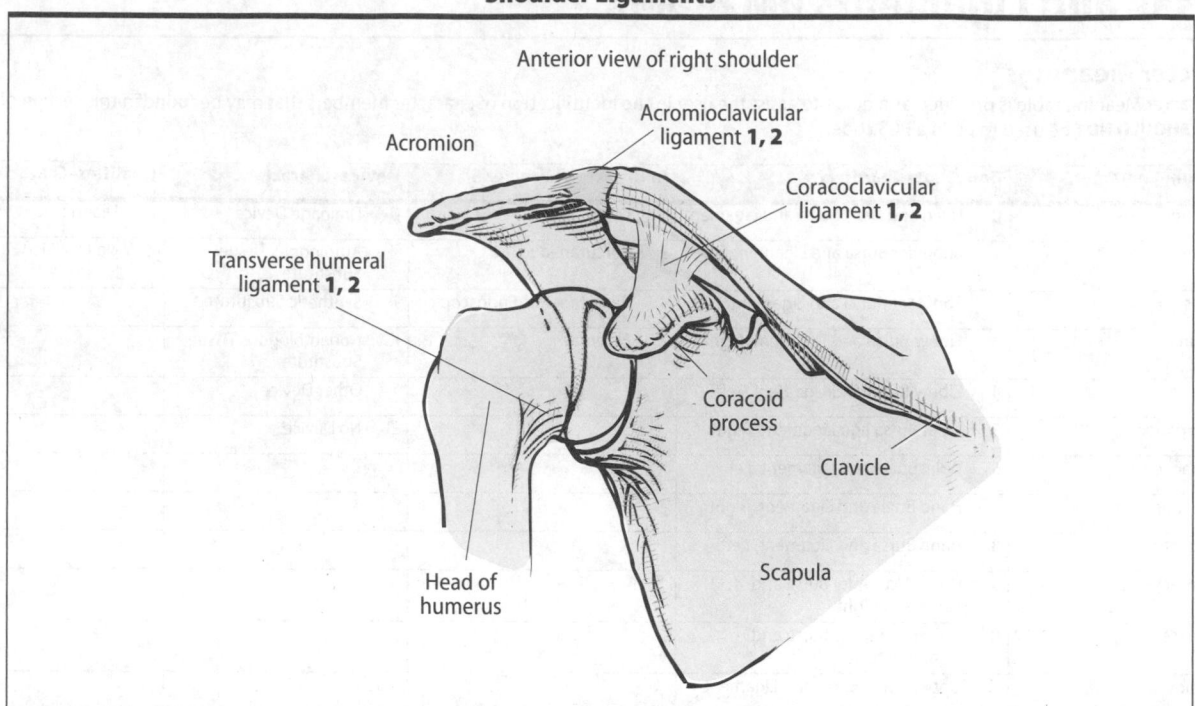

Anterior view of right shoulder

Acromion

Acromioclavicular ligament **1, 2**

Coracoclavicular ligament **1, 2**

Transverse humeral ligament **1, 2**

Coracoid process

Clavicle

Head of humerus

Scapula

Knee Bursae

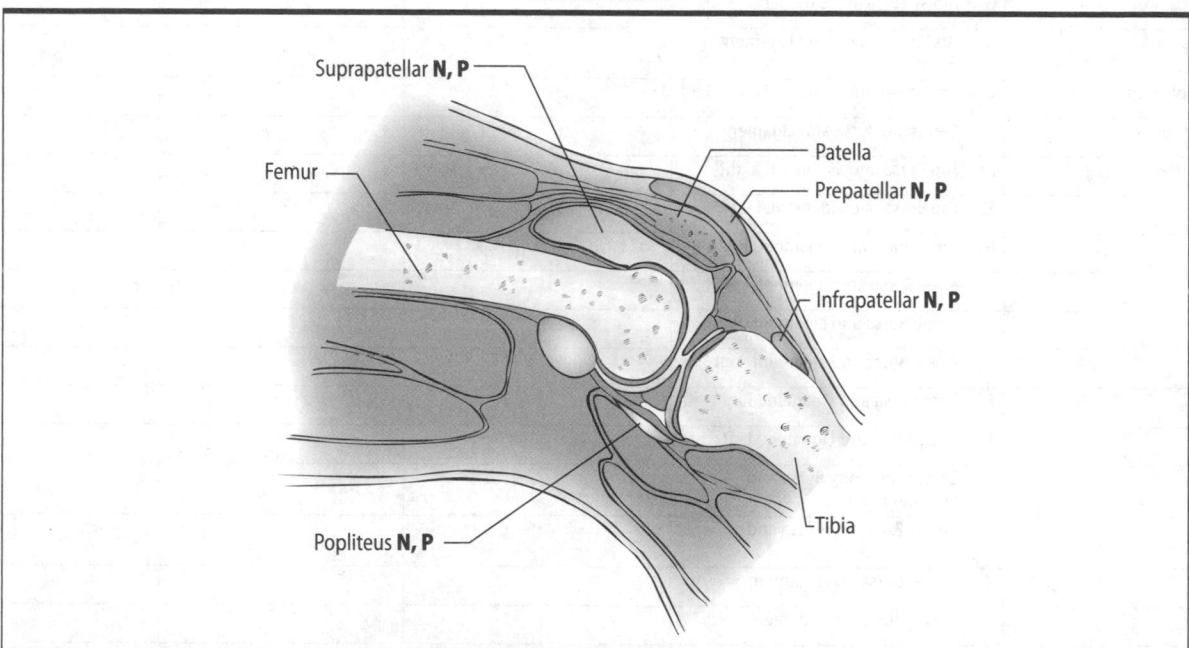

Suprapatellar **N, P**

Femur

Patella

Prepatellar **N, P**

Infrapatellar **N, P**

Popliteus **N, P**

Tibia

Knee Ligaments

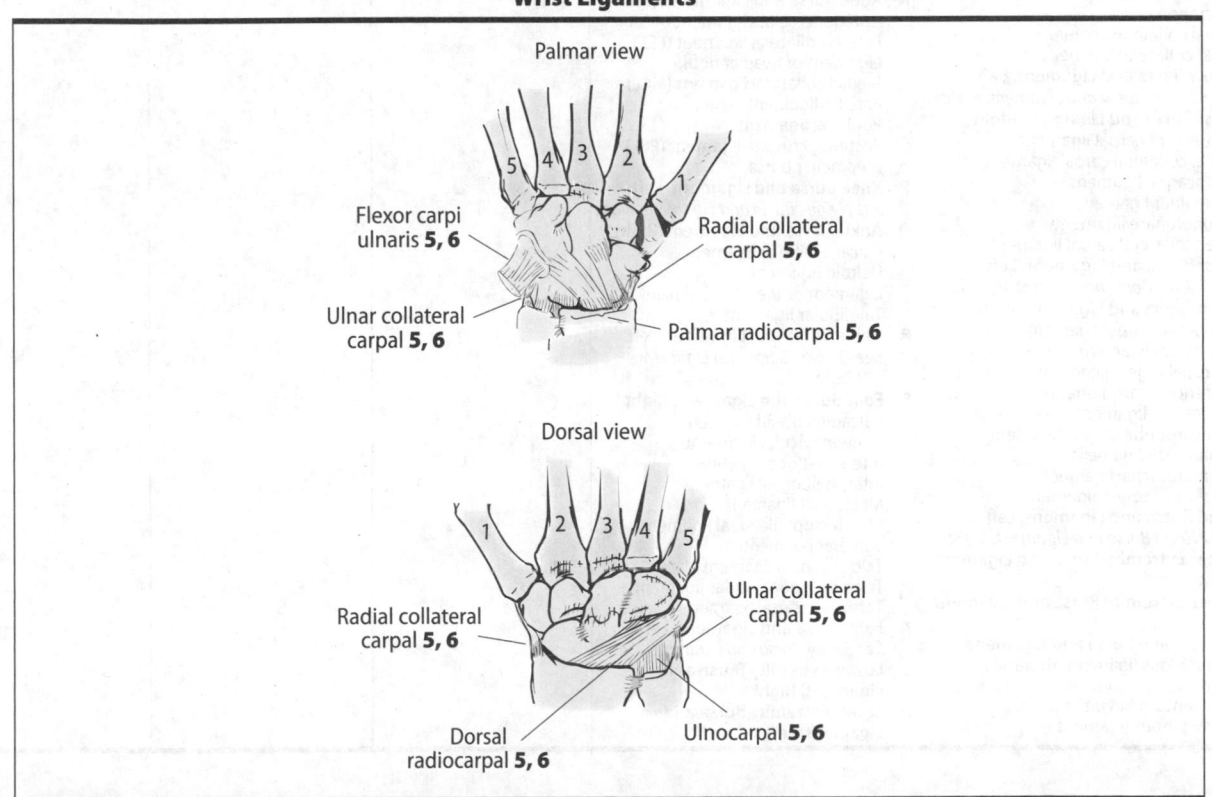

Anterior view

Lateral collateral ligament **N, P**

Medial collateral ligament **N, P**

Patella

Posterior cruciate ligament **N, P**
(Behind the Anterior cruciate)

Anterior cruciate ligament **N, P**

Fibula

Tibia

Posterior cruciate
ligament **N, P**

Anterior cruciate ligament **N, P**

Wrist Ligaments

Palmar view

5 4 3 2 1

Flexor carpi
ulnaris **5, 6**

Radial collateral
carpal **5, 6**

Ulnar collateral
carpal **5, 6**

Palmar radiocarpal **5, 6**

Dorsal view

1 2 3 4 5

Radial collateral
carpal **5, 6**

Ulnar collateral
carpal **5, 6**

Dorsal
radiocarpal **5, 6**

Ulnocarpal **5, 6**

Ø　Medical and Surgical
M　Bursae and Ligaments
2　Change　　　　Definition: Taking out or off a device from a body part and putting back an identical or similar device in or on the same body part without cutting or puncturing the skin or a mucous membrane

Explanation: All CHANGE procedures are coded using the approach EXTERNAL

Body Part Character 4	Approach Character 5	Device Character 6	Qualifier Character 7
X Upper Bursa and Ligament **Y** Lower Bursa and Ligament	**X** External	**Ø** Drainage Device **Y** Other Device	**Z** No Qualifier

Non-OR	All body part, approach, device, and qualifier values

Ø　Medical and Surgical
M　Bursae and Ligaments
5　Destruction　　　Definition: Physical eradication of all or a portion of a body part by the direct use of energy, force, or a destructive agent

Explanation: None of the body part is physically taken out

Body Part Character 4		Approach Character 5	Device Character 6	Qualifier Character 7
Ø Head and Neck Bursa and Ligament 　Alar ligament of axis 　Cervical interspinous ligament 　Cervical intertransverse ligament 　Cervical ligamentum flavum 　Interspinous ligament, cervical 　Intertransverse ligament, cervical 　Lateral temporomandibular ligament 　Ligamentum flavum, cervical 　Sphenomandibular ligament 　Stylomandibular ligament 　Transverse ligament of atlas **1** Shoulder Bursa and Ligament, Right 　Acromioclavicular ligament 　Coracoacromial ligament 　Coracoclavicular ligament 　Coracohumeral ligament 　Costoclavicular ligament 　Glenohumeral ligament 　Interclavicular ligament 　Sternoclavicular ligament 　Subacromial bursa 　Transverse humeral ligament 　Transverse scapular ligament **2** Shoulder Bursa and Ligament, Left 　*See 1 Shoulder Bursa and Ligament, Right* **3** Elbow Bursa and Ligfament, Right 　Annular ligament 　Olecranon bursa 　Radial collateral ligament 　Ulnar collateral ligament **4** Elbow Bursa and Ligament, Left 　*See 3 Elbow Bursa and Ligament, Right* **5** Wrist Bursa and Ligament, Right 　Palmar ulnocarpal ligament 　Radial collateral carpal ligament 　Radiocarpal ligament 　Radioulnar ligament 　Scapholunate ligament 　Ulnar collateral carpal ligament **6** Wrist Bursa and Ligament, Left 　*See 5 Wrist Bursa and Ligament, Right* **7** Hand Bursa and Ligament, Right 　Carpometacarpal ligament 　Intercarpal ligament 　Interphalangeal ligament 　Lunotriquetral ligament 　Metacarpal ligament 　Metacarpophalangeal ligament 　Pisohamate ligament 　Pisometacarpal ligament 　Scaphotrapezium ligament **8** Hand Bursa and Ligament, Left 　*See 7 Hand Bursa and Ligament, Right* **9** Upper Extremity Bursa and Ligament, Right **B** Upper Extremity Bursa and Ligament, Left **C** Upper Spine Bursa and Ligament 　Interspinous ligament, thoracic 　Intertransverse ligament, thoracic 　Ligamentum flavum, thoracic 　Supraspinous ligament	**D** Lower Spine Bursa and Ligament 　Iliolumbar ligament 　Interspinous ligament, lumbar 　Intertransverse ligament, lumbar 　Ligamentum flavum, lumbar 　Sacrococcygeal ligament 　Sacroiliac ligament 　Sacrospinous ligament 　Sacrotuberous ligament 　Supraspinous ligament **F** Sternum Bursa and Ligament 　Costoxiphoid ligament 　Sternocostal ligament **G** Rib(s) Bursa and Ligament 　Costotransverse ligament **H** Abdomen Bursa and Ligament, Right **J** Abdomen Bursa and Ligament, Left **K** Perineum Bursa and Ligament **L** Hip Bursa and Ligament, Right 　Iliofemoral ligament 　Ischiofemoral ligament 　Pubofemoral ligament 　Transverse acetabular ligament 　Trochanteric bursa **M** Hip Bursa and Ligament, Left 　*See L Hip Bursa and Ligament, Right* **N** Knee Bursa and Ligament, Right 　Anterior cruciate ligament (ACL) 　Lateral collateral ligament (LCL) 　Ligament of head of fibula 　Medial collateral ligament (MCL) 　Patellar ligament 　Popliteal ligament 　Posterior cruciate ligament (PCL) 　Prepatellar bursa **P** Knee Bursa and Ligament, Left 　*See N Knee Bursa and Ligament, Right* **Q** Ankle Bursa and Ligament, Right 　Calcaneofibular ligament 　Deltoid ligament 　Ligament of the lateral malleolus 　Talofibular ligament **R** Ankle Bursa and Ligament, Left 　*See Q Ankle Bursa and Ligament, Right* **S** Foot Bursa and Ligament, Right 　Calcaneocuboid ligament 　Cuneonavicular ligament 　Intercuneiform ligament 　Interphalangeal ligament 　Metatarsal ligament 　Metatarsophalangeal ligament 　Subtalar ligament 　Talocalcaneal ligament 　Talocalcaneonavicular ligament 　Tarsometatarsal ligament **T** Foot Bursa and Ligament, Left 　*See S Foot Bursa and Ligament, Right* **V** Lower Extremity Bursa and Ligament, Right **W** Lower Extremity Bursa and Ligament, Left	**Ø** Open **3** Percutaneous **4** Percutaneous Endoscopic	**Z** No Device	**Z** No Qualifier

Ø   Medical and Surgical
M   Bursae and Ligaments
8   Division   Definition: Cutting into a body part, without draining fluids and/or gases from the body part, in order to separate or transect a body part
                 Explanation: All or a portion of the body part is separated into two or more portions

Body Part — Character 4		Approach — Character 5	Device — Character 6	Qualifier — Character 7
Ø Head and Neck Bursa and Ligament Alar ligament of axis Cervical interspinous ligament Cervical intertransverse ligament Cervical ligamentum flavum Interspinous ligament, cervical Intertransverse ligament, cervical Lateral temporomandibular ligament Ligamentum flavum, cervical Sphenomandibular ligament Stylomandibular ligament Transverse ligament of atlas **1** Shoulder Bursa and Ligament, Right Acromioclavicular ligament Coracoacromial ligament Coracoclavicular ligament Coracohumeral ligament Costoclavicular ligament Glenohumeral ligament Interclavicular ligament Sternoclavicular ligament Subacromial bursa Transverse humeral ligament Transverse scapular ligament **2** Shoulder Bursa and Ligament, Left *See 1 Shoulder Bursa and Ligament, Right* **3** Elbow Bursa and Ligament, Right Annular ligament Olecranon bursa Radial collateral ligament Ulnar collateral ligament **4** Elbow Bursa and Ligament, Left *See 3 Elbow Bursa and Ligament, Right* **5** Wrist Bursa and Ligament, Right Palmar ulnocarpal ligament Radial collateral carpal ligament Radiocarpal ligament Radioulnar ligament Scapholunate ligament Ulnar collateral carpal ligament **6** Wrist Bursa and Ligament, Left *See 5 Wrist Bursa and Ligament, Right* **7** Hand Bursa and Ligament, Right Carpometacarpal ligament Intercarpal ligament Interphalangeal ligament Lunotriquetral ligament Metacarpal ligament Metacarpophalangeal ligament Pisohamate ligament Pisometacarpal ligament Scaphotrapezium ligament **8** Hand Bursa and Ligament, Left *See 7 Hand Bursa and Ligament, Right* **9** Upper Extremity Bursa and Ligament, Right **B** Upper Extremity Bursa and Ligament, Left **C** Upper Spine Bursa and Ligament Interspinous ligament, thoracic Intertransverse ligament, thoracic Ligamentum flavum, thoracic Supraspinous ligament	**D** Lower Spine Bursa and Ligament Iliolumbar ligament Interspinous ligament, lumbar Intertransverse ligament, lumbar Ligamentum flavum, lumbar Sacrococcygeal ligament Sacroiliac ligament Sacrospinous ligament Sacrotuberous ligament Supraspinous ligament **F** Sternum Bursa and Ligament Costoxiphoid ligament Sternocostal ligament **G** Rib(s) Bursa and Ligament Costotransverse ligament **H** Abdomen Bursa and Ligament, Right **J** Abdomen Bursa and Ligament, Left **K** Perineum Bursa and Ligament **L** Hip Bursa and Ligament, Right Iliofemoral ligament Ischiofemoral ligament Pubofemoral ligament Transverse acetabular ligament Trochanteric bursa **M** Hip Bursa and Ligament, Left *See L Hip Bursa and Ligament, Right* **N** Knee Bursa and Ligament, Right Anterior cruciate ligament (ACL) Lateral collateral ligament (LCL) Ligament of head of fibula Medial collateral ligament (MCL) Patellar ligament Popliteal ligament Posterior cruciate ligament (PCL) Prepatellar bursa **P** Knee Bursa and Ligament, Left *See N Knee Bursa and Ligament, Right* **Q** Ankle Bursa and Ligament, Right Calcaneofibular ligament Deltoid ligament Ligament of the lateral malleolus Talofibular ligament **R** Ankle Bursa and Ligament, Left *See Q Ankle Bursa and Ligament, Right* **S** Foot Bursa and Ligament, Right Calcaneocuboid ligament Cuneonavicular ligament Intercuneiform ligament Interphalangeal ligament Metatarsal ligament Metatarsophalangeal ligament Subtalar ligament Talocalcaneal ligament Talocalcaneonavicular ligament Tarsometatarsal ligament **T** Foot Bursa and Ligament, Left *See S Foot Bursa and Ligament, Right* **V** Lower Extremity Bursa and Ligament, Right **W** Lower Extremity Bursa and Ligament, Left	**Ø** Open **3** Percutaneous **4** Percutaneous Endoscopic	**Z** No Device	**Z** No Qualifier

Bursae and Ligaments

Ø   **Medical and Surgical**
M   **Bursae and Ligaments**
9   **Drainage**   Definition: Taking or letting out fluids and/or gases from a body part
                         Explanation: The qualifier DIAGNOSTIC is used to identify drainage procedures that are biopsies

Body Part Character 4		Approach Character 5	Device Character 6	Qualifier Character 7
Ø Head and Neck Bursa and Ligament Alar ligament of axis Cervical interspinous ligament Cervical intertransverse ligament Cervical ligamentum flavum Interspinous ligament, cervical Intertransverse ligament, cervical Lateral temporomandibular ligament Ligamentum flavum, cervical Sphenomandibular ligament Stylomandibular ligament Transverse ligament of atlas **1 Shoulder Bursa and Ligament, Right** Acromioclavicular ligament Coracoacromial ligament Coracoclavicular ligament Coracohumeral ligament Costoclavicular ligament Glenohumeral ligament Interclavicular ligament Sternoclavicular ligament Subacromial bursa Transverse humeral ligament Transverse scapular ligament **2 Shoulder Bursa and Ligament, Left** *See 1 Shoulder Bursa and Ligament, Right* **3 Elbow Bursa and Ligament, Right** Annular ligament Olecranon bursa Radial collateral ligament Ulnar collateral ligament **4 Elbow Bursa and Ligament, Left** *See 3 Elbow Bursa and Ligament, Right* **5 Wrist Bursa and Ligament, Right** Palmar ulnocarpal ligament Radial collateral carpal ligament Radiocarpal ligament Radioulnar ligament Scapholunate ligament Ulnar collateral carpal ligament **6 Wrist Bursa and Ligament, Left** *See 5 Wrist Bursa and Ligament, Right* **7 Hand Bursa and Ligament, Right** Carpometacarpal ligament Intercarpal ligament Interphalangeal ligament Lunotriquetral ligament Metacarpal ligament Metacarpophalangeal ligament Pisohamate ligament Pisometacarpal ligament Scaphotrapezium ligament **8 Hand Bursa and Ligament, Left** *See 7 Hand Bursa and Ligament, Right* **9 Upper Extremity Bursa and Ligament, Right** **B Upper Extremity Bursa and Ligament, Left** **C Upper Spine Bursa and Ligament** Interspinous ligament, thoracic Intertransverse ligament, thoracic Ligamentum flavum, thoracic Supraspinous ligament	**D Lower Spine Bursa and Ligament** Iliolumbar ligament Interspinous ligament, lumbar Intertransverse ligament, lumbar Ligamentum flavum, lumbar Sacrococcygeal ligament Sacroiliac ligament Sacrospinous ligament Sacrotuberous ligament Supraspinous ligament **F Sternum Bursa and Ligament** Costoxiphoid ligament Sternocostal ligament **G Rib(s) Bursa and Ligament** Costotransverse ligament **H Abdomen Bursa and Ligament, Right** **J Abdomen Bursa and Ligament, Left** **K Perineum Bursa and Ligament** **L Hip Bursa and Ligament, Right** Iliofemoral ligament Ischiofemoral ligament Pubofemoral ligament Transverse acetabular ligament Trochanteric bursa **M Hip Bursa and Ligament, Left** *See L Hip Bursa and Ligament, Right* **N Knee Bursa and Ligament, Right** Anterior cruciate ligament (ACL) Lateral collateral ligament (LCL) Ligament of head of fibula Medial collateral ligament (MCL) Patellar ligament Popliteal ligament Posterior cruciate ligament (PCL) Prepatellar bursa **P Knee Bursa and Ligament, Left** *See N Knee Bursa and Ligament, Right* **Q Ankle Bursa and Ligament, Right** Calcaneofibular ligament Deltoid ligament Ligament of the lateral malleolus Talofibular ligament **R Ankle Bursa and Ligament, Left** *See Q Ankle Bursa and Ligament, Right* **S Foot Bursa and Ligament, Right** Calcaneocuboid ligament Cuneonavicular ligament Intercuneiform ligament Interphalangeal ligament Metatarsal ligament Metatarsophalangeal ligament Subtalar ligament Talocalcaneal ligament Talocalcaneonavicular ligament Tarsometatarsal ligament **T Foot Bursa and Ligament, Left** *See S Foot Bursa and Ligament, Right* **V Lower Extremity Bursa and Ligament, Right** **W Lower Extremity Bursa and Ligament, Left**	**Ø Open** **3 Percutaneous** **4 Percutaneous Endoscopic**	**Ø Drainage Device**	**Z No Qualifier**

Non-OR   ØM9[Ø,1,2,3,4,5,6,7,8,9,B,C,D,F,G,H,J,K,L,M,N,P,Q,R,S,T,V,W]3ØZ
Non-OR   ØM9[1,2,3,4,7,8,9,B,C,D,F,G,H,J,K,L,M,V,W]4ØZ

ØM9 Continued on next page

ØM9 Continued

Ø   **Medical and Surgical**
M   **Bursae and Ligaments**
9   **Drainage**   Definition: Taking or letting out fluids and/or gases from a body part
                Explanation: The qualifier DIAGNOSTIC is used to identify drainage procedures that are biopsies

Body Part Character 4		Approach Character 5	Device Character 6	Qualifier Character 7
Ø Head and Neck Bursa and Ligament Alar ligament of axis Cervical interspinous ligament Cervical intertransverse ligament Cervical ligamentum flavum Interspinous ligament, cervical Intertransverse ligament, cervical Lateral temporomandibular ligament Ligamentum flavum, cervical Sphenomandibular ligament Stylomandibular ligament Transverse ligament of atlas **1 Shoulder Bursa and Ligament, Right** Acromioclavicular ligament Coracoacromial ligament Coracoclavicular ligament Coracohumeral ligament Costoclavicular ligament Glenohumeral ligament Interclavicular ligament Sternoclavicular ligament Subacromial bursa Transverse humeral ligament Transverse scapular ligament **2 Shoulder Bursa and Ligament, Left** *See* 1 Shoulder Bursa and Ligament, Right **3 Elbow Bursa and Ligament, Right** Annular ligament Olecranon bursa Radial collateral ligament Ulnar collateral ligament **4 Elbow Bursa and Ligament, Left** *See* 3 Elbow Bursa and Ligament, Right **5 Wrist Bursa and Ligament, Right** Palmar ulnocarpal ligament Radial collateral carpal ligament Radiocarpal ligament Radioulnar ligament Scapholunate ligament Ulnar collateral carpal ligament **6 Wrist Bursa and Ligament, Left** *See* 5 Wrist Bursa and Ligament, Right **7 Hand Bursa and Ligament, Right** Carpometacarpal ligament Intercarpal ligament Interphalangeal ligament Lunotriquetral ligament Metacarpal ligament Metacarpophalangeal ligament Pisohamate ligament Pisometacarpal ligament Scaphotrapezium ligament **8 Hand Bursa and Ligament, Left** *See* 7 Hand Bursa and Ligament, Right **9 Upper Extremity Bursa and Ligament, Right** **B Upper Extremity Bursa and Ligament, Left** **C Upper Spine Bursa and Ligament** Interspinous ligament, thoracic Intertransverse ligament, thoracic Ligamentum flavum, thoracic Supraspinous ligament	**D Lower Spine Bursa and Ligament** Iliolumbar ligament Interspinous ligament, lumbar Intertransverse ligament, lumbar Ligamentum flavum, lumbar Sacrococcygeal ligament Sacroiliac ligament Sacrospinous ligament Sacrotuberous ligament Supraspinous ligament **F Sternum Bursa and Ligament** Costoxiphoid ligament Sternocostal ligament **G Rib(s) Bursa and Ligament** Costotransverse ligament **H Abdomen Bursa and Ligament, Right** **J Abdomen Bursa and Ligament, Left** **K Perineum Bursa and Ligament** **L Hip Bursa and Ligament, Right** Iliofemoral ligament Ischiofemoral ligament Pubofemoral ligament Transverse acetabular ligament Trochanteric bursa **M Hip Bursa and Ligament, Left** *See* L Hip Bursa and Ligament, Right **N Knee Bursa and Ligament, Right** Anterior cruciate ligament (ACL) Lateral collateral ligament (LCL) Ligament of head of fibula Medial collateral ligament (MCL) Patellar ligament Popliteal ligament Posterior cruciate ligament (PCL) Prepatellar bursa **P Knee Bursa and Ligament, Left** *See* N Knee Bursa and Ligament, Right **Q Ankle Bursa and Ligament, Right** Calcaneofibular ligament Deltoid ligament Ligament of the lateral malleolus Talofibular ligament **R Ankle Bursa and Ligament, Left** *See* Q Ankle Bursa and Ligament, Right **S Foot Bursa and Ligament, Right** Calcaneocuboid ligament Cuneonavicular ligament Intercuneiform ligament Interphalangeal ligament Metatarsal ligament Metatarsophalangeal ligament Subtalar ligament Talocalcaneal ligament Talocalcaneonavicular ligament Tarsometatarsal ligament **T Foot Bursa and Ligament, Left** *See* S Foot Bursa and Ligament, Right **V Lower Extremity Bursa and Ligament, Right** **W Lower Extremity Bursa and Ligament, Left**	**Ø Open** **3 Percutaneous** **4 Percutaneous Endoscopic**	**Z No Device**	**X Diagnostic** **Z No Qualifier**

Non-OR   ØM9[Ø,1,2,3,4,5,6,7,8,C,D,F,G,L,M,N,P,Q,R,S,T][Ø,3,4]ZX
Non-OR   ØM9[Ø,1,2,3,4,5,6,7,8,9,B,C,D,F,G,H,J,K,L,M,N,P,Q,R,S,T,V,W]3ZZ
Non-OR   ØM9[Ø,5,6,7,8,9,B,C,D,F,G,H,J,K,N,P,Q,R,S,T,V,W]4ZZ

NC Noncovered Procedure   LC Limited Coverage   QA Questionable OB Admit   NT New Tech Add-on   ⊞ Combination Member   ♂ Male   ♀ Female

ICD-10-PCS 2022   505

ØM9–ØM9

Ø Medical and Surgical
M Bursae and Ligaments
B Excision   Definition: Cutting out or off, without replacement, a portion of a body part
              Explanation: The qualifier DIAGNOSTIC is used to identify excision procedures that are biopsies

Body Part Character 4		Approach Character 5	Device Character 6	Qualifier Character 7

Ø Head and Neck Bursa and Ligament
  Alar ligament of axis
  Cervical interspinous ligament
  Cervical intertransverse ligament
  Cervical ligamentum flavum
  Interspinous ligament, cervical
  Intertransverse ligament, cervical
  Lateral temporomandibular
    ligament
  Ligamentum flavum, cervical
  Sphenomandibular ligament
  Stylomandibular ligament
  Transverse ligament of atlas
1 Shoulder Bursa and Ligament, Right
  Acromioclavicular ligament
  Coracoacromial ligament
  Coracoclavicular ligament
  Coracohumeral ligament
  Costoclavicular ligament
  Glenohumeral ligament
  Interclavicular ligament
  Sternoclavicular ligament
  Subacromial bursa
  Transverse humeral ligament
  Transverse scapular ligament
2 Shoulder Bursa and Ligament, Left
  See 1 Shoulder Bursa and Ligament, Right
3 Elbow Bursa and Ligament, Right
  Annular ligament
  Olecranon bursa
  Radial collateral ligament
  Ulnar collateral ligament
4 Elbow Bursa and Ligament, Left
  See 3 Elbow Bursa and Ligament, Right
5 Wrist Bursa and Ligament, Right
  Palmar ulnocarpal ligament
  Radial collateral carpal ligament
  Radiocarpal ligament
  Radioulnar ligament
  Scapholunate ligament
  Ulnar collateral carpal ligament
6 Wrist Bursa and Ligament, Left
  See 5 Wrist Bursa and Ligament, Right
7 Hand Bursa and Ligament, Right
  Carpometacarpal ligament
  Intercarpal ligament
  Interphalangeal ligament
  Lunotriquetral ligament
  Metacarpal ligament
  Metacarpophalangeal ligament
  Pisohamate ligament
  Pisometacarpal ligament
  Scaphotrapezium ligament
8 Hand Bursa and Ligament, Left
  See 7 Hand Bursa and Ligament, Right
9 Upper Extremity Bursa and Ligament, Right
B Upper Extremity Bursa and Ligament, Left
C Upper Spine Bursa and Ligament
  Interspinous ligament, thoracic
  Intertransverse ligament, thoracic
  Ligamentum flavum, thoracic
  Supraspinous ligament
	D Lower Spine Bursa and Ligament
	  Iliolumbar ligament
	  Interspinous ligament, lumbar
	  Intertransverse ligament, lumbar
	  Ligamentum flavum, lumbar
	  Sacrococcygeal ligament
	  Sacroiliac ligament
	  Sacrospinous ligament
	  Sacrotuberous ligament
	  Supraspinous ligament
	F Sternum Bursa and Ligament
	  Costoxiphoid ligament
	  Sternocostal ligament
	G Rib(s) Bursa and Ligament
	  Costotransverse ligament
	H Abdomen Bursa and Ligament, Right
	J Abdomen Bursa and Ligament, Left
	K Perineum Bursa and Ligament
	L Hip Bursa and Ligament, Right
	  Iliofemoral ligament
	  Ischiofemoral ligament
	  Pubofemoral ligament
	  Transverse acetabular ligament
	  Trochanteric bursa
	M Hip Bursa and Ligament, Left
	  See L Hip Bursa and Ligament, Right
	N Knee Bursa and Ligament, Right
	  Anterior cruciate ligament (ACL)
	  Lateral collateral ligament (LCL)
	  Ligament of head of fibula
	  Medial collateral ligament (MCL)
	  Patellar ligament
	  Popliteal ligament
	  Posterior cruciate ligament (PCL)
	  Prepatellar bursa
	P Knee Bursa and Ligament, Left
	  See N Knee Bursa and Ligament, Right
	Q Ankle Bursa and Ligament, Right
	  Calcaneofibular ligament
	  Deltoid ligament
	  Ligament of the lateral malleolus
	  Talofibular ligament
	R Ankle Bursa and Ligament, Left
	  See Q Ankle Bursa and Ligament, Right
	S Foot Bursa and Ligament, Right
	  Calcaneocuboid ligament
	  Cuneonavicular ligament
	  Intercuneiform ligament
	  Interphalangeal ligament
	  Metatarsal ligament
	  Metatarsophalangeal ligament
	  Subtalar ligament
	  Talocalcaneal ligament
	  Talocalcaneonavicular ligament
	  Tarsometatarsal ligament
	T Foot Bursa and Ligament, Left
	  See S Foot Bursa and Ligament, Right
	V Lower Extremity Bursa and Ligament, Right
	W Lower Extremity Bursa and Ligament, Left
		Ø Open
		3 Percutaneous
		4 Percutaneous Endoscopic
			Z No Device	**X** Diagnostic
				Z No Qualifier

Non-OR   ØMB[Ø,1,2,3,4,5,6,7,8,B,C,D,F,G,L,M,N,P,Q,R,S,T][Ø,3,4]ZX
Non-OR   ØMB94ZX

Ø   Medical and Surgical
M   Bursae and Ligaments
C   Extirpation   Definition: Taking or cutting out solid matter from a body part

Explanation: The solid matter may be an abnormal byproduct of a biological function or a foreign body; it may be imbedded in a body part or in the lumen of a tubular body part. The solid matter may or may not have been previously broken into pieces.

Body Part Character 4		Approach Character 5	Device Character 6	Qualifier Character 7
Ø Head and Neck Bursa and Ligament Alar ligament of axis Cervical interspinous ligament Cervical intertransverse ligament Cervical ligamentum flavum Interspinous ligament, cervical Intertransverse ligament, cervical Lateral temporomandibular ligament Ligamentum flavum, cervical Sphenomandibular ligament Stylomandibular ligament Transverse ligament of atlas **1 Shoulder Bursa and Ligament, Right** Acromioclavicular ligament Coracoacromial ligament Coracoclavicular ligament Coracohumeral ligament Costoclavicular ligament Glenohumeral ligament Interclavicular ligament Sternoclavicular ligament Subacromial bursa Transverse humeral ligament Transverse scapular ligament **2 Shoulder Bursa and Ligament, Left** *See 1 Shoulder Bursa and Ligament, Right* **3 Elbow Bursa and Ligament, Right** Annular ligament Olecranon bursa Radial collateral ligament Ulnar collateral ligament **4 Elbow Bursa and Ligament, Left** *See 3 Elbow Bursa and Ligament, Right* **5 Wrist Bursa and Ligament, Right** Palmar ulnocarpal ligament Radial collateral carpal ligament Radiocarpal ligament Radioulnar ligament Scapholunate ligament Ulnar collateral carpal ligament **6 Wrist Bursa and Ligament, Left** *See 5 Wrist Bursa and Ligament, Right* **7 Hand Bursa and Ligament, Right** Carpometacarpal ligament Intercarpal ligament Interphalangeal ligament Lunotriquetral ligament Metacarpal ligament Metacarpophalangeal ligament Pisohamate ligament Pisometacarpal ligament Scaphotrapezium ligament **8 Hand Bursa and Ligament, Left** *See 7 Hand Bursa and Ligament, Right* **9 Upper Extremity Bursa and Ligament, Right** **B Upper Extremity Bursa and Ligament, Left** **C Upper Spine Bursa and Ligament** Interspinous ligament, thoracic Intertransverse ligament, thoracic Ligamentum flavum, thoracic Supraspinous ligament	**D Lower Spine Bursa and Ligament** Iliolumbar ligament Interspinous ligament, lumbar Intertransverse ligament, lumbar Ligamentum flavum, lumbar Sacrococcygeal ligament Sacroiliac ligament Sacrospinous ligament Sacrotuberous ligament Supraspinous ligament **F Sternum Bursa and Ligament** Costoxiphoid ligament Sternocostal ligament **G Rib(s) Bursa and Ligament** Costotransverse ligament **H Abdomen Bursa and Ligament, Right** **J Abdomen Bursa and Ligament, Left** **K Perineum Bursa and Ligament** **L Hip Bursa and Ligament, Right** Iliofemoral ligament Ischiofemoral ligament Pubofemoral ligament Transverse acetabular ligament Trochanteric bursa **M Hip Bursa and Ligament, Left** *See L Hip Bursa and Ligament, Right* **N Knee Bursa and Ligament, Right** Anterior cruciate ligament (ACL) Lateral collateral ligament (LCL) Ligament of head of fibula Medial collateral ligament (MCL) Patellar ligament Popliteal ligament Posterior cruciate ligament (PCL) Prepatellar bursa **P Knee Bursa and Ligament, Left** *See N Knee Bursa and Ligament, Right* **Q Ankle Bursa and Ligament, Right** Calcaneofibular ligament Deltoid ligament Ligament of the lateral malleolus Talofibular ligament **R Ankle Bursa and Ligament, Left** *See Q Ankle Bursa and Ligament, Right* **S Foot Bursa and Ligament, Right** Calcaneocuboid ligament Cuneonavicular ligament Intercuneiform ligament Interphalangeal ligament Metatarsal ligament Metatarsophalangeal ligament Subtalar ligament Talocalcaneal ligament Talocalcaneonavicular ligament Tarsometatarsal ligament **T Foot Bursa and Ligament, Left** *See S Foot Bursa and Ligament, Right* **V Lower Extremity Bursa and Ligament, Right** **W Lower Extremity Bursa and Ligament, Left**	**Ø Open** **3 Percutaneous** **4 Percutaneous Endoscopic**	**Z No Device**	**Z No Qualifier**

NC Noncovered Procedure   **LC** Limited Coverage   **QA** Questionable OB Admit   **NT** New Tech Add-on   ⊞ Combination Member   ♂ Male   ♀ Female

ICD-10-PCS 2022   507

Ø   **Medical and Surgical**
M   **Bursae and Ligaments**
D   **Extraction**   Definition: Pulling or stripping out or off all or a portion of a body part by the use of force
                         Explanation: The qualifier DIAGNOSTIC is used to identify extraction procedures that are biopsies

Body Part Character 4		Approach Character 5	Device Character 6	Qualifier Character 7
Ø **Head and Neck Bursa and Ligament** Alar ligament of axis Cervical interspinous ligament Cervical intertransverse ligament Cervical ligamentum flavum Interspinous ligament, cervical Intertransverse ligament, cervical Lateral temporomandibular ligament Ligamentum flavum, cervical Sphenomandibular ligament Stylomandibular ligament Transverse ligament of atlas **1** **Shoulder Bursa and Ligament, Right** Acromioclavicular ligament Coracoacromial ligament Coracoclavicular ligament Coracohumeral ligament Costoclavicular ligament Glenohumeral ligament Interclavicular ligament Sternoclavicular ligament Subacromial bursa Transverse humeral ligament Transverse scapular ligament **2** **Shoulder Bursa and Ligament, Left** *See 1 Shoulder Bursa and Ligament, Right* **3** **Elbow Bursa and Ligament, Right** Annular ligament Olecranon bursa Radial collateral ligament Ulnar collateral ligament **4** **Elbow Bursa and Ligament, Left** *See 3 Elbow Bursa and Ligament, Right* **5** **Wrist Bursa and Ligament, Right** Palmar ulnocarpal ligament Radial collateral carpal ligament Radiocarpal ligament Radioulnar ligament Scapholunate ligament Ulnar collateral carpal ligament **6** **Wrist Bursa and Ligament, Left** *See 5 Wrist Bursa and Ligament, Right* **7** **Hand Bursa and Ligament, Right** Carpometacarpal ligament Intercarpal ligament Interphalangeal ligament Lunotriquetral ligament Metacarpal ligament Metacarpophalangeal ligament Pisohamate ligament Pisometacarpal ligament Scaphotrapezium ligament **8** **Hand Bursa and Ligament, Left** *See 7 Hand Bursa and Ligament, Right* **9** **Upper Extremity Bursa and Ligament, Right** **B** **Upper Extremity Bursa and Ligament, Left** **C** **Upper Spine Bursa and Ligament** Interspinous ligament, thoracic Intertransverse ligament, thoracic Ligamentum flavum, thoracic Supraspinous ligament	**D** **Lower Spine Bursa and Ligament** Iliolumbar ligament Interspinous ligament, lumbar Intertransverse ligament, lumbar Ligamentum flavum, lumbar Sacrococcygeal ligament Sacroiliac ligament Sacrospinous ligament Sacrotuberous ligament Supraspinous ligament **F** **Sternum Bursa and Ligament** Costoxiphoid ligament Sternocostal ligament **G** **Rib(s) Bursa and Ligament** Costotransverse ligament **H** **Abdomen Bursa and Ligament, Right** **J** **Abdomen Bursa and Ligament, Left** **K** **Perineum Bursa and Ligament** **L** **Hip Bursa and Ligament, Right** Iliofemoral ligament Ischiofemoral ligament Pubofemoral ligament Transverse acetabular ligament Trochanteric bursa **M** **Hip Bursa and Ligament, Left** *See L Hip Bursa and Ligament, Right* **N** **Knee Bursa and Ligament, Right** Anterior cruciate ligament (ACL) Lateral collateral ligament (LCL) Ligament of head of fibula Medial collateral ligament (MCL) Patellar ligament Popliteal ligament Posterior cruciate ligament (PCL) Prepatellar bursa **P** **Knee Bursa and Ligament, Left** *See N Knee Bursa and Ligament, Right* **Q** **Ankle Bursa and Ligament, Right** Calcaneofibular ligament Deltoid ligament Ligament of the lateral malleolus Talofibular ligament **R** **Ankle Bursa and Ligament, Left** *See Q Ankle Bursa and Ligament, Right* **S** **Foot Bursa and Ligament, Right** Calcaneocuboid ligament Cuneonavicular ligament Intercuneiform ligament Interphalangeal ligament Metatarsal ligament Metatarsophalangeal ligament Subtalar ligament Talocalcaneal ligament Talocalcaneonavicular ligament Tarsometatarsal ligament **T** **Foot Bursa and Ligament, Left** *See S Foot Bursa and Ligament, Right* **V** **Lower Extremity Bursa and Ligament, Right** **W** **Lower Extremity Bursa and Ligament, Left**	**Ø** Open **3** Percutaneous **4** Percutaneous Endoscopic	**Z** No Device	**Z** No Qualifier

Ø   **Medical and Surgical**
M   **Bursae and Ligaments**
H   **Insertion**   Definition: Putting in a nonbiological appliance that monitors, assists, performs, or prevents a physiological function but does not physically take the place of a body part

Explanation: None

Body Part Character 4	Approach Character 5	Device Character 6	Qualifier Character 7
X Upper Bursa and Ligament **Y** Lower Bursa and Ligament	**Ø** Open **3** Percutaneous **4** Percutaneous Endoscopic	**Y** Other Device	**Z** No Qualifier

Non-OR   ØMH[X,Y][3,4]YZ

Ø   **Medical and Surgical**
M   **Bursae and Ligaments**
J   **Inspection**   Definition: Visually and/or manually exploring a body part

Explanation: Visual exploration may be performed with or without optical instrumentation. Manual exploration may be performed directly or through intervening body layers.

Body Part Character 4	Approach Character 5	Device Character 6	Qualifier Character 7
X Upper Bursa and Ligament **Y** Lower Bursa and Ligament	**Ø** Open **3** Percutaneous **4** Percutaneous Endoscopic **X** External	**Z** No Device	**Z** No Qualifier

Non-OR   ØMJ[X,Y][3,X]ZZ

Bursae and Ligaments

Ø   **Medical and Surgical**
M   **Bursae and Ligaments**
M   **Reattachment**   Definition: Putting back in or on all or a portion of a separated body part to its normal location or other suitable location
                           Explanation: Vascular circulation and nervous pathways may or may not be reestablished

Body Part Character 4	Approach Character 5	Device Character 6	Qualifier Character 7
Ø Head and Neck Bursa and Ligament Alar ligament of axis Cervical interspinous ligament Cervical intertransverse ligament Cervical ligamentum flavum Interspinous ligament, cervical Intertransverse ligament, cervical Lateral temporomandibular ligament Ligamentum flavum, cervical Sphenomandibular ligament Stylomandibular ligament Transverse ligament of atlas **1 Shoulder Bursa and Ligament, Right** Acromioclavicular ligament Coracoacromial ligament Coracoclavicular ligament Coracohumeral ligament Costoclavicular ligament Glenohumeral ligament Interclavicular ligament Sternoclavicular ligament Subacromial bursa Transverse humeral ligament Transverse scapular ligament **2 Shoulder Bursa and Ligament, Left** See 1 Shoulder Bursa and Ligament, Right **3 Elbow Bursa and Ligament, Right** Annular ligament Olecranon bursa Radial collateral ligament Ulnar collateral ligament **4 Elbow Bursa and Ligament, Left** See 3 Elbow Bursa and Ligament, Right **5 Wrist Bursa and Ligament, Right** Palmar ulnocarpal ligament Radial collateral carpal ligament Radiocarpal ligament Radioulnar ligament Scapholunate ligament Ulnar collateral carpal ligament **6 Wrist Bursa and Ligament, Left** See 5 Wrist Bursa and Ligament, Right **7 Hand Bursa and Ligament, Right** Carpometacarpal ligament Intercarpal ligament Interphalangeal ligament Lunotriquetral ligament Metacarpal ligament Metacarpophalangeal ligament Pisohamate ligament Pisometacarpal ligament Scaphotrapezium ligament **8 Hand Bursa and Ligament, Left** See 7 Hand Bursa and Ligament, Right **9 Upper Extremity Bursa and Ligament, Right** **B Upper Extremity Bursa and Ligament, Left** **C Upper Spine Bursa and Ligament** Interspinous ligament, thoracic Intertransverse ligament, thoracic Ligamentum flavum, thoracic Supraspinous ligament **D Lower Spine Bursa and Ligament** Iliolumbar ligament Interspinous ligament, lumbar Intertransverse ligament, lumbar Ligamentum flavum, lumbar Sacrococcygeal ligament Sacroiliac ligament Sacrospinous ligament Sacrotuberous ligament Supraspinous ligament **F Sternum Bursa and Ligament** Costoxiphoid ligament Sternocostal ligament **G Rib(s) Bursa and Ligament** Costotransverse ligament **H Abdomen Bursa and Ligament, Right** **J Abdomen Bursa and Ligament, Left** **K Perineum Bursa and Ligament** **L Hip Bursa and Ligament, Right** Iliofemoral ligament Ischiofemoral ligament Pubofemoral ligament Transverse acetabular ligament Trochanteric bursa **M Hip Bursa and Ligament, Left** See L Hip Bursa and Ligament, Right **N Knee Bursa and Ligament, Right** Anterior cruciate ligament (ACL) Lateral collateral ligament (LCL) Ligament of head of fibula Medial collateral ligament (MCL) Patellar ligament Popliteal ligament Posterior cruciate ligament (PCL) Prepatellar bursa **P Knee Bursa and Ligament, Left** See N Knee Bursa and Ligament, Right **Q Ankle Bursa and Ligament, Right** Calcaneofibular ligament Deltoid ligament Ligament of the lateral malleolus Talofibular ligament **R Ankle Bursa and Ligament, Left** See Q Ankle Bursa and Ligament, Right **S Foot Bursa and Ligament, Right** Calcaneocuboid ligament Cuneonavicular ligament Intercuneiform ligament Interphalangeal ligament Metatarsal ligament Metatarsophalangeal ligament Subtalar ligament Talocalcaneal ligament Talocalcaneonavicular ligament Tarsometatarsal ligament **T Foot Bursa and Ligament, Left** See S Foot Bursa and Ligament, Right **V Lower Extremity Bursa and Ligament, Right** **W Lower Extremity Bursa and Ligament, Left**	Ø Open 4 Percutaneous Endoscopic	Z No Device	Z No Qualifier

Ø   **Medical and Surgical**
M   **Bursae and Ligaments**
N   **Release**   Definition: Freeing a body part from an abnormal physical constraint by cutting or by the use of force
                Explanation: Some of the restraining tissue may be taken out but none of the body part is taken out

Body Part Character 4		Approach Character 5	Device Character 6	Qualifier Character 7
Ø **Head and Neck Bursa and Ligament** Alar ligament of axis Cervical interspinous ligament Cervical intertransverse ligament Cervical ligamentum flavum Interspinous ligament, cervical Intertransverse ligament, cervical Lateral temporomandibular ligament Ligamentum flavum, cervical Sphenomandibular ligament Stylomandibular ligament Transverse ligament of atlas **1** **Shoulder Bursa and Ligament, Right** Acromioclavicular ligament Coracoacromial ligament Coracoclavicular ligament Coracohumeral ligament Costoclavicular ligament Glenohumeral ligament Interclavicular ligament Sternoclavicular ligament Subacromial bursa Transverse humeral ligament Transverse scapular ligament **2** **Shoulder Bursa and Ligament, Left** *See* 1 Shoulder Bursa and Ligament, Right **3** **Elbow Bursa and Ligament, Right** Annular ligament Olecranon bursa Radial collateral ligament Ulnar collateral ligament **4** **Elbow Bursa and Ligament, Left** *See* 3 Elbow Bursa and Ligament, Right **5** **Wrist Bursa and Ligament, Right** Palmar ulnocarpal ligament Radial collateral carpal ligament Radiocarpal ligament Radioulnar ligament Scapholunate ligament Ulnar collateral carpal ligament **6** **Wrist Bursa and Ligament, Left** *See* 5 Wrist Bursa and Ligament, Right **7** **Hand Bursa and Ligament, Right** Carpometacarpal ligament Intercarpal ligament Interphalangeal ligament Lunotriquetral ligament Metacarpal ligament Metacarpophalangeal ligament Pisohamate ligament Pisometacarpal ligament Scaphotrapezium ligament **8** **Hand Bursa and Ligament, Left** *See* 7 Hand Bursa and Ligament, Right **9** **Upper Extremity Bursa and Ligament, Right** **B** **Upper Extremity Bursa and Ligament, Left** **C** **Upper Spine Bursa and Ligament** Interspinous ligament, thoracic Intertransverse ligament, thoracic Ligamentum flavum, thoracic Supraspinous ligament	**D** **Lower Spine Bursa and Ligament** Iliolumbar ligament Interspinous ligament, lumbar Intertransverse ligament, lumbar Ligamentum flavum, lumbar Sacrococcygeal ligament Sacroiliac ligament Sacrospinous ligament Sacrotuberous ligament Supraspinous ligament **F** **Sternum Bursa and Ligament** Costoxiphoid ligament Sternocostal ligament **G** **Rib(s) Bursa and Ligament** Costotransverse ligament **H** **Abdomen Bursa and Ligament, Right** **J** **Abdomen Bursa and Ligament, Left** **K** **Perineum Bursa and Ligament** **L** **Hip Bursa and Ligament, Right** Iliofemoral ligament Ischiofemoral ligament Pubofemoral ligament Transverse acetabular ligament Trochanteric bursa **M** **Hip Bursa and Ligament, Left** *See* L Hip Bursa and Ligament, Right **N** **Knee Bursa and Ligament, Right** Anterior cruciate ligament (ACL) Lateral collateral ligament (LCL) Ligament of head of fibula Medial collateral ligament (MCL) Patellar ligament Popliteal ligament Posterior cruciate ligament (PCL) Prepatellar bursa **P** **Knee Bursa and Ligament, Left** *See* N Knee Bursa and Ligament, Right **Q** **Ankle Bursa and Ligament, Right** Calcaneofibular ligament Deltoid ligament Ligament of the lateral malleolus Talofibular ligament **R** **Ankle Bursa and Ligament, Left** *See* Q Ankle Bursa and Ligament, Right **S** **Foot Bursa and Ligament, Right** Calcaneocuboid ligament Cuneonavicular ligament Intercuneiform ligament Interphalangeal ligament Metatarsal ligament Metatarsophalangeal ligament Subtalar ligament Talocalcaneal ligament Talocalcaneonavicular ligament Tarsometatarsal ligament **T** **Foot Bursa and Ligament, Left** *See* S Foot Bursa and Ligament, Right **V** **Lower Extremity Bursa and Ligament, Right** **W** **Lower Extremity Bursa and Ligament, Left**	**Ø** Open **3** Percutaneous **4** Percutaneous Endoscopic **X** External	**Z** No Device	**Z** No Qualifier

Non-OR   ØMN[Ø,1,2,3,4,5,6,7,8,9,B,C,D,F,G,H,J,K,L,M,N,P,Q,R,S,T,V,W]XZZ

NC Noncovered Procedure   **LC** Limited Coverage   **QA** Questionable OB Admit   **NT** New Tech Add-on   ⊞ Combination Member   ♂ Male   ♀ Female

ICD-10-PCS 2022   **511**

Ø   Medical and Surgical
M   Bursae and Ligaments
P   Removal   Definition: Taking out or off a device from a body part

Explanation: If a device is taken out and a similar device put in without cutting or puncturing the skin or mucous membrane, the procedure is coded to the root operation CHANGE. Otherwise, the procedure for taking out a device is coded to the root operation REMOVAL.

Body Part Character 4	Approach Character 5	Device Character 6	Qualifier Character 7
X Upper Bursa and Ligament **Y** Lower Bursa and Ligament	**Ø** Open **3** Percutaneous **4** Percutaneous Endoscopic	**Ø** Drainage Device **7** Autologous Tissue Substitute **J** Synthetic Substitute **K** Nonautologous Tissue Substitute **Y** Other Device	**Z** No Qualifier
X Upper Bursa and Ligament **Y** Lower Bursa and Ligament	**X** External	**Ø** Drainage Device	**Z** No Qualifier

Non-OR	ØMP[X,Y]3ØZ
Non-OR	ØMP[X,Y][3,4]YZ
Non-OR	ØMP[X,Y]XØZ

Ø   **Medical and Surgical**
M   **Bursae and Ligaments**
Q   **Repair**   Definition: Restoring, to the extent possible, a body part to its normal anatomic structure and function
                     Explanation: Used only when the method to accomplish the repair is not one of the other root operations

Body Part Character 4		Approach Character 5	Device Character 6	Qualifier Character 7

Ø **Head and Neck Bursa and**
     Ligament
     Alar ligament of axis
     Cervical interspinous ligament
     Cervical intertransverse ligament
     Cervical ligamentum flavum
     Interspinous ligament, cervical
     Intertransverse ligament, cervical
     Lateral temporomandibular
       ligament
     Ligamentum flavum, cervical
     Sphenomandibular ligament
     Stylomandibular ligament
     Transverse ligament of atlas
1 **Shoulder Bursa and Ligament,**
     Right
     Acromioclavicular ligament
     Coracoacromial ligament
     Coracoclavicular ligament
     Coracohumeral ligament
     Costoclavicular ligament
     Glenohumeral ligament
     Interclavicular ligament
     Sternoclavicular ligament
     Subacromial bursa
     Transverse humeral ligament
     Transverse scapular ligament
2 **Shoulder Bursa and Ligament,**
     Left
     See 1 Shoulder Bursa and
       Ligament, Right
3 **Elbow Bursa and Ligament,**
     Right
     Annular ligament
     Olecranon bursa
     Radial collateral ligament
     Ulnar collateral ligament
4 **Elbow Bursa and Ligament, Left**
     See 3 Elbow Bursa and Ligament,
       Right
5 **Wrist Bursa and Ligament, Right**
     Palmar ulnocarpal ligament
     Radial collateral carpal ligament
     Radiocarpal ligament
     Radioulnar ligament
     Scapholunate ligament
     Ulnar collateral carpal ligament
6 **Wrist Bursa and Ligament, Left**
     See 5 Wrist Bursa and Ligament,
       Right
7 **Hand Bursa and Ligament, Right**
     Carpometacarpal ligament
     Intercarpal ligament
     Interphalangeal ligament
     Lunotriquetral ligament
     Metacarpal ligament
     Metacarpophalangeal ligament
     Pisohamate ligament
     Pisometacarpal ligament
     Scaphotrapezium ligament
8 **Hand Bursa and Ligament, Left**
     See 7 Hand Bursa and Ligament,
       Right
9 **Upper Extremity Bursa and**
     Ligament, Right
B **Upper Extremity Bursa and**
     Ligament, Left
C **Upper Spine Bursa and Ligament**
     Interspinous ligament, thoracic
     Intertransverse ligament, thoracic
     Ligamentum flavum, thoracic
     Supraspinous ligament
	D **Lower Spine Bursa and Ligament**
	     Iliolumbar ligament
	     Interspinous ligament, lumbar
	     Intertransverse ligament, lumbar
	     Ligamentum flavum, lumbar
	     Sacrococcygeal ligament
	     Sacroiliac ligament
	     Sacrospinous ligament
	     Sacrotuberous ligament
	     Supraspinous ligament
	F **Sternum Bursa and Ligament**
	     Costoxiphoid ligament
	     Sternocostal ligament
	G **Rib(s) Bursa and Ligament**
	     Costotransverse ligament
	H **Abdomen Bursa and Ligament,**
	     Right
	J **Abdomen Bursa and Ligament,**
	     Left
	K **Perineum Bursa and Ligament**
	L **Hip Bursa and Ligament, Right**
	     Iliofemoral ligament
	     Ischiofemoral ligament
	     Pubofemoral ligament
	     Transverse acetabular ligament
	     Trochanteric bursa
	M **Hip Bursa and Ligament, Left**
	     See L Hip Bursa and Ligament,
	       Right
	N **Knee Bursa and Ligament,**
	     Right
	     Anterior cruciate ligament (ACL)
	     Lateral collateral ligament (LCL)
	     Ligament of head of fibula
	     Medial collateral ligament (MCL)
	     Patellar ligament
	     Popliteal ligament
	     Posterior cruciate ligament (PCL)
	     Prepatellar bursa
	P **Knee Bursa and Ligament,**
	     Left
	     See N Knee Bursa and Ligament,
	       Right
	Q **Ankle Bursa and Ligament, Right**
	     Calcaneofibular ligament
	     Deltoid ligament
	     Ligament of the lateral malleolus
	     Talofibular ligament
	R **Ankle Bursa and Ligament, Left**
	     See Q Ankle Bursa and Ligament,
	       Right
	S **Foot Bursa and Ligament,**
	     Right
	     Calcaneocuboid ligament
	     Cuneonavicular ligament
	     Intercuneiform ligament
	     Interphalangeal ligament
	     Metatarsal ligament
	     Metatarsophalangeal ligament
	     Subtalar ligament
	     Talocalcaneal ligament
	     Talocalcaneonavicular ligament
	     Tarsometatarsal ligament
	T **Foot Bursa and Ligament,**
	     Left
	     See S Foot Bursa and Ligament,
	       Right
	V **Lower Extremity Bursa and**
	     Ligament, Right
	W **Lower Extremity Bursa and**
	     Ligament, Left
		Ø Open
		3 Percutaneous
		4 Percutaneous
		    Endoscopic
			Z No Device	**Z** No Qualifier

NC Noncovered Procedure   **LC** Limited Coverage   **QA** Questionable OB Admit   **NT** New Tech Add-on   ⊞ Combination Member   ♂ Male   ♀ Female

ICD-10-PCS 2022   513

Bursae and Ligaments (side tab)

Ø **Medical and Surgical**
M **Bursae and Ligaments**
R **Replacement**   Definition: Putting in or on biological or synthetic material that physically takes the place and/or function of all or a portion of a body part
       Explanation: The body part may have been taken out or replaced, or may be taken out, physically eradicated, or rendered nonfunctional during the REPLACEMENT procedure. A REMOVAL procedure is coded for taking out the device used in a previous replacement procedure.

Body Part Character 4	Approach Character 5	Device Character 6	Qualifier Character 7
Ø Head and Neck Bursa and Ligament Alar ligament of axis Cervical interspinous ligament Cervical intertransverse ligament Cervical ligamentum flavum Interspinous ligament, cervical Intertransverse ligament, cervical Lateral temporomandibular ligament Ligamentum flavum, cervical Sphenomandibular ligament Stylomandibular ligament Transverse ligament of atlas **1 Shoulder Bursa and Ligament, Right** Acromioclavicular ligament Coracoacromial ligament Coracoclavicular ligament Coracohumeral ligament Costoclavicular ligament Glenohumeral ligament Interclavicular ligament Sternoclavicular ligament Subacromial bursa Transverse humeral ligament Transverse scapular ligament **2 Shoulder Bursa and Ligament, Left** *See 1 Shoulder Bursa and Ligament, Right* **3 Elbow Bursa and Ligament, Right** Annular ligament Olecranon bursa Radial collateral ligament Ulnar collateral ligament **4 Elbow Bursa and Ligament, Left** *See 3 Elbow Bursa and Ligament, Right* **5 Wrist Bursa and Ligament, Right** Palmar ulnocarpal ligament Radial collateral carpal ligament Radiocarpal ligament Radioulnar ligament Scapholunate ligament Ulnar collateral carpal ligament **6 Wrist Bursa and Ligament, Left** *See 5 Wrist Bursa and Ligament, Right* **7 Hand Bursa and Ligament, Right** Carpometacarpal ligament Intercarpal ligament Interphalangeal ligament Lunotriquetral ligament Metacarpal ligament Metacarpophalangeal ligament Pisohamate ligament Pisometacarpal ligament Scaphotrapezium ligament **8 Hand Bursa and Ligament, Left** *See 7 Hand Bursa and Ligament, Right* **9 Upper Extremity Bursa and Ligament, Right** **B Upper Extremity Bursa and Ligament, Left** **C Upper Spine Bursa and Ligament** Interspinous ligament, thoracic Intertransverse ligament, thoracic Ligamentum flavum, thoracic Supraspinous ligament	**Ø Open** **4 Percutaneous Endoscopic**	**7 Autologous Tissue Substitute** **J Synthetic Substitute** **K Nonautologous Tissue Substitute**	**Z No Qualifier**
D Lower Spine Bursa and Ligament Iliolumbar ligament Interspinous ligament, lumbar Intertransverse ligament, lumbar Ligamentum flavum, lumbar Sacrococcygeal ligament Sacroiliac ligament Sacrospinous ligament Sacrotuberous ligament Supraspinous ligament **F Sternum Bursa and Ligament** Costoxiphoid ligament Sternocostal ligament **G Rib(s) Bursa and Ligament** Costotransverse ligament **H Abdomen Bursa and Ligament, Right** **J Abdomen Bursa and Ligament, Left** **K Perineum Bursa and Ligament** **L Hip Bursa and Ligament, Right** Iliofemoral ligament Ischiofemoral ligament Pubofemoral ligament Transverse acetabular ligament Trochanteric bursa **M Hip Bursa and Ligament, Left** *See L Hip Bursa and Ligament, Right* **N Knee Bursa and Ligament, Right** Anterior cruciate ligament (ACL) Lateral collateral ligament (LCL) Ligament of head of fibula Medial collateral ligament (MCL) Patellar ligament Popliteal ligament Posterior cruciate ligament (PCL) Prepatellar bursa **P Knee Bursa and Ligament, Left** *See N Knee Bursa and Ligament, Right* **Q Ankle Bursa and Ligament, Right** Calcaneofibular ligament Deltoid ligament Ligament of the lateral malleolus Talofibular ligament **R Ankle Bursa and Ligament, Left** *See Q Ankle Bursa and Ligament, Right* **S Foot Bursa and Ligament, Right** Calcaneocuboid ligament Cuneonavicular ligament Intercuneiform ligament Interphalangeal ligament Metatarsal ligament Metatarsophalangeal ligament Subtalar ligament Talocalcaneal ligament Talocalcaneonavicular ligament Tarsometatarsal ligament **T Foot Bursa and Ligament, Left** *See S Foot Bursa and Ligament, Right* **V Lower Extremity Bursa and Ligament, Right** **W Lower Extremity Bursa and Ligament, Left**			

Non-OR Procedure   DRG Non-OR Procedure   Valid OR Procedure   HAC Associated Procedure   Combination Only   New/Revised GREEN

Ø   Medical and Surgical
M   Bursae and Ligaments
S   Reposition   Definition: Moving to its normal location, or other suitable location, all or a portion of a body part

Explanation: The body part is moved to a new location from an abnormal location, or from a normal location where it is not functioning correctly. The body part may or may not be cut out or off to be moved to the new location.

Body Part Character 4		Approach Character 5	Device Character 6	Qualifier Character 7
Ø **Head and Neck Bursa and Ligament** Alar ligament of axis Cervical interspinous ligament Cervical intertransverse ligament Cervical ligamentum flavum Interspinous ligament, cervical Intertransverse ligament, cervical Lateral temporomandibular ligament Ligamentum flavum, cervical Sphenomandibular ligament Stylomandibular ligament Transverse ligament of atlas **1** **Shoulder Bursa and Ligament, Right** Acromioclavicular ligament Coracoacromial ligament Coracoclavicular ligament Coracohumeral ligament Costoclavicular ligament Glenohumeral ligament Interclavicular ligament Sternoclavicular ligament Subacromial bursa Transverse humeral ligament Transverse scapular ligament **2** **Shoulder Bursa and Ligament, Left** *See* 1 Shoulder Bursa and Ligament, Right **3** **Elbow Bursa and Ligament, Right** Annular ligament Olecranon bursa Radial collateral ligament Ulnar collateral ligament **4** **Elbow Bursa and Ligament, Left** *See* 3 Elbow Bursa and Ligament, Right **5** **Wrist Bursa and Ligament, Right** Palmar ulnocarpal ligament Radial collateral carpal ligament Radiocarpal ligament Radioulnar ligament Scapholunate ligament Ulnar collateral carpal ligament **6** **Wrist Bursa and Ligament, Left** *See* 5 Wrist Bursa and Ligament, Right **7** **Hand Bursa and Ligament, Right** Carpometacarpal ligament Intercarpal ligament Interphalangeal ligament Lunotriquetral ligament Metacarpal ligament Metacarpophalangeal ligament Pisohamate ligament Pisometacarpal ligament Scaphotrapezium ligament **8** **Hand Bursa and Ligament, Left** *See* 7 Hand Bursa and Ligament, Right **9** **Upper Extremity Bursa and Ligament, Right** **B** **Upper Extremity Bursa and Ligament, Left** **C** **Upper Spine Bursa and Ligament** Interspinous ligament, thoracic Intertransverse ligament, thoracic Ligamentum flavum, thoracic Supraspinous ligament	**D** **Lower Spine Bursa and Ligament** Iliolumbar ligament Interspinous ligament, lumbar Intertransverse ligament, lumbar Ligamentum flavum, lumbar Sacrococcygeal ligament Sacroiliac ligament Sacrospinous ligament Sacrotuberous ligament Supraspinous ligament **F** **Sternum Bursa and Ligament** Costoxiphoid ligament Sternocostal ligament **G** **Rib(s) Bursa and Ligament** Costotransverse ligament **H** **Abdomen Bursa and Ligament, Right** **J** **Abdomen Bursa and Ligament, Left** **K** **Perineum Bursa and Ligament** **L** **Hip Bursa and Ligament, Right** Iliofemoral ligament Ischiofemoral ligament Pubofemoral ligament Transverse acetabular ligament Trochanteric bursa **M** **Hip Bursa and Ligament, Left** *See* L Hip Bursa and Ligament, Right **N** **Knee Bursa and Ligament, Right** Anterior cruciate ligament (ACL) Lateral collateral ligament (LCL) Ligament of head of fibula Medial collateral ligament (MCL) Patellar ligament Popliteal ligament Posterior cruciate ligament (PCL) Prepatellar bursa **P** **Knee Bursa and Ligament, Left** *See* N Knee Bursa and Ligament, Right **Q** **Ankle Bursa and Ligament, Right** Calcaneofibular ligament Deltoid ligament Ligament of the lateral malleolus Talofibular ligament **R** **Ankle Bursa and Ligament, Left** *See* Q Ankle Bursa and Ligament, Right **S** **Foot Bursa and Ligament, Right** Calcaneocuboid ligament Cuneonavicular ligament Intercuneiform ligament Interphalangeal ligament Metatarsal ligament Metatarsophalangeal ligament Subtalar ligament Talocalcaneal ligament Talocalcaneonavicular ligament Tarsometatarsal ligament **T** **Foot Bursa and Ligament, Left** *See* S Foot Bursa and Ligament, Right **V** **Lower Extremity Bursa and Ligament, Right** **W** **Lower Extremity Bursa and Ligament, Left**	**Ø** Open **4** Percutaneous Endoscopic	**Z** No Device	**Z** No Qualifier

NC Noncovered Procedure   **LC** Limited Coverage   **QA** Questionable OB Admit   **NT** New Tech Add-on   ⊞ Combination Member   ♂ Male   ♀ Female

ICD-10-PCS 2022   515

Bursae and Ligaments

Ø   **Medical and Surgical**
M   **Bursae and Ligaments**
T   **Resection**   Definition: Cutting out or off, without replacement, all of a body part
                 Explanation: None

Body Part Character 4		Approach Character 5	Device Character 6	Qualifier Character 7
Ø Head and Neck Bursa and Ligament Alar ligament of axis Cervical interspinous ligament Cervical intertransverse ligament Cervical ligamentum flavum Interspinous ligament, cervical Intertransverse ligament, cervical Lateral temporomandibular ligament Ligamentum flavum, cervical Sphenomandibular ligament Stylomandibular ligament Transverse ligament of atlas **1 Shoulder Bursa and Ligament, Right** Acromioclavicular ligament Coracoacromial ligament Coracoclavicular ligament Coracohumeral ligament Costoclavicular ligament Glenohumeral ligament Interclavicular ligament Sternoclavicular ligament Subacromial bursa Transverse humeral ligament Transverse scapular ligament **2 Shoulder Bursa and Ligament, Left** *See 1 Shoulder Bursa and Ligament, Right* **3 Elbow Bursa and Ligament, Right** Annular ligament Olecranon bursa Radial collateral ligament Ulnar collateral ligament **4 Elbow Bursa and Ligament, Left** *See 3 Elbow Bursa and Ligament, Right* **5 Wrist Bursa and Ligament, Right** Palmar ulnocarpal ligament Radial collateral carpal ligament Radiocarpal ligament Radioulnar ligament Scapholunate ligament Ulnar collateral carpal ligament **6 Wrist Bursa and Ligament, Left** *See 5 Wrist Bursa and Ligament, Right* **7 Hand Bursa and Ligament, Right** Carpometacarpal ligament Intercarpal ligament Interphalangeal ligament Lunotriquetral ligament Metacarpal ligament Metacarpophalangeal ligament Pisohamate ligament Pisometacarpal ligament Scaphotrapezium ligament **8 Hand Bursa and Ligament, Left** *See 7 Hand Bursa and Ligament, Right* **9 Upper Extremity Bursa and Ligament, Right** **B Upper Extremity Bursa and Ligament, Left** **C Upper Spine Bursa and Ligament** Interspinous ligament, thoracic Intertransverse ligament, thoracic Ligamentum flavum, thoracic Supraspinous ligament	**D Lower Spine Bursa and Ligament** Iliolumbar ligament Interspinous ligament, lumbar Intertransverse ligament, lumbar Ligamentum flavum, lumbar Sacrococcygeal ligament Sacroiliac ligament Sacrospinous ligament Sacrotuberous ligament Supraspinous ligament **F Sternum Bursa and Ligament** Costoxiphoid ligament Sternocostal ligament **G Rib(s) Bursa and Ligament** Costotransverse ligament **H Abdomen Bursa and Ligament, Right** **J Abdomen Bursa and Ligament, Left** **K Perineum Bursa and Ligament** **L Hip Bursa and Ligament, Right** Iliofemoral ligament Ischiofemoral ligament Pubofemoral ligament Transverse acetabular ligament Trochanteric bursa **M Hip Bursa and Ligament, Left** *See L Hip Bursa and Ligament, Right* **N Knee Bursa and Ligament, Right** Anterior cruciate ligament (ACL) Lateral collateral ligament (LCL) Ligament of head of fibula Medial collateral ligament (MCL) Patellar ligament Popliteal ligament Posterior cruciate ligament (PCL) Prepatellar bursa **P Knee Bursa and Ligament, Left** *See N Knee Bursa and Ligament, Right* **Q Ankle Bursa and Ligament, Right** Calcaneofibular ligament Deltoid ligament Ligament of the lateral malleolus Talofibular ligament **R Ankle Bursa and Ligament, Left** *See Q Ankle Bursa and Ligament, Right* **S Foot Bursa and Ligament, Right** Calcaneocuboid ligament Cuneonavicular ligament Intercuneiform ligament Interphalangeal ligament Metatarsal ligament Metatarsophalangeal ligament Subtalar ligament Talocalcaneal ligament Talocalcaneonavicular ligament Tarsometatarsal ligament **T Foot Bursa and Ligament, Left** *See S Foot Bursa and Ligament, Right* **V Lower Extremity Bursa and Ligament, Right** **W Lower Extremity Bursa and Ligament, Left**	**Ø Open** **4 Percutaneous Endoscopic**	**Z No Device**	**Z No Qualifier**

Ø Medical and Surgical
M Bursae and Ligaments
U Supplement   Definition: Putting in or on biological or synthetic material that physically reinforces and/or augments the function of a portion of a body part
       Explanation: The biological material is non-living, or is living and from the same individual. The body part may have been previously replaced, and the SUPPLEMENT procedure is performed to physically reinforce and/or augment the function of the replaced body part.

Body Part Character 4		Approach Character 5	Device Character 6	Qualifier Character 7
Ø Head and Neck Bursa and Ligament Alar ligament of axis Cervical interspinous ligament Cervical intertransverse ligament Cervical ligamentum flavum Interspinous ligament, cervical Intertransverse ligament, cervical Lateral temporomandibular ligament Ligamentum flavum, cervical Sphenomandibular ligament Stylomandibular ligament Transverse ligament of atlas	**D Lower Spine Bursa and Ligament** Iliolumbar ligament Interspinous ligament, lumbar Intertransverse ligament, lumbar Ligamentum flavum, lumbar Sacrococcygeal ligament Sacroiliac ligament Sacrospinous ligament Sacrotuberous ligament Supraspinous ligament	**Ø Open** **4 Percutaneous Endoscopic**	**7 Autologous Tissue Substitute** **J Synthetic Substitute** **K Nonautologous Tissue Substitute**	**Z No Qualifier**
1 Shoulder Bursa and Ligament, Right Acromioclavicular ligament Coracoacromial ligament Coracoclavicular ligament Coracohumeral ligament Costoclavicular ligament Glenohumeral ligament Interclavicular ligament Sternoclavicular ligament Subacromial bursa Transverse humeral ligament Transverse scapular ligament	**F Sternum Bursa and Ligament** Costoxiphoid ligament Sternocostal ligament **G Rib(s) Bursa and Ligament** Costotransverse ligament **H Abdomen Bursa and Ligament, Right** **J Abdomen Bursa and Ligament, Left**			
2 Shoulder Bursa and Ligament, Left *See 1 Shoulder Bursa and Ligament, Right*	**K Perineum Bursa and Ligament** **L Hip Bursa and Ligament, Right** Iliofemoral ligament Ischiofemoral ligament Pubofemoral ligament Transverse acetabular ligament Trochanteric bursa			
3 Elbow Bursa and Ligament, Right Annular ligament Olecranon bursa Radial collateral ligament Ulnar collateral ligament	**M Hip Bursa and Ligament, Left** *See L Hip Bursa and Ligament, Right*			
4 Elbow Bursa and Ligament, Left *See 3 Elbow Bursa and Ligament, Right*	**N Knee Bursa and Ligament, Right** Anterior cruciate ligament (ACL) Lateral collateral ligament (LCL) Ligament of head of fibula Medial collateral ligament (MCL) Patellar ligament Popliteal ligament Posterior cruciate ligament (PCL) Prepatellar bursa			
5 Wrist Bursa and Ligament, Right Palmar ulnocarpal ligament Radial collateral carpal ligament Radiocarpal ligament Radioulnar ligament Scapholunate ligament Ulnar collateral carpal ligament	**P Knee Bursa and Ligament, Left** *See N Knee Bursa and Ligament, Right*			
6 Wrist Bursa and Ligament, Left *See 5 Wrist Bursa and Ligament, Right*	**Q Ankle Bursa and Ligament, Right** Calcaneofibular ligament Deltoid ligament Ligament of the lateral malleolus Talofibular ligament			
7 Hand Bursa and Ligament, Right Carpometacarpal ligament Intercarpal ligament Interphalangeal ligament Lunotriquetral ligament Metacarpal ligament Metacarpophalangeal ligament Pisohamate ligament Pisometacarpal ligament Scaphotrapezium ligament	**R Ankle Bursa and Ligament, Left** *See Q Ankle Bursa and Ligament, Right* **S Foot Bursa and Ligament, Right** Calcaneocuboid ligament Cuneonavicular ligament Intercuneiform ligament Interphalangeal ligament Metatarsal ligament Metatarsophalangeal ligament Subtalar ligament Talocalcaneal ligament Talocalcaneonavicular ligament Tarsometatarsal ligament			
8 Hand Bursa and Ligament, Left *See 7 Hand Bursa and Ligament, Right*				
9 Upper Extremity Bursa and Ligament, Right				
B Upper Extremity Bursa and Ligament, Left	**T Foot Bursa and Ligament, Left** *See S Foot Bursa and Ligament, Right*			
C Upper Spine Bursa and Ligament Interspinous ligament, thoracic Intertransverse ligament, thoracic Ligamentum flavum, thoracic Supraspinous ligament	**V Lower Extremity Bursa and Ligament, Right** **W Lower Extremity Bursa and Ligament, Left**			

NC Noncovered Procedure   **LC** Limited Coverage   **QA** Questionable OB Admit   **NT** New Tech Add-on   ⊞ Combination Member   ♂ Male   ♀ Female

Bursae and Ligaments

Ø   **Medical and Surgical**
M   **Bursae and Ligaments**
W   **Revision**   Definition: Correcting, to the extent possible, a portion of a malfunctioning device or the position of a displaced device

Explanation: Revision can include correcting a malfunctioning or displaced device by taking out or putting in components of the device such as a screw or pin

Body Part Character 4		Approach Character 5		Device Character 6		Qualifier Character 7	
X	Upper Bursa and Ligament	Ø	Open	Ø	Drainage Device	Z	No Qualifier
Y	Lower Bursa and Ligament	3	Percutaneous	7	Autologous Tissue Substitute		
		4	Percutaneous Endoscopic	J	Synthetic Substitute		
				K	Nonautologous Tissue Substitute		
				Y	Other Device		
X	Upper Bursa and Ligament	X	External	Ø	Drainage Device	Z	No Qualifier
Y	Lower Bursa and Ligament			7	Autologous Tissue Substitute		
				J	Synthetic Substitute		
				K	Nonautologous Tissue Substitute		

Non-OR   ØMW[X,Y][3,4]YZ
Non-OR   ØMW[X,Y]X[Ø,7,J,K]Z

Ø   Medical and Surgical
M   Bursae and Ligaments
X   Transfer   Definition: Moving, without taking out, all or a portion of a body part to another location to take over the function of all or a portion of a body part
                Explanation: The body part transferred remains connected to its vascular and nervous supply

Body Part Character 4		Approach Character 5	Device Character 6	Qualifier Character 7
Ø Head and Neck Bursa and Ligament Alar ligament of axis Cervical interspinous ligament Cervical intertransverse ligament Cervical ligamentum flavum Interspinous ligament, cervical Intertransverse ligament, cervical Lateral temporomandibular ligament Ligamentum flavum, cervical Sphenomandibular ligament Stylomandibular ligament Transverse ligament of atlas	**D Lower Spine Bursa and Ligament** Iliolumbar ligament Interspinous ligament, lumbar Intertransverse ligament, lumbar Ligamentum flavum, lumbar Sacrococcygeal ligament Sacroiliac ligament Sacrospinous ligament Sacrotuberous ligament Supraspinous ligament	**Ø Open** **4 Percutaneous Endoscopic**	**Z No Device**	**Z No Qualifier**
1 Shoulder Bursa and Ligament, Right Acromioclavicular ligament Coracoacromial ligament Coracoclavicular ligament Coracohumeral ligament Costoclavicular ligament Glenohumeral ligament Interclavicular ligament Sternoclavicular ligament Subacromial bursa Transverse humeral ligament Transverse scapular ligament	**F Sternum Bursa and Ligament** Costoxiphoid ligament Sternocostal ligament **G Rib(s) Bursa and Ligament** Costotransverse ligament **H Abdomen Bursa and Ligament, Right** **J Abdomen Bursa and Ligament, Left** **K Perineum Bursa and Ligament** **L Hip Bursa and Ligament, Right** Iliofemoral ligament Ischiofemoral ligament Pubofemoral ligament Transverse acetabular ligament Trochanteric bursa			
2 Shoulder Bursa and Ligament, Left *See* 1 Shoulder Bursa and Ligament, Right	**M Hip Bursa and Ligament, Left** *See* L Hip Bursa and Ligament, Right			
3 Elbow Bursa and Ligament, Right Annular ligament Olecranon bursa Radial collateral ligament Ulnar collateral ligament	**N Knee Bursa and Ligament, Right** Anterior cruciate ligament (ACL) Lateral collateral ligament (LCL) Ligament of head of fibula Medial collateral ligament (MCL) Patellar ligament Popliteal ligament Posterior cruciate ligament (PCL) Prepatellar bursa			
4 Elbow Bursa and Ligament, Left *See* 3 Elbow Bursa and Ligament, Right	**P Knee Bursa and Ligament, Left** *See* N Knee Bursa and Ligament, Right			
5 Wrist Bursa and Ligament, Right Palmar ulnocarpal ligament Radial collateral carpal ligament Radiocarpal ligament Radioulnar ligament Scapholunate ligament Ulnar collateral carpal ligament	**Q Ankle Bursa and Ligament, Right** Calcaneofibular ligament Deltoid ligament Ligament of the lateral malleolus Talofibular ligament			
6 Wrist Bursa and Ligament, Left *See* 5 Wrist Bursa and Ligament, Right	**R Ankle Bursa and Ligament, Left** *See* Q Ankle Bursa and Ligament, Right			
7 Hand Bursa and Ligament, Right Carpometacarpal ligament Intercarpal ligament Interphalangeal ligament Lunotriquetral ligament Metacarpal ligament Metacarpophalangeal ligament Pisohamate ligament Pisometacarpal ligament Scaphotrapezium ligament	**S Foot Bursa and Ligament, Right** Calcaneocuboid ligament Cuneonavicular ligament Intercuneiform ligament Interphalangeal ligament Metatarsal ligament Metatarsophalangeal ligament Subtalar ligament Talocalcaneal ligament Talocalcaneonavicular ligament Tarsometatarsal ligament			
8 Hand Bursa and Ligament, Left *See* 7 Hand Bursa and Ligament, Right	**T Foot Bursa and Ligament, Left** *See* S Foot Bursa and Ligament, Right			
9 Upper Extremity Bursa and Ligament, Right **B Upper Extremity Bursa and Ligament, Left** **C Upper Spine Bursa and Ligament** Interspinous ligament, thoracic Intertransverse ligament, thoracic Ligamentum flavum, thoracic Supraspinous ligament	**V Lower Extremity Bursa and Ligament, Right** **W Lower Extremity Bursa and Ligament, Left**			

Head and Facial Bones ØN2–ØNW

Character Meanings

This Character Meaning table is provided as a guide to assist the user in the identification of character members that may be found in this section of code tables. It **SHOULD NOT** be used to build a PCS code.

Operation–Character 3	Body Part–Character 4	Approach–Character 5	Device–Character 6	Qualifier–Character 7
2　Change	Ø　Skull	Ø　Open	Ø　Drainage Device	X　Diagnostic
5　Destruction	1　Frontal Bone	3　Percutaneous	3　Infusion Device	Z　No Qualifier
8　Division	3　Parietal Bone, Right	4　Percutaneous Endoscopic	4　Internal Fixation Device	
9　Drainage	4　Parietal Bone, Left	X　External	5　External Fixation Device	
B　Excision	5　Temporal Bone, Right		7　Autologous Tissue Substitute	
C　Extirpation	6　Temporal Bone, Left		J　Synthetic Substitute	
D　Extraction	7　Occipital Bone		K　Nonautologous Tissue Substitute	
H　Insertion	B　Nasal Bone		M　Bone Growth Stimulator	
J　Inspection	C　Sphenoid Bone		N　Neurostimulator Generator	
N　Release	F　Ethmoid Bone, Right		S　Hearing Device	
P　Removal	G　Ethmoid Bone, Left		Y　Other Device	
Q　Repair	H　Lacrimal Bone, Right		Z　No Device	
R　Replacement	J　Lacrimal Bone, Left			
S　Reposition	K　Palatine Bone, Right			
T　Resection	L　Palatine Bone, Left			
U　Supplement	M　Zygomatic Bone, Right			
W　Revision	N　Zygomatic Bone, Left			
	P　Orbit, Right			
	Q　Orbit, Left			
	R　Maxilla			
	T　Mandible, Right			
	V　Mandible, Left			
	W　Facial Bone			
	X　Hyoid Bone			

AHA Coding Clinic for table ØNB
2021, 1Q, 21	Maxillectomy with reconstruction of maxilla
2017, 1Q, 20	Preparatory nasal adhesion repair before definitive cleft palate repair
2015, 3Q, 3-8	Excisional and nonexcisional debridement
2015, 2Q, 12	Orbital exenteration

AHA Coding Clinic for table ØND
2017, 4Q, 41	Extraction procedures

AHA Coding Clinic for table ØNH
2015, 3Q, 13	Nonexcisional debridement of cranial wound with removal and replacement of hardware

AHA Coding Clinic for table ØNP
2015, 3Q, 13	Nonexcisional debridement of cranial wound with removal and replacement of hardware

AHA Coding Clinic for table ØNQ
2016, 3Q, 29	Closure of bilateral alveolar clefts

AHA Coding Clinic for table ØNR
2021, 1Q, 21	Maxillectomy with reconstruction of maxilla
2017, 3Q, 17	Resection of schwannoma and placement of DuraGen and Lorenz cranial plating system
2017, 3Q, 22	Replacement of native skull bone flap
2017, 1Q, 23	Reconstruction of mandible using titanium and bone
2014, 3Q, 7	Hemi-cranioplasty for repair of cranial defect

AHA Coding Clinic for table ØNS
2017, 3Q, 22	Replacement of native skull bone flap
2017, 1Q, 20	Preparatory nasal adhesion repair before definitive cleft palate repair
2016, 2Q, 30	Clipping (occlusion) of cerebral artery, decompressive craniectomy and storage of bone flap in abdominal wall
2015, 3Q, 17	Craniosynostosis with cranial vault reconstruction
2015, 3Q, 27	Moyamoya disease and hemispheric pial synagiosis with craniotomy
2014, 3Q, 23	Le Fort I osteotomy
2013, 3Q, 24	Distraction osteogenesis
2013, 3Q, 25	Fracture of frontal bone with repair and coagulation for hemostasis

AHA Coding Clinic for table ØNU
2016, 3Q, 29	Closure of bilateral alveolar clefts
2013, 3Q, 24	Distraction osteogenesis

Head and Facial Bones

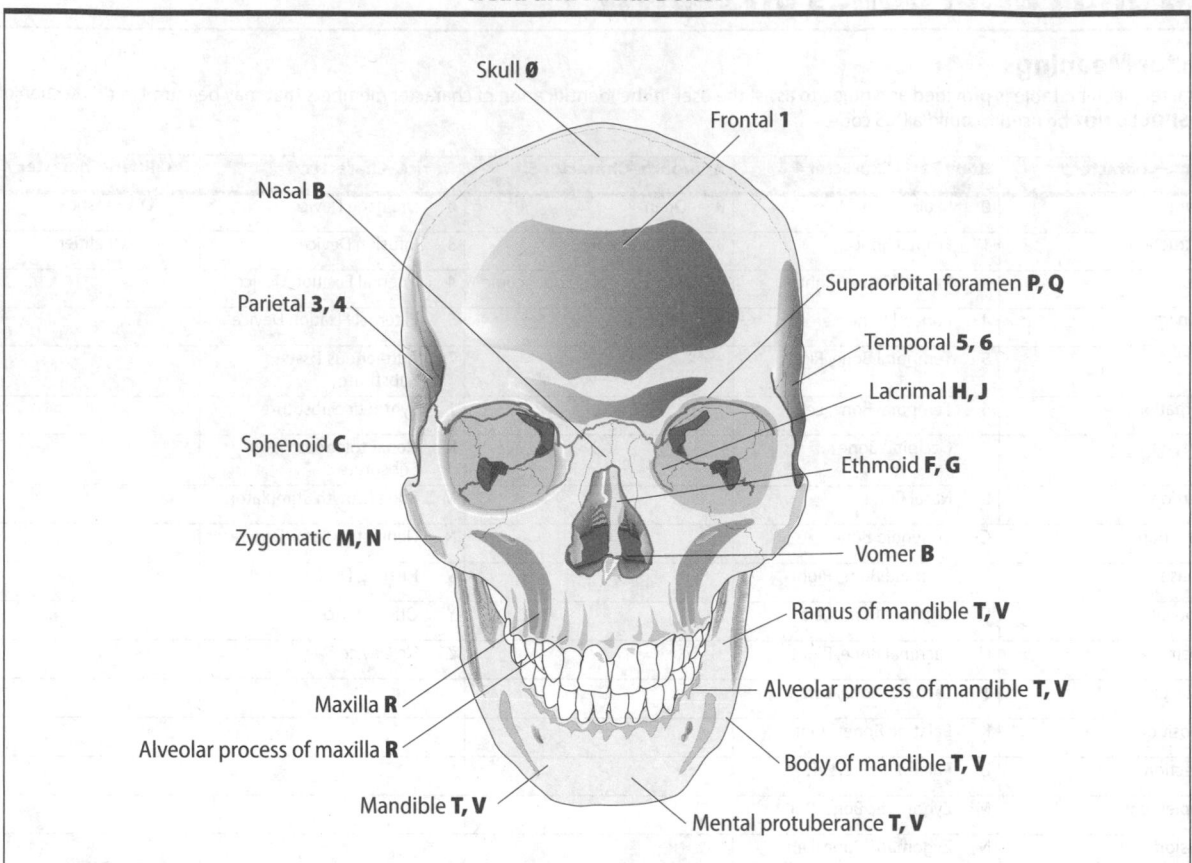

Skull Ø
Frontal 1
Nasal B
Supraorbital foramen P, Q
Parietal 3, 4
Temporal 5, 6
Lacrimal H, J
Sphenoid C
Ethmoid F, G
Zygomatic M, N
Vomer B
Ramus of mandible T, V
Alveolar process of mandible T, V
Maxilla R
Body of mandible T, V
Alveolar process of maxilla R
Mandible T, V
Mental protuberance T, V

Skull Bones

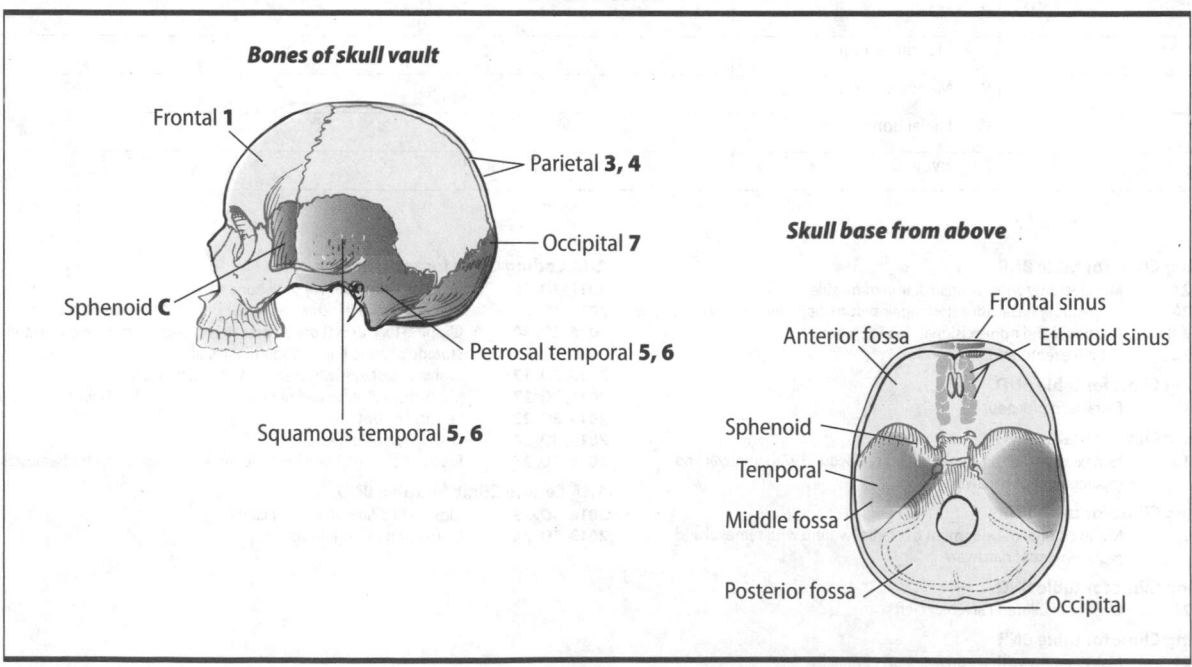

Bones of skull vault

Frontal 1
Parietal 3, 4
Occipital 7
Sphenoid C
Petrosal temporal 5, 6
Squamous temporal 5, 6

Skull base from above

Frontal sinus
Anterior fossa
Ethmoid sinus
Sphenoid
Temporal
Middle fossa
Posterior fossa
Occipital

Head and Facial Bones

Ø   **Medical and Surgical**
N   **Head and Facial Bones**
2   **Change**   Definition: Taking out or off a device from a body part and putting back an identical or similar device in or on the same body part without cutting or puncturing the skin or a mucous membrane
               Explanation: All CHANGE procedures are coded using the approach EXTERNAL

Body Part Character 4	Approach Character 5	Device Character 6	Qualifier Character 7
Ø Skull B Nasal Bone Vomer of nasal septum W Facial Bone	X External	Ø Drainage Device Y Other Device	Z No Qualifier

   Non-OR   All body part, approach, device, and qualifier values

Ø   **Medical and Surgical**
N   **Head and Facial Bones**
5   **Destruction**   Definition: Physical eradication of all or a portion of a body part by the direct use of energy, force, or a destructive agent
               Explanation: None of the body part is physically taken out

Body Part Character 4	Approach Character 5	Device Character 6	Qualifier Character 7

Ø Skull
1 Frontal Bone
   Zygomatic process of frontal bone
3 Parietal Bone, Right
4 Parietal Bone, Left
5 Temporal Bone, Right
   Mastoid process
   Petrous part of temporal bone
   Tympanic part of temporal bone
   Zygomatic process of temporal bone
6 Temporal Bone, Left
   See 5 Temporal Bone, Right
7 Occipital Bone
   Foramen magnum
B Nasal Bone
   Vomer of nasal septum
C Sphenoid Bone
   Greater wing
   Lesser wing
   Optic foramen
   Pterygoid process
   Sella turcica
F Ethmoid Bone, Right
   Cribriform plate
G Ethmoid Bone, Left
   See F Ethmoid Bone, Right
H Lacrimal Bone, Right
J Lacrimal Bone, Left
K Palatine Bone, Right
L Palatine Bone, Left
M Zygomatic Bone, Right
N Zygomatic Bone, Left
P Orbit, Right
   Bony orbit
   Orbital portion of ethmoid bone
   Orbital portion of frontal bone
   Orbital portion of lacrimal bone
   Orbital portion of maxilla
   Orbital portion of palatine bone
   Orbital portion of sphenoid bone
   Orbital portion of zygomatic bone
Q Orbit, Left
   See P Orbit, Right
R Maxilla
   Alveolar process of maxilla
T Mandible, Right
   Alveolar process of mandible
   Condyloid process
   Mandibular notch
   Mental foramen
V Mandible, Left
   See T Mandible, Right
X Hyoid Bone
	Ø Open
	3 Percutaneous
	4 Percutaneous Endoscopic
		Z No Device	Z No Qualifier

NC Noncovered Procedure   LC Limited Coverage   QA Questionable OB Admit   NT New Tech Add-on   ⊞ Combination Member   ♂ Male   ♀ Female

ICD-10-PCS 2022   523

Head and Facial Bones

Ø   **Medical and Surgical**
N   **Head and Facial Bones**
8   **Division**   Definition: Cutting into a body part, without draining fluids and/or gases from the body part, in order to separate or transect a body part
                 Explanation: All or a portion of the body part is separated into two or more portions

Body Part Character 4	Approach Character 5	Device Character 6	Qualifier Character 7
Ø Skull	Ø Open	Z No Device	Z No Qualifier
1 Frontal Bone	3 Percutaneous		
Zygomatic process of frontal bone	4 Percutaneous Endoscopic		
3 Parietal Bone, Right			
4 Parietal Bone, Left			
5 Temporal Bone, Right			
Mastoid process			
Petrous part of temporal bone			
Tympanic part of temporal bone			
Zygomatic process of temporal bone			
6 Temporal Bone, Left			
See 5 Temporal Bone, Right			
7 Occipital Bone			
Foramen magnum			
B Nasal Bone			
Vomer of nasal septum			
C Sphenoid Bone			
Greater wing			
Lesser wing			
Optic foramen			
Pterygoid process			
Sella turcica			
F Ethmoid Bone, Right			
Cribriform plate			
G Ethmoid Bone, Left			
See F Ethmoid Bone, Right			
H Lacrimal Bone, Right			
J Lacrimal Bone, Left			
K Palatine Bone, Right			
L Palatine Bone, Left			
M Zygomatic Bone, Right			
N Zygomatic Bone, Left			
P Orbit, Right			
Bony orbit			
Orbital portion of ethmoid bone			
Orbital portion of frontal bone			
Orbital portion of lacrimal bone			
Orbital portion of maxilla			
Orbital portion of palatine bone			
Orbital portion of sphenoid bone			
Orbital portion of zygomatic bone			
Q Orbit, Left			
See P Orbit, Right			
R Maxilla			
Alveolar process of maxilla			
T Mandible, Right			
Alveolar process of mandible			
Condyloid process			
Mandibular notch			
Mental foramen			
V Mandible, Left			
See T Mandible, Right			
X Hyoid Bone			

Non-OR   ØN8B[Ø,3,4]ZZ

Ø   **Medical and Surgical**
N   **Head and Facial Bones**
9   **Drainage**   Definition: Taking or letting out fluids and/or gases from a body part

                           Explanation: The qualifier DIAGNOSTIC is used to identify drainage procedures that are biopsies

Body Part Character 4	Approach Character 5	Device Character 6	Qualifier Character 7
Ø Skull	Ø Open	Ø Drainage Device	Z No Qualifier
1 Frontal Bone	3 Percutaneous		
Zygomatic process of frontal bone	4 Percutaneous Endoscopic		
3 Parietal Bone, Right			
4 Parietal Bone, Left			
5 Temporal Bone, Right			
Mastoid process			
Petrous part of temporal bone			
Tympanic part of temporal bone			
Zygomatic process of temporal bone			
6 Temporal Bone, Left			
See 5 Temporal Bone, Right			
7 Occipital Bone			
Foramen magnum			
B Nasal Bone			
Vomer of nasal septum			
C Sphenoid Bone			
Greater wing			
Lesser wing			
Optic foramen			
Pterygoid process			
Sella turcica			
F Ethmoid Bone, Right			
Cribriform plate			
G Ethmoid Bone, Left			
See F Ethmoid Bone, Right			
H Lacrimal Bone, Right			
J Lacrimal Bone, Left			
K Palatine Bone, Right			
L Palatine Bone, Left			
M Zygomatic Bone, Right			
N Zygomatic Bone, Left			
P Orbit, Right			
Bony orbit			
Orbital portion of ethmoid bone			
Orbital portion of frontal bone			
Orbital portion of lacrimal bone			
Orbital portion of maxilla			
Orbital portion of palatine bone			
Orbital portion of sphenoid bone			
Orbital portion of zygomatic bone			
Q Orbit, Left			
See P Orbit, Right			
R Maxilla			
Alveolar process of maxilla			
T Mandible, Right			
Alveolar process of mandible			
Condyloid process			
Mandibular notch			
Mental foramen			
V Mandible, Left			
See T Mandible, Right			
X Hyoid Bone			

Non-OR   ØN9[Ø,1,3,4,5,6,7,C,F,G,H,J,K,L,M,N,P,Q,X]3ØZ
Non-OR   ØN9[B,R,T,V][Ø,3,4]ØZ

ØN9 Continued on next page

NC Noncovered Procedure   **LC** Limited Coverage   **QA** Questionable OB Admit   **NT** New Tech Add-on   ⊞ Combination Member   ♂ Male   ♀ Female

ICD-10-PCS 2022   525

Head and Facial Bones

Ø　**Medical and Surgical**　　　　　　　　　　　　　　　　　　　　　　　　　　　　　　*ØN9 Continued*
N　**Head and Facial Bones**
9　**Drainage**　　　Definition: Taking or letting out fluids and/or gases from a body part
　　　　　　　　　　　　Explanation: The qualifier DIAGNOSTIC is used to identify drainage procedures that are biopsies

Body Part Character 4	Approach Character 5	Device Character 6	Qualifier Character 7
Ø　**Skull**	Ø　Open	Z　No Device	X　Diagnostic
1　**Frontal Bone**	3　Percutaneous		Z　No Qualifier
Zygomatic process of frontal bone	4　Percutaneous Endoscopic		
3　**Parietal Bone, Right**			
4　**Parietal Bone, Left**			
5　**Temporal Bone, Right**			
Mastoid process			
Petrous part of temporal bone			
Tympanic part of temporal bone			
Zygomatic process of temporal bone			
6　**Temporal Bone, Left**			
See 5 Temporal Bone, Right			
7　**Occipital Bone**			
Foramen magnum			
B　**Nasal Bone**			
Vomer of nasal septum			
C　**Sphenoid Bone**			
Greater wing			
Lesser wing			
Optic foramen			
Pterygoid process			
Sella turcica			
F　**Ethmoid Bone, Right**			
Cribriform plate			
G　**Ethmoid Bone, Left**			
See F Ethmoid Bone, Right			
H　**Lacrimal Bone, Right**			
J　**Lacrimal Bone, Left**			
K　**Palatine Bone, Right**			
L　**Palatine Bone, Left**			
M　**Zygomatic Bone, Right**			
N　**Zygomatic Bone, Left**			
P　**Orbit, Right**			
Bony orbit			
Orbital portion of ethmoid bone			
Orbital portion of frontal bone			
Orbital portion of lacrimal bone			
Orbital portion of maxilla			
Orbital portion of palatine bone			
Orbital portion of sphenoid bone			
Orbital portion of zygomatic bone			
Q　**Orbit, Left**			
See P Orbit, Right			
R　**Maxilla**			
Alveolar process of maxilla			
T　**Mandible, Right**			
Alveolar process of mandible			
Condyloid process			
Mandibular notch			
Mental foramen			
V　**Mandible, Left**			
See T Mandible, Right			
X　**Hyoid Bone**			

Non-OR　ØN9[Ø,1,3,4,5,6,7,C,F,G,H,J,K,L,M,N,P,Q,X]3ZZ
Non-OR　ØN9B[Ø,3,4]Z[X,Z]
Non-OR　ØN9[R,T,V][Ø,3,4]ZZ

Non-OR Procedure　　　DRG Non-OR Procedure　　　Valid OR Procedure　　　HAC Associated Procedure　　　Combination Only　　　New/Revised GREEN

Ø   **Medical and Surgical**
N   **Head and Facial Bones**
B   **Excision**   Definition: Cutting out or off, without replacement, a portion of a body part
                      Explanation: The qualifier DIAGNOSTIC is used to identify excision procedures that are biopsies

Body Part Character 4	Approach Character 5	Device Character 6	Qualifier Character 7
Ø Skull	**Ø** Open	**Z** No Device	**X** Diagnostic
1 Frontal Bone	**3** Percutaneous		**Z** No Qualifier
Zygomatic process of frontal bone	**4** Percutaneous Endoscopic		
3 Parietal Bone, Right			
4 Parietal Bone, Left			
5 Temporal Bone, Right			
Mastoid process			
Petrous part of temporal bone			
Tympanic part of temporal bone			
Zygomatic process of temporal bone			
6 Temporal Bone, Left			
See 5 Temporal Bone, Right			
7 Occipital Bone			
Foramen magnum			
B Nasal Bone			
Vomer of nasal septum			
C Sphenoid Bone			
Greater wing			
Lesser wing			
Optic foramen			
Pterygoid process			
Sella turcica			
F Ethmoid Bone, Right			
Cribriform plate			
G Ethmoid Bone, Left			
See F Ethmoid Bone, Right			
H Lacrimal Bone, Right			
J Lacrimal Bone, Left			
K Palatine Bone, Right			
L Palatine Bone, Left			
M Zygomatic Bone, Right			
N Zygomatic Bone, Left			
P Orbit, Right			
Bony orbit			
Orbital portion of ethmoid bone			
Orbital portion of frontal bone			
Orbital portion of lacrimal bone			
Orbital portion of maxilla			
Orbital portion of palatine bone			
Orbital portion of sphenoid bone			
Orbital portion of zygomatic bone			
Q Orbit, Left			
See P Orbit, Right			
R Maxilla			
Alveolar process of maxilla			
T Mandible, Right			
Alveolar process of mandible			
Condyloid process			
Mandibular notch			
Mental foramen			
V Mandible, Left			
See T Mandible, Right			
X Hyoid Bone			

Non-OR   ØNB[B,R,T,V][Ø,3,4]ZX

NC Noncovered Procedure   **LC** Limited Coverage   **QA** Questionable OB Admit   **NT** New Tech Add-on   ✚ Combination Member   ♂ Male   ♀ Female

ICD-10-PCS 2022   527

Head and Facial Bones

Ø   **Medical and Surgical**
N   **Head and Facial Bones**
C   **Extirpation**   Definition: Taking or cutting out solid matter from a body part

                      Explanation: The solid matter may be an abnormal byproduct of a biological function or a foreign body; it may be imbedded in a body part or in the lumen of a tubular body part. The solid matter may or may not have been previously broken into pieces.

Body Part Character 4	Approach Character 5	Device Character 6	Qualifier Character 7

1 **Frontal Bone**
    Zygomatic process of frontal bone
3 **Parietal Bone, Right**
4 **Parietal Bone, Left**
5 **Temporal Bone, Right**
    Mastoid process
    Petrous part of temporal bone
    Tympanic part of temporal bone
    Zygomatic process of temporal bone
6 **Temporal Bone, Left**
    See 5 Temporal Bone, Right
7 **Occipital Bone**
    Foramen magnum
B **Nasal Bone**
    Vomer of nasal septum
C **Sphenoid Bone**
    Greater wing
    Lesser wing
    Optic foramen
    Pterygoid process
    Sella turcica
F **Ethmoid Bone, Right**
    Cribriform plate
G **Ethmoid Bone, Left**
    See F Ethmoid Bone, Right
H **Lacrimal Bone, Right**
J **Lacrimal Bone, Left**
K **Palatine Bone, Right**
L **Palatine Bone, Left**
M **Zygomatic Bone, Right**
N **Zygomatic Bone, Left**
P **Orbit, Right**
    Bony orbit
    Orbital portion of ethmoid bone
    Orbital portion of frontal bone
    Orbital portion of lacrimal bone
    Orbital portion of maxilla
    Orbital portion of palatine bone
    Orbital portion of sphenoid bone
    Orbital portion of zygomatic bone
Q **Orbit, Left**
    See P Orbit, Right
R **Maxilla**
    Alveolar process of maxilla
T **Mandible, Right**
    Alveolar process of mandible
    Condyloid process
    Mandibular notch
    Mental foramen
V **Mandible, Left**
    See T Mandible, Right
X **Hyoid Bone**
	Ø **Open**
	3 **Percutaneous**
	4 **Percutaneous Endoscopic**
		Z **No Device**	**Z** **No Qualifier**

Non-OR   ØNC[B,R,T,V][Ø,3,4]ZZ

Ø Medical and Surgical
N Head and Facial Bones
D Extraction   Definition: Pulling or stripping out or off all or a portion of a body part by the use of force
               Explanation: The qualifier DIAGNOSTIC is used to identify extraction procedures that are biopsies

Body Part Character 4	Approach Character 5	Device Character 6	Qualifier Character 7
Ø Skull	**Ø Open**	**Z No Device**	**Z No Qualifier**
1 Frontal Bone Zygomatic process of frontal bone			
3 Parietal Bone, Right			
4 Parietal Bone, Left			
5 Temporal Bone, Right Mastoid process Petrous part of temporal bone Tympanic part of temporal bone Zygomatic process of temporal bone			
6 Temporal Bone, Left *See 5 Temporal Bone, Right*			
7 Occipital Bone Foramen magnum			
B Nasal Bone Vomer of nasal septum			
C Sphenoid Bone Greater wing Lesser wing Optic foramen Pterygoid process Sella turcica			
F Ethmoid Bone, Right Cribriform plate			
G Ethmoid Bone, Left *See F Ethmoid Bone, Right*			
H Lacrimal Bone, Right			
J Lacrimal Bone, Left			
K Palatine Bone, Right			
L Palatine Bone, Left			
M Zygomatic Bone, Right			
N Zygomatic Bone, Left			
P Orbit, Right Bony orbit Orbital portion of ethmoid bone Orbital portion of frontal bone Orbital portion of lacrimal bone Orbital portion of maxilla Orbital portion of palatine bone Orbital portion of sphenoid bone Orbital portion of zygomatic bone			
Q Orbit, Left *See P Orbit, Right*			
R Maxilla Alveolar process of maxilla			
T Mandible, Right Alveolar process of mandible Condyloid process Mandibular notch Mental foramen			
V Mandible, Left *See T Mandible, Right*			
X Hyoid Bone			

NC Noncovered Procedure   LC Limited Coverage   QA Questionable OB Admit   NT New Tech Add-on   ⊞ Combination Member   ♂ Male   ♀ Female

ICD-10-PCS 2022   529

ØND–ØND

Head and Facial Bones

Ø   **Medical and Surgical**
N   **Head and Facial Bones**
H   **Insertion**   Definition: Putting in a nonbiological appliance that monitors, assists, performs, or prevents a physiological function but does not physically take the place of a body part
               Explanation: None

Body Part Character 4	Approach Character 5	Device Character 6	Qualifier Character 7
Ø Skull ⊞	Ø Open	3 Infusion Device 4 Internal Fixation Device 5 External Fixation Device M Bone Growth Stimulator N Neurostimulator Generator	Z No Qualifier
Ø Skull	3 Percutaneous 4 Percutaneous Endoscopic	3 Infusion Device 4 Internal Fixation Device 5 External Fixation Device M Bone Growth Stimulator	Z No Qualifier

1   **Frontal Bone**
    Zygomatic process of frontal bone
3   **Parietal Bone, Right**
4   **Parietal Bone, Left**
7   **Occipital Bone**
    Foramen magnum
C   **Sphenoid Bone**
    Greater wing
    Lesser wing
    Optic foramen
    Pterygoid process
    Sella turcica
F   **Ethmoid Bone, Right**
    Cribriform plate
G   **Ethmoid Bone, Left**
    See F Ethmoid Bone, Right
H   **Lacrimal Bone, Right**
J   **Lacrimal Bone, Left**
K   **Palatine Bone, Right**
L   **Palatine Bone, Left**
M   **Zygomatic Bone, Right**
N   **Zygomatic Bone, Left**
P   **Orbit, Right**
    Bony orbit
    Orbital portion of ethmoid bone
    Orbital portion of frontal bone
    Orbital portion of lacrimal bone
    Orbital portion of maxilla
    Orbital portion of palatine bone
    Orbital portion of sphenoid bone
    Orbital portion of zygomatic bone
Q   **Orbit, Left**
    See P Orbit, Right
X   **Hyoid Bone**
	Ø Open
	3 Percutaneous
	4 Percutaneous Endoscopic
		4 Internal Fixation Device	Z No Qualifier

5   **Temporal Bone, Right**
    Mastoid process
    Petrous part of temporal bone
    Tympanic part of temporal bone
    Zygomatic process of temporal bone
6   **Temporal Bone, Left**
    See 5 Temporal Bone, Right
	Ø Open
	3 Percutaneous
	4 Percutaneous Endoscopic
		4 Internal Fixation Device
		S Hearing Device
			Z No Qualifier

B **Nasal Bone** Vomer of nasal septum	Ø Open 3 Percutaneous 4 Percutaneous Endoscopic	4 Internal Fixation Device M Bone Growth Stimulator	Z No Qualifier

R   **Maxilla**
    Alveolar process of maxilla
T   **Mandible, Right**
    Alveolar process of mandible
    Condyloid process
    Mandibular notch
    Mental foramen
V   **Mandible, Left**
    See T Mandible, Right
	Ø Open
	3 Percutaneous
	4 Percutaneous Endoscopic
		4 Internal Fixation Device
		5 External Fixation Device
			Z No Qualifier

W **Facial Bone**	Ø Open 3 Percutaneous 4 Percutaneous Endoscopic	M Bone Growth Stimulator	Z No Qualifier

Non-OR   ØNHØØ5Z
Non-OR   ØNHØ[3,4]5Z
Non-OR   ØNHB[Ø,3,4][4,M]Z

See Appendix L for Procedure Combinations
   ⊞   ØNHØØNZ

Ø   **Medical and Surgical**
N   **Head and Facial Bones**
J   **Inspection**   Definition: Visually and/or manually exploring a body part

                         Explanation: Visual exploration may be performed with or without optical instrumentation. Manual exploration may be performed directly or through intervening body layers.

Body Part Character 4	Approach Character 5	Device Character 6	Qualifier Character 7
Ø **Skull** **B** **Nasal Bone** Vomer of nasal septum **W** **Facial Bone**	**Ø** Open **3** Percutaneous **4** Percutaneous Endoscopic **X** External	**Z** No Device	**Z** No Qualifier

     Non-OR   ØNJ[Ø,B,W][3,X]ZZ

Ø   **Medical and Surgical**
N   **Head and Facial Bones**
N   **Release**   Definition: Freeing a body part from an abnormal physical constraint by cutting or by the use of force

                         Explanation: Some of the restraining tissue may be taken out but none of the body part is taken out

Body Part Character 4	Approach Character 5	Device Character 6	Qualifier Character 7

1   **Frontal Bone**
     Zygomatic process of frontal bone
3   **Parietal Bone, Right**
4   **Parietal Bone, Left**
5   **Temporal Bone, Right**
     Mastoid process
     Petrous part of temporal bone
     Tympanic part of temporal bone
     Zygomatic process of temporal bone
6   **Temporal Bone, Left**
     See 5 Temporal Bone, Right
7   **Occipital Bone**
     Foramen magnum
B   **Nasal Bone**
     Vomer of nasal septum
C   **Sphenoid Bone**
     Greater wing
     Lesser wing
     Optic foramen
     Pterygoid process
     Sella turcica
F   **Ethmoid Bone, Right**
     Cribriform plate
G   **Ethmoid Bone, Left**
     See F Ethmoid Bone, Right
H   **Lacrimal Bone, Right**
J   **Lacrimal Bone, Left**
K   **Palatine Bone, Right**
L   **Palatine Bone, Left**
M   **Zygomatic Bone, Right**
N   **Zygomatic Bone, Left**
P   **Orbit, Right**
     Bony orbit
     Orbital portion of ethmoid bone
     Orbital portion of frontal bone
     Orbital portion of lacrimal bone
     Orbital portion of maxilla
     Orbital portion of palatine bone
     Orbital portion of sphenoid bone
     Orbital portion of zygomatic bone
Q   **Orbit, Left**
     See P Orbit, Right
R   **Maxilla**
     Alveolar process of maxilla
T   **Mandible, Right**
     Alveolar process of mandible
     Condyloid process
     Mandibular notch
     Mental foramen
V   **Mandible, Left**
     See T Mandible, Right
X   **Hyoid Bone**
	Ø Open
	3 Percutaneous
	4 Percutaneous Endoscopic
		Z No Device	**Z** No Qualifier

     Non-OR   ØNNB[Ø,3,4]ZZ

NC Noncovered Procedure   **LC** Limited Coverage   **QA** Questionable OB Admit   **NT** New Tech Add-on   ⊞ Combination Member   ♂ Male   ♀ Female

ICD-10-PCS 2022   531

Ø   Medical and Surgical
N   Head and Facial Bones
P   Removal   Definition: Taking out or off a device from a body part

Explanation: If a device is taken out and a similar device put in without cutting or puncturing the skin or mucous membrane, the procedure is coded to the root operation CHANGE. Otherwise, the procedure for taking out a device is coded to the root operation REMOVAL.

Body Part Character 4	Approach Character 5	Device Character 6	Qualifier Character 7
Ø Skull	Ø Open	Ø Drainage Device 4 Internal Fixation Device 5 External Fixation Device 7 Autologous Tissue Substitute J Synthetic Substitute K Nonautologous Tissue Substitute M Bone Growth Stimulator N Neurostimulator Generator S Hearing Device	Z No Qualifier
Ø Skull	3 Percutaneous 4 Percutaneous Endoscopic	Ø Drainage Device 4 Internal Fixation Device 5 External Fixation Device 7 Autologous Tissue Substitute J Synthetic Substitute K Nonautologous Tissue Substitute M Bone Growth Stimulator S Hearing Device	Z No Qualifier
Ø Skull	X External	Ø Drainage Device 4 Internal Fixation Device 5 External Fixation Device M Bone Growth Stimulator S Hearing Device	Z No Qualifier
B Nasal Bone Vomer of nasal septum W Facial Bone	Ø Open 3 Percutaneous 4 Percutaneous Endoscopic	Ø Drainage Device 4 Internal Fixation Device 7 Autologous Tissue Substitute J Synthetic Substitute K Nonautologous Tissue Substitute M Bone Growth Stimulator	Z No Qualifier
B Nasal Bone Vomer of nasal septum W Facial Bone	X External	Ø Drainage Device 4 Internal Fixation Device M Bone Growth Stimulator	Z No Qualifier

Non-OR   ØNPØ[3,4]5Z
Non-OR   ØNPØX[Ø,5]Z
Non-OR   ØNPB[Ø,3,4][Ø,4,7,J,K,M]Z
Non-OR   ØNPBX[Ø,4,M]Z
Non-OR   ØNPWX[Ø,M]Z

Ø   **Medical and Surgical**
N   **Head and Facial Bones**
Q   **Repair**   Definition: Restoring, to the extent possible, a body part to its normal anatomic structure and function
                       Explanation: Used only when the method to accomplish the repair is not one of the other root operations

Body Part Character 4	Approach Character 5	Device Character 6	Qualifier Character 7
Ø Skull	Ø Open	Z No Device	Z No Qualifier
1 Frontal Bone Zygomatic process of frontal bone	3 Percutaneous		
3 Parietal Bone, Right	4 Percutaneous Endoscopic		
4 Parietal Bone, Left	X External		

5 Temporal Bone, Right
    Mastoid process
    Petrous part of temporal bone
    Tympanic part of temporal bone
    Zygomatic process of temporal bone			

6 Temporal Bone, Left *See 5 Temporal Bone, Right*			
7 Occipital Bone Foramen magnum			
B Nasal Bone Vomer of nasal septum			

C Sphenoid Bone
    Greater wing
    Lesser wing
    Optic foramen
    Pterygoid process
    Sella turcica			

F Ethmoid Bone, Right Cribriform plate			
G Ethmoid Bone, Left *See F Ethmoid Bone, Right*			
H Lacrimal Bone, Right			
J Lacrimal Bone, Left			
K Palatine Bone, Right			
L Palatine Bone, Left			
M Zygomatic Bone, Right			
N Zygomatic Bone, Left			

P Orbit, Right
    Bony orbit
    Orbital portion of ethmoid bone
    Orbital portion of frontal bone
    Orbital portion of lacrimal bone
    Orbital portion of maxilla
    Orbital portion of palatine bone
    Orbital portion of sphenoid bone
    Orbital portion of zygomatic bone			

Q Orbit, Left *See P Orbit, Right*			
R Maxilla Alveolar process of maxilla			

T Mandible, Right
    Alveolar process of mandible
    Condyloid process
    Mandibular notch
    Mental foramen			

V Mandible, Left *See T Mandible, Right*			
X Hyoid Bone			

Non-OR   ØNQ[Ø,1,3,4,5,6,7,B,C,F,G,H,J,K,L,M,N,P,Q,R,T,V,X]XZZ

Head and Facial Bones

Ø **Medical and Surgical**
N **Head and Facial Bones**
R **Replacement**   Definition: Putting in or on biological or synthetic material that physically takes the place and/or function of all or a portion of a body part

Explanation: The body part may have been taken out or replaced, or may be taken out, physically eradicated, or rendered nonfunctional during the REPLACEMENT procedure. A REMOVAL procedure is coded for taking out the device used in a previous replacement procedure.

Body Part Character 4	Approach Character 5	Device Character 6	Qualifier Character 7

Ø Skull
1 Frontal Bone
    Zygomatic process of frontal bone
3 Parietal Bone, Right
4 Parietal Bone, Left
5 Temporal Bone, Right
    Mastoid process
    Petrous part of temporal bone
    Tympanic part of temporal bone
    Zygomatic process of temporal bone
6 Temporal Bone, Left
    See 5 Temporal Bone, Right
7 Occipital Bone
    Foramen magnum
B Nasal Bone
    Vomer of nasal septum
C Sphenoid Bone
    Greater wing
    Lesser wing
    Optic foramen
    Pterygoid process
    Sella turcica
F Ethmoid Bone, Right
    Cribriform plate
G Ethmoid Bone, Left
    See F Ethmoid Bone, Right
H Lacrimal Bone, Right
J Lacrimal Bone, Left
K Palatine Bone, Right
L Palatine Bone, Left
M Zygomatic Bone, Right
N Zygomatic Bone, Left
P Orbit, Right
    Bony orbit
    Orbital portion of ethmoid bone
    Orbital portion of frontal bone
    Orbital portion of lacrimal bone
    Orbital portion of maxilla
    Orbital portion of palatine bone
    Orbital portion of sphenoid bone
    Orbital portion of zygomatic bone
Q Orbit, Left
    See P Orbit, Right
R Maxilla
    Alveolar process of maxilla
T Mandible, Right
    Alveolar process of mandible
    Condyloid process
    Mandibular notch
    Mental foramen
V Mandible, Left
    See T Mandible, Right
X Hyoid Bone
	Ø Open
	3 Percutaneous
	4 Percutaneous Endoscopic
		7 Autologous Tissue Substitute
		J Synthetic Substitute
		K Nonautologous Tissue Substitute
			Z No Qualifier

Non-OR Procedure   DRG Non-OR Procedure   Valid OR Procedure   HAC Associated Procedure   Combination Only   New/Revised GREEN

Ø   Medical and Surgical
N   Head and Facial Bones
S   Reposition   Definition: Moving to its normal location, or other suitable location, all or a portion of a body part

Explanation: The body part is moved to a new location from an abnormal location, or from a normal location where it is not functioning correctly. The body part may or may not be cut out or off to be moved to the new location.

Body Part Character 4	Approach Character 5	Device Character 6	Qualifier Character 7

Ø Skull
R Maxilla
    Alveolar process of maxilla
T Mandible, Right
    Alveolar process of mandible
    Condyloid process
    Mandibular notch
    Mental foramen
V Mandible, Left
    See T Mandible, Right
	Ø Open
	3 Percutaneous
	4 Percutaneous Endoscopic
		4 Internal Fixation Device
		5 External Fixation Device
		Z No Device
			Z No Qualifier

Ø Skull
R Maxilla
    Alveolar process of maxilla
T Mandible, Right
    Alveolar process of mandible
    Condyloid process
    Mandibular notch
    Mental foramen
V Mandible, Left
    See T Mandible, Right
	X External	**Z** No Device	**Z** No Qualifier

1 Frontal Bone
    Zygomatic process of frontal bone
3 Parietal Bone, Right
4 Parietal Bone, Left
5 Temporal Bone, Right
    Mastoid process
    Petrous part of temporal bone
    Tympanic part of temporal bone
    Zygomatic process of temporal bone
6 Temporal Bone, Left
    See 5 Temporal Bone, Right
7 Occipital Bone
    Foramen magnum
B Nasal Bone
    Vomer of nasal septum
C Sphenoid Bone
    Greater wing
    Lesser wing
    Optic foramen
    Pterygoid process
    Sella turcica
F Ethmoid Bone, Right
    Cribriform plate
G Ethmoid Bone, Left
    See F Ethmoid Bone, Right
H Lacrimal Bone, Right
J Lacrimal Bone, Left
K Palatine Bone, Right
L Palatine Bone, Left
M Zygomatic Bone, Right
N Zygomatic Bone, Left
P Orbit, Right
    Bony orbit
    Orbital portion of ethmoid bone
    Orbital portion of frontal bone
    Orbital portion of lacrimal bone
    Orbital portion of maxilla
    Orbital portion of palatine bone
    Orbital portion of sphenoid bone
    Orbital portion of zygomatic bone
Q Orbit, Left
    See P Orbit, Right
X Hyoid Bone
	Ø Open
	3 Percutaneous
	4 Percutaneous Endoscopic
		4 Internal Fixation Device
		Z No Device
			Z No Qualifier

Non-OR	ØNS[R,T,V][3,4][4,5,Z]Z
Non-OR	ØNS[Ø,R,T,V]XZZ
Non-OR	ØNS[B,C,F,G,H,J,K,L,M,N,P,Q,X][3,4][4,Z]Z

ØNS Continued on next page

Head and Facial Bones

Ø   **Medical and Surgical**   *ØNS Continued*
N   **Head and Facial Bones**
S   **Reposition**   Definition: Moving to its normal location, or other suitable location, all or a portion of a body part
                            Explanation: The body part is moved to a new location from an abnormal location, or from a normal location where it is not functioning
                            correctly. The body part may or may not be cut out or off to be moved to the new location.

Body Part Character 4	Approach Character 5	Device Character 6	Qualifier Character 7

1 **Frontal Bone**
    Zygomatic process of frontal bone
3 **Parietal Bone, Right**
4 **Parietal Bone, Left**
5 **Temporal Bone, Right**
    Mastoid process
    Petrous part of temporal bone
    Tympanic part of temporal bone
    Zygomatic process of temporal bone
6 **Temporal Bone, Left**
    See 5 Temporal Bone, Right
7 **Occipital Bone**
    Foramen magnum
B **Nasal Bone**
    Vomer of nasal septum
C **Sphenoid Bone**
    Greater wing
    Lesser wing
    Optic foramen
    Pterygoid process
    Sella turcica
F **Ethmoid Bone, Right**
    Cribriform plate
G **Ethmoid Bone, Left**
    See F Ethmoid Bone, Right
H **Lacrimal Bone, Right**
J **Lacrimal Bone, Left**
K **Palatine Bone, Right**
L **Palatine Bone, Left**
M **Zygomatic Bone, Right**
N **Zygomatic Bone, Left**
P **Orbit, Right**
    Bony orbit
    Orbital portion of ethmoid bone
    Orbital portion of frontal bone
    Orbital portion of lacrimal bone
    Orbital portion of maxilla
    Orbital portion of palatine bone
    Orbital portion of sphenoid bone
    Orbital portion of zygomatic bone
Q **Orbit, Left**
    See P Orbit, Right
X **Hyoid Bone**
	X External	**Z** No Device	**Z** No Qualifier

Non-OR   ØNS[1,3,4,5,6,7,B,C,F,G,H,J,K,L,M,N,P,Q,X]XZZ

Ø **Medical and Surgical**
N **Head and Facial Bones**
T **Resection**   Definition: Cutting out or off, without replacement, all of a body part
               Explanation: None

Body Part Character 4	Approach Character 5	Device Character 6	Qualifier Character 7
1 Frontal Bone Zygomatic process of frontal bone	**Ø Open**	**Z No Device**	**Z No Qualifier**
3 Parietal Bone, Right			
4 Parietal Bone, Left			
5 Temporal Bone, Right Mastoid process Petrous part of temporal bone Tympanic part of temporal bone Zygomatic process of temporal bone			
6 Temporal Bone, Left *See 5 Temporal Bone, Right*			
7 Occipital Bone Foramen magnum			
B Nasal Bone Vomer of nasal septum			
C Sphenoid Bone Greater wing Lesser wing Optic foramen Pterygoid process Sella turcica			
F Ethmoid Bone, Right Cribriform plate			
G Ethmoid Bone, Left *See F Ethmoid Bone, Right*			
H Lacrimal Bone, Right			
J Lacrimal Bone, Left			
K Palatine Bone, Right			
L Palatine Bone, Left			
M Zygomatic Bone, Right			
N Zygomatic Bone, Left			
P Orbit, Right Bony orbit Orbital portion of ethmoid bone Orbital portion of frontal bone Orbital portion of lacrimal bone Orbital portion of maxilla Orbital portion of palatine bone Orbital portion of sphenoid bone Orbital portion of zygomatic bone			
Q Orbit, Left *See P Orbit, Right*			
R Maxilla Alveolar process of maxilla			
T Mandible, Right Alveolar process of mandible Condyloid process Mandibular notch Mental foramen			
V Mandible, Left *See T Mandible, Right*			
X Hyoid Bone			

NC Noncovered Procedure   **LC** Limited Coverage   **QA** Questionable OB Admit   **NT** New Tech Add-on   ⊞ Combination Member   ♂ Male   ♀ Female

ICD-10-PCS 2022   537

ØNT–ØNT

Head and Facial Bones

Ø **Medical and Surgical**
N **Head and Facial Bones**
U **Supplement**   Definition: Putting in or on biological or synthetic material that physically reinforces and/or augments the function of a portion of a body part
                   Explanation: The biological material is non-living, or is living and from the same individual. The body part may have been previously replaced, and the SUPPLEMENT procedure is performed to physically reinforce and/or augment the function of the replaced body part.

Body Part Character 4	Approach Character 5	Device Character 6	Qualifier Character 7
Ø Skull	Ø Open	7 Autologous Tissue Substitute	Z No Qualifier
1 Frontal Bone	3 Percutaneous	J Synthetic Substitute	
Zygomatic process of frontal bone	4 Percutaneous Endoscopic	K Nonautologous Tissue Substitute	
3 Parietal Bone, Right			
4 Parietal Bone, Left			
5 Temporal Bone, Right			
Mastoid process			
Petrous part of temporal bone			
Tympanic part of temporal bone			
Zygomatic process of temporal bone			
6 Temporal Bone, Left			
See 5 Temporal Bone, Right			
7 Occipital Bone			
Foramen magnum			
B Nasal Bone			
Vomer of nasal septum			
C Sphenoid Bone			
Greater wing			
Lesser wing			
Optic foramen			
Pterygoid process			
Sella turcica			
F Ethmoid Bone, Right			
Cribriform plate			
G Ethmoid Bone, Left			
See F Ethmoid Bone, Right			
H Lacrimal Bone, Right			
J Lacrimal Bone, Left			
K Palatine Bone, Right			
L Palatine Bone, Left			
M Zygomatic Bone, Right			
N Zygomatic Bone, Left			
P Orbit, Right			
Bony orbit			
Orbital portion of ethmoid bone			
Orbital portion of frontal bone			
Orbital portion of lacrimal bone			
Orbital portion of maxilla			
Orbital portion of palatine bone			
Orbital portion of sphenoid bone			
Orbital portion of zygomatic bone			
Q Orbit, Left			
See P Orbit, Right			
R Maxilla			
Alveolar process of maxilla			
T Mandible, Right			
Alveolar process of mandible			
Condyloid process			
Mandibular notch			
Mental foramen			
V Mandible, Left			
See T Mandible, Right			
X Hyoid Bone			

Ø   **Medical and Surgical**
N   **Head and Facial Bones**
W   **Revision**   Definition: Correcting, to the extent possible, a portion of a malfunctioning device or the position of a displaced device

                          Explanation: Revision can include correcting a malfunctioning or displaced device by taking out or putting in components of the device such as a screw or pin

Body Part Character 4	Approach Character 5	Device Character 6	Qualifier Character 7
Ø Skull	Ø Open	Ø Drainage Device 4 Internal Fixation Device 5 External Fixation Device 7 Autologous Tissue Substitute J Synthetic Substitute K Nonautologous Tissue Substitute M Bone Growth Stimulator N Neurostimulator Generator S Hearing Device	Z No Qualifier
Ø Skull	3 Percutaneous 4 Percutaneous Endoscopic X External	Ø Drainage Device 4 Internal Fixation Device 5 External Fixation Device 7 Autologous Tissue Substitute J Synthetic Substitute K Nonautologous Tissue Substitute M Bone Growth Stimulator S Hearing Device	Z No Qualifier
B Nasal Bone Vomer of nasal septum W Facial Bone	Ø Open 3 Percutaneous 4 Percutaneous Endoscopic X External	Ø Drainage Device 4 Internal Fixation Device 7 Autologous Tissue Substitute J Synthetic Substitute K Nonautologous Tissue Substitute M Bone Growth Stimulator	Z No Qualifier

Non-OR   ØNWØX[Ø,4,5,7,J,K,M,S]Z
Non-OR   ØNWB[Ø,3,4,X][Ø,4,7,J,K,M]Z
Non-OR   ØNWWX[Ø,4,7,J,K,M]Z

Upper Bones ØP2–ØPW

Character Meanings

This Character Meaning table is provided as a guide to assist the user in the identification of character members that may be found in this section of code tables. It **SHOULD NOT** be used to build a PCS code.

Operation–Character 3	Body Part–Character 4	Approach–Character 5	Device–Character 6	Qualifier–Character 7
2 Change	Ø Sternum	Ø Open	Ø Drainage Device OR Internal Fixation Device, Rigid Plate	X Diagnostic
5 Destruction	1 Ribs, 1 to 2	3 Percutaneous	3 Spinal Stabilization Device, Vertebral Body Tether	Z No Qualifier
8 Division	2 Ribs, 3 or more	4 Percutaneous Endoscopic	4 Internal Fixation Device	
9 Drainage	3 Cervical Vertebra	X External	5 External Fixation Device	
B Excision	4 Thoracic Vertebra		6 Internal Fixation Device, Intramedullary	
C Extirpation	5 Scapula, Right		7 Autologous Tissue Substitute OR Internal Fixation Device, Intramedullary Limb Lengthening	
D Extraction	6 Scapula, Left		8 External Fixation Device, Limb Lengthening	
H Insertion	7 Glenoid Cavity, Right		B External Fixation Device, Monoplanar	
J Inspection	8 Glenoid Cavity, Left		C External Fixation Device, Ring	
N Release	9 Clavicle, Right		D External Fixation Device, Hybrid	
P Removal	B Clavicle, Left		J Synthetic Substitute	
Q Repair	C Humeral Head, Right		K Nonautologous Tissue Substitute	
R Replacement	D Humeral Head, Left		M Bone Growth Stimulator	
S Reposition	F Humeral Shaft, Right		Y Other Device	
T Resection	G Humeral Shaft, Left		Z No Device	
U Supplement	H Radius, Right			
W Revision	J Radius, Left			
	K Ulna, Right			
	L Ulna, Left			
	M Carpal, Right			
	N Carpal, Left			
	P Metacarpal, Right			
	Q Metacarpal, Left			
	R Thumb Phalanx, Right			
	S Thumb Phalanx, Left			
	T Finger Phalanx, Right			
	V Finger Phalanx, Left			
	Y Upper Bone			

AHA Coding Clinic for table ØPB
2015, 3Q, 3-8 Excisional and nonexcisional debridement
2015, 2Q, 34 Decompressive laminectomy
2013, 4Q, 109 Separating conjoined twins
2013, 4Q, 116 Spinal decompression
2013, 3Q, 20 Superior labrum anterior posterior (SLAP) repair and subacromialdecompression
2012, 4Q, 101 Rib resection with reconstruction of anterior chest wall
2012, 2Q, 19 Multiple decompressive cervical laminectomies

AHA Coding Clinic for table ØPC
2019, 3Q, 19 Removal of sternal wire

AHA Coding Clinic for table ØPD
2017, 4Q, 41 Extraction procedures

AHA Coding Clinic for table ØPH
2020, 1Q, 29 Repair of sternal dehiscence using Sternal Talon® device
2019, 4Q, 34 Intramedullary limb lengthening internal fixation device
2019, 2Q, 40 Decompression of spinal cord and placement of instrumentation
2018, 3Q, 26 Anterior vertebral tethering using Dynesys Tethering System
2017, 2Q, 20 Exchange of intramedullary antibiotic impregnated spacer
2016, 4Q, 117 Placement of magnetic growth rods
2014, 4Q, 28 Removal and replacement of displaced growing rods

AHA Coding Clinic for table ØPP
2019, 3Q, 19 Removal of sternal wire
2017, 2Q, 20 Exchange of intramedullary antibiotic impregnated spacer
2016, 4Q, 117 Placement of magnetic growth rods
2014, 4Q, 28 Removal and replacement of displaced growing rods

AHA Coding Clinic for table ØPR
2018, 4Q, 92 Radial head arthroplasty

AHA Coding Clinic for table ØPS
2020, 1Q, 33 Spinal fusion without use of bone graft
2018, 3Q, 26 Anterior vertebral tethering using Dynesys Tethering System
2017, 4Q, 53 New and revised body part values - Ribs
2016, 1Q, 21 Elongation derotation flexion casting
2015, 4Q, 33 Ravitch operation
2015, 2Q, 35 Application of tongs to reduce and stabilize cervical fracture
2014, 4Q, 26 Placement of vertical expandable prosthetic titanium rib (VEPTR)
2014, 4Q, 32 Open reduction internal fixation of fracture with debridement
2014, 3Q, 33 Radial fracture treatment with open reduction internal fixation, and release of carpal ligament

AHA Coding Clinic for table ØPT
2015, 3Q, 26 Thumb arthroplasty with resection of trapezium

AHA Coding Clinic for table ØPU
2015, 2Q, 20 Cervical laminoplasty
2013, 4Q, 109 Separating conjoined twins

AHA Coding Clinic for table ØPW
2014, 4Q, 26 Adjustment of VEPTR lengthening mechanism
2014, 4Q, 27 Bilateral lengthening of growing rods

Upper Bones

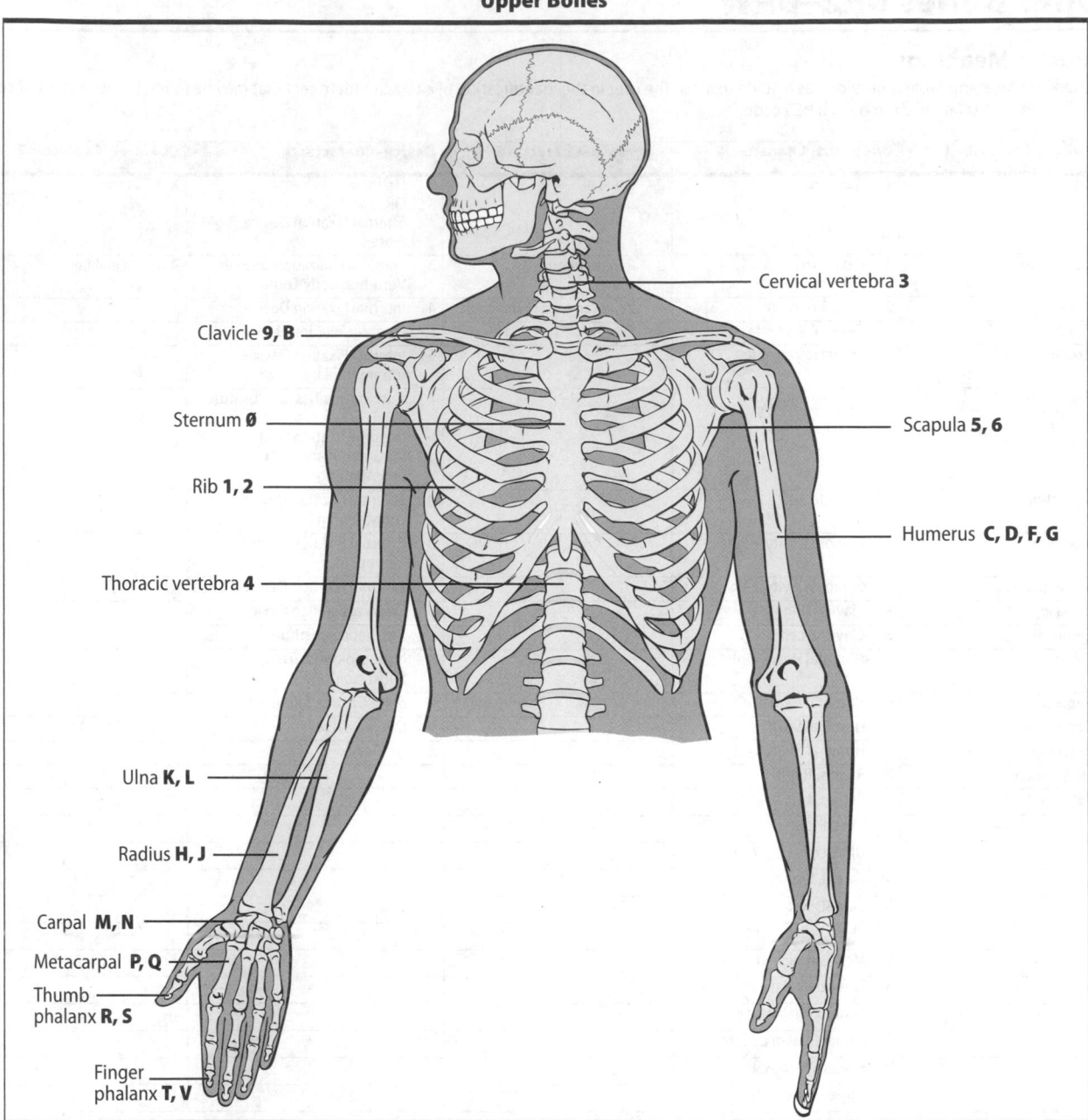

Cervical vertebra **3**

Clavicle **9, B**

Sternum **Ø**

Scapula **5, 6**

Rib **1, 2**

Humerus **C, D, F, G**

Thoracic vertebra **4**

Ulna **K, L**

Radius **H, J**

Carpal **M, N**

Metacarpal **P, Q**

Thumb phalanx **R, S**

Finger phalanx **T, V**

Humerus and Scapula

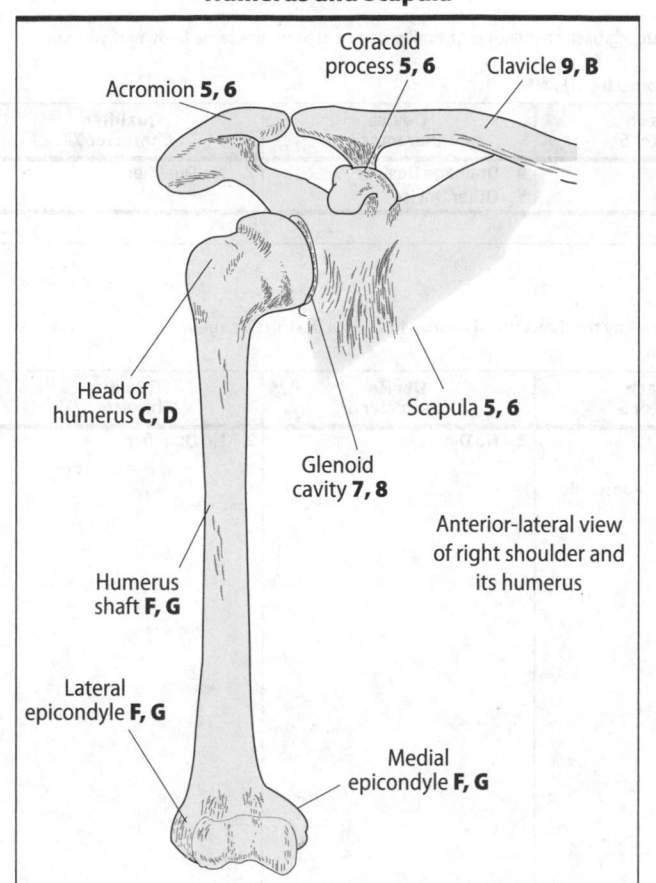

Acromion **5, 6**

Coracoid process **5, 6**

Clavicle **9, B**

Head of humerus **C, D**

Glenoid cavity **7, 8**

Scapula **5, 6**

Humerus shaft **F, G**

Lateral epicondyle **F, G**

Medial epicondyle **F, G**

Anterior-lateral view of right shoulder and its humerus

Radius and Ulna

Radius **H, J**

Olecranon process **K, L**

Coronoid process **K, L**

Ulna **K, L**

Shaft **H, J**

Shaft **K, L**

Radial styloid process **H, J**

Ulnar styloid process **K, L**

Carpal **M, N**

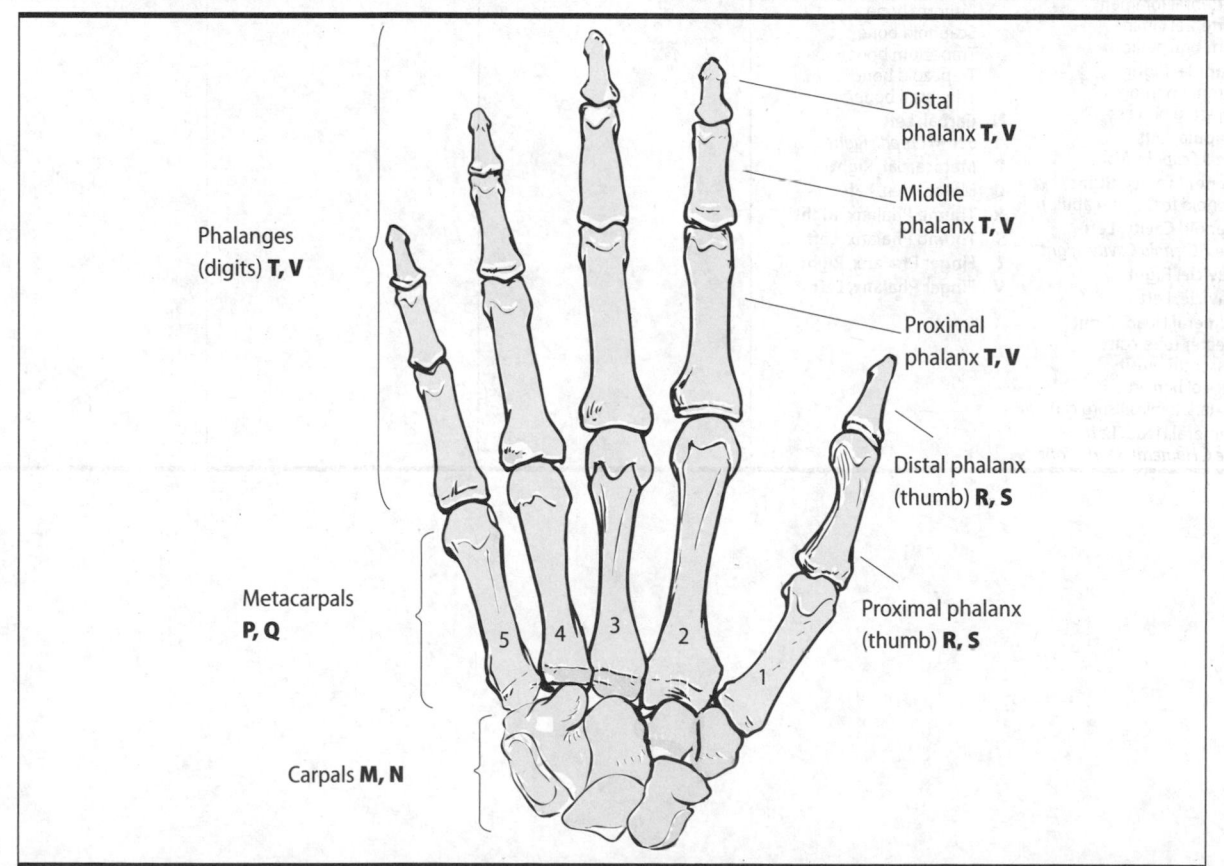

Phalanges (digits) **T, V**

Distal phalanx **T, V**

Middle phalanx **T, V**

Proximal phalanx **T, V**

Distal phalanx (thumb) **R, S**

Proximal phalanx (thumb) **R, S**

Metacarpals **P, Q**

Carpals **M, N**

Ø   **Medical and Surgical**
P   **Upper Bones**
2   **Change**   Definition: Taking out or off a device from a body part and putting back an identical or similar device in or on the same body part without cutting or puncturing the skin or a mucous membrane

                 Explanation: All CHANGE procedures are coded using the approach EXTERNAL

Body Part Character 4	Approach Character 5	Device Character 6	Qualifier Character 7
Y Upper Bone	**X** External	**Ø** Drainage Device **Y** Other Device	**Z** No Qualifier

Non-OR   All body part, approach, device, and qualifier values

---

Ø   **Medical and Surgical**
P   **Upper Bones**
5   **Destruction**   Definition: Physical eradication of all or a portion of a body part by the direct use of energy, force, or a destructive agent

                   Explanation: None of the body part is physically taken out

Body Part Character 4	Approach Character 5	Device Character 6	Qualifier Character 7

Ø   Sternum
    Manubrium
    Suprasternal notch
    Xiphoid process
1   Ribs, 1 to 2
2   Ribs, 3 or More
3   Cervical Vertebra
    Dens
    Odontoid process
    Spinous process
    Transverse foramen
    Transverse process
    Vertebral arch
    Vertebral body
    Vertebral foramen
    Vertebral lamina
    Vertebral pedicle
4   Thoracic Vertebra
    Spinous process
    Transverse process
    Vertebral arch
    Vertebral body
    Vertebral foramen
    Vertebral lamina
    Vertebral pedicle
5   Scapula, Right
    Acromion (process)
    Coracoid process
6   Scapula, Left
    See 5 Scapula, Right
7   Glenoid Cavity, Right
    Glenoid fossa (of scapula)
8   Glenoid Cavity, Left
    See 7 Glenoid Cavity, Right
9   Clavicle, Right
B   Clavicle, Left
C   Humeral Head, Right
    Greater tuberosity
    Lesser tuberosity
    Neck of humerus
      (anatomical)(surgical)
D   Humeral Head, Left
    See C Humeral Head, Right
	F Humeral Shaft, Right
	    Distal humerus
	    Humerus, distal
	    Lateral epicondyle of
	      humerus
	    Medial epicondyle of
	      humerus
	G Humeral Shaft, Left
	    See F Humeral Shaft, Right
	H Radius, Right
	    Ulnar notch
	J Radius, Left
	    See H Radius, Right
	K Ulna, Right
	    Olecranon process
	    Radial notch
	L Ulna, Left
	    See K Ulna, Right
	M Carpal, Right
	    Capitate bone
	    Hamate bone
	    Lunate bone
	    Pisiform bone
	    Scaphoid bone
	    Trapezium bone
	    Trapezoid bone
	    Triquetral bone
	N Carpal, Left
	    See M Carpal, Right
	P Metacarpal, Right
	Q Metacarpal, Left
	R Thumb Phalanx, Right
	S Thumb Phalanx, Left
	T Finger Phalanx, Right
	V Finger Phalanx, Left
		Ø Open
		3 Percutaneous
		4 Percutaneous Endoscopic
			Z No Device	**Z** No Qualifier

Ø   Medical and Surgical
P   Upper Bones
8   Division   Definition: Cutting into a body part, without draining fluids and/or gases from the body part, in order to separate or transect a body part
                 Explanation: All or a portion of the body part is separated into two or more portions

Body Part Character 4	Approach Character 5	Device Character 6	Qualifier Character 7
Ø Sternum Manubrium Suprasternal notch Xiphoid process	**Ø Open** **3 Percutaneous** **4 Percutaneous Endoscopic**	**Z No Device**	**Z No Qualifier**
1 Ribs, 1 to 2			
2 Ribs, 3 or More			
3 Cervical Vertebra Dens Odontoid process Spinous process Transverse foramen Transverse process Vertebral arch Vertebral body Vertebral foramen Vertebral lamina Vertebral pedicle			
4 Thoracic Vertebra Spinous process Transverse process Vertebral arch Vertebral body Vertebral foramen Vertebral lamina Vertebral pedicle			
5 Scapula, Right Acromion (process) Coracoid process			
6 Scapula, Left *See 5 Scapula, Right*			
7 Glenoid Cavity, Right Glenoid fossa (of scapula)			
8 Glenoid Cavity, Left *See 7 Glenoid Cavity, Right*			
9 Clavicle, Right			
B Clavicle, Left			
C Humeral Head, Right Greater tuberosity Lesser tuberosity Neck of humerus (anatomical)(surgical)			
D Humeral Head, Left *See C Humeral Head, Right*			
F Humeral Shaft, Right Distal humerus Humerus, distal Lateral epicondyle of humerus Medial epicondyle of humerus			
G Humeral Shaft, Left *See F Humeral Shaft, Right*			
H Radius, Right Ulnar notch			
J Radius, Left *See H Radius, Right*			
K Ulna, Right Olecranon process Radial notch			
L Ulna, Left *See K Ulna, Right*			
M Carpal, Right Capitate bone Hamate bone Lunate bone Pisiform bone Scaphoid bone Trapezium bone Trapezoid bone Triquetral bone			
N Carpal, Left *See M Carpal, Right*			
P Metacarpal, Right			
Q Metacarpal, Left			
R Thumb Phalanx, Right			
S Thumb Phalanx, Left			
T Finger Phalanx, Right			
V Finger Phalanx, Left			

NC Noncovered Procedure   **LC** Limited Coverage   **UA** Questionable OB Admit   **NT** New Tech Add-on   ⊞ Combination Member   ♂ Male   ♀ Female

Ø   **Medical and Surgical**
P   **Upper Bones**
9   **Drainage**

Definition: Taking or letting out fluids and/or gases from a body part
Explanation: The qualifier DIAGNOSTIC is used to identify drainage procedures that are biopsies

Body Part Character 4		Approach Character 5	Device Character 6	Qualifier Character 7
Ø **Sternum** Manubrium Suprasternal notch Xiphoid process	**D** **Humeral Head, Left** *See C Humeral Head, Right*	**Ø** Open **3** Percutaneous **4** Percutaneous Endoscopic	**Ø** Drainage Device	**Z** No Qualifier
1 **Ribs, 1 to 2**	**F** **Humeral Shaft, Right** Distal humerus Humerus, distal Lateral epicondyle of humerus Medial epicondyle of humerus			
2 **Ribs, 3 or More**				
3 **Cervical Vertebra** Dens Odontoid process Spinous process Transverse foramen Transverse process Vertebral arch Vertebral body Vertebral foramen Vertebral lamina Vertebral pedicle	**G** **Humeral Shaft, Left** *See F Humeral Shaft, Right*			
	H **Radius, Right** Ulnar notch			
	J **Radius, Left** *See H Radius, Right*			
4 **Thoracic Vertebra** Spinous process Transverse process Vertebral arch Vertebral body Vertebral foramen Vertebral lamina Vertebral pedicle	**K** **Ulna, Right** Olecranon process Radial notch			
	L **Ulna, Left** *See K Ulna, Right*			
	M **Carpal, Right** Capitate bone Hamate bone Lunate bone Pisiform bone Scaphoid bone Trapezium bone Trapezoid bone Triquetral bone			
5 **Scapula, Right** Acromion (process) Coracoid process				
6 **Scapula, Left** *See 5 Scapula, Right*	**N** **Carpal, Left** *See M Carpal, Right*			
7 **Glenoid Cavity, Right** Glenoid fossa (of scapula)	**P** **Metacarpal, Right**			
8 **Glenoid Cavity, Left** *See 7 Glenoid Cavity, Right*	**Q** **Metacarpal, Left**			
	R **Thumb Phalanx, Right**			
9 **Clavicle, Right**	**S** **Thumb Phalanx, Left**			
B **Clavicle, Left**	**T** **Finger Phalanx, Right**			
C **Humeral Head, Right** Greater tuberosity Lesser tuberosity Neck of humerus (anatomical)(surgical)	**V** **Finger Phalanx, Left**			

Non-OR   ØP9[Ø,1,2,3,4,5,6,7,8,9,B,C,D,F,G,H,J,K,L,M,N,P,Q,R,S,T,V]3ØZ

ØP9 Continued on next page

Ø   **Medical and Surgical**   ***ØP9 Continued***
P   **Upper Bones**
9   **Drainage**   Definition: Taking or letting out fluids and/or gases from a body part

                            Explanation: The qualifier DIAGNOSTIC is used to identify drainage procedures that are biopsies

Body Part Character 4		Approach Character 5	Device Character 6	Qualifier Character 7

Ø **Sternum**
  Manubrium
  Suprasternal notch
  Xiphoid process
1 **Ribs, 1 to 2**
2 **Ribs, 3 or More**
3 **Cervical Vertebra**
  Dens
  Odontoid process
  Spinous process
  Transverse foramen
  Transverse process
  Vertebral arch
  Vertebral body
  Vertebral foramen
  Vertebral lamina
  Vertebral pedicle
4 **Thoracic Vertebra**
  Spinous process
  Transverse process
  Vertebral arch
  Vertebral body
  Vertebral foramen
  Vertebral lamina
  Vertebral pedicle
5 **Scapula, Right**
  Acromion (process)
  Coracoid process
6 **Scapula, Left**
  See 5 Scapula, Right
7 **Glenoid Cavity, Right**
  Glenoid fossa (of scapula)
8 **Glenoid Cavity, Left**
  See 7 Glenoid Cavity, Right
9 **Clavicle, Right**
B **Clavicle, Left**
C **Humeral Head, Right**
  Greater tuberosity
  Lesser tuberosity
  Neck of humerus
    (anatomical)(surgical)
	D **Humeral Head, Left**
	  See C Humeral Head, Right
	F **Humeral Shaft, Right**
	  Distal humerus
	  Humerus, distal
	  Lateral epicondyle of
	    humerus
	  Medial epicondyle of
	    humerus
	G **Humeral Shaft, Left**
	  See F Humeral Shaft, Right
	H **Radius, Right**
	  Ulnar notch
	J **Radius, Left**
	  See H Radius, Right
	K **Ulna, Right**
	  Olecranon process
	  Radial notch
	L **Ulna, Left**
	  See K Ulna, Right
	M **Carpal, Right**
	  Capitate bone
	  Hamate bone
	  Lunate bone
	  Pisiform bone
	  Scaphoid bone
	  Trapezium bone
	  Trapezoid bone
	  Triquetral bone
	N **Carpal, Left**
	  See M Carpal, Right
	P **Metacarpal, Right**
	Q **Metacarpal, Left**
	R **Thumb Phalanx, Right**
	S **Thumb Phalanx, Left**
	T **Finger Phalanx, Right**
	V **Finger Phalanx, Left**
		Ø **Open**
		3 **Percutaneous**
		4 **Percutaneous Endoscopic**
			Z **No Device**	X **Diagnostic**
				Z **No Qualifier**

Non-OR	ØP9[Ø,1,2,3,4,5,6,7,8,9,B,C,D,F,G,H,J,K,L,M,N,P,Q,R,S,T,V]3ZZ

NC Noncovered Procedure   **LC** Limited Coverage   **QA** Questionable OB Admit   **NT** New Tech Add-on   ⊞ Combination Member   ♂ Male   ♀ Female

ICD-10-PCS 2022   547

ØP9–ØP9

Ø **Medical and Surgical**
P **Upper Bones**
B **Excision**　　Definition: Cutting out or off, without replacement, a portion of a body part
　　　　　　　　　　Explanation: The qualifier DIAGNOSTIC is used to identify excision procedures that are biopsies

Body Part Character 4	Approach Character 5	Device Character 6	Qualifier Character 7
Ø **Sternum** 　Manubrium 　Suprasternal notch 　Xiphoid process	**Ø** Open **3** Percutaneous **4** Percutaneous Endoscopic	**Z** No Device	**X** Diagnostic **Z** No Qualifier
1 **Ribs, 1 to 2**			
2 **Ribs, 3 or More**			
3 **Cervical Vertebra** 　Dens 　Odontoid process 　Spinous process 　Transverse foramen 　Transverse process 　Vertebral arch 　Vertebral body 　Vertebral foramen 　Vertebral lamina 　Vertebral pedicle			
4 **Thoracic Vertebra** 　Spinous process 　Transverse process 　Vertebral arch 　Vertebral body 　Vertebral foramen 　Vertebral lamina 　Vertebral pedicle			
5 **Scapula, Right** 　Acromion (process) 　Coracoid process			
6 **Scapula, Left** 　*See 5 Scapula, Right*			
7 **Glenoid Cavity, Right** 　Glenoid fossa (of scapula)			
8 **Glenoid Cavity, Left** 　*See 7 Glenoid Cavity, Right*			
9 **Clavicle, Right**			
B **Clavicle, Left**			
C **Humeral Head, Right** 　Greater tuberosity 　Lesser tuberosity 　Neck of humerus (anatomical)(surgical)			
D **Humeral Head, Left** 　*See C Humeral Head, Right*			
F **Humeral Shaft, Right** 　Distal humerus 　Humerus, distal 　Lateral epicondyle of humerus 　Medial epicondyle of humerus			
G **Humeral Shaft, Left** 　*See F Humeral Shaft, Right*			
H **Radius, Right** 　Ulnar notch			
J **Radius, Left** 　*See H Radius, Right*			
K **Ulna, Right** 　Olecranon process 　Radial notch			
L **Ulna, Left** 　*See K Ulna, Right*			
M **Carpal, Right** 　Capitate bone 　Hamate bone 　Lunate bone 　Pisiform bone 　Scaphoid bone 　Trapezium bone 　Trapezoid bone 　Triquetral bone			
N **Carpal, Left** 　*See M Carpal, Right*			
P **Metacarpal, Right**			
Q **Metacarpal, Left**			
R **Thumb Phalanx, Right**			
S **Thumb Phalanx, Left**			
T **Finger Phalanx, Right**			
V **Finger Phalanx, Left**			

Ø   **Medical and Surgical**
P   **Upper Bones**
C   **Extirpation**   Definition: Taking or cutting out solid matter from a body part

Explanation: The solid matter may be an abnormal byproduct of a biological function or a foreign body; it may be imbedded in a body part or in the lumen of a tubular body part. The solid matter may or may not have been previously broken into pieces.

Body Part Character 4	Approach Character 5	Device Character 6	Qualifier Character 7

Ø **Sternum**
   Manubrium
   Suprasternal notch
   Xiphoid process
	Ø **Open**
	3 **Percutaneous**
	4 **Percutaneous Endoscopic**
		Z **No Device**	**Z** **No Qualifier**

1 **Ribs, 1 to 2**			
2 **Ribs, 3 or More**			

3 **Cervical Vertebra**
   Dens
   Odontoid process
   Spinous process
   Transverse foramen
   Transverse process
   Vertebral arch
   Vertebral body
   Vertebral foramen
   Vertebral lamina
   Vertebral pedicle			

4 **Thoracic Vertebra**
   Spinous process
   Transverse process
   Vertebral arch
   Vertebral body
   Vertebral foramen
   Vertebral lamina
   Vertebral pedicle			

5 **Scapula, Right**
   Acromion (process)
   Coracoid process			

6 **Scapula, Left** *See 5 Scapula, Right*			
7 **Glenoid Cavity, Right** Glenoid fossa (of scapula)			
8 **Glenoid Cavity, Left** *See 7 Glenoid Cavity, Right*			
9 **Clavicle, Right**			
B **Clavicle, Left**			

C **Humeral Head, Right**
   Greater tuberosity
   Lesser tuberosity
   Neck of humerus (anatomical)(surgical)			

D **Humeral Head, Left** *See C Humeral Head, Right*			

F **Humeral Shaft, Right**
   Distal humerus
   Humerus, distal
   Lateral epicondyle of humerus
   Medial epicondyle of humerus			

G **Humeral Shaft, Left** *See F Humeral Shaft, Right*			
H **Radius, Right** Ulnar notch			
J **Radius, Left** *See H Radius, Right*			

K **Ulna, Right**
   Olecranon process
   Radial notch			

L **Ulna, Left** *See K Ulna, Right*			

M **Carpal, Right**
   Capitate bone
   Hamate bone
   Lunate bone
   Pisiform bone
   Scaphoid bone
   Trapezium bone
   Trapezoid bone
   Triquetral bone			

N **Carpal, Left** *See M Carpal, Right*			
P **Metacarpal, Right**			
Q **Metacarpal, Left**			
R **Thumb Phalanx, Right**			
S **Thumb Phalanx, Left**			
T **Finger Phalanx, Right**			
V **Finger Phalanx, Left**			

NC Noncovered Procedure   **LC** Limited Coverage   **QA** Questionable OB Admit   **NT** New Tech Add-on   ⊞ Combination Member   ♂ Male   ♀ Female

Upper Bones

Ø   **Medical and Surgical**
P   **Upper Bones**
D   **Extraction**   Definition: Pulling or stripping out or off all or a portion of a body part by the use of force
                       Explanation: The qualifier DIAGNOSTIC is used to identify extraction procedures that are biopsies

Body Part Character 4	Approach Character 5	Device Character 6	Qualifier Character 7
Ø Sternum Manubrium Suprasternal notch Xiphoid process	**Ø Open**	**Z No Device**	**Z No Qualifier**
1 Ribs, 1 to 2			
2 Ribs, 3 or More			
3 Cervical Vertebra Dens Odontoid process Spinous process Transverse foramen Transverse process Vertebral arch Vertebral body Vertebral foramen Vertebral lamina Vertebral pedicle			
4 Thoracic Vertebra Spinous process Transverse process Vertebral arch Vertebral body Vertebral foramen Vertebral lamina Vertebral pedicle			
5 Scapula, Right Acromion (process) Coracoid process			
6 Scapula, Left *See 5 Scapula, Right*			
7 Glenoid Cavity, Right Glenoid fossa (of scapula)			
8 Glenoid Cavity, Left *See 7 Glenoid Cavity, Right*			
9 Clavicle, Right			
B Clavicle, Left			
C Humeral Head, Right Greater tuberosity Lesser tuberosity Neck of humerus (anatomical)(surgical)			
D Humeral Head, Left *See C Humeral Head, Right*			
F Humeral Shaft, Right Distal humerus Humerus, distal Lateral epicondyle of humerus Medial epicondyle of humerus			
G Humeral Shaft, Left *See F Humeral Shaft, Right*			
H Radius, Right Ulnar notch			
J Radius, Left *See H Radius, Right*			
K Ulna, Right Olecranon process Radial notch			
L Ulna, Left *See K Ulna, Right*			
M Carpal, Right Capitate bone Hamate bone Lunate bone Pisiform bone Scaphoid bone Trapezium bone Trapezoid bone Triquetral bone			
N Carpal, Left *See M Carpal, Right*			
P Metacarpal, Right			
Q Metacarpal, Left			
R Thumb Phalanx, Right			
S Thumb Phalanx, Left			
T Finger Phalanx, Right			
V Finger Phalanx, Left			

Non-OR Procedure   DRG Non-OR Procedure   Valid OR Procedure   HAC Associated Procedure   Combination Only   New/Revised GREEN

Ø   Medical and Surgical
P   Upper Bones
H   Insertion   Definition: Putting in a nonbiological appliance that monitors, assists, performs, or prevents a physiological function but does not physically take the place of a body part

Explanation: None

Body Part Character 4		Approach Character 5	Device Character 6	Qualifier Character 7

Ø   **Sternum**
    Manubrium
    Suprasternal notch
    Xiphoid process
		Ø Open
		3 Percutaneous
		4 Percutaneous Endoscopic
			Ø Internal Fixation Device,
			    Rigid Plate
			4 Internal Fixation Device
				Z No Qualifier

1   **Ribs, 1 to 2**
2   **Ribs, 3 or More**
3   **Cervical Vertebra**
    Dens
    Odontoid process
    Spinous process
    Transverse foramen
    Transverse process
    Vertebral arch
    Vertebral body
    Vertebral foramen
    Vertebral lamina
    Vertebral pedicle
4   **Thoracic Vertebra**
    Spinous process
    Transverse process
    Vertebral arch
    Vertebral body
    Vertebral foramen
    Vertebral lamina
    Vertebral pedicle
	5 **Scapula, Right**
	    Acromion (process)
	    Coracoid process
	6 **Scapula, Left**
	    See 5 Scapula, Right
	7 **Glenoid Cavity, Right**
	    Glenoid fossa (of scapula)
	8 **Glenoid Cavity, Left**
	    See 7 Glenoid Cavity, Right
	9 **Clavicle, Right**
	B **Clavicle, Left**
		Ø Open
		3 Percutaneous
		4 Percutaneous Endoscopic
			4 Internal Fixation Device	**Z** No Qualifier

C   **Humeral Head, Right**
    Greater tuberosity
    Lesser tuberosity
    Neck of humerus
        (anatomical)(surgical)
D   **Humeral Head, Left**
    See C Humeral Head, Right
	H **Radius, Right**
	    Ulnar notch
	J **Radius, Left**
	    See H Radius, Right
	K **Ulna, Right**
	    Olecranon process
	    Radial notch
	L **Ulna, Left**
	    See K Ulna, Right
		Ø Open
		3 Percutaneous
		4 Percutaneous Endoscopic
			4 Internal Fixation Device
			5 External Fixation Device
			6 Internal Fixation Device,
			    Intramedullary
			8 External Fixation Device,
			    Limb Lengthening
			B External Fixation Device,
			    Monoplanar
			C External Fixation Device, Ring
			D External Fixation Device,
			    Hybrid
				Z No Qualifier

F   **Humeral Shaft, Right**
    Distal humerus
    Humerus, distal
    Lateral epicondyle of
        humerus
    Medial epicondyle of
        humerus
	G **Humeral Shaft, Left**
	    See F Humeral Shaft, Right
		Ø Open
		3 Percutaneous
		4 Percutaneous Endoscopic
			4 Internal Fixation Device
			5 External Fixation Device
			6 Internal Fixation Device,
			    Intramedullary
			7 Internal Fixation Device,
			    Intramedullary Limb
			    Lengthening
			8 External Fixation Device,
			    Limb Lengthening
			B External Fixation Device,
			    Monoplanar
			C External Fixation Device, Ring
			D External Fixation Device,
			    Hybrid
				Z No Qualifier

M   **Carpal, Right**
    Capitate bone
    Hamate bone
    Lunate bone
    Pisiform bone
    Scaphoid bone
    Trapezium bone
    Trapezoid bone
    Triquetral bone
N   **Carpal, Left**
    See M Carpal, Right
	P **Metacarpal, Right**
	Q **Metacarpal, Left**
	R **Thumb Phalanx, Right**
	S **Thumb Phalanx, Left**
	T **Finger Phalanx, Right**
	V **Finger Phalanx, Left**
		Ø Open
		3 Percutaneous
		4 Percutaneous Endoscopic
			4 Internal Fixation Device
			5 External Fixation Device
				Z No Qualifier

Y **Upper Bone**		**Ø** Open **3** Percutaneous **4** Percutaneous Endoscopic	**M** Bone Growth Stimulator	**Z** No Qualifier

Non-OR	ØPH[C,D,H,J,K,L][Ø,3,4]8Z
Non-OR	ØPH[F,G][Ø,3,4]8Z

NC Noncovered Procedure   **LC** Limited Coverage   **QA** Questionable OB Admit   **NT** New Tech Add-on   ⊞ Combination Member   ♂ Male   ♀ Female

ICD-10-PCS 2022   551

ØPH–ØPH

Ø Medical and Surgical
P Upper Bones
J Inspection

Definition: Visually and/or manually exploring a body part

Explanation: Visual exploration may be performed with or without optical instrumentation. Manual exploration may be performed directly or through intervening body layers.

Body Part Character 4	Approach Character 5	Device Character 6	Qualifier Character 7
Y Upper Bone	Ø Open 3 Percutaneous 4 Percutaneous Endoscopic X External	Z No Device	Z No Qualifier

Non-OR ØPJY[3,X]ZZ

Ø Medical and Surgical
P Upper Bones
N Release

Definition: Freeing a body part from an abnormal physical constraint by cutting or by the use of force

Explanation: Some of the restraining tissue may be taken out but none of the body part is taken out

Body Part Character 4		Approach Character 5	Device Character 6	Qualifier Character 7

Ø Sternum
  Manubrium
  Suprasternal notch
  Xiphoid process
1 Ribs, 1 to 2
2 Ribs, 3 or More
3 Cervical Vertebra
  Dens
  Odontoid process
  Spinous process
  Transverse foramen
  Transverse process
  Vertebral arch
  Vertebral body
  Vertebral foramen
  Vertebral lamina
  Vertebral pedicle
4 Thoracic Vertebra
  Spinous process
  Transverse process
  Vertebral arch
  Vertebral body
  Vertebral foramen
  Vertebral lamina
  Vertebral pedicle
5 Scapula, Right
  Acromion (process)
  Coracoid process
6 Scapula, Left
  See 5 Scapula, Right
7 Glenoid Cavity, Right
  Glenoid fossa (of scapula)
8 Glenoid Cavity, Left
  See 7 Glenoid Cavity, Right
9 Clavicle, Right
B Clavicle, Left
C Humeral Head, Right
  Greater tuberosity
  Lesser tuberosity
  Neck of humerus
    (anatomical) (surgical)
D Humeral Head, Left
  See C Humeral Head, Right
	F Humeral Shaft, Right
	  Distal humerus
	  Humerus, distal
	  Lateral epicondyle of
	    humerus
	  Medial epicondyle of
	    humerus
	G Humeral Shaft, Left
	  See F Humeral Shaft, Right
	H Radius, Right
	  Ulnar notch
	J Radius, Left
	  See H Radius, Right
	K Ulna, Right
	  Olecranon process
	  Radial notch
	L Ulna, Left
	  See K Ulna, Right
	M Carpal, Right
	  Capitate bone
	  Hamate bone
	  Lunate bone
	  Pisiform bone
	  Scaphoid bone
	  Trapezium bone
	  Trapezoid bone
	  Triquetral bone
	N Carpal, Left
	  See M Carpal, Right
	P Metacarpal, Right
	Q Metacarpal, Left
	R Thumb Phalanx, Right
	S Thumb Phalanx, Left
	T Finger Phalanx, Right
	V Finger Phalanx, Left
		Ø Open
		3 Percutaneous
		4 Percutaneous Endoscopic
			Z No Device	Z No Qualifier

Ø	**Medical and Surgical**
P	**Upper Bones**
P	**Removal**

Definition: Taking out or off a device from a body part

Explanation: If a device is taken out and a similar device put in without cutting or puncturing the skin or mucous membrane, the procedure is coded to the root operation CHANGE. Otherwise, the procedure for taking out a device is coded to the root operation REMOVAL.

Body Part Character 4		Approach Character 5	Device Character 6	Qualifier Character 7
Ø **Sternum** Manubrium Suprasternal notch Xiphoid process 1 **Ribs, 1 to 2** 2 **Ribs, 3 or More** 3 **Cervical Vertebra** Dens Odontoid process Spinous process Transverse foramen Transverse process Vertebral arch Vertebral body Vertebral foramen Vertebral lamina Vertebral pedicle	4 **Thoracic Vertebra** Spinous process Transverse process Vertebral arch Vertebral body Vertebral foramen Vertebral lamina Vertebral pedicle 5 **Scapula, Right** Acromion (process) Coracoid process 6 **Scapula, Left** *See 5 Scapula, Right* 7 **Glenoid Cavity, Right** Glenoid fossa (of scapula) 8 **Glenoid Cavity, Left** *See 7 Glenoid Cavity, Right* 9 **Clavicle, Right** B **Clavicle, Left**	Ø **Open** 3 **Percutaneous** 4 **Percutaneous Endoscopic**	4 **Internal Fixation Device** 7 **Autologous Tissue Substitute** J **Synthetic Substitute** K **Nonautologous Tissue Substitute**	Z **No Qualifier**
Ø Sternum Manubrium Suprasternal notch Xiphoid process 1 Ribs, 1 to 2 2 Ribs, 3 or More 3 Cervical Vertebra Dens Odontoid process Spinous process Transverse foramen Transverse process Vertebral arch Vertebral body Vertebral foramen Vertebral lamina Vertebral pedicle	4 Thoracic Vertebra Spinous process Transverse process Vertebral arch Vertebral body Vertebral foramen Vertebral lamina Vertebral pedicle 5 Scapula, Right Acromion (process) Coracoid process 6 Scapula, Left *See 5 Scapula, Right* 7 Glenoid Cavity, Right Glenoid fossa (of scapula) 8 Glenoid Cavity, Left *See 7 Glenoid Cavity, Right* 9 Clavicle, Right B Clavicle, Left	X **External**	4 **Internal Fixation Device**	Z **No Qualifier**

C **Humeral Head, Right**
Greater tuberosity
Lesser tuberosity
Neck of humerus
  (anatomical) (surgical)
D **Humeral Head, Left**
See C Humeral Head, Right
F **Humeral Shaft, Right**
Distal humerus
Humerus, distal
Lateral epicondyle of
  humerus
Medial epicondyle of
  humerus
G **Humeral Shaft, Left**
See F Humeral Shaft, Right
H **Radius, Right**
Ulnar notch
J **Radius, Left**
See H Radius, Right
K **Ulna, Right**
Olecranon process
Radial notch
	L **Ulna, Left**
	See K Ulna, Right
	M **Carpal, Right**
	Capitate bone
	Hamate bone
	Lunate bone
	Pisiform bone
	Scaphoid bone
	Trapezium bone
	Trapezoid bone
	Triquetral bone
	N **Carpal, Left**
	See M Carpal, Right
	P **Metacarpal, Right**
	Q **Metacarpal, Left**
	R **Thumb Phalanx, Right**
	S **Thumb Phalanx, Left**
	T **Finger Phalanx, Right**
	V **Finger Phalanx, Left**
		Ø **Open**
		3 **Percutaneous**
		4 **Percutaneous Endoscopic**
			4 **Internal Fixation Device**
			5 **External Fixation Device**
			7 **Autologous Tissue Substitute**
			J **Synthetic Substitute**
			K **Nonautologous Tissue Substitute**
				Z **No Qualifier**

Non-OR   ØPP[Ø,1,2,3,4,5,6,7,8,9,B]X4Z

ØPP Continued on next page

Ø   Medical and Surgical   *ØPP Continued*
P   Upper Bones
P   Removal   Definition: Taking out or off a device from a body part

Explanation: If a device is taken out and a similar device put in without cutting or puncturing the skin or mucous membrane, the procedure is coded to the root operation CHANGE. Otherwise, the procedure for taking out a device is coded to the root operation REMOVAL.

Body Part Character 4		Approach Character 5	Device Character 6	Qualifier Character 7
C Humeral Head, Right Greater tuberosity Lesser tuberosity Neck of humerus (anatomical) (surgical) **D Humeral Head, Left** *See C Humeral Head, Right* **F Humeral Shaft, Right** Distal humerus Humerus, distal Lateral epicondyle of humerus Medial epicondyle of humerus **G Humeral Shaft, Left** *See F Humeral Shaft, Right* **H Radius, Right** Ulnar notch **J Radius, Left** *See H Radius, Right* **K Ulna, Right** Olecranon process Radial notch	**L Ulna, Left** *See K Ulna, Right* **M Carpal, Right** Capitate bone Hamate bone Lunate bone Pisiform bone Scaphoid bone Trapezium bone Trapezoid bone Triquetral bone **N Carpal, Left** *See M Carpal, Right* **P Metacarpal, Right** **Q Metacarpal, Left** **R Thumb Phalanx, Right** **S Thumb Phalanx, Left** **T Finger Phalanx, Right** **V Finger Phalanx, Left**	**X External**	**4 Internal Fixation Device** **5 External Fixation Device**	**Z No Qualifier**
Y Upper Bone		**Ø Open** **3 Percutaneous** **4 Percutaneous Endoscopic** **X External**	**Ø Drainage Device** **M Bone Growth Stimulator**	**Z No Qualifier**

Non-OR	ØPP[C,D,F,G,H,J,K,L,M,N,P,Q,R,S,T,V]X[4,5]Z
Non-OR	ØPPY3ØZ
Non-OR	ØPPYX[Ø,M]Z

Ø Medical and Surgical
P Upper Bones
Q Repair   Definition: Restoring, to the extent possible, a body part to its normal anatomic structure and function
           Explanation: Used only when the method to accomplish the repair is not one of the other root operations

Body Part		Approach	Device	Qualifier
Character 4		**Character 5**	**Character 6**	**Character 7**
Ø Sternum	**F Humeral Shaft, Right**	**Ø Open**	**Z No Device**	**Z No Qualifier**
Manubrium	Distal humerus	**3 Percutaneous**		
Suprasternal notch	Humerus, distal	**4 Percutaneous Endoscopic**		
Xiphoid process	Lateral epicondyle of	**X External**		
1 Ribs, 1 to 2	humerus			
2 Ribs, 3 or More	Medial epicondyle of			
3 Cervical Vertebra	humerus			
Dens	**G Humeral Shaft, Left**			
Odontoid process	*See F Humeral Shaft, Right*			
Spinous process	**H Radius, Right**			
Transverse foramen	Ulnar notch			
Transverse process	**J Radius, Left**			
Vertebral arch	*See H Radius, Right*			
Vertebral body	**K Ulna, Right**			
Vertebral foramen	Olecranon process			
Vertebral lamina	Radial notch			
Vertebral pedicle	**L Ulna, Left**			
4 Thoracic Vertebra	*See K Ulna, Right*			
Spinous process	**M Carpal, Right**			
Transverse process	Capitate bone			
Vertebral arch	Hamate bone			
Vertebral body	Lunate bone			
Vertebral foramen	Pisiform bone			
Vertebral lamina	Scaphoid bone			
Vertebral pedicle	Trapezium bone			
5 Scapula, Right	Trapezoid bone			
Acromion (process)	Triquetral bone			
Coracoid process	**N Carpal, Left**			
6 Scapula, Left	*See M Carpal, Right*			
See 5 Scapula, Right	**P Metacarpal, Right**			
7 Glenoid Cavity, Right	**Q Metacarpal, Left**			
Glenoid fossa (of scapula)	**R Thumb Phalanx, Right**			
8 Glenoid Cavity, Left	**S Thumb Phalanx, Left**			
See 7 Glenoid Cavity, Right	**T Finger Phalanx, Right**			
9 Clavicle, Right	**V Finger Phalanx, Left**			
B Clavicle, Left				
C Humeral Head, Right				
Greater tuberosity				
Lesser tuberosity				
Neck of humerus				
(anatomical)(surgical)				
D Humeral Head, Left				
See C Humeral Head, Right				

Non-OR   ØPQ[Ø,1,2,3,4,5,6,7,8,9,B,C,D,F,G,H,J,K,L,M,N,P,Q,R,S,T,V]XZZ

🅽🅲 Noncovered Procedure   🅛🅒 Limited Coverage   🆀🅰 Questionable OB Admit   🅽🆃 New Tech Add-on   ⊞ Combination Member   ♂ Male   ♀ Female

ICD-10-PCS 2022   555

ØPQ–ØPQ

Ø **Medical and Surgical**
P **Upper Bones**
R **Replacement**　　Definition: Putting in or on biological or synthetic material that physically takes the place and/or function of all or a portion of a body part

　　　　　　　　　　　　Explanation: The body part may have been taken out or replaced, or may be taken out, physically eradicated, or rendered nonfunctional during the REPLACEMENT procedure. A REMOVAL procedure is coded for taking out the device used in a previous replacement procedure.

Body Part Character 4		Approach Character 5	Device Character 6	Qualifier Character 7
Ø **Sternum** 　Manubrium 　Suprasternal notch 　Xiphoid process **1** **Ribs, 1 to 2** **2** **Ribs, 3 or More** **3** **Cervical Vertebra** 　Dens 　Odontoid process 　Spinous process 　Transverse foramen 　Transverse process 　Vertebral arch 　Vertebral body 　Vertebral foramen 　Vertebral lamina 　Vertebral pedicle **4** **Thoracic Vertebra** 　Spinous process 　Transverse process 　Vertebral arch 　Vertebral body 　Vertebral foramen 　Vertebral lamina 　Vertebral pedicle **5** **Scapula, Right** 　Acromion (process) 　Coracoid process **6** **Scapula, Left** 　*See 5 Scapula, Right* **7** **Glenoid Cavity, Right** 　Glenoid fossa (of scapula) **8** **Glenoid Cavity, Left** 　*See 7 Glenoid Cavity, Right* **9** **Clavicle, Right** **B** **Clavicle, Left** **C** **Humeral Head, Right** 　Greater tuberosity 　Lesser tuberosity 　Neck of humerus 　　(anatomical)(surgical) **D** **Humeral Head, Left** 　*See C Humeral Head, Right*	**F** **Humeral Shaft, Right** 　Distal humerus 　Humerus, distal 　Lateral epicondyle of 　　humerus 　Medial epicondyle of 　　humerus **G** **Humeral Shaft, Left** 　*See F Humeral Shaft, Right* **H** **Radius, Right** 　Ulnar notch **J** **Radius, Left** 　*See H Radius, Right* **K** **Ulna, Right** 　Olecranon process 　Radial notch **L** **Ulna, Left** 　*See K Ulna, Right* **M** **Carpal, Right** 　Capitate bone 　Hamate bone 　Lunate bone 　Pisiform bone 　Scaphoid bone 　Trapezium bone 　Trapezoid bone 　Triquetral bone **N** **Carpal, Left** 　*See M Carpal, Right* **P** **Metacarpal, Right** **Q** **Metacarpal, Left** **R** **Thumb Phalanx, Right** **S** **Thumb Phalanx, Left** **T** **Finger Phalanx, Right** **V** **Finger Phalanx, Left**	**Ø** **Open** **3** **Percutaneous** **4** **Percutaneous Endoscopic**	**7** **Autologous Tissue** 　**Substitute** **J** **Synthetic Substitute** **K** **Nonautologous Tissue** 　**Substitute**	**Z** **No Qualifier**

Ø   **Medical and Surgical**
P   **Upper Bones**
S   **Reposition**   Definition: Moving to its normal location, or other suitable location, all or a portion of a body part

Explanation: The body part is moved to a new location from an abnormal location, or from a normal location where it is not functioning correctly. The body part may or may not be cut out or off to be moved to the new location.

Body Part Character 4		Approach Character 5	Device Character 6	Qualifier Character 7
Ø Sternum Manubrium Suprasternal notch Xiphoid process		**Ø** Open **3** Percutaneous **4** Percutaneous Endoscopic	**Ø** Internal Fixation Device, Rigid Plate **4** Internal Fixation Device **Z** No Device	**Z** No Qualifier
Ø Sternum Manubrium Suprasternal notch Xiphoid process		**X** External	**Z** No Device	**Z** No Qualifier
1 Ribs, 1 to 2 **2 Ribs, 3 or More** **3 Cervical Vertebra** ⊞ Dens Odontoid process Spinous process Transverse foramen Transverse process Vertebral arch Vertebral body Vertebral foramen Vertebral lamina Vertebral pedicle	**5 Scapula, Right** Acromion (process) Coracoid process **6 Scapula, Left** *See 5 Scapula, Right* **7 Glenoid Cavity, Right** Glenoid fossa (of scapula) **8 Glenoid Cavity, Left** *See 7 Glenoid Cavity, Right* **9 Clavicle, Right** **B Clavicle, Left**	**Ø** Open **3** Percutaneous **4** Percutaneous Endoscopic	**4** Internal Fixation Device **Z** No Device	**Z** No Qualifier
1 Ribs, 1 to 2 **2 Ribs, 3 or More** **3 Cervical Vertebra** Dens Odontoid process Spinous process Transverse foramen Transverse process Vertebral arch Vertebral body Vertebral foramen Vertebral lamina Vertebral pedicle	**5 Scapula, Right** Acromion (process) Coracoid process **6 Scapula, Left** *See 5 Scapula, Right* **7 Glenoid Cavity, Right** Glenoid fossa (of scapula) **8 Glenoid Cavity, Left** *See 7 Glenoid Cavity, Right* **9 Clavicle, Right** **B Clavicle, Left**	**X** External	**Z** No Device	**Z** No Qualifier
4 Thoracic Vertebra ⊞ Spinous process Transverse process Vertebral arch Vertebral body Vertebral foramen Vertebral lamina Vertebral pedicle		**Ø** Open **4** Percutaneous Endoscopic	**3** Spinal Stabilization Device, Vertebral Body Tether **4** Internal Fixation Device **Z** No Device	**Z** No Qualifier
4 Thoracic Vertebra Spinous process Transverse process Vertebral arch Vertebral body Vertebral foramen Vertebral lamina Vertebral pedicle		**3** Percutaneous	**4** Internal Fixation Device **Z** No Device	**Z** No Qualifier
4 Thoracic Vertebra Spinous process Transverse process Vertebral arch Vertebral body Vertebral foramen Vertebral lamina Vertebral pedicle		**X** External	**Z** No Device	**Z** No Qualifier
C Humeral Head, Right Greater tuberosity Lesser tuberosity Neck of humerus (anatomical)(surgical) **D Humeral Head, Left** *See C Humeral Head, Right* **F Humeral Shaft, Right** Distal humerus Humerus, distal Lateral epicondyle of humerus Medial epicondyle of humerus	**G Humeral Shaft, Left** *See F Humeral Shaft, Right* **H Radius, Right** Ulnar notch **J Radius, Left** *See H Radius, Right* **K Ulna, Right** Olecranon process Radial notch **L Ulna, Left** *See K Ulna, Right*	**Ø** Open **3** Percutaneous **4** Percutaneous Endoscopic	**4** Internal Fixation Device **5** External Fixation Device **6** Internal Fixation Device, Intramedullary **B** External Fixation Device, Monoplanar **C** External Fixation Device, Ring **D** External Fixation Device, Hybrid **Z** No Device	**Z** No Qualifier

Non-OR	ØPSØ[3,4]ZZ	Non-OR	ØPS[1,2,3,5,6,7,8,9,B]XZZ	**See Appendix L for Procedure Combinations**
Non-OR	ØPSØXZZ	Non-OR	ØPS4XZZ	⊞ ØPS[3,4]3ZZ
Non-OR	ØPS[1,2,5,6,7,8,9,B][3,4]ZZ	Non-OR	ØPS[C,D,F,G,H,J,K,L][3,4]ZZ	

ØPS Continued on next page

NC Noncovered Procedure   **LC** Limited Coverage   **OA** Questionable OB Admit   **NT** New Tech Add-on   ⊞ Combination Member   ♂ Male   ♀ Female

Ø   **Medical and Surgical**   *ØPS Continued*
P   **Upper Bones**
S   **Reposition**   Definition: Moving to its normal location, or other suitable location, all or a portion of a body part

Explanation: The body part is moved to a new location from an abnormal location, or from a normal location where it is not functioning correctly. The body part may or may not be cut out or off to be moved to the new location.

Body Part Character 4		Approach Character 5	Device Character 6	Qualifier Character 7

C **Humeral Head, Right**
   Greater tuberosity
   Lesser tuberosity
   Neck of humerus
      (anatomical)(surgical)
D **Humeral Head, Left**
   See C Humeral Head, Right
F **Humeral Shaft, Right**
   Distal humerus
   Humerus, distal
   Lateral epicondyle of humerus
   Medial epicondyle of humerus
	G **Humeral Shaft, Left**
	   See F Humeral Shaft, Right
	H **Radius, Right**
	   Ulnar notch
	J **Radius, Left**
	   See H Radius, Right
	K **Ulna, Right**
	   Olecranon process
	   Radial notch
	L **Ulna, Left**
	   See K Ulna, Right
		X External	**Z** No Device	**Z** No Qualifier

M **Carpal, Right**
   Capitate bone
   Hamate bone
   Lunate bone
   Pisiform bone
   Scaphoid bone
   Trapezium bone
   Trapezoid bone
   Triquetral bone
	N **Carpal, Left**
	   See M Carpal, Right
	P **Metacarpal, Right**
	Q **Metacarpal, Left**
	R **Thumb Phalanx, Right**
	S **Thumb Phalanx, Left**
	T **Finger Phalanx, Right**
	V **Finger Phalanx, Left**
		Ø Open
		3 Percutaneous
		4 Percutaneous Endoscopic
			4 Internal Fixation Device
			5 External Fixation Device
			Z No Device
				Z No Qualifier

M **Carpal, Right**
   Capitate bone
   Hamate bone
   Lunate bone
   Pisiform bone
   Scaphoid bone
   Trapezium bone
   Trapezoid bone
   Triquetral bone
	N **Carpal, Left**
	   See M Carpal, Right
	P **Metacarpal, Right**
	Q **Metacarpal, Left**
	R **Thumb Phalanx, Right**
	S **Thumb Phalanx, Left**
	T **Finger Phalanx, Right**
	V **Finger Phalanx, Left**
		X External	**Z** No Device	**Z** No Qualifier

Non-OR   ØPS[C,D,F,G,H,J,K,L]XZZ
Non-OR   ØPS[M,N,P,Q,R,S,T,V][3,4]ZZ
Non-OR   ØPS[M,N,P,Q,R,S,T,V]XZZ

Ø   **Medical and Surgical**
P   **Upper Bones**
T   **Resection**   Definition: Cutting out or off, without replacement, all of a body part

Explanation: None

Body Part Character 4		Approach Character 5	Device Character 6	Qualifier Character 7

Ø **Sternum**
   Manubrium
   Suprasternal notch
   Xiphoid process
1 **Ribs, 1 to 2**
2 **Ribs, 3 or More**
5 **Scapula, Right**
   Acromion (process)
   Coracoid process
6 **Scapula, Left**
   See 5 Scapula, Right
7 **Glenoid Cavity, Right**
   Glenoid fossa (of scapula)
8 **Glenoid Cavity, Left**
   See 7 Glenoid Cavity, Right
9 **Clavicle, Right**
B **Clavicle, Left**
C **Humeral Head, Right**
   Greater tuberosity
   Lesser tuberosity
   Neck of humerus
      (anatomical) (surgical)
D **Humeral Head, Left**
   See C Humeral Head, Right
F **Humeral Shaft, Right**
   Distal humerus
   Humerus, distal
   Lateral epicondyle of humerus
   Medial epicondyle of humerus
	G **Humeral Shaft, Left**
	   See F Humeral Shaft, Right
	H **Radius, Right**
	   Ulnar notch
	J **Radius, Left**
	   See H Radius, Right
	K **Ulna, Right**
	   Olecranon process
	   Radial notch
	L **Ulna, Left**
	   See K Ulna, Right
	M **Carpal, Right**
	   Capitate bone
	   Hamate bone
	   Lunate bone
	   Pisiform bone
	   Scaphoid bone
	   Trapezium bone
	   Trapezoid bone
	   Triquetral bone
	N **Carpal, Left**
	   See M Carpal, Right
	P **Metacarpal, Right**
	Q **Metacarpal, Left**
	R **Thumb Phalanx, Right**
	S **Thumb Phalanx, Left**
	T **Finger Phalanx, Right**
	V **Finger Phalanx, Left**
		Ø Open	**Z** No Device	**Z** No Qualifier

Ø　**Medical and Surgical**
P　**Upper Bones**
U　**Supplement**　Definition: Putting in or on biological or synthetic material that physically reinforces and/or augments the function of a portion of a body part
Explanation: The biological material is non-living, or is living and from the same individual. The body part may have been previously replaced, and the SUPPLEMENT procedure is performed to physically reinforce and/or augment the function of the replaced body part.

Body Part Character 4		Approach Character 5	Device Character 6	Qualifier Character 7
Ø **Sternum** 　　Manubrium 　　Suprasternal notch 　　Xiphoid process **1** **Ribs, 1 to 2** **2** **Ribs, 3 or More** **3** **Cervical Vertebra** ⊞ 　　Dens 　　Odontoid process 　　Spinous process 　　Transverse foramen 　　Transverse process 　　Vertebral arch 　　Vertebral body 　　Vertebral foramen 　　Vertebral lamina 　　Vertebral pedicle **4** **Thoracic Vertebra** ⊞ 　　Spinous process 　　Transverse process 　　Vertebral arch 　　Vertebral body 　　Vertebral foramen 　　Vertebral lamina 　　Vertebral pedicle **5** **Scapula, Right** 　　Acromion (process) 　　Coracoid process **6** **Scapula, Left** 　　*See 5 Scapula, Right* **7** **Glenoid Cavity, Right** 　　Glenoid fossa (of scapula) **8** **Glenoid Cavity, Left** 　　*See 7 Glenoid Cavity, Right* **9** **Clavicle, Right** **B** **Clavicle, Left** **C** **Humeral Head, Right** 　　Greater tuberosity 　　Lesser tuberosity 　　Neck of humerus 　　　(anatomical) (surgical)	**D** **Humeral Head, Left** 　　*See C Humeral Head, Right* **F** **Humeral Shaft, Right** 　　Distal humerus 　　Humerus, distal 　　Lateral epicondyle of humerus 　　Medial epicondyle of humerus **G** **Humeral Shaft, Left** 　　*See F Humeral Shaft, Right* **H** **Radius, Right** 　　Ulnar notch **J** **Radius, Left** 　　*See H Radius, Right* **K** **Ulna, Right** 　　Olecranon process 　　Radial notch **L** **Ulna, Left** 　　*See K Ulna, Right* **M** **Carpal, Right** 　　Capitate bone 　　Hamate bone 　　Lunate bone 　　Pisiform bone 　　Scaphoid bone 　　Trapezium bone 　　Trapezoid bone 　　Triquetral bone **N** **Carpal, Left** 　　*See M Carpal, Right* **P** **Metacarpal, Right** **Q** **Metacarpal, Left** **R** **Thumb Phalanx, Right** **S** **Thumb Phalanx, Left** **T** **Finger Phalanx, Right** **V** **Finger Phalanx, Left**	**Ø** **Open** **3** **Percutaneous** **4** **Percutaneous Endoscopic**	**7** **Autologous Tissue** 　　**Substitute** **J** **Synthetic Substitute** **K** **Nonautologous Tissue** 　　**Substitute**	**Z** **No Qualifier**

See Appendix L for Procedure Combinations
⊞　　ØPU[3,4]3JZ

Ø   Medical and Surgical
P   Upper Bones
W   Revision

Definition: Correcting, to the extent possible, a portion of a malfunctioning device or the position of a displaced device

Explanation: Revision can include correcting a malfunctioning or displaced device by taking out or putting in components of the device such as a screw or pin

Body Part Character 4		Approach Character 5	Device Character 6	Qualifier Character 7
Ø Sternum 　Manubrium 　Suprasternal notch 　Xiphoid process **1** Ribs, 1 to 2 **2** Ribs, 3 or More **3** Cervical Vertebra 　Dens 　Odontoid process 　Spinous process 　Transverse foramen 　Transverse process 　Vertebral arch 　Vertebral body 　Vertebral foramen 　Vertebral lamina 　Vertebral pedicle **4** Thoracic Vertebra 　Spinous process 　Transverse process 　Vertebral arch 　Vertebral body 　Vertebral foramen 　Vertebral lamina 　Vertebral pedicle	**5** Scapula, Right 　Acromion (process) 　Coracoid process **6** Scapula, Left 　*See 5 Scapula, Right* **7** Glenoid Cavity, Right 　Glenoid fossa (of scapula) **8** Glenoid Cavity, Left 　*See 7 Glenoid Cavity, Right* **9** Clavicle, Right **B** Clavicle, Left	**Ø** Open **3** Percutaneous **4** Percutaneous Endoscopic **X** External	**4** Internal Fixation Device **7** Autologous Tissue 　Substitute **J** Synthetic Substitute **K** Nonautologous Tissue 　Substitute	**Z** No Qualifier
C Humeral Head, Right 　Greater tuberosity 　Lesser tuberosity 　Neck of humerus 　　(anatomical)(surgical) **D** Humeral Head, Left 　*See C Humeral Head, Right* **F** Humeral Shaft, Right 　Distal humerus 　Humerus, distal 　Lateral epicondyle of 　　humerus 　Medial epicondyle of 　　humerus **G** Humeral Shaft, Left 　*See F Humeral Shaft, Right* **H** Radius, Right 　Ulnar notch **J** Radius, Left 　*See H Radius, Right* **K** Ulna, Right 　Olecranon process 　Radial notch	**L** Ulna, Left 　*See K Ulna, Right* **M** Carpal, Right 　Capitate bone 　Hamate bone 　Lunate bone 　Pisiform bone 　Scaphoid bone 　Trapezium bone 　Trapezoid bone 　Triquetral bone **N** Carpal, Left 　*See M Carpal, Right* **P** Metacarpal, Right **Q** Metacarpal, Left **R** Thumb Phalanx, Right **S** Thumb Phalanx, Left **T** Finger Phalanx, Right **V** Finger Phalanx, Left	**Ø** Open **3** Percutaneous **4** Percutaneous Endoscopic **X** External	**4** Internal Fixation Device **5** External Fixation Device **7** Autologous Tissue 　Substitute **J** Synthetic Substitute **K** Nonautologous Tissue 　Substitute	**Z** No Qualifier
Y Upper Bone		**Ø** Open **3** Percutaneous **4** Percutaneous Endoscopic **X** External	**Ø** Drainage Device **M** Bone Growth Stimulator	**Z** No Qualifier

Non-OR	ØPW[Ø,1,2,3,4,5,6,7,8,9,B]X[4,7,J,K]Z
Non-OR	ØPW[C,D,F,G,H,J,K,L,M,N,P,Q,R,S,T,V]X[4,5,7,J,K]Z
Non-OR	ØPWYX[Ø,M]Z

Non-OR Procedure　　　DRG Non-OR Procedure　　　Valid OR Procedure　　　HAC Associated Procedure　　　Combination Only　　　New/Revised GREEN

Lower Bones ØQ2–ØQW

Character Meanings

This Character Meaning table is provided as a guide to assist the user in the identification of character members that may be found in this section of code tables. It **SHOULD NOT** be used to build a PCS code.

Operation–Character 3	Body Part–Character 4	Approach–Character 5	Device–Character 6	Qualifier–Character 7
2 Change	Ø Lumbar Vertebra	Ø Open	Ø Drainage Device	2 Sesamoid Bone(s) 1st Toe
5 Destruction	1 Sacrum	3 Percutaneous	3 Spinal Stabilization Device, Vertebral Body Tether	X Diagnostic
8 Division	2 Pelvic Bone, Right	4 Percutaneous Endoscopic	4 Internal Fixation Device	Z No Qualifier
9 Drainage	3 Pelvic Bone, Left	X External	5 External Fixation Device	
B Excision	4 Acetabulum, Right		6 Internal Fixation Device, Intramedullary	
C Extirpation	5 Acetabulum, Left		7 Autologous Tissue Substitute OR Internal Fixation Device, Intramedullary Limb Lengthening	
D Extraction	6 Upper Femur, Right		8 External Fixation Device, Limb Lengthening	
H Insertion	7 Upper Femur, Left		B External Fixation Device, Monoplanar	
J Inspection	8 Femoral Shaft, Right		C External Fixation Device, Ring	
N Release	9 Femoral Shaft, Left		D External Fixation Device, Hybrid	
P Removal	B Lower Femur, Right		J Synthetic Substitute	
Q Repair	C Lower Femur, Left		K Nonautologous Tissue Substitute	
R Replacement	D Patella, Right		M Bone Growth Stimulator	
S Reposition	F Patella, Left		Y Other Device	
T Resection	G Tibia, Right		Z No Device	
U Supplement	H Tibia, Left			
W Revision	J Fibula, Right			
	K Fibula, Left			
	L Tarsal, Right			
	M Tarsal, Left			
	N Metatarsal, Right			
	P Metatarsal, Left			
	Q Toe Phalanx, Right			
	R Toe Phalanx, Left			
	S Coccyx			
	Y Lower Bone			

AHA Coding Clinic for table ØQ8
2018, 1Q, 25   Periacetabular osteotomy for repair of congenital hip dysplasia
2016, 2Q, 31   Periacetabular ostectomy for repair of congenital hip dysplasia

AHA Coding Clinic for table ØQB
2021, 2Q, 18   Excision of tibial sesamoid
2020, 2Q, 26   Sacral Pressure Ulcer with Excisional and Nonexcisional Debridement of Same Site
2019, 2Q, 19   Cervical spinal fusion, decompression and placement of interfacet stabilization device
2018, 3Q, 17   Excisional debridement of periosteum
2017, 1Q, 23   Reconstruction of mandible using titanium and bone
2016, 3Q, 30   Resection of femur with interposition arthroplasty
2015, 3Q, 3-8   Excisional and nonexcisional debridement
2015, 3Q, 26   Femoral head resection
2015, 2Q, 34   Decompressive laminectomy
2014, 4Q, 25   Femoroacetabular impingement and labral tear with repair
2014, 2Q, 6   Posterior lumbar fusion with discectomy
2013, 4Q, 116   Spinal decompression
2013, 2Q, 39   Ankle fusion, osteotomy, and removal of hardware
2012, 2Q, 19   Multiple decompressive cervical laminectomies

AHA Coding Clinic for table ØQD
2017, 4Q, 41   Extraction procedures

AHA Coding Clinic for table ØQH
2019, 4Q, 34   Intramedullary limb lengthening internal fixation device
2017, 1Q, 21   Staged scoliosis surgery with iliac fixation and spinal fusion
2016, 3Q, 34   Tibial/fibula epiphysiodesis

AHA Coding Clinic for table ØQP
2020, 4Q, 56   Removal of external fixation device
2017, 4Q, 74-75 Magnetic growth rods
2015, 2Q, 6   Planned implant break

AHA Coding Clinic for table ØQQ
2018, 1Q, 15   Pubic symphysis fusion
2014, 3Q, 24   Repair of lipomyelomeningocele and tethered cord

AHA Coding Clinic for table ØQR
2017, 4Q, 22   Total knee replacement and patellar component
2016, 3Q, 30   Resection of femur with interposition arthroplasty

AHA Coding Clinic for table ØQS
2020, 1Q, 33   Spinal fusion without use of bone graft
2019, 3Q, 26   Open reduction with internal fixation and placement of strut allograft
2018, 1Q, 13   Bilateral cuboid osteotomy for repair of congenital talipes equinovarus
2018, 1Q, 25   Periacetabular osteotomy for repair of congenital hip dysplasia
2016, 3Q, 34   Tibial/fibula epiphysiodesis
2014, 4Q, 29   Rotational osteosynthesis
2014, 4Q, 31   Reposition of femur for correction of valgus and recurvatum deformities

AHA Coding Clinic for table ØQT
2017, 1Q, 22   Chopart amputation of foot
2016, 3Q, 30   Resection of femur with interposition arthroplasty
2015, 3Q, 26   Femoral head resection
2014, 4Q, 29   Rotational osteosynthesis

AHA Coding Clinic for table ØQU
2019, 3Q, 26   Open reduction with internal fixation and placement of strut allograft
2019, 2Q, 35   Kiva® kyphoplasty
2015, 3Q, 18   Total hip replacement with acetabular reconstruction
2014, 4Q, 31   Reposition of femur for correction of valgus and recurvatum deformities
2014, 2Q, 12   Percutaneous vertebroplasty using cement
2013, 2Q, 35   Use of bone void filler in grafting

AHA Coding Clinic for table ØQW
2017, 4Q, 74-75 Magnetic growth rods

Lower Bones

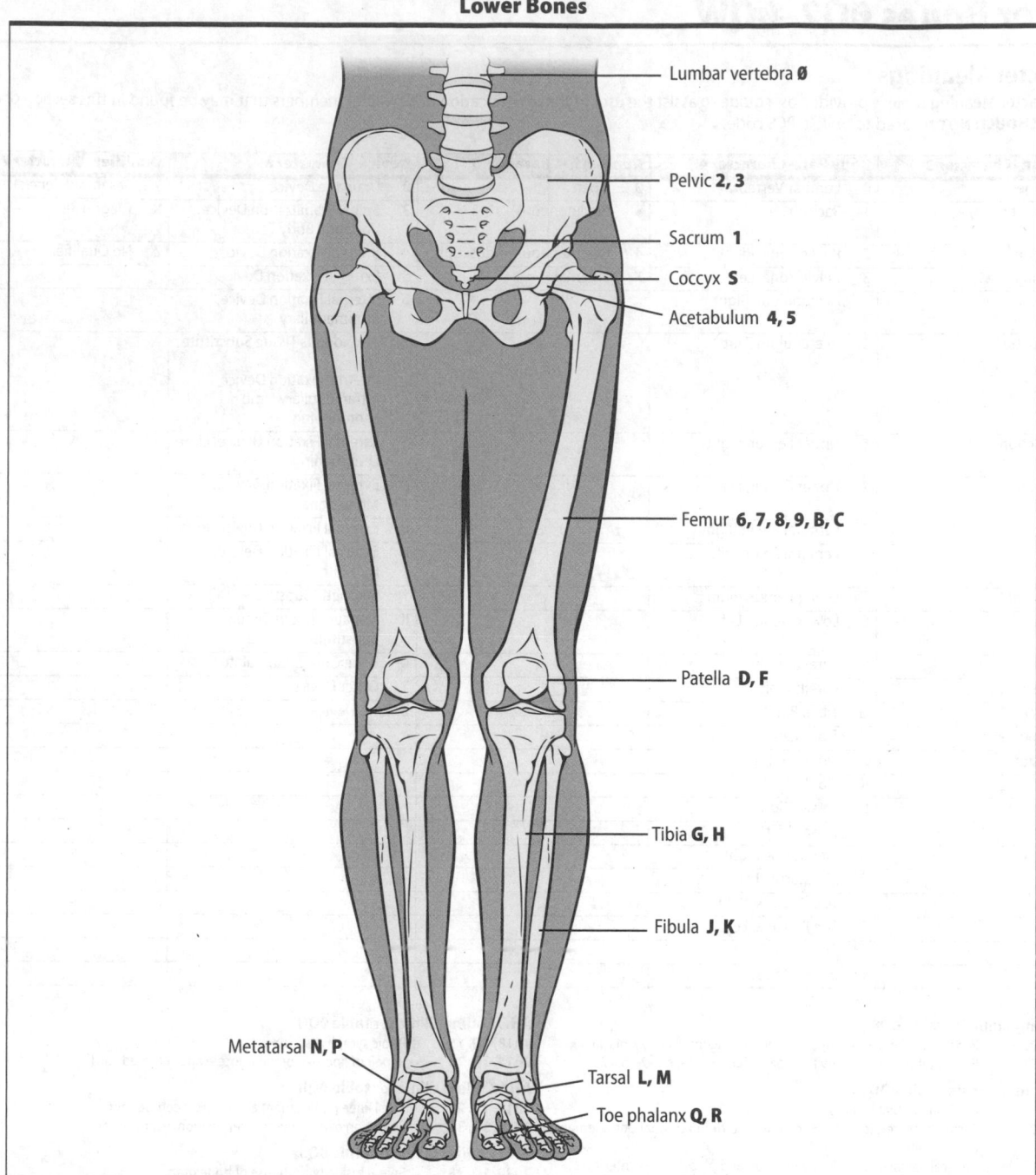

Lumbar vertebra **Ø**

Pelvic **2, 3**

Sacrum **1**

Coccyx **S**

Acetabulum **4, 5**

Femur **6, 7, 8, 9, B, C**

Patella **D, F**

Tibia **G, H**

Fibula **J, K**

Metatarsal **N, P**

Tarsal **L, M**

Toe phalanx **Q, R**

Hip Bone Anatomy

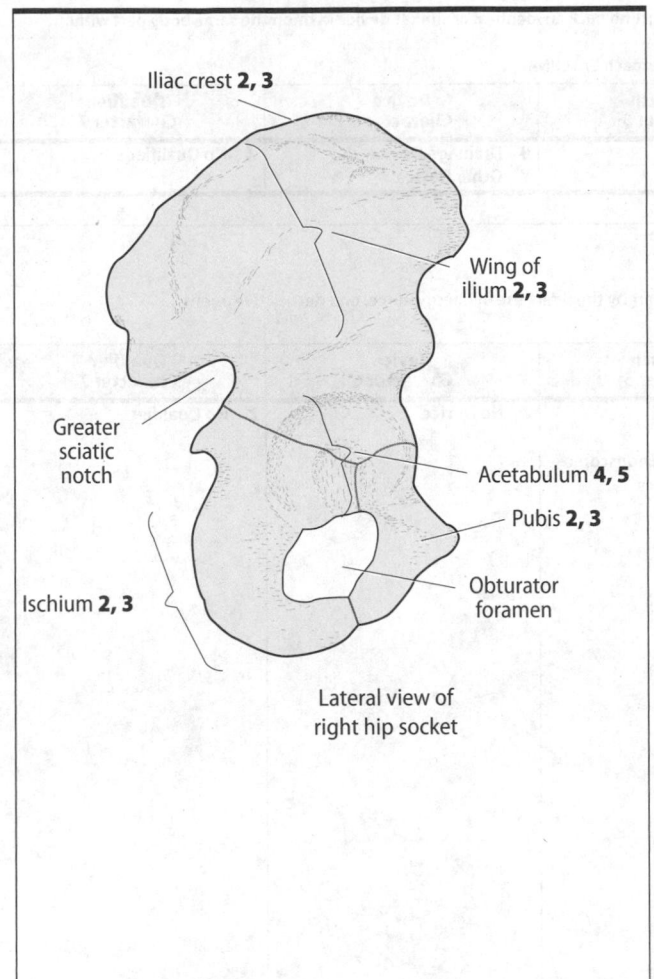

Iliac crest **2, 3**

Wing of ilium **2, 3**

Greater sciatic notch

Acetabulum **4, 5**

Pubis **2, 3**

Obturator foramen

Ischium **2, 3**

Lateral view of right hip socket

Pelvic and Lower Extremity Bones

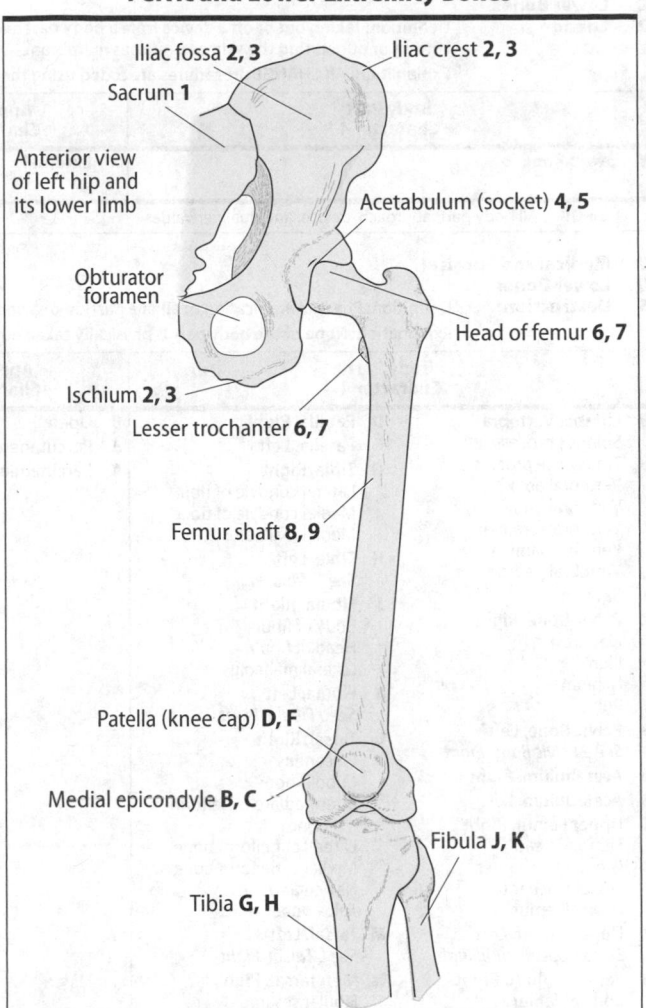

Iliac fossa **2, 3**

Iliac crest **2, 3**

Sacrum **1**

Anterior view of left hip and its lower limb

Acetabulum (socket) **4, 5**

Obturator foramen

Head of femur **6, 7**

Ischium **2, 3**

Lesser trochanter **6, 7**

Femur shaft **8, 9**

Patella (knee cap) **D, F**

Medial epicondyle **B, C**

Fibula **J, K**

Tibia **G, H**

Foot Bones

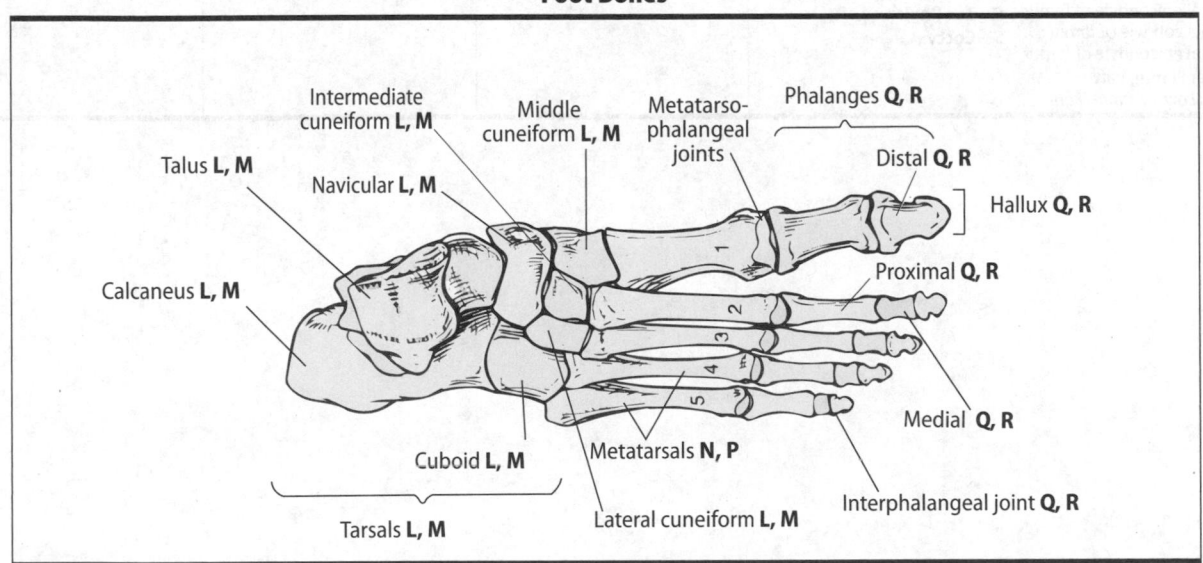

Intermediate cuneiform **L, M**

Middle cuneiform **L, M**

Metatarso-phalangeal joints

Phalanges **Q, R**

Talus **L, M**

Navicular **L, M**

Distal **Q, R**

Hallux **Q, R**

Calcaneus **L, M**

Proximal **Q, R**

Medial **Q, R**

Cuboid **L, M**

Metatarsals **N, P**

Interphalangeal joint **Q, R**

Tarsals **L, M**

Lateral cuneiform **L, M**

Ø　Medical and Surgical
Q　Lower Bones
2　Change　　　Definition: Taking out or off a device from a body part and putting back an identical or similar device in or on the same body part without cutting or puncturing the skin or a mucous membrane

Explanation: All CHANGE procedures are coded using the approach EXTERNAL

Body Part Character 4	Approach Character 5	Device Character 6	Qualifier Character 7
Y　Lower Bone	X　External	Ø　Drainage Device Y　Other Device	Z　No Qualifier

Non-OR	All body part, approach, device, and qualifier values

Ø　Medical and Surgical
Q　Lower Bones
5　Destruction　　　Definition: Physical eradication of all or a portion of a body part by the direct use of energy, force, or a destructive agent

Explanation: None of the body part is physically taken out

Body Part Character 4		Approach Character 5	Device Character 6	Qualifier Character 7
Ø　Lumbar Vertebra 　　Spinous process 　　Transverse process 　　Vertebral arch 　　Vertebral body 　　Vertebral foramen 　　Vertebral lamina 　　Vertebral pedicle 1　Sacrum 2　Pelvic Bone, Right 　　Iliac crest 　　Ilium 　　Ischium 　　Pubis 3　Pelvic Bone, Left 　　*See 2 Pelvic Bone, Right* 4　Acetabulum, Right 5　Acetabulum, Left 6　Upper Femur, Right 　　Femoral head 　　Greater trochanter 　　Lesser trochanter 　　Neck of femur 7　Upper Femur, Left 　　*See 6 Upper Femur, Right* 8　Femoral Shaft, Right 　　Body of femur 9　Femoral Shaft, Left 　　*See 8 Femoral Shaft, Right* B　Lower Femur, Right 　　Lateral condyle of femur 　　Lateral epicondyle of femur 　　Medial condyle of femur 　　Medial epicondyle of femur C　Lower Femur, Left 　　*See B Lower Femur, Right*	D　Patella, Right F　Patella, Left G　Tibia, Right 　　Lateral condyle of tibia 　　Medial condyle of tibia 　　Medial malleolus H　Tibia, Left 　　*See G Tibia, Right* J　Fibula, Right 　　Body of fibula 　　Head of fibula 　　Lateral malleolus K　Fibula, Left 　　*See J Fibula, Right* L　Tarsal, Right 　　Calcaneus 　　Cuboid bone 　　Intermediate cuneiform 　　　bone 　　Lateral cuneiform bone 　　Medial cuneiform bone 　　Navicular bone 　　Talus bone M　Tarsal, Left 　　*See L Tarsal, Right* N　Metatarsal, Right 　　Fibular sesamoid 　　Tibial sesamoid P　Metatarsal, Left 　　*See N Metatarsal, Right* Q　Toe Phalanx, Right R　Toe Phalanx, Left S　Coccyx	Ø　Open 3　Percutaneous 4　Percutaneous Endoscopic	Z　No Device	Z　No Qualifier

0   **Medical and Surgical**
Q   **Lower Bones**
8   **Division**   Definition: Cutting into a body part, without draining fluids and/or gases from the body part, in order to separate or transect a body part
                  Explanation: All or a portion of the body part is separated into two or more portions

Body Part Character 4	Approach Character 5	Device Character 6	Qualifier Character 7

0 **Lumbar Vertebra**
   Spinous process
   Transverse process
   Vertebral arch
   Vertebral body
   Vertebral foramen
   Vertebral lamina
   Vertebral pedicle
1 **Sacrum**
2 **Pelvic Bone, Right**
   Iliac crest
   Ilium
   Ischium
   Pubis
3 **Pelvic Bone, Left**
   See 2 Pelvic Bone, Right
4 **Acetabulum, Right**
5 **Acetabulum, Left**
6 **Upper Femur, Right**
   Femoral head
   Greater trochanter
   Lesser trochanter
   Neck of femur
7 **Upper Femur, Left**
   See 6 Upper Femur, Right
8 **Femoral Shaft, Right**
   Body of femur
9 **Femoral Shaft, Left**
   See 8 Femoral Shaft, Right
B **Lower Femur, Right**
   Lateral condyle of femur
   Lateral epicondyle of femur
   Medial condyle of femur
   Medial epicondyle of femur
C **Lower Femur, Left**
   See B Lower Femur, Right
D **Patella, Right**
F **Patella, Left**
G **Tibia, Right**
   Lateral condyle of tibia
   Medial condyle of tibia
   Medial malleolus
H **Tibia, Left**
   See G Tibia, Right
J **Fibula, Right**
   Body of fibula
   Head of fibula
   Lateral malleolus
K **Fibula, Left**
   See J Fibula, Right
L **Tarsal, Right**
   Calcaneus
   Cuboid bone
   Intermediate cuneiform bone
   Lateral cuneiform bone
   Medial cuneiform bone
   Navicular bone
   Talus bone
M **Tarsal, Left**
   See L Tarsal, Right
N **Metatarsal, Right**
   Fibular sesamoid
   Tibial sesamoid
P **Metatarsal, Left**
   See N Metatarsal, Right
Q **Toe Phalanx, Right**
R **Toe Phalanx, Left**
S **Coccyx**
	0 Open
	3 Percutaneous
	4 Percutaneous Endoscopic
		Z No Device	**Z** No Qualifier

NC Noncovered Procedure   **LC** Limited Coverage   **QA** Questionable OB Admit   **NT** New Tech Add-on   ✚ Combination Member   ♂ Male   ♀ Female

ICD-10-PCS 2022   **565**

0Q8–0Q8

Lower Bones

0   **Medical and Surgical**
Q   **Lower Bones**
9   **Drainage**   Definition: Taking or letting out fluids and/or gases from a body part

Explanation: The qualifier DIAGNOSTIC is used to identify drainage procedures that are biopsies

Body Part Character 4		Approach Character 5	Device Character 6	Qualifier Character 7
0 **Lumbar Vertebra** Spinous process Transverse process Vertebral arch Vertebral body Vertebral foramen Vertebral lamina Vertebral pedicle **1** **Sacrum** **2** **Pelvic Bone, Right** Iliac crest Ilium Ischium Pubis **3** **Pelvic Bone, Left** *See 2 Pelvic Bone, Right* **4** **Acetabulum, Right** **5** **Acetabulum, Left** **6** **Upper Femur, Right** Femoral head Greater trochanter Lesser trochanter Neck of femur **7** **Upper Femur, Left** *See 6 Upper Femur, Right* **8** **Femoral Shaft, Right** Body of femur **9** **Femoral Shaft, Left** *See 8 Femoral Shaft, Right* **B** **Lower Femur, Right** Lateral condyle of femur Lateral epicondyle of femur Medial condyle of femur Medial epicondyle of femur	**C** **Lower Femur, Left** *See B Lower Femur, Right* **D** **Patella, Right** **F** **Patella, Left** **G** **Tibia, Right** Lateral condyle of tibia Medial condyle of tibia Medial malleolus **H** **Tibia, Left** *See G Tibia, Right* **J** **Fibula, Right** Body of fibula Head of fibula Lateral malleolus **K** **Fibula, Left** *See J Fibula, Right* **L** **Tarsal, Right** Calcaneus Cuboid bone Intermediate cuneiform bone Lateral cuneiform bone Medial cuneiform bone Navicular bone Talus bone **M** **Tarsal, Left** *See L Tarsal, Right* **N** **Metatarsal, Right** Fibular sesamoid Tibial sesamoid **P** **Metatarsal, Left** *See N Metatarsal, Right* **Q** **Toe Phalanx, Right** **R** **Toe Phalanx, Left** **S** **Coccyx**	**0** Open **3** Percutaneous **4** Percutaneous Endoscopic	**0** Drainage Device	**Z** No Qualifier
0 **Lumbar Vertebra** Spinous process Transverse process Vertebral arch Vertebral body Vertebral foramen Vertebral lamina Vertebral pedicle **1** **Sacrum** **2** **Pelvic Bone, Right** Iliac crest Ilium Ischium Pubis **3** **Pelvic Bone, Left** *See 2 Pelvic Bone, Right* **4** **Acetabulum, Right** **5** **Acetabulum, Left** **6** **Upper Femur, Right** Femoral head Greater trochanter Lesser trochanter Neck of femur **7** **Upper Femur, Left** *See 6 Upper Femur, Right* **8** **Femoral Shaft, Right** Body of femur **9** **Femoral Shaft, Left** *See 8 Femoral Shaft, Right* **B** **Lower Femur, Right** Lateral condyle of femur Lateral epicondyle of femur Medial condyle of femur Medial epicondyle of femur	**C** **Lower Femur, Left** *See B Lower Femur, Right* **D** **Patella, Right** **F** **Patella, Left** **G** **Tibia, Right** Lateral condyle of tibia Medial condyle of tibia Medial malleolus **H** **Tibia, Left** *See G Tibia, Right* **J** **Fibula, Right** Body of fibula Head of fibula Lateral malleolus **K** **Fibula, Left** *See J Fibula, Right* **L** **Tarsal, Right** Calcaneus Cuboid bone Intermediate cuneiform bone Lateral cuneiform bone Medial cuneiform bone Navicular bone Talus bone **M** **Tarsal, Left** *See L Tarsal, Right* **N** **Metatarsal, Right** Fibular sesamoid Tibial sesamoid **P** **Metatarsal, Left** *See N Metatarsal, Right* **Q** **Toe Phalanx, Right** **R** **Toe Phalanx, Left** **S** Coccyx	**0** Open **3** Percutaneous **4** Percutaneous Endoscopic	**Z** No Device	**X** Diagnostic **Z** No Qualifier

Non-OR   0Q9[0,1,2,3,4,5,6,7,8,9,B,C,D,F,G,H,J,K,L,M,P,Q,R,S]30Z
Non-OR   0Q9[0,1,2,3,4,5,6,7,8,9,B,C,D,F,G,H,J,K,L,M,P,Q,R,S]3ZZ

Non-OR Procedure   DRG Non-OR Procedure   Valid OR Procedure   HAC Associated Procedure   Combination Only   New/Revised GREEN

Ø   **Medical and Surgical**
Q   **Lower Bones**
B   **Excision**   Definition: Cutting out or off, without replacement, a portion of a body part
                 Explanation: The qualifier DIAGNOSTIC is used to identify excision procedures that are biopsies

Body Part Character 4	Approach Character 5	Device Character 6	Qualifier Character 7

Ø   **Lumbar Vertebra**
    Spinous process
    Transverse process
    Vertebral arch
    Vertebral body
    Vertebral foramen
    Vertebral lamina
    Vertebral pedicle
1   **Sacrum**
2   **Pelvic Bone, Right**
    Iliac crest
    Ilium
    Ischium
    Pubis
3   **Pelvic Bone, Left**
    See 2 Pelvic Bone, Right
4   **Acetabulum, Right**
5   **Acetabulum, Left**
6   **Upper Femur, Right**
    Femoral head
    Greater trochanter
    Lesser trochanter
    Neck of femur
7   **Upper Femur, Left**
    See 6 Upper Femur, Right
8   **Femoral Shaft, Right**
    Body of femur
9   **Femoral Shaft, Left**
    See 8 Femoral Shaft, Right
B   **Lower Femur, Right**
    Lateral condyle of femur
    Lateral epicondyle of femur
    Medial condyle of femur
    Medial epicondyle of femur
C   **Lower Femur, Left**
    See B Lower Femur, Right
D   **Patella, Right**
F   **Patella, Left**
G   **Tibia, Right**
    Lateral condyle of tibia
    Medial condyle of tibia
    Medial malleolus
H   **Tibia, Left**
    See G Tibia, Right
J   **Fibula, Right**
    Body of fibula
    Head of fibula
    Lateral malleolus
K   **Fibula, Left**
    See J Fibula, Right
L   **Tarsal, Right**
    Calcaneus
    Cuboid bone
    Intermediate cuneiform bone
    Lateral cuneiform bone
    Medial cuneiform bone
    Navicular bone
    Talus bone
M   **Tarsal, Left**
    See L Tarsal, Right
Q   **Toe Phalanx, Right**
R   **Toe Phalanx, Left**
S   **Coccyx**
	Ø Open
	3 Percutaneous
	4 Percutaneous Endoscopic
		Z No Device	**X** Diagnostic
			Z No Qualifier

N   **Metatarsal, Right**
    Fibular sesamoid
    Tibial sesamoid
P   **Metatarsal, Left**
    See N Metatarsal, Right
	Ø Open
	3 Percutaneous
	4 Percutaneous Endoscopic
		Z No Device	**2** Sesamoid Bone(s) 1st Toe
			X Diagnostic
			Z No Qualifier

NC Noncovered Procedure   **LC** Limited Coverage   **QA** Questionable OB Admit   **NT** New Tech Add-on   ⊞ Combination Member   ♂ Male   ♀ Female

ICD-10-PCS 2022   567

Lower Bones

Ø Medical and Surgical
Q Lower Bones
C Extirpation

Definition: Taking or cutting out solid matter from a body part

Explanation: The solid matter may be an abnormal byproduct of a biological function or a foreign body; it may be imbedded in a body part or in the lumen of a tubular body part. The solid matter may or may not have been previously broken into pieces.

Body Part Character 4	Approach Character 5	Device Character 6	Qualifier Character 7

Ø Lumbar Vertebra
  Spinous process
  Transverse process
  Vertebral arch
  Vertebral body
  Vertebral foramen
  Vertebral lamina
  Vertebral pedicle
1 Sacrum
2 Pelvic Bone, Right
  Iliac crest
  Ilium
  Ischium
  Pubis
3 Pelvic Bone, Left
  See 2 Pelvic Bone, Right
4 Acetabulum, Right
5 Acetabulum, Left
6 Upper Femur, Right
  Femoral head
  Greater trochanter
  Lesser trochanter
  Neck of femur
7 Upper Femur, Left
  See 6 Upper Femur, Right
8 Femoral Shaft, Right
  Body of femur
9 Femoral Shaft, Left
  See 8 Femoral Shaft, Right
B Lower Femur, Right
  Lateral condyle of femur
  Lateral epicondyle of femur
  Medial condyle of femur
  Medial epicondyle of femur
C Lower Femur, Left
  See B Lower Femur, Right
D Patella, Right
F Patella, Left
G Tibia, Right
  Lateral condyle of tibia
  Medial condyle of tibia
  Medial malleolus
H Tibia, Left
  See G Tibia, Right
J Fibula, Right
  Body of fibula
  Head of fibula
  Lateral malleolus
K Fibula, Left
  See J Fibula, Right
L Tarsal, Right
  Calcaneus
  Cuboid bone
  Intermediate cuneiform bone
  Lateral cuneiform bone
  Medial cuneiform bone
  Navicular bone
  Talus bone
M Tarsal, Left
  See L Tarsal, Right
N Metatarsal, Right
  Fibular sesamoid
  Tibial sesamoid
P Metatarsal, Left
  See N Metatarsal, Right
Q Toe Phalanx, Right
R Toe Phalanx, Left
S Coccyx
	Ø Open
	3 Percutaneous
	4 Percutaneous Endoscopic
		Z No Device	Z No Qualifier

0   **Medical and Surgical**
Q   **Lower Bones**
D   **Extraction**   Definition: Pulling or stripping out or off all or a portion of a body part by the use of force

                     Explanation: The qualifier DIAGNOSTIC is used to identify extraction procedures that are biopsies

Body Part Character 4	Approach Character 5	Device Character 6	Qualifier Character 7

0   **Lumbar Vertebra**
    Spinous process
    Transverse process
    Vertebral arch
    Vertebral body
    Vertebral foramen
    Vertebral lamina
    Vertebral pedicle
	0 Open	**Z** No Device	**Z** No Qualifier

1 **Sacrum**			

2   **Pelvic Bone, Right**
    Iliac crest
    Ilium
    Ischium
    Pubis			

3 **Pelvic Bone, Left** *See* 2 Pelvic Bone, Right			
4 **Acetabulum, Right**			
5 **Acetabulum, Left**			

6   **Upper Femur, Right**
    Femoral head
    Greater trochanter
    Lesser trochanter
    Neck of femur			

7 **Upper Femur, Left** *See* 6 Upper Femur, Right			
8 **Femoral Shaft, Right** Body of femur			
9 **Femoral Shaft, Left** *See* 8 Femoral Shaft, Right			

B   **Lower Femur, Right**
    Lateral condyle of femur
    Lateral epicondyle of femur
    Medial condyle of femur
    Medial epicondyle of femur			

C **Lower Femur, Left** *See* B Lower Femur, Right			
D **Patella, Right**			
F **Patella, Left**			

G   **Tibia, Right**
    Lateral condyle of tibia
    Medial condyle of tibia
    Medial malleolus			

H **Tibia, Left** *See* G Tibia, Right			

J   **Fibula, Right**
    Body of fibula
    Head of fibula
    Lateral malleolus			

K **Fibula, Left** *See* J Fibula, Right			

L   **Tarsal, Right**
    Calcaneus
    Cuboid bone
    Intermediate cuneiform bone
    Lateral cuneiform bone
    Medial cuneiform bone
    Navicular bone
    Talus bone			

M **Tarsal, Left** *See* L Tarsal, Right			

N   **Metatarsal, Right**
    Fibular sesamoid
    Tibial sesamoid			

P **Metatarsal, Left** *See* N Metatarsal, Right			
Q **Toe Phalanx, Right**			
R **Toe Phalanx, Left**			
S **Coccyx**			

Lower Bones

Ø   **Medical and Surgical**
Q   **Lower Bones**
H   **Insertion**   Definition: Putting in a nonbiological appliance that monitors, assists, performs, or prevents a physiological function but does not physically take the place of a body part

                Explanation: None

Body Part Character 4		Approach Character 5	Device Character 6	Qualifier Character 7
Ø **Lumbar Vertebra** Spinous process Transverse process Vertebral arch Vertebral body Vertebral foramen Vertebral lamina Vertebral pedicle **1** **Sacrum** **2** **Pelvic Bone, Right** Iliac crest Ilium Ischium Pubis **3** **Pelvic Bone, Left** *See 2 Pelvic Bone, Right* **4** **Acetabulum, Right** **5** **Acetabulum, Left**	**D** **Patella, Right** **F** **Patella, Left** **L** **Tarsal, Right** Calcaneus Cuboid bone Intermediate cuneiform bone Lateral cuneiform bone Medial cuneiform bone Navicular bone Talus bone **M** **Tarsal, Left** *See L Tarsal, Right* **N** **Metatarsal, Right** Fibular sesamoid Tibial sesamoid **P** **Metatarsal, Left** *See N Metatarsal, Right* **Q** **Toe Phalanx, Right** **R** **Toe Phalanx, Left** **S** **Coccyx**	**Ø** Open **3** Percutaneous **4** Percutaneous Endoscopic	**4** Internal Fixation Device **5** External Fixation Device	**Z** No Qualifier
6 **Upper Femur, Right** Femoral head Greater trochanter Lesser trochanter Neck of femur **7** **Upper Femur, Left** *See 6 Upper Femur, Right* **B** **Lower Femur, Right** Lateral condyle of femur Lateral epicondyle of femur Medial condyle of femur Medial epicondyle of femur	**C** **Lower Femur, Left** *See B Lower Femur, Right* **J** **Fibula, Right** Body of fibula Head of fibula Lateral malleolus **K** **Fibula, Left** *See J Fibula, Right*	**Ø** Open **3** Percutaneous **4** Percutaneous Endoscopic	**4** Internal Fixation Device **5** External Fixation Device **6** Internal Fixation Device, Intramedullary **8** External Fixation Device, Limb Lengthening **B** External Fixation Device, Monoplanar **C** External Fixation Device, Ring **D** External Fixation Device, Hybrid	**Z** No Qualifier
8 **Femoral Shaft, Right** Body of femur **9** **Femoral Shaft, Left** *See 8 Femoral Shaft, Right*	**G** **Tibia, Right** Lateral condyle of tibia Medial condyle of tibia Medial malleolus **H** **Tibia, Left** *See G Tibia, Right*	**Ø** Open **3** Percutaneous **4** Percutaneous Endoscopic	**4** Internal Fixation Device **5** External Fixation Device **6** Internal Fixation Device, Intramedullary **7** Internal Fixation Device, Intramedullary Limb Lengthening **8** External Fixation Device, Limb Lengthening **B** External Fixation Device, Monoplanar **C** External Fixation Device, Ring **D** External Fixation Device, Hybrid	**Z** No Qualifier
Y Lower Bone		**Ø** Open **3** Percutaneous **4** Percutaneous Endoscopic	**M** Bone Growth Stimulator	**Z** No Qualifier

Non-OR   ØQH[6,7,B,C,J,K][Ø,3,4]8Z
Non-OR   ØQH[8,9,G,H][Ø,3,4]8Z

Ø   **Medical and Surgical**
Q   **Lower Bones**
J   **Inspection**   Definition: Visually and/or manually exploring a body part

                Explanation: Visual exploration may be performed with or without optical instrumentation. Manual exploration may be performed directly or through intervening body layers.

Body Part Character 4	Approach Character 5	Device Character 6	Qualifier Character 7
Y Lower Bone	**Ø** Open **3** Percutaneous **4** Percutaneous Endoscopic **X** External	**Z** No Device	**Z** No Qualifier

Non-OR   ØQJY[3,X]ZZ

Lower Bones

Ø   **Medical and Surgical**
Q   **Lower Bones**
N   **Release**   Definition: Freeing a body part from an abnormal physical constraint by cutting or by the use of force
                         Explanation: Some of the restraining tissue may be taken out but none of the body part is taken out

Body Part Character 4	Approach Character 5	Device Character 6	Qualifier Character 7
Ø Lumbar Vertebra Spinous process Transverse process Vertebral arch Vertebral body Vertebral foramen Vertebral lamina Vertebral pedicle **1 Sacrum** **2 Pelvic Bone, Right** Iliac crest Ilium Ischium Pubis **3 Pelvic Bone, Left** *See 2 Pelvic Bone, Right* **4 Acetabulum, Right** **5 Acetabulum, Left** **6 Upper Femur, Right** Femoral head Greater trochanter Lesser trochanter Neck of femur **7 Upper Femur, Left** *See 6 Upper Femur, Right* **8 Femoral Shaft, Right** Body of femur **9 Femoral Shaft, Left** *See 8 Femoral Shaft, Right* **B Lower Femur, Right** Lateral condyle of femur Lateral epicondyle of femur Medial condyle of femur Medial epicondyle of femur **C Lower Femur, Left** *See B Lower Femur, Right* **D Patella, Right** **F Patella, Left** **G Tibia, Right** Lateral condyle of tibia Medial condyle of tibia Medial malleolus **H Tibia, Left** *See G Tibia, Right* **J Fibula, Right** Body of fibula Head of fibula Lateral malleolus **K Fibula, Left** *See J Fibula, Right* **L Tarsal, Right** Calcaneus Cuboid bone Intermediate cuneiform bone Lateral cuneiform bone Medial cuneiform bone Navicular bone Talus bone **M Tarsal, Left** *See L Tarsal, Right* **N Metatarsal, Right** Fibular sesamoid Tibial sesamoid **P Metatarsal, Left** *See N Metatarsal, Right* **Q Toe Phalanx, Right** **R Toe Phalanx, Left** **S Coccyx**	**Ø Open** **3 Percutaneous** **4 Percutaneous Endoscopic**	**Z No Device**	**Z No Qualifier**

NC Noncovered Procedure   **LC** Limited Coverage   **QA** Questionable OB Admit   **NT** New Tech Add-on   ⊞ Combination Member   ♂ Male   ♀ Female

ICD-10-PCS 2022   571

Ø Medical and Surgical
Q Lower Bones
P Removal

Definition: Taking out or off a device from a body part

Explanation: If a device is taken out and a similar device put in without cutting or puncturing the skin or mucous membrane, the procedure is coded to the root operation CHANGE. Otherwise, the procedure for taking out a device is coded to the root operation REMOVAL.

Body Part Character 4		Approach Character 5	Device Character 6	Qualifier Character 7
Ø Lumbar Vertebra Spinous process Transverse process Vertebral arch Vertebral body Vertebral foramen Vertebral lamina Vertebral pedicle **1 Sacrum** **2 Pelvic Bone, Right** Iliac crest Ilium Ischium Pubis **3 Pelvic Bone, Left** See 2 Pelvic Bone, Right **4 Acetabulum, Right** **5 Acetabulum, Left** **6 Upper Femur, Right** Femoral head Greater trochanter Lesser trochanter Neck of femur **7 Upper Femur, Left** See 6 Upper Femur, Right **8 Femoral Shaft, Right** Body of femur **9 Femoral Shaft, Left** See 8 Femoral Shaft, Right **B Lower Femur, Right** Lateral condyle of femur Lateral epicondyle of femur Medial condyle of femur Medial epicondyle of femur	**C Lower Femur, Left** See B Lower Femur, Right **D Patella, Right** **F Patella, Left** **G Tibia, Right** Lateral condyle of tibia Medial condyle of tibia Medial malleolus **H Tibia, Left** See G Tibia, Right **J Fibula, Right** Body of fibula Head of fibula Lateral malleolus **K Fibula, Left** See J Fibula, Right **L Tarsal, Right** Calcaneus Cuboid bone Intermediate cuneiform bone Lateral cuneiform bone Medial cuneiform bone Navicular bone Talus bone **M Tarsal, Left** See L Tarsal, Right **N Metatarsal, Right** Fibular sesamoid Tibial sesamoid **P Metatarsal, Left** See N Metatarsal, Right **Q Toe Phalanx, Right** **R Toe Phalanx, Left** **S Coccyx**	**Ø Open** **3 Percutaneous** **4 Percutaneous Endoscopic**	**4 Internal Fixation Device** **5 External Fixation Device** **7 Autologous Tissue Substitute** **J Synthetic Substitute** **K Nonautologous Tissue Substitute**	**Z No Qualifier**
Ø Lumbar Vertebra Spinous process Transverse process Vertebral arch Vertebral body Vertebral foramen Vertebral lamina Vertebral pedicle **1 Sacrum** **2 Pelvic Bone, Right** Iliac crest Ilium Ischium Pubis **3 Pelvic Bone, Left** See 2 Pelvic Bone, Right **4 Acetabulum, Right** **5 Acetabulum, Left** **6 Upper Femur, Right** Femoral head Greater trochanter Lesser trochanter Neck of femur **7 Upper Femur, Left** See 6 Upper Femur, Right **8 Femoral Shaft, Right** Body of femur **9 Femoral Shaft, Left** See 8 Femoral Shaft, Right **B Lower Femur, Right** Lateral condyle of femur Lateral epicondyle of femur Medial condyle of femur Medial epicondyle of femur	**C Lower Femur, Left** See B Lower Femur, Right **D Patella, Right** **F Patella, Left** **G Tibia, Right** Lateral condyle of tibia Medial condyle of tibia Medial malleolus **H Tibia, Left** See G Tibia, Right **J Fibula, Right** Body of fibula Head of fibula Lateral malleolus **K Fibula, Left** See J Fibula, Right **L Tarsal, Right** Calcaneus Cuboid bone Intermediate cuneiform bone Lateral cuneiform bone Medial cuneiform bone Navicular bone Talus bone **M Tarsal, Left** See L Tarsal, Right **N Metatarsal, Right** Fibular sesamoid Tibial sesamoid **P Metatarsal, Left** See N Metatarsal, Right **Q Toe Phalanx, Right** **R Toe Phalanx, Left** **S Coccyx**	**X External**	**4 Internal Fixation Device** **5 External Fixation Device**	**Z No Qualifier**
Y Lower Bone		**Ø Open** **3 Percutaneous** **4 Percutaneous Endoscopic** **X External**	**Ø Drainage Device** **M Bone Growth Stimulator**	**Z No Qualifier**

Non-OR ØQPYX[Ø,M]Z	Non-OR ØQPY3ØZ	Non-OR ØQP[Ø,1,2,3,4,5,6,7,8,9,B,C,D,F,G,H,J,K,L,M,N,P,Q,R,S]X[4,5]Z

Ø   **Medical and Surgical**
Q   **Lower Bones**
Q   **Repair**   Definition: Restoring, to the extent possible, a body part to its normal anatomic structure and function

                         Explanation: Used only when the method to accomplish the repair is not one of the other root operations

Body Part Character 4	Approach Character 5	Device Character 6	Qualifier Character 7

Ø Lumbar Vertebra
   Spinous process
   Transverse process
   Vertebral arch
   Vertebral body
   Vertebral foramen
   Vertebral lamina
   Vertebral pedicle
1 Sacrum
2 Pelvic Bone, Right
   Iliac crest
   Ilium
   Ischium
   Pubis
3 Pelvic Bone, Left
   See 2 Pelvic Bone, Right
4 Acetabulum, Right
5 Acetabulum, Left
6 Upper Femur, Right
   Femoral head
   Greater trochanter
   Lesser trochanter
   Neck of femur
7 Upper Femur, Left
   See 6 Upper Femur, Right
8 Femoral Shaft, Right
   Body of femur
9 Femoral Shaft, Left
   See 8 Femoral Shaft, Right
B Lower Femur, Right
   Lateral condyle of femur
   Lateral epicondyle of femur
   Medial condyle of femur
   Medial epicondyle of femur
C Lower Femur, Left
   See B Lower Femur, Right
D Patella, Right
F Patella, Left
G Tibia, Right
   Lateral condyle of tibia
   Medial condyle of tibia
   Medial malleolus
H Tibia, Left
   See G Tibia, Right
J Fibula, Right
   Body of fibula
   Head of fibula
   Lateral malleolus
K Fibula, Left
   See J Fibula, Right
L Tarsal, Right
   Calcaneus
   Cuboid bone
   Intermediate cuneiform bone
   Lateral cuneiform bone
   Medial cuneiform bone
   Navicular bone
   Talus bone
M Tarsal, Left
   See L Tarsal, Right
N Metatarsal, Right
   Fibular sesamoid
   Tibial sesamoid
P Metatarsal, Left
   See N Metatarsal, Right
Q Toe Phalanx, Right
R Toe Phalanx, Left
S Coccyx
	Ø Open
	3 Percutaneous
	4 Percutaneous Endoscopic
	X External
		Z No Device	**Z** No Qualifier

Non-OR   ØQQ[Ø,1,2,3,4,5,6,7,8,9,B,C,D,F,G,H,J,K,L,M,N,P,Q,R,S]XZZ

NC Noncovered Procedure   LC Limited Coverage   QA Questionable OB Admit   NT New Tech Add-on   ⊞ Combination Member   ♂ Male   ♀ Female

ICD-10-PCS 2022   573

ØQQ–ØQQ

Lower Bones

Ø   **Medical and Surgical**
Q   **Lower Bones**
R   **Replacement**   Definition: Putting in or on biological or synthetic material that physically takes the place and/or function of all or a portion of a body part

Explanation: The body part may have been taken out or replaced, or may be taken out, physically eradicated, or rendered nonfunctional during the REPLACEMENT procedure. A REMOVAL procedure is coded for taking out the device used in a previous replacement procedure.

Body Part Character 4	Approach Character 5	Device Character 6	Qualifier Character 7
Ø **Lumbar Vertebra** Spinous process Transverse process Vertebral arch Vertebral body Vertebral foramen Vertebral lamina Vertebral pedicle **1** **Sacrum** **2** **Pelvic Bone, Right** Iliac crest Ilium Ischium Pubis **3** **Pelvic Bone, Left** *See 2 Pelvic Bone, Right* **4** **Acetabulum, Right** **5** **Acetabulum, Left** **6** **Upper Femur, Right** Femoral head Greater trochanter Lesser trochanter Neck of femur **7** **Upper Femur, Left** *See 6 Upper Femur, Right* **8** **Femoral Shaft, Right** Body of femur **9** **Femoral Shaft, Left** *See 8 Femoral Shaft, Right* **B** **Lower Femur, Right** Lateral condyle of femur Lateral epicondyle of femur Medial condyle of femur Medial epicondyle of femur **C** **Lower Femur, Left** *See B Lower Femur, Right* **D** **Patella, Right** **F** **Patella, Left** **G** **Tibia, Right** Lateral condyle of tibia Medial condyle of tibia Medial malleolus **H** **Tibia, Left** *See G Tibia, Right* **J** **Fibula, Right** Body of fibula Head of fibula Lateral malleolus **K** **Fibula, Left** *See J Fibula, Right* **L** **Tarsal, Right** Calcaneus Cuboid bone Intermediate cuneiform bone Lateral cuneiform bone Medial cuneiform bone Navicular bone Talus bone **M** **Tarsal, Left** *See L Tarsal, Right* **N** **Metatarsal, Right** Fibular sesamoid Tibial sesamoid **P** **Metatarsal, Left** *See N Metatarsal, Right* **Q** **Toe Phalanx, Right** **R** **Toe Phalanx, Left** **S** **Coccyx**	**Ø** Open **3** Percutaneous **4** Percutaneous Endoscopic	**7** Autologous Tissue Substitute **J** Synthetic Substitute **K** Nonautologous Tissue Substitute	**Z** No Qualifier

Non-OR Procedure   DRG Non-OR Procedure   Valid OR Procedure   HAC Associated Procedure   Combination Only   New/Revised GREEN

0   **Medical and Surgical**
Q   **Lower Bones**
S   **Reposition**   Definition: Moving to its normal location, or other suitable location, all or a portion of a body part

Explanation: The body part is moved to a new location from an abnormal location, or from a normal location where it is not functioning correctly. The body part may or may not be cut out or off to be moved to the new location.

Body Part — Character 4	Approach — Character 5	Device — Character 6	Qualifier — Character 7
0 Lumbar Vertebra Spinous process Transverse process Vertebral arch Vertebral body Vertebral foramen Vertebral lamina Vertebral pedicle	**0** Open **4** Percutaneous Endoscopic	**3** Spinal Stabilization Device, Vertebral Body Tether **4** Internal Fixation Device **Z** No Device	**Z** No Qualifier
0 Lumbar Vertebra ⊞ Spinous process Transverse process Vertebral arch Vertebral body Vertebral foramen Vertebral lamina Vertebral pedicle	**3** Percutaneous	**4** Internal Fixation Device **Z** No Device	**Z** No Qualifier
0 Lumbar Vertebra Spinous process Transverse process Vertebral arch Vertebral body Vertebral foramen Vertebral lamina Vertebral pedicle	**X** External	**Z** No Device	**Z** No Qualifier
1 Sacrum ⊞ **4** Acetabulum, Right **5** Acetabulum, Left **S** Coccyx ⊞	**0** Open **3** Percutaneous **4** Percutaneous Endoscopic	**4** Internal Fixation Device **Z** No Device	**Z** No Qualifier
1 Sacrum **4** Acetabulum, Right **5** Acetabulum, Left **S** Coccyx	**X** External	**Z** No Device	**Z** No Qualifier
2 Pelvic Bone, Right Iliac crest Ilium Ischium Pubis **3** Pelvic Bone, Left See 2 Pelvic Bone, Right **D** Patella, Right **F** Patella, Left **L** Tarsal, Right Calcaneus Cuboid bone Intermediate cuneiform bone Lateral cuneiform bone Medial cuneiform bone Navicular bone Talus bone **M** Tarsal, Left See L Tarsal, Right **Q** Toe Phalanx, Right **R** Toe Phalanx, Left	**0** Open **3** Percutaneous **4** Percutaneous Endoscopic	**4** Internal Fixation Device **5** External Fixation Device **Z** No Device	**Z** No Qualifier
2 Pelvic Bone, Right Iliac crest Ilium Ischium Pubis **3** Pelvic Bone, Left See 2 Pelvic Bone, Right **D** Patella, Right **F** Patella, Left **L** Tarsal, Right Calcaneus Cuboid bone Intermediate cuneiform bone Lateral cuneiform bone Medial cuneiform bone Navicular bone Talus bone **M** Tarsal, Left See L Tarsal, Right **Q** Toe Phalanx, Right **R** Toe Phalanx, Left	**X** External	**Z** No Device	**Z** No Qualifier

Non-OR   0QS0XZZ
Non-OR   0QS[4,5][3,4]ZZ
Non-OR   0QS[1,4,5,S]XZZ
Non-OR   0QS[2,3,D,F,L,M,Q,R][3,4]ZZ
Non-OR   0QS[2,3,D,F,L,M,Q,R]XZZ

See Appendix L for Procedure Combinations
⊞   0QS03ZZ
⊞   0QS[1,S]3ZZ

0QS Continued on next page

NC Noncovered Procedure   LC Limited Coverage   QA Questionable OB Admit   NT New Tech Add-on   ⊞ Combination Member   ♂ Male   ♀ Female

ICD-10-PCS 2022   575   0QS–0QS

Lower Bones

Ø **Medical and Surgical**
Q **Lower Bones**
S **Reposition**

ØQS Continued

Definition: Moving to its normal location, or other suitable location, all or a portion of a body part

Explanation: The body part is moved to a new location from an abnormal location, or from a normal location where it is not functioning correctly. The body part may or may not be cut out or off to be moved to the new location.

Body Part Character 4	Approach Character 5	Device Character 6	Qualifier Character 7
6 Upper Femur, Right Femoral head Greater trochanter Lesser trochanter Neck of femur **7 Upper Femur, Left** *See 6 Upper Femur, Right* **8 Femoral Shaft, Right** Body of femur **9 Femoral Shaft, Left** *See 8 Femoral Shaft, Right* **B Lower Femur, Right** Lateral condyle of femur Lateral epicondyle of femur Medial condyle of femur Medial epicondyle of femur **C Lower Femur, Left** *See B Lower Femur, Right* **G Tibia, Right** Lateral condyle of tibia Medial condyle of tibia Medial malleolus **H Tibia, Left** *See G Tibia, Right* **J Fibula, Right** Body of fibula Head of fibula Lateral malleolus **K Fibula, Left** *See J Fibula, Right*	**Ø Open** **3 Percutaneous** **4 Percutaneous Endoscopic**	**4 Internal Fixation Device** **5 External Fixation Device** **6 Internal Fixation Device, Intramedullary** **B External Fixation Device, Monoplanar** **C External Fixation Device, Ring** **D External Fixation Device, Hybrid** **Z No Device**	**Z No Qualifier**
6 Upper Femur, Right Femoral head Greater trochanter Lesser trochanter Neck of femur **7 Upper Femur, Left** *See 6 Upper Femur, Right* **8 Femoral Shaft, Right** Body of femur **9 Femoral Shaft, Left** *See 8 Femoral Shaft, Right* **B Lower Femur, Right** Lateral condyle of femur Lateral epicondyle of femur Medial condyle of femur Medial epicondyle of femur **C Lower Femur, Left** *See B Lower Femur, Right* **G Tibia, Right** Lateral condyle of tibia Medial condyle of tibia Medial malleolus **H Tibia, Left** *See G Tibia, Right* **J Fibula, Right** Body of fibula Head of fibula Lateral malleolus **K Fibula, Left** *See J Fibula, Right*	**X External**	**Z No Device**	**Z No Qualifier**
N Metatarsal, Right Fibular sesamoid Tibial sesamoid **P Metatarsal, Left** *See N Metatarsal, Right*	**Ø Open** **3 Percutaneous** **4 Percutaneous Endoscopic**	**4 Internal Fixation Device** **5 External Fixation Device** **Z No Device**	**2 Sesamoid Bone(s) 1st Toe** **Z No Qualifier**
N Metatarsal, Right Fibular sesamoid Tibial sesamoid **P Metatarsal, Left** *See N Metatarsal, Right*	**X External**	**Z No Device**	**2 Sesamoid Bone(s) 1st Toe** **Z No Qualifier**

Non-OR ØQS[6,7,8,9,B,C,G,H,J,K][3,4]ZZ
Non-OR ØQS[6,7,8,9,B,C,G,H,J,K]XZZ
Non-OR ØQS[N,P][3,4]Z[2,Z]
Non-OR ØQS[N,P]XZ[2,Z]

Non-OR Procedure   DRG Non-OR Procedure   Valid OR Procedure   HAC Associated Procedure   Combination Only   New/Revised GREEN

Ø Medical and Surgical
Q Lower Bones
T Resection   Definition: Cutting out or off, without replacement, all of a body part
               Explanation: None

Body Part – Character 4	Approach – Character 5	Device – Character 6	Qualifier – Character 7
2 Pelvic Bone, Right Iliac crest Ilium Ischium Pubis **3 Pelvic Bone, Left** *See 2 Pelvic Bone, Right* **4 Acetabulum, Right** **5 Acetabulum, Left** **6 Upper Femur, Right** Femoral head Greater trochanter Lesser trochanter Neck of femur **7 Upper Femur, Left** *See 6 Upper Femur, Right* **8 Femoral Shaft, Right** Body of femur **9 Femoral Shaft, Left** *See 8 Femoral Shaft, Right* **B Lower Femur, Right** Lateral condyle of femur Lateral epicondyle of femur Medial condyle of femur Medial epicondyle of femur **C Lower Femur, Left** *See B Lower Femur, Right* **D Patella, Right**	**F Patella, Left** **G Tibia, Right** Lateral condyle of tibia Medial condyle of tibia Medial malleolus **H Tibia, Left** *See G Tibia, Right* **J Fibula, Right** Body of fibula Head of fibula Lateral malleolus **K Fibula, Left** *See J Fibula, Right* **L Tarsal, Right** Calcaneus Cuboid bone Intermediate cuneiform bone Lateral cuneiform bone Medial cuneiform bone Navicular bone Talus bone **M Tarsal, Left** *See L Tarsal, Right* **N Metatarsal, Right** Fibular sesamoid Tibial sesamoid **P Metatarsal, Left** *See N Metatarsal, Right* **Q Toe Phalanx, Right** **R Toe Phalanx, Left** **S Coccyx**	**Ø Open**	**Z No Device**	**Z No Qualifier**

Ø Medical and Surgical
Q Lower Bones
U Supplement   Definition: Putting in or on biological or synthetic material that physically reinforces and/or augments the function of a portion of a body part
               Explanation: The biological material is non-living, or is living and from the same individual. The body part may have been previously replaced, and the SUPPLEMENT procedure is performed to physically reinforce and/or augment the function of the replaced body part.

Body Part – Character 4	Approach – Character 5	Device – Character 6	Qualifier – Character 7
Ø Lumbar Vertebra ⊞ Spinous process Transverse process Vertebral arch Vertebral body Vertebral foramen Vertebral lamina Vertebral pedicle **1 Sacrum** ⊞ **2 Pelvic Bone, Right** Iliac crest Ilium Ischium Pubis **3 Pelvic Bone, Left** *See 2 Pelvic Bone, Right* **4 Acetabulum, Right** **5 Acetabulum, Left** **6 Upper Femur, Right** Femoral head Greater trochanter Lesser trochanter Neck of femur **7 Upper Femur, Left** *See 6 Upper Femur, Right* **8 Femoral Shaft, Right** Body of femur **9 Femoral Shaft, Left** *See 8 Femoral Shaft, Right* **B Lower Femur, Right** Lateral condyle of femur Lateral epicondyle of femur Medial condyle of femur Medial epicondyle of femur	**C Lower Femur, Left** *See B Lower Femur, Right* **D Patella, Right** **F Patella, Left** **G Tibia, Right** Lateral condyle of tibia Medial condyle of tibia Medial malleolus **H Tibia, Left** *See G Tibia, Right* **J Fibula, Right** Body of fibula Head of fibula Lateral malleolus **K Fibula, Left** *See J Fibula, Right* **L Tarsal, Right** Calcaneus Cuboid bone Intermediate cuneiform bone Lateral cuneiform bone Medial cuneiform bone Navicular bone Talus bone **M Tarsal, Left** *See L Tarsal, Right* **N Metatarsal, Right** Fibular sesamoid Tibial sesamoid **P Metatarsal, Left** *See N Metatarsal, Right* **Q Toe Phalanx, Right** **R Toe Phalanx, Left** **S Coccyx** ⊞	**Ø Open** **3 Percutaneous** **4 Percutaneous Endoscopic**	**7 Autologous Tissue Substitute** **J Synthetic Substitute** **K Nonautologous Tissue Substitute**	**Z No Qualifier**

See Appendix L for Procedure Combinations
⊞   ØQU[Ø,1,S]3JZ

NC Noncovered Procedure   **LC** Limited Coverage   **QA** Questionable OB Admit   **NT** New Tech Add-on   ⊞ Combination Member   ♂ Male   ♀ Female

ICD-10-PCS 2022   577

ØQT–ØQU

Lower Bones

ØQW–ØQW

Ø   Medical and Surgical
Q   Lower Bones
W   Revision   Definition: Correcting, to the extent possible, a portion of a malfunctioning device or the position of a displaced device

Explanation: Revision can include correcting a malfunctioning or displaced device by taking out or putting in components of the device such as a screw or pin

Body Part Character 4	Approach Character 5	Device Character 6	Qualifier Character 7
Ø **Lumbar Vertebra** Spinous process Transverse process Vertebral arch Vertebral body Vertebral foramen Vertebral lamina Vertebral pedicle **1** **Sacrum** **4** **Acetabulum, Right** **5** **Acetabulum, Left** **S** **Coccyx**	**Ø** Open **3** Percutaneous **4** Percutaneous Endoscopic **X** External	**4** Internal Fixation Device **7** Autologous Tissue Substitute **J** Synthetic Substitute **K** Nonautologous Tissue Substitute	**Z** No Qualifier
2 **Pelvic Bone, Right** Iliac crest Ilium Ischium Pubis **3** **Pelvic Bone, Left** *See 2 Pelvic Bone, Right* **6** **Upper Femur, Right** Femoral head Greater trochanter Lesser trochanter Neck of femur **7** **Upper Femur, Left** *See 6 Upper Femur, Right* **8** **Femoral Shaft, Right** Body of femur **9** **Femoral Shaft, Left** *See 8 Femoral Shaft, Right* **B** **Lower Femur, Right** Lateral condyle of femur Lateral epicondyle of femur Medial condyle of femur Medial epicondyle of femur **C** **Lower Femur, Left** *See B Lower Femur, Right* **D** **Patella, Right** **F** **Patella, Left** **G** **Tibia, Right** Lateral condyle of tibia Medial condyle of tibia Medial malleolus **H** **Tibia, Left** *See G Tibia, Right* **J** **Fibula, Right** Body of fibula Head of fibula Lateral malleolus **K** **Fibula, Left** *See J Fibula, Right* **L** **Tarsal, Right** Calcaneus Cuboid bone Intermediate cuneiform bone Lateral cuneiform bone Medial cuneiform bone Navicular bone Talus bone **M** **Tarsal, Left** *See L Tarsal, Right* **N** **Metatarsal, Right** Fibular sesamoid Tibial sesamoid **P** **Metatarsal, Left** *See N Metatarsal, Right* **Q** **Toe Phalanx, Right** **R** **Toe Phalanx, Left**	**Ø** Open **3** Percutaneous **4** Percutaneous Endoscopic **X** External	**4** Internal Fixation Device **5** External Fixation Device **7** Autologous Tissue Substitute **J** Synthetic Substitute **K** Nonautologous Tissue Substitute	**Z** No Qualifier
Y **Lower Bone**	**Ø** Open **3** Percutaneous **4** Percutaneous Endoscopic **X** External	**Ø** Drainage Device **M** Bone Growth Stimulator	**Z** No Qualifier

Non-OR ØQW[Ø,1,4,5,S]X[4,7,J,K]Z	**Non-OR** ØQWYX[Ø,M]Z
Non-OR ØQW[2,3,6,7,8,9,B,C,D,F,G,H,J,K,L,M,N,P,Q,R]X[4,5,7,J,K]Z	

Non-OR Procedure   DRG Non-OR Procedure   Valid OR Procedure   HAC Associated Procedure   Combination Only   New/Revised GREEN

Upper Joints ØR2–ØRW

Character Meanings*

This Character Meaning table is provided as a guide to assist the user in the identification of character members that may be found in this section of code tables. It **SHOULD NOT** be used to build a PCS code.

Operation–Character 3	Body Part–Character 4	Approach–Character 5	Device–Character 6	Qualifier–Character 7
2 Change	Ø Occipital-cervical Joint	Ø Open	Ø Drainage Device OR Synthetic Substitute, Reverse Ball and Socket	Ø Anterior Approach, Anterior Column
5 Destruction	1 Cervical Vertebral Joint	3 Percutaneous	3 Infusion Device OR Internal Fixation Device, Sustained Compression	1 Posterior Approach, Posterior Column
9 Drainage	2 Cervical Vertebral Joint, 2 or more	4 Percutaneous Endoscopic	4 Internal Fixation Device	6 Humeral Surface
B Excision	3 Cervical Vertebral Disc	X External	5 External Fixation Device	7 Glenoid Surface
C Extirpation	4 Cervicothoracic Vertebral Joint		7 Autologous Tissue Substitute	J Posterior Approach, Anterior Column
G Fusion	5 Cervicothoracic Vertebral Disc		8 Spacer	X Diagnostic
H Insertion	6 Thoracic Vertebral Joint		A Interbody Fusion Device	Z No Qualifier
J Inspection	7 Thoracic Vertebral Joint, 2 to 7		B Spinal Stabilization Device, Interspinous Process	
N Release	8 Thoracic Vertebral Joint, 8 or more		C Spinal Stabilization Device, Pedicle-Based	
P Removal	9 Thoracic Vertebral Disc		D Spinal Stabilization Device, Facet Replacement	
Q Repair	A Thoracolumbar Vertebral Joint		J Synthetic Substitute	
R Replacement	B Thoracolumbar Vertebral Disc		K Nonautologous Tissue Substitute	
S Reposition	C Temporomandibular Joint, Right		Y Other Device	
T Resection	D Temporomandibular Joint, Left		Z No Device	
U Supplement	E Sternoclavicular Joint, Right			
W Revision	F Sternoclavicular Joint, Left			
	G Acromioclavicular Joint, Right			
	H Acromioclavicular Joint, Left			
	J Shoulder Joint, Right			
	K Shoulder Joint, Left			
	L Elbow Joint, Right			
	M Elbow Joint, Left			
	N Wrist Joint, Right			
	P Wrist Joint, Left			
	Q Carpal Joint, Right			
	R Carpal Joint, Left			
	S Carpometacarpal Joint, Right			
	T Carpometacarpal Joint, Left			
	U Metacarpophalangeal Joint, Right			
	V Metacarpophalangeal Joint, Left			
	W Finger Phalangeal Joint, Right			
	X Finger Phalangeal Joint, Left			
	Y Upper Joint			

* Includes synovial membrane.

AHA Coding Clinic for table ØRB

2019, 3Q, 26	Acromioclavicular joint reconstruction using allograft

AHA Coding Clinic for table ØRG

2021, 1Q, 18	Placement of interspinous distraction device (spacer) for decompression
2021, 1Q, 53	Official guidelines for coding and reporting for interbody fusion device B3.10c
2020, 4Q, 56-58	Intramedullary sustained compression joint fusion
2020, 2Q, 27	Spinal Fusion with NuVasive® VersaTie®
2020, 1Q, 33	Spinal fusion without use of bone graft
2019, 3Q, 28	Use of VERTE-STACK™ implant with fusion
2019, 3Q, 35	Fusion procedures of the spine (guideline B3.10c)
2019, 2Q, 19	Cervical spinal fusion, decompression and placement of interfacet stabilization device
2019, 1Q, 30	Spinal fusion performed at same level as decompressive laminectomy
2018, 4Q, 43	Joint fusion device value
2018, 1Q, 22	Spinal fusion procedures without bone graft
2017, 4Q, 62	Added and revised device values - Nerve substitutes
2017, 4Q, 76	Radiolucent porous interbody fusion device
2017, 2Q, 23	Decompression of spinal cord and placement of instrumentation
2014, 3Q, 30	Spinal fusion and fixation instrumentation
2014, 2Q, 7	Anterior cervical thoracic fusion with total discectomy
2013, 1Q, 21-23	Spinal fusion of thoracic and lumbar vertebrae
2013, 1Q, 29	Cervical and thoracic spinal fusion

AHA Coding Clinic for table ØRH

2021, 1Q, 18	Placement of interspinous distraction device (spacer) for decompression
2019, 2Q, 40	Decompression of spinal cord and placement of instrumentation
2018, 3Q, 26	Anterior vertebral tethering using Dynesys Tethering System
2017, 2Q, 23	Decompression of spinal cord and placement of instrumentation
2016, 3Q, 32	Rotator cuff repair, tenodesis, decompression, acromioplasty and coracoplasty

AHA Coding Clinic for table ØRN

2019, 1Q, 30	Spinal fusion performed at same level as decompressive laminectomy
2016, 3Q, 32	Rotator cuff repair, tenodesis, decompression, acromioplasty and coracoplasty
2015, 2Q, 22	Arthroscopic subacromial decompression
2015, 2Q, 23	Arthroscopic release of shoulder joint

AHA Coding Clinic for table ØRP

2017, 4Q, 107	Total ankle replacement versus revision

AHA Coding Clinic for table ØRQ

2016, 1Q, 30	Thermal capsulorrhapy of shoulder

AHA Coding Clinic for table ØRR

2018, 4Q, 92	Radial head arthroplasty
2017, 4Q, 107	Total ankle replacement versus revision
2015, 3Q, 14	Endoprosthetic replacement of humerus and tendon reattachment
2015, 1Q, 27	Reverse total shoulder arthroplasty

AHA Coding Clinic for table ØRS

2019, 3Q, 26	Acromioclavicular joint reconstruction using allograft
2018, 3Q, 26	Anterior vertebral tethering using Dynesys Tethering System
2015, 2Q, 35	Application of tongs to reduce and stabilize cervical fracture
2014, 4Q, 32	Open reduction internal fixation of fracture with debridement
2014, 3Q, 33	Radial fracture treatment with open reduction internal fixation, and release of carpal ligament
2013, 2Q, 39	Application of cervical tongs for reduction of cervical fracture

AHA Coding Clinic for table ØRT

2019, 3Q, 26	Acromioclavicular joint reconstruction using allograft
2014, 2Q, 7	Anterior cervical thoracic fusion with total discectomy

AHA Coding Clinic for table ØRU

2019, 3Q, 26	Acromioclavicular joint reconstruction using allograft
2015, 3Q, 26	Thumb arthroplasty with resection of trapezium

AHA Coding Clinic for table ØRW

2017, 4Q, 107	Total ankle replacement versus revision

Upper Joints

Temporomandibular **C, D**

Acromioclavicular **G, H**

Sternoclavicular **E, F**

Shoulder **J, K**

Elbow **L, M**

Wrist: Radiocarpal **N, P**

Wrist: Midcarpal **N, P**

Carpometacarpal **S, T**

Metacarpophalangeal **U, V**

Hand Joints

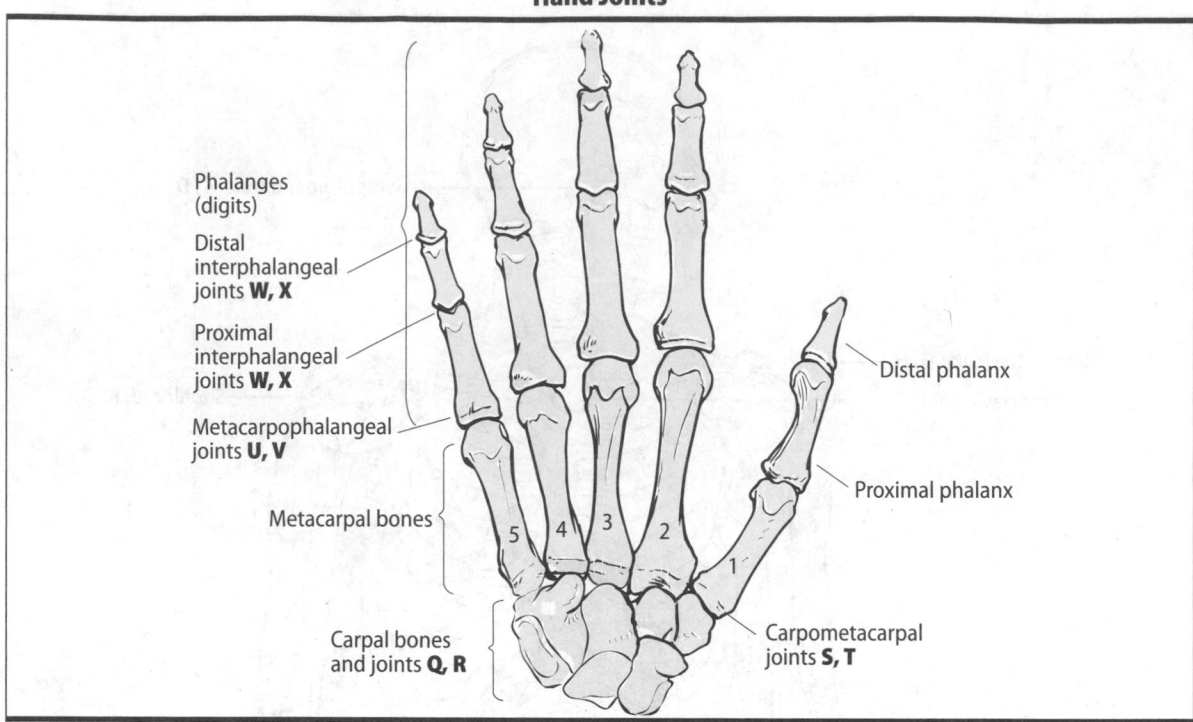

Phalanges (digits)

Distal interphalangeal joints **W, X**

Proximal interphalangeal joints **W, X**

Metacarpophalangeal joints **U, V**

Metacarpal bones

Carpal bones and joints **Q, R**

Distal phalanx

Proximal phalanx

Carpometacarpal joints **S, T**

Shoulder Joints

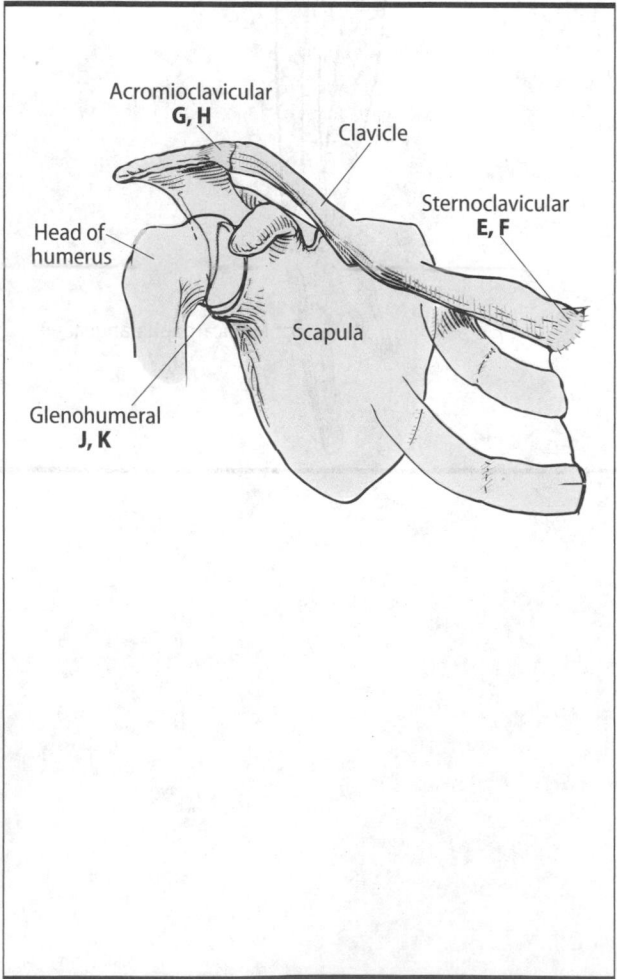

Acromioclavicular **G, H**

Clavicle

Sternoclavicular **E, F**

Head of humerus

Scapula

Glenohumeral **J, K**

Upper Vertebral Joints

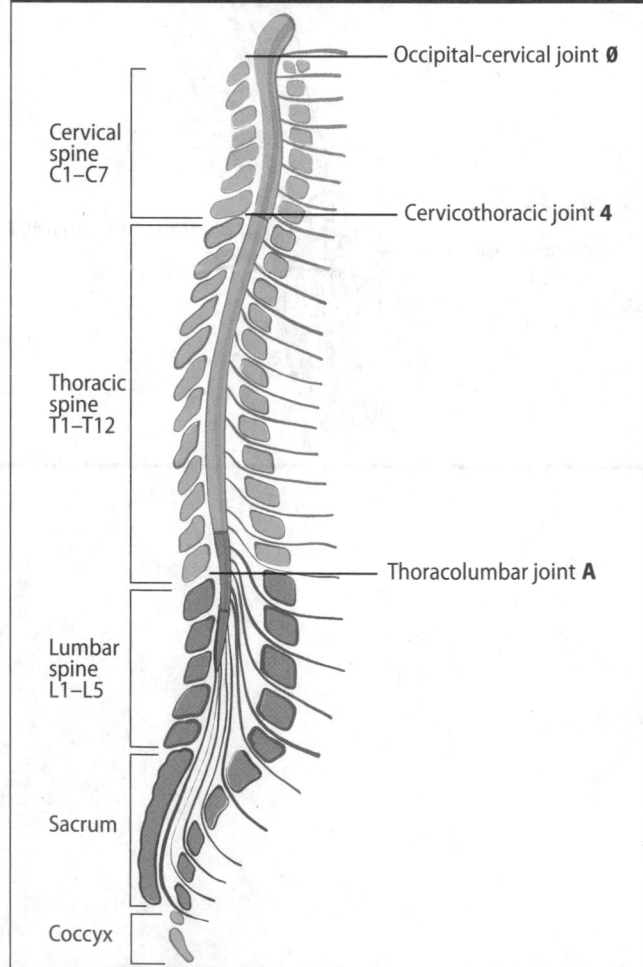

Occipital-cervical joint **Ø**

Cervical spine C1–C7

Cervicothoracic joint **4**

Thoracic spine T1–T12

Thoracolumbar joint **A**

Lumbar spine L1–L5

Sacrum

Coccyx

Ø   Medical and Surgical
R   Upper Joints
2   Change   Definition: Taking out or off a device from a body part and putting back an identical or similar device in or on the same body part without cutting or puncturing the skin or a mucous membrane

                Explanation: All CHANGE procedures are coded using the approach EXTERNAL

Body Part Character 4	Approach Character 5	Device Character 6	Qualifier Character 7
Y Upper Joint	X External	Ø Drainage Device Y Other Device	Z No Qualifier

Non-OR   All body part, approach, device, and qualifier values

---

Ø   Medical and Surgical
R   Upper Joints
5   Destruction   Definition: Physical eradication of all or a portion of a body part by the direct use of energy, force, or a destructive agent

                       Explanation: None of the body part is physically taken out

Body Part Character 4	Approach Character 5	Device Character 6	Qualifier Character 7

Ø   Occipital-cervical Joint
1   Cervical Vertebral Joint
    Atlantoaxial joint
    Cervical facet joint
3   Cervical Vertebral Disc
4   Cervicothoracic Vertebral Joint
    Cervicothoracic facet joint
5   Cervicothoracic Vertebral Disc
6   Thoracic Vertebral Joint
    Costotransverse joint
    Costovertebral joint
    Thoracic facet joint
9   Thoracic Vertebral Disc
A   Thoracolumbar Vertebral Joint
    Thoracolumbar facet joint
B   Thoracolumbar Vertebral Disc
C   Temporomandibular Joint, Right
D   Temporomandibular Joint, Left
E   Sternoclavicular Joint, Right
F   Sternoclavicular Joint, Left
G   Acromioclavicular Joint, Right
H   Acromioclavicular Joint, Left
J   Shoulder Joint, Right
    Glenohumeral joint
    Glenoid ligament (labrum)
K   Shoulder Joint, Left
    See J Shoulder Joint, Right
L   Elbow Joint, Right
    Distal humerus, involving joint
    Humeroradial joint
    Humeroulnar joint
    Proximal radioulnar joint
M   Elbow Joint, Left
    See L Elbow Joint, Right
N   Wrist Joint, Right
    Distal radioulnar joint
    Radiocarpal joint
P   Wrist Joint, Left
    See N Wrist Joint, Right
Q   Carpal Joint, Right
    Intercarpal joint
    Midcarpal joint
R   Carpal Joint, Left
    See Q Carpal Joint, Right
S   Carpometacarpal Joint, Right
T   Carpometacarpal Joint, Left
U   Metacarpophalangeal Joint, Right
V   Metacarpophalangeal Joint, Left
W   Finger Phalangeal Joint, Right
    Interphalangeal (IP) joint
X   Finger Phalangeal Joint, Left
    See W Finger Phalangeal Joint, Right
	Ø Open
	3 Percutaneous
	4 Percutaneous Endoscopic
		Z No Device	Z No Qualifier

Non-OR   ØR5[3,5,9,B][3,4]ZZ

NC Noncovered Procedure   **LC** Limited Coverage   **QA** Questionable OB Admit   **NT** New Tech Add-on   ⊞ Combination Member   ♂ Male   ♀ Female

ICD-10-PCS 2022   **583**

ØR2–ØR5

Ø　**Medical and Surgical**
R　**Upper Joints**
9　**Drainage**　　Definition: Taking or letting out fluids and/or gases from a body part

Explanation: The qualifier DIAGNOSTIC is used to identify drainage procedures that are biopsies

Body Part Character 4		Approach Character 5	Device Character 6	Qualifier Character 7
Ø Occipital-cervical Joint 1 Cervical Vertebral Joint 　Atlantoaxial joint 　Cervical facet joint 3 Cervical Vertebral Disc 4 Cervicothoracic Vertebral 　Joint 　Cervicothoracic facet joint 5 Cervicothoracic Vertebral 　Disc 6 Thoracic Vertebral Joint 　Costotransverse joint 　Costovertebral joint 　Thoracic facet joint 9 Thoracic Vertebral Disc A Thoracolumbar Vertebral 　Joint 　Thoracolumbar facet joint B Thoracolumbar Vertebral 　Disc C Temporomandibular Joint, 　Right D Temporomandibular Joint, 　Left E Sternoclavicular Joint, Right F Sternoclavicular Joint, Left G Acromioclavicular Joint, 　Right H Acromioclavicular Joint, Left J Shoulder Joint, Right 　Glenohumeral joint 　Glenoid ligament (labrum) K Shoulder Joint, Left 　See J Shoulder Joint, Right	L Elbow Joint, Right 　Distal humerus, involving 　　joint 　Humeroradial joint 　Humeroulnar joint 　Proximal radioulnar joint M Elbow Joint, Left 　See L Elbow Joint, Right N Wrist Joint, Right 　Distal radioulnar joint 　Radiocarpal joint P Wrist Joint, Left 　See N Wrist Joint, Right Q Carpal Joint, Right 　Intercarpal joint 　Midcarpal joint R Carpal Joint, Left 　See Q Carpal Joint, Right S Carpometacarpal Joint, 　Right T Carpometacarpal Joint, Left U Metacarpophalangeal Joint, 　Right V Metacarpophalangeal Joint, 　Left W Finger Phalangeal Joint, 　Right 　Interphalangeal (IP) joint X Finger Phalangeal Joint, Left 　See W Finger Phalangeal Joint, 　　Right	Ø Open 3 Percutaneous 4 Percutaneous Endoscopic	Ø Drainage Device	Z No Qualifier
Ø Occipital-cervical Joint 1 Cervical Vertebral Joint 　Atlantoaxial joint 　Cervical facet joint 3 Cervical Vertebral Disc 4 Cervicothoracic Vertebral 　Joint 　Cervicothoracic facet joint 5 Cervicothoracic Vertebral 　Disc 6 Thoracic Vertebral Joint 　Costotransverse joint 　Costovertebral joint 　Thoracic facet joint 9 Thoracic Vertebral Disc A Thoracolumbar Vertebral 　Joint 　Thoracolumbar facet joint B Thoracolumbar Vertebral 　Disc C Temporomandibular Joint, 　Right D Temporomandibular Joint, 　Left E Sternoclavicular Joint, Right F Sternoclavicular Joint, Left G Acromioclavicular Joint, 　Right H Acromioclavicular Joint, Left J Shoulder Joint, Right 　Glenohumeral joint 　Glenoid ligament (labrum) K Shoulder Joint, Left 　See J Shoulder Joint, Right	L Elbow Joint, Right 　Distal humerus, involving 　　joint 　Humeroradial joint 　Humeroulnar joint 　Proximal radioulnar joint M Elbow Joint, Left 　See L Elbow Joint, Right N Wrist Joint, Right 　Distal radioulnar joint 　Radiocarpal joint P Wrist Joint, Left 　See N Wrist Joint, Right Q Carpal Joint, Right 　Intercarpal joint 　Midcarpal joint R Carpal Joint, Left 　See Q Carpal Joint, Right S Carpometacarpal Joint, 　Right T Carpometacarpal Joint, Left U Metacarpophalangeal Joint, 　Right V Metacarpophalangeal Joint, 　Left W Finger Phalangeal Joint, 　Right 　Interphalangeal (IP) joint X Finger Phalangeal Joint, Left 　See W Finger Phalangeal Joint, 　　Right	Ø Open 3 Percutaneous 4 Percutaneous Endoscopic	Z No Device	X Diagnostic Z No Qualifier

Non-OR　ØR9[Ø,1,3,4,5,6,9,A,B,E,F,G,H,J,K,L,M,N,P,Q,R,S,T,U,V,W,X][3,4]ØZ
Non-OR　ØR9[C,D]3ØZ
Non-OR　ØR9[Ø,1,3,4,5,6,9,A,B,E,F,G,H,J,K,L,M,N,P,Q,R,S,T,U,V,W,X][Ø,3,4]ZX
Non-OR　ØR9[Ø,1,3,4,5,6,9,A,B,E,F,G,H,J,K,L,M,N,P,Q,R,S,T,U,V,W,X][3,4]ZZ
Non-OR　ØR9[C,D]3ZZ

Non-OR Procedure　　　DRG Non-OR Procedure　　　Valid OR Procedure　　　HAC Associated Procedure　　　Combination Only　　　New/Revised GREEN

Ø   **Medical and Surgical**
R   **Upper Joints**
B   **Excision**   Definition: Cutting out or off, without replacement, a portion of a body part
                        Explanation: The qualifier DIAGNOSTIC is used to identify excision procedures that are biopsies

Body Part Character 4	Approach Character 5	Device Character 6	Qualifier Character 7
Ø Occipital-cervical Joint	**Ø** Open	**Z** No Device	**X** Diagnostic
1 Cervical Vertebral Joint	**3** Percutaneous		**Z** No Qualifier
Atlantoaxial joint	**4** Percutaneous Endoscopic		
Cervical facet joint			
3 Cervical Vertebral Disc			
4 Cervicothoracic Vertebral Joint			
Cervicothoracic facet joint			
5 Cervicothoracic Vertebral Disc			
6 Thoracic Vertebral Joint			
Costotransverse joint			
Costovertebral joint			
Thoracic facet joint			
9 Thoracic Vertebral Disc			
A Thoracolumbar Vertebral Joint			
Thoracolumbar facet joint			
B Thoracolumbar Vertebral Disc			
C Temporomandibular Joint, Right			
D Temporomandibular Joint, Left			
E Sternoclavicular Joint, Right			
F Sternoclavicular Joint, Left			
G Acromioclavicular Joint, Right			
H Acromioclavicular Joint, Left			
J Shoulder Joint, Right			
Glenohumeral joint			
Glenoid ligament (labrum)			
K Shoulder Joint, Left			
See J Shoulder Joint, Right			
L Elbow Joint, Right			
Distal humerus, involving joint			
Humeroradial joint			
Humeroulnar joint			
Proximal radioulnar joint			
M Elbow Joint, Left			
See L Elbow Joint, Right			
N Wrist Joint, Right			
Distal radioulnar joint			
Radiocarpal joint			
P Wrist Joint, Left			
See N Wrist Joint, Right			
Q Carpal Joint, Right			
Intercarpal joint			
Midcarpal joint			
R Carpal Joint, Left			
See Q Carpal Joint, Right			
S Carpometacarpal Joint, Right			
T Carpometacarpal Joint, Left			
U Metacarpophalangeal Joint, Right			
V Metacarpophalangeal Joint, Left			
W Finger Phalangeal Joint, Right			
Interphalangeal (IP) joint			
X Finger Phalangeal Joint, Left			
See W Finger Phalangeal Joint, Right			

Non-OR   ØRB[Ø,1,3,4,5,6,9,A,B,E,F,G,H,J,K,L,M,N,P,Q,R,S,T,U,V,W,X][Ø,3,4]ZX

Upper Joints

Ø **Medical and Surgical**
R **Upper Joints**
C **Extirpation**   Definition: Taking or cutting out solid matter from a body part

Explanation: The solid matter may be an abnormal byproduct of a biological function or a foreign body; it may be imbedded in a body part or in the lumen of a tubular body part. The solid matter may or may not have been previously broken into pieces.

Body Part Character 4	Approach Character 5	Device Character 6	Qualifier Character 7
Ø **Occipital-cervical Joint**	**Ø** **Open**	**Z** **No Device**	**Z** **No Qualifier**
1 **Cervical Vertebral Joint**	**3** **Percutaneous**		
Atlantoaxial joint	**4** **Percutaneous Endoscopic**		
Cervical facet joint			
3 **Cervical Vertebral Disc**			
4 **Cervicothoracic Vertebral Joint**			
Cervicothoracic facet joint			
5 **Cervicothoracic Vertebral Disc**			
6 **Thoracic Vertebral Joint**			
Costotransverse joint			
Costovertebral joint			
Thoracic facet joint			
9 **Thoracic Vertebral Disc**			
A **Thoracolumbar Vertebral Joint**			
Thoracolumbar facet joint			
B **Thoracolumbar Vertebral Disc**			
C **Temporomandibular Joint, Right**			
D **Temporomandibular Joint, Left**			
E **Sternoclavicular Joint, Right**			
F **Sternoclavicular Joint, Left**			
G **Acromioclavicular Joint, Right**			
H **Acromioclavicular Joint, Left**			
J **Shoulder Joint, Right**			
Glenohumeral joint			
Glenoid ligament (labrum)			
K **Shoulder Joint, Left**			
See J Shoulder Joint, Right			
L **Elbow Joint, Right**			
Distal humerus, involving joint			
Humeroradial joint			
Humeroulnar joint			
Proximal radioulnar joint			
M **Elbow Joint, Left**			
See L Elbow Joint, Right			
N **Wrist Joint, Right**			
Distal radioulnar joint			
Radiocarpal joint			
P **Wrist Joint, Left**			
See N Wrist Joint, Right			
Q **Carpal Joint, Right**			
Intercarpal joint			
Midcarpal joint			
R **Carpal Joint, Left**			
See Q Carpal Joint, Right			
S **Carpometacarpal Joint, Right**			
T **Carpometacarpal Joint, Left**			
U **Metacarpophalangeal Joint, Right**			
V **Metacarpophalangeal Joint, Left**			
W **Finger Phalangeal Joint, Right**			
Interphalangeal (IP) joint			
X **Finger Phalangeal Joint, Left**			
See W Finger Phalangeal Joint, Right			

Ø   **Medical and Surgical**
R   **Upper Joints**
G   **Fusion**   Definition: Joining together portions of an articular body part rendering the articular body part immobile
                   Explanation: The body part is joined together by fixation device, bone graft, or other means

Body Part Character 4		Approach Character 5	Device Character 6	Qualifier Character 7

Ø **Occipital-cervical Joint**
1 **Cervical Vertebral Joint**
    Atlantoaxial joint
    Cervical facet joint
2 **Cervical Vertebral Joints, 2 or more**
    Cervical facet joint
4 **Cervicothoracic Vertebral Joint**
    Cervicothoracic facet joint
6 **Thoracic Vertebral Joint**
    Costotransverse joint
    Costovertebral joint
    Thoracic facet joint
7 **Thoracic Vertebral Joints, 2 to 7** ⊞
8 **Thoracic Vertebral Joints, 8 or more**
A **Thoracolumbar Vertebral Joint**
    Thoracolumbar facet joint
		Ø Open
		3 Percutaneous
		4 Percutaneous Endoscopic
			7 Autologous Tissue
			    Substitute
			J Synthetic Substitute
			K Nonautologous Tissue
			    Substitute
				Ø Anterior Approach, Anterior
				    Column
				1 Posterior Approach,
				    Posterior Column
				J Posterior Approach,
				    Anterior Column

Ø **Occipital-cervical Joint**
1 **Cervical Vertebral Joint**
    Atlantoaxial joint
    Cervical facet joint
2 **Cervical Vertebral Joints, 2 or more**
    Cervical facet joint
4 **Cervicothoracic Vertebral Joint**
    Cervicothoracic facet joint
6 **Thoracic Vertebral Joint**
    Costotransverse joint
    Costovertebral joint
    Thoracic facet joint
7 **Thoracic Vertebral Joints, 2 to 7** ⊞
8 **Thoracic Vertebral Joints, 8 or more**
A **Thoracolumbar Vertebral Joint**
    Thoracolumbar facet joint
		Ø Open
		3 Percutaneous
		4 Percutaneous Endoscopic
			A Interbody Fusion Device	Ø Anterior Approach, Anterior
				    Column
				J Posterior Approach,
				    Anterior Column

C **Temporomandibular Joint, Right**
D **Temporomandibular Joint, Left**
E **Sternoclavicular Joint, Right**
F **Sternoclavicular Joint, Left**
G **Acromioclavicular Joint, Right**
H **Acromioclavicular Joint, Left**
J **Shoulder Joint, Right**
    Glenohumeral joint
    Glenoid ligament (labrum)
K **Shoulder Joint, Left**
    See J Shoulder Joint, Right
		Ø Open
		3 Percutaneous
		4 Percutaneous Endoscopic
			4 Internal Fixation Device
			7 Autologous Tissue
			    Substitute
			J Synthetic Substitute
			K Nonautologous Tissue
			    Substitute
				Z No Qualifier

L **Elbow Joint, Right**
    Distal humerus, involving
       joint
    Humeroradial joint
    Humeroulnar joint
    Proximal radioulnar joint
M **Elbow Joint, Left**
    See L Elbow Joint, Right
N **Wrist Joint, Right**
    Distal radioulnar joint
    Radiocarpal joint
P **Wrist Joint, Left**
    See N Wrist Joint, Right
Q **Carpal Joint, Right**
    Intercarpal joint
    Midcarpal joint
	R **Carpal Joint, Left**
	    See Q Carpal Joint, Right
	S **Carpometacarpal Joint,**
	    Right
	T **Carpometacarpal Joint,**
	    Left
	U **Metacarpophalangeal**
	    Joint, Right
	V **Metacarpophalangeal**
	    Joint, Left
	W **Finger Phalangeal Joint,**
	    Right
	    Interphalangeal (IP) joint
	X **Finger Phalangeal Joint,**
	    Left
	    See W Finger Phalangeal
	    Joint, Right
		Ø Open
		3 Percutaneous
		4 Percutaneous Endoscopic
			3 Internal Fixation Device,
			    Sustained Compression
			4 Internal Fixation Device
			5 External Fixation Device
			7 Autologous Tissue
			    Substitute
			J Synthetic Substitute
			K Nonautologous Tissue
			    Substitute
				Z No Qualifier

HAC   ØRG[Ø,1,2,4,6,7,8,A][Ø,3,4][7,J,K][Ø,1,J] when reported with SDx K68.11 or
       T81.40–T81.49, T84.60-T84.619, T84.63 T84.7 with 7th character A
HAC   ØRG[Ø,1,2,4,6,7,8,A][Ø,3,4]A[Ø,J] when reported with SDx K68.11 or T81.40–T81.49,
       T84.60-T84.619, T84.63-T84.7 with 7th character A
HAC   ØRG[E,F,G,H,J,K][Ø,3,4][4,7,J,K]Z when reported with SDx K68.11 or T81.40–T81.49,
       T84.60-T84.619, T84.63-T84.7 with 7th character A
HAC   ØRG[L,M][Ø,3,4][3,4,5,7,J,K]Z when reported with SDx K68.11 or T81.40–T81.49,
       T84.60-T84.619, T84.63-T84.7 with 7th character A
	See Appendix L for Procedure Combinations
	⊞ ØRG7[Ø,3,4][7,J,K][Ø,1,J]
	⊞ ØRG7[Ø,3,4]A[Ø,J]

NC Noncovered Procedure	**LC** Limited Coverage	**QA** Questionable OB Admit	**NT** New Tech Add-on	⊞ Combination Member	♂ Male	♀ Female

Ø   Medical and Surgical
R   Upper Joints
H   Insertion   Definition: Putting in a nonbiological appliance that monitors, assists, performs, or prevents a physiological function but does not physically take the place of a body part

Explanation: None

Body Part Character 4		Approach Character 5	Device Character 6	Qualifier Character 7
Ø	**Occipital-cervical Joint**	**Ø** Open	**3** Infusion Device	**Z** No Qualifier
1	**Cervical Vertebral Joint**	**3** Percutaneous	**4** Internal Fixation Device	
	Atlantoaxial joint	**4** Percutaneous Endoscopic	**8** Spacer	
	Cervical facet joint		**B** Spinal Stabilization Device, Interspinous Process	
4	**Cervicothoracic Vertebral Joint**		**C** Spinal Stabilization Device, Pedicle-Based	
	Cervicothoracic facet joint		**D** Spinal Stabilization Device, Facet Replacement	
6	**Thoracic Vertebral Joint**			
	Costotransverse joint			
	Costovertebral joint			
	Thoracic facet joint			
A	**Thoracolumbar Vertebral Joint**			
	Thoracolumbar facet joint			
3	**Cervical Vertebral Disc**	**Ø** Open	**3** Infusion Device	**Z** No Qualifier
5	**Cervicothoracic Vertebral Disc**	**3** Percutaneous		
9	**Thoracic Vertebral Disc**	**4** Percutaneous Endoscopic		
B	**Thoracolumbar Vertebral Disc**			
C	**Temporomandibular Joint, Right**	**Ø** Open	**3** Infusion Device	**Z** No Qualifier
D	**Temporomandibular Joint, Left**	**3** Percutaneous	**4** Internal Fixation Device	
E	**Sternoclavicular Joint, Right**	**4** Percutaneous Endoscopic	**8** Spacer	
F	**Sternoclavicular Joint, Left**			
G	**Acromioclavicular Joint, Right**			
H	**Acromioclavicular Joint, Left**			
J	**Shoulder Joint, Right**			
	Glenohumeral joint			
	Glenoid ligament (labrum)			
K	**Shoulder Joint, Left**			
	See J Shoulder Joint, Right			
L	**Elbow Joint, Right**	**Ø** Open	**3** Infusion Device	**Z** No Qualifier
	Distal humerus, involving joint	**3** Percutaneous	**4** Internal Fixation Device	
	Humeroradial joint	**4** Percutaneous Endoscopic	**5** External Fixation Device	
	Humeroulnar joint		**8** Spacer	
	Proximal radioulnar joint			
M	**Elbow Joint, Left**			
	See L Elbow Joint, Right			
N	**Wrist Joint, Right**			
	Distal radioulnar joint			
	Radiocarpal joint			
P	**Wrist Joint, Left**			
	See N Wrist Joint, Right			
Q	**Carpal Joint, Right**			
	Intercarpal joint			
	Midcarpal joint			
R	**Carpal Joint, Left**			
	See Q Carpal Joint, Right			
S	**Carpometacarpal Joint, Right**			
T	**Carpometacarpal Joint, Left**			
U	**Metacarpophalangeal Joint, Right**			
V	**Metacarpophalangeal Joint, Left**			
W	**Finger Phalangeal Joint, Right**			
	Interphalangeal (IP) joint			
X	**Finger Phalangeal Joint, Left**			
	See W Finger Phalangeal Joint, Right			

Non-OR	ØRH[Ø,1,4,6,A][Ø,3,4][3,8]Z
Non-OR	ØRH[3,5,9,B][Ø,3,4]3Z
Non-OR	ØRH[C,D][Ø,4]8Z
Non-OR	ØRH[C,D]3[3,8]Z
Non-OR	ØRH[E,F,G,H,J,K][Ø,3,4][3,8]Z
Non-OR	ØRH[L,M,N,P,Q,R,S,T,U,V,W,X][Ø,3,4][3,8]Z

Upper Joints

Ø   **Medical and Surgical**
R   **Upper Joints**
J   **Inspection**   Definition: Visually and/or manually exploring a body part
                    Explanation: Visual exploration may be performed with or without optical instrumentation. Manual exploration may be performed directly or through intervening body layers.

Body Part Character 4	Approach Character 5	Device Character 6	Qualifier Character 7

Ø   Occipital-cervical Joint
1   Cervical Vertebral Joint
    Atlantoaxial joint
    Cervical facet joint
3   Cervical Vertebral Disc
4   Cervicothoracic Vertebral Joint
    Cervicothoracic facet joint
5   Cervicothoracic Vertebral Disc
6   Thoracic Vertebral Joint
    Costotransverse joint
    Costovertebral joint
    Thoracic facet joint
9   Thoracic Vertebral Disc
A   Thoracolumbar Vertebral Joint
    Thoracolumbar facet joint
B   Thoracolumbar Vertebral Disc
C   Temporomandibular Joint, Right
D   Temporomandibular Joint, Left
E   Sternoclavicular Joint, Right
F   Sternoclavicular Joint, Left
G   Acromioclavicular Joint, Right
H   Acromioclavicular Joint, Left
J   Shoulder Joint, Right
    Glenohumeral joint
    Glenoid ligament (labrum)
K   Shoulder Joint, Left
    See J Shoulder Joint, Right
L   Elbow Joint, Right
    Distal humerus, involving joint
    Humeroradial joint
    Humeroulnar joint
    Proximal radioulnar joint
M   Elbow Joint, Left
    See L Elbow Joint, Right
N   Wrist Joint, Right
    Distal radioulnar joint
    Radiocarpal joint
P   Wrist Joint, Left
    See N Wrist Joint, Right
Q   Carpal Joint, Right
    Intercarpal joint
    Midcarpal joint
R   Carpal Joint, Left
    See Q Carpal Joint, Right
S   Carpometacarpal Joint, Right
T   Carpometacarpal Joint, Left
U   Metacarpophalangeal Joint, Right
V   Metacarpophalangeal Joint, Left
W   Finger Phalangeal Joint, Right
    Interphalangeal (IP) joint
X   Finger Phalangeal Joint, Left
    See W Finger Phalangeal Joint, Right
	Ø Open
	3 Percutaneous
	4 Percutaneous Endoscopic
	X External
		Z No Device	Z No Qualifier

Non-OR   ØRJ[Ø,1,3,4,5,6,9,A,B,C,D,E,F,G,H,J,K,L,M,N,P,Q,R,S,T,U,V,W,X][3,X]ZZ

NC Noncovered Procedure   **LC** Limited Coverage   **OA** Questionable OB Admit   **NT** New Tech Add-on   ⊞ Combination Member   ♂ Male   ♀ Female

ICD-10-PCS 2022   589

Upper Joints

Ø   **Medical and Surgical**
R   **Upper Joints**
N   **Release**   Definition: Freeing a body part from an abnormal physical constraint by cutting or by the use of force
                   Explanation: Some of the restraining tissue may be taken out but none of the body part is taken out

Body Part Character 4	Approach Character 5	Device Character 6	Qualifier Character 7

Ø Occipital-cervical Joint
1 Cervical Vertebral Joint
    Atlantoaxial joint
    Cervical facet joint
3 Cervical Vertebral Disc
4 Cervicothoracic Vertebral Joint
    Cervicothoracic facet joint
5 Cervicothoracic Vertebral Disc
6 Thoracic Vertebral Joint
    Costotransverse joint
    Costovertebral joint
    Thoracic facet joint
9 Thoracic Vertebral Disc
A Thoracolumbar Vertebral Joint
    Thoracolumbar facet joint
B Thoracolumbar Vertebral Disc
C Temporomandibular Joint, Right
D Temporomandibular Joint, Left
E Sternoclavicular Joint, Right
F Sternoclavicular Joint, Left
G Acromioclavicular Joint, Right
H Acromioclavicular Joint, Left
J Shoulder Joint, Right
    Glenohumeral joint
    Glenoid ligament (labrum)
K Shoulder Joint, Left
    See J Shoulder Joint, Right
L Elbow Joint, Right
    Distal humerus, involving joint
    Humeroradial joint
    Humeroulnar joint
    Proximal radioulnar joint
M Elbow Joint, Left
    See L Elbow Joint, Right
N Wrist Joint, Right
    Distal radioulnar joint
    Radiocarpal joint
P Wrist Joint, Left
    See N Wrist Joint, Right
Q Carpal Joint, Right
    Intercarpal joint
    Midcarpal joint
R Carpal Joint, Left
    See Q Carpal Joint, Right
S Carpometacarpal Joint, Right
T Carpometacarpal Joint, Left
U Metacarpophalangeal Joint, Right
V Metacarpophalangeal Joint, Left
W Finger Phalangeal Joint, Right
    Interphalangeal (IP) joint
X Finger Phalangeal Joint, Left
    See W Finger Phalangeal Joint, Right
	Ø Open
	3 Percutaneous
	4 Percutaneous Endoscopic
	X External
		Z No Device	**Z** No Qualifier

Non-OR   ØRN[Ø,1,3,4,5,6,9,A,B,C,D,E,F,G,H,J,K,L,M,N,P,Q,R,S,T,U,V,W,X]XZZ

Ø Medical and Surgical
R Upper Joints
P Removal   Definition: Taking out or off a device from a body part

Explanation: If a device is taken out and a similar device put in without cutting or puncturing the skin or mucous membrane, the procedure is coded to the root operation CHANGE. Otherwise, the procedure for taking out the device is coded to the root operation REMOVAL.

Body Part Character 4	Approach Character 5	Device Character 6	Qualifier Character 7

Ø **Occipital-cervical Joint**
1 **Cervical Vertebral Joint**
  Atlantoaxial joint
  Cervical facet joint
4 **Cervicothoracic Vertebral Joint**
  Cervicothoracic facet joint
6 **Thoracic Vertebral Joint**
  Costotransverse joint
  Costovertebral joint
  Thoracic facet joint
A **Thoracolumbar Vertebral Joint**
  Thoracolumbar facet joint
	Ø Open
	3 Percutaneous
	4 Percutaneous Endoscopic
		Ø Drainage Device
		3 Infusion Device
		4 Internal Fixation Device
		7 Autologous Tissue Substitute
		8 Spacer
		A Interbody Fusion Device
		J Synthetic Substitute
		K Nonautologous Tissue Substitute
			Z No Qualifier

Ø **Occipital-cervical Joint**
1 **Cervical Vertebral Joint**
  Atlantoaxial joint
  Cervical facet joint
4 **Cervicothoracic Vertebral Joint**
  Cervicothoracic facet joint
6 **Thoracic Vertebral Joint**
  Costotransverse joint
  Costovertebral joint
  Thoracic facet joint
A **Thoracolumbar Vertebral Joint**
  Thoracolumbar facet joint
	X External	**Ø** Drainage Device
		3 Infusion Device
		4 Internal Fixation Device
			Z No Qualifier

3 **Cervical Vertebral Disc** **5** **Cervicothoracic Vertebral Disc** **9** **Thoracic Vertebral Disc** **B** **Thoracolumbar Vertebral Disc**	**Ø** Open **3** Percutaneous **4** Percutaneous Endoscopic	**Ø** Drainage Device **3** Infusion Device **7** Autologous Tissue Substitute **J** Synthetic Substitute **K** Nonautologous Tissue Substitute	**Z** No Qualifier
3 **Cervical Vertebral Disc** **5** **Cervicothoracic Vertebral Disc** **9** **Thoracic Vertebral Disc** **B** **Thoracolumbar Vertebral Disc**	**X** External	**Ø** Drainage Device **3** Infusion Device	**Z** No Qualifier
C **Temporomandibular Joint, Right** **D** **Temporomandibular Joint, Left** **E** **Sternoclavicular Joint, Right** **F** **Sternoclavicular Joint, Left** **G** **Acromioclavicular Joint, Right** **H** **Acromioclavicular Joint, Left**	**Ø** Open **3** Percutaneous **4** Percutaneous Endoscopic	**Ø** Drainage Device **3** Infusion Device **4** Internal Fixation Device **7** Autologous Tissue Substitute **8** Spacer **J** Synthetic Substitute **K** Nonautologous Tissue Substitute	**Z** No Qualifier
C Temporomandibular Joint, Right **D** Temporomandibular Joint, Left **E** Sternoclavicular Joint, Right **F** Sternoclavicular Joint, Left **G** Acromioclavicular Joint, Right **H** Acromioclavicular Joint, Left	**X** External	**Ø** Drainage Device **3** Infusion Device **4** Internal Fixation Device	**Z** No Qualifier

J **Shoulder Joint, Right**
  Glenohumeral joint
  Glenoid ligament (labrum)
K **Shoulder Joint, Left**
  See J Shoulder Joint, Right
	Ø Open
	3 Percutaneous
	4 Percutaneous Endoscopic
		Ø Drainage Device
		3 Infusion Device
		4 Internal Fixation Device
		7 Autologous Tissue Substitute
		8 Spacer
		K Nonautologous Tissue Substitute
			Z No Qualifier

J Shoulder Joint, Right
  Glenohumeral joint
  Glenoid ligament (labrum)
K Shoulder Joint, Left
  See J Shoulder Joint, Right
	Ø Open
	3 Percutaneous
	4 Percutaneous Endoscopic
		J Synthetic Substitute	**6** Humeral Surface
			7 Glenoid Surface
			Z No Qualifier

J Shoulder Joint, Right
  Glenohumeral joint
  Glenoid ligament (labrum)
K Shoulder Joint, Left
  See J Shoulder Joint, Right
	X External	**Ø** Drainage Device
		3 Infusion Device
		4 Internal Fixation Device
			Z No Qualifier

Non-OR ØRP[Ø,1,4,6,A]3[Ø,3,8]Z		**Non-OR** ØRP[C,D,E,F,G,H][Ø,4]8Z	
Non-OR ØRP[Ø,1,4,6,A][Ø,4]8Z		**Non-OR** ØRP[C,D]X[Ø,3]Z	
Non-OR ØRP[Ø,1,4,6,A]X[Ø,3,4]Z		**Non-OR** ØRP[E,F,G,H,J,K]X[Ø,3,4]Z	
Non-OR ØRP[3,5,9,B]3[Ø,3]Z		**Non-OR** ØRP[J,K]3[Ø,3,8]Z	
Non-OR ØRP[3,5,9,B]X[Ø,3]Z		**Non-OR** ØRP[J,K][Ø,4]8Z	
Non-OR ØRP[C,D,E,F,G,H]3[Ø,3,8]Z		**Non-OR** ØRP[J,K]X[Ø,3,4]Z	

ØRP Continued on next page

NC Noncovered Procedure   **LC** Limited Coverage   **QA** Questionable OB Admit   **NT** New Tech Add-on   ⊞ Combination Member   ♂ Male   ♀ Female

Upper Joints

Ø   **Medical and Surgical**   *ØRP Continued*

R   **Upper Joints**

P   **Removal**   Definition: Taking out or off a device from a body part

Explanation: If a device is taken out and a similar device put in without cutting or puncturing the skin or mucous membrane, the procedure is coded to the root operation CHANGE. Otherwise, the procedure for taking out the device is coded to the root operation REMOVAL.

Body Part Character 4	Approach Character 5	Device Character 6	Qualifier Character 7

L **Elbow Joint, Right**
   Distal humerus, involving joint
   Humeroradial joint
   Humeroulnar joint
   Proximal radioulnar joint
M **Elbow Joint, Left**
   See L Elbow Joint, Right
N **Wrist Joint, Right**
   Distal radioulnar joint
   Radiocarpal joint
P **Wrist Joint, Left**
   See N Wrist Joint, Right
Q **Carpal Joint, Right**
   Intercarpal joint
   Midcarpal joint
R **Carpal Joint, Left**
   See Q Carpal Joint, Right
S **Carpometacarpal Joint, Right**
T **Carpometacarpal Joint, Left**
U **Metacarpophalangeal Joint, Right**
V **Metacarpophalangeal Joint, Left**
W **Finger Phalangeal Joint, Right**
   Interphalangeal (IP) joint
X **Finger Phalangeal Joint, Left**
   See W Finger Phalangeal Joint, Right
	Ø Open
	3 Percutaneous
	4 Percutaneous Endoscopic
		Ø Drainage Device
		3 Infusion Device
		4 Internal Fixation Device
		5 External Fixation Device
		7 Autologous Tissue Substitute
		8 Spacer
		J Synthetic Substitute
		K Nonautologous Tissue Substitute
			Z No Qualifier

L **Elbow Joint, Right**
   Distal humerus, involving joint
   Humeroradial joint
   Humeroulnar joint
   Proximal radioulnar joint
M **Elbow Joint, Left**
   See L Elbow Joint, Right
N **Wrist Joint, Right**
   Distal radioulnar joint
   Radiocarpal joint
P **Wrist Joint, Left**
   See N Wrist Joint, Right
Q **Carpal Joint, Right**
   Intercarpal joint
   Midcarpal joint
R **Carpal Joint, Left**
   See Q Carpal Joint, Right
S **Carpometacarpal Joint, Right**
T **Carpometacarpal Joint, Left**
U **Metacarpophalangeal Joint, Right**
V **Metacarpophalangeal Joint, Left**
W **Finger Phalangeal Joint, Right**
   Interphalangeal (IP) joint
X **Finger Phalangeal Joint, Left**
   See W Finger Phalangeal Joint, Right
	X External	**Ø** Drainage Device
		3 Infusion Device
		4 Internal Fixation Device
		5 External Fixation Device
			Z No Qualifier

Non-OR   ØRP[L,M,N,P,Q,R,S,T,U,V,W,X]3[Ø,3,8]Z
Non-OR   ØRP[L,M,N,P,Q,R,S,T,U,V,W,X][Ø,4]8Z
Non-OR   ØRP[L,M,N,P,Q,R,S,T,U,V,W,X]X[Ø,3,4,5]Z

Ø   **Medical and Surgical**
R   **Upper Joints**
Q   **Repair**   Definition: Restoring, to the extent possible, a body part to its normal anatomic structure and function
                   Explanation: Used only when the method to accomplish the repair is not one of the other root operations

Body Part Character 4	Approach Character 5	Device Character 6	Qualifier Character 7

Ø   Occipital-cervical Joint
1   Cervical Vertebral Joint
    Atlantoaxial joint
    Cervical facet joint
3   Cervical Vertebral Disc
4   Cervicothoracic Vertebral Joint
    Cervicothoracic facet joint
5   Cervicothoracic Vertebral Disc
6   Thoracic Vertebral Joint
    Costotransverse joint
    Costovertebral joint
    Thoracic facet joint
9   Thoracic Vertebral Disc
A   Thoracolumbar Vertebral Joint
    Thoracolumbar facet joint
B   Thoracolumbar Vertebral Disc
C   Temporomandibular Joint, Right
D   Temporomandibular Joint, Left
E   Sternoclavicular Joint, Right
F   Sternoclavicular Joint, Left
G   Acromioclavicular Joint, Right
H   Acromioclavicular Joint, Left
J   Shoulder Joint, Right
    Glenohumeral joint
    Glenoid ligament (labrum)
K   Shoulder Joint, Left
    See J Shoulder Joint, Right
L   Elbow Joint, Right
    Distal humerus, involving joint
    Humeroradial joint
    Humeroulnar joint
    Proximal radioulnar joint
M   Elbow Joint, Left
    See L Elbow Joint, Right
N   Wrist Joint, Right
    Distal radioulnar joint
    Radiocarpal joint
P   Wrist Joint, Left
    See N Wrist Joint, Right
Q   Carpal Joint, Right
    Intercarpal joint
    Midcarpal joint
R   Carpal Joint, Left
    See Q Carpal Joint, Right
S   Carpometacarpal Joint, Right
T   Carpometacarpal Joint, Left
U   Metacarpophalangeal Joint, Right
V   Metacarpophalangeal Joint, Left
W   Finger Phalangeal Joint, Right
    Interphalangeal (IP) joint
X   Finger Phalangeal Joint, Left
    See W Finger Phalangeal Joint, Right
	Ø Open
	3 Percutaneous
	4 Percutaneous Endoscopic
	X External
		Z No Device	Z No Qualifier

Non-OR   ØRQ[Ø,1,3,4,5,6,9,A,B,C,D,E,F,G,H,J,K,L,M,N,P,Q,R,S,T,U,V,W,X]XZZ
HAC   ØRQ[E,F,G,H,J,K,L,M][Ø,3,4]ZZ when reported with SDx K68.11 or T81.4Ø–T81.49, T84.6Ø-T84.619, T84.63-T84.7 with 7th character A

NC Noncovered Procedure   LC Limited Coverage   QA Questionable OB Admit   NT New Tech Add-on   ⊞ Combination Member   ♂ Male   ♀ Female

ICD-10-PCS 2022   593

ØRQ–ØRQ

Upper Joints

Ø Medical and Surgical
R Upper Joints
R Replacement

Definition: Putting in or on biological or synthetic material that physically takes the place and/or function of all or a portion of a body part

Explanation: The body part may have been taken out or replaced, or may be taken out, physically eradicated, or rendered nonfunctional during the REPLACEMENT procedure. A REMOVAL procedure is coded for taking out the device used in a previous replacement procedure.

Body Part Character 4	Approach Character 5	Device Character 6	Qualifier Character 7

Ø Occipital-cervical Joint
1 Cervical Vertebral Joint
  Atlantoaxial joint
  Cervical facet joint
3 Cervical Vertebral Disc
4 Cervicothoracic Vertebral Joint
  Cervicothoracic facet joint
5 Cervicothoracic Vertebral Disc
6 Thoracic Vertebral Joint
  Costotransverse joint
  Costovertebral joint
  Thoracic facet joint
9 Thoracic Vertebral Disc
A Thoracolumbar Vertebral Joint
  Thoracolumbar facet joint
B Thoracolumbar Vertebral Disc
C Temporomandibular Joint, Right
D Temporomandibular Joint, Left
E Sternoclavicular Joint, Right
F Sternoclavicular Joint, Left
G Acromioclavicular Joint, Right
H Acromioclavicular Joint, Left
L Elbow Joint, Right
  Distal humerus, involving joint
  Humeroradial joint
  Humeroulnar joint
  Proximal radioulnar joint
M Elbow Joint, Left
  See L Elbow Joint, Right
N Wrist Joint, Right
  Distal radioulnar joint
  Radiocarpal joint
P Wrist Joint, Left
  See N Wrist Joint, Right
Q Carpal Joint, Right
  Intercarpal joint
  Midcarpal joint
R Carpal Joint, Left
  See Q Carpal Joint, Right
S Carpometacarpal Joint, Right
T Carpometacarpal Joint, Left
U Metacarpophalangeal Joint, Right
V Metacarpophalangeal Joint, Left
W Finger Phalangeal Joint, Right
  Interphalangeal (IP) joint
X Finger Phalangeal Joint, Left
  See W Finger Phalangeal Joint, Right
	Ø Open	7 Autologous Tissue Substitute
		J Synthetic Substitute
		K Nonautologous Tissue Substitute
			Z No Qualifier

J Shoulder Joint, Right
  Glenohumeral joint
  Glenoid ligament (labrum)
K Shoulder Joint, Left
  See J Shoulder Joint, Right
	Ø Open	Ø Synthetic Substitute, Reverse Ball and Socket
		7 Autologous Tissue Substitute
		K Nonautologous Tissue Substitute
			Z No Qualifier

J Shoulder Joint, Right
  Glenohumeral joint
  Glenoid ligament (labrum)
K Shoulder Joint, Left
  See J Shoulder Joint, Right
	Ø Open	J Synthetic Substitute	6 Humeral Surface
			7 Glenoid Surface
			Z No Qualifier

Ø   **Medical and Surgical**
R   **Upper Joints**
S   **Reposition**   Definition: Moving to its normal location, or other suitable location, all or a portion of a body part

                Explanation: The body part is moved to a new location from an abnormal location, or from a normal location where it is not functioning correctly. The body part may or may not be cut out or off to be moved to the new location.

Body Part Character 4	Approach Character 5	Device Character 6	Qualifier Character 7

Ø   **Occipital-cervical Joint**
1   **Cervical Vertebral Joint**
     Atlantoaxial joint
     Cervical facet joint
4   **Cervicothoracic Vertebral Joint**
     Cervicothoracic facet joint
6   **Thoracic Vertebral Joint**
     Costotransverse joint
     Costovertebral joint
     Thoracic facet joint
A   **Thoracolumbar Vertebral Joint**
     Thoracolumbar facet joint
C   **Temporomandibular Joint, Right**
D   **Temporomandibular Joint, Left**
E   **Sternoclavicular Joint, Right**
F   **Sternoclavicular Joint, Left**
G   **Acromioclavicular Joint, Right**
H   **Acromioclavicular Joint, Left**
J   **Shoulder Joint, Right**
     Glenohumeral joint
     Glenoid ligament (labrum)
K   **Shoulder Joint, Left**
     See J Shoulder Joint, Right
	Ø Open
	3 Percutaneous
	4 Percutaneous Endoscopic
	X External
		4 Internal Fixation Device
		Z No Device
			Z No Qualifier

L   **Elbow Joint, Right**
     Distal humerus, involving joint
     Humeroradial joint
     Humeroulnar joint
     Proximal radioulnar joint
M   **Elbow Joint, Left**
     See L Elbow Joint, Right
N   **Wrist Joint, Right**
     Distal radioulnar joint
     Radiocarpal joint
P   **Wrist Joint, Left**
     See N Wrist Joint, Right
Q   **Carpal Joint, Right**
     Intercarpal joint
     Midcarpal joint
R   **Carpal Joint, Left**
     See Q Carpal Joint, Right
S   **Carpometacarpal Joint, Right**
T   **Carpometacarpal Joint, Left**
U   **Metacarpophalangeal Joint, Right**
V   **Metacarpophalangeal Joint, Left**
W   **Finger Phalangeal Joint, Right**
     Interphalangeal (IP) joint
X   **Finger Phalangeal Joint, Left**
     See W Finger Phalangeal Joint, Right
	Ø Open
	3 Percutaneous
	4 Percutaneous Endoscopic
	X External
		4 Internal Fixation Device
		5 External Fixation Device
		Z No Device
			Z No Qualifier

Non-OR   ØRS[Ø,1,4,6,A,C,D,E,F,G,H,J,K][3,4,X][4,Z]Z
Non-OR   ØRS[L,M,N,P,Q,R,S,T,U,V,W,X][3,4,X][4,5,Z]Z

NC Noncovered Procedure   LC Limited Coverage   QA Questionable OB Admit   NT New Tech Add-on   ⊞ Combination Member   ♂ Male   ♀ Female

ICD-10-PCS 2022   595

ØRS–ØRS

Upper Joints

Ø   **Medical and Surgical**
R   **Upper Joints**
T   **Resection**   Definition: Cutting out or off, without replacement, all of a body part
                    Explanation: None

Body Part Character 4	Approach Character 5	Device Character 6	Qualifier Character 7
3 Cervical Vertebral Disc	**Ø** Open	**Z** No Device	**Z** No Qualifier
4 Cervicothoracic Vertebral Joint Cervicothoracic facet joint			
5 Cervicothoracic Vertebral Disc			
9 Thoracic Vertebral Disc			
B Thoracolumbar Vertebral Disc			
C Temporomandibular Joint, Right			
D Temporomandibular Joint, Left			
E Sternoclavicular Joint, Right			
F Sternoclavicular Joint, Left			
G Acromioclavicular Joint, Right			
H Acromioclavicular Joint, Left			

J Shoulder Joint, Right
    Glenohumeral joint
    Glenoid ligament (labrum)			

K Shoulder Joint, Left *See J Shoulder Joint, Right*			

L Elbow Joint, Right
    Distal humerus, involving joint
    Humeroradial joint
    Humeroulnar joint
    Proximal radioulnar joint			

M Elbow Joint, Left *See L Elbow Joint, Right*			

N Wrist Joint, Right
    Distal radioulnar joint
    Radiocarpal joint			

P Wrist Joint, Left *See N Wrist Joint, Right*			

Q Carpal Joint, Right
    Intercarpal joint
    Midcarpal joint			

R Carpal Joint, Left *See Q Carpal Joint, Right*			
S Carpometacarpal Joint, Right			
T Carpometacarpal Joint, Left			
U Metacarpophalangeal Joint, Right			
V Metacarpophalangeal Joint, Left			
W Finger Phalangeal Joint, Right Interphalangeal (IP) joint			
X Finger Phalangeal Joint, Left *See W Finger Phalangeal Joint, Right*			

Ø   **Medical and Surgical**
R   **Upper Joints**
U   **Supplement**   Definition: Putting in or on biological or synthetic material that physically reinforces and/or augments the function of a portion of a body part
                      Explanation: The biological material is non-living, or is living and from the same individual. The body part may have been previously replaced, and the SUPPLEMENT procedure is performed to physically reinforce and/or augment the function of the replaced body part.

Body Part Character 4	Approach Character 5	Device Character 6	Qualifier Character 7
Ø **Occipital-cervical Joint**	**Ø** Open	**7** Autologous Tissue Substitute	**Z** No Qualifier

1 **Cervical Vertebral Joint**
    Atlantoaxial joint
    Cervical facet joint
	3 Percutaneous
	4 Percutaneous Endoscopic
		J Synthetic Substitute
		K Nonautologous Tissue
		     Substitute	

3 **Cervical Vertebral Disc**			
4 **Cervicothoracic Vertebral Joint** Cervicothoracic facet joint			
5 **Cervicothoracic Vertebral Disc**			

6 **Thoracic Vertebral Joint**
    Costotransverse joint
    Costovertebral joint
    Thoracic facet joint			

9 **Thoracic Vertebral Disc**			
A **Thoracolumbar Vertebral Joint** Thoracolumbar facet joint			
B **Thoracolumbar Vertebral Disc**			
C **Temporomandibular Joint, Right**			
D **Temporomandibular Joint, Left**			
E **Sternoclavicular Joint, Right**			
F **Sternoclavicular Joint, Left**			
G **Acromioclavicular Joint, Right**			
H **Acromioclavicular Joint, Left**			

J **Shoulder Joint, Right**
    Glenohumeral joint
    Glenoid ligament (labrum)			

K **Shoulder Joint, Left** *See J Shoulder Joint, Right*			

L **Elbow Joint, Right**
    Distal humerus, involving joint
    Humeroradial joint
    Humeroulnar joint
    Proximal radioulnar joint			

M **Elbow Joint, Left** *See L Elbow Joint, Right*			

N **Wrist Joint, Right**
    Distal radioulnar joint
    Radiocarpal joint			

P **Wrist Joint, Left** *See N Wrist Joint, Right*			

Q **Carpal Joint, Right**
    Intercarpal joint
    Midcarpal joint			

R **Carpal Joint, Left** *See Q Carpal Joint, Right*			
S **Carpometacarpal Joint, Right**			
T **Carpometacarpal Joint, Left**			
U **Metacarpophalangeal Joint, Right**			
V **Metacarpophalangeal Joint, Left**			
W **Finger Phalangeal Joint, Right** Interphalangeal (IP) joint			
X **Finger Phalangeal Joint, Left** *See W Finger Phalangeal Joint, Right*			

HAC   ØRU[E,F,G,H,J,K,L,M][Ø,3,4][7,J,K]Z when reported with SDx K68.11 or T81.40–T81.49, T84.60-T84.619, T84.63-T84.7 with 7th character A

NC Noncovered Procedure   **LC** Limited Coverage   **OA** Questionable OB Admit   **NT** New Tech Add-on   ⊞ Combination Member   ♂ Male   ♀ Female

ICD-10-PCS 2022   **597**

ØRU–ØRU

Ø   **Medical and Surgical**
R   **Upper Joints**
W   **Revision**   Definition: Correcting, to the extent possible, a portion of a malfunctioning device or the position of a displaced device

Explanation: Revision can include correcting a malfunctioning or displaced device by taking out or putting in components of the device such as a screw or pin

Body Part Character 4	Approach Character 5	Device Character 6	Qualifier Character 7
Ø **Occipital-cervical Joint** **1** **Cervical Vertebral Joint** Atlantoaxial joint Cervical facet joint **4** **Cervicothoracic Vertebral Joint** Cervicothoracic facet joint **6** **Thoracic Vertebral Joint** Costotransverse joint Costovertebral joint Thoracic facet joint **A** **Thoracolumbar Vertebral Joint** Thoracolumbar facet joint	**Ø** Open **3** Percutaneous **4** Percutaneous Endoscopic **X** External	**Ø** Drainage Device **3** Infusion Device **4** Internal Fixation Device **7** Autologous Tissue Substitute **8** Spacer **A** Interbody Fusion Device **J** Synthetic Substitute **K** Nonautologous Tissue Substitute	**Z** No Qualifier
3 **Cervical Vertebral Disc** **5** **Cervicothoracic Vertebral Disc** **9** **Thoracic Vertebral Disc** **B** **Thoracolumbar Vertebral Disc**	**Ø** Open **3** Percutaneous **4** Percutaneous Endoscopic **X** External	**Ø** Drainage Device **3** Infusion Device **7** Autologous Tissue Substitute **J** Synthetic Substitute **K** Nonautologous Tissue Substitute	**Z** No Qualifier
C **Temporomandibular Joint, Right** **D** **Temporomandibular Joint, Left** **E** **Sternoclavicular Joint, Right** **F** **Sternoclavicular Joint, Left** **G** **Acromioclavicular Joint, Right** **H** **Acromioclavicular Joint, Left**	**Ø** Open **3** Percutaneous **4** Percutaneous Endoscopic **X** External	**Ø** Drainage Device **3** Infusion Device **4** Internal Fixation Device **7** Autologous Tissue Substitute **8** Spacer **J** Synthetic Substitute **K** Nonautologous Tissue Substitute	**Z** No Qualifier
J **Shoulder Joint, Right** Glenohumeral joint Glenoid ligament (labrum) **K** **Shoulder Joint, Left** *See J Shoulder Joint, Right*	**Ø** Open **3** Percutaneous **4** Percutaneous Endoscopic **X** External	**Ø** Drainage Device **3** Infusion Device **4** Internal Fixation Device **7** Autologous Tissue Substitute **8** Spacer **J** Synthetic Substitute **K** Nonautologous Tissue Substitute	**Z** No Qualifier
J **Shoulder Joint, Right** Glenohumeral joint Glenoid ligament (labrum) **K** **Shoulder Joint, Left** *See J Shoulder Joint, Right*	**Ø** Open **3** Percutaneous **4** Percutaneous Endoscopic **X** External	**J** Synthetic Substitute	**6** Humeral Surgace **7** Glenoid Surface **Z** No Qualifier
L **Elbow Joint, Right** Distal humerus, involving joint Humeroradial joint Humeroulnar joint Proximal radioulnar joint **M** **Elbow Joint, Left** *See L Elbow Joint, Right* **N** **Wrist Joint, Right** Distal radioulnar joint Radiocarpal joint **P** **Wrist Joint, Left** *See N Wrist Joint, Right* **Q** **Carpal Joint, Right** Intercarpal joint Midcarpal joint **R** **Carpal Joint, Left** *See Q Carpal Joint, Right* **S** **Carpometacarpal Joint, Right** **T** **Carpometacarpal Joint, Left** **U** **Metacarpophalangeal Joint, Right** **V** **Metacarpophalangeal Joint, Left** **W** **Finger Phalangeal Joint, Right** Interphalangeal (IP) joint **X** **Finger Phalangeal Joint, Left** *See W Finger Phalangeal Joint, Right*	**Ø** Open **3** Percutaneous **4** Percutaneous Endoscopic **X** External	**Ø** Drainage Device **3** Infusion Device **4** Internal Fixation Device **5** External Fixation Device **7** Autologous Tissue Substitute **8** Spacer **J** Synthetic Substitute **K** Nonautologous Tissue Substitute	**Z** No Qualifier

Non-OR	ØRW[Ø,1,4,6,A]X[Ø,3,4,7,8,A,J,K]Z
Non-OR	ØRW[3,5,9,B]X[Ø,3,7,J,K]Z
Non-OR	ØRW[C,D,E,F,G,H]X[Ø,3,4,7,8,J,K]Z
Non-OR	ØRW[J,K]X[Ø,3,4,7,8,J,K]Z
Non-OR	ØRW[J,K]XJ[6,7]
Non-OR	ØRW[L,M,N,P,Q,R,S,T,U,V,W,X]X[Ø,3,4,5,7,8,J,K]Z

Lower Joints ØS2–ØSW

Character Meanings*

This Character Meaning table is provided as a guide to assist the user in the identification of character members that may be found in this section of code tables. It **SHOULD NOT** be used to build a PCS code.

Operation–Character 3	Body Part–Character 4	Approach–Character 5	Device–Character 6	Qualifier–Character 7
2 Change	Ø Lumbar Vertebral Joint	Ø Open	Ø Drainage Device OR Synthetic Substitute, Polyethylene	Ø Anterior Approach, Anterior Column
5 Destruction	1 Lumbar Vertebral Joint, 2 or more	3 Percutaneous	1 Synthetic Substitute, Metal	1 Posterior Approach, Posterior Column
9 Drainage	2 Lumbar Vertebral Disc	4 Percutaneous Endoscopic	2 Synthetic Substitute, Metal on Polyethylene	9 Cemented
B Excision	3 Lumbosacral Joint	X External	3 Infusion Device OR Internal Fixation Device, Sustained Compression OR Synthetic Substitute, Ceramic	A Uncemented
C Extirpation	4 Lumbosacral Disc		4 Internal Fixation Device OR Synthetic Substitute, Ceramic on Polyethylene	C Patellar Surface
G Fusion	5 Sacrococcygeal Joint		5 External Fixation Device	J Posterior Approach, Anterior Column
H Insertion	6 Coccygeal Joint		6 Synthetic Substitute, Oxidized Zirconium on Polyethylene	X Diagnostic
J Inspection	7 Sacroiliac Joint, Right		7 Autologous Tissue Substitute	Z No Qualifier
N Release	8 Sacroiliac Joint, Left		8 Spacer	
P Removal	9 Hip Joint, Right		9 Liner	
Q Repair	A Hip Joint, Acetabular Surface, Right		A Interbody Fusion Device	
R Replacement	B Hip Joint, Left		B Resurfacing Device OR Spinal Stabilization Device, Interspinous Process	
S Reposition	C Knee Joint, Right		C Spinal Stabilization Device, Pedicle-Based	
T Resection	D Knee Joint, Left		D Spinal Stabilization Device, Facet Replacement	
U Supplement	E Hip Joint, Acetabular Surface, Left		E Articulating Spacer	
W Revision	F Ankle Joint, Right		J Synthetic Substitute	
	G Ankle Joint, Left		K Nonautologous Tissue Substitute	
	H Tarsal Joint, Right		L Synthetic Substitute, Unicondylar Medial	
	J Tarsal Joint, Left		M Synthetic Substitute, Unicondylar Lateral	
	K Tarsometatarsal Joint, Right		N Synthetic Substitute, Patellofemoral	
	L Tarsometatarsal Joint, Left		Y Other Device	
	M Metatarsal-Phalangeal Joint, Right		Z No Device	
	N Metatarsal-Phalangeal Joint, Left			
	P Toe Phalangeal Joint, Right			
	Q Toe Phalangeal Joint, Left			
	R Hip Joint, Femoral Surface, Right			
	S Hip Joint, Femoral Surface, Left			
	T Knee Joint, Femoral Surface, Right			
	U Knee Joint, Femoral Surface, Left			
	V Knee Joint, Tibial Surface, Right			
	W Knee Joint, Tibial Surface, Left			
	Y Lower Joint			

* Includes synovial membrane.

AHA Coding Clinic for table ØS9

| 2018, 2Q, 17 | Arthroscopic drainage of knee and nonexcisional debridement |
| 2017, 1Q, 50 | Dry aspiration of ankle joint |

AHA Coding Clinic for table ØSB

2017, 4Q, 76	Radiolucent porous interbody fusion device
2016, 2Q, 16	Decompressive laminectomy/foraminotomy and lumbar discectomy
2016, 1Q, 20	Metatarsophalangeal joint resection arthroplasty
2015, 1Q, 34	Arthroscopic meniscectomy with debridement and abrasion chondroplasty
2014, 2Q, 6	Posterior lumbar fusion with discectomy

AHA Coding Clinic for table ØSG

2021, 1Q, 18	Placement of interspinous distraction device (spacer) for decompression
2021, 1Q, 53	Official guidelines for coding and reporting for interbody fusion device B3.10c
2020, 4Q, 56-58	Intramedullary sustained compression joint fusion
2020, 2Q, 27	Spinal Fusion with NuVasive® VersaTie®
2020, 1Q, 33	Spinal fusion without use of bone graft
2019, 3Q, 35	Fusion procedures of the spine (guideline B3.10c)
2019, 1Q, 30	Spinal fusion performed at same level as decompressive laminectomy
2018, 4Q, 43	Joint fusion device value
2018, 1Q, 22	Spinal fusion procedures without bone graft
2017, 4Q, 76	Radiolucent porous interbody fusion device
2017, 2Q, 23	Decompression of spinal cord and placement of instrumentation
2014, 3Q, 30	Spinal fusion and fixation instrumentation
2014, 3Q, 36	Lumbar interbody fusion of two vertebral levels
2014, 2Q, 6	Posterior lumbar fusion with discectomy
2013, 3Q, 25	360-degree spinal fusion
2013, 2Q, 39	Ankle fusion, osteotomy, and removal of hardware
2013, 1Q, 21-23	Spinal fusion of thoracic and lumbar vertebrae

AHA Coding Clinic for table ØSH

| 2021, 1Q, 18 | Placement of interspinous distraction device (spacer) for decompression |
| 2017, 2Q, 23 | Decompression of spinal cord and placement of instrumentation |

AHA Coding Clinic for table ØSJ

| 2017, 1Q, 50 | Dry aspiration of ankle joint |

AHA Coding Clinic for table ØSN

| 2020, 2Q, 26 | Arthroscopic Manipulation and Nonexcisional Debridement of Knee Joint |
| 2019, 1Q, 30 | Spinal fusion performed at same level as decompressive laminectomy |

AHA Coding Clinic for table ØSP

2021, 1Q, 17	Revision of ankle arthroplasty with placement of tibial insert
2018, 4Q, 43	Articulating spacer for hip and knee joint
2018, 2Q, 16	Exchange of tibial polyethylene component with stabilizing insert (tibial tray)
2017, 4Q, 107	Total ankle replacement versus revision
2016, 4Q, 110-112	Removal and revision of hip and knee devices
2015, 2Q, 18	Total knee revision
2015, 2Q, 19	Revision of femoral head and acetabular liner
2013, 2Q, 39	Ankle fusion, osteotomy, and removal of hardware

AHA Coding Clinic for table ØSQ

| 2014, 4Q, 25 | Femoroacetabular impingement and labral tear with repair |

AHA Coding Clinic for table ØSR

2021, 1Q, 17	Revision of ankle arthroplasty with placement of tibial insert
2020, 3Q, 33	Total hip arthroplasty using dual mobility components
2018, 4Q, 43	Articulating spacer for hip and knee joint
2018, 2Q, 16	Exchange of tibial polyethylene component with stabilizing insert (tibial tray)
2017, 4Q, 38-39	Oxidized zirconium on polyethylene bearing surface
2017, 4Q, 107	Total ankle replacement versus revision
2017, 1Q, 22	Total knee replacement and patellar component
2016, 4Q, 110-111	Partial (unicondylar) knee replacement
2016, 4Q, 111-112	Removal and revision of hip and knee devices
2016, 1Q, 20	Use of cemented versus uncemented qualifier for joint replacement
2015, 3Q, 18	Total hip replacement with acetabular reconstruction
2015, 2Q, 18	Total knee revision
2015, 2Q, 19	Revision of femoral head and acetabular liner

AHA Coding Clinic for table ØSS

| 2016, 2Q, 31 | Periacetabular ostectomy for repair of congenital hip dysplasia |

AHA Coding Clinic for table ØST

| 2016, 1Q, 20 | Metatarsophalangeal joint resection arthroplasty |
| 2014, 4Q, 29 | Rotational osteosynthesis |

AHA Coding Clinic for table ØSU

2021, 1Q, 17	Revision of ankle arthroplasty with placement of tibial insert
2018, 2Q, 16	Exchange of tibial polyethylene component with stabilizing insert (tibial tray)
2016, 4Q, 111	Removal and revision of hip and knee devices
2015, 2Q, 19	Revision of femoral head and acetabular liner

AHA Coding Clinic for table ØSW

2017, 4Q, 107	Total ankle replacement versus revision
2016, 4Q, 110-112	Removal and revision of hip and knee devices
2015, 2Q, 18	Total knee revision
2015, 2Q, 19	Revision of femoral head and acetabular liner

Lower Joints

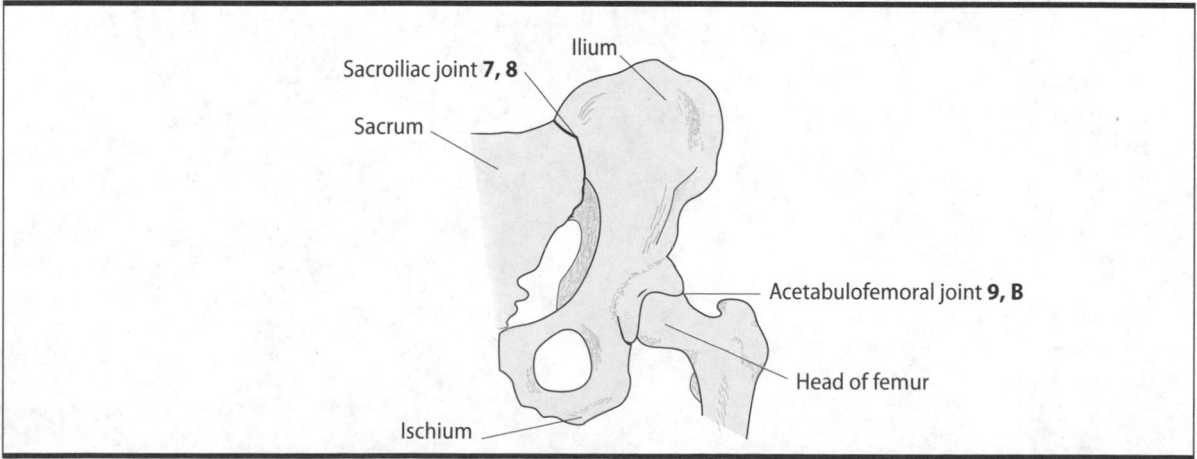

Sacroiliac **7, 8**

Lumbosacral **3**

Sacrococcygeal joint **5**

Hip **9, B**

Knee **C, D**

(Transverse) tarsal **H, J**

Metatarsal-phalangeal **M, N**

Ankle **F, G**

Hip Joint

Sacroiliac joint **7, 8**

Ilium

Sacrum

Acetabulofemoral joint **9, B**

Head of femur

Ischium

Knee Joint

Anterior view

Patella

Medial meniscus
cartilage

Lateral meniscus
cartilage

Lateral view

Femur

Synovial cavity

Patella

Tibia

Foot Joints

Phalanges

Metatarso-phalangeal
joints **M, N**

Tarsal joints **H, J**

Tarsometatarsal joints **K, L**

Distal
interphalangeal
joint **P, Q**

Proximal
interphalangeal
joint **P, Q**

Tarsals

Metatarsals

Ø   **Medical and Surgical**
S   **Lower Joints**
2   **Change**   Definition: Taking out or off a device from a body part and putting back an identical or similar device in or on the same body part without cutting or puncturing the skin or a mucous membrane
                          Explanation: All CHANGE procedures are coded using the approach EXTERNAL

Body Part Character 4	Approach Character 5	Device Character 6	Qualifier Character 7
Y Lower Joint	X External	Ø Drainage Device Y Other Device	Z No Qualifier

Non-OR	All body part, approach, device, and qualifier values

Ø   **Medical and Surgical**
S   **Lower Joints**
5   **Destruction**   Definition: Physical eradication of all or a portion of a body part by the direct use of energy, force, or a destructive agent
                          Explanation: None of the body part is physically taken out

Body Part Character 4	Approach Character 5	Device Character 6	Qualifier Character 7
Ø **Lumbar Vertebral Joint** 　　Lumbar facet joint 2 **Lumbar Vertebral Disc** 3 **Lumbosacral Joint** 　　Lumbosacral facet joint 4 **Lumbosacral Disc** 5 **Sacrococcygeal Joint** 　　Sacrococcygeal symphysis 6 **Coccygeal Joint** 7 **Sacroiliac Joint, Right** 8 **Sacroiliac Joint, Left** 9 **Hip Joint, Right** 　　Acetabulofemoral joint B **Hip Joint, Left** 　　*See 9 Hip Joint, Right* C **Knee Joint, Right** 　　Femoropatellar joint 　　Femorotibial joint 　　Lateral meniscus 　　Medial meniscus 　　Patellofemoral joint 　　Tibiofemoral joint D **Knee Joint, Left** 　　*See C Knee Joint, Right* F **Ankle Joint, Right** 　　Inferior tibiofibular joint 　　Talocrural joint G **Ankle Joint, Left** 　　*See F Ankle Joint, Right* H **Tarsal Joint, Right** 　　Calcaneocuboid joint 　　Cuboideonavicular joint 　　Cuneonavicular joint 　　Intercuneiform joint 　　Subtalar (talocalcaneal) joint 　　Talocalcaneal (subtalar) joint 　　Talocalcaneonavicular joint J **Tarsal Joint, Left** 　　*See H Tarsal Joint, Right* K **Tarsometatarsal Joint, Right** L **Tarsometatarsal Joint, Left** M **Metatarsal-Phalangeal Joint, Right** 　　Metatarsophalangeal (MTP) joint N **Metatarsal-Phalangeal Joint, Left** 　　*See M Metatarsal-Phalangeal Joint, Right* P **Toe Phalangeal Joint, Right** 　　Interphalangeal (IP) joint Q **Toe Phalangeal Joint, Left** 　　*See P Toe Phalangeal Joint, Right*	Ø Open 3 Percutaneous 4 Percutaneous Endoscopic	Z No Device	Z No Qualifier

NC Noncovered Procedure   LC Limited Coverage   QA Questionable OB Admit   NT New Tech Add-on   ⊞ Combination Member   ♂ Male   ♀ Female

ICD-10-PCS 2022   603

Ø **Medical and Surgical**
S **Lower Joints**
9 **Drainage**　　Definition: Taking or letting out fluids and/or gases from a body part

Explanation: The qualifier DIAGNOSTIC is used to identify drainage procedures that are biopsies

Body Part Character 4		Approach Character 5	Device Character 6	Qualifier Character 7
Ø **Lumbar Vertebral Joint** Lumbar facet joint **2** **Lumbar Vertebral Disc** **3** **Lumbosacral Joint** Lumbosacral facet joint **4** **Lumbosacral Disc** **5** **Sacrococcygeal Joint** Sacrococcygeal symphysis **6** **Coccygeal Joint** **7** **Sacroiliac Joint, Right** **8** **Sacroiliac Joint, Left** **9** **Hip Joint, Right** Acetabulofemoral joint **B** **Hip Joint, Left** *See 9 Hip Joint, Right* **C** **Knee Joint, Right** Femoropatellar joint Femorotibial joint Lateral meniscus Medial meniscus Patellofemoral joint Tibiofemoral joint **D** **Knee Joint, Left** *See C Knee Joint, Right* **F** **Ankle Joint, Right** Inferior tibiofibular joint Talocrural joint **G** **Ankle Joint, Left** *See F Ankle Joint, Right*	**H** **Tarsal Joint, Right** Calcaneocuboid joint Cuboideonavicular joint Cuneonavicular joint Intercuneiform joint Subtalar (talocalcaneal) joint Talocalcaneal (subtalar) joint Talocalcaneonavicular joint **J** **Tarsal Joint, Left** *See H Tarsal Joint, Right* **K** **Tarsometatarsal Joint, Right** **L** **Tarsometatarsal Joint, Left** **M** **Metatarsal-Phalangeal Joint, Right** Metatarsophalangeal (MTP) joint **N** **Metatarsal-Phalangeal Joint, Left** *See M Metatarsal-Phalangeal Joint, Right* **P** **Toe Phalangeal Joint, Right** Interphalangeal (IP) joint **Q** **Toe Phalangeal Joint, Left** *See P Toe Phalangeal Joint, Right*	**Ø** Open **3** Percutaneous **4** Percutaneous Endoscopic	**Ø** Drainage Device	**Z** No Qualifier
Ø **Lumbar Vertebral Joint** Lumbar facet joint **2** **Lumbar Vertebral Disc** **3** **Lumbosacral Joint** Lumbosacral facet joint **4** **Lumbosacral Disc** **5** **Sacrococcygeal Joint** Sacrococcygeal symphysis **6** **Coccygeal Joint** **7** **Sacroiliac Joint, Right** **8** **Sacroiliac Joint, Left** **9** **Hip Joint, Right** Acetabulofemoral joint **B** **Hip Joint, Left** *See 9 Hip Joint, Right* **C** **Knee Joint, Right** Femoropatellar joint Femorotibial joint Lateral meniscus Medial meniscus Patellofemoral joint Tibiofemoral joint **D** **Knee Joint, Left** *See C Knee Joint, Right* **F** **Ankle Joint, Right** Inferior tibiofibular joint Talocrural joint **G** **Ankle Joint, Left** *See F Ankle Joint, Right*	**H** **Tarsal Joint, Right** Calcaneocuboid joint Cuboideonavicular joint Cuneonavicular joint Intercuneiform joint Subtalar (talocalcaneal) joint Talocalcaneal (subtalar) joint Talocalcaneonavicular joint **J** **Tarsal Joint, Left** *See H Tarsal Joint, Right* **K** **Tarsometatarsal Joint, Right** **L** **Tarsometatarsal Joint, Left** **M** **Metatarsal-Phalangeal Joint, Right** Metatarsophalangeal (MTP) joint **N** **Metatarsal-Phalangeal Joint, Left** *See M Metatarsal-Phalangeal Joint, Right* **P** **Toe Phalangeal Joint, Right** Interphalangeal (IP) joint **Q** **Toe Phalangeal Joint, Left** *See P Toe Phalangeal Joint, Right*	**Ø** Open **3** Percutaneous **4** Percutaneous Endoscopic	**Z** No Device	**X** Diagnostic **Z** No Qualifier

Non-OR　　ØS9[Ø,2,3,4,5,6,7,8,9,B,C,D,F,G,H,J,K,L,M,N,P,Q][3,4]ØZ
Non-OR　　ØS9[Ø,2,3,4,5,6,7,8,9,B,C,D,F,G,H,J,K,L,M,N,P,Q][Ø,3,4]ZX
Non-OR　　ØS9[Ø,2,3,4,5,6,7,8,9,B,C,D,F,G,H,J,K,L,M,N,P,Q][3,4]ZZ

Non-OR Procedure　　DRG Non-OR Procedure　　Valid OR Procedure　　HAC Associated Procedure　　Combination Only　　New/Revised GREEN
604　　　ICD-10-PCS 2022

ØS9–ØS9

Ø   **Medical and Surgical**
S   **Lower Joints**
B   **Excision**   Definition: Cutting out or off, without replacement, a portion of a body part
                 Explanation: The qualifier DIAGNOSTIC is used to identify excision procedures that are biopsies

Body Part Character 4	Approach Character 5	Device Character 6	Qualifier Character 7

Ø   **Lumbar Vertebral Joint**
    Lumbar facet joint
2   **Lumbar Vertebral Disc**
3   **Lumbosacral Joint**
    Lumbosacral facet joint
4   **Lumbosacral Disc**
5   **Sacrococcygeal Joint**
    Sacrococcygeal symphysis
6   **Coccygeal Joint**
7   **Sacroiliac Joint, Right**
8   **Sacroiliac Joint, Left**
9   **Hip Joint, Right**
    Acetabulofemoral joint
B   **Hip Joint, Left**
    See 9 Hip Joint, Right
C   **Knee Joint, Right**
    Femoropatellar joint
    Femorotibial joint
    Lateral meniscus
    Medial meniscus
    Patellofemoral joint
    Tibiofemoral joint
D   **Knee Joint, Left**
    See C Knee Joint, Right
F   **Ankle Joint, Right**
    Inferior tibiofibular joint
    Talocrural joint
G   **Ankle Joint, Left**
    See F Ankle Joint, Right
H   **Tarsal Joint, Right**
    Calcaneocuboid joint
    Cuboideonavicular joint
    Cuneonavicular joint
    Intercuneiform joint
    Subtalar (talocalcaneal) joint
    Talocalcaneal (subtalar) joint
    Talocalcaneonavicular joint
J   **Tarsal Joint, Left**
    See H Tarsal Joint, Right
K   **Tarsometatarsal Joint, Right**
L   **Tarsometatarsal Joint, Left**
M   **Metatarsal-Phalangeal Joint, Right**
    Metatarsophalangeal (MTP) joint
N   **Metatarsal-Phalangeal Joint, Left**
    See M Metatarsal-Phalangeal Joint, Right
P   **Toe Phalangeal Joint, Right**
    Interphalangeal (IP) joint
Q   **Toe Phalangeal Joint, Left**
    See P Toe Phalangeal Joint, Right
	Ø Open
	3 Percutaneous
	4 Percutaneous Endoscopic
		Z No Device	X Diagnostic
			Z No Qualifier

Non-OR   ØSB[Ø,2,3,4,5,6,7,8,9,B,C,D,F,G,H,J,K,L,M,N,P,Q][Ø,3,4]ZX

NC Noncovered Procedure   LC Limited Coverage   QA Questionable OB Admit   NT New Tech Add-on   ⊞ Combination Member   ♂ Male   ♀ Female

ICD-10-PCS 2022   605

ØSB-ØSB

Ø   Medical and Surgical
S   Lower Joints
C   Extirpation   Definition: Taking or cutting out solid matter from a body part

Explanation: The solid matter may be an abnormal byproduct of a biological function or a foreign body; it may be imbedded in a body part or in the lumen of a tubular body part. The solid matter may or may not have been previously broken into pieces.

Body Part Character 4	Approach Character 5	Device Character 6	Qualifier Character 7

Ø Lumbar Vertebral Joint
    Lumbar facet joint
2 Lumbar Vertebral Disc
3 Lumbosacral Joint
    Lumbosacral facet joint
4 Lumbosacral Disc
5 Sacrococcygeal Joint
    Sacrococcygeal symphysis
6 Coccygeal Joint
7 Sacroiliac Joint, Right
8 Sacroiliac Joint, Left
9 Hip Joint, Right
    Acetabulofemoral joint
B Hip Joint, Left
    See 9 Hip Joint, Right
C Knee Joint, Right
    Femoropatellar joint
    Femorotibial joint
    Lateral meniscus
    Medial meniscus
    Patellofemoral joint
    Tibiofemoral joint
D Knee Joint, Left
    See C Knee Joint, Right
F Ankle Joint, Right
    Inferior tibiofibular joint
    Talocrural joint
G Ankle Joint, Left
    See F Ankle Joint, Right
H Tarsal Joint, Right
    Calcaneocuboid joint
    Cuboideonavicular joint
    Cuneonavicular joint
    Intercuneiform joint
    Subtalar (talocalcaneal) joint
    Talocalcaneal (subtalar) joint
    Talocalcaneonavicular joint
J Tarsal Joint, Left
    See H Tarsal Joint, Right
K Tarsometatarsal Joint, Right
L Tarsometatarsal Joint, Left
M Metatarsal-Phalangeal Joint, Right
    Metatarsophalangeal (MTP) joint
N Metatarsal-Phalangeal Joint, Left
    See M Metatarsal-Phalangeal Joint, Right
P Toe Phalangeal Joint, Right
    Interphalangeal (IP) joint
Q Toe Phalangeal Joint, Left
    See P Toe Phalangeal Joint, Right
	Ø Open
	3 Percutaneous
	4 Percutaneous Endoscopic
		Z No Device	**Z** No Qualifier

Lower Joints

Ø   Medical and Surgical
S   Lower Joints
G   Fusion   Definition: Joining together portions of an articular body part rendering the articular body part immobile
                   Explanation: The body part is joined together by fixation device, bone graft, or other means

Body Part Character 4	Approach Character 5	Device Character 6	Qualifier Character 7

Ø **Lumbar Vertebral Joint**
   Lumbar facet joint
1 **Lumbar Vertebral Joints, 2 or more** ⊞
3 **Lumbosacral Joint**
   Lumbosacral facet joint
	Ø Open
	3 Percutaneous
	4 Percutaneous Endoscopic
		7 Autologous Tissue Substitute
		J Synthetic Substitute
		K Nonautologous Tissue Substitute
			Ø Anterior Approach, Anterior Column
			1 Posterior Approach, Posterior Column
			J Posterior Approach, Anterior Column

Ø **Lumbar Vertebral Joint**
   Lumbar facet joint
1 **Lumbar Vertebral Joints, 2 or more** ⊞
3 **Lumbosacral Joint**
   Lumbosacral facet joint
	Ø Open
	3 Percutaneous
	4 Percutaneous Endoscopic
		A Interbody Fusion Device	**Ø** Anterior Approach, Anterior Column
			J Posterior Approach, Anterior Column

5 **Sacrococcygeal Joint** Sacrococcygeal symphysis **6** **Coccygeal Joint** **7** **Sacroiliac Joint, Right** **8** **Sacroiliac Joint, Left**	**Ø** Open **3** Percutaneous **4** Percutaneous Endoscopic	**4** Internal Fixation Device **7** Autologous Tissue Substitute **J** Synthetic Substitute **K** Nonautologous Tissue Substitute	**Z** No Qualifier

9 **Hip Joint, Right**
   Acetabulofemoral joint
B **Hip Joint, Left**
   See 9 Hip Joint, Right
C **Knee Joint, Right**
   Femoropatellar joint
   Femorotibial joint
   Lateral meniscus
   Medial meniscus
   Patellofemoral joint
   Tibiofemoral joint
D **Knee Joint, Left**
   See C Knee Joint, Right
F **Ankle Joint, Right**
   Inferior tibiofibular joint
   Talocrural joint
G **Ankle Joint, Left**
   See F Ankle Joint, Right
H **Tarsal Joint, Right**
   Calcaneocuboid joint
   Cuboideonavicular joint
   Cuneonavicular joint
   Intercuneiform joint
   Subtalar (talocalcaneal) joint
   Talocalcaneal (subtalar) joint
   Talocalcaneonavicular joint
J **Tarsal Joint, Left**
   See H Tarsal Joint, Right
K **Tarsometatarsal Joint, Right**
L **Tarsometatarsal Joint, Left**
M **Metatarsal-Phalangeal Joint, Right**
   Metatarsophalangeal (MTP) joint
N **Metatarsal-Phalangeal Joint, Left**
   See M Metatarsal-Phalangeal Joint, Right
P **Toe Phalangeal Joint, Right**
   Interphalangeal (IP) joint
Q **Toe Phalangeal Joint, Left**
   See P Toe Phalangeal Joint, Right
	Ø Open
	3 Percutaneous
	4 Percutaneous Endoscopic
		3 Internal Fixation Device, Sustained Compression
		4 Internal Fixation Device
		5 External Fixation Device
		7 Autologous Tissue Substitute
		J Synthetic Substitute
		K Nonautologous Tissue Substitute
			Z No Qualifier

HAC   ØSG[Ø,1,3][Ø,3,4][7,J,K][Ø,1,J] when reported with SDx K68.11 or T81.4Ø–T81.49, T84.6Ø-T84.619, T84.63-T84.7 with 7th character A
HAC   ØSG[Ø,1,3][Ø,3,4]A[Ø,J] when reported with SDx K68.11 or T81.4Ø–T81.49, T84.6Ø-T84.619, T84.63-T84.7 with 7th character A
HAC   ØSG[7,8][Ø,3,4][4,7,J,K]Z when reported with SDx K68.11 or T81.4Ø–T81.49, T84.6Ø-T84.619, T84.63-T84.7 with 7th character A

See Appendix L for Procedure Combinations
⊞   ØSG1[Ø,3,4][7,J,K][Ø,1,J]
⊞   ØSG1[Ø,3,4]A[Ø,J]

NC Noncovered Procedure   LC Limited Coverage   QA Questionable OB Admit   NT New Tech Add-on   ⊞ Combination Member   ♂ Male   ♀ Female

Ø   **Medical and Surgical**
S   **Lower Joints**
H   **Insertion**   Definition: Putting in a nonbiological appliance that monitors, assists, performs, or prevents a physiological function but does not physically take the place of a body part
                 Explanation: None

Body Part Character 4	Approach Character 5	Device Character 6	Qualifier Character 7

Ø Lumbar Vertebral Joint
    Lumbar facet joint
3 Lumbosacral Joint
    Lumbosacral facet joint
	Ø Open
	3 Percutaneous
	4 Percutaneous Endoscopic
		3 Infusion Device
		4 Internal Fixation Device
		8 Spacer
		B Spinal Stabilization Device, Interspinous Process
		C Spinal Stabilization Device, Pedicle-Based
		D Spinal Stabilization Device, Facet Replacement
			Z No Qualifier

2 Lumbar Vertebral Disc **4** Lumbosacral Disc	**Ø** Open **3** Percutaneous **4** Percutaneous Endoscopic	**3** Infusion Device **8** Spacer	**Z** No Qualifier
5 Sacrococcygeal Joint Sacrococcygeal symphysis **6** Coccygeal Joint **7** Sacroiliac Joint, Right **8** Sacroiliac Joint, Left	**Ø** Open **3** Percutaneous **4** Percutaneous Endoscopic	**3** Infusion Device **4** Internal Fixation Device **8** Spacer	**Z** No Qualifier

9 Hip Joint, Right
    Acetabulofemoral joint
B Hip Joint, Left
    See 9 Hip Joint, Right
C Knee Joint, Right
    Femoropatellar joint
    Femorotibial joint
    Lateral meniscus
    Medial meniscus
    Patellofemoral joint
    Tibiofemoral joint
D Knee Joint, Left
    See C Knee Joint, Right
F Ankle Joint, Right
    Inferior tibiofibular joint
    Talocrural joint
G Ankle Joint, Left
    See F Ankle Joint, Right
H Tarsal Joint, Right
    Calcaneocuboid joint
    Cuboideonavicular joint
    Cuneonavicular joint
    Intercuneiform joint
    Subtalar (talocalcaneal) joint
    Talocalcaneal (subtalar) joint
    Talocalcaneonavicular joint
J Tarsal Joint, Left
    See H Tarsal Joint, Right
K Tarsometatarsal Joint, Right
L Tarsometatarsal Joint, Left
M Metatarsal-Phalangeal Joint, Right
    Metatarsophalangeal (MTP) joint
N Metatarsal-Phalangeal Joint, Left
    See M Metatarsal-Phalangeal Joint, Right
P Toe Phalangeal Joint, Right
    Interphalangeal (IP) joint
Q Toe Phalangeal Joint, Left
    See P Toe Phalangeal Joint, Right
	Ø Open
	3 Percutaneous
	4 Percutaneous Endoscopic
		3 Infusion Device
		4 Internal Fixation Device
		5 External Fixation Device
		8 Spacer
			Z No Qualifier

Non-OR	ØSH[Ø,3][Ø,3,4][3,8]Z
Non-OR	ØSH[2,4][Ø,3,4][3,8]Z
Non-OR	ØSH[5,6,7,8][Ø,3,4][3,8]Z
Non-OR	ØSH[9,B,C,D][Ø,3,4]3Z
Non-OR	ØSH[9,B,C,D][3,4]8Z
Non-OR	ØSH[F,G,H,J,K,L,M,N,P,Q][Ø,3,4][3,8]Z

Ø   Medical and Surgical
S   Lower Joints
J   Inspection   Definition: Visually and/or manually exploring a body part

Explanation: Visual exploration may be performed with or without optical instrumentation. Manual exploration may be performed directly or through intervening body layers.

Body Part Character 4	Approach Character 5	Device Character 6	Qualifier Character 7
Ø Lumbar Vertebral Joint Lumbar facet joint **2 Lumbar Vertebral Disc** **3 Lumbosacral Joint** Lumbosacral facet joint **4 Lumbosacral Disc** **5 Sacrococcygeal Joint** Sacrococcygeal symphysis **6 Coccygeal Joint** **7 Sacroiliac Joint, Right** **8 Sacroiliac Joint, Left** **9 Hip Joint, Right** Acetabulofemoral joint **B Hip Joint, Left** *See 9 Hip Joint, Right* **C Knee Joint, Right** Femoropatellar joint Femorotibial joint Lateral meniscus Medial meniscus Patellofemoral joint Tibiofemoral joint **D Knee Joint, Left** *See C Knee Joint, Right* **F Ankle Joint, Right** Inferior tibiofibular joint Talocrural joint **G Ankle Joint, Left** *See F Ankle Joint, Right*	**H Tarsal Joint, Right** Calcaneocuboid joint Cuboideonavicular joint Cuneonavicular joint Intercuneiform joint Subtalar (talocalcaneal) joint Talocalcaneal (subtalar) joint Talocalcaneonavicular joint **J Tarsal Joint, Left** *See H Tarsal Joint, Right* **K Tarsometatarsal Joint, Right** **L Tarsometatarsal Joint, Left** **M Metatarsal-Phalangeal Joint, Right** Metatarsophalangeal (MTP) joint **N Metatarsal-Phalangeal Joint, Left** *See M Metatarsal-Phalangeal Joint, Right* **P Toe Phalangeal Joint, Right** Interphalangeal (IP) joint **Q Toe Phalangeal Joint, Left** *See P Toe Phalangeal Joint, Right*	**Ø Open** **3 Percutaneous** **4 Percutaneous Endoscopic** **X External**	**Z No Device**	**Z No Qualifier**

Non-OR   ØSJ[Ø,2,3,4,5,6,7,8,9,B,C,D,F,G,H,J,K,L,M,N,P,Q][3,X]ZZ

Ø   Medical and Surgical
S   Lower Joints
N   Release   Definition: Freeing a body part from an abnormal physical constraint by cutting or by the use of force

Explanation: Some of the restraining tissue may be taken out but none of the body part is taken out

Body Part Character 4	Approach Character 5	Device Character 6	Qualifier Character 7
Ø Lumbar Vertebral Joint Lumbar facet joint **2 Lumbar Vertebral Disc** **3 Lumbosacral Joint** Lumbosacral facet joint **4 Lumbosacral Disc** **5 Sacrococcygeal Joint** Sacrococcygeal symphysis **6 Coccygeal Joint** **7 Sacroiliac Joint, Right** **8 Sacroiliac Joint, Left** **9 Hip Joint, Right** Acetabulofemoral joint **B Hip Joint, Left** *See 9 Hip Joint, Right* **C Knee Joint, Right** Femoropatellar joint Femorotibial joint Lateral meniscus Medial meniscus Patellofemoral joint Tibiofemoral joint **D Knee Joint, Left** *See C Knee Joint, Right* **F Ankle Joint, Right** Inferior tibiofibular joint Talocrural joint **G Ankle Joint, Left** *See F Ankle Joint, Right*	**H Tarsal Joint, Right** Calcaneocuboid joint Cuboideonavicular joint Cuneonavicular joint Intercuneiform joint Subtalar (talocalcaneal) joint Talocalcaneal (subtalar) joint Talocalcaneonavicular joint **J Tarsal Joint, Left** *See H Tarsal Joint, Right* **K Tarsometatarsal Joint, Right** **L Tarsometatarsal Joint, Left** **M Metatarsal-Phalangeal Joint, Right** Metatarsophalangeal (MTP) joint **N Metatarsal-Phalangeal Joint, Left** *See M Metatarsal-Phalangeal Joint, Right* **P Toe Phalangeal Joint, Right** Interphalangeal (IP) joint **Q Toe Phalangeal Joint, Left** *See P Toe Phalangeal Joint, Right*	**Ø Open** **3 Percutaneous** **4 Percutaneous Endoscopic** **X External**	**Z No Device**	**Z No Qualifier**

Non-OR   ØSN[Ø,2,3,4,5,6,7,8,9,B,C,D,F,G,H,J,K,L,M,N,P,Q]XZZ

NC Noncovered Procedure   LC Limited Coverage   QA Questionable OB Admit   NT New Tech Add-on   ⊞ Combination Member   ♂ Male   ♀ Female

Lower Joints

Ø **Medical and Surgical**
S **Lower Joints**
P **Removal**

Definition: Taking out or off a device from a body part

Explanation: If a device is taken out and a similar device put in without cutting or puncturing the skin or mucous membrane, the procedure is coded to the root operation CHANGE. Otherwise, the procedure for taking out the device is coded to the root operation REMOVAL.

Body Part Character 4	Approach Character 5	Device Character 6	Qualifier Character 7
Ø Lumbar Vertebral Joint Lumbar facet joint 3 Lumbosacral Joint Lumbosacral facet joint	Ø Open 3 Percutaneous 4 Percutaneous Endoscopic	Ø Drainage Device 3 Infusion Device 4 Internal Fixation Device 7 Autologous Tissue Substitute 8 Spacer A Interbody Fusion Device J Synthetic Substitute K Nonautologous Tissue Substitute	Z No Qualifier
Ø Lumbar Vertebral Joint Lumbar facet joint 3 Lumbosacral Joint Lumbosacral facet joint	X External	Ø Drainage Device 3 Infusion Device 4 Internal Fixation Device	Z No Qualifier
2 Lumbar Vertebral Disc 4 Lumbosacral Disc	Ø Open 3 Percutaneous 4 Percutaneous Endoscopic	Ø Drainage Device 3 Infusion Device 7 Autologous Tissue Substitute J Synthetic Substitute K Nonautologous Tissue Substitute	Z No Qualifier
2 Lumbar Vertebral Disc 4 Lumbosacral Disc	X External	Ø Drainage Device 3 Infusion Device	Z No Qualifier
5 Sacrococcygeal Joint Sacrococcygeal symphysis 6 Coccygeal Joint 7 Sacroiliac Joint, Right 8 Sacroiliac Joint, Left	Ø Open 3 Percutaneous 4 Percutaneous Endoscopic	Ø Drainage Device 3 Infusion Device 4 Internal Fixation Device 7 Autologous Tissue Substitute 8 Spacer J Synthetic Substitute K Nonautologous Tissue Substitute	Z No Qualifier
5 Sacrococcygeal Joint Sacrococcygeal symphysis 6 Coccygeal Joint 7 Sacroiliac Joint, Right 8 Sacroiliac Joint, Left	X External	Ø Drainage Device 3 Infusion Device 4 Internal Fixation Device	Z No Qualifier
9 Hip Joint, Right ⊞ Acetabulofemoral joint B Hip Joint, Left ⊞ See 9 Hip Joint, Right	Ø Open	Ø Drainage Device 3 Infusion Device 4 Internal Fixation Device 5 External Fixation Device 7 Autologous Tissue Substitute 8 Spacer 9 Liner B Resurfacing Device E Articulating Spacer J Synthetic Substitute K Nonautologous Tissue Substitute	Z No Qualifier
9 Hip Joint, Right ⊞ Acetabulofemoral joint B Hip Joint, Left ⊞ See 9 Hip Joint, Right	3 Percutaneous 4 Percutaneous Endoscopic	Ø Drainage Device 3 Infusion Device 4 Internal Fixation Device 5 External Fixation Device 7 Autologous Tissue Substitute 8 Spacer J Synthetic Substitute K Nonautologous Tissue Substitute	Z No Qualifier
9 Hip Joint, Right Acetabulofemoral joint B Hip Joint, Left See 9 Hip Joint, Right	X External	Ø Drainage Device 3 Infusion Device 4 Internal Fixation Device 5 External Fixation Device	Z No Qualifier

Non-OR	ØSP[Ø,3][Ø,3,4]8Z
Non-OR	ØSP[Ø,3]3[Ø,3]Z
Non-OR	ØSP[Ø,3]X[Ø,3,4]Z
Non-OR	ØSP[2,4]3[Ø,3]Z
Non-OR	ØSP[2,4]X[Ø,3]Z
Non-OR	ØSP[5,6,7,8][Ø,3,4]8Z
Non-OR	ØSP[5,6,7,8]3[Ø,3]Z
Non-OR	ØSP[5,6,7,8]X[Ø,3,4]Z
Non-OR	ØSP[9,B]3[Ø,3,8]Z
Non-OR	ØSP[9,B]X[Ø,3,4,5]Z

See Appendix L for Procedure Combinations

Combo-only	ØSP[9,B]48Z
⊞	ØSP[9,B]Ø[8,9,B,E,J]Z
⊞	ØSP[9,B]4JZ

ØSP Continued on next page

Non-OR Procedure   DRG Non-OR Procedure   Valid OR Procedure   HAC Associated Procedure   Combination Only   New/Revised GREEN

Ø   **Medical and Surgical**   ***ØSP Continued***
S   **Lower Joints**
P   **Removal**   Definition: Taking out or off a device from a body part

                      Explanation: If a device is taken out and a similar device put in without cutting or puncturing the skin or mucous membrane, the procedure is coded to the root operation CHANGE. Otherwise, the procedure for taking out the device is coded to the root operation REMOVAL.

Body Part Character 4	Approach Character 5	Device Character 6	Qualifier Character 7

A Hip Joint, Acetabular Surface, ⊞
    Right
E Hip Joint, Acetabular Surface, ⊞
    Left
R Hip Joint, Femoral Surface, ⊞
    Right
S Hip Joint, Femoral Surface, Left ⊞
T Knee Joint, Femoral Surface, ⊞
    Right
    Femoropatellar joint
    Patellofemoral joint
U Knee Joint, Femoral Surface, ⊞
    Left
    See T Knee Joint, Femoral Surface,
       Right
V Knee Joint, Tibial Surface, Right ⊞
    Femorotibial joint
    Tibiofemoral joint
W Knee Joint, Tibial Surface, Left ⊞
    See V Knee Joint, Tibial Surface, Right
	Ø Open
	3 Percutaneous
	4 Percutaneous Endoscopic
		J Synthetic Substitute	**Z** No Qualifier

C Knee Joint, Right ⊞
    Femoropatellar joint
    Femorotibial joint
    Lateral meniscus
    Medial meniscus
    Patellofemoral joint
    Tibiofemoral joint
D Knee Joint, Left ⊞
    See C Knee Joint, Right
	Ø Open	**Ø** Drainage Device
		3 Infusion Device
		4 Internal Fixation Device
		5 External Fixation Device
		7 Autologous Tissue Substitute
		8 Spacer
		9 Liner
		E Articulating Spacer
		K Nonautologous Tissue Substitute
		L Synthetic Substitute, Unicondylar
		    Medial
		M Synthetic Substitute, Unicondylar
		    Lateral
		N Synthetic Substitute, Patellofemoral
			Z No Qualifier

C Knee Joint, Right ⊞
    Femoropatellar joint
    Femorotibial joint
    Lateral meniscus
    Medial meniscus
    Patellofemoral joint
    Tibiofemoral joint
D Knee Joint, Left ⊞
    See C Knee Joint, Right
	Ø Open	**J** Synthetic Substitute	**C** Patellar Surface
			Z No Qualifier

C Knee Joint, Right ⊞
    Femoropatellar joint
    Femorotibial joint
    Lateral meniscus
    Medial meniscus
    Patellofemoral joint
    Tibiofemoral joint
D Knee Joint, Left ⊞
    See C Knee Joint, Right
	3 Percutaneous
	4 Percutaneous Endoscopic
		Ø Drainage Device
		3 Infusion Device
		4 Internal Fixation Device
		5 External Fixation Device
		7 Autologous Tissue Substitute
		8 Spacer
		K Nonautologous Tissue Substitute
		L Synthetic Substitute, Unicondylar
		    Medial
		M Synthetic Substitute, Unicondylar
		    Lateral
		N Synthetic Substitute, Patellofemoral
			Z No Qualifier

C Knee Joint, Right ⊞
    Femoropatellar joint
    Femorotibial joint
    Lateral meniscus
    Medial meniscus
    Patellofemoral joint
    Tibiofemoral joint
D Knee Joint, Left ⊞
    See C Knee Joint, Right
	3 Percutaneous
	4 Percutaneous Endoscopic
		J Synthetic Substitute	**C** Patellar Surface
			Z No Qualifier

Non-OR   ØSP[C,D]3[Ø,3]Z

See Appendix L for Procedure Combinations
Combo-only   ØSP[C,D][3,4]8Z   ⊞   ØSP[C,D]ØJ[C,Z]
⊞   ØSP[A,E,R,S,T,U,V,W][Ø,4]JZ   ⊞   ØSP[C,D]4[L,M,N]Z
⊞   ØSP[C,D]Ø[8,9,E,L,M,N]Z   ⊞   ØSP[C,D]4J[C,Z]

ØSP Continued on next page

NC Noncovered Procedure   **LC** Limited Coverage   **OA** Questionable OB Admit   **NT** New Tech Add-on   ⊞ Combination Member   ♂ Male   ♀ Female

Lower Joints

Ø Medical and Surgical
S Lower Joints
P Removal

ØSP Continued

Definition: Taking out or off a device from a body part

Explanation: If a device is taken out and a similar device put in without cutting or puncturing the skin or mucous membrane, the procedure is coded to the root operation CHANGE. Otherwise, the procedure for taking out the device is coded to the root operation REMOVAL.

Body Part Character 4	Approach Character 5	Device Character 6	Qualifier Character 7
C Knee Joint, Right Femoropatellar joint Femorotibial joint Lateral meniscus Medial meniscus Patellofemoral joint Tibiofemoral joint **D Knee Joint, Left** *See C Knee Joint, Right*	**X External**	**Ø Drainage Device** **3 Infusion Device** **4 Internal Fixation Device** **5 External Fixation Device**	**Z No Qualifier**
F Ankle Joint, Right Inferior tibiofibular joint Talocrural joint **G Ankle Joint, Left** *See F Ankle Joint, Right* **H Tarsal Joint, Right** Calcaneocuboid joint Cuboideonavicular joint Cuneonavicular joint Intercuneiform joint Subtalar (talocalcaneal) joint Talocalcaneal (subtalar) joint Talocalcaneonavicular joint **J Tarsal Joint, Left** *See H Tarsal Joint, Right* **K Tarsometatarsal Joint, Right** **L Tarsometatarsal Joint, Left** **M Metatarsal-Phalangeal Joint, Right** Metatarsophalangeal (MTP) joint **N Metatarsal-Phalangeal Joint, Left** *See M Metatarsal-Phalangeal Joint, Right* **P Toe Phalangeal Joint, Right** Interphalangeal (IP) joint **Q Toe Phalangeal Joint, Left** *See P Toe Phalangeal Joint, Right*	**Ø Open** **3 Percutaneous** **4 Percutaneous Endoscopic**	**Ø Drainage Device** **3 Infusion Device** **4 Internal Fixation Device** **5 External Fixation Device** **7 Autologous Tissue Substitute** **8 Spacer** **J Synthetic Substitute** **K Nonautologous Tissue Substitute**	**Z No Qualifier**
F Ankle Joint, Right Inferior tibiofibular joint Talocrural joint **G Ankle Joint, Left** *See F Ankle Joint, Right* **H Tarsal Joint, Right** Calcaneocuboid joint Cuboideonavicular joint Cuneonavicular joint Intercuneiform joint Subtalar (talocalcaneal) joint Talocalcaneal (subtalar) joint Talocalcaneonavicular joint **J Tarsal Joint, Left** *See H Tarsal Joint, Right* **K Tarsometatarsal Joint, Right** **L Tarsometatarsal Joint, Left** **M Metatarsal-Phalangeal Joint, Right** Metatarsophalangeal (MTP) joint **N Metatarsal-Phalangeal Joint, Left** *See M Metatarsal-Phalangeal Joint, Right* **P Toe Phalangeal Joint, Right** Interphalangeal (IP) joint **Q Toe Phalangeal Joint, Left** *See P Toe Phalangeal Joint, Right*	**X External**	**Ø Drainage Device** **3 Infusion Device** **4 Internal Fixation Device** **5 External Fixation Device**	**Z No Qualifier**

Non-OR ØSP[C,D]X[Ø,3,4,5]Z
Non-OR ØSP[F,G,H,J,K,L,M,N,P,Q]3[Ø,3,8]Z
Non-OR ØSP[F,G,H,J,K,L,M,N,P,Q][Ø,4]8Z
Non-OR ØSP[F,G,H,J,K,L,M,N,P,Q]X[Ø,3,4,5]Z

Ø   Medical and Surgical
S   Lower Joints
Q   Repair   Definition: Restoring, to the extent possible, a body part to its normal anatomic structure and function
                   Explanation: Used only when the method to accomplish the repair is not one of the other root operations

Body Part Character 4	Approach Character 5	Device Character 6	Qualifier Character 7

Ø   **Lumbar Vertebral Joint**
    Lumbar facet joint
2   **Lumbar Vertebral Disc**
3   **Lumbosacral Joint**
    Lumbosacral facet joint
4   **Lumbosacral Disc**
5   **Sacrococcygeal Joint**
    Sacrococcygeal symphysis
6   **Coccygeal Joint**
7   **Sacroiliac Joint, Right**
8   **Sacroiliac Joint, Left**
9   **Hip Joint, Right**
    Acetabulofemoral joint
B   **Hip Joint, Left**
    See 9 Hip Joint, Right
C   **Knee Joint, Right**
    Femoropatellar joint
    Femorotibial joint
    Lateral meniscus
    Medial meniscus
    Patellofemoral joint
    Tibiofemoral joint
D   **Knee Joint, Left**
    See C Knee Joint, Right
F   **Ankle Joint, Right**
    Inferior tibiofibular joint
    Talocrural joint
G   **Ankle Joint, Left**
    See F Ankle Joint, Right
H   **Tarsal Joint, Right**
    Calcaneocuboid joint
    Cuboideonavicular joint
    Cuneonavicular joint
    Intercuneiform joint
    Subtalar (talocalcaneal) joint
    Talocalcaneal (subtalar) joint
    Talocalcaneonavicular joint
J   **Tarsal Joint, Left**
    See H Tarsal Joint, Right
K   **Tarsometatarsal Joint, Right**
L   **Tarsometatarsal Joint, Left**
M   **Metatarsal-Phalangeal Joint, Right**
    Metatarsophalangeal (MTP) joint
N   **Metatarsal-Phalangeal Joint, Left**
    See M Metatarsal-Phalangeal Joint, Right
P   **Toe Phalangeal Joint, Right**
    Interphalangeal (IP) joint
Q   **Toe Phalangeal Joint, Left**
    See P Toe Phalangeal Joint, Right
	Ø Open
	3 Percutaneous
	4 Percutaneous Endoscopic
	X External
		Z No Device	**Z** No Qualifier

Non-OR   ØSQ[Ø,2,3,4,5,6,7,8,9,B,C,D,F,G,H,J,K,L,M,N,P,Q]XZZ

Ø   **Medical and Surgical**
S   **Lower Joints**
R   **Replacement**   Definition: Putting in or on biological or synthetic material that physically takes the place and/or function of all or a portion of a body part
                             Explanation: The body part may have been taken out or replaced, or may be taken out, physically eradicated, or rendered nonfunctional during
                             the REPLACEMENT procedure. A REMOVAL procedure is coded for taking out the device used in a previous replacement procedure.

Body Part Character 4	Approach Character 5	Device Character 6	Qualifier Character 7

Ø **Lumbar Vertebral Joint**
    Lumbar facet joint
2 **Lumbar Vertebral Disc**   NC
3 **Lumbosacral Joint**
    Lumbosacral facet joint
4 **Lumbosacral Disc**   NC
5 **Sacrococcygeal Joint**
    Sacrococcygeal symphysis
6 **Coccygeal Joint**
7 **Sacroiliac Joint, Right**
8 **Sacroiliac Joint, Left**
H **Tarsal Joint, Right**
    Calcaneocuboid joint
    Cuboideonavicular joint
    Cuneonavicular joint
    Intercuneiform joint
    Subtalar (talocalcaneal) joint
    Talocalcaneal (subtalar) joint
    Talocalcaneonavicular joint
J **Tarsal Joint, Left**
    See H Tarsal Joint, Right
K **Tarsometatarsal Joint, Right**
L **Tarsometatarsal Joint, Left**
M **Metatarsal-Phalangeal Joint, Right**
    Metatarsophalangeal (MTP) joint
N **Metatarsal-Phalangeal Joint, Left**
    See M Metatarsal-Phalangeal Joint, Right
P **Toe Phalangeal Joint, Right**
    Interphalangeal (IP) joint
Q **Toe Phalangeal Joint, Left**
    See P Toe Phalangeal Joint, Right
	Ø Open	**7** Autologous Tissue Substitute
		J Synthetic Substitute
		K Nonautologous Tissue Substitute
			Z No Qualifier

9 **Hip Joint, Right** ⊞
    Acetabulofemoral joint
B **Hip Joint, Left** ⊞
    See 9 Hip Joint, Right
	Ø Open	**1** Synthetic Substitute, Metal
		2 Synthetic Substitute, Metal on
		    Polyethylene
		3 Synthetic Substitute, Ceramic
		4 Synthetic Substitute, Ceramic on
		    Polyethylene
		6 Synthetic Substitute, Oxidized
		    Zirconium on Polyethylene
		J Synthetic Substitute
			9 Cemented
			A Uncemented
			Z No Qualifier

9 **Hip Joint, Right** ⊞
    Acetabulofemoral joint
B **Hip Joint, Left** ⊞
    See 9 Hip Joint, Right
	Ø Open	**7** Autologous Tissue Substitute
		E Articulating Spacer
		K Nonautologous Tissue Substitute
			Z No Qualifier

A **Hip Joint, Acetabular Surface,
    Right** ⊞
E **Hip Joint, Acetabular Surface,
    Left** ⊞
	Ø Open	**Ø** Synthetic Substitute, Polyethylene
		1 Synthetic Substitute, Metal
		3 Synthetic Substitute, Ceramic
		J Synthetic Substitute
			9 Cemented
			A Uncemented
			Z No Qualifier

A **Hip Joint, Acetabular Surface, Right** **E** **Hip Joint, Acetabular Surface, Left**	**Ø** Open	**7** Autologous Tissue Substitute **K** Nonautologous Tissue Substitute	**Z** No Qualifier

HAC   ØSR[9,B]Ø[1,2,3,4,6,J][9,A,Z] when reported with SDx of I26.Ø2-I26.Ø9,
             I26.92-I26.99, or I82.4Ø1-I82.4Z9
HAC   ØSR[9,B]Ø[7,E,K]Z when reported with SDx of I26.Ø2-I26.Ø9, I26.92-I26.99,
             or I82.4Ø1-I82.4Z9
HAC   ØSR[A,E]Ø[Ø,1,3,J][9,A,Z] when reported with SDx of I26.Ø2-I26.Ø9,
             I26.92-I26.99, or I82.4Ø1-I82.4Z9
HAC   ØSR[A,E]Ø[7,K]Z when reported with SDx of I26.Ø2-I26.Ø9, I26.92-I26.99,
             or I82.4Ø1-I82.4Z9
NC   ØSR[2,4]ØJZ when beneficiary age is over 6Ø

See Appendix L for Procedure Combinations
⊞ ØSR[9,B]Ø[1,2,3,4,6,J][9,A,Z]
⊞ ØSR[9,B]ØEZ
⊞ ØSR[A,E]Ø[Ø,1,3,J][9,A,Z]

ØSR Continued on next page

Ø Medical and Surgical
S Lower Joints
R Replacement

ØSR Continued

Definition: Putting in or on biological or synthetic material that physically takes the place and/or function of all or a portion of a body part

Explanation: The body part may have been taken out or replaced, or may be taken out, physically eradicated, or rendered nonfunctional during the REPLACEMENT procedure. A REMOVAL procedure is coded for taking out the device used in a previous replacement procedure.

Body Part Character 4	Approach Character 5	Device Character 6	Qualifier Character 7
C Knee Joint, Right ⊞ Femoropatellar joint Femorotibial joint Lateral meniscus Medial meniscus Patellofemoral joint Tibiofemoral joint **D Knee Joint, Left** ⊞ *See C Knee Joint, Right*	Ø Open	6 Synthetic Substitute, Oxidized Zirconium on Polyethylene J Synthetic Substitute L Synthetic Substitute, Unicondylar Medial M Synthetic Substitute, Unicondylar Lateral N Synthetic Substitute, Patellofemoral	9 Cemented A Uncemented Z No Qualifier
C Knee Joint, Right ⊞ Femoropatellar joint Femorotibial joint Lateral meniscus Medial meniscus Patellofemoral joint Tibiofemoral joint **D Knee Joint, Left** ⊞ *See C Knee Joint, Right*	Ø Open	7 Autologous Tissue Substitute E Articulating Spacer K Nonautologous Tissue Substitute	Z No Qualifier
F Ankle Joint, Right Inferior tibiofibular joint Talocrural joint **G Ankle Joint, Left** *See F Ankle Joint, Right* **T Knee Joint, Femoral Surface, Right** Femoropatellar joint Patellofemoral joint **U Knee Joint, Femoral Surface, Left** *See T Knee Joint, Femoral Surface, Right* **V Knee Joint, Tibial Surface, Right** Femorotibial joint Tibiofemoral joint **W Knee Joint, Tibial Surface, Left** *See V Knee Joint, Tibial Surface, Right*	Ø Open	7 Autologous Tissue Substitute K Nonautologous Tissue Substitute	Z No Qualifier
F Ankle Joint, Right Inferior tibiofibular joint Talocrural joint **G Ankle Joint, Left** *See F Ankle Joint, Right* **T Knee Joint, Femoral Surface, Right** ⊞ Femoropatellar joint Patellofemoral joint **U Knee Joint, Femoral Surface, Left** ⊞ *See T Knee Joint, Femoral Surface, Right* **V Knee Joint, Tibial Surface, Right** ⊞ Femorotibial joint Tibiofemoral joint **W Knee Joint, Tibial Surface, Left** ⊞ *See V Knee Joint, Tibial Surface, Right*	Ø Open	J Synthetic Substitute	9 Cemented A Uncemented Z No Qualifier
R Hip Joint, Femoral Surface, Right ⊞ **S Hip Joint, Femoral Surface, Left** ⊞	Ø Open	1 Synthetic Substitute, Metal 3 Synthetic Substitute, Ceramic J Synthetic Substitute	9 Cemented A Uncemented Z No Qualifier
R Hip Joint, Femoral Surface, Right **S Hip Joint, Femoral Surface, Left**	Ø Open	7 Autologous Tissue Substitute K Nonautologous Tissue Substitute	Z No Qualifier

HAC	ØSR[C,D]Ø[6,J,L,M,N][9,A,Z] when reported with SDx of I26.Ø2-I26.Ø9, I26.92-I26.99 or I82.4Ø1-I82.4Z9
HAC	ØSR[C,D]Ø[7,E,K]Z when reported with SDx of I26.Ø2-I26.Ø9, I26.92-I26.99 or I82.4Ø1-I82.4Z9
HAC	ØSR[T,U,V,W]Ø[7,K]Z when reported with SDx of I26.Ø2-I26.Ø9, I26.92-I26.99 or I82.4Ø1-I82.4Z9
HAC	ØSR[T,U,V,W]ØJ[9,A,Z] when reported with SDx of I26.Ø2-I26.Ø9, I26.92-I26.99 or I82.4Ø1-I82.4Z9
HAC	ØSR[R,S]Ø[1,3,J][9,A,Z] when reported with SDx of I26.Ø2-I26.Ø9, I26.92-I26.99, or I82.4Ø1-I82.4Z9
HAC	ØSR[R,S]Ø[7,K]Z when reported with SDx of I26.Ø2-I26.Ø9, I26.92-I26.99, or I82.4Ø1-I82.4Z9

See Appendix L for Procedure Combinations
⊞ ØSR[C,D]Ø[6,J,L,M,N][9,A,Z]
⊞ ØSR[C,D]ØEZ
⊞ ØSR[T,U,V,W]ØJ[9,A,Z]
⊞ ØSR[R,S]Ø[1,3,J][9,A,Z]

NC Noncovered Procedure   LC Limited Coverage   QA Questionable OB Admit   NT New Tech Add-on   ⊞ Combination Member   ♂ Male   ♀ Female

ICD-10-PCS 2022   ØSR–ØSR   615

Ø   Medical and Surgical
S   Lower Joints
S   Reposition   Definition: Moving to its normal location, or other suitable location, all or a portion of a body part

Explanation: The body part is moved to a new location from an abnormal location, or from a normal location where it is not functioning correctly. The body part may or may not be cut out or off to be moved to the new location.

Body Part Character 4		Approach Character 5	Device Character 6	Qualifier Character 7

Ø **Lumbar Vertebral Joint**
    Lumbar facet joint
3 **Lumbosacral Joint**
    Lumbosacral facet joint
5 **Sacrococcygeal Joint**
    Sacrococcygeal symphysis
6 **Coccygeal Joint**
7 **Sacroiliac Joint, Right**
8 **Sacroiliac Joint, Left**
		Ø Open
		3 Percutaneous
		4 Percutaneous Endoscopic
		X External
			4 Internal Fixation Device
			Z No Device
				Z No Qualifier

9 **Hip Joint, Right**
    Acetabulofemoral joint
B **Hip Joint, Left**
    See 9 Hip Joint, Right
C **Knee Joint, Right**
    Femoropatellar joint
    Femorotibial joint
    Lateral meniscus
    Medial meniscus
    Patellofemoral joint
    Tibiofemoral joint
D **Knee Joint, Left**
    See C Knee Joint, Right
F **Ankle Joint, Right**
    Inferior tibiofibular joint
    Talocrural joint
G **Ankle Joint, Left**
    See F Ankle Joint, Right
H **Tarsal Joint, Right**
    Calcaneocuboid joint
    Cuboideonavicular joint
    Cuneonavicular joint
    Intercuneiform joint
    Subtalar (talocalcaneal) joint
    Talocalcaneal (subtalar)
       joint
    Talocalcaneonavicular joint
	J **Tarsal Joint, Left**
	    See H Tarsal Joint, Right
	K **Tarsometatarsal Joint,**
	    Right
	L **Tarsometatarsal Joint, Left**
	M **Metatarsal-Phalangeal**
	    Joint, Right
	    Metatarsophalangeal (MTP)
	       joint
	N **Metatarsal-Phalangeal**
	    Joint, Left
	    See M Metatarsal-Phalangeal
	    Joint, Right
	P **Toe Phalangeal Joint, Right**
	    Interphalangeal (IP) joint
	Q **Toe Phalangeal Joint, Left**
	    See P Toe Phalangeal Joint,
	    Right
		Ø Open
		3 Percutaneous
		4 Percutaneous Endoscopic
		X External
			4 Internal Fixation Device
			5 External Fixation Device
			Z No Device
				Z No Qualifier

Non-OR   ØSS[Ø,3,5,6,7,8][3,4,X][4,Z]Z
Non-OR   ØSS[9,B,C,D,F,G,H,J,K,L,M,N,P,Q][3,4,X][4,5,Z]Z

Ø   Medical and Surgical
S   Lower Joints
T   Resection   Definition: Cutting out or off, without replacement, all of a body part

Explanation: None

Body Part Character 4		Approach Character 5	Device Character 6	Qualifier Character 7

2 **Lumbar Vertebral Disc**
4 **Lumbosacral Disc**
5 **Sacrococcygeal Joint**
    Sacrococcygeal symphysis
6 **Coccygeal Joint**
7 **Sacroiliac Joint, Right**
8 **Sacroiliac Joint, Left**
9 **Hip Joint, Right**
    Acetabulofemoral joint
B **Hip Joint, Left**
    See 9 Hip Joint, Right
C **Knee Joint, Right**
    Femoropatellar joint
    Femorotibial joint
    Lateral meniscus
    Medial meniscus
    Patellofemoral joint
    Tibiofemoral joint
D **Knee Joint, Left**
    See C Knee Joint, Right
F **Ankle Joint, Right**
    Inferior tibiofibular joint
    Talocrural joint
G **Ankle Joint, Left**
    See F Ankle Joint, Right
	H **Tarsal Joint, Right**
	    Calcaneocuboid joint
	    Cuboideonavicular joint
	    Cuneonavicular joint
	    Intercuneiform joint
	    Subtalar (talocalcaneal) joint
	    Talocalcaneal (subtalar) joint
	    Talocalcaneonavicular joint
	J **Tarsal Joint, Left**
	    See H Tarsal Joint, Right
	K **Tarsometatarsal Joint,**
	    Right
	L **Tarsometatarsal Joint, Left**
	M **Metatarsal-Phalangeal**
	    Joint, Right
	    Metatarsophalangeal (MTP)
	       joint
	N **Metatarsal-Phalangeal**
	    Joint, Left
	    See M Metatarsal-Phalangeal
	    Joint, Right
	P **Toe Phalangeal Joint, Right**
	    Interphalangeal (IP) joint
	Q **Toe Phalangeal Joint, Left**
	    See P Toe Phalangeal Joint,
	    Right
		Ø Open	Z No Device	Z No Qualifier

Ø   Medical and Surgical
S   Lower Joints
U   Supplement

Definition: Putting in or on biological or synthetic material that physically reinforces and/or augments the function of a portion of a body part

Explanation: The biological material is non-living, or is living and from the same individual. The body part may have been previously replaced, and the SUPPLEMENT procedure is performed to physically reinforce and/or augment the function of the replaced body part.

Body Part Character 4	Approach Character 5	Device Character 6	Qualifier Character 7
Ø Lumbar Vertebral Joint Lumbar facet joint **2 Lumbar Vertebral Disc** **3 Lumbosacral Joint** Lumbosacral facet joint **4 Lumbosacral Disc** **5 Sacrococcygeal Joint** Sacrococcygeal symphysis **6 Coccygeal Joint** **7 Sacroiliac Joint, Right** **8 Sacroiliac Joint, Left** **F Ankle Joint, Right** Inferior tibiofibular joint Talocrural joint **G Ankle Joint, Left** *See F Ankle Joint, Right* **H Tarsal Joint, Right** Calcaneocuboid joint Cuboideonavicular joint Cuneonavicular joint Intercuneiform joint Subtalar (talocalcaneal) joint Talocalcaneal (subtalar) joint Talocalcaneonavicular joint **J Tarsal Joint, Left** *See H Tarsal Joint, Right* **K Tarsometatarsal Joint, Right** **L Tarsometatarsal Joint, Left** **M Metatarsal-Phalangeal Joint, Right** Metatarsophalangeal (MTP) joint **N Metatarsal-Phalangeal Joint, Left** *See M Metatarsal-Phalangeal Joint, Right* **P Toe Phalangeal Joint, Right** Interphalangeal (IP) joint **Q Toe Phalangeal Joint, Left** *See P Toe Phalangeal Joint, Right*	**Ø Open** **3 Percutaneous** **4 Percutaneous Endoscopic**	**7 Autologous Tissue Substitute** **J Synthetic Substitute** **K Nonautologous Tissue Substitute**	**Z No Qualifier**
9 Hip Joint, Right ⊞ Acetabulofemoral joint **B Hip Joint, Left** ⊞ *See 9 Hip Joint, Right*	**Ø Open**	**7 Autologous Tissue Substitute** **9 Liner** **B Resurfacing Device** **J Synthetic Substitute** **K Nonautologous Tissue Substitute**	**Z No Qualifier**
9 Hip Joint, Right Acetabulofemoral joint **B Hip Joint, Left** *See 9 Hip Joint, Right*	**3 Percutaneous** **4 Percutaneous Endoscopic**	**7 Autologous Tissue Substitute** **J Synthetic Substitute** **K Nonautologous Tissue Substitute**	**Z No Qualifier**
A Hip Joint, Acetabular Surface, Right ⊞ **E Hip Joint, Acetabular Surface, Left** ⊞ **R Hip Joint, Femoral Surface, Right** ⊞ **S Hip Joint, Femoral Surface, Left** ⊞	**Ø Open**	**9 Liner** **B Resurfacing Device**	**Z No Qualifier**
C Knee Joint, Right Femoropatellar joint Femorotibial joint Lateral meniscus Medial meniscus Patellofemoral joint Tibiofemoral joint **D Knee Joint, Left** *See C Knee Joint, Right*	**Ø Open**	**7 Autologous Tissue Substitute** **J Synthetic Substitute** **K Nonautologous Tissue Substitute**	**Z No Qualifier**
C Knee Joint, Right Femoropatellar joint Femorotibial joint Lateral meniscus Medial meniscus Patellofemoral joint Tibiofemoral joint **D Knee Joint, Left** *See C Knee Joint, Right*	**Ø Open**	**9 Liner**	**C Patellar Surface** **Z No Qualifier**

HAC   ØSU[9,B]ØBZ when reported with SDx of I26.02-I26.09,
      I26.92-I26.99, or I82.401-I82.4Z9

HAC   ØSU[A,E,R,S]ØBZ when reported with SDx of I26.02-I26.09,
      I26.92-I26.99, or I82.401-I82.4Z9

See Appendix L for Procedure Combinations
⊞   ØSU[9,B]Ø9Z
⊞   ØSU[A,E,R,S]Ø9Z

ØSU Continued on next page

NC Noncovered Procedure   LC Limited Coverage   QA Questionable OB Admit   NT New Tech Add-on   ⊞ Combination Member   ♂ Male   ♀ Female

Lower Joints

Ø   Medical and Surgical   *ØSU Continued*
S   Lower Joints
U   Supplement   Definition: Putting in or on biological or synthetic material that physically reinforces and/or augments the function of a portion of a body part
Explanation: The biological material is non-living, or is living and from the same individual. The body part may have been previously replaced, and the SUPPLEMENT procedure is performed to physically reinforce and/or augment the function of the replaced body part.

Body Part Character 4	Approach Character 5	Device Character 6	Qualifier Character 7

C Knee Joint, Right
    Femoropatellar joint
    Femorotibial joint
    Lateral meniscus
    Medial meniscus
    Patellofemoral joint
    Tibiofemoral joint
D Knee Joint, Left
    See C Knee Joint, Right
	3 Percutaneous
	4 Percutaneous Endoscopic
		7 Autologous Tissue Substitute
		J Synthetic Substitute
		K Nonautologous Tissue Substitute
			Z No Qualifier

T Knee Joint, Femoral Surface, Right
    Femoropatellar joint
    Patellofemoral joint
U Knee Joint, Femoral Surface, Left
    See T Knee Joint, Femoral Surface, Right
V Knee Joint, Tibial Surface, Right ⊞
    Femorotibial joint
    Tibiofemoral joint
W Knee Joint, Tibial Surface, Left ⊞
    See V Knee Joint, Tibial Surface, Right
	Ø Open	**9** Liner	**Z** No Qualifier

See Appendix L for Procedure Combinations
⊞   ØSU[V,W]Ø9Z

Ø   Medical and Surgical
S   Lower Joints
W   Revision

Definition: Correcting, to the extent possible, a portion of a malfunctioning device or the position of a displaced device

Explanation: Revision can include correcting a malfunctioning or displaced device by taking out or putting in components of the device such as a screw or pin

Body Part Character 4	Approach Character 5	Device Character 6	Qualifier Character 7
Ø Lumbar Vertebral Joint Lumbar facet joint **3 Lumbosacral Joint** Lumbosacral facet joint	**Ø** Open **3** Percutaneous **4** Percutaneous Endoscopic **X** External	**Ø** Drainage Device **3** Infusion Device **4** Internal Fixation Device **7** Autologous Tissue Substitute **8** Spacer **A** Interbody Fusion Device **J** Synthetic Substitute **K** Nonautologous Tissue Substitute	**Z** No Qualifier
2 Lumbar Vertebral Disc **4 Lumbosacral Disc**	**Ø** Open **3** Percutaneous **4** Percutaneous Endoscopic **X** External	**Ø** Drainage Device **3** Infusion Device **7** Autologous Tissue Substitute **J** Synthetic Substitute **K** Nonautologous Tissue Substitute	**Z** No Qualifier
5 Sacrococcygeal Joint Sacrococcygeal symphysis **6 Coccygeal Joint** **7 Sacroiliac Joint, Right** **8 Sacroiliac Joint, Left**	**Ø** Open **3** Percutaneous **4** Percutaneous Endoscopic **X** External	**Ø** Drainage Device **3** Infusion Device **4** Internal Fixation Device **7** Autologous Tissue Substitute **8** Spacer **J** Synthetic Substitute **K** Nonautologous Tissue Substitute	**Z** No Qualifier
9 Hip Joint, Right Acetabulofemoral joint **B Hip Joint, Left** *See 9 Hip Joint, Right*	**Ø** Open	**Ø** Drainage Device **3** Infusion Device **4** Internal Fixation Device **5** External Fixation Device **7** Autologous Tissue Substitute **8** Spacer **9** Liner **B** Resurfacing Device **J** Synthetic Substitute **K** Nonautologous Tissue Substitute	**Z** No Qualifier
9 Hip Joint, Right Acetabulofemoral joint **B Hip Joint, Left** *See 9 Hip Joint, Right*	**3** Percutaneous **4** Percutaneous Endoscopic **X** External	**Ø** Drainage Device **3** Infusion Device **4** Internal Fixation Device **5** External Fixation Device **7** Autologous Tissue Substitute **8** Spacer **J** Synthetic Substitute **K** Nonautologous Tissue Substitute	**Z** No Qualifier
A Hip Joint, Acetabular Surface, Right **E Hip Joint, Acetabular Surface, Left** **R Hip Joint, Femoral Surface, Right** **S Hip Joint, Femoral Surface, Left** **T Knee Joint, Femoral Surface, Right** Femoropatellar joint Patellofemoral joint **U Knee Joint, Femoral Surface, Left** *See T Knee Joint, Femoral Surface, Right* **V Knee Joint, Tibial Surface, Right** Femorotibial joint Tibiofemoral joint **W Knee Joint, Tibial Surface, Left** *See V Knee Joint, Tibial Surface, Right*	**Ø** Open **3** Percutaneous **4** Percutaneous Endoscopic **X** External	**J** Synthetic Substitute	**Z** No Qualifier
C Knee Joint, Right Femoropatellar joint Femorotibial joint Lateral meniscus Medial meniscus Patellofemoral joint Tibiofemoral joint **D Knee Joint, Left** *See C Knee Joint, Right*	**Ø** Open	**Ø** Drainage Device **3** Infusion Device **4** Internal Fixation Device **5** External Fixation Device **7** Autologous Tissue Substitute **8** Spacer **9** Liner **K** Nonautologous Tissue Substitute	**Z** No Qualifier

Non-OR	ØSW[Ø,3]X[Ø,3,4,7,8,A,J,K]Z
Non-OR	ØSW[2,4]X[Ø,3,7,J,K]Z
Non-OR	ØSW[5,6,7,8]X[Ø,3,4,7,8,J,K]Z
Non-OR	ØSW[9,B]X[Ø,3,4,5,7,8,J,K]Z
Non-OR	ØSW[A,E,R,S,T,U,V,W]XJZ

ØSW Continued on next page

NC Noncovered Procedure   **LC** Limited Coverage   **QA** Questionable OB Admit   **NT** New Tech Add-on   ⊞ Combination Member   ♂ Male   ♀ Female

Ø Medical and Surgical
S Lower Joints
W Revision

ØSW Continued

Definition: Correcting, to the extent possible, a portion of a malfunctioning device or the position of a displaced device

Explanation: Revision can include correcting a malfunctioning or displaced device by taking out or putting in components of the device such as a screw or pin

Body Part Character 4	Approach Character 5	Device Character 6	Qualifier Character 7
C Knee Joint, Right Femoropatellar joint Femorotibial joint Lateral meniscus Medial meniscus Patellofemoral joint Tibiofemoral joint **D Knee Joint, Left** *See C Knee Joint, Right*	**Ø Open**	**J Synthetic Substitute**	**C Patellar Surface** **Z No Qualifier**
C Knee Joint, Right Femoropatellar joint Femorotibial joint Lateral meniscus Medial meniscus Patellofemoral joint Tibiofemoral joint **D Knee Joint, Left** *See C Knee Joint, Right*	**3 Percutaneous** **4 Percutaneous Endoscopic** **X External**	**Ø Drainage Device** **3 Infusion Device** **4 Internal Fixation Device** **5 External Fixation Device** **7 Autologous Tissue Substitute** **8 Spacer** **K Nonautologous Tissue Substitute**	**Z No Qualifier**
C Knee Joint, Right Femoropatellar joint Femorotibial joint Lateral meniscus Medial meniscus Patellofemoral joint Tibiofemoral joint **D Knee Joint, Left** *See C Knee Joint, Right*	**3 Percutaneous** **4 Percutaneous Endoscopic** **X External**	**J Synthetic Substitute**	**C Patellar Surface** **Z No Qualifier**
F Ankle Joint, Right Inferior tibiofibular joint Talocrural joint **G Ankle Joint, Left** *See F Ankle Joint, Right* **H Tarsal Joint, Right** Calcaneocuboid joint Cuboideonavicular joint Cuneonavicular joint Intercuneiform joint Subtalar (talocalcaneal) joint Talocalcaneal (subtalar) joint Talocalcaneonavicular joint **J Tarsal Joint, Left** *See H Tarsal Joint, Right* **K Tarsometatarsal Joint, Right** **L Tarsometatarsal Joint, Left** **M Metatarsal-Phalangeal Joint, Right** Metatarsophalangeal (MTP) joint **N Metatarsal-Phalangeal Joint, Left** *See M Metatarsal-Phalangeal Joint, Right* **P Toe Phalangeal Joint, Right** Interphalangeal (IP) joint **Q Toe Phalangeal Joint, Left** *See P Toe Phalangeal Joint, Right*	**Ø Open** **3 Percutaneous** **4 Percutaneous Endoscopic** **X External**	**Ø Drainage Device** **3 Infusion Device** **4 Internal Fixation Device** **5 External Fixation Device** **7 Autologous Tissue Substitute** **8 Spacer** **J Synthetic Substitute** **K Nonautologous Tissue Substitute**	**Z No Qualifier**

Non-OR   ØSW[C,D]X[Ø,3,4,5,7,8,K]Z
Non-OR   ØSW[C,D]XJ[C,Z]
Non-OR   ØSW[F,G,H,J,K,L,M,N,P,Q]X[Ø,3,4,5,7,8,J,K]Z

Urinary System ØT1–ØTY

Character Meanings

This Character Meaning table is provided as a guide to assist the user in the identification of character members that may be found in this section of code tables. It **SHOULD NOT** be used to build a PCS code.

Operation–Character 3	Body Part–Character 4	Approach–Character 5	Device–Character 6	Qualifier–Character 7
1 Bypass	Ø Kidney, Right	Ø Open	Ø Drainage Device	Ø Allogeneic
2 Change	1 Kidney, Left	3 Percutaneous	1 Radioactive Element	1 Syngeneic
5 Destruction	2 Kidneys, Bilateral	4 Percutaneous Endoscopic	2 Monitoring Device	2 Zooplastic
7 Dilation	3 Kidney Pelvis, Right	7 Via Natural or Artificial Opening	3 Infusion Device	3 Kidney Pelvis, Right
8 Division	4 Kidney Pelvis, Left	8 Via Natural or Artificial Opening Endoscopic	7 Autologous Tissue Substitute	4 Kidney Pelvis, Left
9 Drainage	5 Kidney	X External	C Extraluminal Device	6 Ureter, Right
B Excision	6 Ureter, Right		D Intraluminal Device	7 Ureter, Left
C Extirpation	7 Ureter, Left		J Synthetic Substitute	8 Colon
D Extraction	8 Ureters, Bilateral		K Nonautologous Tissue Substitute	9 Colocutaneous
F Fragmentation	9 Ureter		L Artificial Sphincter	A Ileum
H Insertion	B Bladder		M Stimulator Lead	B Bladder
J Inspection	C Bladder Neck		Y Other Device	C Ileocutaneous
L Occlusion	D Urethra		Z No Device	D Cutaneous
M Reattachment				X Diagnostic
N Release				Z No Qualifier
P Removal				
Q Repair				
R Replacement				
S Reposition				
T Resection				
U Supplement				
V Restriction				
W Revision				
Y Transplantation				

AHA Coding Clinic for table ØT1
2017, 3Q, 20   Creation of Indiana pouch
2017, 3Q, 21   Augmentation cystoplasty with Indiana pouch and continent urinary diversion
2017, 1Q, 37   Perineal urethrostomy
2015, 3Q, 34   Redo urinary diversion surgery via left ureteral reimplantation

AHA Coding Clinic for table ØT7
2019, 2Q, 16   Reimplantation of ureters with insertion of tubes
2017, 4Q, 111   Exchange of ureteral stent
2016, 2Q, 27   Exchange of ureteral stents
2015, 2Q, 8   Urinary calculi fragmentation and evacuation
2013, 4Q, 123   Urolift® procedure

AHA Coding Clinic for table ØT9
2017, 3Q, 19   Ureteral stent placement for urinary leakage
2017, 3Q, 20   Creation of Indiana pouch
2017, 3Q, 21   Augmentation cystoplasty with Indiana pouch and continent urinary diversion

AHA Coding Clinic for table ØTB
2016, 1Q, 19   Biopsy of neobladder malignancy
2015, 3Q, 34   Excision of Mitrofanoff polyp
2014, 2Q, 8   Ileoscopy with excision of polyp of Ileal loop urinary diversion

AHA Coding Clinic for table ØTC
2019, 3Q, 4   Evacuation of clots from bladder dome
2016, 3Q, 23   Ureteral stone migrating into bladder
2015, 2Q, 7   Urinary calculi fragmentation and evacuation
2015, 2Q, 8   Urinary calculi fragmentation and evacuation
2013, 4Q, 122   Laser lithotripsy with removal of fragments

AHA Coding Clinic for table ØTF
2015, 2Q, 7   Urinary calculi fragmentation and evacuation
2013, 4Q, 122   Extracorporeal shock wave lithotripsy
2013, 4Q, 122   Laser lithotripsy with removal of fragments

AHA Coding Clinic for table ØTH
2020, 4Q, 43-44 Insertion of radioactive element
2019, 2Q, 16   Reimplantation of ureters with insertion of tubes

AHA Coding Clinic for table ØTP
2017, 4Q, 111   Exchange of ureteral stent
2016, 2Q, 27   Exchange of ureteral stents

AHA Coding Clinic for table ØTQ
2018, 2Q, 27   Dismembered pyeloplasty
2017, 1Q, 37   Perineal urethrostomy

AHA Coding Clinic for table ØTR
2017, 3Q, 20   Creation of Indiana pouch

AHA Coding Clinic for table ØTS
2019, 1Q, 29   Young-Dees-Leadbetter bladder neck reconstruction
2018, 2Q, 27   Dismembered pyeloplasty
2017, 1Q, 36   Dismembered pyeloplasty
2016, 1Q, 15   Pubovaginal sling placement

AHA Coding Clinic for table ØTT
2014, 3Q, 16   Hand-assisted laparoscopy nephroureterectomy

AHA Coding Clinic for table ØTU
2019, 1Q, 29   Young-Dees-Leadbetter bladder neck reconstruction
2017, 3Q, 21   Augmentation cystoplasty with Indiana pouch and continent urinary diversion

AHA Coding Clinic for table ØTV
2015, 2Q, 11   Cystourethroscopic Deflux® injection

Urinary System

- Inferior vena cava
- Aorta
- Right kidney Ø
- Left kidney **1**
- Left ureter **7**
- Right ureter **6**
- Urinary bladder **B**
- Ureteral orifice **6, 7, 8, 9**
- Bladder neck **C**
- Urethra **D**
- Urogenital diaphragm

Kidney

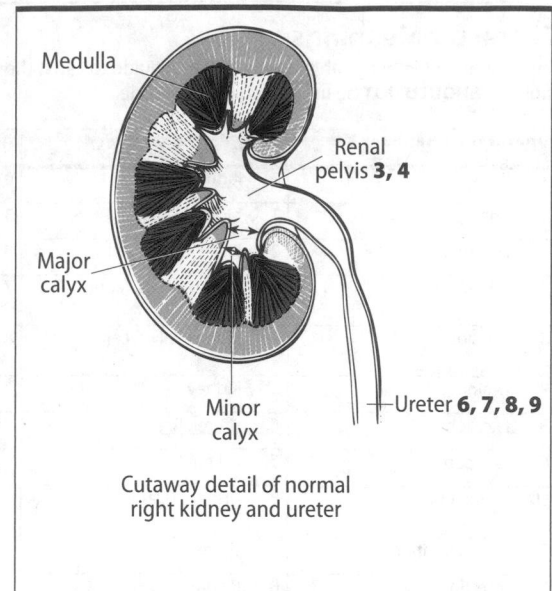

- Medulla
- Renal pelvis **3, 4**
- Major calyx
- Minor calyx
- Ureter **6, 7, 8, 9**

Cutaway detail of normal right kidney and ureter

Bladder

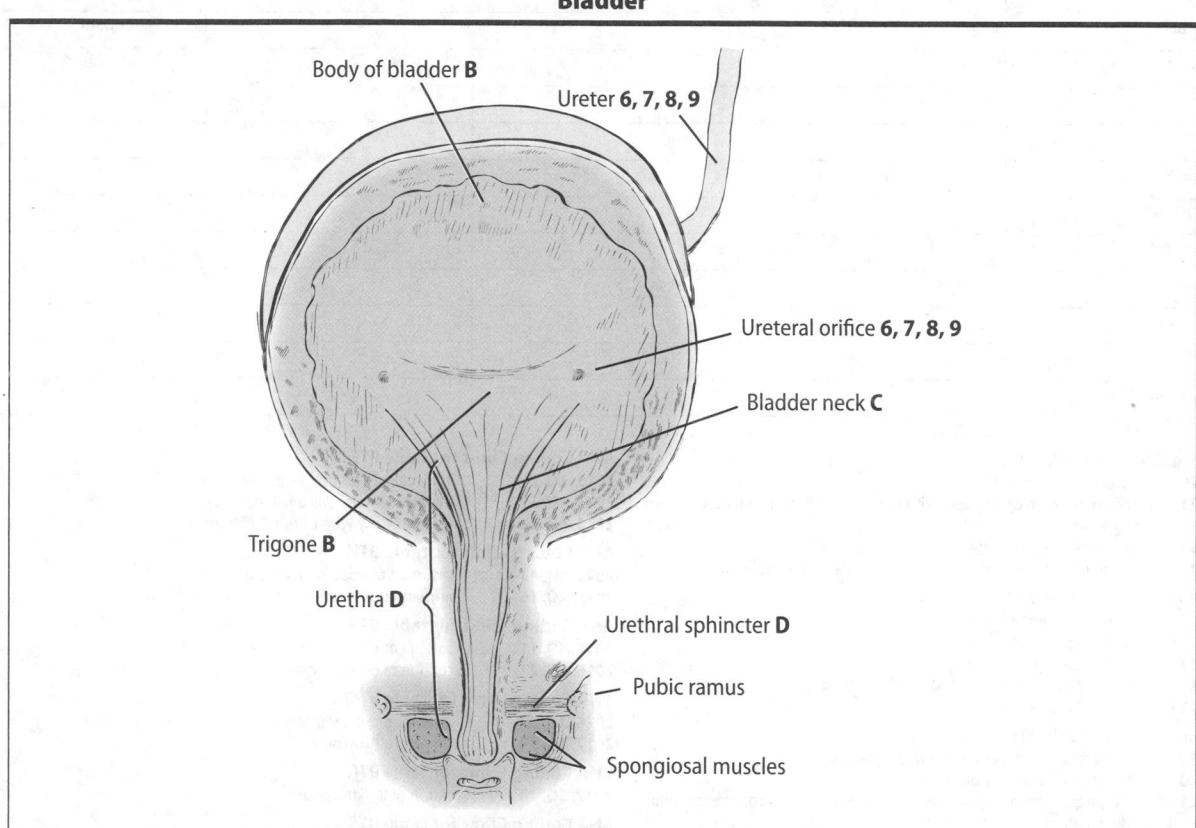

- Body of bladder **B**
- Ureter **6, 7, 8, 9**
- Ureteral orifice **6, 7, 8, 9**
- Bladder neck **C**
- Trigone **B**
- Urethra **D**
- Urethral sphincter **D**
- Pubic ramus
- Spongiosal muscles

0   Medical and Surgical
T   Urinary System
1   Bypass   Definition: Altering the route of passage of the contents of a tubular body part

Explanation: Rerouting contents of a body part to a downstream area of the normal route, to a similar route and body part, or to an abnormal route and dissimilar body part. Includes one or more anastomoses, with or without the use of a device.

Body Part Character 4	Approach Character 5	Device Character 6	Qualifier Character 7
3 Kidney Pelvis, Right Ureteropelvic junction (UPJ) **4** Kidney Pelvis, Left *See 3 Kidney Pelvis, Right*	**0** Open **4** Percutaneous Endoscopic	**7** Autologous Tissue Substitute **J** Synthetic Substitute **K** Nonautologous Tissue Substitute **Z** No Device	**3** Kidney Pelvis, Right **4** Kidney Pelvis, Left **6** Ureter, Right **7** Ureter, Left **8** Colon **9** Colocutaneous **A** Ileum **B** Bladder **C** Ileocutaneous **D** Cutaneous
3 Kidney Pelvis, Right Ureteropelvic junction (UPJ) **4** Kidney Pelvis, Left *See 3 Kidney Pelvis, Right*	**3** Percutaneous	**J** Synthetic Substitute	**D** Cutaneous
6 Ureter, Right Ureteral orifice Ureterovesical orifice **7** Ureter, Left *See 6 Ureter, Right* **8** Ureters, Bilateral *See 6 Ureter, Right*	**0** Open **4** Percutaneous Endoscopic	**7** Autologous Tissue Substitute **J** Synthetic Substitute **K** Nonautologous Tissue Substitute **Z** No Device	**6** Ureter, Right **7** Ureter, Left **8** Colon **9** Colocutaneous **A** Ileum **B** Bladder **C** Ileocutaneous **D** Cutaneous
6 Ureter, Right Ureteral orifice Ureterovesical orifice **7** Ureter, Left *See 6 Ureter, Right* **8** Ureters, Bilateral *See 6 Ureter, Right*	**3** Percutaneous	**J** Synthetic Substitute	**D** Cutaneous
B Bladder Trigone of bladder	**0** Open **4** Percutaneous Endoscopic	**7** Autologous Tissue Substitute **J** Synthetic Substitute **K** Nonautologous Tissue Substitute **Z** No Device	**9** Colocutaneous **C** Ileocutaneous **D** Cutaneous
B Bladder Trigone of bladder	**3** Percutaneous	**J** Synthetic Substitute	**D** Cutaneous

0   Medical and Surgical
T   Urinary System
2   Change   Definition: Taking out or off a device from a body part and putting back an identical or similar device in or on the same body part without cutting or puncturing the skin or a mucous membrane

Explanation: All CHANGE procedures are coded using the approach EXTERNAL

Body Part Character 4	Approach Character 5	Device Character 6	Qualifier Character 7
5 Kidney Renal calyx Renal capsule Renal cortex Renal segment **9** Ureter Ureteral orifice Ureterovesical orifice **B** Bladder Trigone of bladder **D** Urethra Bulbourethral (Cowper's) gland Cowper's (bulbourethral) gland External urethral sphincter Internal urethral sphincter Membranous urethra Penile urethra Prostatic urethra	**X** External	**0** Drainage Device **Y** Other Device	**Z** No Qualifier

Non-OR   All body part, approach, device, and qualifier values

NC Noncovered Procedure   LC Limited Coverage   OA Questionable OB Admit   NT New Tech Add-on   ⊞ Combination Member   ♂ Male   ♀ Female

ICD-10-PCS 2022   623

0T1–0T2

Ø   **Medical and Surgical**
T   **Urinary System**
5   **Destruction**   Definition: Physical eradication of all or a portion of a body part by the direct use of energy, force, or a destructive agent

                    Explanation: None of the body part is physically taken out

Body Part Character 4	Approach Character 5	Device Character 6	Qualifier Character 7
Ø **Kidney, Right** Renal calyx Renal capsule Renal cortex Renal segment **1** **Kidney, Left** *See Ø Kidney, Right* **3** **Kidney Pelvis, Right** Ureteropelvic junction (UPJ) **4** **Kidney Pelvis, Left** *See 3 Kidney Pelvis, Right* **6** **Ureter, Right** Ureteral orifice Ureterovesical orifice **7** **Ureter, Left** *See 6 Ureter, Right* **B** **Bladder** Trigone of bladder **C** **Bladder Neck**	**Ø** **Open** **3** **Percutaneous** **4** **Percutaneous Endoscopic** **7** **Via Natural or Artificial Opening** **8** **Via Natural or Artificial Opening Endoscopic**	**Z** No Device	**Z** No Qualifier
D **Urethra** Bulbourethral (Cowper's) gland Cowper's (bulbourethral) gland External urethral sphincter Internal urethral sphincter Membranous urethra Penile urethra Prostatic urethra	**Ø** **Open** **3** **Percutaneous** **4** **Percutaneous Endoscopic** **7** **Via Natural or Artificial Opening** **8** **Via Natural or Artificial Opening Endoscopic** **X** **External**	**Z** No Device	**Z** No Qualifier

Non-OR   ØT5D[Ø,3,4,7,8,X]ZZ

Ø   **Medical and Surgical**
T   **Urinary System**
7   **Dilation**   Definition: Expanding an orifice or the lumen of a tubular body part

                    Explanation: The orifice can be a natural orifice or an artificially created orifice. Accomplished by stretching a tubular body part using intraluminal pressure or by cutting part of the orifice or wall of the tubular body part.

Body Part Character 4	Approach Character 5	Device Character 6	Qualifier Character 7
3 **Kidney Pelvis, Right** Ureteropelvic junction (UPJ) **4** **Kidney Pelvis, Left** *See 3 Kidney Pelvis, Right* **6** **Ureter, Right** Ureteral orifice Ureterovesical orifice **7** **Ureter, Left** *See 6 Ureter, Right* **8** **Ureters, Bilateral** *See 6 Ureter, Right* **B** **Bladder** Trigone of bladder **C** **Bladder Neck** **D** **Urethra** Bulbourethral (Cowper's) gland Cowper's (bulbourethral) gland External urethral sphincter Internal urethral sphincter Membranous urethra Penile urethra Prostatic urethra	**Ø** **Open** **3** **Percutaneous** **4** **Percutaneous Endoscopic** **7** **Via Natural or Artificial Opening** **8** **Via Natural or Artificial Opening Endoscopic**	**D** Intraluminal Device **Z** No Device	**Z** No Qualifier

Non-OR   ØT7[6,7,8][Ø,3,4,7]DZ   Non-OR   ØT7B7[D,Z]Z   Non-OR   ØT7[C,D][7,8][D,Z]Z
Non-OR   ØT7[6,7,8]7ZZ   Non-OR   ØT7C[Ø,3,4]ZZ
Non-OR   ØT788ZZ   Non-OR   ØT7[C,D][Ø,3,4]DZ

Ø   **Medical and Surgical**
T   **Urinary System**
8   **Division**   Definition: Cutting into a body part, without draining fluids and/or gases from the body part, in order to separate or transect a body part

                    Explanation: All or a portion of the body part is separated into two or more portions

Body Part Character 4	Approach Character 5	Device Character 6	Qualifier Character 7
2 **Kidneys, Bilateral** Renal calyx Renal capsule Renal cortex Renal segment **C** **Bladder Neck**	**Ø** **Open** **3** **Percutaneous** **4** **Percutaneous Endoscopic**	**Z** No Device	**Z** No Qualifier

Ø   Medical and Surgical
T   Urinary System
9   Drainage   Definition: Taking or letting out fluids and/or gases from a body part

                     Explanation: The qualifier DIAGNOSTIC is used to identify drainage procedures that are biopsies

Body Part Character 4	Approach Character 5	Device Character 6	Qualifier Character 7

Ø   Kidney, Right
   Renal calyx
   Renal capsule
   Renal cortex
   Renal segment
1   Kidney, Left
   See Ø Kidney, Right
3   Kidney Pelvis, Right
   Ureteropelvic junction (UPJ)
4   Kidney Pelvis, Left
   See 3 Kidney Pelvis, Right
6   Ureter, Right
   Ureteral orifice
   Ureterovesical orifice
7   Ureter, Left
   See 6 Ureter, Right
8   Ureters, Bilateral
   See 6 Ureter, Right
B   Bladder
   Trigone of bladder
C   Bladder Neck
	Ø Open
	3 Percutaneous
	4 Percutaneous Endoscopic
	7 Via Natural or Artificial Opening
	**8 Via Natural or Artificial Opening
	   Endoscopic**
		Ø Drainage Device	**Z No Qualifier**

Ø   Kidney, Right
   Renal calyx
   Renal capsule
   Renal cortex
   Renal segment
1   Kidney, Left
   See Ø Kidney, Right
3   Kidney Pelvis, Right
   Ureteropelvic junction (UPJ)
4   Kidney Pelvis, Left
   See 3 Kidney Pelvis, Right
6   Ureter, Right
   Ureteral orifice
   Ureterovesical orifice
7   Ureter, Left
   See 6 Ureter, Right
8   Ureters, Bilateral
   See 6 Ureter, Right
B   Bladder
   Trigone of bladder
C   Bladder Neck
	Ø Open
	3 Percutaneous
	4 Percutaneous Endoscopic
	7 Via Natural or Artificial Opening
	**8 Via Natural or Artificial Opening
	   Endoscopic**
		Z No Device	**X Diagnostic**
			Z No Qualifier

D   Urethra
   Bulbourethral (Cowper's) gland
   Cowper's (bulbourethral) gland
   External urethral sphincter
   Internal urethral sphincter
   Membranous urethra
   Penile urethra
   Prostatic urethra
	Ø Open
	3 Percutaneous
	4 Percutaneous Endoscopic
	7 Via Natural or Artificial Opening
	**8 Via Natural or Artificial Opening
	   Endoscopic**
	X External
		Ø Drainage Device	**Z No Qualifier**

D   Urethra
   Bulbourethral (Cowper's) gland
   Cowper's (bulbourethral) gland
   External urethral sphincter
   Internal urethral sphincter
   Membranous urethra
   Penile urethra
   Prostatic urethra
	Ø Open
	3 Percutaneous
	4 Percutaneous Endoscopic
	7 Via Natural or Artificial Opening
	**8 Via Natural or Artificial Opening
	   Endoscopic**
	X External
		Z No Device	**X Diagnostic**
			Z No Qualifier

Non-OR	ØT9[Ø,1,3,4]3ØZ
Non-OR	ØT9[6,7,8][Ø,3,4,7,8]ØZ
Non-OR	ØT9[B,C][3,4,7,8]ØZ
Non-OR	ØT9[Ø,1,3,4,6,7,8][3,4,7,8]ZX
Non-OR	ØT9[Ø,1,3,4][3,4]ZZ
Non-OR	ØT9[6,7,8]3ZZ
Non-OR	ØT9[B,C][3,4,7,8]ZZ
Non-OR	ØT9DØZ
Non-OR	ØT9D[Ø,3,4,7,8,X]ZX
Non-OR	ØT9D3ZZ

NC Noncovered Procedure   **LC** Limited Coverage   **QA** Questionable OB Admit   **NT** New Tech Add-on   ⊞ Combination Member   ♂ Male   ♀ Female

ICD-10-PCS 2022   625

Urinary System

Ø Medical and Surgical
T Urinary System
B Excision

Definition: Cutting out or off, without replacement, a portion of a body part

Explanation: The qualifier DIAGNOSTIC is used to identify excision procedures that are biopsies

Body Part Character 4	Approach Character 5	Device Character 6	Qualifier Character 7

Ø Kidney, Right
  Renal calyx
  Renal capsule
  Renal cortex
  Renal segment
1 Kidney, Left
  See Ø Kidney, Right
3 Kidney Pelvis, Right
  Ureteropelvic junction (UPJ)
4 Kidney Pelvis, Left
  See 3 Kidney Pelvis, Right
6 Ureter, Right
  Ureteral orifice
  Ureterovesical orifice
7 Ureter, Left
  See 6 Ureter, Right
B Bladder
  Trigone of bladder
C Bladder Neck
	Ø Open
	3 Percutaneous
	4 Percutaneous Endoscopic
	7 Via Natural or Artificial Opening
	8 Via Natural or Artificial Opening Endoscopic
		Z No Device	X Diagnostic
			Z No Qualifier

D Urethra
  Bulbourethral (Cowper's) gland
  Cowper's (bulbourethral) gland
  External urethral sphincter
  Internal urethral sphincter
  Membranous urethra
  Penile urethra
  Prostatic urethra
	Ø Open
	3 Percutaneous
	4 Percutaneous Endoscopic
	7 Via Natural or Artificial Opening
	8 Via Natural or Artificial Opening Endoscopic
	X External
		Z No Device	X Diagnostic
			Z No Qualifier

Non-OR ØTB[Ø,1,3,4,6,7][3,4,7,8]ZX
Non-OR ØTBD[Ø,3,4,7,8,X]ZX

Ø Medical and Surgical
T Urinary System
C Extirpation

Definition: Taking or cutting out solid matter from a body part

Explanation: The solid matter may be an abnormal byproduct of a biological function or a foreign body; it may be imbedded in a body part or in the lumen of a tubular body part. The solid matter may or may not have been previously broken into pieces.

Body Part Character 4	Approach Character 5	Device Character 6	Qualifier Character 7

Ø Kidney, Right
  Renal calyx
  Renal capsule
  Renal cortex
  Renal segment
1 Kidney, Left
  See Ø Kidney, Right
3 Kidney Pelvis, Right
  Ureteropelvic junction (UPJ)
4 Kidney Pelvis, Left
  See 3 Kidney Pelvis, Right
6 Ureter, Right
  Ureteral orifice
  Ureterovesical orifice
7 Ureter, Left
  See 6 Ureter, Right
B Bladder
  Trigone of bladder
C Bladder Neck
	Ø Open
	3 Percutaneous
	4 Percutaneous Endoscopic
	7 Via Natural or Artificial Opening
	8 Via Natural or Artificial Opening Endoscopic
		Z No Device	Z No Qualifier

D Urethra
  Bulbourethral (Cowper's) gland
  Cowper's (bulbourethral) gland
  External urethral sphincter
  Internal urethral sphincter
  Membranous urethra
  Penile urethra
  Prostatic urethra
	Ø Open
	3 Percutaneous
	4 Percutaneous Endoscopic
	7 Via Natural or Artificial Opening
	8 Via Natural or Artificial Opening Endoscopic
	X External
		Z No Device	Z No Qualifier

Non-OR ØTC[B,C][7,8]ZZ
Non-OR ØTCD[7,8,X]ZZ

Ø   **Medical and Surgical**
T   **Urinary System**
D   **Extraction**   Definition: Pulling or stripping out or off all or a portion of a body part by the use of force

                  Explanation: The qualifier DIAGNOSTIC is used to identify extraction procedures that are biopsies

Body Part Character 4	Approach Character 5	Device Character 6	Qualifier Character 7

Ø   **Kidney, Right**
     Renal calyx
     Renal capsule
     Renal cortex
     Renal segment
1   **Kidney, Left**
     See Ø Kidney, Right
	Ø Open
	3 Percutaneous
	4 Percutaneous Endoscopic
		Z No Device	**Z** No Qualifier

Ø   **Medical and Surgical**
T   **Urinary System**
F   **Fragmentation**   Definition: Breaking solid matter in a body part into pieces

                  Explanation: Physical force (e.g., manual, ultrasonic) applied directly or indirectly is used to break the solid matter into pieces. The solid matter may be an abnormal byproduct of a biological function or a foreign body. The pieces of solid matter are not taken out.

Body Part Character 4	Approach Character 5	Device Character 6	Qualifier Character 7

3   **Kidney Pelvis, Right**
     Ureteropelvic junction (UPJ)
4   **Kidney Pelvis, Left**
     See 3 Kidney Pelvis, Right
6   **Ureter, Right**
     Ureteral orifice
     Ureterovesical orifice
7   **Ureter, Left**
     See 6 Ureter, Right
B   **Bladder**
     Trigone of bladder
C   **Bladder Neck**
D   **Urethra**   **NC**
     Bulbourethral (Cowper's) gland
     Cowper's (bulbourethral) gland
     External urethral sphincter
     Internal urethral sphincter
     Membranous urethra
     Penile urethra
     Prostatic urethra
	Ø Open
	3 Percutaneous
	4 Percutaneous Endoscopic
	7 Via Natural or Artificial Opening
	8 Via Natural or Artificial Opening
	     Endoscopic
	X External
		Z No Device	**Z** No Qualifier

Non-OR	ØTF[3,4][Ø,7,8]ZZ
Non-OR	ØTF[6,7,B,C,D][Ø,3,4,7,8]ZZ
Non-OR	ØTF[3,4,6,7,B,C,D]XZZ
NC	ØTFDXZZ

NC Noncovered Procedure   **LC** Limited Coverage   **QA** Questionable OB Admit   **NT** New Tech Add-on   ⊞ Combination Member   ♂ Male   ♀ Female

ICD-10-PCS 2022   **627**

ØTD–ØTF

Urinary System

Ø   Medical and Surgical
T   Urinary System
H   Insertion   Definition: Putting in a nonbiological appliance that monitors, assists, performs, or prevents a physiological function but does not physically take the place of a body part
               Explanation: None

Body Part Character 4	Approach Character 5	Device Character 6	Qualifier Character 7
5 Kidney Renal calyx Renal capsule Renal cortex Renal segment	Ø Open 3 Percutaneous 4 Percutaneous Endoscopic 7 Via Natural or Artificial Opening 8 Via Natural or Artificial Opening Endoscopic	1 Radioactive Element 2 Monitoring Device 3 Infusion Device Y Other Device	Z No Qualifier
9 Ureter Ureteral orifice Ureterovesical orifice	Ø Open 3 Percutaneous 4 Percutaneous Endoscopic 7 Via Natural or Artificial Opening 8 Via Natural or Artificial Opening Endoscopic	1 Radioactive Element 2 Monitoring Device 3 Infusion Device M Stimulator Lead Y Other Device	Z No Qualifier
B Bladder NC Trigone of bladder	Ø Open 3 Percutaneous 4 Percutaneous Endoscopic 7 Via Natural or Artificial Opening 8 Via Natural or Artificial Opening Endoscopic	1 Radioactive Element 2 Monitoring Device 3 Infusion Device L Artificial Sphincter M Stimulator Lead Y Other Device	Z No Qualifier
C Bladder Neck	Ø Open 3 Percutaneous 4 Percutaneous Endoscopic 7 Via Natural or Artificial Opening 8 Via Natural or Artificial Opening Endoscopic	L Artificial Sphincter	Z No Qualifier
D Urethra Bulbourethral (Cowper's) gland Cowper's (bulbourethral) gland External urethral sphincter Internal urethral sphincter Membranous urethra Penile urethra Prostatic urethra	Ø Open 3 Percutaneous 4 Percutaneous Endoscopic 7 Via Natural or Artificial Opening 8 Via Natural or Artificial Opening Endoscopic	1 Radioactive Element 2 Monitoring Device 3 Infusion Device L Artificial Sphincter Y Other Device	Z No Qualifier
D Urethra Bulbourethral (Cowper's) gland Cowper's (bulbourethral) gland External urethral sphincter Internal urethral sphincter Membranous urethra Penile urethra Prostatic urethra	X External	2 Monitoring Device 3 Infusion Device L Artificial Sphincter	Z No Qualifier

Non-OR   ØTH5Ø3Z
Non-OR   ØTH53[1,3,Y]Z
Non-OR   ØTH54[3,Y]Z
Non-OR   ØTH57[1,2,3,Y]Z
Non-OR   ØTH58[2,3]Z
Non-OR   ØTH9Ø3Z
Non-OR   ØTH93[1,3,Y]Z
Non-OR   ØTH94[3,Y]Z
Non-OR   ØTH97[1,2,3,Y]Z
Non-OR   ØTH98[2,3]Z
Non-OR   ØTHBØ3Z

Non-OR   ØTHB3[1,3,Y]Z
Non-OR   ØTHB4[3,Y]Z
Non-OR   ØTHB7[1,2,3,Y]Z
Non-OR   ØTHB8[2,3]Z
Non-OR   ØTHDØ3Z
Non-OR   ØTHD3[1,3,Y]Z
Non-OR   ØTHD4[3,Y]Z
Non-OR   ØTHD7[1,2,3,Y]Z
Non-OR   ØTHD8[2,3,Y]Z
Non-OR   ØTHDX3Z
NC   ØTHB[Ø,3,4,7,8]MZ

Non-OR Procedure   DRG Non-OR Procedure   Valid OR Procedure   HAC Associated Procedure   Combination Only   New/Revised GREEN
628   ICD-10-PCS 2022

ØTH–ØTH

0 Medical and Surgical
T Urinary System
J Inspection   Definition: Visually and/or manually exploring a body part

Explanation: Visual exploration may be performed with or without optical instrumentation. Manual exploration may be performed directly or through intervening body layers.

Body Part Character 4	Approach Character 5	Device Character 6	Qualifier Character 7
5 Kidney Renal calyx Renal capsule Renal cortex Renal segment **9 Ureter** Ureteral orifice Ureterovesical orifice **B Bladder** Trigone of bladder **D Urethra** Bulbourethral (Cowper's) gland Cowper's (bulbourethral) gland External urethral sphincter Internal urethral sphincter Membranous urethra Penile urethra Prostatic urethra	**0** Open **3** Percutaneous **4** Percutaneous Endoscopic **7** Via Natural or Artificial Opening **8** Via Natural or Artificial Opening Endoscopic **X** External	**Z** No Device	**Z** No Qualifier

Non-OR   0TJ[5,9,D][3,4,7,8,X]ZZ
Non-OR   0TJB[3,7,8,X]ZZ

0 Medical and Surgical
T Urinary System
L Occlusion   Definition: Completely closing an orifice or the lumen of a tubular body part

Explanation: The orifice can be a natural orifice or an artificially created orifice

Body Part Character 4	Approach Character 5	Device Character 6	Qualifier Character 7
3 Kidney Pelvis, Right Ureteropelvic junction (UPJ) **4 Kidney Pelvis, Left** *See 3 Kidney Pelvis, Right* **6 Ureter, Right** Ureteral orifice Ureterovesical orifice **7 Ureter, Left** *See 6 Ureter, Right* **B Bladder** Trigone of bladder **C Bladder Neck**	**0** Open **3** Percutaneous **4** Percutaneous Endoscopic	**C** Extraluminal Device **D** Intraluminal Device **Z** No Device	**Z** No Qualifier
3 Kidney Pelvis, Right Ureteropelvic junction (UPJ) **4 Kidney Pelvis, Left** *See 3 Kidney Pelvis, Right* **6 Ureter, Right** Ureteral orifice Ureterovesical orifice **7 Ureter, Left** *See 6 Ureter, Right* **B Bladder** Trigone of bladder **C Bladder Neck**	**7** Via Natural or Artificial Opening **8** Via Natural or Artificial Opening Endoscopic	**D** Intraluminal Device **Z** No Device	**Z** No Qualifier
D Urethra Bulbourethral (Cowper's) gland Cowper's (bulbourethral) gland External urethral sphincter Internal urethral sphincter Membranous urethra Penile urethra Prostatic urethra	**0** Open **3** Percutaneous **4** Percutaneous Endoscopic **X** External	**C** Extraluminal Device **D** Intraluminal Device **Z** No Device	**Z** No Qualifier
D Urethra Bulbourethral (Cowper's) gland Cowper's (bulbourethral) gland External urethral sphincter Internal urethral sphincter Membranous urethra Penile urethra Prostatic urethra	**7** Via Natural or Artificial Opening **8** Via Natural or Artificial Opening Endoscopic	**D** Intraluminal Device **Z** No Device	**Z** No Qualifier

NC Noncovered Procedure   **LC** Limited Coverage   **QA** Questionable OB Admit   **NT** New Tech Add-on   ⊞ Combination Member   ♂ Male   ♀ Female

ICD-10-PCS 2022   629

0TJ–0TL

Urinary System

Ø   **Medical and Surgical**
T   **Urinary System**
M   **Reattachment**   Definition: Putting back in or on all or a portion of a separated body part to its normal location or other suitable location
                      Explanation: Vascular circulation and nervous pathways may or may not be reestablished

Body Part Character 4	Approach Character 5	Device Character 6	Qualifier Character 7

Ø   **Kidney, Right**
     Renal calyx
     Renal capsule
     Renal cortex
     Renal segment
1   **Kidney, Left**
     See Ø Kidney, Right
2   **Kidneys, Bilateral**
     See Ø Kidney, Right
3   **Kidney Pelvis, Right**
     Ureteropelvic junction (UPJ)
4   **Kidney Pelvis, Left**
     See 3 Kidney Pelvis, Right
6   **Ureter, Right**
     Ureteral orifice
     Ureterovesical orifice
7   **Ureter, Left**
     See 6 Ureter, Right
8   **Ureters, Bilateral**
     See 6 Ureter, Right
B   **Bladder**
     Trigone of bladder
C   **Bladder Neck**
D   **Urethra**
     Bulbourethral (Cowper's) gland
     Cowper's (bulbourethral) gland
     External urethral sphincter
     Internal urethral sphincter
     Membranous urethra
     Penile urethra
     Prostatic urethra
	Ø Open
	4 Percutaneous Endoscopic
		Z No Device	**Z** No Qualifier

Ø   **Medical and Surgical**
T   **Urinary System**
N   **Release**   Definition: Freeing a body part from an abnormal physical constraint by cutting or by the use of force
                      Explanation: Some of the restraining tissue may be taken out but none of the body part is taken out

Body Part Character 4	Approach Character 5	Device Character 6	Qualifier Character 7

Ø   **Kidney, Right**
     Renal calyx
     Renal capsule
     Renal cortex
     Renal segment
1   **Kidney, Left**
     See Ø Kidney, Right
3   **Kidney Pelvis, Right**
     Ureteropelvic junction (UPJ)
4   **Kidney Pelvis, Left**
     See 3 Kidney Pelvis, Right
6   **Ureter, Right**
     Ureteral orifice
     Ureterovesical orifice
7   **Ureter, Left**
     See 6 Ureter, Right
B   **Bladder**
     Trigone of bladder
C   **Bladder Neck**
	Ø Open
	3 Percutaneous
	4 Percutaneous Endoscopic
	7 Via Natural or Artificial Opening
	8 Via Natural or Artificial Opening
	     Endoscopic
		Z No Device	**Z** No Qualifier

D   **Urethra**
     Bulbourethral (Cowper's) gland
     Cowper's (bulbourethral) gland
     External urethral sphincter
     Internal urethral sphincter
     Membranous urethra
     Penile urethra
     Prostatic urethra
	Ø Open
	3 Percutaneous
	4 Percutaneous Endoscopic
	7 Via Natural or Artificial Opening
	8 Via Natural or Artificial Opening
	     Endoscopic
	X External
		Z No Device	**Z** No Qualifier

Ø   Medical and Surgical
T   Urinary System
P   Removal   Definition: Taking out or off a device from a body part

Explanation: If a device is taken out and a similar device put in without cutting or puncturing the skin or mucous membrane, the procedure is coded to the root operation CHANGE. Otherwise, the procedure for taking out the device is coded to the root operation REMOVAL.

Body Part Character 4	Approach Character 5	Device Character 6	Qualifier Character 7
5 Kidney Renal calyx Renal capsule Renal cortex Renal segment	Ø Open 3 Percutaneous 4 Percutaneous Endoscopic 7 Via Natural or Artificial Opening 8 Via Natural or Artificial Opening Endoscopic	Ø Drainage Device 2 Monitoring Device 3 Infusion Device 7 Autologous Tissue Substitute C Extraluminal Device D Intraluminal Device J Synthetic Substitute K Nonautologous Tissue Substitute Y Other Device	Z No Qualifier
5 Kidney Renal calyx Renal capsule Renal cortex Renal segment	X External	Ø Drainage Device 2 Monitoring Device 3 Infusion Device D Intraluminal Device	Z No Qualifier
9 Ureter Ureteral orifice Ureterovesical orifice	Ø Open 3 Percutaneous 4 Percutaneous Endoscopic 7 Via Natural or Artificial Opening 8 Via Natural or Artificial Opening Endoscopic	Ø Drainage Device 2 Monitoring Device 3 Infusion Device 7 Autologous Tissue Substitute C Extraluminal Device D Intraluminal Device J Synthetic Substitute K Nonautologous Tissue Substitute M Stimulator Lead Y Other Device	Z No Qualifier
9 Ureter Ureteral orifice Ureterovesical orifice	X External	Ø Drainage Device 2 Monitoring Device 3 Infusion Device D Intraluminal Device M Stimulator Lead	Z No Qualifier
B Bladder **NC** Trigone of bladder	Ø Open 3 Percutaneous 4 Percutaneous Endoscopic 7 Via Natural or Artificial Opening 8 Via Natural or Artificial Opening Endoscopic	Ø Drainage Device 2 Monitoring Device 3 Infusion Device 7 Autologous Tissue Substitute C Extraluminal Device D Intraluminal Device J Synthetic Substitute K Nonautologous Tissue Substitute L Artificial Sphincter M Stimulator Lead Y Other Device	Z No Qualifier
B Bladder Trigone of bladder	X External	Ø Drainage Device 2 Monitoring Device 3 Infusion Device D Intraluminal Device L Artificial Sphincter M Stimulator Lead	Z No Qualifier
D Urethra Bulbourethral (Cowper's) gland Cowper's (bulbourethral) gland External urethral sphincter Internal urethral sphincter Membranous urethra Penile urethra Prostatic urethra	Ø Open 3 Percutaneous 4 Percutaneous Endoscopic 7 Via Natural or Artificial Opening 8 Via Natural or Artificial Opening Endoscopic	Ø Drainage Device 2 Monitoring Device 3 Infusion Device 7 Autologous Tissue Substitute C Extraluminal Device D Intraluminal Device J Synthetic Substitute K Nonautologous Tissue Substitute L Artificial Sphincter Y Other Device	Z No Qualifier
D Urethra Bulbourethral (Cowper's) gland Cowper's (bulbourethral) gland External urethral sphincter Internal urethral sphincter Membranous urethra Penile urethra Prostatic urethra	X External	Ø Drainage Device 2 Monitoring Device 3 Infusion Device D Intraluminal Device L Artificial Sphincter	Z No Qualifier

Non-OR ØTP5[3,4,7]YZ	**Non-OR** ØTP9[7,8][Ø,2,3,D]Z	**Non-OR** ØTPB[7,8][Ø,2,3,D]Z	**Non-OR** ØTPD[7,8][Ø,2,3,D,Y]Z
Non-OR ØTP5[7,8][Ø,2,3,D]Z	**Non-OR** ØTP9X[Ø,2,3,D]Z	**Non-OR** ØTPBX[Ø,2,3,D,L]Z	**Non-OR** ØTPDX[Ø,2,3,D]Z
Non-OR ØTP5X[Ø,2,3,D]Z	**Non-OR** ØTPB[3,4,7]YZ	**Non-OR** ØTPD[3,4]YZ	**NC** ØTPB[Ø,3,4,7,8]MZ
Non-OR ØTP9[3,4,7]YZ			

NC Noncovered Procedure   **LC** Limited Coverage   **QA** Questionable OB Admit   **NT** New Tech Add-on   ⊞ Combination Member   ♂ Male   ♀ Female

ICD-10-PCS 2022   631

ØTP–ØTP

Ø Medical and Surgical
T Urinary System
Q Repair

Definition: Restoring, to the extent possible, a body part to its normal anatomic structure and function
Explanation: Used only when the method to accomplish the repair is not one of the other root operations

Body Part Character 4	Approach Character 5	Device Character 6	Qualifier Character 7
Ø Kidney, Right Renal calyx Renal capsule Renal cortex Renal segment **1 Kidney, Left** *See Ø Kidney, Right* **3 Kidney Pelvis, Right** Ureteropelvic junction (UPJ) **4 Kidney Pelvis, Left** *See 3 Kidney Pelvis, Right* **6 Ureter, Right** Ureteral orifice Ureterovesical orifice **7 Ureter, Left** *See 6 Ureter, Right* **B Bladder** ⊞ Trigone of bladder **C Bladder Neck**	**Ø Open** **3 Percutaneous** **4 Percutaneous Endoscopic** **7 Via Natural or Artificial Opening** **8 Via Natural or Artificial Opening Endoscopic**	**Z No Device**	**Z No Qualifier**
D Urethra Bulbourethral (Cowper's) gland Cowper's (bulbourethral) gland External urethral sphincter Internal urethral sphincter Membranous urethra Penile urethra Prostatic urethra	**Ø Open** **3 Percutaneous** **4 Percutaneous Endoscopic** **7 Via Natural or Artificial Opening** **8 Via Natural or Artificial Opening Endoscopic** **X External**	**Z No Device**	**Z No Qualifier**

See Appendix L for Procedure Combinations
  ⊞   ØTQB[Ø,3,4]ZZ

Ø Medical and Surgical
T Urinary System
R Replacement

Definition: Putting in or on biological or synthetic material that physically takes the place and/or function of all or a portion of a body part
Explanation: The body part may have been taken out or replaced, or may be taken out, physically eradicated, or rendered nonfunctional during the REPLACEMENT procedure. A REMOVAL procedure is coded for taking out the device used in a previous replacement procedure.

Body Part Character 4	Approach Character 5	Device Character 6	Qualifier Character 7
3 Kidney Pelvis, Right Ureteropelvic junction (UPJ) **4 Kidney Pelvis, Left** *See 3 Kidney Pelvis, Right* **6 Ureter, Right** Ureteral orifice Ureterovesical orifice **7 Ureter, Left** *See 6 Ureter, Right* **B Bladder** Trigone of bladder **C Bladder Neck**	**Ø Open** **4 Percutaneous Endoscopic** **7 Via Natural or Artificial Opening** **8 Via Natural or Artificial Opening Endoscopic**	**7 Autologous Tissue Substitute** **J Synthetic Substitute** **K Nonautologous Tissue Substitute**	**Z No Qualifier**
D Urethra Bulbourethral (Cowper's) gland Cowper's (bulbourethral) gland External urethral sphincter Internal urethral sphincter Membranous urethra Penile urethra Prostatic urethra	**Ø Open** **4 Percutaneous Endoscopic** **7 Via Natural or Artificial Opening** **8 Via Natural or Artificial Opening Endoscopic** **X External**	**7 Autologous Tissue Substitute** **J Synthetic Substitute** **K Nonautologous Tissue Substitute**	**Z No Qualifier**

Ø   Medical and Surgical
T   Urinary System
S   Reposition   Definition: Moving to its normal location, or other suitable location, all or a portion of a body part

Explanation: The body part is moved to a new location from an abnormal location, or from a normal location where it is not functioning correctly. The body part may or may not be cut out or off to be moved to the new location.

Body Part Character 4	Approach Character 5	Device Character 6	Qualifier Character 7
Ø Kidney, Right Renal calyx Renal capsule Renal cortex Renal segment **1 Kidney, Left** *See Ø Kidney, Right* **2 Kidneys, Bilateral** *See Ø Kidney, Right* **3 Kidney Pelvis, Right** Ureteropelvic junction (UPJ) **4 Kidney Pelvis, Left** *See 3 Kidney Pelvis, Right* **6 Ureter, Right** Ureteral orifice Ureterovesical orifice **7 Ureter, Left** *See 6 Ureter, Right* **8 Ureters, Bilateral** *See 6 Ureter, Right* **B Bladder** Trigone of bladder **C Bladder Neck** **D Urethra** Bulbourethral (Cowper's) gland Cowper's (bulbourethral) gland External urethral sphincter Internal urethral sphincter Membranous urethra Penile urethra Prostatic urethra	**Ø Open** **4 Percutaneous Endoscopic**	**Z No Device**	**Z No Qualifier**

Ø   Medical and Surgical
T   Urinary System
T   Resection   Definition: Cutting out or off, without replacement, all of a body part

Explanation: None

Body Part Character 4	Approach Character 5	Device Character 6	Qualifier Character 7
Ø Kidney, Right Renal calyx Renal capsule Renal cortex Renal segment **1 Kidney, Left** *See Ø Kidney, Right* **2 Kidneys, Bilateral** *See Ø Kidney, Right*	**Ø Open** **4 Percutaneous Endoscopic**	**Z No Device**	**Z No Qualifier**
3 Kidney Pelvis, Right Ureteropelvic junction (UPJ) **4 Kidney Pelvis, Left** *See 3 Kidney Pelvis, Right* **6 Ureter, Right** Ureteral orifice Ureterovesical orifice **7 Ureter, Left** *See 6 Ureter, Right* **B Bladder** ⊞ Trigone of bladder **C Bladder Neck** **D Urethra** Bulbourethral (Cowper's) gland Cowper's (bulbourethral) gland External urethral sphincter Internal urethral sphincter Membranous urethra Penile urethra Prostatic urethra	**Ø Open** **4 Percutaneous Endoscopic** **7 Via Natural or Artificial Opening** **8 Via Natural or Artificial Opening Endoscopic**	**Z No Device**	**Z No Qualifier**

Non-OR   ØTTD[4,7,8]ZZ

See Appendix L for Procedure Combinations
   Combo-only   ØTTDØZZ
   ⊞   ØTTBØZZ

NC Noncovered Procedure   **LC** Limited Coverage   **QA** Questionable OB Admit   **NT** New Tech Add-on   ⊞ Combination Member   ♂ Male   ♀ Female

ICD-10-PCS 2022   **633**

Urinary System

Ø Medical and Surgical
T Urinary System
U Supplement   Definition: Putting in or on biological or synthetic material that physically reinforces and/or augments the function of a portion of a body part

Explanation: The biological material is non-living, or is living and from the same individual. The body part may have been previously replaced, and the SUPPLEMENT procedure is performed to physically reinforce and/or augment the function of the replaced body part.

Body Part Character 4	Approach Character 5	Device Character 6	Qualifier Character 7
3 Kidney Pelvis, Right Ureteropelvic junction (UPJ) 4 Kidney Pelvis, Left *See 3 Kidney Pelvis, Right* 6 Ureter, Right Ureteral orifice Ureterovesical orifice 7 Ureter, Left *See 6 Ureter, Right* B Bladder Trigone of bladder C Bladder Neck	Ø Open 4 Percutaneous Endoscopic 7 Via Natural or Artificial Opening 8 Via Natural or Artificial Opening Endoscopic	7 Autologous Tissue Substitute J Synthetic Substitute K Nonautologous Tissue Substitute	Z No Qualifier
D Urethra Bulbourethral (Cowper's) gland Cowper's (bulbourethral) gland External urethral sphincter Internal urethral sphincter Membranous urethra Penile urethra Prostatic urethra	Ø Open 4 Percutaneous Endoscopic 7 Via Natural or Artificial Opening 8 Via Natural or Artificial Opening Endoscopic X External	7 Autologous Tissue Substitute J Synthetic Substitute K Nonautologous Tissue Substitute	Z No Qualifier

Ø Medical and Surgical
T Urinary System
V Restriction   Definition: Partially closing an orifice or the lumen of a tubular body part

Explanation: The orifice can be a natural orifice or an artificially created orifice

Body Part Character 4	Approach Character 5	Device Character 6	Qualifier Character 7
3 Kidney Pelvis, Right Ureteropelvic junction (UPJ) 4 Kidney Pelvis, Left *See 3 Kidney Pelvis, Right* 6 Ureter, Right Ureteral orifice Ureterovesical orifice 7 Ureter, Left *See 6 Ureter, Right* B Bladder Trigone of bladder C Bladder Neck	Ø Open 3 Percutaneous 4 Percutaneous Endoscopic	C Extraluminal Device D Intraluminal Device Z No Device	Z No Qualifier
3 Kidney Pelvis, Right Ureteropelvic junction (UPJ) 4 Kidney Pelvis, Left *See 3 Kidney Pelvis, Right* 6 Ureter, Right Ureteral orifice Ureterovesical orifice 7 Ureter, Left *See 6 Ureter, Right* B Bladder Trigone of bladder C Bladder Neck	7 Via Natural or Artificial Opening 8 Via Natural or Artificial Opening Endoscopic	D Intraluminal Device Z No Device	Z No Qualifier
D Urethra Bulbourethral (Cowper's) gland Cowper's (bulbourethral) gland External urethral sphincter Internal urethral sphincter Membranous urethra Penile urethra Prostatic urethra	Ø Open 3 Percutaneous 4 Percutaneous Endoscopic	C Extraluminal Device D Intraluminal Device Z No Device	Z No Qualifier
D Urethra Bulbourethral (Cowper's) gland Cowper's (bulbourethral) gland External urethral sphincter Internal urethral sphincter Membranous urethra Penile urethra Prostatic urethra	7 Via Natural or Artificial Opening 8 Via Natural or Artificial Opening Endoscopic	D Intraluminal Device Z No Device	Z No Qualifier
D Urethra Bulbourethral (Cowper's) gland Cowper's (bulbourethral) gland External urethral sphincter Internal urethral sphincter Membranous urethra Penile urethra Prostatic urethra	X External	Z No Device	Z No Qualifier

Non-OR Procedure   DRG Non-OR Procedure   Valid OR Procedure   HAC Associated Procedure   Combination Only   New/Revised GREEN

Ø   **Medical and Surgical**
T   **Urinary System**
W   **Revision**   Definition: Correcting, to the extent possible, a portion of a malfunctioning device or the position of a displaced device

                      Explanation: Revision can include correcting a malfunctioning or displaced device by taking out or putting in components of the device such as a screw or pin

Body Part Character 4	Approach Character 5	Device Character 6	Qualifier Character 7
5 **Kidney** Renal calyx Renal capsule Renal cortex Renal segment	**Ø** Open **3** Percutaneous **4** Percutaneous Endoscopic **7** Via Natural or Artificial Opening **8** Via Natural or Artificial Opening Endoscopic	**Ø** Drainage Device **2** Monitoring Device **3** Infusion Device **7** Autologous Tissue Substitute **C** Extraluminal Device **D** Intraluminal Device **J** Synthetic Substitute **K** Nonautologous Tissue Substitute **Y** Other Device	**Z** No Qualifier
5 **Kidney** Renal calyx Renal capsule Renal cortex Renal segment	**X** External	**Ø** Drainage Device **2** Monitoring Device **3** Infusion Device **7** Autologous Tissue Substitute **C** Extraluminal Device **D** Intraluminal Device **J** Synthetic Substitute **K** Nonautologous Tissue Substitute	**Z** No Qualifier
9 **Ureter** Ureteral orifice Ureterovesical orifice	**Ø** Open **3** Percutaneous **4** Percutaneous Endoscopic **7** Via Natural or Artificial Opening **8** Via Natural or Artificial Opening Endoscopic	**Ø** Drainage Device **2** Monitoring Device **3** Infusion Device **7** Autologous Tissue Substitute **C** Extraluminal Device **D** Intraluminal Device **J** Synthetic Substitute **K** Nonautologous Tissue Substitute **M** Stimulator Lead **Y** Other Device	**Z** No Qualifier
9 **Ureter** Ureteral orifice Ureterovesical orifice	**X** External	**Ø** Drainage Device **2** Monitoring Device **3** Infusion Device **7** Autologous Tissue Substitute **C** Extraluminal Device **D** Intraluminal Device **J** Synthetic Substitute **K** Nonautologous Tissue Substitute **M** Stimulator Lead	**Z** No Qualifier
B **Bladder** Trigone of bladder	**Ø** Open **3** Percutaneous **4** Percutaneous Endoscopic **7** Via Natural or Artificial Opening **8** Via Natural or Artificial Opening Endoscopic	**Ø** Drainage Device **2** Monitoring Device **3** Infusion Device **7** Autologous Tissue Substitute **C** Extraluminal Device **D** Intraluminal Device **J** Synthetic Substitute **K** Nonautologous Tissue Substitute **L** Artificial Sphincter **M** Stimulator Lead **Y** Other Device	**Z** No Qualifier
B **Bladder** Trigone of bladder	**X** External	**Ø** Drainage Device **2** Monitoring Device **3** Infusion Device **7** Autologous Tissue Substitute **C** Extraluminal Device **D** Intraluminal Device **J** Synthetic Substitute **K** Nonautologous Tissue Substitute **L** Artificial Sphincter **M** Stimulator Lead	**Z** No Qualifier

Non-OR ØTW5[3,4,7]YZ	**Non-OR** ØTW9X[Ø,2,3,7,C,D,J,K,M]Z
Non-OR ØTW5X[Ø,2,3,7,C,D,J,K]Z	**Non-OR** ØTWB[3,4,7]YZ
Non-OR ØTW9[3,4,7]YZ	**Non-OR** ØTWBX[Ø,2,3,7,C,D,J,K,L,M]Z

ØTW Continued on next page

NC Noncovered Procedure   **LC** Limited Coverage   **QA** Questionable OB Admit   **NT** New Tech Add-on   ⊞ Combination Member   ♂ Male   ♀ Female

Urinary System

Ø **Medical and Surgical**
T **Urinary System**
W **Revision**

ØTW Continued

Definition: Correcting, to the extent possible, a portion of a malfunctioning device or the position of a displaced device

Explanation: Revision can include correcting a malfunctioning or displaced device by taking out or putting in components of the device such as a screw or pin

Body Part Character 4	Approach Character 5	Device Character 6	Qualifier Character 7
D Urethra Bulbourethral (Cowper's) gland Cowper's (bulbourethral) gland External urethral sphincter Internal urethral sphincter Membranous urethra Penile urethra Prostatic urethra	**Ø** Open **3** Percutaneous **4** Percutaneous Endoscopic **7** Via Natural or Artificial Opening **8** Via Natural or Artificial Opening Endoscopic	**Ø** Drainage Device **2** Monitoring Device **3** Infusion Device **7** Autologous Tissue Substitute **C** Extraluminal Device **D** Intraluminal Device **J** Synthetic Substitute **K** Nonautologous Tissue Substitute **L** Artificial Sphincter **Y** Other Device	**Z** No Qualifier
D Urethra Bulbourethral (Cowper's) gland Cowper's (bulbourethral) gland External urethral sphincter Internal urethral sphincter Membranous urethra Penile urethra Prostatic urethra	**X** External	**Ø** Drainage Device **2** Monitoring Device **3** Infusion Device **7** Autologous Tissue Substitute **C** Extraluminal Device **D** Intraluminal Device **J** Synthetic Substitute **K** Nonautologous Tissue Substitute **L** Artificial Sphincter	**Z** No Qualifier

Non-OR ØTWD[3,4,7,8]YZ
Non-OR ØTWDX[Ø,2,3,7,C,D,J,K,L]Z

Ø **Medical and Surgical**
T **Urinary System**
Y **Transplantation**

Definition: Putting in or on all or a portion of a living body part taken from another individual or animal to physically take the place and/or function of all or a portion of a similar body part

Explanation: The native body part may or may not be taken out, and the transplanted body part may take over all or a portion of its function

Body Part Character 4	Approach Character 5	Device Character 6	Qualifier Character 7
Ø Kidney, Right LC ⊞ Renal calyx Renal capsule Renal cortex Renal segment **1** Kidney, Left LC ⊞ *See Ø Kidney, Right*	**Ø** Open	**Z** No Device	**Ø** Allogeneic **1** Syngeneic **2** Zooplastic

LC ØTY[Ø,1]ØZ[Ø,1,2]

See Appendix L for Procedure Combinations
⊞ ØTY[Ø,1]ØZ[Ø,1,2]

Female Reproductive System 0U1–0UY

Character Meanings

This Character Meaning table is provided as a guide to assist the user in the identification of character members that may be found in this section of code tables. It **SHOULD NOT** be used to build a PCS code.

Operation–Character 3		Body Part–Character 4		Approach–Character 5		Device–Character 6		Qualifier–Character 7	
1	Bypass	0	Ovary, Right	0	Open	0	Drainage Device	0	Allogeneic
2	Change	1	Ovary, Left	3	Percutaneous	1	Radioactive Element	1	Syngeneic
5	Destruction	2	Ovaries, Bilateral	4	Percutaneous Endoscopic	3	Infusion Device	2	Zooplastic
7	Dilation	3	Ovary	7	Via Natural or Artificial Opening	7	Autologous Tissue Substitute	5	Fallopian Tube, Right
8	Division	4	Uterine Supporting Structure	8	Via Natural or Artificial Opening Endoscopic	C	Extraluminal Device	6	Fallopian Tube, Left
9	Drainage	5	Fallopian Tube, Right	F	Via Natural or Artificial Opening With Percutaneous Endoscopic Assistance	D	Intraluminal Device	9	Uterus
B	Excision	6	Fallopian Tube, Left	X	External	G	Intraluminal Device, Pessary	L	Supracervical
C	Extirpation	7	Fallopian Tubes, Bilateral			H	Contraceptive Device	X	Diagnostic
D	Extraction	8	Fallopian Tube			J	Synthetic Substitute	Z	No Qualifier
F	Fragmentation	9	Uterus			K	Nonautologous Tissue Substitute		
H	Insertion	B	Endometrium			Y	Other Device		
J	Inspection	C	Cervix			Z	No Device		
L	Occlusion	D	Uterus and Cervix						
M	Reattachment	F	Cul-de-sac						
N	Release	G	Vagina						
P	Removal	H	Vagina and Cul-de-sac						
Q	Repair	J	Clitoris						
S	Reposition	K	Hymen						
T	Resection	L	Vestibular Gland						
U	Supplement	M	Vulva						
V	Restriction	N	Ova						
W	Revision								
Y	Transplantation								

AHA Coding Clinic for table 0U5
2015, 3Q, 31   Tubal ligation for sterilization

AHA Coding Clinic for table 0U7
2020, 2Q, 30   Duhrssen Cervical Incision

AHA Coding Clinic for table 0U9
2016, 4Q, 58   Longitudinal vaginal septum

AHA Coding Clinic for table 0UB
2018, 1Q, 23   Tubal ligation procedure
2015, 3Q, 31   Laparoscopic partial salpingectomy for ectopic pregnancy
2015, 3Q, 31   Tubal ligation for sterilization
2014, 4Q, 16   Excision of multiple uterine fibroids
2014, 3Q, 12   Excision of skin tag from labia majora

AHA Coding Clinic for table 0UC
2015, 3Q, 30   Removal of cervical cerclage
2013, 2Q, 38   Evacuation of clot post-partum

AHA Coding Clinic for table 0UH
2020, 4Q, 43-44   Insertion of radioactive element
2018, 1Q, 25   Intrauterine brachytherapy & placement of tandems & ovoids
2013, 2Q, 34   Placement of intrauterine device via open approach

AHA Coding Clinic for table 0UJ
2015, 1Q, 33   Robotic-assisted laparoscopic hysterectomy converted to open procedure

AHA Coding Clinic for table 0UL
2018, 1Q, 23   Tubal ligation procedure
2015, 3Q, 31   Tubal ligation for sterilization

AHA Coding Clinic for table 0UQ
2020, 4Q, 59-60   Extraction of ectopic products of conception
2014, 4Q, 18   Obstetrical periurethral laceration
2013, 4Q, 120   Repair of clitoral obstetric laceration

AHA Coding Clinic for table 0US
2016, 1Q, 9   Anteversion of retroverted pregnant uterus

AHA Coding Clinic for table 0UT
2017, 4Q, 68   New qualifier values - Supracervical hysterectomy
2015, 1Q, 33   Robotic-assisted laparoscopic hysterectomy converted to open procedure
2013, 3Q, 28   Total hysterectomy
2013, 1Q, 24   Excision versus Resection of remaining ovarian remnant following previous excision

AHA Coding Clinic for table 0UV
2015, 3Q, 30   Insertion of cervical cerclage

AHA Coding Clinic for table 0UY
2018, 4Q, 40   Uterus transplant

Female Reproductive System

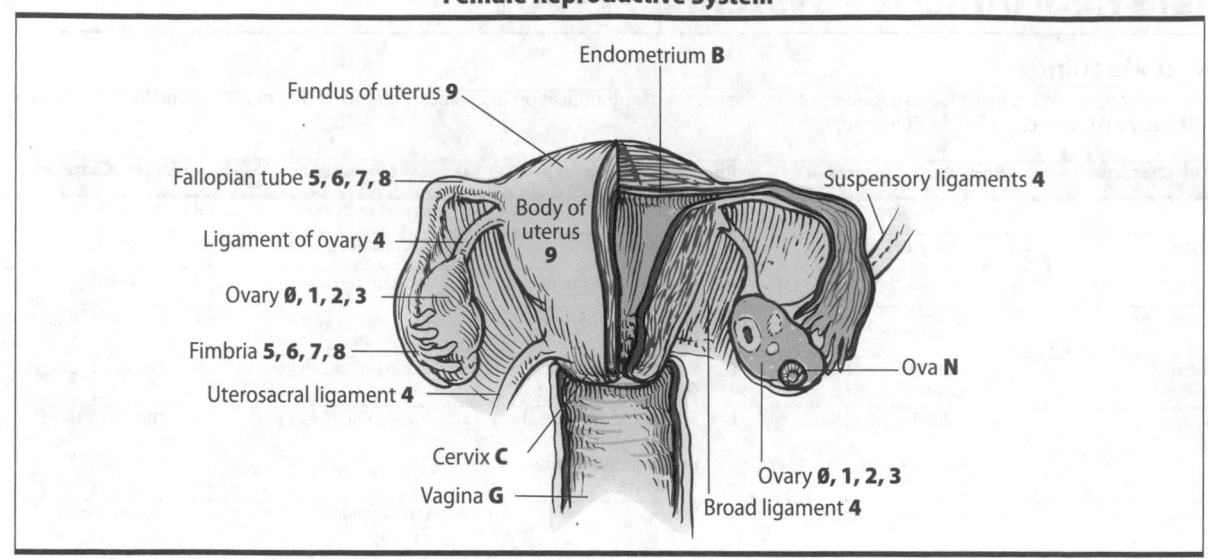

Fundus of uterus **9**

Endometrium **B**

Fallopian tube **5, 6, 7, 8**

Body of uterus **9**

Suspensory ligaments **4**

Ligament of ovary **4**

Ovary **Ø, 1, 2, 3**

Fimbria **5, 6, 7, 8**

Ova **N**

Uterosacral ligament **4**

Cervix **C**

Ovary **Ø, 1, 2, 3**

Vagina **G**

Broad ligament **4**

Female Internal/External Structures

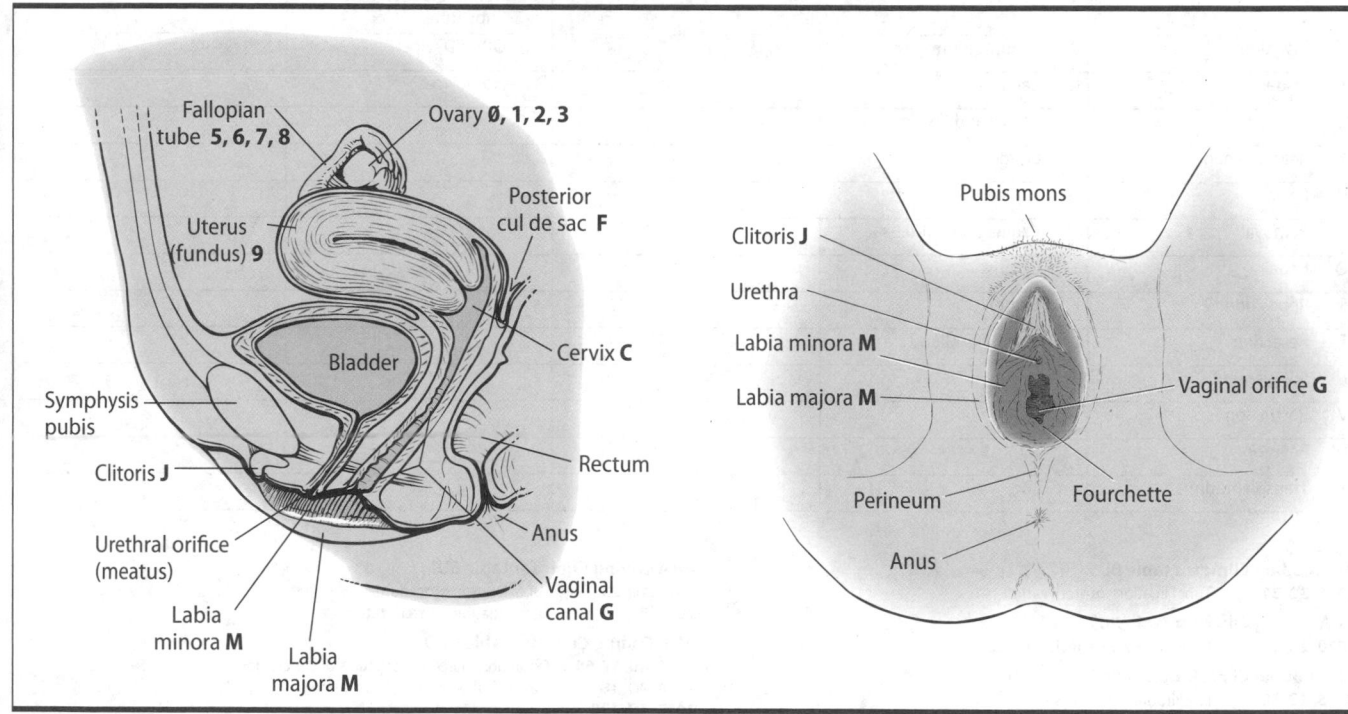

Fallopian tube **5, 6, 7, 8**

Ovary **Ø, 1, 2, 3**

Uterus (fundus) **9**

Posterior cul de sac **F**

Bladder

Cervix **C**

Symphysis pubis

Clitoris **J**

Rectum

Urethral orifice (meatus)

Anus

Labia minora **M**

Vaginal canal **G**

Labia majora **M**

Pubis mons

Clitoris **J**

Urethra

Labia minora **M**

Labia majora **M**

Vaginal orifice **G**

Perineum

Fourchette

Anus

Ø Medical and Surgical
U Female Reproductive System
1 Bypass   Definition: Altering the route of passage of the contents of a tubular body part

             Explanation: Rerouting contents of a body part to a downstream area of the normal route, to a similar route and body part, or to an abnormal route and dissimilar body part. Includes one or more anastomoses, with or without the use of a device.

Body Part Character 4		Approach Character 5	Device Character 6	Qualifier Character 7

5 Fallopian Tube, Right ♀
  Oviduct
  Salpinx
  Uterine tube
6 Fallopian Tube, Left ♀
  See 5 Fallopian Tube, Right
		Ø Open
		4 Percutaneous Endoscopic
			7 Autologous Tissue Substitute
			J Synthetic Substitute
			K Nonautologous Tissue Substitute
			Z No Device
				5 Fallopian Tube, Right
				6 Fallopian Tube, Left
				9 Uterus

   ♀   All body part, approach, device, and qualifier values

Ø Medical and Surgical
U Female Reproductive System
2 Change   Definition: Taking out or off a device from a body part and putting back an identical or similar device in or on the same body part without cutting or puncturing the skin or a mucous membrane

             Explanation: All CHANGE procedures are coded using the approach EXTERNAL

Body Part Character 4		Approach Character 5	Device Character 6	Qualifier Character 7

3 Ovary ♀
8 Fallopian Tube ♀
M Vulva ♀
  Labia majora
  Labia minora
		X External	**Ø** Drainage Device
			Y Other Device
				Z No Qualifier

D Uterus and Cervix ♀		**X** External	**Ø** Drainage Device **H** Contraceptive Device **Y** Other Device	**Z** No Qualifier
H Vagina and Cul-de-sac ♀		**X** External	**Ø** Drainage Device **G** Intraluminal Device, Pessary **Y** Other Device	**Z** No Qualifier

   Non-OR   All body part, approach, device, and qualifier values   ♀   All body part, approach, device, and qualifier values

Female Reproductive System

Ø   **Medical and Surgical**
U   **Female Reproductive System**
5   **Destruction**   Definition: Physical eradication of all or a portion of a body part by the direct use of energy, force, or a destructive agent
                     Explanation: None of the body part is physically taken out

Body Part Character 4	Approach Character 5	Device Character 6	Qualifier Character 7

Ø   Ovary, Right   ♀
1   Ovary, Left   ♀
2   Ovaries, Bilateral   ♀
4   Uterine Supporting Structure   ♀
     Broad ligament
     Infundibulopelvic ligament
     Ovarian ligament
     Round ligament of uterus
	Ø Open
	3 Percutaneous
	4 Percutaneous Endoscopic
	8 Via Natural or Artificial Opening
	     Endoscopic
		Z No Device	Z No Qualifier

5   Fallopian Tube, Right   ♀
     Oviduct
     Salpinx
     Uterine tube
6   Fallopian Tube, Left   ♀
     See 5 Fallopian Tube, Right
7   Fallopian Tubes, Bilateral   **NC** ♀
9   Uterus   ♀
     Fundus uteri
     Myometrium
     Perimetrium
     Uterine cornu
B   Endometrium   ♀
C   Cervix   ♀
F   Cul-de-sac   ♀
	Ø Open
	3 Percutaneous
	4 Percutaneous Endoscopic
	7 Via Natural or Artificial Opening
	8 Via Natural or Artificial Opening
	     Endoscopic
		Z No Device	Z No Qualifier

G Vagina ♀ K Hymen ♀	Ø Open 3 Percutaneous 4 Percutaneous Endoscopic 7 Via Natural or Artificial Opening 8 Via Natural or Artificial Opening Endoscopic X External	Z No Device	Z No Qualifier

J   Clitoris   ♀
L   Vestibular Gland   ♀
     Bartholin's (greater vestibular) gland
     Greater vestibular (Bartholin's) gland
     Paraurethral (Skene's) gland
     Skene's (paraurethral) gland
M   Vulva   ♀
     Labia majora
     Labia minora
	Ø Open
	X External
		Z No Device	Z No Qualifier

     NC   ØU57[Ø,3,4,7,8]ZZ with principal or secondary diagnosis of Z30.2   ♀   All body part, approach, device, and qualifier values

0   **Medical and Surgical**
U   **Female Reproductive System**
7   **Dilation**   Definition: Expanding an orifice or the lumen of a tubular body part

              Explanation: The orifice can be a natural orifice or an artificially created orifice. Accomplished by stretching a tubular body part using intraluminal pressure or by cutting part of the orifice or wall of the tubular body part.

Body Part Character 4		Approach Character 5	Device Character 6	Qualifier Character 7

5 Fallopian Tube, Right ♀
   Oviduct
   Salpinx
   Uterine tube
6 Fallopian Tube, Left ♀
   See 5 Fallopian Tube, Right
7 Fallopian Tubes, Bilateral ♀
9 Uterus ♀
   Fundus uteri
   Myometrium
   Perimetrium
   Uterine cornu
C Cervix ♀
G Vagina ♀
		0 Open
		3 Percutaneous
		4 Percutaneous Endoscopic
		7 Via Natural or Artificial Opening
		8 Via Natural or Artificial Opening
		   Endoscopic
			D Intraluminal Device
			Z No Device
				Z No Qualifier

K Hymen ♀		**0** Open **3** Percutaneous **4** Percutaneous Endoscopic **7** Via Natural or Artificial Opening **8** Via Natural or Artificial Opening Endoscopic **X** External	**D** Intraluminal Device **Z** No Device	**Z** No Qualifier

Non-OR	0U7C[0,3,4,7,8][D,Z]Z	♀	All body part, approach, device, and qualifier values
Non-OR	0U7G[7,8][D,Z]Z		

0   **Medical and Surgical**
U   **Female Reproductive System**
8   **Division**   Definition: Cutting into a body part, without draining fluids and/or gases from the body part, in order to separate or transect a body part

              Explanation: All or a portion of the body part is separated into two or more portions

Body Part Character 4		Approach Character 5	Device Character 6	Qualifier Character 7

0 Ovary, Right ♀
1 Ovary, Left ♀
2 Ovaries, Bilateral ♀
4 Uterine Supporting Structure ♀
   Broad ligament
   Infundibulopelvic ligament
   Ovarian ligament
   Round ligament of uterus
		0 Open
		3 Percutaneous
		4 Percutaneous Endoscopic
			Z No Device	**Z** No Qualifier

K Hymen ♀		**7** Via Natural or Artificial Opening **8** Via Natural or Artificial Opening Endoscopic **X** External	**Z** No Device	**Z** No Qualifier

Non-OR	0U8K[7,8,X]ZZ	♀	All body part, approach, device, and qualifier values

Female Reproductive System

ØU9–ØU9

Ø   Medical and Surgical
U   Female Reproductive System
9   Drainage   Definition: Taking or letting out fluids and/or gases from a body part
                    Explanation: The qualifier DIAGNOSTIC is used to identify drainage procedures that are biopsies

Body Part — Character 4	Approach — Character 5	Device — Character 6	Qualifier — Character 7
Ø Ovary, Right ♀ 1 Ovary, Left ♀ 2 Ovaries, Bilateral ♀	Ø Open 3 Percutaneous 4 Percutaneous Endoscopic 8 Via Natural or Artificial Opening Endoscopic	Ø Drainage Device	Z No Qualifier
Ø Ovary, Right ♀ 1 Ovary, Left ♀ 2 Ovaries, Bilateral ♀	Ø Open 3 Percutaneous 4 Percutaneous Endoscopic 8 Via Natural or Artificial Opening Endoscopic	Z No Device	X Diagnostic Z No Qualifier
Ø Ovary, Right ♀ 1 Ovary, Left ♀ 2 Ovaries, Bilateral ♀	X External	Z No Device	Z No Qualifier

4 Uterine Supporting Structure ♀
    Broad ligament
    Infundibulopelvic ligament
    Ovarian ligament
    Round ligament of uterus
	Ø Open
	 3 Percutaneous
	 4 Percutaneous Endoscopic
	 8 Via Natural or Artificial Opening Endoscopic
		Ø Drainage Device	Z No Qualifier

4 Uterine Supporting Structure ♀
    Broad ligament
    Infundibulopelvic ligament
    Ovarian ligament
    Round ligament of uterus
	Ø Open
	 3 Percutaneous
	 4 Percutaneous Endoscopic
	 8 Via Natural or Artificial Opening Endoscopic
		Z No Device	X Diagnostic
			 Z No Qualifier

5 Fallopian Tube, Right ♀
    Oviduct
    Salpinx
    Uterine tube
 6 Fallopian Tube, Left ♀
    See 5 Fallopian Tube, Right
 7 Fallopian Tubes, Bilateral ♀
 9 Uterus ♀
    Fundus uteri
    Myometrium
    Perimetrium
    Uterine cornu
 C Cervix ♀
 F Cul-de-sac ♀
	Ø Open
	 3 Percutaneous
	 4 Percutaneous Endoscopic
	 7 Via Natural or Artificial Opening
	 8 Via Natural or Artificial Opening Endoscopic
		Ø Drainage Device	Z No Qualifier

5 Fallopian Tube, Right ♀
    Oviduct
    Salpinx
    Uterine tube
 6 Fallopian Tube, Left ♀
    See 5 Fallopian Tube, Right
 7 Fallopian Tubes, Bilateral ♀
 9 Uterus ♀
    Fundus uteri
    Myometrium
    Perimetrium
    Uterine cornu
 C Cervix ♀
 F Cul-de-sac ♀
	Ø Open
	 3 Percutaneous
	 4 Percutaneous Endoscopic
	 7 Via Natural or Artificial Opening
	 8 Via Natural or Artificial Opening Endoscopic
		Z No Device	X Diagnostic
			 Z No Qualifier

Non-OR ØU9[Ø,1,2][3,8]ØZ		**Non-OR** ØU9[5,6,7,9,C]3ØZ	
Non-OR ØU9[Ø,1,2][3,8]ZZ		**Non-OR** ØU9F[3,4]ØZ	
Non-OR ØU9[Ø,1,2]8ZX		**Non-OR** ØU9[5,6,7][3,4,7,8]ZZ	
Non-OR ØU94[3,8]ØZ		**Non-OR** ØU9[9,C]3ZZ	
Non-OR ØU94[3,8]ZZ		**Non-OR** ØU9F[3,4]ZZ	
Non-OR ØU948ZX		♀ All body part, approach, device, and qualifier values	

ØU9 Continued on next page

Female Reproductive System

0   **Medical and Surgical**
U   **Female Reproductive System**
9   **Drainage**   Definition: Taking or letting out fluids and/or gases from a body part

0U9 Continued

                                Explanation: The qualifier DIAGNOSTIC is used to identify drainage procedures that are biopsies

Body Part Character 4	Approach Character 5	Device Character 6	Qualifier Character 7
G Vagina ♀ **K** Hymen ♀	**0** Open **3** Percutaneous **4** Percutaneous Endoscopic **7** Via Natural or Artificial Opening **8** Via Natural or Artificial Opening Endoscopic **X** External	**0** Drainage Device	**Z** No Qualifier
G Vagina ♀ **K** Hymen ♀	**0** Open **3** Percutaneous **4** Percutaneous Endoscopic **7** Via Natural or Artificial Opening **8** Via Natural or Artificial Opening Endoscopic **X** External	**Z** No Device	**X** Diagnostic **Z** No Qualifier

J Clitoris ♀
L Vestibular Gland ♀
    Bartholin's (greater vestibular) gland
    Greater vestibular (Bartholin's) gland
    Paraurethral (Skene's) gland
    Skene's (paraurethral) gland
M Vulva ♀
    Labia majora
    Labia minora
	0 Open
	X External
		0 Drainage Device	**Z** No Qualifier

J Clitoris ♀
L Vestibular Gland ♀
    Bartholin's (greater vestibular) gland
    Greater vestibular (Bartholin's) gland
    Paraurethral (Skene's) gland
    Skene's (paraurethral) gland
M Vulva ♀
    Labia majora
    Labia minora
	0 Open
	X External
		Z No Device	**X** Diagnostic
			Z No Qualifier

Non-OR 0U9G30Z		**Non-OR** 0U9L[0,X]0Z	
Non-OR 0U9K[0,3,4,7,8,X]0Z		**Non-OR** 0U9L[0,X]ZZ	
Non-OR 0U9G3ZZ		♀ All body part, approach, device, and qualifier values	
Non-OR 0U9K[0,3,4,7,8,X]ZZ			

NC Noncovered Procedure   LC Limited Coverage   QA Questionable OB Admit   NT New Tech Add-on   ⊞ Combination Member   ♂ Male   ♀ Female

ICD-10-PCS 2022   643

0U9–0U9

Female Reproductive System

Ø   **Medical and Surgical**
U   **Female Reproductive System**
B   **Excision**   Definition: Cutting out or off, without replacement, a portion of a body part

                      Explanation: The qualifier DIAGNOSTIC is used to identify excision procedures that are biopsies

Body Part Character 4	Approach Character 5	Device Character 6	Qualifier Character 7

Ø Ovary, Right ♀
1 Ovary, Left ♀
2 Ovaries, Bilateral ♀
4 Uterine Supporting Structure ♀
    Broad ligament
    Infundibulopelvic ligament
    Ovarian ligament
    Round ligament of uterus
5 Fallopian Tube, Right ♀
    Oviduct
    Salpinx
    Uterine tube
6 Fallopian Tube, Left ♀
    See 5 Fallopian Tube, Right
7 Fallopian Tubes, Bilateral ♀
9 Uterus ♀
    Fundus uteri
    Myometrium
    Perimetrium
    Uterine cornu
C Cervix ♀
F Cul-de-sac ♀
	Ø Open
	3 Percutaneous
	4 Percutaneous Endoscopic
	7 Via Natural or Artificial Opening
	8 Via Natural or Artificial Opening
	    Endoscopic
		Z No Device	X Diagnostic
			Z No Qualifier

G Vagina ♀ K Hymen ♀	Ø Open 3 Percutaneous 4 Percutaneous Endoscopic 7 Via Natural or Artificial Opening 8 Via Natural or Artificial Opening Endoscopic X External	Z No Device	X Diagnostic Z No Qualifier

J Clitoris ♀
L Vestibular Gland ♀
    Bartholin's (greater vestibular) gland
    Greater vestibular (Bartholin's) gland
    Paraurethral (Skene's) gland
    Skene's (paraurethral) gland
M Vulva ♀
    Labia majora
    Labia minora
	Ø Open
	X External
		Z No Device	X Diagnostic
			Z No Qualifier

♀   All body part, approach, device, and qualifier values

Ø   Medical and Surgical
U   Female Reproductive System
C   Extirpation   Definition: Taking or cutting out solid matter from a body part

Explanation: The solid matter may be an abnormal byproduct of a biological function or a foreign body; it may be imbedded in a body part or in the lumen of a tubular body part. The solid matter may or may not have been previously broken into pieces.

Body Part Character 4	Approach Character 5	Device Character 6	Qualifier Character 7

Ø Ovary, Right ♀
1 Ovary, Left ♀
2 Ovaries, Bilateral ♀
4 Uterine Supporting Structure ♀
  Broad ligament
  Infundibulopelvic ligament
  Ovarian ligament
  Round ligament of uterus
	Ø Open
	3 Percutaneous
	4 Percutaneous Endoscopic
	8 Via Natural or Artificial Opening
	  Endoscopic
		Z No Device	**Z** No Qualifier

5 Fallopian Tube, Right ♀
  Oviduct
  Salpinx
  Uterine tube
6 Fallopian Tube, Left ♀
  See 5 Fallopian Tube, Right
7 Fallopian Tubes, Bilateral ♀
9 Uterus ♀
  Fundus uteri
  Myometrium
  Perimetrium
  Uterine cornu
B Endometrium ♀
C Cervix ♀
F Cul-de-sac ♀
	Ø Open
	3 Percutaneous
	4 Percutaneous Endoscopic
	7 Via Natural or Artificial Opening
	8 Via Natural or Artificial Opening
	  Endoscopic
		Z No Device	**Z** No Qualifier

G Vagina ♀ **K** Hymen ♀	**Ø** Open **3** Percutaneous **4** Percutaneous Endoscopic **7** Via Natural or Artificial Opening **8** Via Natural or Artificial Opening Endoscopic **X** External	**Z** No Device	**Z** No Qualifier

J Clitoris ♀
L Vestibular Gland ♀
  Bartholin's (greater vestibular) gland
  Greater vestibular (Bartholin's) gland
  Paraurethral (Skene's) gland
  Skene's (paraurethral) gland
M Vulva ♀
  Labia majora
  Labia minora
	Ø Open
	X External
		Z No Device	**Z** No Qualifier

Non-OR ØUC9[7,8]ZZ		**Non-OR** ØUCMXZZ	
Non-OR ØUCG[7,8,X]ZZ		♀ All body part, approach, device, and qualifier values	
Non-OR ØUCK[Ø,3,4,7,8,X]ZZ			

Ø   Medical and Surgical
U   Female Reproductive System
D   Extraction   Definition: Pulling or stripping out or off all or a portion of a body part by the use of force

Explanation: The qualifier DIAGNOSTIC is used to identify extraction procedures that are biopsies

Body Part Character 4	Approach Character 5	Device Character 6	Qualifier Character 7
B Endometrium ♀	**7** Via Natural or Artificial Opening **8** Via Natural or Artificial Opening Endoscopic	**Z** No Device	**X** Diagnostic **Z** No Qualifier
N Ova ♀	**Ø** Open **3** Percutaneous **4** Percutaneous Endoscopic	**Z** No Device	**Z** No Qualifier

♀ All body part, approach, device, and qualifier values			

NC Noncovered Procedure **LC** Limited Coverage **QA** Questionable OB Admit **NT** New Tech Add-on ⊞ Combination Member ♂ Male ♀ Female	

Female Reproductive System

Ø   **Medical and Surgical**
U   **Female Reproductive System**
F   **Fragmentation**   Definition: Breaking solid matter in a body part into pieces

Explanation: Physical force (e.g., manual, ultrasonic) applied directly or indirectly is used to break the solid matter into pieces. The solid matter may be an abnormal byproduct of a biological function or a foreign body. The pieces of solid matter are not taken out.

Body Part Character 4	Approach Character 5	Device Character 6	Qualifier Character 7

5 **Fallopian Tube, Right** NC ♀
   Oviduct
   Salpinx
   Uterine tube
6 **Fallopian Tube, Left** NC ♀
   See 5 Fallopian Tube, Right
7 **Fallopian Tubes, Bilateral** NC ♀
9 **Uterus** NC ♀
   Fundus uteri
   Myometrium
   Perimetrium
   Uterine cornu
	Ø Open
	3 Percutaneous
	4 Percutaneous Endoscopic
	7 Via Natural or Artificial Opening
	8 Via Natural or Artificial Opening
	   Endoscopic
	X External
		Z No Device	**Z** No Qualifier

Non-OR   ØUF[5,6,7,9]XZZ
NC   ØUF[5,6,7,9]XZZ

♀   All body part, approach, device, and qualifier values

Ø   **Medical and Surgical**
U   **Female Reproductive System**
H   **Insertion**   Definition: Putting in a nonbiological appliance that monitors, assists, performs, or prevents a physiological function but does not physically take the place of a body part

Explanation: None

Body Part Character 4	Approach Character 5	Device Character 6	Qualifier Character 7
3 Ovary ♀	**Ø** Open **3** Percutaneous **4** Percutaneous Endoscopic	**1** Radioactive Element **3** Infusion Device **Y** Other Device	**Z** No Qualifier
3 Ovary ♀	**7** Via Natural or Artificial Opening **8** Via Natural or Artificial Opening Endoscopic	**1** Radioactive Element **Y** Other Device	**Z** No Qualifier
8 Fallopian Tube ♀ **D** Uterus and Cervix ♀ **H** Vagina and Cul-de-sac ♀	**Ø** Open **3** Percutaneous **4** Percutaneous Endoscopic **7** Via Natural or Artificial Opening **8** Via Natural or Artificial Opening Endoscopic	**3** Infusion Device **Y** Other Device	**Z** No Qualifier

9 Uterus ♀
   Fundus uteri
   Myometrium
   Perimetrium
   Uterine cornu
	Ø Open
	7 Via Natural or Artificial Opening
	8 Via Natural or Artificial Opening
	   Endoscopic
		1 Radioactive Element
		H Contraceptive Device
			Z No Qualifier

C Cervix ♀	**Ø** Open **3** Percutaneous **4** Percutaneous Endoscopic	**1** Radioactive Element	**Z** No Qualifier
C Cervix ♀	**7** Via Natural or Artificial Opening **8** Via Natural or Artificial Opening Endoscopic	**1** Radioactive Element **H** Contraceptive Device	**Z** No Qualifier
F Cul-de-sac ♀	**7** Via Natural or Artificial Opening **8** Via Natural or Artificial Opening Endoscopic	**G** Intraluminal Device, Pessary	**Z** No Qualifier
G Vagina ♀	**Ø** Open **3** Percutaneous **4** Percutaneous Endoscopic **X** External	**1** Radioactive Element	**Z** No Qualifier
G Vagina ♀	**7** Via Natural or Artificial Opening **8** Via Natural or Artificial Opening Endoscopic	**1** Radioactive Element **G** Intraluminal Device, Pessary	**Z** No Qualifier

Non-OR   ØUH3[Ø,4][3,Y]Z
Non-OR   ØUH33[1,3,Y]Z
Non-OR   ØUH3[7,8][1,Y]Z
Non-OR   ØUH[8,D][Ø,3,4,7,8][3,Y]Z
Non-OR   ØUHH[3,4]YZ
Non-OR   ØUHH[7,8][3,Y]Z

Non-OR   ØUH9[Ø,7,8][1,H]Z
Non-OR   ØUHC[7,8]HZ
Non-OR   ØUHF[7,8]HZ
Non-OR   ØUHG[7,8]HZ
♀   All body part, approach, device, and qualifier values

Ø   Medical and Surgical
U   Female Reproductive System
J   Inspection   Definition: Visually and/or manually exploring a body part

Explanation: Visual exploration may be performed with or without optical instrumentation. Manual exploration may be performed directly or through intervening body layers.

Body Part Character 4		Approach Character 5	Device Character 6	Qualifier Character 7
3 Ovary	♀	**Ø** Open **3** Percutaneous **4** Percutaneous Endoscopic **8** Via Natural or Artificial Opening Endoscopic **X** External	**Z** No Device	**Z** No Qualifier
8 Fallopian Tube **D** Uterus and Cervix **H** Vagina and Cul-de-sac	♀ ♀ ♀	**Ø** Open **3** Percutaneous **4** Percutaneous Endoscopic **7** Via Natural or Artificial Opening **8** Via Natural or Artificial Opening Endoscopic **X** External	**Z** No Device	**Z** No Qualifier

M   Vulva
     Labia majora
     Labia minora
	♀	**Ø** Open
		X External
			Z No Device	**Z** No Qualifier

Non-OR	ØUJ3[3,8,X]ZZ		Non-OR	ØUJMXZZ
Non-OR	ØUJ[8,D,H][3,7,8,X]ZZ		♀	All body part, approach, device, and qualifier values

Ø   Medical and Surgical
U   Female Reproductive System
L   Occlusion   Definition: Completely closing an orifice or the lumen of a tubular body part

Explanation: The orifice can be a natural orifice or an artificially created orifice

Body Part Character 4		Approach Character 5	Device Character 6	Qualifier Character 7

5   Fallopian Tube, Right
     Oviduct
     Salpinx
     Uterine tube
6   Fallopian Tube, Left
     See 5 Fallopian Tube, Right
7   Fallopian Tubes, Bilateral   **NC**
	♀
	
	♀
	
	♀
		Ø Open
		3 Percutaneous
		4 Percutaneous Endoscopic
			C Extraluminal Device
			D Intraluminal Device
			Z No Device
				Z No Qualifier

5   Fallopian Tube, Right
     Oviduct
     Salpinx
     Uterine tube
6   Fallopian Tube, Left
     See 5 Fallopian Tube, Right
7   Fallopian Tubes, Bilateral   **NC**
	♀
	
	♀
	
	♀
		7 Via Natural or Artificial Opening
		8 Via Natural or Artificial Opening
		     Endoscopic
			D Intraluminal Device
			Z No Device
				Z No Qualifier

F Cul-de-sac **G** Vagina	♀ ♀	**7** Via Natural or Artificial Opening **8** Via Natural or Artificial Opening Endoscopic	**D** Intraluminal Device **Z** No Device	**Z** No Qualifier

NC	ØUL7[Ø,3,4][C,D,Z]Z with principal or secondary diagnosis of Z3Ø.2		♀	All body part, approach, device, and qualifier values
NC	ØUL7[7,8][D,Z]Z with principal or secondary diagnosis of Z3Ø.2			

NC Noncovered Procedure   **LC** Limited Coverage   **QA** Questionable OB Admit   **NT** New Tech Add-on   ⊞ Combination Member   ♂ Male   ♀ Female

ICD-10-PCS 2022   647

ØUJ–ØUL

Female Reproductive System

Ø   **Medical and Surgical**
U   **Female Reproductive System**
M   **Reattachment**   Definition: Putting back in or on all or a portion of a separated body part to its normal location or other suitable location
                   Explanation: Vascular circulation and nervous pathways may or may not be reestablished

Body Part Character 4		Approach Character 5	Device Character 6	Qualifier Character 7

Ø   Ovary, Right
1   Ovary, Left
2   Ovaries, Bilateral
4   **Uterine Supporting Structure**
      Broad ligament
      Infundibulopelvic ligament
      Ovarian ligament
      Round ligament of uterus
5   **Fallopian Tube, Right**
      Oviduct
      Salpinx
      Uterine tube
6   **Fallopian Tube, Left**
      See 5 Fallopian Tube, Right
7   **Fallopian Tubes, Bilateral**
9   **Uterus**
      Fundus uteri
      Myometrium
      Perimetrium
      Uterine cornu
C   **Cervix**
F   **Cul-de-sac**
G   **Vagina**
	♀
	♀
	♀
	♀
	
	♀
	
	♀
	
	♀
	♀
	
	♀
	♀
	♀
		Ø Open
		4 Percutaneous Endoscopic
			Z No Device	Z No Qualifier

J   **Clitoris**
M   **Vulva**
      Labia majora
      Labia minora
	♀
	♀
		X External	Z No Device	Z No Qualifier

K **Hymen**	♀	Ø Open 4 Percutaneous Endoscopic X External	Z No Device	Z No Qualifier

♀   All body part, approach, device, and qualifier values

Ø   **Medical and Surgical**
U   **Female Reproductive System**
N   **Release**   Definition: Freeing a body part from an abnormal physical constraint by cutting or by the use of force
                          Explanation: Some of the restraining tissue may be taken out but none of the body part is taken out

Body Part Character 4	Approach Character 5	Device Character 6	Qualifier Character 7

Ø Ovary, Right ♀
1 Ovary, Left ♀
2 Ovaries, Bilateral ♀
4 Uterine Supporting Structure ♀
     Broad ligament
     Infundibulopelvic ligament
     Ovarian ligament
     Round ligament of uterus
	Ø Open
	3 Percutaneous
	4 Percutaneous Endoscopic
	8 Via Natural or Artificial Opening
	     Endoscopic
		Z No Device	**Z** No Qualifier

5 Fallopian Tube, Right ♀
     Oviduct
     Salpinx
     Uterine tube
6 Fallopian Tube, Left ♀
     See 5 Fallopian Tube, Right
7 Fallopian Tubes, Bilateral ♀
9 Uterus ♀
     Fundus uteri
     Myometrium
     Perimetrium
     Uterine cornu
C Cervix ♀
F Cul-de-sac ♀
	Ø Open
	3 Percutaneous
	4 Percutaneous Endoscopic
	7 Via Natural or Artificial Opening
	8 Via Natural or Artificial Opening
	     Endoscopic
		Z No Device	**Z** No Qualifier

G Vagina ♀ **K** Hymen ♀	**Ø** Open **3** Percutaneous **4** Percutaneous Endoscopic **7** Via Natural or Artificial Opening **8** Via Natural or Artificial Opening Endoscopic **X** External	**Z** No Device	**Z** No Qualifier

J Clitoris ♀
L Vestibular Gland ♀
     Bartholin's (greater vestibular) gland
     Greater vestibular (Bartholin's) gland
     Paraurethral (Skene's) gland
     Skene's (paraurethral) gland
M Vulva ♀
     Labia majora
     Labia minora
	Ø Open
	X External
		Z No Device	**Z** No Qualifier

♀   All body part, approach, device, and qualifier values

Female Reproductive System

Ø **Medical and Surgical**
U **Female Reproductive System**
P **Removal** Definition: Taking out or off a device from a body part
Explanation: If a device is taken out and a similar device put in without cutting or puncturing the skin or mucous membrane, the procedure is coded to the root operation CHANGE. Otherwise, the procedure for taking out the device is coded to the root operation REMOVAL.

Body Part Character 4		Approach Character 5	Device Character 6	Qualifier Character 7
3 Ovary	♀	Ø Open 3 Percutaneous 4 Percutaneous Endoscopic	Ø Drainage Device 3 Infusion Device Y Other Device	Z No Qualifier
3 Ovary	♀	7 Via Natural or Artificial Opening 8 Via Natural or Artificial Opening Endoscopic	Y Other Device	Z No Qualifier
3 Ovary	♀	X External	Ø Drainage Device 3 Infusion Device	Z No Qualifier
8 Fallopian Tube	♀	Ø Open 3 Percutaneous 4 Percutaneous Endoscopic 7 Via Natural or Artificial Opening 8 Via Natural or Artificial Opening Endoscopic	Ø Drainage Device 3 Infusion Device 7 Autologous Tissue Substitute C Extraluminal Device D Intraluminal Device J Synthetic Substitute K Nonautologous Tissue Substitute Y Other Device	Z No Qualifier
8 Fallopian Tube	♀	X External	Ø Drainage Device 3 Infusion Device D Intraluminal Device	Z No Qualifier
D Uterus and Cervix	♀	Ø Open 3 Percutaneous 4 Percutaneous Endoscopic 7 Via Natural or Artificial Opening 8 Via Natural or Artificial Opening Endoscopic	Ø Drainage Device 1 Radioactive Element 3 Infusion Device 7 Autologous Tissue Substitute C Extraluminal Device D Intraluminal Device H Contraceptive Device J Synthetic Substitute K Nonautologous Tissue Substitute Y Other Device	Z No Qualifier
D Uterus and Cervix	♀	X External	Ø Drainage Device 3 Infusion Device D Intraluminal Device H Contraceptive Device	Z No Qualifier
H Vagina and Cul-de-sac	♀	Ø Open 3 Percutaneous 4 Percutaneous Endoscopic 7 Via Natural or Artificial Opening 8 Via Natural or Artificial Opening Endoscopic	Ø Drainage Device 1 Radioactive Element 3 Infusion Device 7 Autologous Tissue Substitute D Intraluminal Device J Synthetic Substitute K Nonautologous Tissue Substitute Y Other Device	Z No Qualifier
H Vagina and Cul-de-sac	♀	X External	Ø Drainage Device 1 Radioactive Element 3 Infusion Device D Intraluminal Device	Z No Qualifier
M Vulva Labia majora Labia minora	♀	Ø Open	Ø Drainage Device 7 Autologous Tissue Substitute J Synthetic Substitute K Nonautologous Tissue Substitute	Z No Qualifier
M Vulva Labia majora Labia minora	♀	X External	Ø Drainage Device	Z No Qualifier

Non-OR	ØUP3[3,4]YZ		Non-OR	ØUPD[7,8][Ø,3,C,D,H,Y]Z
Non-OR	ØUP3[7,8]YZ		Non-OR	ØUPDX[Ø,3,D,H]Z
Non-OR	ØUP3X[Ø,3]Z		Non-OR	ØUPH[3,4]YZ
Non-OR	ØUP8[3,4]YZ		Non-OR	ØUPH[7,8][Ø,3,D,Y]Z
Non-OR	ØUP8[7,8][Ø,3,D,Y]Z		Non-OR	ØUPHX[Ø,1,3,D]Z
Non-OR	ØUP8X[Ø,3,D]Z		Non-OR	ØUPMXØZ
Non-OR	ØUPD[3,4][C,Y]Z		♀	All body part, approach, device, and qualifier values

Non-OR Procedure   DRG Non-OR Procedure   Valid OR Procedure   HAC Associated Procedure   Combination Only   New/Revised GREEN

Ø   Medical and Surgical
U   Female Reproductive System
Q   Repair   Definition: Restoring, to the extent possible, a body part to its normal anatomic structure and function

         Explanation: Used only when the method to accomplish the repair is not one of the other root operations

Body Part Character 4	Approach Character 5	Device Character 6	Qualifier Character 7

Ø   Ovary, Right   ♀
1   Ovary, Left   ♀
2   Ovaries, Bilateral   ♀
4   Uterine Supporting Structure   ♀
     Broad ligament
     Infundibulopelvic ligament
     Ovarian ligament
     Round ligament of uterus
	Ø Open
	3 Percutaneous
	4 Percutaneous Endoscopic
	8 Via Natural or Artificial Opening
	     Endoscopic
		Z No Device	Z No Qualifier

5   Fallopian Tube, Right   ♀
     Oviduct
     Salpinx
     Uterine tube
6   Fallopian Tube, Left   ♀
     See 5 Fallopian Tube, Right
7   Fallopian Tubes, Bilateral   ♀
9   Uterus   ♀
     Fundus uteri
     Myometrium
     Perimetrium
     Uterine cornu
C   Cervix   ♀
F   Cul-de-sac   ♀
	Ø Open
	3 Percutaneous
	4 Percutaneous Endoscopic
	7 Via Natural or Artificial Opening
	8 Via Natural or Artificial Opening
	     Endoscopic
		Z No Device	Z No Qualifier

G Vagina ♀ K Hymen ♀	Ø Open 3 Percutaneous 4 Percutaneous Endoscopic 7 Via Natural or Artificial Opening 8 Via Natural or Artificial Opening Endoscopic X External	Z No Device	Z No Qualifier

J   Clitoris   ♀
L   Vestibular Gland   ♀
     Bartholin's (greater vestibular) gland
     Greater vestibular (Bartholin's) gland
     Paraurethral (Skene's) gland
     Skene's (paraurethral) gland
M   Vulva   ♀
     Labia majora
     Labia minora
	Ø Open
	X External
		Z No Device	Z No Qualifier

Non-OR ØUQG[7,X]ZZ		**Non-OR** ØUQMXZZ	
Non-OR ØUQKXZZ		♀ All body part, approach, device, and qualifier values	

Ø   Medical and Surgical
U   Female Reproductive System
S   Reposition   Definition: Moving to its normal location, or other suitable location, all or a portion of a body part

         Explanation: The body part is moved to a new location from an abnormal location, or from a normal location where it is not functioning correctly. The body part may or may not be cut out or off to be moved to the new location.

Body Part Character 4	Approach Character 5	Device Character 6	Qualifier Character 7

Ø   Ovary, Right   ♀
1   Ovary, Left   ♀
2   Ovaries, Bilateral   ♀
4   Uterine Supporting Structure   ♀
     Broad ligament
     Infundibulopelvic ligament
     Ovarian ligament
     Round ligament of uterus
5   Fallopian Tube, Right   ♀
     Oviduct
     Salpinx
     Uterine tube
6   Fallopian Tube, Left   ♀
     See 5 Fallopian Tube, Right
7   Fallopian Tubes, Bilateral   ♀
C   Cervix   ♀
F   Cul-de-sac   ♀
	Ø Open
	4 Percutaneous Endoscopic
	8 Via Natural or Artificial Opening
	     Endoscopic
		Z No Device	Z No Qualifier

9   Uterus   ♀
     Fundus uteri
     Myometrium
     Perimetrium
     Uterine cornu
G   Vagina   ♀
	Ø Open
	4 Percutaneous Endoscopic
	7 Via Natural or Artificial Opening
	8 Via Natural or Artificial Opening
	     Endoscopic
	X External
		Z No Device	Z No Qualifier

Non-OR ØUS9XZZ	♀ All body part, approach, device, and qualifier values	

NC Noncovered Procedure   **LC** Limited Coverage   **QA** Questionable OB Admit   **NT** New Tech Add-on   ⊞ Combination Member   ♂ Male   ♀ Female

ICD-10-PCS 2022   651

ØUQ–ØUS

Ø   **Medical and Surgical**
U   **Female Reproductive System**
T   **Resection**   Definition: Cutting out or off, without replacement, all of a body part
                Explanation: None

Body Part Character 4	Approach Character 5	Device Character 6	Qualifier Character 7

Ø Ovary, Right ♀
1 Ovary, Left ♀
2 Ovaries, Bilateral ⊞♀
5 Fallopian Tube, Right ♀
    Oviduct
    Salpinx
    Uterine tube
6 Fallopian Tube, Left ♀
    See 5 Fallopian Tube, Right
7 Fallopian Tubes, Bilateral ⊞♀
	Ø Open
	4 Percutaneous Endoscopic
	7 Via Natural or Artificial Opening
	8 Via Natural or Artificial Opening
	    Endoscopic
	F Via Natural or Artificial Opening
	    With Percutaneous Endoscopic
	    Assistance
		Z No Device	**Z** No Qualifier

4 Uterine Supporting Structure ⊞♀
    Broad ligament
    Infundibulopelvic ligament
    Ovarian ligament
    Round ligament of uterus
C Cervix ⊞♀
F Cul-de-sac ♀
G Vagina ⊞♀
	Ø Open
	4 Percutaneous Endoscopic
	7 Via Natural or Artificial Opening
	8 Via Natural or Artificial Opening
	    Endoscopic
		Z No Device	**Z** No Qualifier

9 Uterus ⊞♀
    Fundus uteri
    Myometrium
    Perimetrium
    Uterine cornu
	Ø Open
	4 Percutaneous Endoscopic
	7 Via Natural or Artificial Opening
	8 Via Natural or Artificial Opening
	    Endoscopic
	F Via Natural or Artificial Opening
	    With Percutaneous Endoscopic
	    Assistance
		Z No Device	**L** Supracervical
			Z No Qualifier

J Clitoris ♀
L Vestibular Gland ♀
    Bartholin's (greater vestibular)
        gland
    Greater vestibular (Bartholin's)
        gland
    Paraurethral (Skene's) gland
    Skene's (paraurethral) gland
M Vulva ⊞♀
    Labia majora
    Labia minora
	Ø Open
	X External
		Z No Device	**Z** No Qualifier

K Hymen ♀	**Ø** Open **4** Percutaneous Endoscopic **7** Via Natural or Artificial Opening **8** Via Natural or Artificial Opening Endoscopic **X** External	**Z** No Device	**Z** No Device

♀   All body part, approach, device, and qualifier values

See Appendix L for Procedure Combinations
⊞   ØUT[2,7]ØZZ
⊞   ØUT[4,C][Ø,4,7,8]ZZ
⊞   ØUTGØZZ
⊞   ØUT9[Ø,4,7,8,F]ZZ
⊞   ØUTM[Ø,X]ZZ

Ø   **Medical and Surgical**
U   **Female Reproductive System**
U   **Supplement**   Definition: Putting in or on biological or synthetic material that physically reinforces and/or augments the function of a portion of a body part

               Explanation: The biological material is non-living, or is living and from the same individual. The body part may have been previously replaced, and the SUPPLEMENT procedure is performed to physically reinforce and/or augment the function of the replaced body part.

Body Part Character 4	Approach Character 5	Device Character 6	Qualifier Character 7

4 Uterine Supporting Structure ♀
    Broad ligament
    Infundibulopelvic ligament
    Ovarian ligament
    Round ligament of uterus
	Ø Open
	4 Percutaneous Endoscopic
		7 Autologous Tissue Substitute
		J Synthetic Substitute
		K Nonautologous Tissue Substitute
			Z No Qualifier

5 Fallopian Tube, Right ♀
    Oviduct
    Salpinx
    Uterine tube
6 Fallopian Tube, Left ♀
    See 5 Fallopian Tube, Right
7 Fallopian Tubes, Bilateral ♀
F Cul-de-sac ♀
	Ø Open
	4 Percutaneous Endoscopic
	7 Via Natural or Artificial Opening
	8 Via Natural or Artificial Opening Endoscopic
		7 Autologous Tissue Substitute
		J Synthetic Substitute
		K Nonautologous Tissue Substitute
			Z No Qualifier

G Vagina ♀ **K** Hymen ♀	**Ø** Open **4** Percutaneous Endoscopic **7** Via Natural or Artificial Opening **8** Via Natural or Artificial Opening Endoscopic **X** External	**7** Autologous Tissue Substitute **J** Synthetic Substitute **K** Nonautologous Tissue Substitute	**Z** No Qualifier

J Clitoris ♀
M Vulva ♀
    Labia majora
    Labia minora
	Ø Open
	X External
		7 Autologous Tissue Substitute
		J Synthetic Substitute
		K Nonautologous Tissue Substitute
			Z No Qualifier

♀   All body part, approach, device, and qualifier values

Ø   **Medical and Surgical**
U   **Female Reproductive System**
V   **Restriction**   Definition: Partially closing an orifice or the lumen of a tubular body part

               Explanation: The orifice can be a natural orifice or an artificially created orifice

Body Part Character 4	Approach Character 5	Device Character 6	Qualifier Character 7
C Cervix ♀	**Ø** Open **3** Percutaneous **4** Percutaneous Endoscopic	**C** Extraluminal Device **D** Intraluminal Device **Z** No Device	**Z** No Qualifier
C Cervix ♀	**7** Via Natural or Artificial Opening **8** Via Natural or Artificial Opening Endoscopic	**D** Intraluminal Device **Z** No Device	**Z** No Qualifier

♀   All body part, approach, device, and qualifier values

NC Noncovered Procedure   **LC** Limited Coverage   **QA** Questionable OB Admit   **NT** New Tech Add-on   ⊞ Combination Member   ♂ Male   ♀ Female

ICD-10-PCS 2022   653

Female Reproductive System (sidebar)

Ø   **Medical and Surgical**
U   **Female Reproductive System**
W   **Revision**   Definition: Correcting, to the extent possible, a portion of a malfunctioning device or the position of a displaced device
                             Explanation: Revision can include correcting a malfunctioning or displaced device by taking out or putting in components of the device such as a screw or pin

Body Part Character 4		Approach Character 5	Device Character 6	Qualifier Character 7
3 Ovary ♀		**Ø** Open **3** Percutaneous **4** Percutaneous Endoscopic	**Ø** Drainage Device **3** Infusion Device **Y** Other Device	**Z** No Qualifier
3 Ovary ♀		**7** Via Natural or Artificial Opening **8** Via Natural or Artificial Opening Endoscopic	**Y** Other Device	**Z** No Qualifier
3 Ovary ♀		**X** External	**Ø** Drainage Device **3** Infusion Device	**Z** No Qualifier
8 Fallopian Tube ♀		**Ø** Open **3** Percutaneous **4** Percutaneous Endoscopic **7** Via Natural or Artificial Opening **8** Via Natural or Artificial Opening Endoscopic	**Ø** Drainage Device **3** Infusion Device **7** Autologous Tissue Substitute **C** Extraluminal Device **D** Intraluminal Device **J** Synthetic Substitute **K** Nonautologous Tissue Substitute **Y** Other Device	**Z** No Qualifier
8 Fallopian Tube ♀		**X** External	**Ø** Drainage Device **3** Infusion Device **7** Autologous Tissue Substitute **C** Extraluminal Device **D** Intraluminal Device **J** Synthetic Substitute **K** Nonautologous Tissue Substitute	**Z** No Qualifier
D Uterus and Cervix ♀		**Ø** Open **3** Percutaneous **4** Percutaneous Endoscopic **7** Via Natural or Artificial Opening **8** Via Natural or Artificial Opening Endoscopic	**Ø** Drainage Device **1** Radioactive Element **3** Infusion Device **7** Autologous Tissue Substitute **C** Extraluminal Device **D** Intraluminal Device **H** Contraceptive Device **J** Synthetic Substitute **K** Nonautologous Tissue Substitute **Y** Other Device	**Z** No Qualifier
D Uterus and Cervix ♀		**X** External	**Ø** Drainage Device **3** Infusion Device **7** Autologous Tissue Substitute **C** Extraluminal Device **D** Intraluminal Device **H** Contraceptive Device **J** Synthetic Substitute **K** Nonautologous Tissue Substitute	**Z** No Qualifier
H Vagina and Cul-de-sac ♀		**Ø** Open **3** Percutaneous **4** Percutaneous Endoscopic **7** Via Natural or Artificial Opening **8** Via Natural or Artificial Opening Endoscopic	**Ø** Drainage Device **1** Radioactive Element **3** Infusion Device **7** Autologous Tissue Substitute **D** Intraluminal Device **J** Synthetic Substitute **K** Nonautologous Tissue Substitute **Y** Other Device	**Z** No Qualifier
H Vagina and Cul-de-sac ♀		**X** External	**Ø** Drainage Device **3** Infusion Device **7** Autologous Tissue Substitute **D** Intraluminal Device **J** Synthetic Substitute **K** Nonautologous Tissue Substitute	**Z** No Qualifier

M   Vulva ♀
      Labia majora
      Labia minora
		Ø Open
		X External
			Ø Drainage Device
			7 Autologous Tissue Substitute
			J Synthetic Substitute
			K Nonautologous Tissue Substitute
				Z No Qualifier

Non-OR	ØUW3[3,4]YZ		**Non-OR**	ØUWDX[Ø,3,7,C,D,H,J,K]Z
Non-OR	ØUW3[7,8]YZ		**Non-OR**	ØUWH[3,4,7,8]YZ
Non-OR	ØUW3X[Ø,3]Z		**Non-OR**	ØUWHX[Ø,3,7,D,J,K]Z
Non-OR	ØUW8[3,4,7,8]YZ		**Non-OR**	ØUWMX[Ø,7,J,K]Z
Non-OR	ØUW8X[Ø,3,7,C,D,J,K]Z		♀	All body part, approach, device, and qualifier values
Non-OR	ØUWD[3,4,7,8]YZ			

Ø   **Medical and Surgical**
U   **Female Reproductive System**
Y   **Transplantation**   Definition: Putting in or on all or a portion of a living body part taken from another individual or animal to physically take the place and/or function of all or a portion of a similar body part

                         Explanation: The native body part may or may not be taken out, and the transplanted body part may take over all or a portion of its function

Body Part Character 4		Approach Character 5	Device Character 6	Qualifier Character 7
Ø Ovary, Right	♀	**Ø** Open	**Z** No Device	**Ø** Allogeneic
1 Ovary, Left	♀			**1** Syngeneic
9 Uterus	♀			**2** Zooplastic
♀ All body part, approach, device, and qualifier values				

NC Noncovered Procedure   **LC** Limited Coverage   **QA** Questionable OB Admit   **NT** New Tech Add-on   ⊞ Combination Member   ♂ Male   ♀ Female

ICD-10-PCS 2022   655

Male Reproductive System ØV1–ØVX

Character Meanings

This Character Meaning table is provided as a guide to assist the user in the identification of character members that may be found in this section of code tables. It **SHOULD NOT** be used to build a PCS code.

Operation–Character 3		Body Part–Character 4		Approach–Character 5		Device–Character 6		Qualifier–Character 7	
1	Bypass	Ø	Prostate	Ø	Open	Ø	Drainage Device	Ø	Allogeneic
2	Change	1	Seminal Vesicle, Right	3	Percutaneous	1	Radioactive Element	1	Syngeneic
5	Destruction	2	Seminal Vesicle, Left	4	Percutaneous Endoscopic	3	Infusion Device	2	Zooplastic
7	Dilation	3	Seminal Vesicles, Bilateral	7	Via Natural or Artificial Opening	7	Autologous Tissue Substitute	D	Urethra
9	Drainage	4	Prostate and Seminal Vesicles	8	Via Natural or Artificial Opening Endoscopic	C	Extraluminal Device	J	Epididymis, Right
B	Excision	5	Scrotum	X	External	D	Intraluminal Device	K	Epididymis, Left
C	Extirpation	6	Tunica Vaginalis, Right			J	Synthetic Substitute	N	Vas Deferens, Right
H	Insertion	7	Tunica Vaginalis, Left			K	Nonautologous Tissue Substitute	P	Vas Deferens, Left
J	Inspection	8	Scrotum and Tunica Vaginalis			Y	Other Device	S	Penis
L	Occlusion	9	Testis, Right			Z	No Device	X	Diagnostic
M	Reattachment	B	Testis, Left					Z	No Qualifier
N	Release	C	Testes, Bilateral						
P	Removal	D	Testis						
Q	Repair	F	Spermatic Cord, Right						
R	Replacement	G	Spermatic Cord, Left						
S	Reposition	H	Spermatic Cords, Bilateral						
T	Resection	J	Epididymis, Right						
U	Supplement	K	Epididymis, Left						
W	Revision	L	Epididymis, Bilateral						
X	Transfer	M	Epididymis and Spermatic Cord						
Y	Transplantation	N	Vas Deferens, Right						
		P	Vas Deferens, Left						
		Q	Vas Deferens, Bilateral						
		R	Vas Deferens						
		S	Penis						
		T	Prepuce						

AHA Coding Clinic for table ØV1
2018, 3Q, 12   Al-Ghorab distal penile shunt surgery

AHA Coding Clinic for table ØV9
2018, 3Q, 12   Al-Ghorab distal penile shunt surgery

AHA Coding Clinic for table ØVB
2020, 1Q, 31   Repair of buried penis
2019, 3Q, 18   Radical prostatectomy and lymph node dissection with biopsy of neurovascular bundle
2016, 1Q, 23   Transurethral resection of ejaculatory ducts
2014, 4Q, 33   Radical prostatectomy

AHA Coding Clinic for table ØVH
2020, 4Q, 43-44   Insertion of radioactive element

AHA Coding Clinic for table ØVP
2016, 2Q, 28   Removal of multi-component inflatable penile prosthesis with placement of new malleable device

AHA Coding Clinic for table ØVQ
2018, 3Q, 12   Al-Ghorab distal penile shunt surgery

AHA Coding Clinic for table ØVT
2020, 4Q, 99   Robotic-assisted prostatectomy with extension of incision for specimen removal
2019, 3Q, 18   Radical prostatectomy and lymph node dissection with biopsy of neurovascular bundle
2014, 4Q, 33   Radical prostatectomy

AHA Coding Clinic for table ØVU
2020, 1Q, 31   Repair of buried penis
2016, 2Q, 28   Removal of multi-component inflatable penile prosthesis with placement of new malleable device
2015, 3Q, 25   Placement of inflatable penile prosthesis

AHA Coding Clinic for table ØVX
2018, 4Q, 40   Transfer of prepuce

AHA Coding Clinic for table ØVY
2020, 4Q, 58   Male reproductive organ transplant

Male Reproductive System

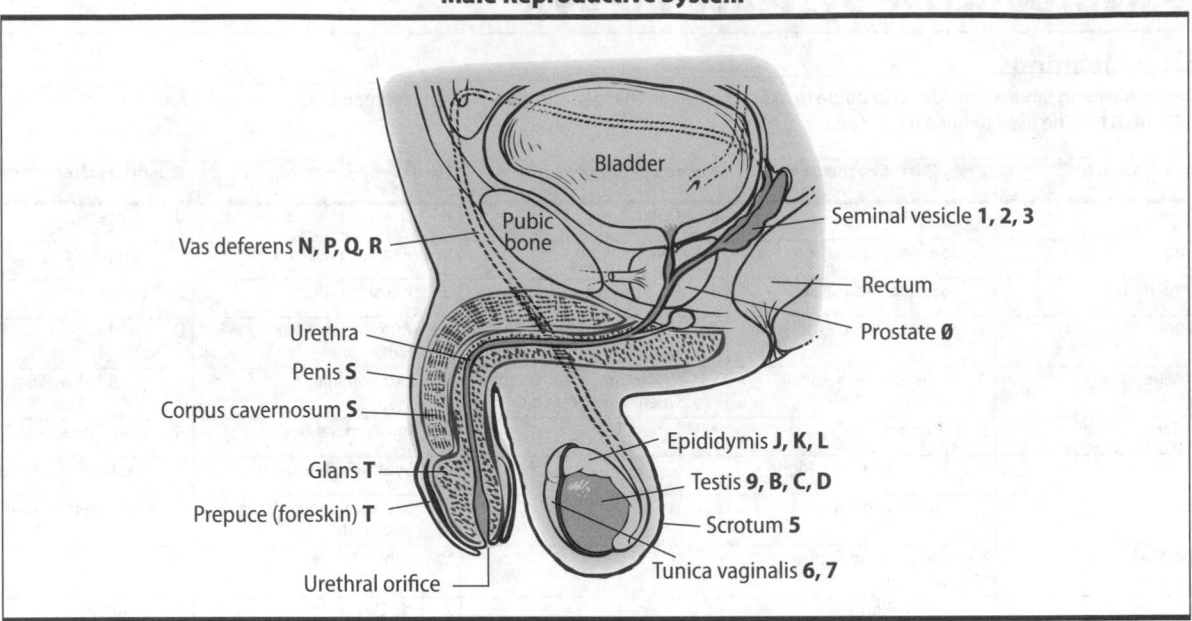

- Bladder
- Pubic bone
- Vas deferens **N, P, Q, R**
- Urethra
- Penis **S**
- Corpus cavernosum **S**
- Glans **T**
- Prepuce (foreskin) **T**
- Urethral orifice
- Seminal vesicle **1, 2, 3**
- Rectum
- Prostate **Ø**
- Epididymis **J, K, L**
- Testis **9, B, C, D**
- Scrotum **5**
- Tunica vaginalis **6, 7**

Penis

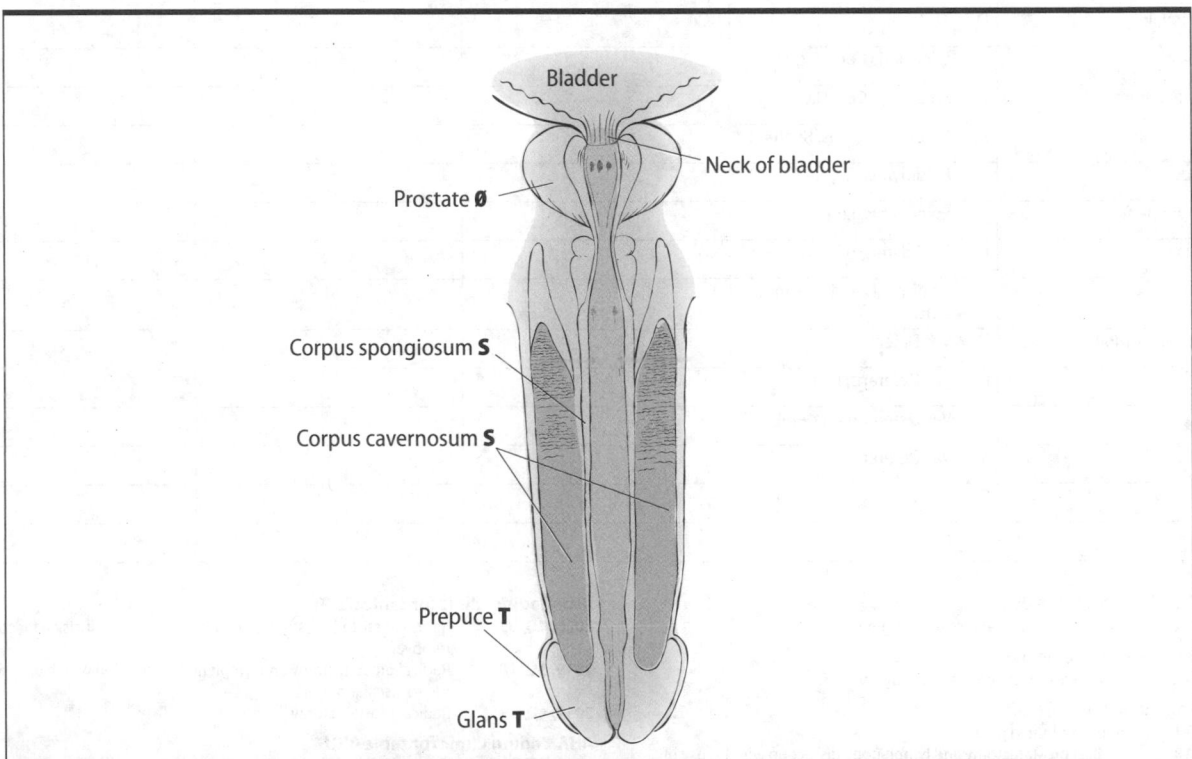

- Bladder
- Prostate **Ø**
- Neck of bladder
- Corpus spongiosum **S**
- Corpus cavernosum **S**
- Prepuce **T**
- Glans **T**

Ø Medical and Surgical
V Male Reproductive System
1 Bypass   Definition: Altering the route of passage of the contents of a tubular body part

Explanation: Rerouting contents of a body part to a downstream area of the normal route, to a similar route and body part, or to an abnormal route and dissimilar body part. Includes one or more anastomoses, with or without the use of a device.

Body Part Character 4	Approach Character 5	Device Character 6	Qualifier Character 7

N Vas Deferens, Right ♂
  Ductus deferens
  Ejaculatory duct
P Vas Deferens, Left ♂
  See N Vas Deferens, Right
Q Vas Deferens, Bilateral ♂
  See N Vas Deferens, Right
	Ø Open
	4 Percutaneous Endoscopic
		7 Autologous Tissue Substitute
		J Synthetic Substitute
		K Nonautologous Tissue Substitute
		Z No Device
			J Epididymis, Right
			K Epididymis, Left
			N Vas Deferens, Right
			P Vas Deferens, Left

♂   All body part, approach, device, and qualifier values

Ø Medical and Surgical
V Male Reproductive System
2 Change   Definition: Taking out or off a device from a body part and putting back an identical or similar device in or on the same body part without cutting or puncturing the skin or a mucous membrane

Explanation: All CHANGE procedures are coded using the approach EXTERNAL

Body Part Character 4	Approach Character 5	Device Character 6	Qualifier Character 7

4 Prostate and Seminal Vesicles ♂
8 Scrotum and Tunica Vaginalis ♂
D Testis ♂
M Epididymis and Spermatic Cord ♂
R Vas Deferens ♂
  Ductus deferens
  Ejaculatory duct
S Penis ♂
  Corpus cavernosum
  Corpus spongiosum
	X External	Ø Drainage Device
		Y Other Device
			Z No Qualifier

Non-OR   All body part, approach, device, and qualifier values   ♂   All body part, approach, device, and qualifier values

---

Ø Medical and Surgical
V Male Reproductive System
5 Destruction   Definition: Physical eradication of all or a portion of a body part by the direct use of energy, force, or a destructive agent

Explanation: None of the body part is physically taken out

Body Part Character 4	Approach Character 5	Device Character 6	Qualifier Character 7
Ø Prostate ♂	Ø Open 3 Percutaneous 4 Percutaneous Endoscopic 7 Via Natural or Artificial Opening 8 Via Natural or Artificial Opening Endoscopic	Z No Device	Z No Qualifier
1 Seminal Vesicle, Right ♂ 2 Seminal Vesicle, Left ♂ 3 Seminal Vesicles, Bilateral ♂ 6 Tunica Vaginalis, Right ♂ 7 Tunica Vaginalis, Left ♂ 9 Testis, Right ♂ B Testis, Left ♂ C Testes, Bilateral ♂	Ø Open 3 Percutaneous 4 Percutaneous Endoscopic	Z No Device	Z No Qualifier

5 Scrotum ♂
S Penis ♂
  Corpus cavernosum
  Corpus spongiosum
T Prepuce ♂
  Foreskin
  Glans penis
	Ø Open
	3 Percutaneous
	4 Percutaneous Endoscopic
	X External
		Z No Device	Z No Qualifier

F Spermatic Cord, Right ♂
G Spermatic Cord, Left ♂
H Spermatic Cords, Bilateral ♂
J Epididymis, Right ♂
K Epididymis, Left ♂
L Epididymis, Bilateral ♂
N Vas Deferens, Right NC ♂
  Ductus deferens
  Ejaculatory duct
P Vas Deferens, Left NC ♂
  See N Vas Deferens, Right
Q Vas Deferens, Bilateral NC ♂
  See N Vas Deferens, Right
	Ø Open
	3 Percutaneous
	4 Percutaneous Endoscopic
	8 Via Natural or Artificial Opening Endoscopic
		Z No Device	Z No Qualifier

Non-OR   ØV55[Ø,3,4,X]ZZ
Non-OR   ØV5[N,P,Q][Ø,3,4,8]ZZ   NC ØV5[N,P,Q][Ø,3,4]ZZ with principal or secondary diagnosis of Z3Ø.2
    ♂   All body part, approach, device, and qualifier values

---

NC Noncovered Procedure   LC Limited Coverage   QA Questionable OB Admit   NT New Tech Add-on   ⊞ Combination Member   ♂ Male   ♀ Female

Male Reproductive System

Ø   Medical and Surgical
V   Male Reproductive System
7   Dilation   Definition: Expanding an orifice or the lumen of a tubular body part

Explanation: The orifice can be a natural orifice or an artificially created orifice. Accomplished by stretching a tubular body part using intraluminal pressure or by cutting part of the orifice or wall of the tubular body part.

Body Part Character 4	Approach Character 5	Device Character 6	Qualifier Character 7

N Vas Deferens, Right ♂
  Ductus deferens
  Ejaculatory duct
P Vas Deferens, Left ♂
  See N Vas Deferens, Right
Q Vas Deferens, Bilateral ♂
  See N Vas Deferens, Right
	Ø Open
	3 Percutaneous
	4 Percutaneous Endoscopic
		D Intraluminal Device
		Z No Device
			Z No Qualifier

♂   All body part, approach, device, and qualifier values

Ø   Medical and Surgical
V   Male Reproductive System
9   Drainage   Definition: Taking or letting out fluids and/or gases from a body part

Explanation: The qualifier DIAGNOSTIC is used to identify drainage procedures that are biopsies

Body Part Character 4	Approach Character 5	Device Character 6	Qualifier Character 7
Ø Prostate ♂	**Ø Open** **3 Percutaneous** **4 Percutaneous Endoscopic** **7 Via Natural or Artificial Opening** **8 Via Natural or Artificial Opening Endoscopic**	**Ø Drainage Device**	**Z No Qualifier**
Ø Prostate ♂	**Ø Open** **3 Percutaneous** **4 Percutaneous Endoscopic** **7 Via Natural or Artificial Opening** **8 Via Natural or Artificial Opening Endoscopic**	**Z No Device**	**X Diagnostic** **Z No Qualifier**

1 Seminal Vesicle, Right ♂
2 Seminal Vesicle, Left ♂
3 Seminal Vesicles, Bilateral ♂
6 Tunica Vaginalis, Right ♂
7 Tunica Vaginalis, Left ♂
9 Testis, Right ♂
B Testis, Left ♂
C Testes, Bilateral ♂
F Spermatic Cord, Right ♂
G Spermatic Cord, Left ♂
H Spermatic Cords, Bilateral ♂
J Epididymis, Right ♂
K Epididymis, Left ♂
L Epididymis, Bilateral ♂
N Vas Deferens, Right ♂
  Ductus deferens
  Ejaculatory duct
P Vas Deferens, Left ♂
  See N Vas Deferens, Right
Q Vas Deferens, Bilateral ♂
  See N Vas Deferens, Right
	Ø Open
	3 Percutaneous
	4 Percutaneous Endoscopic
		Ø Drainage Device	**Z No Qualifier**

Non-OR ØV9Ø[3,4]ØZ	**Non-OR** ØV9[6,7,F,G,H,N,P,Q][Ø,3,4]ØZ
Non-OR ØV9Ø[3,4]Z[X,Z]	**Non-OR** ØV9[J,K,L]3ØZ
Non-OR ØV9Ø[7,8]ZX	♂ All body part, approach, device, and qualifier values
Non-OR ØV9[1,2,3,9,B,C][3,4]ØZ	

ØV9 Continued on next page

Ø **Medical and Surgical**
V **Male Reproductive System**
9 **Drainage**

Definition: Taking or letting out fluids and/or gases from a body part

Explanation: The qualifier DIAGNOSTIC is used to identify drainage procedures that are biopsies

Body Part Character 4	Approach Character 5	Device Character 6	Qualifier Character 7

1 Seminal Vesicle, Right ♂
2 Seminal Vesicle, Left ♂
3 Seminal Vesicles, Bilateral ♂
6 Tunica Vaginalis, Right ♂
7 Tunica Vaginalis, Left ♂
9 Testis, Right ♂
B Testis, Left ♂
C Testes, Bilateral ♂
F Spermatic Cord, Right ♂
G Spermatic Cord, Left ♂
H Spermatic Cords, Bilateral ♂
J Epididymis, Right ♂
K Epididymis, Left ♂
L Epididymis, Bilateral ♂
N Vas Deferens, Right ♂
   Ductus deferens
   Ejaculatory duct
P Vas Deferens, Left ♂
   See N Vas Deferens, Right
Q Vas Deferens, Bilateral ♂
   See N Vas Deferens, Right
	Ø Open
	3 Percutaneous
	4 Percutaneous Endoscopic
		Z No Device	**X** Diagnostic
			Z No Qualifier

5 Scrotum ♂
S Penis ♂
   Corpus cavernosum
   Corpus spongiosum
T Prepuce ♂
   Foreskin
   Glans penis
	Ø Open
	3 Percutaneous
	4 Percutaneous Endoscopic
	X External
		Ø Drainage Device	**Z** No Qualifier

5 Scrotum ♂
S Penis ♂
   Corpus cavernosum
   Corpus spongiosum
T Prepuce ♂
   Foreskin
   Glans penis
	Ø Open
	3 Percutaneous
	4 Percutaneous Endoscopic
	X External
		Z No Device	**X** Diagnostic
			Z No Qualifier

Non-OR	ØV9[1,2,3,9,B,C][3,4]Z[X,Z]	
Non-OR	ØV9[6,7,F,G,H,J,K,L,N,P,Q][Ø,3,4]ZX	
Non-OR	ØV9[6,7,F,G,H,N,P,Q][Ø,3,4]ZZ	
Non-OR	ØV9[J,K,L]3ZZ	
Non-OR	ØV95[Ø,3,4,X]ØZ	

Non-OR	ØV9[S,T]3ØZ
Non-OR	ØV95ØZX
Non-OR	ØV95[3,4,X]Z[X,Z]
Non-OR	ØV9[S,T]3ZZ
♂	All body part, approach, device, and qualifier values

Male Reproductive System

Ø **Medical and Surgical**
V **Male Reproductive System**
B **Excision**   Definition: Cutting out or off, without replacement, a portion of a body part
                            Explanation: The qualifier DIAGNOSTIC is used to identify excision procedures that are biopsies

Body Part Character 4	Approach Character 5	Device Character 6	Qualifier Character 7
Ø Prostate ♂	**Ø** Open **3** Percutaneous **4** Percutaneous Endoscopic **7** Via Natural or Artificial Opening **8** Via Natural or Artificial Opening Endoscopic	**Z** No Device	**X** Diagnostic **Z** No Qualifier
1 Seminal Vesicle, Right ♂ **2** Seminal Vesicle, Left ♂ **3** Seminal Vesicles, Bilateral ♂ **6** Tunica Vaginalis, Right ♂ **7** Tunica Vaginalis, Left ♂ **9** Testis, Right ♂ **B** Testis, Left ♂ **C** Testes, Bilateral ♂	**Ø** Open **3** Percutaneous **4** Percutaneous Endoscopic	**Z** No Device	**X** Diagnostic **Z** No Qualifier

5 Scrotum ♂
S Penis ♂
   Corpus cavernosum
   Corpus spongiosum
T Prepuce ♂
   Foreskin
   Glans penis
	Ø Open
	3 Percutaneous
	4 Percutaneous Endoscopic
	X External
		Z No Device	**X** Diagnostic
			Z No Qualifier

F Spermatic Cord, Right ♂
G Spermatic Cord, Left ♂
H Spermatic Cords, Bilateral ♂
J Epididymis, Right ♂
K Epididymis, Left ♂
L Epididymis, Bilateral ♂
N Vas Deferens, Right NC ♂
   Ductus deferens
   Ejaculatory duct
P Vas Deferens, Left NC ♂
   See N Vas Deferens, Right
Q Vas Deferens, Bilateral NC ♂
   See N Vas Deferens, Right
	Ø Open
	3 Percutaneous
	4 Percutaneous Endoscopic
	8 Via Natural or Artificial Opening Endoscopic
		Z No Device	**X** Diagnostic
			Z No Qualifier

Non-OR ØVBØ[3,4,7,8]ZX	**Non-OR** ØVB[F,G,H,J,K,L][Ø,3,4,8]ZX
Non-OR ØVB[1,2,3,9,B,C][3,4]ZX	**Non-OR** ØVB[N,P,Q][Ø,3,4,8]Z[X,Z]
Non-OR ØVB[6,7][Ø,3,4]ZX	**NC** ØVB[N,P,Q][Ø,3,4]ZZ with principal or secondary diagnosis of Z3Ø.2
Non-OR ØVB5ØZX	♂ All body part, approach, device, and qualifier values
Non-OR ØVB5[3,4,X]Z[X,Z]	

Ø   **Medical and Surgical**
V   **Male Reproductive System**
C   **Extirpation**   Definition: Taking or cutting out solid matter from a body part

                Explanation: The solid matter may be an abnormal byproduct of a biological function or a foreign body; it may be imbedded in a body part or in the lumen of a tubular body part. The solid matter may or may not have been previously broken into pieces.

Body Part Character 4	Approach Character 5	Device Character 6	Qualifier Character 7
Ø Prostate ♂	**Ø** Open **3** Percutaneous **4** Percutaneous Endoscopic **7** Via Natural or Artificial Opening **8** Via Natural or Artificial Opening Endoscopic	**Z** No Device	**Z** No Qualifier

1 Seminal Vesicle, Right   ♂
2 Seminal Vesicle, Left   ♂
3 Seminal Vesicles, Bilateral   ♂
6 Tunica Vaginalis, Right   ♂
7 Tunica Vaginalis, Left   ♂
9 Testis, Right   ♂
B Testis, Left   ♂
C Testes, Bilateral   ♂
F Spermatic Cord, Right   ♂
G Spermatic Cord, Left   ♂
H Spermatic Cords, Bilateral   ♂
J Epididymis, Right   ♂
K Epididymis, Left   ♂
L Epididymis, Bilateral   ♂
N Vas Deferens, Right   ♂
      Ductus deferens
      Ejaculatory duct
P Vas Deferens, Left   ♂
      See N Vas Deferens, Right
Q Vas Deferens, Bilateral   ♂
      See N Vas Deferens, Right
	Ø Open
	3 Percutaneous
	4 Percutaneous Endoscopic
		Z No Device	**Z** No Qualifier

5 Scrotum   ♂
S Penis   ♂
      Corpus cavernosum
      Corpus spongiosum
T Prepuce   ♂
      Foreskin
      Glans penis
	Ø Open
	3 Percutaneous
	4 Percutaneous Endoscopic
	X External
		Z No Device	**Z** No Qualifier

Non-OR ØVC[6,7,N,P,Q][Ø,3,4]ZZ	**Non-OR** ØVCSXZZ	
Non-OR ØVC5[3,4,X]ZZ	♂ All body part, approach, device, and qualifier values	

NC Noncovered Procedure   **LC** Limited Coverage   **QA** Questionable OB Admit   **NT** New Tech Add-on   ⊞ Combination Member   ♂ Male   ♀ Female

ICD-10-PCS 2022   663

Male Reproductive System

Ø   **Medical and Surgical**
V   **Male Reproductive System**
H   **Insertion**   Definition: Putting in a nonbiological appliance that monitors, assists, performs, or prevents a physiological function but does not physically take the place of a body part
                 Explanation: None

Body Part Character 4		Approach Character 5	Device Character 6	Qualifier Character 7
Ø Prostate	♂	Ø Open 3 Percutaneous 4 Percutaneous Endoscopic 7 Via Natural or Artificial Opening 8 Via Natural or Artificial Opening Endoscopic	1 Radioactive Element	Z No Qualifier

4   Prostate and Seminal Vesicles
8   Scrotum and Tunica Vaginalis
M   Epididymis and Spermatic Cord
R   Vas Deferens
     Ductus deferens
     Ejaculatory duct
	♂
	♂
	♂
	♂
		Ø Open
		3 Percutaneous
		4 Percutaneous Endoscopic
		7 Via Natural or Artificial Opening
		8 Via Natural or Artificial Opening Endoscopic
			3 Infusion Device
			Y Other Device
				Z No Qualifier

D Testis	♂	Ø Open 3 Percutaneous 4 Percutaneous Endoscopic 7 Via Natural or Artificial Opening 8 Via Natural or Artificial Opening Endoscopic	1 Radioactive Element 3 Infusion Device Y Other Device	Z No Qualifier

S   Penis
     Corpus cavernosum
     Corpus spongiosum
	♂	Ø Open
		3 Percutaneous
		4 Percutaneous Endoscopic
			3 Infusion Device
			Y Other Device
				Z No Qualifier

S   Penis
     Corpus cavernosum
     Corpus spongiosum
	♂	7 Via Natural or Artificial Opening
		8 Via Natural or Artificial Opening Endoscopic
			Y Other Device	Z No Qualifier

S   Penis
     Corpus cavernosum
     Corpus spongiosum
	♂	X External	3 Infusion Device	Z No Qualifier

Non-OR   ØVH[4,8,M,R][Ø,3,4,7,8][3,Y]Z
Non-OR   ØVHD[Ø,3,4,7,8][1,3,Y]Z
Non-OR   ØVHS[Ø,3,4][3,Y]Z
Non-OR   ØVHS[7,8]YZ

Non-OR   ØVHSX3Z
♂   All body part, approach, device, and qualifier values

Ø   **Medical and Surgical**
V   **Male Reproductive System**
J   **Inspection**   Definition: Visually and/or manually exploring a body part •
                Explanation: Visual exploration may be performed with or without optical instrumentation. Manual exploration may be performed directly or through intervening body layers.

Body Part Character 4		Approach Character 5	Device Character 6	Qualifier Character 7

4   Prostate and Seminal Vesicles
8   Scrotum and Tunica Vaginalis
D   Testis
M   Epididymis and Spermatic Cord
R   Vas Deferens
     Ductus deferens
     Ejaculatory duct
S   Penis
     Corpus cavernosum
     Corpus spongiosum
	♂
	♂
	♂
	♂
	♂
	
	♂
		Ø Open
		3 Percutaneous
		4 Percutaneous Endoscopic
		X External
			Z No Device	Z No Qualifier

Non-OR   ØVJ[4,D,M,R][3,X]ZZ
Non-OR   ØVJ8[Ø,3,4,X]ZZ
Non-OR   ØVJS[3,4,X]ZZ

♂   All body part, approach, device, and qualifier values

Ø   **Medical and Surgical**
V   **Male Reproductive System**
L   **Occlusion**   Definition: Completely closing an orifice or the lumen of a tubular body part

                         Explanation: The orifice can be a natural orifice or an artificially created orifice

Body Part Character 4	Approach Character 5	Device Character 6	Qualifier Character 7

F Spermatic Cord, Right ᴺᶜ♂
G Spermatic Cord, Left ᴺᶜ♂
H Spermatic Cords, Bilateral ᴺᶜ♂
N Vas Deferens, Right ᴺᶜ♂
     Ductus deferens
     Ejaculatory duct
P Vas Deferens, Left ᴺᶜ♂
     See N Vas Deferens, Right
Q Vas Deferens, Bilateral ᴺᶜ♂
     See N Vas Deferens, Right
	Ø Open
	3 Percutaneous
	4 Percutaneous Endoscopic
	8 Via Natural or Artificial Opening
	     Endoscopic
		C Extraluminal Device
		D Intraluminal Device
		Z No Device
			Z No Qualifier

Non-OR ØVL[F,G,H][Ø,3,4,8][C,D,Z]Z Non-OR ØVL[N,P,Q][Ø,3,4,8][C,Z]Z		ᴺᶜ ØVL[F,G,H][Ø,3,4][C,D,Z]Z with principal or secondary diagnosis of Z3Ø.2 ᴺᶜ ØVL[N,P,Q][Ø,3,4][C,Z]Z with principal or secondary diagnosis of Z3Ø.2 ♂ All body part, approach, device, and qualifier values	

Ø   **Medical and Surgical**
V   **Male Reproductive System**
M   **Reattachment**   Definition: Putting back in or on all or a portion of a separated body part to its normal location or other suitable location

                          Explanation: Vascular circulation and nervous pathways may or may not be reestablished

Body Part Character 4	Approach Character 5	Device Character 6	Qualifier Character 7

5 Scrotum ♂
S Penis ♂
     Corpus cavernosum
     Corpus spongiosum
	X External	**Z** No Device	**Z** No Qualifier

6 Tunica Vaginalis, Right ♂ **7** Tunica Vaginalis, Left ♂ **9** Testis, Right ♂ **B** Testis, Left ♂ **C** Testes, Bilateral ♂ **F** Spermatic Cord, Right ♂ **G** Spermatic Cord, Left ♂ **H** Spermatic Cords, Bilateral ♂	**Ø** Open **4** Percutaneous Endoscopic	**Z** No Device	**Z** No Qualifier

♂	All body part, approach, device, and qualifier values

Ø   Medical and Surgical
V   Male Reproductive System
N   Release   Definition: Freeing a body part from an abnormal physical constraint by cutting or by the use of force
                          Explanation: Some of the restraining tissue may be taken out but none of the body part is taken out

Body Part Character 4		Approach Character 5	Device Character 6	Qualifier Character 7
Ø Prostate	♂	Ø Open 3 Percutaneous 4 Percutaneous Endoscopic 7 Via Natural or Artificial Opening 8 Via Natural or Artificial Opening Endoscopic	Z No Device	Z No Qualifier
1 Seminal Vesicle, Right 2 Seminal Vesicle, Left 3 Seminal Vesicles, Bilateral 6 Tunica Vaginalis, Right 7 Tunica Vaginalis, Left 9 Testis, Right B Testis, Left C Testes, Bilateral	♂ ♂ ♂ ♂ ♂ ♂ ♂ ♂	Ø Open 3 Percutaneous 4 Percutaneous Endoscopic	Z No Device	Z No Qualifier

5 Scrotum
S Penis
   Corpus cavernosum
   Corpus spongiosum
T Prepuce
   Foreskin
   Glans penis
	♂
	♂
	
	♂
		Ø Open
		3 Percutaneous
		4 Percutaneous Endoscopic
		X External
			Z No Device	Z No Qualifier

F Spermatic Cord, Right
G Spermatic Cord, Left
H Spermatic Cords, Bilateral
J Epididymis, Right
K Epididymis, Left
L Epididymis, Bilateral
N Vas Deferens, Right
   Ductus deferens
   Ejaculatory duct
P Vas Deferens, Left
   See N Vas Deferens, Right
Q Vas Deferens, Bilateral
   See N Vas Deferens, Right
	♂
	♂
	♂
	♂
	♂
	♂
	♂
	
	♂
	
	♂
		Ø Open
		3 Percutaneous
		4 Percutaneous Endoscopic
		8 Via Natural or Artificial Opening Endoscopic
			Z No Device	Z No Qualifier

Non-OR	ØVN[9,B,C][Ø,3,4]ZZ		♂	All body part, approach, device, and qualifier values
Non-OR	ØVNT[Ø,3,4,X]ZZ			

Ø **Medical and Surgical**
V **Male Reproductive System**
P **Removal**   Definition: Taking out or off a device from a body part

Explanation: If a device is taken out and a similar device put in without cutting or puncturing the skin or mucous membrane, the procedure is coded to the root operation CHANGE. Otherwise, the procedure for taking out the device is coded to the root operation REMOVAL.

Body Part Character 4		Approach Character 5	Device Character 6	Qualifier Character 7
4 Prostate and Seminal Vesicles ♂		**Ø** Open **3** Percutaneous **4** Percutaneous Endoscopic **7** Via Natural or Artificial Opening **8** Via Natural or Artificial Opening Endoscopic	**Ø** Drainage Device **1** Radioactive Element **3** Infusion Device **7** Autologous Tissue Substitute **J** Synthetic Substitute **K** Nonautologous Tissue Substitute **Y** Other Device	**Z** No Qualifier
4 Prostate and Seminal Vesicles ♂		**X** External	**Ø** Drainage Device **1** Radioactive Element **3** Infusion Device	**Z** No Qualifier
8 Scrotum and Tunica Vaginalis ♂ **D** Testis ♂ **S** Penis ♂ Corpus cavernosum Corpus spongiosum		**Ø** Open **3** Percutaneous **4** Percutaneous Endoscopic **7** Via Natural or Artificial Opening **8** Via Natural or Artificial Opening Endoscopic	**Ø** Drainage Device **3** Infusion Device **7** Autologous Tissue Substitute **J** Synthetic Substitute **K** Nonautologous Tissue Substitute **Y** Other Device	**Z** No Qualifier
8 Scrotum and Tunica Vaginalis ♂ **D** Testis ♂ **S** Penis ♂ Corpus cavernosum Corpus spongiosum		**X** External	**Ø** Drainage Device **3** Infusion Device	**Z** No Qualifier
M Epididymis and Spermatic Cord ♂		**Ø** Open **3** Percutaneous **4** Percutaneous Endoscopic **7** Via Natural or Artificial Opening **8** Via Natural or Artificial Opening Endoscopic	**Ø** Drainage Device **3** Infusion Device **7** Autologous Tissue Substitute **C** Extraluminal Device **J** Synthetic Substitute **K** Nonautologous Tissue Substitute **Y** Other Device	**Z** No Qualifier
M Epididymis and Spermatic Cord ♂		**X** External	**Ø** Drainage Device **3** Infusion Device	**Z** No Qualifier
R Vas Deferens ♂ Ductus deferens Ejaculatory duct		**Ø** Open **3** Percutaneous **4** Percutaneous Endoscopic **7** Via Natural or Artificial Opening **8** Via Natural or Artificial Opening Endoscopic	**Ø** Drainage Device **3** Infusion Device **7** Autologous Tissue Substitute **C** Extraluminal Device **D** Intraluminal Device **J** Synthetic Substitute **K** Nonautologous Tissue Substitute **Y** Other Device	**Z** No Qualifier
R Vas Deferens ♂ Ductus deferens Ejaculatory duct		**X** External	**Ø** Drainage Device **3** Infusion Device **D** Intraluminal Device	**Z** No Qualifier

Non-OR	ØVP4[3,4]YZ		Non-OR	ØVPM[3,4]YZ
Non-OR	ØVP4[7,8][Ø,3,Y]Z		Non-OR	ØVPM[7,8][Ø,3,Y]Z
Non-OR	ØVP4X[Ø,1,3]Z		Non-OR	ØVPMX[Ø,3]Z
Non-OR	ØVP8[Ø,3,4,7,8][Ø,3,7,J,K,Y]Z		Non-OR	ØVPR[Ø,3,4][Ø,3,7,C,J,K,Y]Z
Non-OR	ØVP[D,S][3,4]YZ		Non-OR	ØVPR[7,8][Ø,3,7,C,D,J,K,Y]Z
Non-OR	ØVP[D,S][7,8][Ø,3,Y]Z		Non-OR	ØVPRX[Ø,3,D]Z
Non-OR	ØVP[8,D,S]X[Ø,3]Z		♂	All body part, approach, device, and qualifier values

Ø Medical and Surgical
V Male Reproductive System
Q Repair Definition: Restoring, to the extent possible, a body part to its normal anatomic structure and function

Explanation: Used only when the method to accomplish the repair is not one of the other root operations

Body Part Character 4		Approach Character 5	Device Character 6	Qualifier Character 7
Ø Prostate	♂	**Ø** Open **3** Percutaneous **4** Percutaneous Endoscopic **7** Via Natural or Artificial Opening **8** Via Natural or Artificial Opening Endoscopic	**Z** No Device	**Z** No Qualifier
1 Seminal Vesicle, Right **2** Seminal Vesicle, Left **3** Seminal Vesicles, Bilateral **6** Tunica Vaginalis, Right **7** Tunica Vaginalis, Left **9** Testis, Right **B** Testis, Left **C** Testes, Bilateral	♂ ♂ ♂ ♂ ♂ ♂ ♂ ♂	**Ø** Open **3** Percutaneous **4** Percutaneous Endoscopic	**Z** No Device	**Z** No Qualifier

5 Scrotum
S Penis
  Corpus cavernosum
  Corpus spongiosum
T Prepuce
  Foreskin
  Glans penis
	♂
	♂
	
	♂
		Ø Open
		3 Percutaneous
		4 Percutaneous Endoscopic
		X External
			Z No Device	**Z** No Qualifier

F Spermatic Cord, Right
G Spermatic Cord, Left
H Spermatic Cords, Bilateral
J Epididymis, Right
K Epididymis, Left
L Epididymis, Bilateral
N Vas Deferens, Right
  Ductus deferens
  Ejaculatory duct
P Vas Deferens, Left
  See N Vas Deferens, Right
Q Vas Deferens, Bilateral
  See N Vas Deferens, Right
	♂
	♂
	♂
	♂
	♂
	♂
	♂
	
	♂
	
	♂
		Ø Open
		3 Percutaneous
		4 Percutaneous Endoscopic
		8 Via Natural or Artificial Opening Endoscopic
			Z No Device	**Z** No Qualifier

Non-OR ØVQ[6,7][Ø,3,4]ZZ   ♂   All body part, approach, device, and qualifier values
Non-OR ØVQ5[Ø,3,4,X]ZZ

Ø Medical and Surgical
V Male Reproductive System
R Replacement Definition: Putting in or on biological or synthetic material that physically takes the place and/or function of all or a portion of a body part

Explanation: The body part may have been taken out or replaced, or may be taken out, physically eradicated, or rendered nonfunctional during the REPLACEMENT procedure. A REMOVAL procedure is coded for taking out the device used in a previous replacement procedure.

Body Part Character 4		Approach Character 5	Device Character 6	Qualifier Character 7
9 Testis, Right **B** Testis, Left **C** Testes, Bilateral	♂ ♂ ♂	**Ø** Open	**J** Synthetic Substitute	**Z** No Qualifier

♂   All body part, approach, device, and qualifier values

Ø Medical and Surgical
V Male Reproductive System
S Reposition Definition: Moving to its normal location, or other suitable location, all or a portion of a body part

Explanation: The body part is moved to a new location from an abnormal location, or from a normal location where it is not functioning correctly. The body part may or may not be cut out or off to be moved to the new location.

Body Part Character 4		Approach Character 5	Device Character 6	Qualifier Character 7
9 Testis, Right **B** Testis, Left **C** Testes, Bilateral **F** Spermatic Cord, Right **G** Spermatic Cord, Left **H** Spermatic Cords, Bilateral	♂ ♂ ♂ ♂ ♂ ♂	**Ø** Open **3** Percutaneous **4** Percutaneous Endoscopic **8** Via Natural or Artificial Opening Endoscopic	**Z** No Device	**Z** No Qualifier

♂   All body part, approach, device, and qualifier values

Ø   **Medical and Surgical**
V   **Male Reproductive System**
T   **Resection**   Definition: Cutting out or off, without replacement, all of a body part
                     Explanation: None

Body Part Character 4		Approach Character 5	Device Character 6	Qualifier Character 7
Ø Prostate	⊞♂	**Ø** Open **4** Percutaneous Endoscopic **7** Via Natural or Artificial Opening **8** Via Natural or Artificial Opening Endoscopic	**Z** No Device	**Z** No Qualifier

1 Seminal Vesicle, Right
2 Seminal Vesicle, Left
3 Seminal Vesicles, Bilateral
6 Tunica Vaginalis, Right
7 Tunica Vaginalis, Left
9 Testis, Right
B Testis, Left
C Testes, Bilateral
F Spermatic Cord, Right
G Spermatic Cord, Left
H Spermatic Cords, Bilateral
J Epididymis, Right
K Epididymis, Left
L Epididymis, Bilateral
N Vas Deferens, Right
    Ductus deferens
    Ejaculatory duct
P Vas Deferens, Left
    See N Vas Deferens, Right
Q Vas Deferens, Bilateral
    See N Vas Deferens, Right
	♂
	♂
	⊞♂
	♂
	♂
	♂
	♂
	♂
	♂
	♂
	♂
	♂
	♂
	♂
	NC♂
	
	NC♂
	
	NC♂
		Ø Open
		4 Percutaneous Endoscopic
			Z No Device	**Z** No Qualifier

5 Scrotum
S Penis
    Corpus cavernosum
    Corpus spongiosum
T Prepuce
    Foreskin
    Glans penis
	♂
	♂
	
	♂
		Ø Open
		4 Percutaneous Endoscopic
		X External
			Z No Device	**Z** No Qualifier

Non-OR ØVT[N,P,Q][Ø,4]ZZ	
Non-OR ØVT[5,T][Ø,4,X]ZZ	**See Appendix L for Procedure Combinations**
NC ØVT[N,P,Q][Ø,4]ZZ with principal or secondary diagnosis of Z3Ø.2	⊞ ØVTØ[Ø,4,7,8]ZZ
♂ All body part, approach, device, and qualifier values	⊞ ØVT3[Ø,4]ZZ

Male Reproductive System

Ø   **Medical and Surgical**
V   **Male Reproductive System**
U   **Supplement**   Definition: Putting in or on biological or synthetic material that physically reinforces and/or augments the function of a portion of a body part
           Explanation: The biological material is non-living, or is living and from the same individual. The body part may have been previously replaced, and the SUPPLEMENT procedure is performed to physically reinforce and/or augment the function of the replaced body part.

Body Part Character 4		Approach Character 5	Device Character 6	Qualifier Character 7

1   Seminal Vesicle, Right   ♂
2   Seminal Vesicle, Left   ♂
3   Seminal Vesicles, Bilateral   ♂
6   Tunica Vaginalis, Right   ♂
7   Tunica Vaginalis, Left   ♂
F   Spermatic Cord, Right   ♂
G   Spermatic Cord, Left   ♂
H   Spermatic Cords, Bilateral   ♂
J   Epididymis, Right   ♂
K   Epididymis, Left   ♂
L   Epididymis, Bilateral   ♂
N   Vas Deferens, Right   ♂
     Ductus deferens
     Ejaculatory duct
P   Vas Deferens, Left   ♂
     See N Vas Deferens, Right
Q   Vas Deferens, Bilateral   ♂
     See N Vas Deferens, Right
		Ø Open
		4 Percutaneous Endoscopic
		8 Via Natural or Artificial Opening
		     Endoscopic
			7 Autologous Tissue Substitute
			J Synthetic Substitute
			K Nonautologous Tissue Substitute
				Z No Qualifier

5   Scrotum   ♂
S   Penis   ♂
     Corpus cavernosum
     Corpus spongiosum
T   Prepuce   ♂
     Foreskin
     Glans penis
		Ø Open
		4 Percutaneous Endoscopic
		X External
			7 Autologous Tissue Substitute
			J Synthetic Substitute
			K Nonautologous Tissue Substitute
				Z No Qualifier

9 Testis, Right ♂ B Testis, Left ♂ C Testes, Bilateral ♂		Ø Open	7 Autologous Tissue Substitute J Synthetic Substitute K Nonautologous Tissue Substitute	Z No Qualifier

Non-OR   ØVUSX[7,J,K]Z   ♂   All body part, approach, device, and qualifier values

Ø   Medical and Surgical
V   Male Reproductive System
W   Revision   Definition: Correcting, to the extent possible, a portion of a malfunctioning device or the position of a displaced device

Explanation: Revision can include correcting a malfunctioning or displaced device by taking out or putting in components of the device such as a screw or pin

Body Part Character 4	Approach Character 5	Device Character 6	Qualifier Character 7

4   **Prostate and Seminal Vesicles** ♂
8   **Scrotum and Tunica Vaginalis** ♂
D   **Testis** ♂
S   **Penis** ♂
     Corpus cavernosum
     Corpus spongiosum
	Ø Open
	3 Percutaneous
	4 Percutaneous Endoscopic
	7 Via Natural or Artificial Opening
	8 Via Natural or Artificial Opening
	     Endoscopic
		Ø Drainage Device
		3 Infusion Device
		7 Autologous Tissue Substitute
		J Synthetic Substitute
		K Nonautologous Tissue Substitute
		Y Other Device
			Z No Qualifier

4   **Prostate and Seminal Vesicles** ♂
8   **Scrotum and Tunica Vaginalis** ♂
D   **Testis** ♂
S   **Penis** ♂
     Corpus cavernosum
     Corpus spongiosum
	X External	**Ø** Drainage Device
		3 Infusion Device
		7 Autologous Tissue Substitute
		J Synthetic Substitute
		K Nonautologous Tissue Substitute
			Z No Qualifier

M **Epididymis and Spermatic Cord** ♂	**Ø** Open **3** Percutaneous **4** Percutaneous Endoscopic **7** Via Natural or Artificial Opening **8** Via Natural or Artificial Opening Endoscopic	**Ø** Drainage Device **3** Infusion Device **7** Autologous Tissue Substitute **C** Extraluminal Device **J** Synthetic Substitute **K** Nonautologous Tissue Substitute **Y** Other Device	**Z** No Qualifier
M **Epididymis and Spermatic Cord** ♂	**X** External	**Ø** Drainage Device **3** Infusion Device **7** Autologous Tissue Substitute **C** Extraluminal Device **J** Synthetic Substitute **K** Nonautologous Tissue Substitute	**Z** No Qualifier

R   **Vas Deferens** ♂
     Ductus deferens
     Ejaculatory duct
	Ø Open
	3 Percutaneous
	4 Percutaneous Endoscopic
	7 Via Natural or Artificial Opening
	8 Via Natural or Artificial Opening
	     Endoscopic
		Ø Drainage Device
		3 Infusion Device
		7 Autologous Tissue Substitute
		C Extraluminal Device
		D Intraluminal Device
		J Synthetic Substitute
		K Nonautologous Tissue Substitute
		Y Other Device
			Z No Qualifier

R   **Vas Deferens** ♂
     Ductus deferens
     Ejaculatory duct
	X External	**Ø** Drainage Device
		3 Infusion Device
		7 Autologous Tissue Substitute
		C Extraluminal Device
		D Intraluminal Device
		J Synthetic Substitute
		K Nonautologous Tissue Substitute
			Z No Qualifier

Non-OR	ØVW[4,D,S][3,4,7,8]YZ	**Non-OR**	ØVWMX[Ø,3,7,C,J,K]Z
Non-OR	ØVW8[Ø,3,4,7,8][Ø,3,7,J,K,Y]Z	**Non-OR**	ØVWR[Ø,3,4,7,8][Ø,3,7,C,D,J,K,Y]Z
Non-OR	ØVW[4,8,D,S]X[Ø,3,7,J,K]Z	**Non-OR**	ØVWRX[Ø,3,7,C,D,J,K]Z
Non-OR	ØVWM[3,4,7,8]YZ	♂	All body part, approach, device, and qualifier values

Ø   Medical and Surgical
V   Male Reproductive System
X   Transfer   Definition: Moving, without taking out, all or a portion of a body part to another location to take over the function of all or a portion of a body part

Explanation: The body part transferred remains connected to its vascular and nervous supply

Body Part Character 4	Approach Character 5	Device Character 6	Qualifier Character 7

T   Prepuce
     Foreskin
     Glans penis
	Ø Open
	X External
		Z No Device	**D** Urethra
			S Penis

NC Noncovered Procedure   **LC** Limited Coverage   **QA** Questionable OB Admit   **NT** New Tech Add-on   ✛ Combination Member   ♂ Male   ♀ Female

ICD-10-PCS 2022   **671**

ØVW–ØVX

Ø   **Medical and Surgical**
V   **Male Reproductive System**
Y   **Transplantation**   Definition: Putting in or on all or a portion of a living body part taken from another individual or animal to physically take the place and/or function of all or a portion of a similar body part
Explanation: The native body part may or may not be taken out, and the transplanted body part may take over all or a portion of its function

Body Part Character 4		Approach Character 5	Device Character 6	Qualifier Character 7

5   Scrotum   ♂
S   Penis   ♂
      Corpus cavernosum
      Corpus spongiosum
		Ø Open	Z No Device	Ø Allogeneic
				1 Syngeneic
				2 Zooplastic

♂ All body part, approach, device, and qualifier values				

Anatomical Regions, General ØWØ–ØWY

Character Meanings

This Character Meaning table is provided as a guide to assist the user in the identification of character members that may be found in this section of code tables. It **SHOULD NOT** be used to build a PCS code.

Operation–Character 3		Body Region–Character 4		Approach–Character 5		Device–Character 6		Qualifier–Character 7	
Ø	Alteration	Ø	Head	Ø	Open	Ø	Drainage Device	Ø	Vagina OR Allogeneic
1	Bypass	1	Cranial Cavity	3	Percutaneous	1	Radioactive Element	1	Penis OR Syngeneic
2	Change	2	Face	4	Percutaneous Endoscopic	3	Infusion Device	2	Stoma
3	Control	3	Oral Cavity and Throat	7	Via Natural or Artificial Opening	7	Autologous Tissue Substitute	4	Cutaneous
4	Creation	4	Upper Jaw	8	Via Natural or Artificial Opening Endoscopic	J	Synthetic Substitute	6	Bladder
8	Division	5	Lower Jaw	X	External	K	Nonautologous Tissue Substitute	9	Pleural Cavity, Right
9	Drainage	6	Neck			Y	Other Device	B	Pleural Cavity, Left
B	Excision	8	Chest Wall			Z	No Device	G	Peritoneal Cavity
C	Extirpation	9	Pleural Cavity, Right					J	Pelvic Cavity
F	Fragmentation	B	Pleural Cavity, Left					W	Upper Vein
H	Insertion	C	Mediastinum					X	Diagnostic
J	Inspection	D	Pericardial Cavity					Y	Lower Vein
M	Reattachment	F	Abdominal Wall					Z	No Qualifier
P	Removal	G	Peritoneal Cavity						
Q	Repair	H	Retroperitoneum						
U	Supplement	J	Pelvic Cavity						
W	Revision	K	Upper Back						
Y	Transplantation	L	Lower Back						
		M	Perineum, Male						
		N	Perineum, Female						
		P	Gastrointestinal Tract						
		Q	Respiratory Tract						
		R	Genitourinary Tract						

AHA Coding Clinic for table ØWØ
2015, 1Q, 31   Bilateral browpexy

AHA Coding Clinic for table ØW1
2020, 4Q, 55   Insertion of subcutaneous pump system for ascites drainage
2018, 4Q, 41-42   Anatomical regions bypass qualifiers
2015, 2Q, 36   Insertion of infusion device into peritoneal cavity
2013, 4Q, 126-127   Creation of percutaneous cutaneoperitoneal fistula

AHA Coding Clinic for table ØW3
2019, 3Q, 4   Evacuation of subdural hematoma and control of bleeding artery
2018, 4Q, 38   Control of epistaxis
2018, 1Q, 19   Argon plasma coagulation of duodenal arteriovenous malformation
2018, 1Q, 19   Control of epistaxis via silver nitrate cauterization
2017, 4Q, 57-58   Added approach values - Transorifice esophageal vein banding
2017, 4Q, 105   Control of gastrointestinal bleeding
2017, 4Q, 106   Control of bleeding of external naris using suture
2017, 4Q, 106   Nasal packing for epistaxis
2016, 4Q, 99-100   Root operation Control
2014, 4Q, 44   Bakri balloon for control of postpartum hemorrhage
2013, 3Q, 23   Control of intraoperative bleeding

AHA Coding Clinic for table ØW4
2019, 4Q, 30   Transfer large intestine to vagina
2016, 4Q, 101   Root operation Creation

AHA Coding Clinic for table ØW9
2020, 4Q, 56   Transvaginal drainage of pelvis
2017, 3Q, 12   Therapeutic and diagnostic paracentesis
2017, 2Q, 16   Incision and drainage of floor of mouth

AHA Coding Clinic for table ØWB
2019, 1Q, 27   Excision of pelvic sidewall mass
2017, 2Q, 16   Excision of floor of mouth
2016, 1Q, 21   Excision of urachal mass
2013, 4Q, 119   Excision of inclusion cyst of perineum

AHA Coding Clinic for table ØWC
2019, 4Q, 35   Extirpation of jaw
2017, 2Q, 16   Excision of floor of mouth

AHA Coding Clinic for table ØWH
2021, 2Q, 14   Peritoneal dialysis catheter placement
2019, 4Q, 43   Unidirectional source brachytherapy
2018, 1Q, 25   Intrauterine brachytherapy & placement of tandems & ovoids
2017, 4Q, 104   Intrauterine brachytherapy & placement of tandems & ovoids
2016, 2Q, 14   Insertion of peritoneal totally implantable venous access device
2015, 2Q, 36   Insertion of infusion device into peritoneal cavity

AHA Coding Clinic for table ØWJ
2021, 2Q, 19   Electromagnetic stealth guided ventriculoperitoneal shunt insertion with endoscopy
2019, 1Q, 3-8   Whipple procedure
2019, 1Q, 25   Laparoscopic appendectomy converted to open procedure
2018, 3Q, 29   Decommissioning of left ventricular assist device with exploration of mediastinum
2016, 4Q, 58   Longitudinal vaginal septum
2013, 2Q, 36   Insertion of ventriculoperitoneal shunt with laparoscopic assistance

AHA Coding Clinic for table ØWP
2021, 2Q, 14   Removal of peritoneal dialysis catheter

AHA Coding Clinic for table ØWQ
2017, 4Q, 106   Control of bleeding of external naris using suture
2017, 3Q, 8   Removal of silo and closure of gastroschisis
2016, 3Q, 3-7   Stoma creation & takedown procedures
2014, 4Q, 38   Abdominoplasty and abdominal wall plication for hernia repair
2014, 3Q, 28   Ileostomy takedown and parastomal hernia repair

AHA Coding Clinic for table ØWU
2017, 3Q, 8   First stage of gastroschisis repair with silo placement
2016, 3Q, 40   Omentoplasty
2015, 2Q, 29   Placement of Ioban™ antimicrobial drape over surgical wound
2014, 4Q, 39   Abdominal component release with placement of mesh for hernia repair
2012, 4Q, 101   Rib resection with reconstruction of anterior chest wall

AHA Coding Clinic for table ØWW
2015, 2Q, 9   Revision of ventriculoperitoneal (VP) shunt

AHA Coding Clinic for table ØWY
2016, 4Q, 112-113   Transplantation

Ø   **Medical and Surgical**
W   **Anatomical Regions, General**
Ø   **Alteration**   Definition: Modifying the anatomic structure of a body part without affecting the function of the body part

Explanation: Principal purpose is to improve appearance

Body Part Character 4	Approach Character 5	Device Character 6	Qualifier Character 7

Ø Head
2 Face
4 Upper Jaw
5 Lower Jaw
6 Neck
    Parapharyngeal space
    Retropharyngeal space
8 Chest Wall
F Abdominal Wall
K Upper Back
L Lower Back
M Perineum, Male   ♂
N Perineum, Female   ♀
	Ø Open
	3 Percutaneous
	4 Percutaneous Endoscopic
		7 Autologous Tissue Substitute
		J Synthetic Substitute
		K Nonautologous Tissue Substitute
		Z No Device
			Z No Qualifier

♂   ØWØM[Ø,3,4][7,J,K,Z]Z
♀   ØWØN[Ø,3,4][7,J,K,Z]Z

Ø   **Medical and Surgical**
W   **Anatomical Regions, General**
1   **Bypass**   Definition: Altering the route of passage of the contents of a tubular body part

Explanation: Rerouting contents of a body part to a downstream area of the normal route, to a similar route and body part, or to an abnormal route and dissimilar body part. Includes one or more anastomoses, with or without the use of a device.

Body Part Character 4	Approach Character 5	Device Character 6	Qualifier Character 7
1 Cranial Cavity	**Ø** Open	**J** Synthetic Substitute	**9** Pleural Cavity, Right **B** Pleural Cavity, Left **G** Peritoneal Cavity **J** Pelvic Cavity
9 Pleural Cavity, Right **B** Pleural Cavity, Left **J** Pelvic Cavity Retropubic space	**Ø** Open **3** Percutaneous **4** Percutaneous Endoscopic	**J** Synthetic Substitute	**4** Cutaneous **9** Pleural Cavity, Right **B** Pleural Cavity, Left **G** Peritoneal Cavity **J** Pelvic Cavity **W** Upper Vein **Y** Lower Vein
G Peritoneal Cavity	**Ø** Open **3** Percutaneous **4** Percutaneous Endoscopic	**J** Synthetic Substitute	**4** Cutaneous **6** Bladder **9** Pleural Cavity, Right **B** Pleural Cavity, Left **G** Peritoneal Cavity **J** Pelvic Cavity **W** Upper Vein **Y** Lower Vein

Non-OR   ØW1[9,B][Ø,3,4]J[4,G,W,Y]
Non-OR   ØW1J[Ø,3,4]J[4,W,Y]
Non-OR   ØW1G[Ø,3,4]J[9,B,G,J]

Ø   **Medical and Surgical**
W   **Anatomical Regions, General**
2   **Change**   Definition: Taking out or off a device from a body part and putting back an identical or similar device in or on the same body part without cutting or puncturing the skin or a mucous membrane

                        Explanation: All CHANGE procedures are coded using the approach EXTERNAL

Body Part Character 4	Approach Character 5	Device Character 6	Qualifier Character 7
Ø Head	X External	Ø Drainage Device	Z No Qualifier
1 Cranial Cavity		Y Other Device	
2 Face			
4 Upper Jaw			
5 Lower Jaw			
6 Neck			
Parapharyngeal space			
Retropharyngeal space			
8 Chest Wall			
9 Pleural Cavity, Right			
B Pleural Cavity, Left			
C Mediastinum			
Mediastinal cavity			
Mediastinal space			
D Pericardial Cavity			
F Abdominal Wall			
G Peritoneal Cavity			
H Retroperitoneum			
Retroperitoneal cavity			
Retroperitoneal space			
J Pelvic Cavity			
Retropubic space			
K Upper Back			
L Lower Back			
M Perineum, Male ♂			
N Perineum, Female ♀			

Non-OR	All body part, approach, device, and qualifier values	♂	ØW2MX[Ø,Y]Z
		♀	ØW2NX[Ø,Y]Z

NC Noncovered Procedure   LC Limited Coverage   QA Questionable OB Admit   NT New Tech Add-on   ⊞ Combination Member   ♂ Male   ♀ Female

ICD-10-PCS 2022   675

Ø **Medical and Surgical**
W **Anatomical Regions, General**
3 **Control** Definition: Stopping, or attempting to stop, postprocedural or other acute bleeding
  Explanation: None

Body Part Character 4	Approach Character 5	Device Character 6	Qualifier Character 7

Ø Head
1 Cranial Cavity
2 Face
4 Upper Jaw
5 Lower Jaw
6 Neck
  Parapharyngeal space
  Retropharyngeal space
8 Chest Wall
9 Pleural Cavity, Right
B Pleural Cavity, Left
C Mediastinum
  Mediastinal cavity
  Mediastinal space
D Pericardial Cavity
F Abdominal Wall
G Peritoneal Cavity
H Retroperitoneum
  Retroperitoneal cavity
  Retroperitoneal space
J Pelvic Cavity
  Retropubic space
K Upper Back
L Lower Back
M Perineum, Male ♂
N Perineum, Female ♀
	Ø Open
	3 Percutaneous
	4 Percutaneous Endoscopic
		Z No Device	Z No Qualifier

3 Oral Cavity and Throat	Ø Open 3 Percutaneous 4 Percutaneous Endoscopic 7 Via Natural or Artificial Opening 8 Via Natural or Artificial Opening Endoscopic X External	Z No Device	Z No Qualifier
P Gastrointestinal Tract Q Respiratory Tract R Genitourinary Tract	Ø Open 3 Percutaneous 4 Percutaneous Endoscopic 7 Via Natural or Artificial Opening 8 Via Natural or Artificial Opening Endoscopic	Z No Device	Z No Qualifier

Non-OR ØW3P8ZZ
  ♂ ØW3M[Ø,3,4]ZZ
  ♀ ØW3N[Ø,3,4]ZZ

Ø **Medical and Surgical**
W **Anatomical Regions, General**
4 **Creation** Definition: Putting in or on biological or synthetic material to form a new body part that to the extent possible replicates the anatomic structure or function of an absent body part
  Explanation: Used for gender reassignment surgery and corrective procedures in individuals with congenital anomalies

Body Part Character 4	Approach Character 5	Device Character 6	Qualifier Character 7
M Perineum, Male ♂	Ø Open	7 Autologous Tissue Substitute J Synthetic Substitute K Nonautologous Tissue Substitute	Ø Vagina
N Perineum, Female ♀	Ø Open	7 Autologous Tissue Substitute J Synthetic Substitute K Nonautologous Tissue Substitute	1 Penis

  ♂ ØW4MØ[7,J,K]Ø
  ♀ ØW4NØ[7,J,K]1

Ø **Medical and Surgical**
W **Anatomical Regions, General**
8 **Division** Definition: Cutting into a body part, without draining fluids and/or gases from the body part, in order to separate or transect a body part
  Explanation: All or a portion of the body part is separated into two or more portions

Body Part Character 4	Approach Character 5	Device Character 6	Qualifier Character 7
N Perineum, Female ♀	X External	Z No Device	Z No Qualifier

Non-OR ØW8NXZZ
  ♀ ØW8NXZZ

Non-OR Procedure   DRG Non-OR Procedure   Valid OR Procedure   HAC Associated Procedure   Combination Only   New/Revised GREEN

0   **Medical and Surgical**
W   **Anatomical Regions, General**
9   **Drainage**   Definition: Taking or letting out fluids and/or gases from a body part
                          Explanation: The qualifier DIAGNOSTIC is used to identify drainage procedures that are biopsies

Body Part Character 4	Approach Character 5	Device Character 6	Qualifier Character 7

0 Head
1 Cranial Cavity
2 Face
3 Oral Cavity and Throat
4 Upper Jaw
5 Lower Jaw
6 Neck
   Parapharyngeal space
   Retropharyngeal space
8 Chest Wall
9 Pleural Cavity, Right
B Pleural Cavity, Left
C Mediastinum
   Mediastinal cavity
   Mediastinal space
D Pericardial Cavity
F Abdominal Wall
G Peritoneal Cavity
H Retroperitoneum
   Retroperitoneal cavity
   Retroperitoneal space
K Upper Back
L Lower Back
M Perineum, Male   ♂
N Perineum, Female   ♀
	0 Open
	3 Percutaneous
	4 Percutaneous Endoscopic
		0 Drainage Device	**Z** No Qualifier

0 Head
1 Cranial Cavity
2 Face
3 Oral Cavity and Throat
4 Upper Jaw
5 Lower Jaw
6 Neck
   Parapharyngeal space
   Retropharyngeal space
8 Chest Wall
9 Pleural Cavity, Right
B Pleural Cavity, Left
C Mediastinum
   Mediastinal cavity
   Mediastinal space
D Pericardial Cavity
F Abdominal Wall
G Peritoneal Cavity
H Retroperitoneum
   Retroperitoneal cavity
   Retroperitoneal space
K Upper Back
L Lower Back
M Perineum, Male   ♂
N Perineum, Female   ♀
	0 Open
	3 Percutaneous
	4 Percutaneous Endoscopic
		Z No Device	**X** Diagnostic
			Z No Qualifier

J Pelvic Cavity
   Retropubic space
	0 Open
	3 Percutaneous
	4 Percutaneous Endoscopic
	7 Via Natural or Artificial Opening
	8 Via Natural or Artificial Opening
	   Endoscopic
		0 Drainage Device	**Z** No Qualifier

J Pelvic Cavity
   Retropubic space
	0 Open
	3 Percutaneous
	4 Percutaneous Endoscopic
	7 Via Natural or Artificial Opening
	8 Via Natural or Artificial Opening
	   Endoscopic
		Z No Device	**X** Diagnostic
			Z No Qualifier

Non-OR	0W9[0,8,9,B,K,L,M]00Z	Non-OR	0W9[0,1,8,F,K,L,M]4ZZ
Non-OR	0W9[0,1,2,3,4,5,6,8,9,B,C,D,F,G,H,K,L,M,N]30Z	Non-OR	0W9J[3,7,8]0Z
Non-OR	0W9[0,1,8,F,K,L,M]40Z	Non-OR	0W9J[3,7,8]Z[X,Z]
Non-OR	0W9[0,2,3,4,5,6,8,9,B,K,L,M,N]0ZX		
Non-OR	0W9[0,1,2,3,4,5,6,8,9,B,C,D,G,K,L,M,N]3ZX	♂	0W9M[0,3,4]0Z
Non-OR	0W9[0,1,2,3,4,5,6,8,C,K,L,M,N]4ZX	♂	0W9M[0,3,4]Z[X,Z]
Non-OR	0W9[0,8,9,B,K,L,M]0ZZ	♀	0W9N[0,3,4]0Z
Non-OR	0W9[0,1,2,3,4,5,6,8,9,B,C,D,F,G,H,K,L,M,N]3ZZ	♀	0W9N[0,3]Z[X,Z]
		♀	0W9N4ZZ

NC Noncovered Procedure   **LC** Limited Coverage   **QA** Questionable OB Admit   **NT** New Tech Add-on   ✚ Combination Member   ♂ Male   ♀ Female

Ø   **Medical and Surgical**
W   **Anatomical Regions, General**
B   **Excision**   Definition: Cutting out or off, without replacement, a portion of a body part
                     Explanation: The qualifier DIAGNOSTIC is used to identify excision procedures that are biopsies

Body Part Character 4	Approach Character 5	Device Character 6	Qualifier Character 7
Ø Head **2** Face **3** Oral Cavity and Throat **4** Upper Jaw **5** Lower Jaw **8** Chest Wall **K** Upper Back **L** Lower Back **M** Perineum, Male ♂ **N** Perineum, Female ♀	**Ø** Open **3** Percutaneous **4** Percutaneous Endoscopic **X** External	**Z** No Device	**X** Diagnostic **Z** No Qualifier

6 Neck
    Parapharyngeal space
    Retropharyngeal space
F Abdominal Wall
	Ø Open
	3 Percutaneous
	4 Percutaneous Endoscopic
		Z No Device	**X** Diagnostic
			Z No Qualifier

6 Neck
    Parapharyngeal space
    Retropharyngeal space
F Abdominal Wall
	X External	**Z** No Device	**2** Stoma
			X Diagnostic
			Z No Qualifier

C Mediastinum
    Mediastinal cavity
    Mediastinal space
H Retroperitoneum
    Retroperitoneal cavity
    Retroperitoneal space
	Ø Open
	3 Percutaneous
	4 Percutaneous Endoscopic
		Z No Device	**X** Diagnostic
			Z No Qualifier

Non-OR ØWB[Ø,2,4,5,8,K,L,M][Ø,3,4,X]ZX		♂	ØWBM[Ø,3,4,X]Z[X,Z]
Non-OR ØWB6[Ø,3,4]ZX		♀	ØWBN[Ø,3,4,X]Z[X,Z]
Non-OR ØWB6XZX			
Non-OR ØWBH[3,4]ZX			

Ø   **Medical and Surgical**
W   **Anatomical Regions, General**
C   **Extirpation**   Definition: Taking or cutting out solid matter from a body part
                     Explanation: The solid matter may be an abnormal byproduct of a biological function or a foreign body; it may be imbedded in a body part or in
                     the lumen of a tubular body part. The solid matter may or may not have been previously broken into pieces.

Body Part Character 4	Approach Character 5	Device Character 6	Qualifier Character 7

1 Cranial Cavity
3 Oral Cavity and Throat
9 Pleural Cavity, Right
B Pleural Cavity, Left
C Mediastinum
    Mediastinal cavity
    Mediastinal space
D Pericardial Cavity
G Peritoneal Cavity
H Retroperitoneum
    Retroperitoneal cavity
    Retroperitoneal space
J Pelvic Cavity
    Retropubic space
	Ø Open
	3 Percutaneous
	4 Percutaneous Endoscopic
	X External
		Z No Device	**Z** No Qualifier

4 Upper Jaw **5** Lower Jaw	**Ø** Open **3** Percutaneous **4** Percutaneous Endoscopic	**Z** No Device	**Z** No Qualifier
P Gastrointestinal Tract **Q** Respiratory Tract **R** Genitourinary Tract	**Ø** Open **3** Percutaneous **4** Percutaneous Endoscopic **7** Via Natural or Artificial Opening **8** Via Natural or Artificial Opening Endoscopic **X** External	**Z** No Device	**Z** No Qualifier

Non-OR	ØWC[1,3]XZZ
Non-OR	ØWC[9,B][Ø,3,4,X]ZZ
Non-OR	ØWC[C,D,G,H,J]XZZ
Non-OR	ØWC[4,5][Ø,3,4]ZZ
Non-OR	ØWC[P,R][7,8,X]ZZ
Non-OR	ØWCQ[Ø,3,4,X]ZZ

Ø   **Medical and Surgical**
W   **Anatomical Regions, General**
F   **Fragmentation**   Definition: Breaking solid matter in a body part into pieces

Explanation: Physical force (e.g., manual, ultrasonic) applied directly or indirectly is used to break the solid matter into pieces. The solid matter may be an abnormal byproduct of a biological function or a foreign body. The pieces of solid matter are not taken out.

Body Part Character 4		Approach Character 5	Device Character 6	Qualifier Character 7
1 Cranial Cavity	NC	Ø Open	Z No Device	Z No Qualifier
3 Oral Cavity and Throat	NC	3 Percutaneous		
9 Pleural Cavity, Right	NC	4 Percutaneous Endoscopic		
B Pleural Cavity, Left	NC	X External		
C Mediastinum	NC			
Mediastinal cavity				
Mediastinal space				
D Pericardial Cavity				
G Peritoneal Cavity	NC			
J Pelvic Cavity	NC			
Retropubic space				
P Gastrointestinal Tract	NC	Ø Open	Z No Device	Z No Qualifier
Q Respiratory Tract	NC	3 Percutaneous		
R Genitourinary Tract		4 Percutaneous Endoscopic		
		7 Via Natural or Artificial Opening		
		8 Via Natural or Artificial Opening Endoscopic		
		X External		

Non-OR	ØWF[1,3,9,B,C,G]XZZ	NC	ØWF[1,3,9,B,C,G,J]XZZ
Non-OR	ØWFJ[Ø,3,4,X]ZZ	NC	ØWF[P,Q]XZZ
Non-OR	ØWFP[Ø,3,4,7,8,X]ZZ		
Non-OR	ØWFQXZZ		
Non-OR	ØWFR[Ø,3,4,7,8,X]ZZ		

Ø   **Medical and Surgical**
W   **Anatomical Regions, General**
H   **Insertion**   Definition: Putting in a nonbiological appliance that monitors, assists, performs, or prevents a physiological function but does not physically take the place of a body part

Explanation: None

Body Part Character 4	Approach Character 5	Device Character 6	Qualifier Character 7
Ø Head	Ø Open	1 Radioactive Element	Z No Qualifier
1 Cranial Cavity	3 Percutaneous	3 Infusion Device	
2 Face	4 Percutaneous Endoscopic	Y Other Device	
3 Oral Cavity and Throat			
4 Upper Jaw			
5 Lower Jaw			
6 Neck			
Parapharyngeal space			
Retropharyngeal space			
8 Chest Wall			
9 Pleural Cavity, Right			
B Pleural Cavity, Left			
C Mediastinum			
Mediastinal cavity			
Mediastinal space			
D Pericardial Cavity			
F Abdominal Wall			
G Peritoneal Cavity			
H Retroperitoneum			
Retroperitoneal cavity			
Retroperitoneal space			
J Pelvic Cavity			
Retropubic space			
K Upper Back			
L Lower Back			
M Perineum, Male			
N Perineum, Female ♀			
P Gastrointestinal Tract	Ø Open	1 Radioactive Element	Z No Qualifier
Q Respiratory Tract	3 Percutaneous	3 Infusion Device	
R Genitourinary Tract	4 Percutaneous Endoscopic	Y Other Device	
	7 Via Natural or Artificial Opening		
	8 Via Natural or Artificial Opening Endoscopic		

DRG Non-OR	ØWH[Ø,2,4,5,6,K,L,M][Ø,3,4][3,Y]Z	Non-OR	ØWHP[3,4,7,8][3,Y]Z
Non-OR	ØWH1[Ø,3,4]3Z	Non-OR	ØWHQ[Ø,7,8][3,Y]Z
Non-OR	ØWH[8,9,B][Ø,3,4][3,Y]Z	Non-OR	ØWHR[Ø,3,4,7,8][3,Y]Z
Non-OR	ØWHPØYZ	♀	ØWHN[Ø,3,4][3,Y]Z

NC Noncovered Procedure   LC Limited Coverage   QA Questionable OB Admit   NT New Tech Add-on   ⊞ Combination Member   ♂ Male   ♀ Female

Ø Medical and Surgical
W Anatomical Regions, General
J Inspection   Definition: Visually and/or manually exploring a body part

Explanation: Visual exploration may be performed with or without optical instrumentation. Manual exploration may be performed directly or through intervening body layers.

Body Part Character 4	Approach Character 5	Device Character 6	Qualifier Character 7

Ø Head
2 Face
3 Oral Cavity and Throat
4 Upper Jaw
5 Lower Jaw
6 Neck
  Parapharyngeal space
  Retropharyngeal space
8 Chest Wall
F Abdominal Wall
K Upper Back
L Lower Back
M Perineum, Male ♂
N Perineum, Female ♀
	Ø Open
	3 Percutaneous
	4 Percutaneous Endoscopic
	X External
		Z No Device	Z No Qualifier

1 Cranial Cavity
9 Pleural Cavity, Right
B Pleural Cavity, Left
C Mediastinum
  Mediastinal cavity
  Mediastinal space
D Pericardial Cavity
G Peritoneal Cavity
H Retroperitoneum
  Retroperitoneal cavity
  Retroperitoneal space
J Pelvic Cavity
  Retropubic space
	Ø Open
	3 Percutaneous
	4 Percutaneous Endoscopic
		Z No Device	Z No Qualifier

P Gastrointestinal Tract Q Respiratory Tract R Genitourinary Tract	Ø Open 3 Percutaneous 4 Percutaneous Endoscopic 7 Via Natural or Artificial Opening 8 Via Natural or Artificial Opening Endoscopic	Z No Device	Z No Qualifier

DRG Non-OR ØWJ[Ø,2,4,5,K,L]ØZZ
DRG Non-OR ØWJM[Ø,4]ZZ
Non-OR ØWJ3ØZZ
Non-OR ØWJ[Ø,2,3,4,5,6,8,F,K,L,M,N][3,X]ZZ
Non-OR ØWJ[Ø,2,3,4,5,K,L]4ZZ
Non-OR ØWJDØZZ
Non-OR ØWJ[1,9,B,C,D,G,H,J]3ZZ
Non-OR ØWJ[P,Q,R][3,7,8]ZZ
♂ ØWJM[Ø,3,4,X]ZZ
♀ ØWJN[Ø,3,4,X]ZZ

Ø Medical and Surgical
W Anatomical Regions, General
M Reattachment   Definition: Putting back in or on all or a portion of a separated body part to its normal location or other suitable location

Explanation: Vascular circulation and nervous pathways may or may not be reestablished

Body Part Character 4	Approach Character 5	Device Character 6	Qualifier Character 7

2 Face
4 Upper Jaw
5 Lower Jaw
6 Neck
  Parapharyngeal space
  Retropharyngeal space
8 Chest Wall
F Abdominal Wall
K Upper Back
L Lower Back
M Perineum, Male ♂
N Perineum, Female ♀
	Ø Open	Z No Device	Z No Qualifier

♂ ØWMMØZZ
♀ ØWMNØZZ

Ø   Medical and Surgical
W   Anatomical Regions, General
P   Removal   Definition: Taking out or off a device from a body part

        Explanation: If a device is taken out and a similar device put in without cutting or puncturing the skin or mucous membrane, the procedure is coded to the root operation CHANGE. Otherwise, the procedure for taking out the device is coded to the root operation REMOVAL.

Body Part Character 4	Approach Character 5	Device Character 6	Qualifier Character 7

Ø Head
2 Face
4 Upper Jaw
5 Lower Jaw
6 Neck
     Parapharyngeal space
     Retropharyngeal space
8 Chest Wall
C Mediastinum
     Mediastinal cavity
     Mediastinal space
F Abdominal Wall
K Upper Back
L Lower Back
M Perineum, Male   ♂
N Perineum, Female   ♀
	Ø Open
	3 Percutaneous
	4 Percutaneous Endoscopic
	X External
		Ø Drainage Device
		1 Radioactive Element
		3 Infusion Device
		7 Autologous Tissue Substitute
		J Synthetic Substitute
		K Nonautologous Tissue Substitute
		Y Other Device
			Z No Qualifier

1 Cranial Cavity 9 Pleural Cavity, Right B Pleural Cavity, Left G Peritoneal Cavity J Pelvic Cavity Retropubic space	Ø Open 3 Percutaneous 4 Percutaneous Endoscopic	Ø Drainage Device 1 Radioactive Element 3 Infusion Device J Synthetic Substitute Y Other Device	Z No Qualifier
1 Cranial Cavity 9 Pleural Cavity, Right B Pleural Cavity, Left G Peritoneal Cavity J Pelvic Cavity Retropubic space	X External	Ø Drainage Device 1 Radioactive Element 3 Infusion Device	Z No Qualifier

D Pericardial Cavity
H Retroperitoneum
     Retroperitoneal cavity
     Retroperitoneal space
	Ø Open
	3 Percutaneous
	4 Percutaneous Endoscopic
		Ø Drainage Device
		1 Radioactive Element
		3 Infusion Device
		Y Other Device
			Z No Qualifier

D Pericardial Cavity
H Retroperitoneum
     Retroperitoneal cavity
     Retroperitoneal space
	X External	Ø Drainage Device
		1 Radioactive Element
		3 Infusion Device
			Z No Qualifier

P Gastrointestinal Tract Q Respiratory Tract R Genitourinary Tract	Ø Open 3 Percutaneous 4 Percutaneous Endoscopic 7 Via Natural or Artificial Opening 8 Via Natural or Artificial Opening Endoscopic X External	1 Radioactive Element 3 Infusion Device Y Other Device	Z No Qualifier

Non-OR   ØWP[Ø,2,4,5,6,8][Ø,3,4,X][Ø,1,3,7,J,K,Y]Z
Non-OR   ØWP[C,F]X[Ø,1,3,7,J,K,Y]Z
Non-OR   ØWP[K,L][Ø,3,4,X][Ø,1,3,7,J,K,Y]Z
Non-OR   ØWPM[Ø,3,4][Ø,1,3,J,Y]Z
Non-OR   ØWPMX[Ø,1,3,Y]Z
Non-OR   ØWPNX[Ø,1,3,7,J,K,Y]Z
Non-OR   ØWP1[Ø,3,4]3Z
Non-OR   ØWP[9,B,J][Ø,3,4][Ø,1,3,J,Y]Z
Non-OR   ØWP[1,9,B,G,J]X[Ø,1,3]Z
Non-OR   ØWP[D,H]X[Ø,1,3]Z
Non-OR   ØWPP[3,4,7,8,X][1,3,Y]Z
Non-OR   ØWPQ73Z
Non-OR   ØWPQ8[3,Y]Z
Non-OR   ØWPQ[Ø,X][1,3,Y]Z
Non-OR   ØWPR[Ø,3,4,7,8,X][1,3,Y]Z

♂   ØWPM[Ø,3,4,X][Ø,1,3,7,J,K,Y]Z
♀   ØWPN[Ø,3,4,X][Ø,1,3,7,J,K,Y]Z

NC Noncovered Procedure   **LC** Limited Coverage   **QA** Questionable OB Admit   **NT** New Tech Add-on   ⊞ Combination Member   ♂ Male   ♀ Female

ICD-10-PCS 2022   681

Anatomical Regions, General

Ø   Medical and Surgical
W   Anatomical Regions, General
Q   Repair   Definition: Restoring, to the extent possible, a body part to its normal anatomic structure and function

                      Explanation: Used only when the method to accomplish the repair is not one of the other root operations

Body Part Character 4	Approach Character 5	Device Character 6	Qualifier Character 7
Ø Head 2 Face 3 Oral Cavity and Throat 4 Upper Jaw 5 Lower Jaw 8 Chest Wall K Upper Back L Lower Back M Perineum, Male ♂ N Perineum, Female ♀	Ø Open 3 Percutaneous 4 Percutaneous Endoscopic X External	Z No Device	Z No Qualifier

6   Neck
     Parapharyngeal space
     Retropharyngeal space
F   Abdominal Wall
	Ø Open
	3 Percutaneous
	4 Percutaneous Endoscopic
		Z No Device	Z No Qualifier

6   Neck
     Parapharyngeal space
     Retropharyngeal space
F   Abdominal Wall   ⊞
	X External	Z No Device	2 Stoma
			Z No Qualifier

C   Mediastinum
     Mediastinal cavity
     Mediastinal space
	Ø Open
	3 Percutaneous
	4 Percutaneous Endoscopic
		Z No Device	Z No Qualifier

Non-OR   ØWQNXZZ
♂   ØWQM[Ø,3,4,X]ZZ
♀   ØWQN[Ø,3,4,X]ZZ

See Appendix L for Procedure Combinations
⊞   ØWQFXZ[2,Z]

Ø   Medical and Surgical
W   Anatomical Regions, General
U   Supplement   Definition: Putting in or on biological or synthetic material that physically reinforces and/or augments the function of a portion of a body part

                      Explanation: The biological material is non-living, or is living and from the same individual. The body part may have been previously replaced, and the SUPPLEMENT procedure is performed to physically reinforce and/or augment the function of the replaced body part.

Body Part Character 4	Approach Character 5	Device Character 6	Qualifier Character 7

Ø   Head
2   Face
4   Upper Jaw
5   Lower Jaw
6   Neck
     Parapharyngeal space
     Retropharyngeal space
8   Chest Wall
C   Mediastinum
     Mediastinal cavity
     Mediastinal space
F   Abdominal Wall
K   Upper Back
L   Lower Back
M   Perineum, Male   ♂
N   Perineum, Female   ♀
	Ø Open
	4 Percutaneous Endoscopic
		7 Autologous Tissue Substitute
		J Synthetic Substitute
		K Nonautologous Tissue Substitute
			Z No Qualifier

♂   ØWUM[Ø,4][7,J,K]Z
♀   ØWUN[Ø,4][7,J,K]Z

Ø Medical and Surgical
W Anatomical Regions, General
W Revision   Definition: Correcting, to the extent possible, a portion of a malfunctioning device or the position of a displaced device

Explanation: Revision can include correcting a malfunctioning or displaced device by taking out or putting in components of the device such as a screw or pin

Body Part Character 4	Approach Character 5	Device Character 6	Qualifier Character 7

Ø Head
2 Face
4 Upper Jaw
5 Lower Jaw
6 Neck
  Parapharyngeal space
  Retropharyngeal space
8 Chest Wall
C Mediastinum
  Mediastinal cavity
  Mediastinal space
F Abdominal Wall
K Upper Back
L Lower Back
M Perineum, Male ♂
N Perineum, Female ♀
	Ø Open
	3 Percutaneous
	4 Percutaneous Endoscopic
	X External
		Ø Drainage Device
		1 Radioactive Element
		3 Infusion Device
		7 Autologous Tissue Substitute
		J Synthetic Substitute
		K Nonautologous Tissue Substitute
		Y Other Device
			Z No Qualifier

1 Cranial Cavity 9 Pleural Cavity, Right B Pleural Cavity, Left G Peritoneal Cavity J Pelvic Cavity Retropubic space	Ø Open 3 Percutaneous 4 Percutaneous Endoscopic X External	Ø Drainage Device 1 Radioactive Element 3 Infusion Device J Synthetic Substitute Y Other Device	Z No Qualifier

D Pericardial Cavity
H Retroperitoneum
  Retroperitoneal cavity
  Retroperitoneal space
	Ø Open
	3 Percutaneous
	4 Percutaneous Endoscopic
	X External
		Ø Drainage Device
		1 Radioactive Element
		3 Infusion Device
		Y Other Device
			Z No Qualifier

P Gastrointestinal Tract Q Respiratory Tract R Genitourinary Tract	Ø Open 3 Percutaneous 4 Percutaneous Endoscopic 7 Via Natural or Artificial Opening 8 Via Natural or Artificial Opening Endoscopic X External	1 Radioactive Element 3 Infusion Device Y Other Device	Z No Qualifier

DRG Non-OR   ØWW[Ø,2,4,5,6,K,L][Ø,3,4][Ø,1,3,7,J,K,Y]Z   ♂   ØWWM[Ø,3,4,X][Ø,1,3,7,K,Y]Z
DRG Non-OR   ØWWM[Ø,3,4][Ø,1,3,J,Y]Z   ♀   ØWWN[Ø,3,4,X][Ø,1,3,7,K,Y]Z
Non-OR   ØWW[Ø,2,4,5,6,C,F,K,L,M,N]X[Ø,1,3,7,J,K,Y]Z
Non-OR   ØWW8[Ø,3,4,X][Ø,1,3,7,J,K,Y]Z
Non-OR   ØWW[1,G,J]X[Ø,1,3,J,Y]Z
Non-OR   ØWW[9,B][Ø,3,4,X][Ø,1,3,J,Y]Z
Non-OR   ØWW[D,H]X[Ø,1,3,Y]Z
Non-OR   ØWWP[3,4,7,8,X][1,3,Y]Z
Non-OR   ØWWQ[Ø,X][1,3,Y]Z
Non-OR   ØWWR[Ø,3,4,7,8,X][1,3,Y]Z

Ø Medical and Surgical
W Anatomical Regions, General
Y Transplantation   Definition: Putting in or on all or a portion of a living body part taken from another individual or animal to physically take the place and/or function of all or a portion of a similar body part

Explanation: The native body part may or may not be taken out, and the transplanted body part may take over all or a portion of its function

Body Part Character 4	Approach Character 5	Device Character 6	Qualifier Character 7
2 Face	Ø Open	Z No Device	Ø Allogeneic 1 Syngeneic

NC Noncovered Procedure   LC Limited Coverage   QA Questionable OB Admit   NT New Tech Add-on   ⊞ Combination Member   ♂ Male   ♀ Female

ICD-10-PCS 2022   683

Anatomical Regions, Upper Extremities ØXØ–ØXY

Character Meanings

This Character Meaning table is provided as a guide to assist the user in the identification of character members that may be found in this section of code tables. It **SHOULD NOT** be used to build a PCS code.

Operation–Character 3		Body Part–Character 4		Approach–Character 5		Device–Character 6		Qualifier–Character 7	
Ø	Alteration	Ø	Forequarter, Right	Ø	Open	Ø	Drainage Device	Ø	Allogeneic OR Complete
2	Change	1	Forequarter, Left	3	Percutaneous	1	Radioactive Element	1	High OR Syngeneic
3	Control	2	Shoulder Region, Right	4	Percutaneous Endoscopic	3	Infusion Device	2	Mid
6	Detachment	3	Shoulder Region, Left	X	External	7	Autologous Tissue Substitute	3	Low
9	Drainage	4	Axilla, Right			J	Synthetic Substitute	4	Complete 1st Ray
B	Excision	5	Axilla, Left			K	Nonautologous Tissue Substitute	5	Complete 2nd Ray
H	Insertion	6	Upper Extremity, Right			Y	Other Device	6	Complete 3rd Ray
J	Inspection	7	Upper Extremity, Left			Z	No Device	7	Complete 4th Ray
M	Reattachment	8	Upper Arm, Right					8	Complete 5th Ray
P	Removal	9	Upper Arm, Left					9	Partial 1st Ray
Q	Repair	B	Elbow Region, Right					B	Partial 2nd Ray
R	Replacement	C	Elbow Region, Left					C	Partial 3rd Ray
U	Supplement	D	Lower Arm, Right					D	Partial 4th Ray
W	Revision	F	Lower Arm, Left					F	Partial 5th Ray
X	Transfer	G	Wrist Region, Right					L	Thumb, Right
Y	Transplantation	H	Wrist Region, Left					M	Thumb, Left
		J	Hand, Right					N	Toe, Right
		K	Hand, Left					P	Toe, Left
		L	Thumb, Right					X	Diagnostic
		M	Thumb, Left					Z	No Qualifier
		N	Index Finger, Right						
		P	Index Finger, Left						
		Q	Middle Finger, Right						
		R	Middle Finger, Left						
		S	Ring Finger, Right						
		T	Ring Finger, Left						
		V	Little Finger, Right						
		W	Little Finger, Left						

AHA Coding Clinic for table ØX3

2016, 4Q, 99	Root operation Control
2015, 1Q, 35	Evacuation of hematoma for control of postprocedural bleeding
2013, 3Q, 23	Control of intraoperative bleeding

AHA Coding Clinic for table ØX6

2017, 2Q, 3-4	Qualifiers for the root operation detachment
2017, 2Q, 18	Removal of polydactyl digits
2017, 1Q, 52	Further distal phalangeal amputation
2016, 3Q, 33	Traumatic amputation of fingers with further revision amputation

AHA Coding Clinic for table ØXH

2017, 2Q, 20	Exchange of intramedullary antibiotic impregnated spacer

AHA Coding Clinic for table ØXP

2017, 2Q, 20	Exchange of intramedullary antibiotic impregnated spacer

AHA Coding Clinic for table ØXY

2016, 4Q, 112-113	Transplantation

Detachment Qualifier Descriptions

Qualifier Definition	Upper Arm	Lower Arm
1 **High:** Amputation at the proximal portion of the shaft of the:	Humerus	Radius/Ulna
2 **Mid:** Amputation at the middle portion of the shaft of the:	Humerus	Radius/Ulna
3 **Low:** Amputation at the distal portion of the shaft of the:	Humerus	Radius/Ulna

Qualifier Definition	Hand
Ø Complete 1st through 5th Rays Ray: digit of hand or foot with corresponding metacarpus or metatarsus	Through carpo-metacarpal joint, **Wrist**
4 Complete 1st Ray	Through carpo-metacarpal joint, **Thumb**
5 Complete 2nd Ray	Through carpo-metacarpal joint, **Index Finger**
6 Complete 3rd Ray	Through carpo-metacarpal joint, **Middle Finger**
7 Complete 4th Ray	Through carpo-metacarpal joint, **Ring Finger**
8 Complete 5th Ray	Through carpo-metacarpal joint, **Little Finger**
9 Partial 1st Ray	Anywhere along shaft or head of metacarpal bone, **Thumb**
B Partial 2nd Ray	Anywhere along shaft or head of metacarpal bone, **Index Finger**
C Partial 3rd Ray	Anywhere along shaft or head of metacarpal bone, **Middle Finger**
D Partial 4th Ray	Anywhere along shaft or head of metacarpal bone, **Ring Finger**
F Partial 5th Ray	Anywhere along shaft or head of metacarpal bone, **Little Finger**

Qualifier Definition	Thumb/Finger
Ø Complete	At the metacarpophalangeal joint
1 High	Anywhere along the proximal phalanx
2 Mid	Through the proximal interphalangeal joint or anywhere along the middle phalanx
3 Low	Through the distal interphalangeal joint or anywhere along the distal phalanx

Ø **Medical and Surgical**
X **Anatomical Regions, Upper Extremities**
Ø **Alteration** Definition: Modifying the anatomic structure of a body part without affecting the function of the body part
　　　　　　　Explanation: Principal purpose is to improve appearance

Body Part Character 4	Approach Character 5	Device Character 6	Qualifier Character 7
2 Shoulder Region, Right 3 Shoulder Region, Left 4 Axilla, Right 5 Axilla, Left 6 Upper Extremity, Right 7 Upper Extremity, Left 8 Upper Arm, Right 9 Upper Arm, Left B Elbow Region, Right C Elbow Region, Left D Lower Arm, Right F Lower Arm, Left G Wrist Region, Right H Wrist Region, Left	Ø Open 3 Percutaneous 4 Percutaneous Endoscopic	7 Autologous Tissue Substitute J Synthetic Substitute K Nonautologous Tissue Substitute Z No Device	Z No Qualifier

Ø **Medical and Surgical**
X **Anatomical Regions, Upper Extremities**
2 **Change** Definition: Taking out or off a device from a body part and putting back an identical or similar device in or on the same body part without cutting or puncturing the skin or a mucous membrane
　　　　　　　Explanation: All CHANGE procedures are coded using the approach EXTERNAL

Body Part Character 4	Approach Character 5	Device Character 6	Qualifier Character 7
6 Upper Extremity, Right 7 Upper Extremity, Left	X External	Ø Drainage Device Y Other Device	Z No Qualifier

Non-OR　All body part, approach, device, and qualifier values

Ø **Medical and Surgical**
X **Anatomical Regions, Upper Extremities**
3 **Control** Definition: Stopping, or attempting to stop, postprocedural or other acute bleeding
　　　　　　　Explanation: None

Body Part Character 4	Approach Character 5	Device Character 6	Qualifier Character 7
2 Shoulder Region, Right 3 Shoulder Region, Left 4 Axilla, Right 5 Axilla, Left 6 Upper Extremity, Right 7 Upper Extremity, Left 8 Upper Arm, Right 9 Upper Arm, Left B Elbow Region, Right C Elbow Region, Left D Lower Arm, Right F Lower Arm, Left G Wrist Region, Right H Wrist Region, Left J Hand, Right K Hand, Left	Ø Open 3 Percutaneous 4 Percutaneous Endoscopic	Z No Device	Z No Qualifier

Ø   Medical and Surgical
X   Anatomical Regions, Upper Extremities
6   Detachment   Definition: Cutting off all or a portion of the upper or lower extremities

Explanation: The body part value is the site of the detachment, with a qualifier if applicable to further specify the level where the extremity was detached

Body Part Character 4	Approach Character 5	Device Character 6	Qualifier Character 7
Ø Forequarter, Right 1 Forequarter, Left 2 Shoulder Region, Right 3 Shoulder Region, Left B Elbow Region, Right C Elbow Region, Left	Ø Open	Z No Device	Z No Qualifier
8 Upper Arm, Right 9 Upper Arm, Left D Lower Arm, Right F Lower Arm, Left	Ø Open	Z No Device	1 High 2 Mid 3 Low
J Hand, Right K Hand, Left	Ø Open	Z No Device	Ø Complete 4 Complete 1st Ray 5 Complete 2nd Ray 6 Complete 3rd Ray 7 Complete 4th Ray 8 Complete 5th Ray 9 Partial 1st Ray B Partial 2nd Ray C Partial 3rd Ray D Partial 4th Ray F Partial 5th Ray
L Thumb, Right M Thumb, Left N Index Finger, Right P Index Finger, Left Q Middle Finger, Right R Middle Finger, Left S Ring Finger, Right T Ring Finger, Left V Little Finger, Right W Little Finger, Left	Ø Open	Z No Device	Ø Complete 1 High 2 Mid 3 Low

0   Medical and Surgical
X   Anatomical Regions, Upper Extremities
9   Drainage   Definition: Taking or letting out fluids and/or gases from a body part
                          Explanation: The qualifier DIAGNOSTIC is used to identify drainage procedures that are biopsies

Body Part Character 4	Approach Character 5	Device Character 6	Qualifier Character 7
2 Shoulder Region, Right 3 Shoulder Region, Left 4 Axilla, Right 5 Axilla, Left 6 Upper Extremity, Right 7 Upper Extremity, Left 8 Upper Arm, Right 9 Upper Arm, Left B Elbow Region, Right C Elbow Region, Left D Lower Arm, Right F Lower Arm, Left G Wrist Region, Right H Wrist Region, Left J Hand, Right K Hand, Left	0 Open 3 Percutaneous 4 Percutaneous Endoscopic	0 Drainage Device	Z No Qualifier
2 Shoulder Region, Right 3 Shoulder Region, Left 4 Axilla, Right 5 Axilla, Left 6 Upper Extremity, Right 7 Upper Extremity, Left 8 Upper Arm, Right 9 Upper Arm, Left B Elbow Region, Right C Elbow Region, Left D Lower Arm, Right F Lower Arm, Left G Wrist Region, Right H Wrist Region, Left J Hand, Right K Hand, Left	0 Open 3 Percutaneous 4 Percutaneous Endoscopic	Z No Device	X Diagnostic Z No Qualifier

Non-OR   All body part, approach, device, and qualifier values

0   Medical and Surgical
X   Anatomical Regions, Upper Extremities
B   Excision   Definition: Cutting out or off, without replacement, a portion of a body part
                          Explanation: The qualifier DIAGNOSTIC is used to identify excision procedures that are biopsies

Body Part Character 4	Approach Character 5	Device Character 6	Qualifier Character 7
2 Shoulder Region, Right 3 Shoulder Region, Left 4 Axilla, Right 5 Axilla, Left 6 Upper Extremity, Right 7 Upper Extremity, Left 8 Upper Arm, Right 9 Upper Arm, Left B Elbow Region, Right C Elbow Region, Left D Lower Arm, Right F Lower Arm, Left G Wrist Region, Right H Wrist Region, Left J Hand, Right K Hand, Left	0 Open 3 Percutaneous 4 Percutaneous Endoscopic	Z No Device	X Diagnostic Z No Qualifier

Non-OR   0XB[2,3,4,5,6,7,8,9,B,C,D,F,G,H,J,K][0,3,4]ZX

Anatomical Regions, Upper Extremities

Ø **Medical and Surgical**
X **Anatomical Regions, Upper Extremities**
H **Insertion**   Definition: Putting in a nonbiological appliance that monitors, assists, performs, or prevents a physiological function but does not physically take the place of a body part
           Explanation: None

Body Part Character 4	Approach Character 5	Device Character 6	Qualifier Character 7
2 Shoulder Region, Right	Ø Open	1 Radioactive Element	Z No Qualifier
3 Shoulder Region, Left	3 Percutaneous	3 Infusion Device	
4 Axilla, Right	4 Percutaneous Endoscopic	Y Other Device	
5 Axilla, Left			
6 Upper Extremity, Right			
7 Upper Extremity, Left			
8 Upper Arm, Right			
9 Upper Arm, Left			
B Elbow Region, Right			
C Elbow Region, Left			
D Lower Arm, Right			
F Lower Arm, Left			
G Wrist Region, Right			
H Wrist Region, Left			
J Hand, Right			
K Hand, Left			

DRG Non-OR   ØXH[2,3,4,5,6,7,8,9,B,C,D,F,G,H,J,K][Ø,3,4][3,Y]Z

Ø **Medical and Surgical**
X **Anatomical Regions, Upper Extremities**
J **Inspection**   Definition: Visually and/or manually exploring a body part
           Explanation: Visual exploration may be performed with or without optical instrumentation. Manual exploration may be performed directly or through intervening body layers.

Body Part Character 4	Approach Character 5	Device Character 6	Qualifier Character 7
2 Shoulder Region, Right	Ø Open	Z No Device	Z No Qualifier
3 Shoulder Region, Left	3 Percutaneous		
4 Axilla, Right	4 Percutaneous Endoscopic		
5 Axilla, Left	X External		
6 Upper Extremity, Right			
7 Upper Extremity, Left			
8 Upper Arm, Right			
9 Upper Arm, Left			
B Elbow Region, Right			
C Elbow Region, Left			
D Lower Arm, Right			
F Lower Arm, Left			
G Wrist Region, Right			
H Wrist Region, Left			
J Hand, Right			
K Hand, Left			

DRG Non-OR   ØXJ[2,3,4,5,6,7,8,9,B,C,D,F,G,H,J,K]ØZZ
Non-OR   ØXJ[2,3,4,5,6,7,8,9,B,C,D,F,G,H][3,4,X]ZZ
Non-OR   ØXJ[J,K][3,X]ZZ

Ø   **Medical and Surgical**
X   **Anatomical Regions, Upper Extremities**
M   **Reattachment**   Definition: Putting back in or on all or a portion of a separated body part to its normal location or other suitable location

           Explanation: Vascular circulation and nervous pathways may or may not be reestablished

Body Part Character 4	Approach Character 5	Device Character 6	Qualifier Character 7
Ø Forequarter, Right	Ø Open	Z No Device	Z No Qualifier
1 Forequarter, Left			
2 Shoulder Region, Right			
3 Shoulder Region, Left			
4 Axilla, Right			
5 Axilla, Left			
6 Upper Extremity, Right			
7 Upper Extremity, Left			
8 Upper Arm, Right			
9 Upper Arm, Left			
B Elbow Region, Right			
C Elbow Region, Left			
D Lower Arm, Right			
F Lower Arm, Left			
G Wrist Region, Right			
H Wrist Region, Left			
J Hand, Right			
K Hand, Left			
L Thumb, Right			
M Thumb, Left			
N Index Finger, Right			
P Index Finger, Left			
Q Middle Finger, Right			
R Middle Finger, Left			
S Ring Finger, Right			
T Ring Finger, Left			
V Little Finger, Right			
W Little Finger, Left			

Ø   **Medical and Surgical**
X   **Anatomical Regions, Upper Extremities**
P   **Removal**   Definition: Taking out or off a device from a body part

           Explanation: If a device is taken out and a similar device put in without cutting or puncturing the skin or mucous membrane, the procedure is coded to the root operation CHANGE. Otherwise, the procedure for taking out the device is coded to the root operation REMOVAL.

Body Part Character 4	Approach Character 5	Device Character 6	Qualifier Character 7
6 Upper Extremity, Right	Ø Open	Ø Drainage Device	Z No Qualifier
7 Upper Extremity, Left	3 Percutaneous	1 Radioactive Element	
	4 Percutaneous Endoscopic	3 Infusion Device	
	X External	7 Autologous Tissue Substitute	
		J Synthetic Substitute	
		K Nonautologous Tissue Substitute	
		Y Other Device	

Non-OR   All body part, approach, device, and qualifier values

NC Noncovered Procedure   **LC** Limited Coverage   **QA** Questionable OB Admit   **NT** New Tech Add-on   ⊞ Combination Member   ♂ Male   ♀ Female

ICD-10-PCS 2022   **691**

ØXM–ØXP

Anatomical Regions, Upper Extremities

Ø   Medical and Surgical
X   Anatomical Regions, Upper Extremities
Q   Repair   Definition: Restoring, to the extent possible, a body part to its normal anatomic structure and function

           Explanation: Used only when the method to accomplish the repair is not one of the other root operations

Body Part Character 4	Approach Character 5	Device Character 6	Qualifier Character 7
2 Shoulder Region, Right	Ø Open	Z No Device	Z No Qualifier
3 Shoulder Region, Left	3 Percutaneous		
4 Axilla, Right	4 Percutaneous Endoscopic		
5 Axilla, Left	X External		
6 Upper Extremity, Right			
7 Upper Extremity, Left			
8 Upper Arm, Right			
9 Upper Arm, Left			
B Elbow Region, Right			
C Elbow Region, Left			
D Lower Arm, Right			
F Lower Arm, Left			
G Wrist Region, Right			
H Wrist Region, Left			
J Hand, Right			
K Hand, Left			
L Thumb, Right			
M Thumb, Left			
N Index Finger, Right			
P Index Finger, Left			
Q Middle Finger, Right			
R Middle Finger, Left			
S Ring Finger, Right			
T Ring Finger, Left			
V Little Finger, Right			
W Little Finger, Left			

Ø   Medical and Surgical
X   Anatomical Regions, Upper Extremities
R   Replacement   Definition: Putting in or on biological or synthetic material that physically takes the place and/or function of all or a portion of a body part

           Explanation: The body part may have been taken out or replaced, or may be taken out, physically eradicated, or rendered nonfunctional during the REPLACEMENT procedure. A REMOVAL procedure is coded for taking out the device used in a previous replacement procedure.

Body Part Character 4	Approach Character 5	Device Character 6	Qualifier Character 7
L Thumb, Right	Ø Open	7 Autologous Tissue Substitute	N Toe, Right
M Thumb, Left	4 Percutaneous Endoscopic		P Toe, Left

Ø   Medical and Surgical
X   Anatomical Regions, Upper Extremities
U   Supplement   Definition: Putting in or on biological or synthetic material that physically reinforces and/or augments the function of a portion of a body part

Explanation: The biological material is non-living, or is living and from the same individual. The body part may have been previously replaced, and the SUPPLEMENT procedure is performed to physically reinforce and/or augment the function of the replaced body part.

Body Part Character 4	Approach Character 5	Device Character 6	Qualifier Character 7
2 Shoulder Region, Right 3 Shoulder Region, Left 4 Axilla, Right 5 Axilla, Left 6 Upper Extremity, Right 7 Upper Extremity, Left 8 Upper Arm, Right 9 Upper Arm, Left B Elbow Region, Right C Elbow Region, Left D Lower Arm, Right F Lower Arm, Left G Wrist Region, Right H Wrist Region, Left J Hand, Right K Hand, Left L Thumb, Right M Thumb, Left N Index Finger, Right P Index Finger, Left Q Middle Finger, Right R Middle Finger, Left S Ring Finger, Right T Ring Finger, Left V Little Finger, Right W Little Finger, Left	Ø Open 4 Percutaneous Endoscopic	7 Autologous Tissue Substitute J Synthetic Substitute K Nonautologous Tissue Substitute	Z No Qualifier

Ø   Medical and Surgical
X   Anatomical Regions, Upper Extremities
W   Revision   Definition: Correcting, to the extent possible, a portion of a malfunctioning device or the position of a displaced device

Explanation: Revision can include correcting a malfunctioning or displaced device by taking out or putting in components of the device such as a screw or pin

Body Part Character 4	Approach Character 5	Device Character 6	Qualifier Character 7
6 Upper Extremity, Right 7 Upper Extremity, Left	Ø Open 3 Percutaneous 4 Percutaneous Endoscopic X External	Ø Drainage Device 3 Infusion Device 7 Autologous Tissue Substitute J Synthetic Substitute K Nonautologous Tissue Substitute Y Other Device	Z No Qualifier

DRG Non-OR   ØXW[6,7][Ø,3,4][Ø,3,7,J,K,Y]Z
Non-OR   ØXW[6,7]X[Ø,3,7,J,K,Y]Z

Ø   Medical and Surgical
X   Anatomical Regions, Upper Extremities
X   Transfer   Definition: Moving, without taking out, all or a portion of a body part to another location to take over the function of all or a portion of a body part

Explanation: The body part transferred remains connected to its vascular and nervous supply

Body Part Character 4	Approach Character 5	Device Character 6	Qualifier Character 7
N Index Finger, Right	Ø Open	Z No Device	L Thumb, Right
P Index Finger, Left	Ø Open	Z No Device	M Thumb, Left

Ø   Medical and Surgical
X   Anatomical Regions, Upper Extremities
Y   Transplantation   Definition: Putting in or on all or a portion of a living body part taken from another individual or animal to physically take the place and/or function of all or a portion of a similar body part

Explanation: The native body part may or may not be taken out, and the transplanted body part may take over all or a portion of its function

Body Part Character 4	Approach Character 5	Device Character 6	Qualifier Character 7
J Hand, Right	Ø Open	Z No Device	Ø Allogeneic
K Hand, Left			1 Syngeneic

NC Noncovered Procedure   LC Limited Coverage   QA Questionable OB Admit   NT New Tech Add-on   ⊞ Combination Member   ♂ Male   ♀ Female

ICD-10-PCS 2022   693

ØXU–ØXY

Anatomical Regions, Lower Extremities ØYØ–ØYW

Character Meanings

This Character Meaning table is provided as a guide to assist the user in the identification of character members that may be found in this section of code tables. It **SHOULD NOT** be used to build a PCS code.

Operation–Character 3		Body Part–Character 4		Approach–Character 5		Device–Character 6		Qualifier–Character 7	
Ø	Alteration	Ø	Buttock, Right	Ø	Open	Ø	Drainage Device	Ø	Complete
2	Change	1	Buttock, Left	3	Percutaneous	1	Radioactive Element	1	High
3	Control	2	Hindquarter, Right	4	Percutaneous Endoscopic	3	Infusion Device	2	Mid
6	Detachment	3	Hindquarter, Left	X	External	7	Autologous Tissue Substitute	3	Low
9	Drainage	4	Hindquarter, Bilateral			J	Synthetic Substitute	4	Complete 1st Ray
B	Excision	5	Inguinal Region, Right			K	Nonautologous Tissue Substitute	5	Complete 2nd Ray
H	Insertion	6	Inguinal Region, Left			Y	Other Device	6	Complete 3rd Ray
J	Inspection	7	Femoral Region, Right			Z	No Device	7	Complete 4th Ray
M	Reattachment	8	Femoral Region, Left					8	Complete 5th Ray
P	Removal	9	Lower Extremity, Right					9	Partial 1st Ray
Q	Repair	A	Inguinal Region, Bilateral					B	Partial 2nd Ray
U	Supplement	B	Lower Extremity, Left					C	Partial 3rd Ray
W	Revision	C	Upper Leg, Right					D	Partial 4th Ray
		D	Upper Leg, Left					F	Partial 5th Ray
		E	Femoral Region, Bilateral					X	Diagnostic
		F	Knee Region, Right					Z	No Qualifier
		G	Knee Region, Left						
		H	Lower Leg, Right						
		J	Lower Leg, Left						
		K	Ankle Region, Right						
		L	Ankle Region, Left						
		M	Foot, Right						
		N	Foot, Left						
		P	1st Toe, Right						
		Q	1st Toe, Left						
		R	2nd Toe, Right						
		S	2nd Toe, Left						
		T	3rd Toe, Right						
		U	3rd Toe, Left						
		V	4th Toe, Right						
		W	4th Toe, Left						
		X	5th Toe, Right						
		Y	5th Toe, Left						

AHA Coding Clinic for table ØY3
2016, 4Q, 99	Root operation Control
2013, 3Q, 23	Control of intraoperative bleeding

AHA Coding Clinic for table ØY6
2019, 2Q, 17	Cryoamputation of lower leg
2017, 2Q, 3-4	Qualifiers for the root operation detachment
2017, 1Q, 22	Chopart amputation of foot
2015, 2Q, 28	Partial amputation of hallux at interphalangeal Joint
2015, 1Q, 28	Mid-foot amputation

AHA Coding Clinic for table ØY9
2015, 1Q, 22	Incision and drainage of abscess of femoropopliteal bypass site
2015, 1Q, 22	Incision and drainage of groin abscess

Detachment Qualifier Descriptions

Qualifier Definition		Upper Leg	Lower Leg
1	**High:** Amputation at the proximal portion of the shaft of the:	Femur	Tibia/Fibula
2	**Mid:** Amputation at the middle portion of the shaft of the:	Femur	Tibia/Fibula
3	**Low:** Amputation at the distal portion of the shaft of the:	Femur	Tibia/Fibula

Qualifier Definition	Foot
Ø Complete 1st through 5th Rays Ray: digit of hand or foot with corresponding metacarpus or metatarsus	Through tarso-metatarsal Joint, **Ankle**
4 Complete 1st Ray	Through tarso-metatarsal joint, **Great Toe**
5 Complete 2nd Ray	Through tarso-metatarsal joint, **2nd Toe**
6 Complete 3rd Ray	Through tarso-metatarsal joint, **3rd Toe**
7 Complete 4th Ray	Through tarso-metatarsal joint, **4th Toe**
8 Complete 5th Ray	Through tarso-metatarsal joint, **Little Toe**
9 Partial 1st Ray	Anywhere along shaft or head of metatarsal bone, **Great Toe**
B Partial 2nd Ray	Anywhere along shaft or head of metatarsal bone, **2nd Toe**
C Partial 3rd Ray	Anywhere along shaft or head of metatarsal bone, **3rd Toe**
D Partial 4th Ray	Anywhere along shaft or head of metatarsal bone, **4th Toe**
F Partial 5th Ray	Anywhere along shaft or head of metatarsal bone, **Little Toe**

Qualifier Definition	Toe
Ø Complete	At the metatarsal-phalangeal joint
1 High	Anywhere along the proximal phalanx
2 Mid	Through the proximal interphalangeal joint or anywhere along the middle phalanx
3 Low	Through the distal interphalangeal joint or anywhere along the distal phalanx

Ø   **Medical and Surgical**
Y   **Anatomical Regions, Lower Extremities**
Ø   **Alteration**   Definition: Modifying the anatomic structure of a body part without affecting the function of the body part
                         Explanation: Principal purpose is to improve appearance

Body Part Character 4	Approach Character 5	Device Character 6	Qualifier Character 7
Ø Buttock, Right 1 Buttock, Left 9 Lower Extremity, Right B Lower Extremity, Left C Upper Leg, Right D Upper Leg, Left F Knee Region, Right G Knee Region, Left H Lower Leg, Right J Lower Leg, Left K Ankle Region, Right L Ankle Region, Left	Ø Open 3 Percutaneous 4 Percutaneous Endoscopic	7 Autologous Tissue Substitute J Synthetic Substitute K Nonautologous Tissue Substitute Z No Device	Z No Qualifier

Ø   **Medical and Surgical**
Y   **Anatomical Regions, Lower Extremities**
2   **Change**   Definition: Taking out or off a device from a body part and putting back an identical or similar device in or on the same body part without
                         cutting or puncturing the skin or a mucous membrane
                         Explanation: All CHANGE procedures are coded using the approach EXTERNAL

Body Part Character 4	Approach Character 5	Device Character 6	Qualifier Character 7
9 Lower Extremity, Right B Lower Extremity, Left	X External	Ø Drainage Device Y Other Device	Z No Qualifier

Non-OR   All body part, approach, device, and qualifier values

Ø   **Medical and Surgical**
Y   **Anatomical Regions, Lower Extremities**
3   **Control**   Definition: Stopping, or attempting to stop, postprocedural or other acute bleeding
                         Explanation: None

Body Part Character 4	Approach Character 5	Device Character 6	Qualifier Character 7

Ø   Buttock, Right
1   Buttock, Left
5   Inguinal Region, Right
     Inguinal canal
     Inguinal triangle
6   Inguinal Region, Left
     See 5 Inguinal Region, Right
7   Femoral Region, Right
8   Femoral Region, Left
9   Lower Extremity, Right
B   Lower Extremity, Left
C   Upper Leg, Right
D   Upper Leg, Left
F   Knee Region, Right
G   Knee Region, Left
H   Lower Leg, Right
J   Lower Leg, Left
K   Ankle Region, Right
L   Ankle Region, Left
M   Foot, Right
N   Foot, Left
	Ø Open
	3 Percutaneous
	4 Percutaneous Endoscopic
		Z No Device	Z No Qualifier

NC Noncovered Procedure   **LC** Limited Coverage   **QA** Questionable OB Admit   **NT** New Tech Add-on   ⊞ Combination Member   ♂ Male   ♀ Female

ICD-10-PCS 2022   **697**

Anatomical Regions, Lower Extremities

Ø   **Medical and Surgical**
Y   **Anatomical Regions, Lower Extremities**
6   **Detachment**   Definition: Cutting off all or a portion of the upper or lower extremities
                             Explanation: The body part value is the site of the detachment, with a qualifier if applicable to further specify the level where the extremity was detached

Body Part Character 4	Approach Character 5	Device Character 6	Qualifier Character 7
2 Hindquarter, Right 3 Hindquarter, Left 4 Hindquarter, Bilateral 7 Femoral Region, Right 8 Femoral Region, Left F Knee Region, Right G Knee Region, Left	Ø Open	Z No Device	Z No Qualifier
C Upper Leg, Right D Upper Leg, Left H Lower Leg, Right J Lower Leg, Left	Ø Open	Z No Device	1 High 2 Mid 3 Low
M Foot, Right N Foot, Left	Ø Open	Z No Device	Ø Complete 4 Complete 1st Ray 5 Complete 2nd Ray 6 Complete 3rd Ray 7 Complete 4th Ray 8 Complete 5th Ray 9 Partial 1st Ray B Partial 2nd Ray C Partial 3rd Ray D Partial 4th Ray F Partial 5th Ray

P 1st Toe, Right
   Hallux
Q 1st Toe, Left
   See 1st Toe, Right
R 2nd Toe, Right
S 2nd Toe, Left
T 3rd Toe, Right
U 3rd Toe, Left
V 4th Toe, Right
W 4th Toe, Left
X 5th Toe, Right
Y 5th Toe, Left
	Ø Open	Z No Device	Ø Complete
			1 High
			2 Mid
			3 Low

ØY6–ØY6

Non-OR Procedure   DRG Non-OR Procedure   Valid OR Procedure   HAC Associated Procedure   Combination Only   New/Revised GREEN
698   ICD-10-PCS 2022

Ø   Medical and Surgical
Y   Anatomical Regions, Lower Extremities
9   Drainage   Definition: Taking or letting out fluids and/or gases from a body part
                   Explanation: The qualifier DIAGNOSTIC is used to identify drainage procedures that are biopsies

Body Part Character 4	Approach Character 5	Device Character 6	Qualifier Character 7

Ø   Buttock, Right
1   Buttock, Left
5   Inguinal Region, Right
     Inguinal canal
     Inguinal triangle
6   Inguinal Region, Left
     See 5 Inguinal Region, Right
7   Femoral Region, Right
8   Femoral Region, Left
9   Lower Extremity, Right
B   Lower Extremity, Left
C   Upper Leg, Right
D   Upper Leg, Left
F   Knee Region, Right
G   Knee Region, Left
H   Lower Leg, Right
J   Lower Leg, Left
K   Ankle Region, Right
L   Ankle Region, Left
M   Foot, Right
N   Foot, Left
	Ø Open
	3 Percutaneous
	4 Percutaneous Endoscopic
		Ø Drainage Device	Z No Qualifier

Ø   Buttock, Right
1   Buttock, Left
5   Inguinal Region, Right
     Inguinal canal
     Inguinal triangle
6   Inguinal Region, Left
     See 5 Inguinal Region, Right
7   Femoral Region, Right
8   Femoral Region, Left
9   Lower Extremity, Right
B   Lower Extremity, Left
C   Upper Leg, Right
D   Upper Leg, Left
F   Knee Region, Right
G   Knee Region, Left
H   Lower Leg, Right
J   Lower Leg, Left
K   Ankle Region, Right
L   Ankle Region, Left
M   Foot, Right
N   Foot, Left
	Ø Open
	3 Percutaneous
	4 Percutaneous Endoscopic
		Z No Device	X Diagnostic
			Z No Qualifier

Non-OR	ØY9[Ø,1,7,8,9,B,C,D,F,G,H,J,K,L,M,N][Ø,3,4]ØZ
Non-OR	ØY9[5,6]3ØZ
Non-OR	ØY9[Ø,1,7,8,9,B,C,D,F,G,H,J,K,L,M,N][Ø,3,4]Z[X,Z]
Non-OR	ØY9[5,6]3ZZ

NC Noncovered Procedure   LC Limited Coverage   QA Questionable OB Admit   NT New Tech Add-on   ✚ Combination Member   ♂ Male   ♀ Female

ICD-10-PCS 2022   699

Ø   Medical and Surgical
Y   Anatomical Regions, Lower Extremities
B   Excision   Definition: Cutting out or off, without replacement, a portion of a body part

Explanation: The qualifier DIAGNOSTIC is used to identify excision procedures that are biopsies

Body Part Character 4	Approach Character 5	Device Character 6	Qualifier Character 7

Ø   Buttock, Right
1   Buttock, Left
5   Inguinal Region, Right
     Inguinal canal
     Inguinal triangle
6   Inguinal Region, Left
     See 5 Inguinal Region, Right
7   Femoral Region, Right
8   Femoral Region, Left
9   Lower Extremity, Right
B   Lower Extremity, Left
C   Upper Leg, Right
D   Upper Leg, Left
F   Knee Region, Right
G   Knee Region, Left
H   Lower Leg, Right
J   Lower Leg, Left
K   Ankle Region, Right
L   Ankle Region, Left
M   Foot, Right
N   Foot, Left
	Ø Open
	3 Percutaneous
	4 Percutaneous Endoscopic
		Z No Device	X Diagnostic
			Z No Qualifier

Non-OR   ØYB[Ø,1,9,B,C,D,F,G,H,J,K,L,M,N][Ø,3,4]ZX

Ø   Medical and Surgical
Y   Anatomical Regions, Lower Extremities
H   Insertion   Definition: Putting in a nonbiological appliance that monitors, assists, performs, or prevents a physiological function but does not physically take the place of a body part

Explanation: None

Body Part Character 4	Approach Character 5	Device Character 6	Qualifier Character 7

Ø   Buttock, Right
1   Buttock, Left
5   Inguinal Region, Right
     Inguinal canal
     Inguinal triangle
6   Inguinal Region, Left
     See 5 Inguinal Region, Right
7   Femoral Region, Right
8   Femoral Region, Left
9   Lower Extremity, Right
B   Lower Extremity, Left
C   Upper Leg, Right
D   Upper Leg, Left
F   Knee Region, Right
G   Knee Region, Left
H   Lower Leg, Right
J   Lower Leg, Left
K   Ankle Region, Right
L   Ankle Region, Left
M   Foot, Right
N   Foot, Left
	Ø Open
	3 Percutaneous
	4 Percutaneous Endoscopic
		1 Radioactive Element
		3 Infusion Device
		Y Other Device
			Z No Qualifier

DRG Non-OR   ØYH[Ø,1,5,6,7,8,9,B,C,D,F,G,H,J,K,L,M,N][Ø,3,4][3,Y]Z

Ø **Medical and Surgical**
Y **Anatomical Regions, Lower Extremities**
J **Inspection**   Definition: Visually and/or manually exploring a body part

Explanation: Visual exploration may be performed with or without optical instrumentation. Manual exploration may be performed directly or through intervening body layers.

Body Part Character 4	Approach Character 5	Device Character 6	Qualifier Character 7
Ø Buttock, Right	**Ø** Open	**Z** No Device	**Z** No Qualifier
1 Buttock, Left	**3** Percutaneous		
5 Inguinal Region, Right	**4** Percutaneous Endoscopic		
Inguinal canal	**X** External		
Inguinal triangle			
6 Inguinal Region, Left			
See 5 Inguinal Region, Right			
7 Femoral Region, Right			
8 Femoral Region, Left			
9 Lower Extremity, Right			
A Inguinal Region, Bilateral			
See 5 Inguinal Region, Right			
B Lower Extremity, Left			
C Upper Leg, Right			
D Upper Leg, Left			
E Femoral Region, Bilateral			
F Knee Region, Right			
G Knee Region, Left			
H Lower Leg, Right			
J Lower Leg, Left			
K Ankle Region, Right			
L Ankle Region, Left			
M Foot, Right			
N Foot, Left			

DRG Non-OR ØYJ[Ø,1,8,9,B,C,D,E,F,G,H,J,K,L,M,N]ØZZ
Non-OR ØYJ[Ø,1,9,B,C,D,F,G,H,J,K,L,M,N][3,4,X]ZZ
Non-OR ØYJ[5,6,7,8,A,E][3,X]ZZ

Ø   Medical and Surgical
Y   Anatomical Regions, Lower Extremities
M   Reattachment   Definition: Putting back in or on all or a portion of a separated body part to its normal location or other suitable location

            Explanation: Vascular circulation and nervous pathways may or may not be reestablished

Body Part Character 4	Approach Character 5	Device Character 6	Qualifier Character 7

Ø   Buttock, Right
1   Buttock, Left
2   Hindquarter, Right
3   Hindquarter, Left
4   Hindquarter, Bilateral
5   Inguinal Region, Right
     Inguinal canal
     Inguinal triangle
6   Inguinal Region, Left
     See 5 Inguinal Region, Right
7   Femoral Region, Right
8   Femoral Region, Left
9   Lower Extremity, Right
B   Lower Extremity, Left
C   Upper Leg, Right
D   Upper Leg, Left
F   Knee Region, Right
G   Knee Region, Left
H   Lower Leg, Right
J   Lower Leg, Left
K   Ankle Region, Right
L   Ankle Region, Left
M   Foot, Right
N   Foot, Left
P   1st Toe, Right
     Hallux
Q   1st Toe, Left
     See 1st Toe, Right
R   2nd Toe, Right
S   2nd Toe, Left
T   3rd Toe, Right
U   3rd Toe, Left
V   4th Toe, Right
W   4th Toe, Left
X   5th Toe, Right
Y   5th Toe, Left
	Ø Open	Z No Device	Z No Qualifier

Ø   Medical and Surgical
Y   Anatomical Regions, Lower Extremities
P   Removal   Definition: Taking out or off a device from a body part

            Explanation: If a device is taken out and a similar device put in without cutting or puncturing the skin or mucous membrane, the procedure is coded to the root operation CHANGE. Otherwise, the procedure for taking out the device is coded to the root operation REMOVAL.

Body Part Character 4	Approach Character 5	Device Character 6	Qualifier Character 7
9 Lower Extremity, Right B Lower Extremity, Left	Ø Open 3 Percutaneous 4 Percutaneous Endoscopic X External	Ø Drainage Device 1 Radioactive Element 3 Infusion Device 7 Autologous Tissue Substitute J Synthetic Substitute K Nonautologous Tissue Substitute Y Other Device	Z No Qualifier

Non-OR	All body part, approach, device, and qualifier values

Ø   Medical and Surgical
Y   Anatomical Regions, Lower Extremities
Q   Repair   Definition: Restoring, to the extent possible, a body part to its normal anatomic structure and function
                       Explanation: Used only when the method to accomplish the repair is not one of the other root operations

Body Part Character 4	Approach Character 5	Device Character 6	Qualifier Character 7
Ø Buttock, Right	Ø Open	Z No Device	Z No Qualifier
1 Buttock, Left	3 Percutaneous		
5 Inguinal Region, Right	4 Percutaneous Endoscopic		
Inguinal canal	X External		
Inguinal triangle			
6 Inguinal Region, Left			
See 5 Inguinal Region, Right			
7 Femoral Region, Right			
8 Femoral Region, Left			
9 Lower Extremity, Right			
A Inguinal Region, Bilateral			
See 5 Inguinal Region, Right			
B Lower Extremity, Left			
C Upper Leg, Right			
D Upper Leg, Left			
E Femoral Region, Bilateral			
F Knee Region, Right			
G Knee Region, Left			
H Lower Leg, Right			
J Lower Leg, Left			
K Ankle Region, Right			
L Ankle Region, Left			
M Foot, Right			
N Foot, Left			
P 1st Toe, Right			
Hallux			
Q 1st Toe, Left			
See 1st Toe, Right			
R 2nd Toe, Right			
S 2nd Toe, Left			
T 3rd Toe, Right			
U 3rd Toe, Left			
V 4th Toe, Right			
W 4th Toe, Left			
X 5th Toe, Right			
Y 5th Toe, Left			

Non-OR   ØYQ[5,6,7,8,A,E]XZZ

Ø   **Medical and Surgical**
Y   **Anatomical Regions, Lower Extremities**
U   **Supplement**   Definition: Putting in or on biological or synthetic material that physically reinforces and/or augments the function of a portion of a body part
                 Explanation: The biological material is non-living, or is living and from the same individual. The body part may have been previously replaced, and the SUPPLEMENT procedure is performed to physically reinforce and/or augment the function of the replaced body part.

Body Part Character 4	Approach Character 5	Device Character 6	Qualifier Character 7

Ø Buttock, Right
1 Buttock, Left
5 Inguinal Region, Right
     Inguinal canal
     Inguinal triangle
6 Inguinal Region, Left
     See 5 Inguinal Region, Right
7 Femoral Region, Right
8 Femoral Region, Left
9 Lower Extremity, Right
A Inguinal Region, Bilateral
     See 5 Inguinal Region, Right
B Lower Extremity, Left
C Upper Leg, Right
D Upper Leg, Left
E Femoral Region, Bilateral
F Knee Region, Right
G Knee Region, Left
H Lower Leg, Right
J Lower Leg, Left
K Ankle Region, Right
L Ankle Region, Left
M Foot, Right
N Foot, Left
P 1st Toe, Right
     Hallux
Q 1st Toe, Left
     See 1st Toe, Right
R 2nd Toe, Right
S 2nd Toe, Left
T 3rd Toe, Right
U 3rd Toe, Left
V 4th Toe, Right
W 4th Toe, Left
X 5th Toe, Right
Y 5th Toe, Left
	Ø Open
	4 Percutaneous Endoscopic
		7 Autologous Tissue Substitute
		J Synthetic Substitute
		K Nonautologous Tissue Substitute
			Z No Qualifier

Ø   **Medical and Surgical**
Y   **Anatomical Regions, Lower Extremities**
W   **Revision**   Definition: Correcting, to the extent possible, a portion of a malfunctioning device or the position of a displaced device
                Explanation: Revision can include correcting a malfunctioning or displaced device by taking out or putting in components of the device such as a screw or pin

Body Part Character 4	Approach Character 5	Device Character 6	Qualifier Character 7
9 Lower Extremity, Right B Lower Extremity, Left	Ø Open 3 Percutaneous 4 Percutaneous Endoscopic X External	Ø Drainage Device 3 Infusion Device 7 Autologous Tissue Substitute J Synthetic Substitute K Nonautologous Tissue Substitute Y Other Device	Z No Qualifier

DRG Non-OR   ØYW[9,B][Ø,3,4][Ø,3,7,J,K,Y]Z
Non-OR   ØYW[9,B]X[Ø,3,7,J,K,Y]Z

Obstetrics 1Ø2–1ØY

Character Meanings

This Character Meaning table is provided as a guide to assist the user in the identification of character members that may be found in this section of code tables. It **SHOULD NOT** be used to build a PCS code.

Ø: Pregnancy

Operation–Character 3		Body Part–Character 4		Approach–Character 5		Device–Character 6		Qualifier–Character 7	
2	Change	Ø	Products of Conception	Ø	Open	3	Monitoring Electrode	Ø	High
9	Drainage	1	Products of Conception, Retained	3	Percutaneous	Y	Other Device	1	Low
A	Abortion	2	Products of Conception, Ectopic	4	Percutaneous Endoscopic	Z	No Device	2	Extraperitoneal
D	Extraction			7	Via Natural or Artificial Opening			3	Low Forceps
E	Delivery			8	Via Natural or Artificial Opening Endoscopic			4	Mid Forceps
H	Insertion			X	External			5	High Forceps
J	Inspection							6	Vacuum
P	Removal							7	Internal Version
Q	Repair							8	Other
S	Reposition							9	Fetal Blood OR Manual
T	Resection							A	Fetal Cerebrospinal Fluid
Y	Transplantation							B	Fetal Fluid, Other
								C	Amniotic Fluid, Therapeutic
								D	Fluid, Other
								E	Nervous System
								F	Cardiovascular System
								G	Lymphatics & Hemic
								H	Eye
								J	Ear, Nose & Sinus
								K	Respiratory System
								L	Mouth & Throat
								M	Gastrointestinal System
								N	Hepatobiliary & Pancreas
								P	Endocrine System
								Q	Skin
								R	Musculoskeletal System
								S	Urinary System
								T	Female Reproductive System
								U	Amniotic Fluid, Diagnostic
								V	Male Reproductive System
								W	Laminaria
								X	Abortifacient
								Y	Other Body System
								Z	No Qualifier

AHA Coding Clinic for table 1Ø9

| 2014, 3Q, 12 | Fetoscopic laser photocoagulation and laser microseptostomy for twin-twin transfusion syndrome |
| 2014, 2Q, 9 | Pitocin administration to augment labor |

AHA Coding Clinic for table 1ØD

2021, 1Q, 52	Removal of ectopic pregnancy via laparotomy
2020, 4Q, 59-60	Extraction of ectopic products of conception
2018, 4Q, 49-51	Revised qualifier values for root operation "extraction" (cesarean delivery)
2018, 2Q, 17	High transverse cesarean section
2016, 1Q, 9	Vaginal delivery assisted by vacuum and low forceps extraction
2014, 4Q, 43	Cesarean delivery assisted by vacuum extraction
2014, 4Q, 43	Vacuum dilation and curettage for blighted ovum

AHA Coding Clinic for table 1ØE

2017, 3Q, 5	Delivery of placenta
2016, 2Q, 34	Assisted vaginal delivery
2014, 4Q, 17	RH (D) alloimmunization (sensitization)
2014, 2Q, 9	Pitocin administration to augment labor

AHA Coding Clinic for table 1ØH

| 2013, 2Q, 36 | Intrauterine pressure monitor |

AHA Coding Clinic for table 1ØQ

| 2021, 2Q, 21 | Ex Utero intrapartum treatment procedure |
| 2014, 3Q, 12 | Fetoscopic laser photocoagulation and laser microseptostomy for twin-twin transfusion syndrome |

AHA Coding Clinic for table 1ØT

| 2020, 3Q, 47 | Removal of ectopic cornual pregnancy |
| 2015, 3Q, 31 | Laparoscopic partial salpingectomy for ectopic pregnancy |

1 Obstetrics
0 Pregnancy
2 Change

Definition: Taking out or off a device from a body part and putting back an identical or similar device in or on the same body part without cutting or puncturing the skin or a mucous membrane
Explanation: None

Body Part Character 4		Approach Character 5	Device Character 6	Qualifier Character 7
0 Products of Conception ♀		7 Via Natural or Artificial Opening	3 Monitoring Electrode Y Other Device	Z No Qualifier

Non-OR	All body part, approach, device, and qualifier values	♀	All body part, approach, device, and qualifier values

1 Obstetrics
0 Pregnancy
9 Drainage

Definition: Taking or letting out fluids and/or gases from a body part
Explanation: None

Body Part Character 4		Approach Character 5	Device Character 6	Qualifier Character 7
0 Products of Conception ♀		0 Open 3 Percutaneous 4 Percutaneous Endoscopic 7 Via Natural or Artificial Opening 8 Via Natural or Artificial Opening Endoscopic	Z No Device	9 Fetal Blood A Fetal Cerebrospinal Fluid B Fetal Fluid, Other C Amniotic Fluid, Therapeutic D Fluid, Other U Amniotic Fluid, Diagnostic

Non-OR	All body part, approach, device, and qualifier values	♀	All body part, approach, device, and qualifier values

1 Obstetrics
0 Pregnancy
A Abortion

Definition: Artificially terminating a pregnancy
Explanation: None

Body Part Character 4		Approach Character 5	Device Character 6	Qualifier Character 7
0 Products of Conception ♀		0 Open 3 Percutaneous 4 Percutaneous Endoscopic 8 Via Natural or Artificial Opening Endoscopic	Z No Device	Z No Qualifier
0 Products of Conception ♀		7 Via Natural or Artificial Opening	Z No Device	6 Vacuum W Laminaria X Abortifacient Z No Qualifier

Non-OR	10A07Z[6,W,X]	♀	All body part, approach, device, and qualifier values

1 Obstetrics
0 Pregnancy
D Extraction

Definition: Pulling or stripping out or off all or a portion of a body part by the use of force
Explanation: None

Body Part Character 4		Approach Character 5	Device Character 6	Qualifier Character 7
0 Products of Conception `QA` ♀		0 Open	Z No Device	0 High 1 Low 2 Extraperitoneal
0 Products of Conception `QA` ♀		7 Via Natural or Artificial Opening	Z No Device	3 Low Forceps 4 Mid Forceps 5 High Forceps 6 Vacuum 7 Internal Version 8 Other
1 Products of Conception, Retained ♀		7 Via Natural or Artificial Opening 8 Via Natural or Artificial Opening Endoscopic	Z No Device	9 Manual Z No Qualifier
2 Products of Conception, Ectopic ♀		0 Open 4 Percutaneous Endoscopic 7 Via Natural or Artificial Opening 8 Via Natural or Artificial Opening Endoscopic	Z No Device	Z No Qualifier

DRG Non-OR `QA`	10D07Z[3,4,5,6,7,8]	♀	All body part, approach, device, and qualifier values
	10D00Z[0,1,2] except when a corresponding SDX of Z37.0-Z37.9 is also reported		
`QA`	10D07Z[3,4,5,7] except when a corresponding SDX of Z37.0-Z37.9 is also reported		

Non-OR Procedure   DRG Non-OR Procedure   Valid OR Procedure   HAC Associated Procedure   Combination Only   New/Revised GREEN

1 Obstetrics
0 Pregnancy
E Delivery

Definition: Assisting the passage of the products of conception from the genital canal

Explanation: None

Body Part Character 4	Approach Character 5	Device Character 6	Qualifier Character 7
0 Products of Conception **QA**♀	X External	Z No Device	Z No Qualifier

DRG Non-OR **QA**	10E0XZZ 10E0XZZ except when a corresponding SDX of Z37.0-Z37.9 is also reported	♀ All body part, approach, device, and qualifier values

1 Obstetrics
0 Pregnancy
H Insertion

Definition: Putting in a nonbiological appliance that monitors, assists, performs, or prevents a physiological function but does not physically take the place of a body part

Explanation: None

Body Part Character 4	Approach Character 5	Device Character 6	Qualifier Character 7
0 Products of Conception ♀	0 Open 7 Via Natural or Artificial Opening	3 Monitoring Electrode Y Other Device	Z No Qualifier

Non-OR	All body part, approach, device, and qualifier values	♀ All body part, approach, device, and qualifier values

1 Obstetrics
0 Pregnancy
J Inspection

Definition: Visually and/or manually exploring a body part

Explanation: Visual exploration may be performed with or without optical instrumentation. Manual exploration may be performed directly or through intervening body layers.

Body Part Character 4	Approach Character 5	Device Character 6	Qualifier Character 7
0 Products of Conception ♀ 1 Products of Conception, Retained ♀ 2 Products of Conception, Ectopic ♀	0 Open 3 Percutaneous 4 Percutaneous Endoscopic 7 Via Natural or Artificial Opening 8 Via Natural or Artificial Opening Endoscopic X External	Z No Device	Z No Qualifier

Non-OR	All body part, approach, device, and qualifier values	♀ All body part, approach, device, and qualifier values

1 Obstetrics
0 Pregnancy
P Removal

Definition: Taking out or off a device from a body part, region or orifice

Explanation: If a device is taken out and a similar device put in without cutting or puncturing the skin or mucous membrane, the procedure is coded to the root operation CHANGE. Otherwise, the procedure for taking out a device is coded to the root operation REMOVAL.

Body Part Character 4	Approach Character 5	Device Character 6	Qualifier Character 7
0 Products of Conception ♀	0 Open 7 Via Natural or Artificial Opening	3 Monitoring Electrode Y Other Device	Z No Qualifier

Non-OR	All body part, approach, device, and qualifier values	♀ All body part, approach, device, and qualifier values

1 Obstetrics
0 Pregnancy
Q Repair

Definition: Restoring, to the extent possible, a body part to its normal anatomic structure and function

Explanation: Used only when the method to accomplish the repair is not one of the other root operations

Body Part Character 4	Approach Character 5	Device Character 6	Qualifier Character 7
0 Products of Conception ♀	0 Open 3 Percutaneous 4 Percutaneous Endoscopic 7 Via Natural or Artificial Opening 8 Via Natural or Artificial Opening Endoscopic	Y Other Device Z No Device	E Nervous System F Cardiovascular System G Lymphatics and Hemic H Eye J Ear, Nose and Sinus K Respiratory System L Mouth and Throat M Gastrointestinal System N Hepatobiliary and Pancreas P Endocrine System Q Skin R Musculoskeletal System S Urinary System T Female Reproductive System V Male Reproductive System Y Other Body System

Non-OR	All body part, approach, device, and qualifier values	♀ All body part, approach, device, and qualifier values

NC Noncovered Procedure   **LC** Limited Coverage   **QA** Questionable OB Admit   **NT** New Tech Add-on   ⊞ Combination Member   ♂ Male   ♀ Female

1   Obstetrics
Ø   Pregnancy
S   Reposition   Definition: Moving to its normal location, or other suitable location, all or a portion of a body part

Explanation: The body part is moved to a new location from an abnormal location, or from a normal location where it is not functioning correctly. The body part may or may not be cut out or off to be moved to the new location.

Body Part Character 4		Approach Character 5	Device Character 6	Qualifier Character 7
Ø Products of Conception	♀	7 Via Natural or Artificial Opening X External	Z No Device	Z No Qualifier
2 Products of Conception, Ectopic	♀	Ø Open 3 Percutaneous 4 Percutaneous Endoscopic 7 Via Natural or Artificial Opening 8 Via Natural or Artificial Opening Endoscopic	Z No Device	Z No Qualifier

Non-OR	10SØ[7,X]ZZ	♀	All body part, approach, device, and qualifier values

1   Obstetrics
Ø   Pregnancy
T   Resection   Definition: Cutting out or off, without replacement, all of a body part

Explanation: None

Body Part Character 4		Approach Character 5	Device Character 6	Qualifier Character 7
2 Products of Conception, Ectopic	♀	Ø Open 3 Percutaneous 4 Percutaneous Endoscopic 7 Via Natural or Artificial Opening 8 Via Natural or Artificial Opening Endoscopic	Z No Device	Z No Qualifier

	♀	All body part, approach, device, and qualifier values

1   Obstetrics
Ø   Pregnancy
Y   Transplantation   Definition: Putting in or on all or a portion of a living body part taken from another individual or animal to physically take the place and/or function of all or a portion of a similar body part

Explanation: The native body part may or may not be taken out, and the transplanted body part may take over all or a portion of its function

Body Part Character 4		Approach Character 5	Device Character 6	Qualifier Character 7
Ø Products of Conception	♀	3 Percutaneous 4 Percutaneous Endoscopic 7 Via Natural or Artificial Opening	Z No Device	E Nervous System F Cardiovascular System G Lymphatics and Hemic H Eye J Ear, Nose and Sinus K Respiratory System L Mouth and Throat M Gastrointestinal System N Hepatobiliary and Pancreas P Endocrine System Q Skin R Musculoskeletal System S Urinary System T Female Reproductive System V Male Reproductive System Y Other Body System

Non-OR	All body part, approach, device, and qualifier values	♀	All body part, approach, device, and qualifier values

Placement 2W0–2Y5

AHA Coding Clinic for table 2W6

2015, 2Q, 35	Application of tongs to reduce and stabilize cervical fracture
2013, 2Q, 39	Application of cervical tongs for reduction of cervical fracture

AHA Coding Clinic for table 2Y4

2018, 4Q, 38	Control of epistaxis
2017, 4Q, 106	Nasal packing for epistaxis

2   Placement
W   Anatomical Regions
0   Change   Definition: Taking out or off a device from a body part and putting back an identical or similar device in or on the same body part without cutting or puncturing the skin or a mucous membrane

Body Region Character 4	Approach Character 5	Device Character 6	Qualifier Character 7
0 Head 2 Neck 3 Abdominal Wall 4 Chest Wall 5 Back 6 Inguinal Region, Right 7 Inguinal Region, Left 8 Upper Extremity, Right 9 Upper Extremity, Left A Upper Arm, Right B Upper Arm, Left C Lower Arm, Right D Lower Arm, Left E Hand, Right F Hand, Left G Thumb, Right H Thumb, Left J Finger, Right K Finger, Left L Lower Extremity, Right M Lower Extremity, Left N Upper Leg, Right P Upper Leg, Left Q Lower Leg, Right R Lower Leg, Left S Foot, Right T Foot, Left U Toe, Right V Toe, Left	X External	0 Traction Apparatus 1 Splint 2 Cast 3 Brace 4 Bandage 5 Packing Material 6 Pressure Dressing 7 Intermittent Pressure Device Y Other Device	Z No Qualifier
1 Face	X External	0 Traction Apparatus 1 Splint 2 Cast 3 Brace 4 Bandage 5 Packing Material 6 Pressure Dressing 7 Intermittent Pressure Device 9 Wire Y Other Device	Z No Qualifier

NC Noncovered Procedure   LC Limited Coverage   QA Questionable OB Admit   NT New Tech Add-on   ⊞ Combination Member   ♂ Male   ♀ Female

ICD-10-PCS 2022   709

2 Placement
W Anatomical Regions
1 Compression Definition: Putting pressure on a body region

Body Region Character 4	Approach Character 5	Device Character 6	Qualifier Character 7
Ø Head	X External	6 Pressure Dressing	Z No Qualifier
1 Face		7 Intermittent Pressure Device	
2 Neck			
3 Abdominal Wall			
4 Chest Wall			
5 Back			
6 Inguinal Region, Right			
7 Inguinal Region, Left			
8 Upper Extremity, Right			
9 Upper Extremity, Left			
A Upper Arm, Right			
B Upper Arm, Left			
C Lower Arm, Right			
D Lower Arm, Left			
E Hand, Right			
F Hand, Left			
G Thumb, Right			
H Thumb, Left			
J Finger, Right			
K Finger, Left			
L Lower Extremity, Right			
M Lower Extremity, Left			
N Upper Leg, Right			
P Upper Leg, Left			
Q Lower Leg, Right			
R Lower Leg, Left			
S Foot, Right			
T Foot, Left			
U Toe, Right			
V Toe, Left			

2 Placement
W Anatomical Regions
2 Dressing Definition: Putting material on a body region for protection

Body Region Character 4	Approach Character 5	Device Character 6	Qualifier Character 7
Ø Head	X External	4 Bandage	Z No Qualifier
1 Face			
2 Neck			
3 Abdominal Wall			
4 Chest Wall			
5 Back			
6 Inguinal Region, Right			
7 Inguinal Region, Left			
8 Upper Extremity, Right			
9 Upper Extremity, Left			
A Upper Arm, Right			
B Upper Arm, Left			
C Lower Arm, Right			
D Lower Arm, Left			
E Hand, Right			
F Hand, Left			
G Thumb, Right			
H Thumb, Left			
J Finger, Right			
K Finger, Left			
L Lower Extremity, Right			
M Lower Extremity, Left			
N Upper Leg, Right			
P Upper Leg, Left			
Q Lower Leg, Right			
R Lower Leg, Left			
S Foot, Right			
T Foot, Left			
U Toe, Right			
V Toe, Left			

Non-OR Procedure   DRG Non-OR Procedure   Valid OR Procedure   HAC Associated Procedure   Combination Only   New/Revised GREEN

2   Placement
W   Anatomical Regions
3   Immobilization   Definition: Limiting or preventing motion of a body region

Body Region Character 4	Approach Character 5	Device Character 6	Qualifier Character 7
Ø Head 2 Neck 3 Abdominal Wall 4 Chest Wall 5 Back 6 Inguinal Region, Right 7 Inguinal Region, Left 8 Upper Extremity, Right 9 Upper Extremity, Left A Upper Arm, Right B Upper Arm, Left C Lower Arm, Right D Lower Arm, Left E Hand, Right F Hand, Left G Thumb, Right H Thumb, Left J Finger, Right K Finger, Left L Lower Extremity, Right M Lower Extremity, Left N Upper Leg, Right P Upper Leg, Left Q Lower Leg, Right R Lower Leg, Left S Foot, Right T Foot, Left U Toe, Right V Toe, Left	X External	1 Splint 2 Cast 3 Brace Y Other Device	Z No Qualifier
1 Face	X External	1 Splint 2 Cast 3 Brace 9 Wire Y Other Device	Z No Qualifier

2   Placement
W   Anatomical Regions
4   Packing   Definition: Putting material in a body region or orifice

Body Region Character 4	Approach Character 5	Device Character 6	Qualifier Character 7
Ø Head 1 Face 2 Neck 3 Abdominal Wall 4 Chest Wall 5 Back 6 Inguinal Region, Right 7 Inguinal Region, Left 8 Upper Extremity, Right 9 Upper Extremity, Left A Upper Arm, Right B Upper Arm, Left C Lower Arm, Right D Lower Arm, Left E Hand, Right F Hand, Left G Thumb, Right H Thumb, Left J Finger, Right K Finger, Left L Lower Extremity, Right M Lower Extremity, Left N Upper Leg, Right P Upper Leg, Left Q Lower Leg, Right R Lower Leg, Left S Foot, Right T Foot, Left U Toe, Right V Toe, Left	X External	5 Packing Material	Z No Qualifier

NC Noncovered Procedure   **LC** Limited Coverage   **QA** Questionable OB Admit   **NT** New Tech Add-on   ⊞ Combination Member   ♂ Male   ♀ Female

2 Placement
W Anatomical Regions
5 Removal   Definition: Taking out or off a device from a body part

Body Region Character 4	Approach Character 5	Device Character 6	Qualifier Character 7
Ø Head 2 Neck 3 Abdominal Wall 4 Chest Wall 5 Back 6 Inguinal Region, Right 7 Inguinal Region, Left 8 Upper Extremity, Right 9 Upper Extremity, Left A Upper Arm, Right B Upper Arm, Left C Lower Arm, Right D Lower Arm, Left E Hand, Right F Hand, Left G Thumb, Right H Thumb, Left J Finger, Right K Finger, Left L Lower Extremity, Right M Lower Extremity, Left N Upper Leg, Right P Upper Leg, Left Q Lower Leg, Right R Lower Leg, Left S Foot, Right T Foot, Left U Toe, Right V Toe, Left	X External	Ø Traction Apparatus 1 Splint 2 Cast 3 Brace 4 Bandage 5 Packing Material 6 Pressure Dressing 7 Intermittent Pressure Device Y Other Device	Z No Qualifier
1 Face	X External	Ø Traction Apparatus 1 Splint 2 Cast 3 Brace 4 Bandage 5 Packing Material 6 Pressure Dressing 7 Intermittent Pressure Device 9 Wire Y Other Device	Z No Qualifier

2 Placement
W Anatomical Regions
6 Traction   Definition: Exerting a pulling force on a body region in a distal direction

Body Region Character 4	Approach Character 5	Device Character 6	Qualifier Character 7
Ø Head 1 Face 2 Neck 3 Abdominal Wall 4 Chest Wall 5 Back 6 Inguinal Region, Right 7 Inguinal Region, Left 8 Upper Extremity, Right 9 Upper Extremity, Left A Upper Arm, Right B Upper Arm, Left C Lower Arm, Right D Lower Arm, Left E Hand, Right F Hand, Left G Thumb, Right H Thumb, Left J Finger, Right K Finger, Left L Lower Extremity, Right M Lower Extremity, Left N Upper Leg, Right P Upper Leg, Left Q Lower Leg, Right R Lower Leg, Left S Foot, Right T Foot, Left U Toe, Right V Toe, Left	X External	Ø Traction Apparatus Z No Device	Z No Qualifier

2 Placement
Y Anatomical Orifices
Ø Change   Definition: Taking out or off a device from a body part and putting back an identical or similar device in or on the same body part without cutting or puncturing the skin or a mucous membrane

Body Region Character 4	Approach Character 5	Device Character 6	Qualifier Character 7
Ø Mouth and Pharynx 1 Nasal 2 Ear 3 Anorectal 4 Female Genital Tract ♀ 5 Urethra	X External	5 Packing Material	Z No Qualifier

♀   2YØ4X5Z

2 Placement
Y Anatomical Orifices
4 Packing   Definition: Putting material in a body region or orifice

Body Region Character 4	Approach Character 5	Device Character 6	Qualifier Character 7
Ø Mouth and Pharynx 1 Nasal 2 Ear 3 Anorectal 4 Female Genital Tract ♀ 5 Urethra	X External	5 Packing Material	Z No Qualifier

♀   2Y44X5Z

2 Placement
Y Anatomical Orifices
5 Removal   Definition: Taking out or off a device from a body part

Body Region Character 4	Approach Character 5	Device Character 6	Qualifier Character 7
Ø Mouth and Pharynx 1 Nasal 2 Ear 3 Anorectal 4 Female Genital Tract ♀ 5 Urethra	X External	5 Packing Material	Z No Qualifier

♀   2Y54X5Z

NC Noncovered Procedure   LC Limited Coverage   QA Questionable OB Admit   NT New Tech Add-on   ⊞ Combination Member   ♂ Male   ♀ Female

Administration 3Ø2–3E1

AHA Coding Clinic for table 3Ø2

2020, 4Q, 60-61	Transfusion stem cell progenitor cells
2019, 4Q, 35	Transfusion of blood products
2019, 4Q, 36	T-cell depleted hematopoietic stem cells for transplantation
2016, 4Q, 113	Bone marrow and stem cell transfusion (Transplantation)

AHA Coding Clinic for table 3EØ

2021, 1Q, 49	Frequently asked questions regarding ICD-10-CM and ICD-10-PCS coding for COVID-19
2020, 4Q, 49-50	Intravascular ultrasound assisted thrombolysis
2020, 4Q, 95	Frequently Asked Questions Regarding ICD-10-PCS Coding for COVID-19
2020, 3Q, 17-21	New procedure codes for introduction or infusion of therapeutics
2019, 4Q, 36-37	Hyperthermic antineoplastic chemotherapy
2018, 3Q, 7	Coronary brachytherapy with angioplasty
2018, 1Q, 8	Placement of bone morphogenetic protein & spinal fusion surgery
2017, 2Q, 14	Infusion of tPA into pleural cavity
2017, 1Q, 37	Injection of glue into enteric fistula tract
2016, 4Q, 113-114	Substances applied to cranial cavity and brain
2016, 3Q, 29	Closure of bilateral alveolar clefts
2016, 1Q, 20	Metatarsophalangeal joint resection arthroplasty
2015, 3Q, 24	Esophagogastroduodenoscopy with epinephrine injection for control of bleeding

AHA Coding Clinic for table 3EØ (Continued)

2015, 3Q, 29	Placement of adhesion barrier
2015, 2Q, 29	Insertion of nasogastric tube for drainage and feeding
2015, 2Q, 31	Thoracoscopic talc pleurodesis
2015, 1Q, 31	Intrathecal chemotherapy
2015, 1Q, 38	Chemoembolization of the hepatic artery
2014, 4Q, 16	Administration of RH (D) immunoglobulin
2014, 4Q, 17	RH (D) alloimmunization (sensitization)
2014, 4Q, 19	Ultrasound accelerated thrombolysis
2014, 4Q, 34	Resection of brain malignancy with implantation of chemotherapeutic wafer
2014, 4Q, 38	Placement of saline and seprafilm solution into abdominal cavity
2014, 3Q, 26	Coil embolization of gastroduodenal artery with chemoembolization of hepatic artery
2014, 2Q, 8	Medical induction of labor with Cervidil tampon insertion
2014, 2Q, 10	Prophylactic Neulasta injection for infection prevention
2013, 4Q, 124	Administration of tPA for stroke treatment prior to transfer
2013, 1Q, 27	Injection of sclerosing agent into an esophageal varix

AHA Coding Clinic for table 3E1

| 2019, 4Q, 38 | Irrigation of joint using irrigating substance |
| 2017, 3Q, 14 | Bronchoscopy with suctioning and washings for removal of mucus plug |

3   **Administration**
Ø   **Circulatory**
2   **Transfusion**   Definition: Putting in blood or blood products

Body System/Region Character 4	Approach Character 5	Substance Character 6	Qualifier Character 7
3 Peripheral Vein NC **4** Central Vein NC	**3** Percutaneous	**A** Stem Cells, Embryonic	**Z** No Qualifier
3 Peripheral Vein **4** Central Vein	**3** Percutaneous	**C** Hematopoietic Stem/Progenitor Cells, Genetically Modified	**Ø** Autologous
3 Peripheral Vein **4** Central Vein	**3** Percutaneous	**D** Pathogen Reduced Cryoprecipitated Fibrinogen Complex	**1** Nonautologous
3 Peripheral Vein NC **4** Central Vein NC	**3** Percutaneous	**G** Bone Marrow **X** Stem Cells, Cord Blood **Y** Stem Cells, Hematopoietic	**Ø** Autologous **2** Allogeneic, Related **3** Allogeneic, Unrelated **4** Allogeneic, Unspecified
3 Peripheral Vein **4** Central Vein	**3** Percutaneous	**H** Whole Blood **J** Serum Albumin **K** Frozen Plasma **L** Fresh Plasma **M** Plasma Cryoprecipitate **N** Red Blood Cells **P** Frozen Red Cells **Q** White Cells **R** Platelets **S** Globulin **T** Fibrinogen **V** Antihemophilic Factors **W** Factor IX	**Ø** Autologous **1** Nonautologous
3 Peripheral Vein **4** Central Vein	**3** Percutaneous	**U** Stem Cells, T-cell Depleted Hematopoietic	**2** Allogeneic, Related **3** Allogeneic, Unrelated **4** Allogeneic, Unspecified
7 Products of Conception, Circulatory ♀	**3** Percutaneous **7** Via Natural or Artificial Opening	**H** Whole Blood **J** Serum Albumin **K** Frozen Plasma **L** Fresh Plasma **M** Plasma Cryoprecipitate **N** Red Blood Cells **P** Frozen Red Cells **Q** White Cells **R** Platelets **S** Globulin **T** Fibrinogen **V** Antihemophilic Factors **W** Factor IX	**1** Nonautologous
8 Vein	**3** Percutaneous	**B** 4-Factor Prothrombin Complex Concentrate	**1** Nonautologous

DRG Non-OR	3Ø2[3,4]3AZ
DRG Non-OR	3Ø2[3,4]3CØ
DRG Non-OR	3Ø2[3,4]3[G,X,Y][Ø,2,3,4]
DRG Non-OR	3Ø2[3,4]3U[2,3,4]

NC   3Ø2[3,4]3AZ Only when reported with PDx or SDx of C91.ØØ, C92.ØØ, C92.1Ø, C92.11, C92.4Ø, C92.5Ø, C92.6Ø, C92.AØ, C93.ØØ, C94.ØØ, C95.ØØ

NC   3Ø2[3,4]3[G,Y]Ø Only when reported with PDx or SDx of C91.ØØ, C92.ØØ, C92.1Ø, C92.11, C92.4Ø, C92.5Ø, C92.6Ø, C92.AØ, C93.ØØ, C94.ØØ, C95.ØØ

♀   3Ø27[3,7][H,J,K,L,M;N,P,Q,R,S,T,V,W]1

NC Noncovered Procedure   **LC** Limited Coverage   **QA** Questionable OB Admit   **NT** New Tech Add-on   ✛ Combination Member   ♂ Male   ♀ Female

Administration *(side tab)*

3   **Administration**
C   **Indwelling Device**
1   **Irrigation**   Definition: Putting in or on a cleansing substance

Body System/Region Character 4	Approach Character 5	Substance Character 6	Qualifier Character 7
Z None	**X** External	**8** Irrigating Substance	**Z** No Qualifier

3   **Administration**
E   **Physiological Systems and Anatomical Regions**
Ø   **Introduction**   Definition: Putting in or on a therapeutic, diagnostic, nutritional, physiological, or prophylactic substance except blood or blood products

Body System/Region Character 4	Approach Character 5	Substance Character 6	Qualifier Character 7
Ø Skin and Mucous Membranes	**X** External	**Ø** Antineoplastic	**5** Other Antineoplastic **M** Monoclonal Antibody
Ø Skin and Mucous Membranes	**X** External	**2** Anti-infective	**8** Oxazolidinones **9** Other Anti-infective
Ø Skin and Mucous Membranes	**X** External	**3** Anti-inflammatory **4** Serum, Toxoid and Vaccine **B** Anesthetic Agent **K** Other Diagnostic Substance **M** Pigment **N** Analgesics, Hypnotics, Sedatives **T** Destructive Agent	**Z** No Qualifier
Ø Skin and Mucous Membranes	**X** External	**G** Other Therapeutic Substance	**C** Other Substance
1 Subcutaneous Tissue	**Ø** Open	**2** Anti-infective	**A** Anti-Infective Envelope
1 Subcutaneous Tissue	**3** Percutaneous	**Ø** Antineoplastic	**5** Other Antineoplastic **M** Monoclonal Antibody
1 Subcutaneous Tissue	**3** Percutaneous	**2** Anti-infective	**8** Oxazolidinones **9** Other Anti-infective **A** Anti-Infective Envelope
1 Subcutaneous Tissue	**3** Percutaneous	**3** Anti-inflammatory **6** Nutritional Substance **7** Electrolytic and Water Balance Substance **B** Anesthetic Agent **H** Radioactive Substance **K** Other Diagnostic Substance **N** Analgesics, Hypnotics, Sedatives **T** Destructive Agent	**Z** No Qualifier
1 Subcutaneous Tissue	**3** Percutaneous	**4** Serum, Toxoid and Vaccine	**Ø** Influenza Vaccine **Z** No Qualifier
1 Subcutaneous Tissue	**3** Percutaneous	**G** Other Therapeutic Substance	**C** Other Substance
1 Subcutaneous Tissue	**3** Percutaneous	**V** Hormone	**G** Insulin **J** Other Hormone
2 Muscle	**3** Percutaneous	**Ø** Antineoplastic	**5** Other Antineoplastic **M** Monoclonal Antibody
2 Muscle	**3** Percutaneous	**2** Anti-infective	**8** Oxazolidinones **9** Other Anti-infective
2 Muscle	**3** Percutaneous	**3** Anti-inflammatory **6** Nutritional Substance **7** Electrolytic and Water Balance Substance **B** Anesthetic Agent **H** Radioactive Substance **K** Other Diagnostic Substance **N** Analgesics, Hypnotics, Sedatives **T** Destructive Agent	**Z** No Qualifier
2 Muscle	**3** Percutaneous	**4** Serum, Toxoid and Vaccine	**Ø** Influenza Vaccine **Z** No Qualifier
2 Muscle	**3** Percutaneous	**G** Other Therapeutic Substance	**C** Other Substance
3 Peripheral Vein	**Ø** Open	**Ø** Antineoplastic	**2** High-dose Interleukin-2 **3** Low-dose Interleukin-2 **5** Other Antineoplastic **M** Monoclonal Antibody **P** Clofarabine
3 Peripheral Vein	**Ø** Open	**1** Thrombolytic	**6** Recombinant Human- activated Protein C **7** Other Thrombolytic
3 Peripheral Vein	**Ø** Open	**2** Anti-infective	**8** Oxazolidinones **9** Other Anti-infective

DRG Non-OR   3E03002
DRG Non-OR   3E03017

3EØ Continued on next page

*3C1–3EØ (side tab)*

3   **Administration**
E   **Physiological Systems and Anatomical Regions**
Ø   **Introduction**   Definition: Putting in or on a therapeutic, diagnostic, nutritional, physiological, or prophylactic substance except blood or blood products

Body System/Region Character 4	Approach Character 5	Substance Character 6	Qualifier Character 7
3 Peripheral Vein	**Ø** Open	**3** Anti-inflammatory **4** Serum, Toxoid and Vaccine **6** Nutritional Substance **7** Electrolytic and Water Balance Substance **F** Intracirculatory Anesthetic **H** Radioactive Substance **K** Other Diagnostic Substance **N** Analgesics, Hypnotics, Sedatives **P** Platelet Inhibitor **R** Antiarrhythmic **T** Destructive Agent **X** Vasopressor	**Z** No Qualifier
3 Peripheral Vein	**Ø** Open	**G** Other Therapeutic Substance	**C** Other Substance **N** Blood Brain Barrier Disruption
3 Peripheral Vein	**Ø** Open	**U** Pancreatic Islet Cells	**Ø** Autologous **1** Nonautologous
3 Peripheral Vein	**Ø** Open	**V** Hormone	**G** Insulin **H** Human B-type Natriuretic Peptide **J** Other Hormone
3 Peripheral Vein	**Ø** Open	**W** Immunotherapeutic	**K** Immunostimulator **L** Immunosuppressive
3 Peripheral Vein	**3** Percutaneous	**Ø** Antineoplastic	**2** High-dose Interleukin-2 **3** Low-dose Interleukin-2 **5** Other Antineoplastic **M** Monoclonal Antibody **P** Clofarabine
3 Peripheral Vein	**3** Percutaneous	**1** Thrombolytic	**6** Recombinant Human- activated Protein C **7** Other Thrombolytic
3 Peripheral Vein	**3** Percutaneous	**2** Anti-infective	**8** Oxazolidinones **9** Other Anti-infective
3 Peripheral Vein	**3** Percutaneous	**3** Anti-inflammatory **4** Serum, Toxoid and Vaccine **6** Nutritional Substance **7** Electrolytic and Water Balance Substance **F** Intracirculatory Anesthetic **H** Radioactive Substance **K** Other Diagnostic Substance **N** Analgesics, Hypnotics, Sedatives **P** Platelet Inhibitor **R** Antiarrhythmic **T** Destructive Agent **X** Vasopressor	**Z** No Qualifier
3 Peripheral Vein	**3** Percutaneous	**G** Other Therapeutic Substance	**C** Other Substance **N** Blood Brain Barrier Disruption **Q** Glucarpidase
3 Peripheral Vein	**3** Percutaneous	**U** Pancreatic Islet Cells	**Ø** Autologous **1** Nonautologous
3 Peripheral Vein	**3** Percutaneous	**V** Hormone	**G** Insulin **H** Human B-type Natriuretic Peptide **J** Other Hormone
3 Peripheral Vein	**3** Percutaneous	**W** Immunotherapeutic	**K** Immunostimulator **L** Immunosuppressive
4 Central Vein	**Ø** Open	**Ø** Antineoplastic	**2** High-dose Interleukin-2 **3** Low-dose Interleukin-2 **5** Other Antineoplastic **M** Monoclonal Antibody **P** Clofarabine
4 Central Vein	**Ø** Open	**1** Thrombolytic	**6** Recombinant Human- activated Protein C **7** Other Thrombolytic

Valid OR	3EØ3ØTZ	**DRG Non-OR**	3EØ33U[Ø,1]
DRG Non-OR	3EØ3ØU[Ø,1]	**DRG Non-OR**	3EØ4ØØ2
DRG Non-OR	3EØ33Ø2	**DRG Non-OR**	3EØ4Ø17
DRG Non-OR	3EØ3317		

3EØ Continued on next page

NC Noncovered Procedure   LC Limited Coverage   QA Questionable OB Admit   NT New Tech Add-on   ⊞ Combination Member   ♂ Male   ♀ Female

Administration

3   **Administration**
E   **Physiological Systems and Anatomical Regions**
Ø   **Introduction**   Definition: Putting in or on a therapeutic, diagnostic, nutritional, physiological, or prophylactic substance except blood or blood products

3EØ Continued

Body System/Region Character 4		Approach Character 5		Substance Character 6		Qualifier Character 7	
4	Central Vein	Ø	Open	2	Anti-infective	8 9	Oxazolidinones Other Anti-infective
4	Central Vein	Ø	Open	3 4 6 7 F H K N P R T X	Anti-inflammatory Serum, Toxoid and Vaccine Nutritional Substance Electrolytic and Water Balance Substance Intracirculatory Anesthetic Radioactive Substance Other Diagnostic Substance Analgesics, Hypnotics, Sedatives Platelet Inhibitor Antiarrhythmic Destructive Agent Vasopressor	Z	No Qualifier
4	Central Vein	Ø	Open	G	Other Therapeutic Substance	C N	Other Substance Blood Brain Barrier Disruption
4	Central Vein	Ø	Open	V	Hormone	G H J	Insulin Human B-type Natriuretic Peptide Other Hormone
4	Central Vein	Ø	Open	W	Immunotherapeutic	K L	Immunostimulator Immunosuppressive
4	Central Vein	3	Percutaneous	Ø	Antineoplastic	2 3 5 M P	High-dose Interleukin-2 Low-dose Interleukin-2 Other Antineoplastic Monoclonal Antibody Clofarabine
4	Central Vein	3	Percutaneous	1	Thrombolytic	6 7	Recombinant Human- activated Protein C Other Thrombolytic
4	Central Vein	3	Percutaneous	2	Anti-infective	8 9	Oxazolidinones Other Anti-infective
4	Central Vein	3	Percutaneous	3 4 6 7 F H K N P R T X	Anti-inflammatory Serum, Toxoid and Vaccine Nutritional Substance Electrolytic and Water Balance Substance Intracirculatory Anesthetic Radioactive Substance Other Diagnostic Substance Analgesics, Hypnotics, Sedatives Platelet Inhibitor Antiarrhythmic Destructive Agent Vasopressor	Z	No Qualifier
4	Central Vein	3	Percutaneous	G	Other Therapeutic Substance	C N Q	Other Substance Blood Brain Barrier Disruption Glucarpidase
4	Central Vein	3	Percutaneous	V	Hormone	G H J	Insulin Human B-type Natriuretic Peptide Other Hormone
4	Central Vein	3	Percutaneous	W	Immunotherapeutic	K L	Immunostimulator Immunosuppressive
5 6	Peripheral Artery Central Artery	Ø 3	Open Percutaneous	Ø	Antineoplastic	2 3 5 M P	High-dose Interleukin-2 Low-dose Interleukin-2 Other Antineoplastic Monoclonal Antibody Clofarabine
5 6	Peripheral Artery Central Artery	Ø 3	Open Percutaneous	1	Thrombolytic	6 7	Recombinant Human- activated Protein C Other Thrombolytic
5 6	Peripheral Artery Central Artery	Ø 3	Open Percutaneous	2	Anti-infective	8 9	Oxazolidinones Other Anti-infective

Valid OR	3EØ4ØTZ	**DRG Non-OR**	3EØ[5,6][Ø,3]Ø2
DRG Non-OR	3EØ43Ø2	**DRG Non-OR**	3EØ[5,6][Ø,3]17
DRG Non-OR	3EØ4317		

3EØ Continued on next page

Non-OR Procedure   DRG Non-OR Procedure   Valid OR Procedure   HAC Associated Procedure   Combination Only   New/Revised GREEN

3   **Administration**   *3E0 Continued*
E   **Physiological Systems and Anatomical Regions**
0   **Introduction**   Definition: Putting in or on a therapeutic, diagnostic, nutritional, physiological, or prophylactic substance except blood or blood products

Body System/Region Character 4	Approach Character 5	Substance Character 6	Qualifier Character 7
5 Peripheral Artery 6 Central Artery	0 Open 3 Percutaneous	3 Anti-inflammatory 4 Serum, Toxoid and Vaccine 6 Nutritional Substance 7 Electrolytic and Water Balance Substance F Intracirculatory Anesthetic H Radioactive Substance K Other Diagnostic Substance N Analgesics, Hypnotics, Sedatives P Platelet Inhibitor R Antiarrhythmic T Destructive Agent X Vasopressor	Z No Qualifier
5 Peripheral Artery 6 Central Artery	0 Open 3 Percutaneous	G Other Therapeutic Substance	C Other Substance N Blood Brain Barrier Disruption
5 Peripheral Artery 6 Central Artery	0 Open 3 Percutaneous	V Hormone	G Insulin H Human B-type Natriuretic Peptide J Other Hormone
5 Peripheral Artery 6 Central Artery	0 Open 3 Percutaneous	W Immunotherapeutic	K Immunostimulator L Immunosuppressive
7 Coronary Artery 8 Heart	0 Open 3 Percutaneous	1 Thrombolytic	6 Recombinant Human- activated Protein C 7 Other Thrombolytic
7 Coronary Artery 8 Heart	0 Open 3 Percutaneous	G Other Therapeutic Substance	C Other Substance
7 Coronary Artery 8 Heart	0 Open 3 Percutaneous	K Other Diagnostic Substance P Platelet Inhibitor	Z No Qualifier
7 Coronary Artery 8 Heart	4 Percutaneous Endoscopic	G Other Therapeutic Substance	C Other Substance
9 Nose	3 Percutaneous 7 Via Natural or Artificial Opening X External	0 Antineoplastic	5 Other Antineoplastic M Monoclonal Antibody
9 Nose	3 Percutaneous 7 Via Natural or Artificial Opening X External	2 Anti-infective	8 Oxazolidinones 9 Other Anti-infective
9 Nose	3 Percutaneous 7 Via Natural or Artificial Opening X External	3 Anti-inflammatory 4 Serum, Toxoid and Vaccine B Anesthetic Agent H Radioactive Substance K Other Diagnostic Substance N Analgesics, Hypnotics, Sedatives T Destructive Agent	Z No Qualifier
9 Nose	3 Percutaneous 7 Via Natural or Artificial Opening X External	G Other Therapeutic Substance	C Other Substance
A Bone Marrow	3 Percutaneous	0 Antineoplastic	5 Other Antineoplastic M Monoclonal Antibody
A Bone Marrow	3 Percutaneous	G Other Therapeutic Substance	C Other Substance
B Ear	3 Percutaneous 7 Via Natural or Artificial Opening X External	0 Antineoplastic	4 Liquid Brachytherapy Radioisotope 5 Other Antineoplastic M Monoclonal Antibody
B Ear	3 Percutaneous 7 Via Natural or Artificial Opening X External	2 Anti-infective	8 Oxazolidinones 9 Other Anti-infective
B Ear	3 Percutaneous 7 Via Natural or Artificial Opening X External	3 Anti-inflammatory B Anesthetic Agent H Radioactive Substance K Other Diagnostic Substance N Analgesics, Hypnotics, Sedatives T Destructive Agent	Z No Qualifier
B Ear	3 Percutaneous 7 Via Natural or Artificial Opening X External	G Other Therapeutic Substance	C Other Substance

DRG Non-OR   3E08[0,3]17

3E0 Continued on next page

NC Noncovered Procedure   LC Limited Coverage   QA Questionable OB Admit   NT New Tech Add-on   ⊞ Combination Member   ♂ Male   ♀ Female

3E0 Continued

3   **Administration**
E   **Physiological Systems and Anatomical Regions**
Ø   **Introduction**   Definition: Putting in or on a therapeutic, diagnostic, nutritional, physiological, or prophylactic substance except blood or blood products

Body System/Region Character 4	Approach Character 5	Substance Character 6	Qualifier Character 7
C Eye	3 Percutaneous 7 Via Natural or Artificial Opening X External	Ø Antineoplastic	4 Liquid Brachytherapy Radioisotope 5 Other Antineoplastic M Monoclonal Antibody
C Eye	3 Percutaneous 7 Via Natural or Artificial Opening X External	2 Anti-infective	8 Oxazolidinones 9 Other Anti-infective
C Eye	3 Percutaneous 7 Via Natural or Artificial Opening X External	3 Anti-inflammatory B Anesthetic Agent H Radioactive Substance K Other Diagnostic Substance M Pigment N Analgesics, Hypnotics, Sedatives T Destructive Agent	Z No Qualifier
C Eye	3 Percutaneous 7 Via Natural or Artificial Opening X External	G Other Therapeutic Substance	C Other Substance
C Eye	3 Percutaneous 7 Via Natural or Artificial Opening X External	S Gas	F Other Gas
D Mouth and Pharynx	3 Percutaneous 7 Via Natural or Artificial Opening X External	Ø Antineoplastic	4 Liquid Brachytherapy Radioisotope 5 Other Antineoplastic M Monoclonal Antibody
D Mouth and Pharynx	3 Percutaneous 7 Via Natural or Artificial Opening X External	2 Anti-infective	8 Oxazolidinones 9 Other Anti-infective
D Mouth and Pharynx	3 Percutaneous 7 Via Natural or Artificial Opening X External	3 Anti-inflammatory 4 Serum, Toxoid and Vaccine 6 Nutritional Substance 7 Electrolytic and Water Balance Substance B Anesthetic Agent H Radioactive Substance K Other Diagnostic Substance N Analgesics, Hypnotics, Sedatives R Antiarrhythmic T Destructive Agent	Z No Qualifier
D Mouth and Pharynx	3 Percutaneous 7 Via Natural or Artificial Opening X External	G Other Therapeutic Substance	C Other Substance
E Products of Conception ♀ G Upper GI H Lower GI K Genitourinary Tract N Male Reproductive ♂	3 Percutaneous 7 Via Natural or Artificial Opening 8 Via Natural or Artificial Opening Endoscopic	Ø Antineoplastic	4 Liquid Brachytherapy Radioisotope 5 Other Antineoplastic M Monoclonal Antibody
E Products of Conception ♀ G Upper GI H Lower GI K Genitourinary Tract N Male Reproductive ♂	3 Percutaneous 7 Via Natural or Artificial Opening 8 Via Natural or Artificial Opening Endoscopic	2 Anti-infective	8 Oxazolidinones 9 Other Anti-infective
E Products of Conception ♀ G Upper GI H Lower GI K Genitourinary Tract N Male Reproductive ♂	3 Percutaneous 7 Via Natural or Artificial Opening 8 Via Natural or Artificial Opening Endoscopic	3 Anti-inflammatory 6 Nutritional Substance 7 Electrolytic and Water Balance Substance B Anesthetic Agent H Radioactive Substance K Other Diagnostic Substance N Analgesics, Hypnotics, Sedatives T Destructive Agent	Z No Qualifier
E Products of Conception ♀ G Upper GI H Lower GI K Genitourinary Tract N Male Reproductive ♂	3 Percutaneous 7 Via Natural or Artificial Opening 8 Via Natural or Artificial Opening Endoscopic	G Other Therapeutic Substance	C Other Substance

♂   All approach, substance, and qualifier values for body system/region (character 4) with this icon
♀   All approach, substance, and qualifier values for body system/region (character 4) with this icon

3E0 Continued on next page

3   **Administration**
E   **Physiological Systems and Anatomical Regions**
0   **Introduction**   Definition: Putting in or on a therapeutic, diagnostic, nutritional, physiological, or prophylactic substance except blood or blood products

Body System/Region Character 4	Approach Character 5	Substance Character 6	Qualifier Character 7
E Products of Conception ♀ **G** Upper GI **H** Lower GI **K** Genitourinary Tract **N** Male Reproductive ♂	**3** Percutaneous **7** Via Natural or Artificial Opening **8** Via Natural or Artificial Opening Endoscopic	**S** Gas	**F** Other Gas
E Products of Conception ♀ **G** Upper GI **H** Lower GI **K** Genitourinary Tract **N** Male Reproductive ♂	**4** Percutaneous Endoscopic	**G** Other Therapeutic Substance	**C** Other Substance
F Respiratory Tract	**3** Percutaneous **7** Via Natural or Artificial Opening **8** Via Natural or Artificial Opening Endoscopic	**0** Antineoplastic	**4** Liquid Brachytherapy Radioisotope **5** Other Antineoplastic **M** Monoclonal Antibody
F Respiratory Tract	**3** Percutaneous **7** Via Natural or Artificial Opening **8** Via Natural or Artificial Opening Endoscopic	**2** Anti-infective	**8** Oxazolidinones **9** Other Anti-infective
F Respiratory Tract	**3** Percutaneous **7** Via Natural or Artificial Opening **8** Via Natural or Artificial Opening Endoscopic	**3** Anti-inflammatory **6** Nutritional Substance **7** Electrolytic and Water Balance Substance **B** Anesthetic Agent **H** Radioactive Substance **K** Other Diagnostic Substance **N** Analgesics, Hypnotics, Sedatives **T** Destructive Agent	**Z** No Qualifier
F Respiratory Tract	**3** Percutaneous **7** Via Natural or Artificial Opening **8** Via Natural or Artificial Opening Endoscopic	**G** Other Therapeutic Substance	**C** Other Substance
F Respiratory Tract	**3** Percutaneous **7** Via Natural or Artificial Opening **8** Via Natural or Artificial Opening Endoscopic	**S** Gas	**D** Nitric Oxide **F** Other Gas
F Respiratory Tract	**4** Percutaneous Endoscopic	**G** Other Therapeutic Substance	**C** Other Substance
J Biliary and Pancreatic Tract	**3** Percutaneous **7** Via Natural or Artificial Opening **8** Via Natural or Artificial Opening Endoscopic	**0** Antineoplastic	**4** Liquid Brachytherapy Radioisotope **5** Other Antineoplastic **M** Monoclonal Antibody
J Biliary and Pancreatic Tract	**3** Percutaneous **7** Via Natural or Artificial Opening **8** Via Natural or Artificial Opening Endoscopic	**2** Anti-infective	**8** Oxazolidinones **9** Other Anti-infective
J Biliary and Pancreatic Tract	**3** Percutaneous **7** Via Natural or Artificial Opening **8** Via Natural or Artificial Opening Endoscopic	**3** Anti-inflammatory **6** Nutritional Substance **7** Electrolytic and Water Balance Substance **B** Anesthetic Agent **H** Radioactive Substance **K** Other Diagnostic Substance **N** Analgesics, Hypnotics, Sedatives **T** Destructive Agent	**Z** No Qualifier
J Biliary and Pancreatic Tract	**3** Percutaneous **7** Via Natural or Artificial Opening **8** Via Natural or Artificial Opening Endoscopic	**G** Other Therapeutic Substance	**C** Other Substance
J Biliary and Pancreatic Tract	**3** Percutaneous **7** Via Natural or Artificial Opening **8** Via Natural or Artificial Opening Endoscopic	**S** Gas	**F** Other Gas

♂   All approach, substance, and qualifier values for body system/region (character 4) with this icon
♀   All approach, substance, and qualifier values for body system/region (character 4) with this icon

3E0 Continued on next page

NC Noncovered Procedure   **LC** Limited Coverage   **QA** Questionable OB Admit   **NT** New Tech Add-on   ⊞ Combination Member   ♂ Male   ♀ Female

ICD-10-PCS 2022   721

3E0–3E0

Administration

3E0 Continued

3   **Administration**
E   **Physiological Systems and Anatomical Regions**
Ø   **Introduction**   Definition: Putting in or on a therapeutic, diagnostic, nutritional, physiological, or prophylactic substance except blood or blood products

Body System/Region Character 4	Approach Character 5	Substance Character 6	Qualifier Character 7
J Biliary and Pancreatic Tract	3 Percutaneous 7 Via Natural or Artificial Opening 8 Via Natural or Artificial Opening Endoscopic	U Pancreatic Islet Cells	Ø Autologous 1 Nonautologous
J Biliary and Pancreatic Tract	4 Percutaneous Endoscopic	G Other Therapeutic Substance	C Other Substance
L Pleural Cavity	Ø Open	5 Adhesion Barrier	Z No Qualifier
L Pleural Cavity	3 Percutaneous	Ø Antineoplastic	4 Liquid Brachytherapy Radioisotope 5 Other Antineoplastic M Monoclonal Antibody
L Pleural Cavity	3 Percutaneous	2 Anti-infective	8 Oxazolidinones 9 Other Anti-infective
L Pleural Cavity	3 Percutaneous	3 Anti-inflammatory 5 Adhesion Barrier 6 Nutritional Substance 7 Electrolytic and Water Balance Substance B Anesthetic Agent H Radioactive Substance K Other Diagnostic Substance N Analgesics, Hypnotics, Sedatives T Destructive Agent	Z No Qualifier
L Pleural Cavity	3 Percutaneous	G Other Therapeutic Substance	C Other Substance
L Pleural Cavity	3 Percutaneous	S Gas	F Other Gas
L Pleural Cavity	4 Percutaneous Endoscopic	5 Adhesion Barrier	Z No Qualifier
L Pleural Cavity	4 Percutaneous Endoscopic	G Other Therapeutic Substance	C Other Substance
L Pleural Cavity	7 Via Natural or Artificial Opening	Ø Antineoplastic	4 Liquid Brachytherapy Radioisotope 5 Other Antineoplastic M Monoclonal Antibody
L Pleural Cavity	7 Via Natural or Artificial Opening	S Gas	F Other Gas
M Peritoneal Cavity	Ø Open	5 Adhesion Barrier	Z No Qualifier
M Peritoneal Cavity	3 Percutaneous	Ø Antineoplastic	4 Liquid Brachytherapy Radioisotope 5 Other Antineoplastic M Monoclonal Antibody Y Hyperthermic
M Peritoneal Cavity	3 Percutaneous	2 Anti-infective	8 Oxazolidinones 9 Other Anti-infective
M Peritoneal Cavity	3 Percutaneous	3 Anti-inflammatory 5 Adhesion Barrier 6 Nutritional Substance 7 Electrolytic and Water Balance Substance B Anesthetic Agent H Radioactive Substance K Other Diagnostic Substance N Analgesics, Hypnotics, Sedatives T Destructive Agent	Z No Qualifier
M Peritoneal Cavity	3 Percutaneous	G Other Therapeutic Substance	C Other Substance
M Peritoneal Cavity	3 Percutaneous	S Gas	F Other Gas
M Peritoneal Cavity	4 Percutaneous Endoscopic	5 Adhesion Barrier	Z No Qualifier
M Peritoneal Cavity	4 Percutaneous Endoscopic	G Other Therapeutic Substance	C Other Substance
M Peritoneal Cavity	7 Via Natural or Artificial Opening	Ø Antineoplastic	4 Liquid Brachytherapy Radioisotope 5 Other Antineoplastic M Monoclonal Antibody
M Peritoneal Cavity	7 Via Natural or Artificial Opening	S Gas	F Other Gas
P Female Reproductive ♀	Ø Open	5 Adhesion Barrier	Z No Qualifier
P Female Reproductive ♀	3 Percutaneous	Ø Antineoplastic	4 Liquid Brachytherapy Radioisotope 5 Other Antineoplastic M Monoclonal Antibody
P Female Reproductive ♀	3 Percutaneous	2 Anti-infective	8 Oxazolidinones 9 Other Anti-infective

Valid OR   3E0L4GC
DRG Non-OR   3E0J[3,7,8]U[0,1]
♀   All approach, substance, and qualifier values for body system/region (character 4) with this icon

3E0 Continued on next page

3   **Administration**

E   **Physiological Systems and Anatomical Regions**

Ø   **Introduction**   Definition: Putting in or on a therapeutic, diagnostic, nutritional, physiological, or prophylactic substance except blood or blood products

3EØ Continued

Body System/Region Character 4		Approach Character 5	Substance Character 6	Qualifier Character 7
P	Female Reproductive ♀	3 Percutaneous	3 Anti-inflammatory 5 Adhesion Barrier 6 Nutritional Substance 7 Electrolytic and Water Balance Substance B Anesthetic Agent H Radioactive Substance K Other Diagnostic Substance L Sperm N Analgesics, Hypnotics, Sedatives T Destructive Agent V Hormone	Z No Qualifier
P	Female Reproductive ♀	3 Percutaneous	G Other Therapeutic Substance	C Other Substance
P	Female Reproductive ♀	3 Percutaneous	Q Fertilized Ovum	Ø Autologous 1 Nonautologous
P	Female Reproductive ♀	3 Percutaneous	S Gas	F Other Gas
P	Female Reproductive ♀	4 Percutaneous Endoscopic	5 Adhesion Barrier	Z No Qualifier
P	Female Reproductive ♀	4 Percutaneous Endoscopic	G Other Therapeutic Substance	C Other Substance
P	Female Reproductive ♀	7 Via Natural or Artificial Opening	Ø Antineoplastic	4 Liquid Brachytherapy Radioisotope 5 Other Antineoplastic M Monoclonal Antibody
P	Female Reproductive ♀	7 Via Natural or Artificial Opening	2 Anti-infective	8 Oxazolidinones 9 Other Anti-infective
P	Female Reproductive ♀	7 Via Natural or Artificial Opening	3 Anti-inflammatory 6 Nutritional Substance 7 Electrolytic and Water Balance Substance B Anesthetic Agent H Radioactive Substance K Other Diagnostic Substance L Sperm N Analgesics, Hypnotics, Sedatives T Destructive Agent V Hormone	Z No Qualifier
P	Female Reproductive ♀	7 Via Natural or Artificial Opening	G Other Therapeutic Substance	C Other Substance
P	Female Reproductive ♀	7 Via Natural or Artificial Opening	Q Fertilized Ovum	Ø Autologous 1 Nonautologous
P	Female Reproductive ♀	7 Via Natural or Artificial Opening	S Gas	F Other Gas
P	Female Reproductive ♀	8 Via Natural or Artificial Opening Endoscopic	Ø Antineoplastic	4 Liquid Brachytherapy Radioisotope 5 Other Antineoplastic M Monoclonal Antibody
P	Female Reproductive ♀	8 Via Natural or Artificial Opening Endoscopic	2 Anti-infective	8 Oxazolidinones 9 Other Anit-infection
P	Female Reproductive ♀	8 Via Natural or Artificial Opening Endoscopic	3 Anti-inflammatory 6 Nutritional Substance 7 Electrolytic and Water Balance Substance B Anesthetic Agent H Radioactive Substance K Other Diagnostic Substance N Analgesics, Hypnotics, Sedative T Destructive Agent	Z No Qualifier
P	Female Reproductive ♀	8 Via Natural or Artificial Opening Endoscopic	G Other Therapeutic Substance	C Other Substance
P	Female Reproductive ♀	8 Via Natural or Artificial Opening Endoscopic	S Gas	F Other Gas
Q	Cranial Cavity and Brain	Ø Open 3 Percutaneous	Ø Antineoplastic	4 Liquid Brachytherapy Radioisotope 5 Other Antineoplastic M Monoclonal Antibody
Q	Cranial Cavity and Brain	Ø Open 3 Percutaneous	2 Anti-infective	8 Oxazolidinones 9 Other Anti-infective

Valid OR   3EØP3Q[Ø,1]

Valid OR   3EØP7Q[Ø,1]

DRG Non-OR   3EØQ[Ø,3]Ø5

♀   All approach, substance, and qualifier values for body system/region (character 4) with this icon

3EØ Continued on next page

NC Noncovered Procedure   LC Limited Coverage   QA Questionable OB Admit   NT New Tech Add-on   ⊞ Combination Member   ♂ Male   ♀ Female

Administration

3EØ Continued

3   **Administration**
E   **Physiological Systems and Anatomical Regions**
Ø   **Introduction**   Definition: Putting in or on a therapeutic, diagnostic, nutritional, physiological, or prophylactic substance except blood or blood products

Body System/Region Character 4	Approach Character 5	Substance Character 6	Qualifier Character 7
Q Cranial Cavity and Brain	Ø Open 3 Percutaneous	3 Anti-inflammatory 6 Nutritional Substance 7 Electrolytic and Water Balance Substance A Stem Cells, Embryonic B Anesthetic Agent H Radioactive Substance K Other Diagnostic Substance N Analgesics, Hypnotics, Sedatives T Destructive Agent	Z No Qualifier
Q Cranial Cavity and Brain	Ø Open 3 Percutaneous	E Stem Cells, Somatic	Ø Autologous 1 Nonautologous
Q Cranial Cavity and Brain	Ø Open 3 Percutaneous	G Other Therapeutic Substance	C Other Substance
Q Cranial Cavity and Brain	Ø Open 3 Percutaneous	S Gas	F Other Gas
Q Cranial Cavity and Brain	7 Via Natural or Artificial Opening	Ø Antineoplastic	4 Liquid Brachytherapy Radioisotope 5 Other Antineoplastic M Monoclonal Antibody
Q Cranial Cavity and Brain	7 Via Natural or Artificial Opening	S Gas	F Other Gas
R Spinal Canal	Ø Open	A Stem Cells, Embryonic	Z No Qualifier
R Spinal Canal	Ø Open	E Stem Cells, Somatic	Ø Autologous 1 Nonautologous
R Spinal Canal	3 Percutaneous	Ø Antineoplastic	2 High-dose Interleukin-2 3 Low-dose Interleukin-2 4 Liquid Brachytherapy Radioisotope 5 Other Antineoplastic M Monoclonal Antibody
R Spinal Canal	3 Percutaneous	2 Anti-infective	8 Oxazolidinones 9 Other Anti-infective
R Spinal Canal	3 Percutaneous	3 Anti-inflammatory 6 Nutritional Substance 7 Electrolytic and Water Balance Substance A Stem Cells, Embryonic B Anesthetic Agent H Radioactive Substance K Other Diagnostic Substance N Analgesics, Hypnotics, Sedatives T Destructive Agent	Z No Qualifier
R Spinal Canal	3 Percutaneous	E Stem Cells, Somatic	Ø Autologous 1 Nonautologous
R Spinal Canal	3 Percutaneous	G Other Therapeutic Substance	C Other Substance
R Spinal Canal	3 Percutaneous	S Gas	F Other Gas
R Spinal Canal	7 Via Natural or Artificial Opening	S Gas	F Other Gas
S Epidural Space	3 Percutaneous	Ø Antineoplastic	2 High-dose Interleukin-2 3 Low-dose Interleukin-2 4 Liquid Brachytherapy Radioisotope 5 Other Antineoplastic M Monoclonal Antibody
S Epidural Space	3 Percutaneous	2 Anti-infective	8 Oxazolidinones 9 Other Anti-infective
S Epidural Space	3 Percutaneous	3 Anti-inflammatory 6 Nutritional Substance 7 Electrolytic and Water Balance Substance B Anesthetic Agent H Radioactive Substance K Other Diagnostic Substance N Analgesics, Hypnotics, Sedatives T Destructive Agent	Z No Qualifier

DRG Non-OR   3EØQ7Ø5
DRG Non-OR   3EØR3Ø2
DRG Non-OR   3EØS3Ø2

3EØ Continued on next page

Non-OR Procedure   DRG Non-OR Procedure   Valid OR Procedure   HAC Associated Procedure   Combination Only   New/Revised GREEN

3 **Administration**
E **Physiological Systems and Anatomical Regions**   **3E0 Continued**
Ø **Introduction**   Definition: Putting in or on a therapeutic, diagnostic, nutritional, physiological, or prophylactic substance except blood or blood products

Body System/Region Character 4		Approach Character 5		Substance Character 6		Qualifier Character 7	
S	Epidural Space	3	Percutaneous	G	Other Therapeutic Substance	C	Other Substance
S	Epidural Space	3	Percutaneous	S	Gas	F	Other Gas
S	Epidural Space	7	Via Natural or Artificial Opening	S	Gas	F	Other Gas
T	Peripheral Nerves and Plexi	3	Percutaneous	3	Anti-inflammatory	Z	No Qualifier
X	Cranial Nerves			B	Anesthetic Agent		
				T	Destructive Agent		
T	Peripheral Nerves and Plexi	3	Percutaneous	G	Other Therapeutic Substance	C	Other Substance
X	Cranial Nerves						
U	Joints	Ø	Open	2	Anti-infective	8	Oxazolidinones
						9	Other Anti-infective
U	Joints	Ø	Open	G	Other Therapeutic Substance	B	Recombinant Bone Morphogenetic Protein
U	Joints	3	Percutaneous	Ø	Antineoplastic	4	Liquid Brachytherapy Radioisotope
						5	Other Antineoplastic
						M	Monoclonal Antibody
U	Joints	3	Percutaneous	2	Anti-infective	8	Oxazolidinones
						9	Other Anti-infective
U	Joints	3	Percutaneous	3	Anti-inflammatory	Z	No Qualifier
				6	Nutritional Substance		
				7	Electrolytic and Water Balance Substance		
				B	Anesthetic Agent		
				H	Radioactive Substance		
				K	Other Diagnostic Substance		
				N	Analgesics, Hypnotics, Sedatives		
				T	Destructive Agent		
U	Joints	3	Percutaneous	G	Other Therapeutic Substance	B	Recombinant Bone Morphogenetic Protein
						C	Other Substance
U	Joints	3	Percutaneous	S	Gas	F	Other Gas
U	Joints	4	Percutaneous Endoscopic	G	Other Therapeutic Substance	C	Other Substance
V	Bones	Ø	Open	G	Other Therapeutic Substance	B	Recombinant Bone Morphogenetic Protein
V	Bones	3	Percutaneous	Ø	Antineoplastic	5	Other Antineoplastic
						M	Monoclonal Antibody
V	Bones	3	Percutaneous	2	Anti-infective	8	Oxazolidinones
						9	Other Anti-infective
V	Bones	3	Percutaneous	3	Anti-inflammatory	Z	No Qualifier
				6	Nutritional Substance		
				7	Electrolytic and Water Balance Substance		
				B	Anesthetic Agent		
				H	Radioactive Substance		
				K	Other Diagnostic Substance		
				N	Analgesics, Hypnotics, Sedatives		
				T	Destructive Agent		
V	Bones	3	Percutaneous	G	Other Therapeutic Substance	B	Recombinant Bone Morphogenetic Protein
						C	Other Substance
W	Lymphatics	3	Percutaneous	Ø	Antineoplastic	5	Other Antineoplastic
						M	Monoclonal Antibody
W	Lymphatics	3	Percutaneous	2	Anti-infective	8	Oxazolidinones
						9	Other Anti-infective
W	Lymphatics	3	Percutaneous	3	Anti-inflammatory	Z	No Qualifier
				6	Nutritional Substance		
				7	Electrolytic and Water Balance Substance		
				B	Anesthetic Agent		
				H	Radioactive Substance		
				K	Other Diagnostic Substance		
				N	Analgesics, Hypnotics, Sedatives		
				T	Destructive Agent		
W	Lymphatics	3	Percutaneous	G	Other Therapeutic Substance	C	Other Substance

3E0 Continued on next page

NC Noncovered Procedure   LC Limited Coverage   QA Questionable OB Admit   NT New Tech Add-on   ⊞ Combination Member   ♂ Male   ♀ Female

ICD-10-PCS 2022   725

3   **Administration**   ***3E0 Continued***
E   **Physiological Systems and Anatomical Regions**
0   **Introduction**   Definition: Putting in or on a therapeutic, diagnostic, nutritional, physiological, or prophylactic substance except blood or blood products

Body System/Region Character 4	Approach Character 5	Substance Character 6	Qualifier Character 7
Y Pericardial Cavity	3 Percutaneous	0 Antineoplastic	4 Liquid Brachytherapy Radioisotope 5 Other Antineoplastic M Monoclonal Antibody
Y Pericardial Cavity	3 Percutaneous	2 Anti-infective	8 Oxazolidinones 9 Other Anti-infective
Y Pericardial Cavity	3 Percutaneous	3 Anti-inflammatory 6 Nutritional Substance 7 Electrolytic and Water Balance Substance B Anesthetic Agent H Radioactive Substance K Other Diagnostic Substance N Analgesics, Hypnotics, Sedatives T Destructive Agent	Z No Qualifier
Y Pericardial Cavity	3 Percutaneous	G Other Therapeutic Substance	C Other Substance
Y Pericardial Cavity	3 Percutaneous	S Gas	F Other Gas
Y Pericardial Cavity	4 Percutaneous Endoscopic	G Other Therapeutic Substance	C Other Substance
Y Pericardial Cavity	7 Via Natural or Artificial Opening	0 Antineoplastic	4 Liquid Brachytherapy Radioisotope 5 Other Antineoplastic M Monoclonal Antibody
Y Pericardial Cavity	7 Via Natural or Artificial Opening	S Gas	F Other Gas

3   **Administration**
E   **Physiological Systems and Anatomical Regions**
1   **Irrigation**   Definition: Putting in or on a cleansing substance

Body System/Region Character 4	Approach Character 5	Substance Character 6	Qualifier Character 7
0 Skin and Mucous Membranes C Eye	3 Percutaneous X External	8 Irrigating Substance	X Diagnostic Z No Qualifier
9 Nose B Ear F Respiratory Tract G Upper GI H Lower GI J Biliary and Pancreatic Tract K Genitourinary Tract N Male Reproductive ♂ P Female Reproductive ♀	3 Percutaneous 7 Via Natural or Artificial Opening 8 Via Natural or Artificial Opening Endoscopic	8 Irrigating Substance	X Diagnostic Z No Qualifier
L Pleural Cavity Q Cranial Cavity and Brain R Spinal Canal S Epidural Space Y Pericardial Cavity	3 Percutaneous	8 Irrigating Substance	X Diagnostic Z No Qualifier
M Peritoneal Cavity	3 Percutaneous	8 Irrigating Substance	X Diagnostic Z No Qualifier
M Peritoneal Cavity	3 Percutaneous	9 Dialysate	Z No Qualifier
M Peritoneal Cavity	4 Percutaneous Endoscopic	8 Irrigating Substance	X Diagnostic Z No Qualifier
U Joints	3 Percutaneous 4 Percutaneous Endoscopic	8 Irrigating Substance	X Diagnostic Z No Qualifier

♂   3E1N[3,7,8]8[X,Z]
♀   3E1P[3,7,8]8[X,Z]

Non-OR Procedure   DRG Non-OR Procedure   Valid OR Procedure   HAC Associated Procedure   Combination Only   New/Revised GREEN
726   ICD-10-PCS 2022

3E0–3E1

Measurement and Monitoring 4A0–4B0

AHA Coding Clinic for table 4A0

2020, 4Q, 62	Measurement of intracranial arterial flow
2020, 4Q, 62	Percutaneous endoscopic measurement of portal venous pressure
2020, 4Q, 63	Intercompartmental pressure measurement
2019, 3Q, 32	Endomyocardial biopsy and right heart catheterization
2018, 1Q, 12	Percutaneous balloon valvuloplasty & cardiac catheterization with ventriculogram
2016, 3Q, 37	Fractional flow reserve
2015, 3Q, 29	Approach value for esophageal electrophysiology study

AHA Coding Clinic for table 4A1

2019, 4Q, 38-39	Intraoperative fluorescence lymphatic mapping using Indocyanine green dye
2016, 4Q, 114	Fluorescence vascular angiography
2016, 2Q, 29	Decompressive craniectomy with cryopreservation and storage of bone flap
2016, 2Q, 33	Monitoring of arterial pressure & pulse
2015, 3Q, 35	Swan Ganz catheterization
2015, 2Q, 14	Intraoperative EMG monitoring via endotracheal tube
2015, 1Q, 26	Intraoperative monitoring using Sentio MMG®
2014, 4Q, 28	Removal and replacement of displaced growing rods

4   Measurement and Monitoring
A   Physiological Systems
0   Measurement   Definition: Determining the level of a physiological or physical function at a point in time

Body System Character 4	Approach Character 5	Function/Device Character 6	Qualifier Character 7
0 Central Nervous	0 Open	2 Conductivity 4 Electrical Activity B Pressure	Z No Qualifier
0 Central Nervous	3 Percutaneous 7 Via Natural or Artificial Opening 8 Via Natural or Artificial Opening Endoscopic	4 Electrical Activity	Z No Qualifier
0 Central Nervous	3 Percutaneous 7 Via Natural or Artificial Opening 8 Via Natural or Artificial Opening Endoscopic	B Pressure K Temperature R Saturation	D Intracranial
0 Central Nervous	X External	2 Conductivity 4 Electrical Activity	Z No Qualifier
1 Peripheral Nervous	0 Open 3 Percutaneous 7 Via Natural or Artificial Opening 8 Via Natural or Artificial Opening Endoscopic X External	2 Conductivity	9 Sensory B Motor
1 Peripheral Nervous	0 Open 3 Percutaneous 7 Via Natural or Artificial Opening 8 Via Natural or Artificial Opening Endoscopic X External	4 Electrical Activity	Z No Qualifier
2 Cardiac	0 Open 3 Percutaneous 7 Via Natural or Artificial Opening 8 Via Natural or Artificial Opening Endoscopic	4 Electrical Activity 9 Output C Rate F Rhythm H Sound P Action Currents	Z No Qualifier
2 Cardiac	0 Open 3 Percutaneous 7 Via Natural or Artificial Opening 8 Via Natural or Artificial Opening Endoscopic	N Sampling and Pressure	6 Right Heart 7 Left Heart 8 Bilateral
2 Cardiac	X External	4 Electrical Activity	A Guidance Z No Qualifier
2 Cardiac	X External	9 Output C Rate F Rhythm H Sound P Action Currents	Z No Qualifier
2 Cardiac	X External	M Total Activity	4 Stress
3 Arterial	0 Open 3 Percutaneous	5 Flow J Pulse	1 Peripheral 3 Pulmonary C Coronary
3 Arterial	0 Open 3 Percutaneous	B Pressure	1 Peripheral 3 Pulmonary C Coronary F Other Thoracic

DRG Non-OR   4A02[3,7,8]FZ
DRG Non-OR   4A02[0,3,7,8]N[6,7,8]

4A0 Continued on next page

4   Measurement and Monitoring   *4A0 Continued*
A   Physiological Systems
0   Measurement   Definition: Determining the level of a physiological or physical function at a point in time

Body System Character 4	Approach Character 5	Function/Device Character 6	Qualifier Character 7
3 Arterial	Ø Open 3 Percutaneous	H Sound R Saturation	1 Peripheral
3 Arterial	X External	5 Flow **NT**	1 Peripheral D Intracranial
3 Arterial	X External	B Pressure H Sound J Pulse R Saturation	1 Peripheral
4 Venous	Ø Open 3 Percutaneous	5 Flow B Pressure J Pulse	Ø Central 1 Peripheral 2 Portal 3 Pulmonary
4 Venous	Ø Open 3 Percutaneous	R Saturation	1 Peripheral
4 Venous	4 Percutaneous Endoscopic	B Pressure	2 Portal
4 Venous	X External	5 Flow B Pressure J Pulse R Saturation	1 Peripheral
5 Circulatory	X External	L Volume	Z No Qualifier
6 Lymphatic	Ø Open 3 Percutaneous 7 Via Natural or Artificial Opening 8 Via Natural or Artificial Opening Endoscopic	5 Flow B Pressure	Z No Qualifier
7 Visual	X External	Ø Acuity 7 Mobility B Pressure	Z No Qualifier
8 Olfactory	X External	Ø Acuity	Z No Qualifier
9 Respiratory	7 Via Natural or Artificial Opening 8 Via Natural or Artificial Opening Endoscopic X External	1 Capacity 5 Flow C Rate D Resistance L Volume M Total Activity	Z No Qualifier
B Gastrointestinal	7 Via Natural or Artificial Opening 8 Via Natural or Artificial Opening Endoscopic	8 Motility B Pressure G Secretion	Z No Qualifier
C Biliary	3 Percutaneous 4 Percutaneous Endoscopic 7 Via Natural or Artificial Opening 8 Via Natural or Artificial Opening Endoscopic	5 Flow B Pressure	Z No Qualifier
D Urinary	7 Via Natural or Artificial Opening 8 Via Natural or Artificial Opening Endoscopic	3 Contractility 5 Flow B Pressure D Resistance L Volume	Z No Qualifier
F Musculoskeletal	3 Percutaneous	3 Contractility	Z No Qualifier
F Musculoskeletal	3 Percutaneous	B Pressure	E Compartment
F Musculoskeletal	X External	3 Contractility	Z No Qualifier
H Products of Conception, Cardiac ♀	7 Via Natural or Artificial Opening 8 Via Natural or Artificial Opening Endoscopic X External	4 Electrical Activity C Rate F Rhythm H Sound	Z No Qualifier
J Products of Conception, Nervous ♀	7 Via Natural or Artificial Opening 8 Via Natural or Artificial Opening Endoscopic X External	2 Conductivity 4 Electrical Activity B Pressure	Z No Qualifier
Z None	7 Via Natural or Artificial Opening	6 Metabolism K Temperature	Z No Qualifier
Z None	X External	6 Metabolism K Temperature Q Sleep	Z No Qualifier

Valid OR	4A060[5,B]Z	♀	4A0H[7,8,X][4,C,F,H]Z
Valid OR	4A0C4[5,B]Z	♀	4A0J[7,8,X][2,4,B]Z
NT	4A03X5D for use of ContaCT		

4   Measurement and Monitoring
A   Physiological Systems
1   Monitoring   Definition: Determining the level of a physiological or physical function repetitively over a period of time

Body System Character 4	Approach Character 5	Function/Device Character 6	Qualifier Character 7
Ø Central Nervous	Ø Open	2 Conductivity B Pressure	Z No Qualifier
Ø Central Nervous	Ø Open	4 Electrical Activity	G Intraoperative Z No Qualifier
Ø Central Nervous	3 Percutaneous 7 Via Natural or Artificial Opening 8 Via Natural or Artificial Opening Endoscopic	4 Electrical Activity	G Intraoperative Z No Qualifier
Ø Central Nervous	3 Percutaneous 7 Via Natural or Artificial Opening 8 Via Natural or Artificial Opening Endoscopic	B Pressure K Temperature R Saturation	D Intracranial
Ø Central Nervous	X External	2 Conductivity	Z No Qualifier
Ø Central Nervous	X External	4 Electrical Activity	G Intraoperative Z No Qualifier
1 Peripheral Nervous	Ø Open 3 Percutaneous 7 Via Natural or Artificial Opening 8 Via Natural or Artificial Opening Endoscopic X External	2 Conductivity	9 Sensory B Motor
1 Peripheral Nervous	Ø Open 3 Percutaneous 7 Via Natural or Artificial Opening 8 Via Natural or Artificial Opening Endoscopic X External	4 Electrical Activity	G Intraoperative Z No Qualifier
2 Cardiac	Ø Open 3 Percutaneous 7 Via Natural or Artificial Opening 8 Via Natural or Artificial Opening Endoscopic	4 Electrical Activity 9 Output C Rate F Rhythm H Sound	Z No Qualifier
2 Cardiac	X External	4 Electrical Activity	5 Ambulatory Z No Qualifier
2 Cardiac	X External	9 Output C Rate F Rhythm H Sound	Z No Qualifier
2 Cardiac	X External	M Total Activity	4 Stress
2 Cardiac	X External	S Vascular Perfusion	H Indocyanine Green Dye
3 Arterial	Ø Open 3 Percutaneous	5 Flow B Pressure J Pulse	1 Peripheral 3 Pulmonary C Coronary
3 Arterial	Ø Open 3 Percutaneous	H Sound R Saturation	1 Peripheral
3 Arterial	X External	5 Flow B Pressure H Sound J Pulse R Saturation	1 Peripheral
4 Venous	Ø Open 3 Percutaneous	5 Flow B Pressure J Pulse	Ø Central 1 Peripheral 2 Portal 3 Pulmonary
4 Venous	Ø Open 3 Percutaneous	R Saturation	Ø Central 2 Portal 3 Pulmonary
4 Venous	X External	5 Flow B Pressure J Pulse	1 Peripheral
6 Lymphatic	Ø Open 3 Percutaneous 7 Via Natural or Artificial Opening 8 Via Natural or Artificial Opening Endoscopic	5 Flow	H Indocyanine Green Dye Z No Qualifier

Valid OR   4A16Ø5Z

4A1 Continued on next page

NC Noncovered Procedure   LC Limited Coverage   QA Questionable OB Admit   NT New Tech Add-on   ⊞ Combination Member   ♂ Male   ♀ Female

ICD-10-PCS 2022   729

Measurement and Monitoring

4   **Measurement and Monitoring**
A   **Physiological Systems**
1   **Monitoring**   Definition: Determining the level of a physiological or physical function repetitively over a period of time

4A1 Continued

Body System Character 4	Approach Character 5	Function/Device Character 6	Qualifier Character 7
6 Lymphatic	Ø Open 3 Percutaneous 7 Via Natural or Artificial Opening 8 Via Natural or Artificial Opening Endoscopic	B Pressure	Z No Qualifier
9 Respiratory	7 Via Natural or Artificial Opening X External	1 Capacity 5 Flow C Rate D Resistance L Volume	Z No Qualifier
B Gastrointestinal	7 Via Natural or Artificial Opening 8 Via Natural or Artificial Opening Endoscopic	8 Motility B Pressure G Secretion	Z No Qualifier
B Gastrointestinal	X External	S Vascular Perfusion	H Indocyanine Green Dye
D Urinary	7 Via Natural or Artificial Opening 8 Via Natural or Artificial Opening Endoscopic	3 Contractility 5 Flow B Pressure D Resistance L Volume	Z No Qualifier
G Skin and Breast	X External	S Vascular Perfusion	H Indocyanine Green Dye
H Products of Conception, Cardiac ♀	7 Via Natural or Artificial Opening 8 Via Natural or Artificial Opening Endoscopic X External	4 Electrical Activity C Rate F Rhythm H Sound	Z No Qualifier
J Products of Conception, Nervous ♀	7 Via Natural or Artificial Opening 8 Via Natural or Artificial Opening Endoscopic X External	2 Conductivity 4 Electrical Activity B Pressure	Z No Qualifier
Z None	7 Via Natural or Artificial Opening	K Temperature	Z No Qualifier
Z None	X External	K Temperature Q Sleep	Z No Qualifier

Valid OR   4A16ØBZ
♀   4A1H[7,8,X][4,C,F,H]Z
♀   4A1J[7,8,X][2,4,B]Z

4   **Measurement and Monitoring**
B   **Physiological Devices**
Ø   **Measurement**   Definition: Determining the level of a physiological or physical function at a point in time

Body System Character 4	Approach Character 5	Function/Device Character 6	Qualifier Character 7
Ø Central Nervous	X External	V Stimulator	Z No Qualifier
Ø Central Nervous	X External	W Cerebrospinal Fluid Shunt	Ø Wireless Sensor
1 Peripheral Nervous F Musculoskeletal	X External	V Stimulator	Z No Qualifier
2 Cardiac	X External	S Pacemaker T Defibrillator	Z No Qualifier
9 Respiratory	X External	S Pacemaker	Z No Qualifier

Extracorporeal or Systemic Assistance and Performance 5A0–5A2

AHA Coding Clinic for table 5A0
2021, 2Q, 12   Repositioning of displaced intra-aortic balloon pump
2020, 4Q, 64-65   Ventilatory assistance by high flow or high velocity nasal cannula devices
2020, 1Q, 10   Intermittent use of continuous positive airway pressure
2018, 2Q, 3-5   Intra-aortic balloon pump
2017, 4Q, 43-44   Insertion of external heart assist devices
2017, 3Q, 18   Intra-aortic balloon pump removal
2017, 1Q, 10-11   External heart assist device
2017, 1Q, 29   Newborn resuscitation using positive pressure ventilation
2017, 1Q, 29   Newborn noninvasive ventilation
2016, 4Q, 137-139 Heart assist device systems
2014, 4Q, 9   Mechanical ventilation
2014, 3Q, 19   Ablation of ventricular tachycardia with Impella® support
2013, 3Q, 18   Heart transplant surgery

AHA Coding Clinic for table 5A1
2019, 4Q, 39-41   Intraoperative extracorporeal membrane oxygenation
2019, 3Q, 19   Insertion of left ventricular catheter
2019, 3Q, 20   Removal and revision of ECMO component
2019, 3Q, 21   Exchange of extracorporeal membrane oxygenation component (oxygenator)
2019, 2Q, 36   Veno-arterial extracorporeal membrane oxygenation via sternotomy
2019, 3Q, 22   Extracorporeal membrane oxygenation and Centrimag™ pump
2019, 3Q, 22   Extracorporeal membrane oxygenation transfers
2018, 4Q, 52-54   Percutaneous extracorporeal membrane oxygenation
2018, 1Q, 13   Mechanical ventilation using patient's equipment
2017, 4Q, 71-73   Hemodialysis and renal replacement therapy
2017, 3Q, 7   Senning procedure (arterial switch)
2017, 1Q, 19   Norwood Sano procedure
2016, 1Q, 27   Aortocoronary bypass graft utilizing Y-graft
2016, 1Q, 28   Extracorporeal liver assist device
2016, 1Q, 29   Duration of hemodialysis
2015, 4Q, 22-24   Congenital heart corrective procedures
2014, 4Q, 3-10   Mechanical ventilation
2014, 4Q, 11-15   Sequencing of mechanical ventilation with other procedures
2014, 3Q, 16   Repair of Tetralogy of Fallot
2014, 3Q, 20   MAZE procedure performed with coronary artery bypass graft
2014, 1Q, 10   Repair of thoracic aortic aneurysm & coronary artery bypass graft
2013, 3Q, 18   Heart transplant surgery

5   Extracorporeal or Systemic Assistance and Performance
A   Physiological Systems
0   Assistance   Definition: Taking over a portion of a physiological function by extracorporeal means

Body System Character 4	Duration Character 5		Function Character 6		Qualifier Character 7	
2 Cardiac	1	Intermittent	1	Output	0	Balloon Pump
	2	Continuous			5	Pulsatile Compression
					6	Other Pump
					D	Impeller Pump
5 Circulatory	1	Intermittent	2	Oxygenation	1	Hyperbaric
	2	Continuous			C	Supersaturated
9 Respiratory	2	Continuous	0	Filtration	Z	No Qualifier
9 Respiratory	3	Less than 24 Consecutive Hours	5	Ventilation	7	Continuous Positive Airway Pressure
	4	24-96 Consecutive Hours			8	Intermittent Positive Airway Pressure
	5	Greater than 96 Consecutive Hours			9	Continuous Negative Airway Pressure
					A	High Nasal Flow/Velocity
					B	Intermittent Negative Airway Pressure
					Z	No Qualifier

Valid OR   5A02[1,2]1[0,6,D]

Extracorporeal or Systemic Assistance and Performance

5   **Extracorporeal or Systemic Assistance and Performance**
A   **Physiological Systems**
1   **Performance**   Definition: Completely taking over a physiological function by extracorporeal means

Body System Character 4	Duration Character 5	Function Character 6	Qualifier Character 7
2 Cardiac	Ø Single	1 Output	2 Manual
2 Cardiac	1 Intermittent	3 Pacing	Z No Qualifier
2 Cardiac	2 Continuous	1 Output	J Automated Z No Qualifier
2 Cardiac	2 Continuous	3 Pacing	Z No Qualifier
5 Circulatory	2 Continuous A Intraoperative	2 Oxygenation	F Membrane, Central G Membrane, Peripheral Veno-arterial H Membrane, Peripheral Veno-venous
9 Respiratory	Ø Single	5 Ventilation	4 Nonmechanical
9 Respiratory	3 Less than 24 Consecutive Hours 4 24-96 Consecutive Hours 5 Greater than 96 Consecutive Hours	5 Ventilation	Z No Qualifier
C Biliary	Ø Single 6 Multiple	Ø Filtration	Z No Qualifier
D Urinary	7 Intermittent, Less than 6 Hours per day 8 Prolonged Intermittent, 6-18 Hours per day 9 Continuous, Greater than 18 Hours per day	Ø Filtration	Z No Qualifier

Valid OR   5A1522F
DRG Non-OR 5A1522[G,H]
DRG Non-OR 5A19[3,4]5Z
DRG Non-OR 5A1955Z Length of stay must be > 4 consecutive days.
DRG Non-OR 5A1D[7,8,9]ØZ

5   **Extracorporeal or Systemic Assistance and Performance**
A   **Physiological Systems**
2   **Restoration**   Definition: Returning, or attempting to return, a physiological function to its original state by extracorporeal means.

Body System Character 4	Duration Character 5	Function Character 6	Qualifier Character 7
2 Cardiac	Ø Single	4 Rhythm	Z No Qualifier

Extracorporeal or Systemic Therapies 6A0–6AB

AHA Coding Clinic for table 6A4
2019, 2Q, 17   Cryoamputation of lower leg

AHA Coding Clinic for table 6A7
2014, 4Q, 19   Ultrasound accelerated thrombolysis

AHA Coding Clinic for table 6AB
2016, 4Q, 115   Donor organ perfusion

6   Extracorporeal or Systemic Therapies
A   Physiological Systems
0   Atmospheric Control   Definition: Extracorporeal control of atmospheric pressure and composition

Body System Character 4	Duration Character 5	Qualifier Character 6	Qualifier Character 7
Z None	0 Single 1 Multiple	Z No Qualifier	Z No Qualifier

6   Extracorporeal or Systemic Therapies
A   Physiological Systems
1   Decompression   Definition: Extracorporeal elimination of undissolved gas from body fluids

Body System Character 4	Duration Character 5	Qualifier Character 6	Qualifier Character 7
5 Circulatory	0 Single 1 Multiple	Z No Qualifier	Z No Qualifier

6   Extracorporeal or Systemic Therapies
A   Physiological Systems
2   Electromagnetic Therapy   Definition: Extracorporeal treatment by electromagnetic rays

Body System Character 4	Duration Character 5	Qualifier Character 6	Qualifier Character 7
1 Urinary 2 Central Nervous	0 Single 1 Multiple	Z No Qualifier	Z No Qualifier

6   Extracorporeal or Systemic Therapies
A   Physiological Systems
3   Hyperthermia   Definition: Extracorporeal raising of body temperature

Body System Character 4	Duration Character 5	Qualifier Character 6	Qualifier Character 7
Z None	0 Single 1 Multiple	Z No Qualifier	Z No Qualifier

6   Extracorporeal or Systemic Therapies
A   Physiological Systems
4   Hypothermia   Definition: Extracorporeal lowering of body temperature

Body System Character 4	Duration Character 5	Qualifier Character 6	Qualifier Character 7
Z None	0 Single 1 Multiple	Z No Qualifier	Z No Qualifier

6   Extracorporeal or Systemic Therapies
A   Physiological Systems
5   Pheresis   Definition: Extracorporeal separation of blood products

Body System Character 4	Duration Character 5	Qualifier Character 6	Qualifier Character 7
5 Circulatory	0 Single 1 Multiple	Z No Qualifier	0 Erythrocytes 1 Leukocytes 2 Platelets 3 Plasma T Stem Cells, Cord Blood V Stem Cells, Hematopoietic

6   Extracorporeal or Systemic Therapies
A   Physiological Systems
6   Phototherapy   Definition: Extracorporeal treatment by light rays

Body System Character 4	Duration Character 5	Qualifier Character 6	Qualifier Character 7
0 Skin 5 Circulatory	0 Single 1 Multiple	Z No Qualifier	Z No Qualifier

---

NC Noncovered Procedure   **LC** Limited Coverage   **QA** Questionable OB Admit   **NT** New Tech Add-on   ⊞ Combination Member   ♂ Male   ♀ Female

Extracorporeal or Systemic Therapies

6   **Extracorporeal or Systemic Therapies**
A   **Physiological Systems**
7   **Ultrasound Therapy**   Definition: Extracorporeal treatment by ultrasound

Body System Character 4	Duration Character 5	Qualifier Character 6	Qualifier Character 7
5 Circulatory	Ø Single 1 Multiple	Z No Qualifier	4 Head and Neck Vessels 5 Heart 6 Peripheral Vessels 7 Other Vessels Z No Qualifier

6   **Extracorporeal or Systemic Therapies**
A   **Physiological Systems**
8   **Ultraviolet Light Therapy**   Definition: Extracorporeal treatment by ultraviolet light

Body System Character 4	Duration Character 5	Qualifier Character 6	Qualifier Character 7
Ø Skin	Ø Single 1 Multiple	Z No Qualifier	Z No Qualifier

6   **Extracorporeal or Systemic Therapies**
A   **Physiological Systems**
9   **Shock Wave Therapy**   Definition: Extracorporeal treatment by shock waves

Body System Character 4	Duration Character 5	Qualifier Character 6	Qualifier Character 7
3 Musculoskeletal	Ø Single 1 Multiple	Z No Qualifier	Z No Qualifier

6   **Extracorporeal or Systemic Therapies**
A   **Physiological Systems**
B   **Perfusion**   Definition: Extracorporeal treatment by diffusion of therapeutic fluid

Body System Character 4	Duration Character 5	Qualifier Character 6	Qualifier Character 7
5 Circulatory B Respiratory System F Hepatobiliary System and Pancreas T Urinary System	Ø Single	B Donor Organ	Z No Qualifier

Osteopathic 7W0

7　Osteopathic
W　Anatomical Regions
0　Treatment　　Definition: Manual treatment to eliminate or alleviate somatic dysfunction and related disorders

Body Region Character 4	Approach Character 5	Method Character 6	Qualifier Character 7
0　Head 1　Cervical 2　Thoracic 3　Lumbar 4　Sacrum 5　Pelvis 6　Lower Extremities 7　Upper Extremities 8　Rib Cage 9　Abdomen	X　External	0　Articulatory-Raising 1　Fascial Release 2　General Mobilization 3　High Velocity-Low Amplitude 4　Indirect 5　Low Velocity-High Amplitude 6　Lymphatic Pump 7　Muscle Energy-Isometric 8　Muscle Energy-Isotonic 9　Other Method	Z　None

Other Procedures 8C0–8E0

AHA Coding Clinic for table 8E0

2021, 2Q, 19	Electromagnetic stealth guided ventriculoperitoneal shunt insertion with endoscopy
2020, 4Q, 53	Bypass pancreatic duct to stomach
2020, 4Q, 65-66	Near infrared spectroscopy for tissue viability assessment
2020, 4Q, 99	Robotic-assisted prostatectomy with extension of incision for specimen removal
2020, 4Q, 100	Robotic-assisted sigmoid colectomy with extension of incision for specimen removal
2019, 4Q, 41-42	Intraoperative fluorescence guidance
2019, 1Q, 30	Laparoscopic-assisted rectopexy with manual reduction of prolapse
2015, 1Q, 33	Robotic-assisted laparoscopic hysterectomy converted to open procedure
2014, 4Q, 33	Radical prostatectomy

8   **Other Procedures**
C   **Indwelling Device**
0   **Other Procedures**   Definition: Methodologies which attempt to remediate or cure a disorder or disease

Body Region Character 4	Approach Character 5	Method Character 6	Qualifier Character 7
1 Nervous System	X External	6 Collection	J Cerebrospinal Fluid L Other Fluid
2 Circulatory System	X External	6 Collection	K Blood L Other Fluid

8   **Other Procedures**
E   **Physiological Systems and Anatomical Regions**
0   **Other Procedures**   Definition: Methodologies which attempt to remediate or cure a disorder or disease

Body Region Character 4	Approach Character 5	Method Character 6	Qualifier Character 7
1 Nervous System U Female Reproductive System ♀	X External	Y Other Method	7 Examination
2 Circulatory System	3 Percutaneous X External	D Near Infrared Spectroscopy	Z No Qualifier
9 Head and Neck Region	0 Open	C Robotic Assisted Procedure	Z No Qualifier
9 Head and Neck Region	0 Open	E Fluorescence Guided Procedure	M Aminolevulinic Acid Z No Qualifier
9 Head and Neck Region	3 Percutaneous 4 Percutaneous Endoscopic 7 Via Natural or Artificial Opening 8 Via Natural or Artificial Opening Endoscopic	C Robotic Assisted Procedure E Fluorescence Guided Procedure	Z No Qualifier
9 Head and Neck Region	X External	B Computer Assisted Procedure	F With Fluoroscopy G With Computerized Tomography H With Magnetic Resonance Imaging Z No Qualifier
9 Head and Neck Region	X External	C Robotic Assisted Procedure	Z No Qualifier
9 Head and Neck Region	X External	Y Other Method	8 Suture Removal
H Integumentary System and Breast	3 Percutaneous	0 Acupuncture	0 Anesthesia Z No Qualifier
H Integumentary System and Breast ♀	X External	6 Collection	2 Breast Milk
H Integumentary System and Breast	X External	Y Other Method	9 Piercing
K Musculoskeletal System	X External	1 Therapeutic Massage	Z No Qualifier
K Musculoskeletal System	X External	Y Other Method	7 Examination
V Male Reproductive System ♂	X External	1 Therapeutic Massage	C Prostate D Rectum
V Male Reproductive System ♂	X External	6 Collection	3 Sperm
W Trunk Region	0 Open 3 Percutaneous 4 Percutaneous Endoscopic 7 Via Natural or Artificial Opening 8 Via Natural or Artificial Opening Endoscopic	C Robotic Assisted Procedure E Fluorescence Guided Procedure	Z No Qualifier
W Trunk Region	X External	B Computer Assisted Procedure	F With Fluoroscopy G With Computerized Tomography H With Magnetic Resonance Imaging Z No Qualifier
W Trunk Region	X External	C Robotic Assisted Procedure	Z No Qualifier
W Trunk Region	X External	Y Other Method	8 Suture Removal
X Upper Extremity Y Lower Extremity	0 Open 3 Percutaneous 4 Percutaneous Endoscopic	C Robotic Assisted Procedure E Fluorescence Guided Procedure	Z No Qualifier

♂ 8E0VX1C		♀ 8E0UXY7	
♂ 8E0VX63		♀ 8E0HX62	

8E0 Continued on next page

NC Noncovered Procedure   **LC** Limited Coverage   **QA** Questionable OB Admit   **NT** New Tech Add-on   ⊞ Combination Member   ♂ Male   ♀ Female

Other Procedures

8   Other Procedures
E   Physiological Systems and Anatomical Regions
Ø   Other Procedures   Definition: Methodologies which attempt to remediate or cure a disorder or disease

Body Region Character 4	Approach Character 5	Method Character 6	Qualifier Character 7
X Upper Extremity Y Lower Extremity	X External	B Computer Assisted Procedure	F With Fluoroscopy G With Computerized Tomography H With Magnetic Resonance Imaging Z No Qualifier
X Upper Extremity Y Lower Extremity	X External	C Robotic Assisted Procedure	Z No Qualifier
X Upper Extremity Y Lower Extremity	X External	Y Other Method	8 Suture Removal
Z None	X External	Y Other Method	1 In Vitro Fertilization 4 Yoga Therapy 5 Meditation 6 Isolation

Chiropractic 9WB

9   **Chiropractic**
W   **Anatomical Regions**
B   **Manipulation**   Definition: Manual procedure that involves a directed thrust to move a joint past the physiological range of motion, without exceeding the anatomical limit

Body Region Character 4	Approach Character 5	Method Character 6	Qualifier Character 7
Ø Head	**X** External	**B** Non-Manual	**Z** None
1 Cervical		**C** Indirect Visceral	
2 Thoracic		**D** Extra-Articular	
3 Lumbar		**F** Direct Visceral	
4 Sacrum		**G** Long Lever Specific Contact	
5 Pelvis		**H** Short Lever Specific Contact	
6 Lower Extremities		**J** Long and Short Lever Specific Contact	
7 Upper Extremities		**K** Mechanically Assisted	
8 Rib Cage		**L** Other Method	
9 Abdomen			

Imaging B00–BY4

AHA Coding Clinic for table B21
2018, 1Q, 12　　　Percutaneous balloon valvuloplasty & cardiac catheterization with ventriculogram
2016, 3Q, 36　　　Type of contrast medium for angiography (high osmolar, low osmolar, and other)

AHA Coding Clinic for table B41
2015, 3Q, 9　　　Aborted endovascular stenting of superficial femoral artery

AHA Coding Clinic for table B51
2015, 4Q, 30　　　Vascular access devices

AHA Coding Clinic for table BF4
2014, 3Q, 15　　　Drainage of pancreatic pseudocyst
2020, 4Q, 66　　　Other imaging type

AHA Coding Clinic for table BF5
2020, 4Q, 66　　　Other imaging type
2020, 4Q, 66-67　　Fluorescence imaging of hepatobiliary system

AHA Coding Clinic for table BW5
2020, 4Q, 66　　　Other imaging type
2020, 4Q, 68　　　Bacterial autofluorescence detection

B　Imaging
0　Central Nervous System
0　Plain Radiography　　Definition: Planar display of an image developed from the capture of external ionizing radiation on photographic or photoconductive plate

Body Part Character 4	Contrast Character 5	Qualifier Character 6	Qualifier Character 7
B　Spinal Cord	0　High Osmolar 1　Low Osmolar Y　Other Contrast Z　None	Z　None	Z　None

B　Imaging
0　Central Nervous System
1　Fluoroscopy　　Definition: Single plane or bi-plane real time display of an image developed from the capture of external ionizing radioation on a fluorescent screen. The image may also be stored by either digital or analog means.

Body Part Character 4	Contrast Character 5	Qualifier Character 6	Qualifier Character 7
B　Spinal Cord	0　High Osmolar 1　Low Osmolar Y　Other Contrast Z　None	Z　None	Z　None

B　Imaging
0　Central Nervous System
2　Computerized Tomography (CT Scan)　Definition: Computer reformatted digital display of multiplanar images developed from the capture of multiple exposures of external ionizing radiation

Body Part Character 4	Contrast Character 5	Qualifier Character 6	Qualifier Character 7
0　Brain 7　Cisterna 8　Cerebral Ventricle(s) 9　Sella Turcica/Pituitary Gland B　Spinal Cord	0　High Osmolar 1　Low Osmolar Y　Other Contrast	0　Unenhanced and Enhanced Z　None	Z　None
0　Brain 7　Cisterna 8　Cerebral Ventricle(s) 9　Sella Turcica/Pituitary Gland B　Spinal Cord	Z　None	Z　None	Z　None

B　Imaging
0　Central Nervous System
3　Magnetic Resonance Imaging (MRI)　　Definition: Computer reformatted digital display of multiplanar images developed from the capture of radio-frequency signals emitted by nuclei in a body site excited within a magnetic field

Body Part Character 4	Contrast Character 5	Qualifier Character 6	Qualifier Character 7
0　Brain 9　Sella Turcica/Pituitary Gland B　Spinal Cord C　Acoustic Nerves	Y　Other Contrast	0　Unenhanced and Enhanced Z　None	Z　None
0　Brain 9　Sella Turcica/Pituitary Gland B　Spinal Cord C　Acoustic Nerves	Z　None	Z　None	Z　None

---

NC Noncovered Procedure　　**LC** Limited Coverage　　**UA** Questionable OB Admit　　**NT** New Tech Add-on　　⊞ Combination Member　　♂ Male　　♀ Female

B   **Imaging**
Ø   **Central Nervous System**
4   **Ultrasonography**   Definition: Real time display of images of anatomy or flow information developed from the capture of reflected and attenuated high frequency sound waves

Body Part Character 4	Contrast Character 5	Qualifier Character 6	Qualifier Character 7
Ø Brain B Spinal Cord	Z None	Z None	Z None

B   **Imaging**
2   **Heart**
Ø   **Plain Radiography**   Definition: Planar display of an image developed from the capture of external ionizing radiation on photographic or photoconductive plate

Body Part Character 4	Contrast Character 5	Qualifier Character 6	Qualifier Character 7
Ø Coronary Artery, Single 1 Coronary Arteries, Multiple 2 Coronary Artery Bypass Graft, Single 3 Coronary Artery Bypass Grafts, Multiple 4 Heart, Right 5 Heart, Left 6 Heart, Right and Left 7 Internal Mammary Bypass Graft, Right 8 Internal Mammary Bypass Graft, Left F Bypass Graft, Other	Ø High Osmolar 1 Low Osmolar Y Other Contrast	Z None	Z None

DRG Non-OR   All body part, contrast, and qualifier values

B   **Imaging**
2   **Heart**
1   **Fluoroscopy**   Definition: Single plane or bi-plane real time display of an image developed from the capture of external ionizing radioation on a fluorescent screen. The image may also be stored by either digital or analog means.

Body Part Character 4	Contrast Character 5	Qualifier Character 6	Qualifier Character 7
Ø Coronary Artery, Single 1 Coronary Arteries, Multiple 2 Coronary Artery Bypass Graft, Single 3 Coronary Artery Bypass Grafts, Multiple	Ø High Osmolar 1 Low Osmolar Y Other Contrast	1 Laser	Ø Intraoperative
Ø Coronary Artery, Single 1 Coronary Arteries, Multiple 2 Coronary Artery Bypass Graft, Single 3 Coronary Artery Bypass Grafts, Multiple	Ø High Osmolar 1 Low Osmolar Y Other Contrast	Z None	Z None
4 Heart, Right 5 Heart, Left 6 Heart, Right and Left 7 Internal Mammary Bypass Graft, Right 8 Internal Mammary Bypass Graft, Left F Bypass Graft, Other	Ø High Osmolar 1 Low Osmolar Y Other Contrast	Z None	Z None

DRG Non-OR   B21[Ø,1,2,3][Ø,1,Y]ZZ
DRG Non-OR   B21[4,5,6,7,8,F][Ø,1,Y]ZZ

B   **Imaging**
2   **Heart**
2   **Computerized Tomography (CT Scan)**   Definition: Computer reformatted digital display of multiplanar images developed from the capture of multiple exposures of external ionizing radiation

Body Part Character 4	Contrast Character 5	Qualifier Character 6	Qualifier Character 7
1 Coronary Arteries, Multiple 3 Coronary Artery Bypass Grafts, Multiple 6 Heart, Right and Left	Ø High Osmolar 1 Low Osmolar Y Other Contrast	Ø Unenhanced and Enhanced Z None	Z None
1 Coronary Arteries, Multiple 3 Coronary Artery Bypass Grafts, Multiple 6 Heart, Right and Left	Z None	2 Intravascular Optical Coherence Z None	Z None

B   Imaging
2   Heart
3   Magnetic Resonance Imaging (MRI)   Definition: Computer reformatted digital display of multiplanar images developed from the capture of radio-frequency signals emitted by nuclei in a body site excited within a magnetic field

Body Part Character 4	Contrast Character 5	Qualifier Character 6	Qualifier Character 7
1 Coronary Arteries, Multiple **3** Coronary Artery Bypass Grafts, Multiple **6** Heart, Right and Left	**Y** Other Contrast	**Ø** Unenhanced and Enhanced **Z** None	**Z** None
1 Coronary Arteries, Multiple **3** Coronary Artery Bypass Grafts, Multiple **6** Heart, Right and Left	**Z** None	**Z** None	**Z** None

B   Imaging
2   Heart
4   Ultrasonography   Definition: Real time display of images of anatomy or flow information developed from the capture of reflected and attenuated high frequency sound waves

Body Part Character 4	Contrast Character 5	Qualifier Character 6	Qualifier Character 7
Ø Coronary Artery, Single **1** Coronary Arteries, Multiple **4** Heart, Right **5** Heart, Left **6** Heart, Right and Left **B** Heart with Aorta **C** Pericardium **D** Pediatric Heart	**Y** Other Contrast	**Z** None	**Z** None
Ø Coronary Artery, Single **1** Coronary Arteries, Multiple **4** Heart, Right **5** Heart, Left **6** Heart, Right and Left **B** Heart with Aorta **C** Pericardium **D** Pediatric Heart	**Z** None	**Z** None	**3** Intravascular **4** Transesophageal **Z** None

B   Imaging
3   Upper Arteries
Ø   Plain Radiography   Definition: Planar display of an image developed from the capture of external ionizing radiation on photographic or photoconductive plate

Body Part Character 4	Contrast Character 5	Qualifier Character 6	Qualifier Character 7
Ø Thoracic Aorta **1** Brachiocephalic-Subclavian Artery, Right **2** Subclavian Artery, Left **3** Common Carotid Artery, Right **4** Common Carotid Artery, Left **5** Common Carotid Arteries, Bilateral **6** Internal Carotid Artery, Right **7** Internal Carotid Artery, Left **8** Internal Carotid Arteries, Bilateral **9** External Carotid Artery, Right **B** External Carotid Artery, Left **C** External Carotid Arteries, Bilateral **D** Vertebral Artery, Right **F** Vertebral Artery, Left **G** Vertebral Arteries, Bilateral **H** Upper Extremity Arteries, Right **J** Upper Extremity Arteries, Left **K** Upper Extremity Arteries, Bilateral **L** Intercostal and Bronchial Arteries **M** Spinal Arteries **N** Upper Arteries, Other **P** Thoraco-Abdominal Aorta **Q** Cervico-Cerebral Arch **R** Intracranial Arteries **S** Pulmonary Artery, Right **T** Pulmonary Artery, Left	**Ø** High Osmolar **1** Low Osmolar **Y** Other Contrast **Z** None	**Z** None	**Z** None

B   **Imaging**
3   **Upper Arteries**
1   **Fluoroscopy**   Definition: Single plane or bi-plane real time display of an image developed from the capture of external ionizing radiation on a fluorescent screen. The image may also be stored by either digital or analog means.

Body Part Character 4	Contrast Character 5	Qualifier Character 6	Qualifier Character 7
Ø Thoracic Aorta	Ø High Osmolar	1 Laser	Ø Intraoperative
1 Brachiocephalic-Subclavian Artery, Right	1 Low Osmolar		
2 Subclavian Artery, Left	Y Other Contrast		
3 Common Carotid Artery, Right			
4 Common Carotid Artery, Left			
5 Common Carotid Arteries, Bilateral			
6 Internal Carotid Artery, Right			
7 Internal Carotid Artery, Left			
8 Internal Carotid Arteries, Bilateral			
9 External Carotid Artery, Right			
B External Carotid Artery, Left			
C External Carotid Arteries, Bilateral			
D Vertebral Artery, Right			
F Vertebral Artery, Left			
G Vertebral Arteries, Bilateral			
H Upper Extremity Arteries, Right			
J Upper Extremity Arteries, Left			
K Upper Extremity Arteries, Bilateral			
L Intercostal and Bronchial Arteries			
M Spinal Arteries			
N Upper Arteries, Other			
P Thoraco-Abdominal Aorta			
Q Cervico-Cerebral Arch			
R Intracranial Arteries			
S Pulmonary Artery, Right			
T Pulmonary Artery, Left			
U Pulmonary Trunk			
Ø Thoracic Aorta	Ø High Osmolar	Z None	Z None
1 Brachiocephalic-Subclavian Artery, Right	1 Low Osmolar		
2 Subclavian Artery, Left	Y Other Contrast		
3 Common Carotid Artery, Right			
4 Common Carotid Artery, Left			
5 Common Carotid Arteries, Bilateral			
6 Internal Carotid Artery, Right			
7 Internal Carotid Artery, Left			
8 Internal Carotid Arteries, Bilateral			
9 External Carotid Artery, Right			
B External Carotid Artery, Left			
C External Carotid Arteries, Bilateral			
D Vertebral Artery, Right			
F Vertebral Artery, Left			
G Vertebral Arteries, Bilateral			
H Upper Extremity Arteries, Right			
J Upper Extremity Arteries, Left			
K Upper Extremity Arteries, Bilateral			
L Intercostal and Bronchial Arteries			
M Spinal Arteries			
N Upper Arteries, Other			
P Thoraco-Abdominal Aorta			
Q Cervico-Cerebral Arch			
R Intracranial Arteries			
S Pulmonary Artery, Right			
T Pulmonary Artery, Left			
U Pulmonary Trunk			

B31 Continued on next page

B   **Imaging**
3   **Upper Arteries**
1   **Fluoroscopy**   Definition: Single plane or bi-plane real time display of an image developed from the capture of external ionizing radiation on a fluorescent screen. The image may also be stored by either digital or analog means.

Body Part Character 4	Contrast Character 5	Qualifier Character 6	Qualifier Character 7
Ø Thoracic Aorta	Z None	Z None	Z None
1 Brachiocephalic-Subclavian Artery, Right			
2 Subclavian Artery, Left			
3 Common Carotid Artery, Right			
4 Common Carotid Artery, Left			
5 Common Carotid Arteries, Bilateral			
6 Internal Carotid Artery, Right			
7 Internal Carotid Artery, Left			
8 Internal Carotid Arteries, Bilateral			
9 External Carotid Artery, Right			
B External Carotid Artery, Left			
C External Carotid Arteries, Bilateral			
D Vertebral Artery, Right			
F Vertebral Artery, Left			
G Vertebral Arteries, Bilateral			
H Upper Extremity Arteries, Right			
J Upper Extremity Arteries, Left			
K Upper Extremity Arteries, Bilateral			
L Intercostal and Bronchial Arteries			
M Spinal Arteries			
N Upper Arteries, Other			
P Thoraco-Abdominal Aorta			
Q Cervico-Cerebral Arch			
R Intracranial Arteries			
S Pulmonary Artery, Right			
T Pulmonary Artery, Left			
U Pulmonary Trunk			

B   **Imaging**
3   **Upper Arteries**
2   **Computerized Tomography (CT Scan)**   Definition: Computer reformatted digital display of multiplanar images developed from the capture of multiple exposures of external ionizing radiation

Body Part Character 4	Contrast Character 5	Qualifier Character 6	Qualifier Character 7
Ø Thoracic Aorta	Ø High Osmolar	Z None	Z None
5 Common Carotid Arteries, Bilateral	1 Low Osmolar		
8 Internal Carotid Arteries, Bilateral	Y Other Contrast		
G Vertebral Arteries, Bilateral			
R Intracranial Arteries			
S Pulmonary Artery, Right			
T Pulmonary Artery, Left			
Ø Thoracic Aorta	Z None	2 Intravascular Optical Coherence	Z None
5 Common Carotid Arteries, Bilateral		Z None	
8 Internal Carotid Arteries, Bilateral			
G Vertebral Arteries, Bilateral			
R Intracranial Arteries			
S Pulmonary Artery, Right			
T Pulmonary Artery, Left			

Imaging

B   **Imaging**
3   **Upper Arteries**
3   **Magnetic Resonance Imaging (MRI)**   Definition: Computer reformatted digital display of multiplanar images developed from the capture of radio-frequency signals emitted by nuclei in a body site excited within a magnetic field

Body Part Character 4	Contrast Character 5	Qualifier Character 6	Qualifier Character 7
Ø Thoracic Aorta 5 Common Carotid Arteries, Bilateral 8 Internal Carotid Arteries, Bilateral G Vertebral Arteries, Bilateral H Upper Extremity Arteries, Right J Upper Extremity Arteries, Left K Upper Extremity Arteries, Bilateral M Spinal Arteries Q Cervico-Cerebral Arch R Intracranial Arteries	Y Other Contrast	Ø Unenhanced and Enhanced Z None	Z None
Ø Thoracic Aorta 5 Common Carotid Arteries, Bilateral 8 Internal Carotid Arteries, Bilateral G Vertebral Arteries, Bilateral H Upper Extremity Arteries, Right J Upper Extremity Arteries, Left K Upper Extremity Arteries, Bilateral M Spinal Arteries Q Cervico-Cerebral Arch R Intracranial Arteries	Z None	Z None	Z None

B   **Imaging**
3   **Upper Arteries**
4   **Ultrasonography**   Definition: Real time display of images of anatomy or flow information developed from the capture of reflected and attenuated high frequency sound waves

Body Part Character 4	Contrast Character 5	Qualifier Character 6	Qualifier Character 7
Ø Thoracic Aorta 1 Brachiocephalic-Subclavian Artery, Right 2 Subclavian Artery, Left 3 Common Carotid Artery, Right 4 Common Carotid Artery, Left 5 Common Carotid Arteries, Bilateral 6 Internal Carotid Artery, Right 7 Internal Carotid Artery, Left 8 Internal Carotid Arteries, Bilateral H Upper Extremity Arteries, Right J Upper Extremity Arteries, Left K Upper Extremity Arteries, Bilateral R Intracranial Arteries S Pulmonary Artery, Right T Pulmonary Artery, Left V Ophthalmic Arteries	Z None	Z None	3 Intravascular Z None

B   **Imaging**
4   **Lower Arteries**
Ø   **Plain Radiography**   Definition: Planar display of an image developed from the capture of external ionizing radiation on photographic or photoconductive plate

Body Part Character 4	Contrast Character 5	Qualifier Character 6	Qualifier Character 7
Ø Abdominal Aorta 2 Hepatic Artery 3 Splenic Arteries 4 Superior Mesenteric Artery 5 Inferior Mesenteric Artery 6 Renal Artery, Right 7 Renal Artery, Left 8 Renal Arteries, Bilateral 9 Lumbar Arteries B Intra-Abdominal Arteries, Other C Pelvic Arteries D Aorta and Bilateral Lower Extremity Arteries F Lower Extremity Arteries, Right G Lower Extremity Arteries, Left J Lower Arteries, Other M Renal Artery Transplant	Ø High Osmolar 1 Low Osmolar Y Other Contrast	Z None	Z None

B   **Imaging**
4   **Lower Arteries**
1   **Fluoroscopy**   Definition: Single plane or bi-plane real time display of an image developed from the capture of external ionizing radiation on a fluorescent screen. The image may also be stored by either digital or analog means.

Body Part Character 4	Contrast Character 5	Qualifier Character 6	Qualifier Character 7
Ø Abdominal Aorta **2** Hepatic Artery **3** Splenic Arteries **4** Superior Mesenteric Artery **5** Inferior Mesenteric Artery **6** Renal Artery, Right **7** Renal Artery, Left **8** Renal Arteries, Bilateral **9** Lumbar Arteries **B** Intra-Abdominal Arteries, Other **C** Pelvic Arteries **D** Aorta and Bilateral Lower Extremity Arteries **F** Lower Extremity Arteries, Right **G** Lower Extremity Arteries, Left **J** Lower Arteries, Other	**Ø** High Osmolar **1** Low Osmolar **Y** Other Contrast	**1** Laser	**Ø** Intraoperative
Ø Abdominal Aorta **2** Hepatic Artery **3** Splenic Arteries **4** Superior Mesenteric Artery **5** Inferior Mesenteric Artery **6** Renal Artery, Right **7** Renal Artery, Left **8** Renal Arteries, Bilateral **9** Lumbar Arteries **B** Intra-Abdominal Arteries, Other **C** Pelvic Arteries **D** Aorta and Bilateral Lower Extremity Arteries **F** Lower Extremity Arteries, Right **G** Lower Extremity Arteries, Left **J** Lower Arteries, Other	**Ø** High Osmolar **1** Low Osmolar **Y** Other Contrast	**Z** None	**Z** None
Ø Abdominal Aorta **2** Hepatic Artery **3** Splenic Arteries **4** Superior Mesenteric Artery **5** Inferior Mesenteric Artery **6** Renal Artery, Right **7** Renal Artery, Left **8** Renal Arteries, Bilateral **9** Lumbar Arteries **B** Intra-Abdominal Arteries, Other **C** Pelvic Arteries **D** Aorta and Bilateral Lower Extremity Arteries **F** Lower Extremity Arteries, Right **G** Lower Extremity Arteries, Left **J** Lower Arteries, Other	**Z** None	**Z** None	**Z** None

Imaging

B Imaging
4 Lower Arteries
2 Computerized Tomography (CT Scan) Definition: Computer reformatted digital display of multiplanar images developed from the capture of multiple exposures of external ionizing radiation

Body Part Character 4	Contrast Character 5	Qualifier Character 6	Qualifier Character 7
Ø Abdominal Aorta 1 Celiac Artery 4 Superior Mesenteric Artery 8 Renal Arteries, Bilateral C Pelvic Arteries F Lower Extremity Arteries, Right G Lower Extremity Arteries, Left H Lower Extremity Arteries, Bilateral M Renal Artery Transplant	Ø High Osmolar 1 Low Osmolar Y Other Contrast	Z None	Z None
Ø Abdominal Aorta 1 Celiac Artery 4 Superior Mesenteric Artery 8 Renal Arteries, Bilateral C Pelvic Arteries F Lower Extremity Arteries, Right G Lower Extremity Arteries, Left H Lower Extremity Arteries, Bilateral M Renal Artery Transplant	Z None	2 Intravascular Optical Coherence Z None	Z None

B Imaging
4 Lower Arteries
3 Magnetic Resonance Imaging (MRI) Definition: Computer reformatted digital display of multiplanar images developed from the capture of radio-frequency signals emitted by nuclei in a body site excited within a magnetic field

Body Part Character 4	Contrast Character 5	Qualifier Character 6	Qualifier Character 7
Ø Abdominal Aorta 1 Celiac Artery 4 Superior Mesenteric Artery 8 Renal Arteries, Bilateral C Pelvic Arteries F Lower Extremity Arteries, Right G Lower Extremity Arteries, Left H Lower Extremity Arteries, Bilateral	Y Other Contrast	Ø Unenhanced and Enhanced Z None	Z None
Ø Abdominal Aorta 1 Celiac Artery 4 Superior Mesenteric Artery 8 Renal Arteries, Bilateral C Pelvic Arteries F Lower Extremity Arteries, Right G Lower Extremity Arteries, Left H Lower Extremity Arteries, Bilateral	Z None	Z None	Z None

B Imaging
4 Lower Arteries
4 Ultrasonography Definition: Real time display of images of anatomy or flow information developed from the capture of reflected and attenuated high frequency sound waves

Body Part Character 4	Contrast Character 5	Qualifier Character 6	Qualifier Character 7
Ø Abdominal Aorta 4 Superior Mesenteric Artery 5 Inferior Mesenteric Artery 6 Renal Artery, Right 7 Renal Artery, Left 8 Renal Arteries, Bilateral B Intra-Abdominal Arteries, Other F Lower Extremity Arteries, Right G Lower Extremity Arteries, Left H Lower Extremity Arteries, Bilateral K Celiac and Mesenteric Arteries L Femoral Artery N Penile Arteries	Z None	Z None	3 Intravascular Z None

B Imaging
5 Veins
Ø Plain Radiography Definition: Planar display of an image developed from the capture of external ionizing radiation on photographic or photoconductive plate

Body Part Character 4	Contrast Character 5	Qualifier Character 6	Qualifier Character 7
Ø Epidural Veins	Ø High Osmolar	Z None	Z None
1 Cerebral and Cerebellar Veins	1 Low Osmolar		
2 Intracranial Sinuses	Y Other Contrast		
3 Jugular Veins, Right			
4 Jugular Veins, Left			
5 Jugular Veins, Bilateral			
6 Subclavian Vein, Right			
7 Subclavian Vein, Left			
8 Superior Vena Cava			
9 Inferior Vena Cava			
B Lower Extremity Veins, Right			
C Lower Extremity Veins, Left			
D Lower Extremity Veins, Bilateral			
F Pelvic (Iliac) Veins, Right			
G Pelvic (Iliac) Veins, Left			
H Pelvic (Iliac) Veins, Bilateral			
J Renal Vein, Right			
K Renal Vein, Left			
L Renal Veins, Bilateral			
M Upper Extremity Veins, Right			
N Upper Extremity Veins, Left			
P Upper Extremity Veins, Bilateral			
Q Pulmonary Vein, Right			
R Pulmonary Vein, Left			
S Pulmonary Veins, Bilateral			
T Portal and Splanchnic Veins			
V Veins, Other			
W Dialysis Shunt/Fistula			

B Imaging
5 Veins
1 Fluoroscopy Definition: Single plane or bi-plane real time display of an image developed from the capture of external ionizing radioation on a fluorescent screen. The image may also be stored by either digital or analog means.

Body Part Character 4	Contrast Character 5	Qualifier Character 6	Qualifier Character 7
Ø Epidural Veins	Ø High Osmolar	Z None	A Guidance
1 Cerebral and Cerebellar Veins	1 Low Osmolar		Z None
2 Intracranial Sinuses	Y Other Contrast		
3 Jugular Veins, Right	Z None		
4 Jugular Veins, Left			
5 Jugular Veins, Bilateral			
6 Subclavian Vein, Right			
7 Subclavian Vein, Left			
8 Superior Vena Cava			
9 Inferior Vena Cava			
B Lower Extremity Veins, Right			
C Lower Extremity Veins, Left			
D Lower Extremity Veins, Bilateral			
F Pelvic (Iliac) Veins, Right			
G Pelvic (Iliac) Veins, Left			
H Pelvic (Iliac) Veins, Bilateral			
J Renal Vein, Right			
K Renal Vein, Left			
L Renal Veins, Bilateral			
M Upper Extremity Veins, Right			
N Upper Extremity Veins, Left			
P Upper Extremity Veins, Bilateral			
Q Pulmonary Vein, Right			
R Pulmonary Vein, Left			
S Pulmonary Veins, Bilateral			
T Portal and Splanchnic Veins			
V Veins, Other			
W Dialysis Shunt/Fistula			

NC Noncovered Procedure LC Limited Coverage QA Questionable OB Admit NT New Tech Add-on ⊞ Combination Member ♂ Male ♀ Female
ICD-10-PCS 2022 749

B5Ø-B51

Imaging

B   **Imaging**
5   **Veins**
2   **Computerized Tomography (CT Scan)**   Definition: Computer reformatted digital display of multiplanar images developed from the capture of multiple exposures of external ionizing radiation

Body Part Character 4	Contrast Character 5	Qualifier Character 6	Qualifier Character 7
2 Intracranial Sinuses 8 Superior Vena Cava 9 Inferior Vena Cava F Pelvic (Iliac) Veins, Right G Pelvic (Iliac) Veins, Left H Pelvic (Iliac) Veins, Bilateral J Renal Vein, Right K Renal Vein, Left L Renal Veins, Bilateral Q Pulmonary Vein, Right R Pulmonary Vein, Left S Pulmonary Veins, Bilateral T Portal and Splanchnic Veins	Ø High Osmolar 1 Low Osmolar Y Other Contrast	Ø Unenhanced and Enhanced Z None	Z None
2 Intracranial Sinuses 8 Superior Vena Cava 9 Inferior Vena Cava F Pelvic (Iliac) Veins, Right G Pelvic (Iliac) Veins, Left H Pelvic (Iliac) Veins, Bilateral J Renal Vein, Right K Renal Vein, Left L Renal Veins, Bilateral Q Pulmonary Vein, Right R Pulmonary Vein, Left S Pulmonary Veins, Bilateral T Portal and Splanchnic Veins	Z None	2 Intravascular Optical Coherence Z None	Z None

B   **Imaging**
5   **Veins**
3   **Magnetic Resonance Imaging (MRI)**   Definition: Computer reformatted digital display of multiplanar images developed from the capture of radio-frequency signals emitted by nuclei in a body site excited within a magnetic field

Body Part Character 4	Contrast Character 5	Qualifier Character 6	Qualifier Character 7
1 Cerebral and Cerebellar Veins 2 Intracranial Sinuses 5 Jugular Veins, Bilateral 8 Superior Vena Cava 9 Inferior Vena Cava B Lower Extremity Veins, Right C Lower Extremity Veins, Left D Lower Extremity Veins, Bilateral H Pelvic (Iliac) Veins, Bilateral L Renal Veins, Bilateral M Upper Extremity Veins, Right N Upper Extremity Veins, Left P Upper Extremity Veins, Bilateral S Pulmonary Veins, Bilateral T Portal and Splanchnic Veins V Veins, Other	Y Other Contrast	Ø Unenhanced and Enhanced Z None	Z None
1 Cerebral and Cerebellar Veins 2 Intracranial Sinuses 5 Jugular Veins, Bilateral 8 Superior Vena Cava 9 Inferior Vena Cava B Lower Extremity Veins, Right C Lower Extremity Veins, Left D Lower Extremity Veins, Bilateral H Pelvic (Iliac) Veins, Bilateral L Renal Veins, Bilateral M Upper Extremity Veins, Right N Upper Extremity Veins, Left P Upper Extremity Veins, Bilateral S Pulmonary Veins, Bilateral T Portal and Splanchnic Veins V Veins, Other	Z None	Z None	Z None

B   Imaging
5   Veins
4   Ultrasonography   Definition: Real time display of images of anatomy or flow information developed from the capture of reflected and attenuated high frequency sound waves

Body Part Character 4	Contrast Character 5	Qualifier Character 6	Qualifier Character 7
3 Jugular Veins, Right 4 Jugular Veins, Left 6 Subclavian Vein, Right 7 Subclavian Vein, Left 8 Superior Vena Cava 9 Inferior Vena Cava B Lower Extremity Veins, Right C Lower Extremity Veins, Left D Lower Extremity Veins, Bilateral J Renal Vein, Right K Renal Vein, Left L Renal Veins, Bilateral M Upper Extremity Veins, Right N Upper Extremity Veins, Left P Upper Extremity Veins, Bilateral T Portal and Splanchnic Veins	Z None	Z None	3 Intravascular A Guidance Z None

B   Imaging
7   Lymphatic System
0   Plain Radiography   Definition: Planar display of an image developed from the capture of external ionizing radiation on photographic or photoconductive plate

Body Part Character 4	Contrast Character 5	Qualifier Character 6	Qualifier Character 7

0   Abdominal/Retroperitoneal
    Lymphatics, Unilateral
1   Abdominal/Retroperitoneal
    Lymphatics, Bilateral
4   Lymphatics, Head and Neck
5   Upper Extremity Lymphatics, Right
6   Upper Extremity Lymphatics, Left
7   Upper Extremity Lymphatics,
    Bilateral
8   Lower Extremity Lymphatics, Right
9   Lower Extremity Lymphatics, Left
B   Lower Extremity Lymphatics,
    Bilateral
C   Lymphatics, Pelvic
	0 High Osmolar
	1 Low Osmolar
	Y Other Contrast
		Z None	Z None

B   Imaging
8   Eye
0   Plain Radiography   Definition: Planar display of an image developed from the capture of external ionizing radiation on photographic or photoconductive plate

Body Part Character 4	Contrast Character 5	Qualifier Character 6	Qualifier Character 7
0 Lacrimal Duct, Right 1 Lacrimal Duct, Left 2 Lacrimal Ducts, Bilateral	0 High Osmolar 1 Low Osmolar Y Other Contrast	Z None	Z None
3 Optic Foramina, Right 4 Optic Foramina, Left 5 Eye, Right 6 Eye, Left 7 Eyes, Bilateral	Z None	Z None	Z None

B   Imaging
8   Eye
2   Computerized Tomography (CT Scan)   Definition: Computer reformatted digital display of multiplanar images developed from the capture of multiple exposures of external ionizing radiation

Body Part Character 4	Contrast Character 5	Qualifier Character 6	Qualifier Character 7
5 Eye, Right 6 Eye, Left 7 Eyes, Bilateral	0 High Osmolar 1 Low Osmolar Y Other Contrast	0 Unenhanced and Enhanced Z None	Z None
5 Eye, Right 6 Eye, Left 7 Eyes, Bilateral	Z None	Z None	Z None

NC Noncovered Procedure   **LC** Limited Coverage   **QA** Questionable OB Admit   **NT** New Tech Add-on   ⊞ Combination Member   ♂ Male   ♀ Female

ICD-10-PCS 2022   751

B54–B82

B   Imaging
8   Eye
3   Magnetic Resonance Imaging (MRI)   Definition: Computer reformatted digital display of multiplanar images developed from the capture of radio-frequency signals emitted by nuclei in a body site excited within a magnetic field

Body Part Character 4	Contrast Character 5	Qualifier Character 6	Qualifier Character 7
5 Eye, Right 6 Eye, Left 7 Eyes, Bilateral	Y Other Contrast	Ø Unenhanced and Enhanced Z None	Z None
5 Eye, Right 6 Eye, Left 7 Eyes, Bilateral	Z None	Z None	Z None

B   Imaging
8   Eye
4   Ultrasonography   Definition: Real time display of images of anatomy or flow information developed from the capture of reflected and attenuated high frequency sound waves

Body Part Character 4	Contrast Character 5	Qualifier Character 6	Qualifier Character 7
5 Eye, Right 6 Eye, Left 7 Eyes, Bilateral	Z None	Z None	Z None

B   Imaging
9   Ear, Nose, Mouth and Throat
Ø   Plain Radiography   Definition: Planar display of an image developed from the capture of external ionizing radiation on photographic or photoconductive plate

Body Part Character 4	Contrast Character 5	Qualifier Character 6	Qualifier Character 7
2 Paranasal Sinuses F Nasopharynx/Oropharynx H Mastoids	Z None	Z None	Z None
4 Parotid Gland, Right 5 Parotid Gland, Left 6 Parotid Glands, Bilateral 7 Submandibular Gland, Right 8 Submandibular Gland, Left 9 Submandibular Glands, Bilateral B Salivary Gland, Right C Salivary Gland, Left D Salivary Glands, Bilateral	Ø High Osmolar 1 Low Osmolar Y Other Contrast	Z None	Z None

B   Imaging
9   Ear, Nose, Mouth and Throat
1   Fluoroscopy   Definition: Single plane or bi-plane real time display of an image developed from the capture of external ionizing radioation on a fluorescent screen. The image may also be stored by either digital or analog means.

Body Part Character 4	Contrast Character 5	Qualifier Character 6	Qualifier Character 7
G Pharynx and Epiglottis J Larynx	Y Other Contrast Z None	Z None	Z None

B   Imaging
9   Ear, Nose, Mouth and Throat
2   Computerized Tomography (CT Scan)   Definition: Computer reformatted digital display of multiplanar images developed from the capture of multiple exposures of external ionizing radiation

Body Part Character 4	Contrast Character 5	Qualifier Character 6	Qualifier Character 7
Ø Ear 2 Paranasal Sinuses 6 Parotid Glands, Bilateral 9 Submandibular Glands, Bilateral D Salivary Glands, Bilateral F Nasopharynx/Oropharynx J Larynx	Ø High Osmolar 1 Low Osmolar Y Other Contrast	Ø Unenhanced and Enhanced Z None	Z None
Ø Ear 2 Paranasal Sinuses 6 Parotid Glands, Bilateral 9 Submandibular Glands, Bilateral D Salivary Glands, Bilateral F Nasopharynx/Oropharynx J Larynx	Z None	Z None	Z None

B   **Imaging**
9   **Ear, Nose, Mouth and Throat**
3   **Magnetic Resonance Imaging (MRI)**   Definition: Computer reformatted digital display of multiplanar images developed from the capture of radio-frequency signals emitted by nuclei in a body site excited within a magnetic field

Body Part Character 4	Contrast Character 5	Qualifier Character 6	Qualifier Character 7
Ø Ear 2 Paranasal Sinuses 6 Parotid Glands, Bilateral 9 Submandibular Glands, Bilateral D Salivary Glands, Bilateral F Nasopharynx/Oropharynx J Larynx	Y Other Contrast	Ø Unenhanced and Enhanced Z None	Z None
Ø Ear 2 Paranasal Sinuses 6 Parotid Glands, Bilateral 9 Submandibular Glands, Bilateral D Salivary Glands, Bilateral F Nasopharynx/Oropharynx J Larynx	Z None	Z None	Z None

B   **Imaging**
B   **Respiratory System**
Ø   **Plain Radiography**   Definition: Planar display of an image developed from the capture of external ionizing radiation on photographic or photoconductive plate

Body Part Character 4	Contrast Character 5	Qualifier Character 6	Qualifier Character 7
7 Tracheobronchial Tree, Right 8 Tracheobronchial Tree, Left 9 Tracheobronchial Trees, Bilateral	Y Other Contrast	Z None	Z None
D Upper Airways	Z None	Z None	Z None

B   **Imaging**
B   **Respiratory System**
1   **Fluoroscopy**   Definition: Single plane or bi-plane real time display of an image developed from the capture of external ionizing radioation on a fluorescent screen. The image may also be stored by either digital or analog means.

Body Part Character 4	Contrast Character 5	Qualifier Character 6	Qualifier Character 7
2 Lung, Right 3 Lung, Left 4 Lungs, Bilateral 6 Diaphragm C Mediastinum D Upper Airways	Z None	Z None	Z None
7 Tracheobronchial Tree, Right 8 Tracheobronchial Tree, Left 9 Tracheobronchial Trees, Bilateral	Y Other Contrast	Z None	Z None

B   **Imaging**
B   **Respiratory System**
2   **Computerized Tomography (CT Scan)**   Definition: Computer reformatted digital display of multiplanar images developed from the capture of multiple exposures of external ionizing radiation

Body Part Character 4	Contrast Character 5	Qualifier Character 6	Qualifier Character 7
4 Lungs, Bilateral 7 Tracheobronchial Tree, Right 8 Tracheobronchial Tree, Left 9 Tracheobronchial Trees, Bilateral F Trachea/Airways	Ø High Osmolar 1 Low Osmolar Y Other Contrast	Ø Unenhanced and Enhanced Z None	Z None
4 Lungs, Bilateral 7 Tracheobronchial Tree, Right 8 Tracheobronchial Tree, Left 9 Tracheobronchial Trees, Bilateral F Trachea/Airways	Z None	Z None	Z None

NC Noncovered Procedure   LC Limited Coverage   QA Questionable OB Admit   NT New Tech Add-on   ⊞ Combination Member   ♂ Male   ♀ Female

ICD-10-PCS 2022   753

B93–BB2

B   Imaging
B   Respiratory System
3   Magnetic Resonance Imaging (MRI)   Definition: Computer reformatted digital display of multiplanar images developed from the capture of radio-frequency signals emitted by nuclei in a body site excited within a magnetic field

Body Part Character 4	Contrast Character 5	Qualifier Character 6	Qualifier Character 7
G Lung Apices	Y Other Contrast	0 Unenhanced and Enhanced Z None	Z None
G Lung Apices	Z None	Z None	Z None

B   Imaging
B   Respiratory System
4   Ultrasonography   Definition: Real time display of images of anatomy or flow information developed from the capture of reflected and attenuated high frequency sound waves

Body Part Character 4	Contrast Character 5	Qualifier Character 6	Qualifier Character 7
B Pleura C Mediastinum	Z None	Z None	Z None

B   Imaging
D   Gastrointestinal System
1   Fluoroscopy   Definition: Single plane or bi-plane real time display of an image developed from the capture of external ionizing radioation on a fluorescent screen. The image may also be stored by either digital or analog means.

Body Part Character 4	Contrast Character 5	Qualifier Character 6	Qualifier Character 7
1 Esophagus 2 Stomach 3 Small Bowel 4 Colon 5 Upper GI 6 Upper GI and Small Bowel 9 Duodenum B Mouth/Oropharynx	Y Other Contrast Z None	Z None	Z None

B   Imaging
D   Gastrointestinal System
2   Computerized Tomography (CT Scan)   Definition: Computer reformatted digital display of multiplanar images developed from the capture of multiple exposures of external ionizing radiation

Body Part Character 4	Contrast Character 5	Qualifier Character 6	Qualifier Character 7
4 Colon	0 High Osmolar 1 Low Osmolar Y Other Contrast	0 Unenhanced and Enhanced Z None	Z None
4 Colon	Z None	Z None	Z None

B   Imaging
D   Gastrointestinal System
4   Ultrasonography   Definition: Real time display of images of anatomy or flow information developed from the capture of reflected and attenuated high frequency sound waves

Body Part Character 4	Contrast Character 5	Qualifier Character 6	Qualifier Character 7
1 Esophagus 2 Stomach 7 Gastrointestinal Tract 8 Appendix 9 Duodenum C Rectum	Z None	Z None	Z None

B   Imaging
F   Hepatobiliary System and Pancreas
0   Plain Radiography   Definition: Planar display of an image developed from the capture of external ionizing radiation on photographic or photoconductive plate

Body Part Character 4	Contrast Character 5	Qualifier Character 6	Qualifier Character 7
0 Bile Ducts 3 Gallbladder and Bile Ducts C Hepatobiliary System, All	0 High Osmolar 1 Low Osmolar Y Other Contrast	Z None	Z None

B   **Imaging**
F   **Hepatobiliary System and Pancreas**
1   **Fluoroscopy**   Definition: Single plane or bi-plane real time display of an image developed from the capture of external ionizing radioation on a fluorescent screen. The image may also be stored by either digital or analog means.

Body Part Character 4	Contrast Character 5	Qualifier Character 6	Qualifier Character 7
Ø Bile Ducts 1 Biliary and Pancreatic Ducts 2 Gallbladder 3 Gallbladder and Bile Ducts 4 Gallbladder, Bile Ducts and Pancreatic Ducts 8 Pancreatic Ducts	Ø High Osmolar 1 Low Osmolar Y Other Contrast	Z None	Z None
5 Liver	Ø High Osmolar 1 Low Osmolar Y Other Contrast	Z None	Z None
5 Liver	Z None	Z None	A Guidance

B   **Imaging**
F   **Hepatobiliary System and Pancreas**
2   **Computerized Tomography (CT Scan)**   Definition: Computer reformatted digital display of multiplanar images developed from the capture of multiple exposures of external ionizing radiation

Body Part Character 4	Contrast Character 5	Qualifier Character 6	Qualifier Character 7
5 Liver 6 Liver and Spleen 7 Pancreas C Hepatobiliary System, All	Ø High Osmolar 1 Low Osmolar Y Other Contrast	Ø Unenhanced and Enhanced Z None	Z None
5 Liver 6 Liver and Spleen 7 Pancreas C Hepatobiliary System, All	Z None	Z None	Z None

B   **Imaging**
F   **Hepatobiliary System and Pancreas**
3   **Magnetic Resonance Imaging (MRI)**   Definition: Computer reformatted digital display of multiplanar images developed from the capture of radio-frequency signals emitted by nuclei in a body site excited within a magnetic field

Body Part Character 4	Contrast Character 5	Qualifier Character 6	Qualifier Character 7
5 Liver 6 Liver and Spleen 7 Pancreas	Y Other Contrast	Ø Unenhanced and Enhanced Z None	Z None
5 Liver 6 Liver and Spleen 7 Pancreas	Z None	Z None	Z None

B   **Imaging**
F   **Hepatobiliary System and Pancreas**
4   **Ultrasonography**   Definition: Real time display of images of anatomy or flow information developed from the capture of reflected and attenuated high frequency sound waves

Body Part Character 4	Contrast Character 5	Qualifier Character 6	Qualifier Character 7
Ø Bile Ducts 2 Gallbladder 3 Gallbladder and Bile Ducts 5 Liver 6 Liver and Spleen 7 Pancreas C Hepatobiliary System, All	Z None	Z None	Z None

B   **Imaging**
F   **Hepatobiliary System and Pancreas**
5   **Other Imaging**   Definition: Other specified modality for visualizing a body part

Body Part Character 4	Contrast Character 5	Qualifier Character 6	Qualifier Character 7
Ø Bile Ducts 2 Gallbladder 3 Gallbladder and Bile Ducts 5 Liver 6 Liver and Spleen 7 Pancreas C Hepatobiliary System, All	2 Fluorescing Agent	Ø Indocyanine Green Dye Z None	Ø Intraoperative Z None

NC Noncovered Procedure   **LC** Limited Coverage   **QA** Questionable OB Admit   **NT** New Tech Add-on   ⊞ Combination Member   ♂ Male   ♀ Female

B   Imaging
G   Endocrine System
2   Computerized Tomography (CT Scan)   Definition: Computer reformatted digital display of multiplanar images developed from the capture of multiple exposures of external ionizing radiation

Body Part Character 4	Contrast Character 5	Qualifier Character 6	Qualifier Character 7
2 Adrenal Glands, Bilateral 3 Parathyroid Glands 4 Thyroid Gland	Ø High Osmolar 1 Low Osmolar Y Other Contrast	Ø Unenhanced and Enhanced Z None	Z None
2 Adrenal Glands, Bilateral 3 Parathyroid Glands 4 Thyroid Gland	Z None	Z None	Z None

B   Imaging
G   Endocrine System
3   Magnetic Resonance Imaging (MRI)   Definition: Computer reformatted digital display of multiplanar images developed from the capture of radio-frequency signals emitted by nuclei in a body site excited within a magnetic field

Body Part Character 4	Contrast Character 5	Qualifier Character 6	Qualifier Character 7
2 Adrenal Glands, Bilateral 3 Parathyroid Glands 4 Thyroid Gland	Y Other Contrast	Ø Unenhanced and Enhanced Z None	Z None
2 Adrenal Glands, Bilateral 3 Parathyroid Glands 4 Thyroid Gland	Z None	Z None	Z None

B   Imaging
G   Endocrine System
4   Ultrasonography   Definition: Real time display of images of anatomy or flow information developed from the capture of reflected and attenuated high frequency sound waves

Body Part Character 4	Contrast Character 5	Qualifier Character 6	Qualifier Character 7
Ø Adrenal Gland, Right 1 Adrenal Gland, Left 2 Adrenal Glands, Bilateral 3 Parathyroid Glands 4 Thyroid Gland	Z None	Z None	Z None

B   Imaging
H   Skin, Subcutaneous Tissue and Breast
Ø   Plain Radiography   Definition: Planar display of an image developed from the capture of external ionizing radiation on photographic or photoconductive plate

Body Part Character 4	Contrast Character 5	Qualifier Character 6	Qualifier Character 7
Ø Breast, Right 1 Breast, Left 2 Breasts, Bilateral	Z None	Z None	Z None
3 Single Mammary Duct, Right 4 Single Mammary Duct, Left 5 Multiple Mammary Ducts, Right 6 Multiple Mammary Ducts, Left	Ø High Osmolar 1 Low Osmolar Y Other Contrast Z None	Z None	Z None

B   **Imaging**
H   **Skin, Subcutaneous Tissue and Breast**
3   **Magnetic Resonance Imaging (MRI)**   Definition: Computer reformatted digital display of multiplanar images developed from the capture of radio-frequency signals emitted by nuclei in a body site excited within a magnetic field

Body Part Character 4	Contrast Character 5	Qualifier Character 6	Qualifier Character 7

Ø Breast, Right
1 Breast, Left
2 Breasts, Bilateral
D Subcutaneous Tissue, Head/Neck
F Subcutaneous Tissue, Upper
    Extremity
G Subcutaneous Tissue, Thorax
H Subcutaneous Tissue, Abdomen
    and Pelvis
J Subcutaneous Tissue, Lower
    Extremity
	Y Other Contrast	**Ø** Unenhanced and Enhanced
		Z None
			Z None

Ø Breast, Right
1 Breast, Left
2 Breasts, Bilateral
D Subcutaneous Tissue, Head/Neck
F Subcutaneous Tissue, Upper
    Extremity
G Subcutaneous Tissue, Thorax
H Subcutaneous Tissue, Abdomen
    and Pelvis
J Subcutaneous Tissue, Lower
    Extremity
	Z None	**Z** None	**Z** None

B   **Imaging**
H   **Skin, Subcutaneous Tissue and Breast**
4   **Ultrasonography**   Definition: Real time display of images of anatomy or flow information developed from the capture of reflected and attenuated high frequency sound waves

Body Part Character 4	Contrast Character 5	Qualifier Character 6	Qualifier Character 7
Ø Breast, Right **1** Breast, Left **2** Breasts, Bilateral **7** Extremity, Upper **8** Extremity, Lower **9** Abdominal Wall **B** Chest Wall **C** Head and Neck	**Z** None	**Z** None	**Z** None

B   **Imaging**
L   **Connective Tissue**
3   **Magnetic Resonance Imaging (MRI)**   Definition: Computer reformatted digital display of multiplanar images developed from the capture of radio-frequency signals emitted by nuclei in a body site excited within a magnetic field

Body Part Character 4	Contrast Character 5	Qualifier Character 6	Qualifier Character 7
Ø Connective Tissue, Upper Extremity **1** Connective Tissue, Lower Extremity **2** Tendons, Upper Extremity **3** Tendons, Lower Extremity	**Y** Other Contrast	**Ø** Unenhanced and Enhanced **Z** None	**Z** None
Ø Connective Tissue, Upper Extremity **1** Connective Tissue, Lower Extremity **2** Tendons, Upper Extremity **3** Tendons, Lower Extremity	**Z** None	**Z** None	**Z** None

B   **Imaging**
L   **Connective Tissue**
4   **Ultrasonography**   Definition: Real time display of images of anatomy or flow information developed from the capture of reflected and attenuated high frequency sound waves

Body Part Character 4	Contrast Character 5	Qualifier Character 6	Qualifier Character 7
Ø Connective Tissue, Upper Extremity **1** Connective Tissue, Lower Extremity **2** Tendons, Upper Extremity **3** Tendons, Lower Extremity	**Z** None	**Z** None	**Z** None

B **Imaging**
N **Skull and Facial Bones**
0 **Plain Radiography** Definition: Planar display of an image developed from the capture of external ionizing radiation on photographic or photoconductive plate

Body Part Character 4	Contrast Character 5	Qualifier Character 6	Qualifier Character 7
0 Skull **1** Orbit, Right **2** Orbit, Left **3** Orbits, Bilateral **4** Nasal Bones **5** Facial Bones **6** Mandible **B** Zygomatic Arch, Right **C** Zygomatic Arch, Left **D** Zygomatic Arches, Bilateral **G** Tooth, Single **H** Teeth, Multiple **J** Teeth, All	**Z** None	**Z** None	**Z** None
7 Temporomandibular Joint, Right **8** Temporomandibular Joint, Left **9** Temporomandibular Joints, Bilateral	**0** High Osmolar **1** Low Osmolar **Y** Other Contrast **Z** None	**Z** None	**Z** None

B **Imaging**
N **Skull and Facial Bones**
1 **Fluoroscopy** Definition: Single plane or bi-plane real time display of an image developed from the capture of external ionizing radioation on a fluorescent screen. The image may also be stored by either digital or analog means.

Body Part Character 4	Contrast Character 5	Qualifier Character 6	Qualifier Character 7
7 Temporomandibular Joint, Right **8** Temporomandibular Joint, Left **9** Temporomandibular Joints, Bilateral	**0** High Osmolar **1** Low Osmolar **Y** Other Contrast **Z** None	**Z** None	**Z** None

B **Imaging**
N **Skull and Facial Bones**
2 **Computerized Tomography (CT Scan)** Definition: Computer reformatted digital display of multiplanar images developed from the capture of multiple exposures of external ionizing radiation

Body Part Character 4	Contrast Character 5	Qualifier Character 6	Qualifier Character 7
0 Skull **3** Orbits, Bilateral **5** Facial Bones **6** Mandible **9** Temporomandibular Joints, Bilateral **F** Temporal Bones	**0** High Osmolar **1** Low Osmolar **Y** Other Contrast **Z** None	**Z** None	**Z** None

B **Imaging**
N **Skull and Facial Bones**
3 **Magnetic Resonance Imaging (MRI)** Definition: Computer reformatted digital display of multiplanar images developed from the capture of radio-frequency signals emitted by nuclei in a body site excited within a magnetic field

Body Part Character 4	Contrast Character 5	Qualifier Character 6	Qualifier Character 7
9 Temporomandibular Joints, Bilateral	**Y** Other Contrast **Z** None	**Z** None	**Z** None

Non-OR Procedure   DRG Non-OR Procedure   Valid OR Procedure   HAC Associated Procedure   Combination Only   New/Revised GREEN
758   ICD-10-PCS 2022

BN0–BN3

B   **Imaging**
P   **Non-Axial Upper Bones**
0   **Plain Radiography**   Definition: Planar display of an image developed from the capture of external ionizing radiation on photographic or photoconductive plate

Body Part Character 4	Contrast Character 5	Qualifier Character 6	Qualifier Character 7
0 Sternoclavicular Joint, Right 1 Sternoclavicular Joint, Left 2 Sternoclavicular Joints, Bilateral 3 Acromioclavicular Joints, Bilateral 4 Clavicle, Right 5 Clavicle, Left 6 Scapula, Right 7 Scapula, Left A Humerus, Right B Humerus, Left E Upper Arm, Right F Upper Arm, Left J Forearm, Right K Forearm, Left N Hand, Right P Hand, Left R Finger(s), Right S Finger(s), Left X Ribs, Right Y Ribs, Left	Z None	Z None	Z None
8 Shoulder, Right 9 Shoulder, Left C Hand/Finger Joint, Right D Hand/Finger Joint, Left G Elbow, Right H Elbow, Left L Wrist, Right M Wrist, Left	0 High Osmolar 1 Low Osmolar Y Other Contrast Z None	Z None	Z None

B   **Imaging**
P   **Non-Axial Upper Bones**
1   **Fluoroscopy**   Definition: Single plane or bi-plane real time display of an image developed from the capture of external ionizing radioation on a fluorescent screen. The image may also be stored by either digital or analog means.

Body Part Character 4	Contrast Character 5	Qualifier Character 6	Qualifier Character 7
0 Sternoclavicular Joint, Right 1 Sternoclavicular Joint, Left 2 Sternoclavicular Joints, Bilateral 3 Acromioclavicular Joints, Bilateral 4 Clavicle, Right 5 Clavicle, Left 6 Scapula, Right 7 Scapula, Left A Humerus, Right B Humerus, Left E Upper Arm, Right F Upper Arm, Left J Forearm, Right K Forearm, Left N Hand, Right P Hand, Left R Finger(s), Right S Finger(s), Left X Ribs, Right Y Ribs, Left	Z None	Z None	Z None
8 Shoulder, Right 9 Shoulder, Left L Wrist, Right M Wrist, Left	0 High Osmolar 1 Low Osmolar Y Other Contrast Z None	Z None	Z None
C Hand/Finger Joint, Right D Hand/Finger Joint, Left G Elbow, Right H Elbow, Left	0 High Osmolar 1 Low Osmolar Y Other Contrast	Z None	Z None

NC Noncovered Procedure   **LC** Limited Coverage   **QA** Questionable OB Admit   **NT** New Tech Add-on   ⊞ Combination Member   ♂ Male   ♀ Female

ICD-10-PCS 2022   759

BP0–BP1

B   **Imaging**
P   **Non-Axial Upper Bones**
2   **Computerized Tomography (CT Scan)** Definition: Computer reformatted digital display of multiplanar images developed from the capture of multiple exposures of external ionizing radiation

Body Part Character 4	Contrast Character 5	Qualifier Character 6	Qualifier Character 7
Ø Sternoclavicular Joint, Right 1 Sternoclavicular Joint, Left W Thorax	Ø High Osmolar 1 Low Osmolar Y Other Contrast	Z None	Z None
2 Sternoclavicular Joints, Bilateral 3 Acromioclavicular Joints, Bilateral 4 Clavicle, Right 5 Clavicle, Left 6 Scapula, Right 7 Scapula, Left 8 Shoulder, Right 9 Shoulder, Left A Humerus, Right B Humerus, Left E Upper Arm, Right F Upper Arm, Left G Elbow, Right H Elbow, Left J Forearm, Right K Forearm, Left L Wrist, Right M Wrist, Left N Hand, Right P Hand, Left Q Hands and Wrists, Bilateral R Finger(s), Right S Finger(s), Left T Upper Extremity, Right U Upper Extremity, Left V Upper Extremities, Bilateral X Ribs, Right Y Ribs, Left	Ø High Osmolar 1 Low Osmolar Y Other Contrast Z None	Z None	Z None
C Hand/Finger Joint, Right D Hand/Finger Joint, Left	Z None	Z None	Z None

B   **Imaging**
P   **Non-Axial Upper Bones**
3   **Magnetic Resonance Imaging (MRI)**   Definition: Computer reformatted digital display of multiplanar images developed from the capture of radio-frequency signals emitted by nuclei in a body site excited within a magnetic field

Body Part Character 4	Contrast Character 5	Qualifier Character 6	Qualifier Character 7
8 Shoulder, Right 9 Shoulder, Left C Hand/Finger Joint, Right D Hand/Finger Joint, Left E Upper Arm, Right F Upper Arm, Left G Elbow, Right H Elbow, Left J Forearm, Right K Forearm, Left L Wrist, Right M Wrist, Left	Y Other Contrast	Ø Unenhanced and Enhanced Z None	Z None
8 Shoulder, Right 9 Shoulder, Left C Hand/Finger Joint, Right D Hand/Finger Joint, Left E Upper Arm, Right F Upper Arm, Left G Elbow, Right H Elbow, Left J Forearm, Right K Forearm, Left L Wrist, Right M Wrist, Left	Z None	Z None	Z None

B   Imaging
P   Non-Axial Upper Bones
4   Ultrasonography   Definition: Real time display of images of anatomy or flow information developed from the capture of reflected and attenuated high frequency sound waves

Body Part Character 4	Contrast Character 5	Qualifier Character 6	Qualifier Character 7
8 Shoulder, Right 9 Shoulder, Left G Elbow, Right H Elbow, Left L Wrist, Right M Wrist, Left N Hand, Right P Hand, Left	Z None	Z None	1 Densitometry Z None

B   Imaging
Q   Non-Axial Lower Bones
Ø   Plain Radiography   Definition: Planar display of an image developed from the capture of external ionizing radiation on photographic or photoconductive plate

Body Part Character 4	Contrast Character 5	Qualifier Character 6	Qualifier Character 7
Ø Hip, Right 1 Hip, Left	Ø High Osmolar 1 Low Osmolar Y Other Contrast	Z None	Z None
Ø Hip, Right 1 Hip, Left	Z None	Z None	1 Densitometry Z None
3 Femur, Right 4 Femur, Left	Z None	Z None	1 Densitometry Z None
7 Knee, Right 8 Knee, Left G Ankle, Right H Ankle, Left	Ø High Osmolar 1 Low Osmolar Y Other Contrast Z None	Z None	Z None
D Lower Leg, Right F Lower Leg, Left J Calcaneus, Right K Calcaneus, Left L Foot, Right M Foot, Left P Toe(s), Right Q Toe(s), Left V Patella, Right W Patella, Left	Z None	Z None	Z None
X Foot/Toe Joint, Right Y Foot/Toe Joint, Left	Ø High Osmolar 1 Low Osmolar Y Other Contrast	Z None	Z None

B   Imaging
Q   Non-Axial Lower Bones
1   Fluoroscopy   Definition: Single plane or bi-plane real time display of an image developed from the capture of external ionizing radioation on a fluorescent screen. The image may also be stored by either digital or analog means.

Body Part Character 4	Contrast Character 5	Qualifier Character 6	Qualifier Character 7
Ø Hip, Right 1 Hip, Left 7 Knee, Right 8 Knee, Left G Ankle, Right H Ankle, Left X Foot/Toe Joint, Right Y Foot/Toe Joint, Left	Ø High Osmolar 1 Low Osmolar Y Other Contrast Z None	Z None	Z None
3 Femur, Right 4 Femur, Left D Lower Leg, Right F Lower Leg, Left J Calcaneus, Right K Calcaneus, Left L Foot, Right M Foot, Left P Toe(s), Right Q Toe(s), Left V Patella, Right W Patella, Left	Z None	Z None	Z None

NC Noncovered Procedure   LC Limited Coverage   QA Questionable OB Admit   NT New Tech Add-on   ⊞ Combination Member   ♂ Male   ♀ Female

ICD-10-PCS 2022   761

Imaging

BP4–BQ1

B   Imaging
Q   Non-Axial Lower Bones
2   Computerized Tomography (CT Scan) Definition: Computer reformatted digital display of multiplanar images developed from the capture of multiple exposures of external ionizing radiation

Body Part Character 4	Contrast Character 5	Qualifier Character 6	Qualifier Character 7
Ø Hip, Right 1 Hip, Left 3 Femur, Right 4 Femur, Left 7 Knee, Right 8 Knee, Left D Lower Leg, Right F Lower Leg, Left G Ankle, Right H Ankle, Left J Calcaneus, Right K Calcaneus, Left L Foot, Right M Foot, Left P Toe(s), Right Q Toe(s), Left R Lower Extremity, Right S Lower Extremity, Left V Patella, Right W Patella, Left X Foot/Toe Joint, Right Y Foot/Toe Joint, Left	Ø High Osmolar 1 Low Osmolar Y Other Contrast Z None	Z None	Z None
B Tibia/Fibula, Right C Tibia/Fibula, Left	Ø High Osmolar 1 Low Osmolar Y Other Contrast	Z None	Z None

B   Imaging
Q   Non-Axial Lower Bones
3   Magnetic Resonance Imaging (MRI) Definition: Computer reformatted digital display of multiplanar images developed from the capture of radio-frequency signals emitted by nuclei in a body site excited within a magnetic field

Body Part Character 4	Contrast Character 5	Qualifier Character 6	Qualifier Character 7
Ø Hip, Right 1 Hip, Left 3 Femur, Right 4 Femur, Left 7 Knee, Right 8 Knee, Left D Lower Leg, Right F Lower Leg, Left G Ankle, Right H Ankle, Left J Calcaneus, Right K Calcaneus, Left L Foot, Right M Foot, Left P Toe(s), Right Q Toe(s), Left V Patella, Right W Patella, Left	Y Other Contrast	Ø Unenhanced and Enhanced Z None	Z None
Ø Hip, Right 1 Hip, Left 3 Femur, Right 4 Femur, Left 7 Knee, Right 8 Knee, Left D Lower Leg, Right F Lower Leg, Left G Ankle, Right H Ankle, Left J Calcaneus, Right K Calcaneus, Left L Foot, Right M Foot, Left P Toe(s), Right Q Toe(s), Left V Patella, Right W Patella, Left	Z None	Z None	Z None

B   Imaging
Q   Non-Axial Lower Bones
4   Ultrasonography   Definition: Real time display of images of anatomy or flow information developed from the capture of reflected and attenuated high frequency sound waves

Body Part Character 4	Contrast Character 5	Qualifier Character 6	Qualifier Character 7
Ø Hip, Right 1 Hip, Left 2 Hips, Bilateral 7 Knee, Right 8 Knee, Left 9 Knees, Bilateral	Z None	Z None	Z None

B   Imaging
R   Axial Skeleton, Except Skull and Facial Bones
Ø   Plain Radiography   Definition: Planar display of an image developed from the capture of external ionizing radiation on photographic or photoconductive plate

Body Part Character 4	Contrast Character 5	Qualifier Character 6	Qualifier Character 7
Ø Cervical Spine 7 Thoracic Spine 9 Lumbar Spine G Whole Spine	Z None	Z None	1 Densitometry Z None
1 Cervical Disc(s) 2 Thoracic Disc(s) 3 Lumbar Disc(s) 4 Cervical Facet Joint(s) 5 Thoracic Facet Joint(s) 6 Lumbar Facet Joint(s) D Sacroiliac Joints	Ø High Osmolar 1 Low Osmolar Y Other Contrast Z None	Z None	Z None
8 Thoracolumbar Joint B Lumbosacral Joint C Pelvis F Sacrum and Coccyx H Sternum	Z None	Z None	Z None

B   Imaging
R   Axial Skeleton, Except Skull and Facial Bones
1   Fluoroscopy   Definition: Single plane or bi-plane real time display of an image developed from the capture of external ionizing radioation on a fluorescent screen. The image may also be stored by either digital or analog means.

Body Part Character 4	Contrast Character 5	Qualifier Character 6	Qualifier Character 7
Ø Cervical Spine 1 Cervical Disc(s) 2 Thoracic Disc(s) 3 Lumbar Disc(s) 4 Cervical Facet Joint(s) 5 Thoracic Facet Joint(s) 6 Lumbar Facet Joint(s) 7 Thoracic Spine 8 Thoracolumbar Joint 9 Lumbar Spine B Lumbosacral Joint C Pelvis D Sacroiliac Joints F Sacrum and Coccyx G Whole Spine H Sternum	Ø High Osmolar 1 Low Osmolar Y Other Contrast Z None	Z None	Z None

B   Imaging
R   Axial Skeleton, Except Skull and Facial Bones
2   Computerized Tomography (CT Scan)   Definition: Computer reformatted digital display of multiplanar images developed from the capture of multiple exposures of external ionizing radiation

Body Part Character 4	Contrast Character 5	Qualifier Character 6	Qualifier Character 7
Ø Cervical Spine 7 Thoracic Spine 9 Lumbar Spine C Pelvis D Sacroiliac Joints F Sacrum and Coccyx	Ø High Osmolar 1 Low Osmolar Y Other Contrast Z None	Z None	Z None

NC Noncovered Procedure   **LC** Limited Coverage   **QA** Questionable OB Admit   **NT** New Tech Add-on   ⊞ Combination Member   ♂ Male   ♀ Female

ICD-10-PCS 2022   763

BQ4–BR2

B   **Imaging**
R   **Axial Skeleton, Except Skull and Facial Bones**
3   **Magnetic Resonance Imaging (MRI)**   Definition: Computer reformatted digital display of multiplanar images developed from the capture of radio-frequency signals emitted by nuclei in a body site excited within a magnetic field

Body Part Character 4	Contrast Character 5	Qualifier Character 6	Qualifier Character 7
Ø Cervical Spine 1 Cervical Disc(s) 2 Thoracic Disc(s) 3 Lumbar Disc(s) 7 Thoracic Spine 9 Lumbar Spine C Pelvis F Sacrum and Coccyx	Y Other Contrast	Ø Unenhanced and Enhanced Z None	Z None
Ø Cervical Spine 1 Cervical Disc(s) 2 Thoracic Disc(s) 3 Lumbar Disc(s) 7 Thoracic Spine 9 Lumbar Spine C Pelvis F Sacrum and Coccyx	Z None	Z None	Z None

B   **Imaging**
R   **Axial Skeleton, Except Skull and Facial Bones**
4   **Ultrasonography**   Definition: Real time display of images of anatomy or flow information developed from the capture of reflected and attenuated high frequency sound waves

Body Part Character 4	Contrast Character 5	Qualifier Character 6	Qualifier Character 7
Ø Cervical Spine 7 Thoracic Spine 9 Lumbar Spine F Sacrum and Coccyx	Z None	Z None	Z None

B   **Imaging**
T   **Urinary System**
Ø   **Plain Radiography**   Definition: Planar display of an image developed from the capture of external ionizing radiation on photographic or photoconductive plate

Body Part Character 4	Contrast Character 5	Qualifier Character 6	Qualifier Character 7
Ø Bladder 1 Kidney, Right 2 Kidney, Left 3 Kidneys, Bilateral 4 Kidneys, Ureters and Bladder 5 Urethra 6 Ureter, Right 7 Ureter, Left 8 Ureters, Bilateral B Bladder and Urethra C Ileal Diversion Loop	Ø High Osmolar 1 Low Osmolar Y Other Contrast Z None	Z None	Z None

B   **Imaging**
T   **Urinary System**
1   **Fluoroscopy**   Definition: Single plane or bi-plane real time display of an image developed from the capture of external ionizing radioation on a fluorescent screen. The image may also be stored by either digital or analog means.

Body Part Character 4	Contrast Character 5	Qualifier Character 6	Qualifier Character 7
Ø Bladder 1 Kidney, Right 2 Kidney, Left 3 Kidneys, Bilateral 4 Kidneys, Ureters and Bladder 5 Urethra 6 Ureter, Right 7 Ureter, Left B Bladder and Urethra C Ileal Diversion Loop D Kidney, Ureter and Bladder, Right F Kidney, Ureter and Bladder, Left G Ileal Loop, Ureters and Kidneys	Ø High Osmolar 1 Low Osmolar Y Other Contrast Z None	Z None	Z None

B   **Imaging**
T   **Urinary System**
2   **Computerized Tomography (CT Scan)**   Definition: Computer reformatted digital display of multiplanar images developed from the capture of multiple exposures of external ionizing radiation

Body Part Character 4	Contrast Character 5	Qualifier Character 6	Qualifier Character 7
Ø Bladder 1 Kidney, Right 2 Kidney, Left 3 Kidneys, Bilateral 9 Kidney Transplant	Ø High Osmolar 1 Low Osmolar Y Other Contrast	Ø Unenhanced and Enhanced Z None	Z None
Ø Bladder 1 Kidney, Right 2 Kidney, Left 3 Kidneys, Bilateral 9 Kidney Transplant	Z None	Z None	Z None

B   **Imaging**
T   **Urinary System**
3   **Magnetic Resonance Imaging (MRI)**   Definition: Computer reformatted digital display of multiplanar images developed from the capture of radio-frequency signals emitted by nuclei in a body site excited within a magnetic field

Body Part Character 4	Contrast Character 5	Qualifier Character 6	Qualifier Character 7
Ø Bladder 1 Kidney, Right 2 Kidney, Left 3 Kidneys, Bilateral 9 Kidney Transplant	Y Other Contrast	Ø Unenhanced and Enhanced Z None	Z None
Ø Bladder 1 Kidney, Right 2 Kidney, Left 3 Kidneys, Bilateral 9 Kidney Transplant	Z None	Z None	Z None

B   **Imaging**
T   **Urinary System**
4   **Ultrasonography**   Definition: Real time display of images of anatomy or flow information developed from the capture of reflected and attenuated high frequency sound waves

Body Part Character 4	Contrast Character 5	Qualifier Character 6	Qualifier Character 7
Ø Bladder 1 Kidney, Right 2 Kidney, Left 3 Kidneys, Bilateral 5 Urethra 6 Ureter, Right 7 Ureter, Left 8 Ureters, Bilateral 9 Kidney Transplant J Kidneys and Bladder	Z None	Z None	Z None

B   **Imaging**
U   **Female Reproductive System**
Ø   **Plain Radiography**   Definition: Planar display of an image developed from the capture of external ionizing radiation on photographic or photoconductive plate

Body Part Character 4	Contrast Character 5	Qualifier Character 6	Qualifier Character 7
Ø Fallopian Tube, Right ♀ 1 Fallopian Tube, Left ♀ 2 Fallopian Tubes, Bilateral ♀ 6 Uterus ♀ 8 Uterus and Fallopian Tubes ♀ 9 Vagina ♀	Ø High Osmolar 1 Low Osmolar Y Other Contrast	Z None	Z None
♀ All body part, contrast, and qualifier values			

B   **Imaging**
U   **Female Reproductive System**
1   **Fluoroscopy**   Definition: Single plane or bi-plane real time display of an image developed from the capture of external ionizing radioation on a fluorescent screen. The image may also be stored by either digital or analog means.

Body Part Character 4	Contrast Character 5	Qualifier Character 6	Qualifier Character 7
Ø Fallopian Tube, Right ♀	Ø High Osmolar	Z None	Z None
1 Fallopian Tube, Left ♀	1 Low Osmolar		
2 Fallopian Tubes, Bilateral ♀	Y Other Contrast		
6 Uterus ♀	Z None		
8 Uterus and Fallopian Tubes ♀			
9 Vagina ♀			

♀   All body part, contrast, and qualifier values

B   **Imaging**
U   **Female Reproductive System**
3   **Magnetic Resonance Imaging (MRI)**   Definition: Computer reformatted digital display of multiplanar images developed from the capture of radio-frequency signals emitted by nuclei in a body site excited within a magnetic field

Body Part Character 4	Contrast Character 5	Qualifier Character 6	Qualifier Character 7
3 Ovary, Right ♀	Y Other Contrast	Ø Unenhanced and Enhanced	Z None
4 Ovary, Left ♀		Z None	
5 Ovaries, Bilateral ♀			
6 Uterus ♀			
9 Vagina ♀			
B Pregnant Uterus ♀			
C Uterus and Ovaries ♀			
3 Ovary, Right ♀	Z None	Z None	Z None
4 Ovary, Left ♀			
5 Ovaries, Bilateral ♀			
6 Uterus ♀			
9 Vagina ♀			
B Pregnant Uterus ♀			
C Uterus and Ovaries ♀			

♀   All body part, contrast, and qualifier values

B   **Imaging**
U   **Female Reproductive System**
4   **Ultrasonography**   Definition: Real time display of images of anatomy or flow information developed from the capture of reflected and attenuated high frequency sound waves

Body Part Character 4	Contrast Character 5	Qualifier Character 6	Qualifier Character 7
Ø Fallopian Tube, Right ♀	Y Other Contrast	Z None	Z None
1 Fallopian Tube, Left ♀	Z None		
2 Fallopian Tubes, Bilateral ♀			
3 Ovary, Right ♀			
4 Ovary, Left ♀			
5 Ovaries, Bilateral ♀			
6 Uterus ♀			
C Uterus and Ovaries ♀			

♀   All body part, contrast, and qualifier values

B   **Imaging**
V   **Male Reproductive System**
Ø   **Plain Radiography**   Definition: Planar display of an image developed from the capture of external ionizing radiation on photographic or photoconductive plate

Body Part Character 4	Contrast Character 5	Qualifier Character 6	Qualifier Character 7
Ø Corpora Cavernosa ♂	Ø High Osmolar	Z None	Z None
1 Epididymis, Right ♂	1 Low Osmolar		
2 Epididymis, Left ♂	Y Other Contrast		
3 Prostate ♂			
5 Testicle, Right ♂			
6 Testicle, Left ♂			
8 Vasa Vasorum ♂			

♂   All body part, contrast, and qualifier values

B   Imaging
V   Male Reproductive System
1   Fluoroscopy   Definition: Single plane or bi-plane real time display of an image developed from the capture of external ionizing radiation on a fluorescent screen. The image may also be stored by either digital or analog means.

Body Part Character 4	Contrast Character 5	Qualifier Character 6	Qualifier Character 7
Ø Corpora Cavernosa ♂ 8 Vasa Vasorum ♂	Ø High Osmolar 1 Low Osmolar Y Other Contrast Z None	Z None	Z None

    ♂   All body part, contrast, and qualifier values

B   Imaging
V   Male Reproductive System
2   Computerized Tomography (CT Scan)   Definition: Computer reformatted digital display of multiplanar images developed from the capture of multiple exposures of external ionizing radiation

Body Part Character 4	Contrast Character 5	Qualifier Character 6	Qualifier Character 7
3 Prostate ♂	Ø High Osmolar 1 Low Osmolar Y Other Contrast	Ø Unenhanced and Enhanced Z None	Z None
3 Prostate ♂	Z None	Z None	Z None

    ♂   BV23[Ø,Y][Ø,Z]Z   ♂   BV23ZZZ
    ♂   BV231ØZ

B   Imaging
V   Male Reproductive System
3   Magnetic Resonance Imaging (MRI)   Definition: Computer reformatted digital display of multiplanar images developed from the capture of radio-frequency signals emitted by nuclei in a body site excited within a magnetic field

Body Part Character 4	Contrast Character 5	Qualifier Character 6	Qualifier Character 7
Ø Corpora Cavernosa ♂ 3 Prostate ♂ 4 Scrotum ♂ 5 Testicle, Right ♂ 6 Testicle, Left ♂ 7 Testicles, Bilateral ♂	Y Other Contrast	Ø Unenhanced and Enhanced Z None	Z None
Ø Corpora Cavernosa ♂ 3 Prostate ♂ 4 Scrotum ♂ 5 Testicle, Right ♂ 6 Testicle, Left ♂ 7 Testicles, Bilateral ♂	Z None	Z None	Z None

    ♂   All body part, contrast, and qualifier values

B   Imaging
V   Male Reproductive System
4   Ultrasonography   Definition: Real time display of images of anatomy or flow information developed from the capture of reflected and attenuated high frequency sound waves

Body Part Character 4	Contrast Character 5	Qualifier Character 6	Qualifier Character 7
4 Scrotum ♂ 9 Prostate and Seminal Vesicles ♂ B Penis ♂	Z None	Z None	Z None

    ♂   All body part, contrast, and qualifier values

B   Imaging
W   Anatomical Regions
Ø   Plain Radiography   Definition: Planar display of an image developed from the capture of external ionizing radiation on photographic or photoconductive plate

Body Part Character 4	Contrast Character 5	Qualifier Character 6	Qualifier Character 7
Ø Abdomen 1 Abdomen and Pelvis 3 Chest B Long Bones, All C Lower Extremity J Upper Extremity K Whole Body L Whole Skeleton M Whole Body, Infant	Z None	Z None	Z None

---

B　**Imaging**
W　**Anatomical Regions**
1　**Fluoroscopy**　Definition: Single plane or bi-plane real time display of an image developed from the capture of external ionizing radioation on a fluorescent screen. The image may also be stored by either digital or analog means.

Body Part Character 4	Contrast Character 5	Qualifier Character 6	Qualifier Character 7
1 Abdomen and Pelvis	Ø High Osmolar	Z None	Z None
9 Head and Neck	1 Low Osmolar		
C Lower Extremity	Y Other Contrast		
J Upper Extremity	Z None		

B　**Imaging**
W　**Anatomical Regions**
2　**Computerized Tomography (CT Scan)**　Definition: Computer reformatted digital display of multiplanar images developed from the capture of multiple exposures of external ionizing radiation

Body Part Character 4	Contrast Character 5	Qualifier Character 6	Qualifier Character 7
Ø Abdomen	Ø High Osmolar	Ø Unenhanced and Enhanced	Z None
1 Abdomen and Pelvis	1 Low Osmolar	Z None	
4 Chest and Abdomen	Y Other Contrast		
5 Chest, Abdomen and Pelvis			
8 Head			
9 Head and Neck			
F Neck			
G Pelvic Region			
Ø Abdomen	Z None	Z None	Z None
1 Abdomen and Pelvis			
4 Chest and Abdomen			
5 Chest, Abdomen and Pelvis			
8 Head			
9 Head and Neck			
F Neck			
G Pelvic Region			

B　**Imaging**
W　**Anatomical Regions**
3　**Magnetic Resonance Imaging (MRI)**　Definition: Computer reformatted digital display of multiplanar images developed from the capture of radio-frequency signals emitted by nuclei in a body site excited within a magnetic field

Body Part Character 4	Contrast Character 5	Qualifier Character 6	Qualifier Character 7
Ø Abdomen	Y Other Contrast	Ø Unenhanced and Enhanced	Z None
8 Head		Z None	
F Neck			
G Pelvic Region			
H Retroperitoneum			
P Brachial Plexus			
Ø Abdomen	Z None	Z None	Z None
8 Head			
F Neck			
G Pelvic Region			
H Retroperitoneum			
P Brachial Plexus			
3 Chest	Y Other Contrast	Ø Unenhanced and Enhanced	Z None
		Z None	

B　**Imaging**
W　**Anatomical Regions**
4　**Ultrasonography**　Definition: Real time display of images of anatomy or flow information developed from the capture of reflected and attenuated high frequency sound waves

Body Part Character 4	Contrast Character 5	Qualifier Character 6	Qualifier Character 7
Ø Abdomen	Z None	Z None	Z None
1 Abdomen and Pelvis			
F Neck			
G Pelvic Region			

B   **Imaging**
W   **Anatomical Regions**
5   **Other Imaging**   Definition: Other specified modality for visualizing a body part

Body Part Character 4	Contrast Character 5	Qualifier Character 6	Qualifier Character 7
2 Trunk **9** Head and Neck **C** Lower Extremity **J** Upper Extremity	**Z** None	**1** Bacterial Autofluorescence	**Z** None

B   **Imaging**
Y   **Fetus and Obstetrical**
3   **Magnetic Resonance Imaging (MRI)**   Definition: Computer reformatted digital display of multiplanar images developed from the capture of radio-frequency signals emitted by nuclei in a body site excited within a magnetic field

Body Part Character 4	Contrast Character 5	Qualifier Character 6	Qualifier Character 7
Ø Fetal Head ♀ **1** Fetal Heart ♀ **2** Fetal Thorax ♀ **3** Fetal Abdomen ♀ **4** Fetal Spine ♀ **5** Fetal Extremities ♀ **6** Whole Fetus ♀	**Y** Other Contrast	**Ø** Unenhanced and Enhanced **Z** None	**Z** None
Ø Fetal Head ♀ **1** Fetal Heart ♀ **2** Fetal Thorax ♀ **3** Fetal Abdomen ♀ **4** Fetal Spine ♀ **5** Fetal Extremities ♀ **6** Whole Fetus ♀	**Z** None	**Z** None	**Z** None

♀   BY3[Ø,1,2,3,5,6]Y[Ø,Z]Z
♀   BY34YZZ
♀   BY3[Ø,1,2,3,4,5,6]ZZZ

B   **Imaging**
Y   **Fetus and Obstetrical**
4   **Ultrasonography**   Definition: Real time display of images of anatomy or flow information developed from the capture of reflected and attenuated high frequency sound waves

Body Part Character 4	Contrast Character 5	Qualifier Character 6	Qualifier Character 7
7 Fetal Umbilical Cord ♀ **8** Placenta ♀ **9** First Trimester, Single Fetus ♀ **B** First Trimester, Multiple Gestation ♀ **C** Second Trimester, Single Fetus ♀ **D** Second Trimester, Multiple Gestation ♀ **F** Third Trimester, Single Fetus ♀ **G** Third Trimester, Multiple Gestation ♀	**Z** None	**Z** None	**Z** None

♀   All body part, contrast, and qualifier values

NC Noncovered Procedure   **LC** Limited Coverage   **QA** Questionable OB Admit   **NT** New Tech Add-on   ⊞ Combination Member   ♂ Male   ♀ Female

ICD-10-PCS 2022   769

Nuclear Medicine C01–CW7

C   **Nuclear Medicine**
0   **Central Nervous System**
1   **Planar Nuclear Medicine Imaging**   Definition: Introduction of radioactive materials into the body for single plane display of images developed from the capture of radioactive emissions

Body Part Character 4	Radionuclide Character 5	Qualifier Character 6	Qualifier Character 7
0 Brain	1 Technetium 99m (Tc-99m) Y Other Radionuclide	Z None	Z None
5 Cerebrospinal Fluid	D Indium 111 (In-111) Y Other Radionuclide	Z None	Z None
Y Central Nervous System	Y Other Radionuclide	Z None	Z None

C   **Nuclear Medicine**
0   **Central Nervous System**
2   **Tomographic (Tomo) Nuclear Medicine Imaging**   Definition: Introduction of radioactive materials into the body for three dimensional display of images developed from the capture of radioactive emissions

Body Part Character 4	Radionuclide Character 5	Qualifier Character 6	Qualifier Character 7
0 Brain	1 Technetium 99m (Tc-99m) F Iodine 123 (I-123) S Thallium 201 (Tl-201) Y Other Radionuclide	Z None	Z None
5 Cerebrospinal Fluid	D Indium 111 (In-111) Y Other Radionuclide	Z None	Z None
Y Central Nervous System	Y Other Radionuclide	Z None	Z None

C   **Nuclear Medicine**
0   **Central Nervous System**
3   **Positron Emission Tomographic (PET) Imaging**   Definition: Introduction of radioactive materials into the body for three dimensional display of images developed from the simultaneous capture, 180 degrees apart, of radioactive emissions

Body Part Character 4	Radionuclide Character 5	Qualifier Character 6	Qualifier Character 7
0 Brain	B Carbon 11 (C-11) K Fluorine 18 (F-18) M Oxygen 15 (O-15) Y Other Radionuclide	Z None	Z None
Y Central Nervous System	Y Other Radionuclide	Z None	Z None

C   **Nuclear Medicine**
0   **Central Nervous System**
5   **Nonimaging Nuclear Medicine Probe**   Definition: Introduction of radioactive materials into the body for the study of distribution and fate of certain substances by the detection of radioactive emissions; or, alternatively, measurement of absorption of radioactive emissions from an external source

Body Part Character 4	Radionuclide Character 5	Qualifier Character 6	Qualifier Character 7
0 Brain	V Xenon 133 (Xe-133) Y Other Radionuclide	Z None	Z None
Y Central Nervous System	Y Other Radionuclide	Z None	Z None

C   **Nuclear Medicine**
2   **Heart**
1   **Planar Nuclear Medicine Imaging**   Definition: Introduction of radioactive materials into the body for single plane display of images developed from the capture of radioactive emissions

Body Part Character 4	Radionuclide Character 5	Qualifier Character 6	Qualifier Character 7
6 Heart, Right and Left	1 Technetium 99m (Tc-99m) Y Other Radionuclide	Z None	Z None
G Myocardium	1 Technetium 99m (Tc-99m) D Indium 111 (In-111) S Thallium 201 (Tl-201) Y Other Radionuclide Z None	Z None	Z None
Y Heart	Y Other Radionuclide	Z None	Z None

Nuclear Medicine

C   Nuclear Medicine
2   Heart
2   Tomographic (Tomo) Nuclear Medicine Imaging   Definition: Introduction of radioactive materials into the body for three dimensional display of images developed from the capture of radioactive emissions

Body Part Character 4	Radionuclide Character 5	Qualifier Character 6	Qualifier Character 7
6 Heart, Right and Left	1 Technetium 99m (Tc-99m) Y Other Radionuclide	Z None	Z None
G Myocardium	1 Technetium 99m (Tc-99m) D Indium 111 (In-111) K Fluorine 18 (F-18) S Thallium 201 (Tl-201) Y Other Radionuclide Z None	Z None	Z None
Y Heart	Y Other Radionuclide	Z None	Z None

C   Nuclear Medicine
2   Heart
3   Positron Emission Tomographic (PET) Imaging   Definition: Introduction of radioactive materials into the body for three dimensional display of images developed from the simultaneous capture, 180 degrees apart, of radioactive emissions

Body Part Character 4	Radionuclide Character 5	Qualifier Character 6	Qualifier Character 7
G Myocardium	K Fluorine 18 (F-18) M Oxygen 15 (O-15) Q Rubidium 82 (Rb-82) R Nitrogen 13 (N-13) Y Other Radionuclide	Z None	Z None
Y Heart	Y Other Radionuclide	Z None	Z None

C   Nuclear Medicine
2   Heart
5   Nonimaging Nuclear Medicine Probe   Definition: Introduction of radioactive materials into the body for the study of distribution and fate of certain substances by the detection of radioactive emissions; or, alternatively, measurement of absorption of radioactive emissions from an external source

Body Part Character 4	Radionuclide Character 5	Qualifier Character 6	Qualifier Character 7
6 Heart, Right and Left	1 Technetium 99m (Tc-99m) Y Other Radionuclide	Z None	Z None
Y Heart	Y Other Radionuclide	Z None	Z None

C   Nuclear Medicine
5   Veins
1   Planar Nuclear Medicine Imaging   Definition: Introduction of radioactive materials into the body for single plane display of images developed from the capture of radioactive emissions

Body Part Character 4	Radionuclide Character 5	Qualifier Character 6	Qualifier Character 7
B Lower Extremity Veins, Right C Lower Extremity Veins, Left D Lower Extremity Veins, Bilateral N Upper Extremity Veins, Right P Upper Extremity Veins, Left Q Upper Extremity Veins, Bilateral R Central Veins	1 Technetium 99m (Tc-99m) Y Other Radionuclide	Z None	Z None
Y Veins	Y Other Radionuclide	Z None	Z None

C   Nuclear Medicine
7   Lymphatic and Hematologic System
1   Planar Nuclear Medicine Imaging   Definition: Introduction of radioactive materials into the body for single plane display of images developed from the capture of radioactive emissions

Body Part Character 4	Radionuclide Character 5	Qualifier Character 6	Qualifier Character 7
Ø Bone Marrow	1 Technetium 99m (Tc-99m) D Indium 111 (In-111) Y Other Radionuclide	Z None	Z None
2 Spleen 5 Lymphatics, Head and Neck D Lymphatics, Pelvic J Lymphatics, Head K Lymphatics, Neck L Lymphatics, Upper Chest M Lymphatics, Trunk N Lymphatics, Upper Extremity P Lymphatics, Lower Extremity	1 Technetium 99m (Tc-99m) Y Other Radionuclide	Z None	Z None
3 Blood	D Indium 111 (In-111) Y Other Radionuclide	Z None	Z None
Y Lymphatic and Hematologic System	Y Other Radionuclide	Z None	Z None

C   Nuclear Medicine
7   Lymphatic and Hematologic System
2   Tomographic (Tomo) Nuclear Medicine Imaging   Definition: Introduction of radioactive materials into the body for three dimensional display of images developed from the capture of radioactive emissions

Body Part Character 4	Radionuclide Character 5	Qualifier Character 6	Qualifier Character 7
2 Spleen	1 Technetium 99m (Tc-99m) Y Other Radionuclide	Z None	Z None
Y Lymphatic and Hematologic System	Y Other Radionuclide	Z None	Z None

C   Nuclear Medicine
7   Lymphatic and Hematologic System
5   Nonimaging Nuclear Medicine Probe   Definition: Introduction of radioactive materials into the body for the study of distribution and fate of certain substances by the detection of radioactive emissions; or, alternatively, measurement of absorption of radioactive emissions from an external source

Body Part Character 4	Radionuclide Character 5	Qualifier Character 6	Qualifier Character 7
5 Lymphatics, Head and Neck D Lymphatics, Pelvic J Lymphatics, Head K Lymphatics, Neck L Lymphatics, Upper Chest M Lymphatics, Trunk N Lymphatics, Upper Extremity P Lymphatics, Lower Extremity	1 Technetium 99m (Tc-99m) Y Other Radionuclide	Z None	Z None
Y Lymphatic and Hematologic System	Y Other Radionuclide	Z None	Z None

C   Nuclear Medicine
7   Lymphatic and Hematologic System
6   Nonimaging Nuclear Medicine Assay   Definition: Introduction of radioactive materials into the body for the study of body fluids and blood elements, by the detection of radioactive emissions

Body Part Character 4	Radionuclide Character 5	Qualifier Character 6	Qualifier Character 7
3 Blood	1 Technetium 99m (Tc-99m) 7 Cobalt 58 (Co-58) C Cobalt 57 (Co-57) D Indium 111 (In-111) H Iodine 125 (I-125) W Chromium (Cr-51) Y Other Radionuclide	Z None	Z None
Y Lymphatic and Hematologic System	Y Other Radionuclide	Z None	Z None

NC Noncovered Procedure   **LC** Limited Coverage   **QA** Questionable OB Admit   **NT** New Tech Add-on   ⊞ Combination Member   ♂ Male   ♀ Female

ICD-10-PCS 2022   773

C71–C76

Nuclear Medicine

C   **Nuclear Medicine**
8   **Eye**
1   **Planar Nuclear Medicine Imaging**   Definition: Introduction of radioactive materials into the body for single plane display of images developed from the capture of radioactive emissions

Body Part Character 4	Radionuclide Character 5	Qualifier Character 6	Qualifier Character 7
9 Lacrimal Ducts, Bilateral	1 Technetium 99m (Tc-99m) Y Other Radionuclide	Z None	Z None
Y Eye	Y Other Radionuclide	Z None	Z None

C   **Nuclear Medicine**
9   **Ear, Nose, Mouth and Throat**
1   **Planar Nuclear Medicine Imaging**   Definition: Introduction of radioactive materials into the body for single plane display of images developed from the capture of radioactive emissions

Body Part Character 4	Radionuclide Character 5	Qualifier Character 6	Qualifier Character 7
B Salivary Glands, Bilateral	1 Technetium 99m (Tc-99m) Y Other Radionuclide	Z None	Z None
Y Ear, Nose, Mouth and Throat	Y Other Radionuclide	Z None	Z None

C   **Nuclear Medicine**
B   **Respiratory System**
1   **Planar Nuclear Medicine Imaging**   Definition: Introduction of radioactive materials into the body for single plane display of images developed from the capture of radioactive emissions

Body Part Character 4	Radionuclide Character 5	Qualifier Character 6	Qualifier Character 7
2 Lungs and Bronchi	1 Technetium 99m (Tc-99m) 9 Krypton (Kr-81m) T Xenon 127 (Xe-127) V Xenon 133 (Xe-133) Y Other Radionuclide	Z None	Z None
Y Respiratory System	Y Other Radionuclide	Z None	Z None

C   **Nuclear Medicine**
B   **Respiratory System**
2   **Tomographic (Tomo) Nuclear Medicine Imaging**   Definition: Introduction of radioactive materials into the body for three dimensional display of images developed from the capture of radioactive emissions

Body Part Character 4	Radionuclide Character 5	Qualifier Character 6	Qualifier Character 7
2 Lungs and Bronchi	1 Technetium 99m (Tc-99m) 9 Krypton (Kr-81m) Y Other Radionuclide	Z None	Z None
Y Respiratory System	Y Other Radionuclide	Z None	Z None

C   **Nuclear Medicine**
B   **Respiratory System**
3   **Positron Emission Tomographic (PET) Imaging**   Definition: Introduction of radioactive materials into the body for three dimensional display of images developed from the simultaneous capture, 180 degrees apart, of radioactive emissions

Body Part Character 4	Radionuclide Character 5	Qualifier Character 6	Qualifier Character 7
2 Lungs and Bronchi	K Fluorine 18 (F-18) Y Other Radionuclide	Z None	Z None
Y Respiratory System	Y Other Radionuclide	Z None	Z None

C   **Nuclear Medicine**
D   **Gastrointestinal System**
1   **Planar Nuclear Medicine Imaging**   Definition: Introduction of radioactive materials into the body for single plane display of images developed from the capture of radioactive emissions

Body Part Character 4	Radionuclide Character 5	Qualifier Character 6	Qualifier Character 7
5 Upper Gastrointestinal Tract 7 Gastrointestinal Tract	1 Technetium 99m (Tc-99m) D Indium 111 (In-111) Y Other Radionuclide	Z None	Z None
Y Digestive System	Y Other Radionuclide	Z None	Z None

C   Nuclear Medicine
D   Gastrointestinal System
2   Tomographic (Tomo) Nuclear Medicine Imaging   Definition: Introduction of radioactive materials into the body for three dimensional display of images developed from the capture of radioactive emissions

Body Part Character 4	Radionuclide Character 5	Qualifier Character 6	Qualifier Character 7
7 Gastrointestinal Tract	1 Technetium 99m (Tc-99m) D Indium 111 (In-111) Y Other Radionuclide	Z None	Z None
Y Digestive System	Y Other Radionuclide	Z None	Z None

C   Nuclear Medicine
F   Hepatobiliary System and Pancreas
1   Planar Nuclear Medicine Imaging   Definition: Introduction of radioactive materials into the body for single plane display of images developed from the capture of radioactive emissions

Body Part Character 4	Radionuclide Character 5	Qualifier Character 6	Qualifier Character 7
4 Gallbladder 5 Liver 6 Liver and Spleen C Hepatobiliary System, All	1 Technetium 99m (Tc-99m) Y Other Radionuclide	Z None	Z None
Y Hepatobiliary System and Pancreas	Y Other Radionuclide	Z None	Z None

C   Nuclear Medicine
F   Hepatobiliary System and Pancreas
2   Tomographic (Tomo) Nuclear Medicine Imaging   Definition: Introduction of radioactive materials into the body for three dimensional display of images developed from the capture of radioactive emissions

Body Part Character 4	Radionuclide Character 5	Qualifier Character 6	Qualifier Character 7
4 Gallbladder 5 Liver 6 Liver and Spleen	1 Technetium 99m (Tc-99m) Y Other Radionuclide	Z None	Z None
Y Hepatobiliary System and Pancreas	Y Other Radionuclide	Z None	Z None

C   Nuclear Medicine
G   Endocrine System
1   Planar Nuclear Medicine Imaging   Definition: Introduction of radioactive materials into the body for single plane display of images developed from the capture of radioactive emissions

Body Part Character 4	Radionuclide Character 5	Qualifier Character 6	Qualifier Character 7
1 Parathyroid Glands	1 Technetium 99m (Tc-99m) S Thallium 201 (Tl-201) Y Other Radionuclide	Z None	Z None
2 Thyroid Gland	1 Technetium 99m (Tc-99m) F Iodine 123 (I-123) G Iodine 131 (I-131) Y Other Radionuclide	Z None	Z None
4 Adrenal Glands, Bilateral	G Iodine 131 (I-131) Y Other Radionuclide	Z None	Z None
Y Endocrine System	Y Other Radionuclide	Z None	Z None

C   Nuclear Medicine
G   Endocrine System
2   Tomographic (Tomo) Nuclear Medicine Imaging   Definition: Introduction of radioactive materials into the body for three dimensional display of images developed from the capture of radioactive emissions

Body Part Character 4	Radionuclide Character 5	Qualifier Character 6	Qualifier Character 7
1 Parathyroid Glands	1 Technetium 99m (Tc-99m) S Thallium 201 (Tl-201) Y Other Radionuclide	Z None	Z None
Y Endocrine System	Y Other Radionuclide	Z None	Z None

C   Nuclear Medicine
G   Endocrine System
4   Nonimaging Nuclear Medicine Uptake   Definition: Introduction of radioactive materials into the body for measurements of organ function, from the detection of radioactive emmissions

Body Part Character 4	Radionuclide Character 5	Qualifier Character 6	Qualifier Character 7
2 Thyroid Gland	1 Technetium 99m (Tc-99m) F Iodine 123 (I-123) G Iodine 131 (I-131) Y Other Radionuclide	Z None	Z None
Y Endocrine System	Y Other Radionuclide	Z None	Z None

C   Nuclear Medicine
H   Skin, Subcutaneous Tissue and Breast
1   Planar Nuclear Medicine Imaging   Definition: Introduction of radioactive materials into the body for single plane display of images developed from the capture of radioactive emissions

Body Part Character 4	Radionuclide Character 5	Qualifier Character 6	Qualifier Character 7
0 Breast, Right 1 Breast, Left 2 Breasts, Bilateral	1 Technetium 99m (Tc-99m) S Thallium 201 (Tl-201) Y Other Radionuclide	Z None	Z None
Y Skin, Subcutaneous Tissue and Breast	Y Other Radionuclide	Z None	Z None

C   Nuclear Medicine
H   Skin, Subcutaneous Tissue and Breast
2   Tomographic (Tomo) Nuclear Medicine Imaging   Definition: Introduction of radioactive materials into the body for three dimensional display of images developed from the capture of radioactive emissions

Body Part Character 4	Radionuclide Character 5	Qualifier Character 6	Qualifier Character 7
0 Breast, Right 1 Breast, Left 2 Breasts, Bilateral	1 Technetium 99m (Tc-99m) S Thallium 201 (Tl-201) Y Other Radionuclide	Z None	Z None
Y Skin, Subcutaneous Tissue and Breast	Y Other Radionuclide	Z None	Z None

C   Nuclear Medicine
P   Musculoskeletal System
1   Planar Nuclear Medicine Imaging   Definition: Introduction of radioactive materials into the body for single plane display of images developed from the capture of radioactive emissions

Body Part Character 4	Radionuclide Character 5	Qualifier Character 6	Qualifier Character 7
1 Skull 4 Thorax 5 Spine 6 Pelvis 7 Spine and Pelvis 8 Upper Extremity, Right 9 Upper Extremity, Left B Upper Extremities, Bilateral C Lower Extremity, Right D Lower Extremity, Left F Lower Extremities, Bilateral Z Musculoskeletal System, All	1 Technetium 99m (Tc-99m) Y Other Radionuclide	Z None	Z None
Y Musculoskeletal System, Other	Y Other Radionuclide	Z None	Z None

C   **Nuclear Medicine**
P   **Musculoskeletal System**
2   **Tomographic (Tomo) Nuclear Medicine Imaging**   Definition: Introduction of radioactive materials into the body for three dimensional display of images developed from the capture of radioactive emissions

Body Part Character 4	Radionuclide Character 5	Qualifier Character 6	Qualifier Character 7
1 Skull 2 Cervical Spine 3 Skull and Cervical Spine 4 Thorax 6 Pelvis 7 Spine and Pelvis 8 Upper Extremity, Right 9 Upper Extremity, Left B Upper Extremities, Bilateral C Lower Extremity, Right D Lower Extremity, Left F Lower Extremities, Bilateral G Thoracic Spine H Lumbar Spine J Thoracolumbar Spine	1 Technetium 99m (Tc-99m) Y Other Radionuclide	Z None	Z None
Y Musculoskeletal System, Other	Y Other Radionuclide	Z None	Z None

C   **Nuclear Medicine**
P   **Musculoskeletal System**
5   **Nonimaging Nuclear Medicine Probe**   Definition: Introduction of radioactive materials into the body for the study of distribution and fate of certain substances by the detection of radioactive emissions; or, alternatively, measurement of absorption of radioactive emissions from an external source

Body Part Character 4	Radionuclide Character 5	Qualifier Character 6	Qualifier Character 7
5 Spine N Upper Extremities P Lower Extremities	Z None	Z None	Z None
Y Musculoskeletal System, Other	Y Other Radionuclide	Z None	Z None

C   **Nuclear Medicine**
T   **Urinary System**
1   **Planar Nuclear Medicine Imaging**   Definition: Introduction of radioactive materials into the body for single plane display of images developed from the capture of radioactive emissions

Body Part Character 4	Radionuclide Character 5	Qualifier Character 6	Qualifier Character 7
3 Kidneys, Ureters and Bladder	1 Technetium 99m (Tc-99m) F Iodine 123 (I-123) G Iodine 131 (I-131) Y Other Radionuclide	Z None	Z None
H Bladder and Ureters	1 Technetium 99m (Tc-99m) Y Other Radionuclide	Z None	Z None
Y Urinary System	Y Other Radionuclide	Z None	Z None

C   **Nuclear Medicine**
T   **Urinary System**
2   **Tomographic (Tomo) Nuclear Medicine Imaging**   Definition: Introduction of radioactive materials into the body for three dimensional display of images developed from the capture of radioactive emissions

Body Part Character 4	Radionuclide Character 5	Qualifier Character 6	Qualifier Character 7
3 Kidneys, Ureters and Bladder	1 Technetium 99m (Tc-99m) Y Other Radionuclide	Z None	Z None
Y Urinary System	Y Other Radionuclide	Z None	Z None

C   **Nuclear Medicine**
T   **Urinary System**
6   **Nonimaging Nuclear Medicine Assay**   Definition: Introduction of radioactive materials into the body for the study of body fluids and blood elements, by the detection of radioactive emissions

Body Part Character 4	Radionuclide Character 5	Qualifier Character 6	Qualifier Character 7
3 Kidneys, Ureters and Bladder	1 Technetium 99m (Tc-99m) F Iodine 123 (I-123) G Iodine 131 (I-131) H Iodine 125 (I-125) Y Other Radionuclide	Z None	Z None
Y Urinary System	Y Other Radionuclide	Z None	Z None

NC Noncovered Procedure   LC Limited Coverage   OA Questionable OB Admit   NT New Tech Add-on   ⊞ Combination Member   ♂Male   ♀Female

ICD-10-PCS 2022   777

CP2–CT6

C   **Nuclear Medicine**
V   **Male Reproductive System**
1   **Planar Nuclear Medicine Imaging**   Definition: Introduction of radioactive materials into the body for single plane display of images developed from the capture of radioactive emissions

Body Part Character 4	Radionuclide Character 5	Qualifier Character 6	Qualifier Character 7
9 Testicles, Bilateral ♂	1 Technetium 99m (Tc-99m) Y Other Radionuclide	Z None	Z None
Y Male Reproductive System ♂	Y Other Radionuclide	Z None	Z None

♂   All body part, radionuclide, and qualifier values

C   **Nuclear Medicine**
W   **Anatomical Regions**
1   **Planar Nuclear Medicine Imaging**   Definition: Introduction of radioactive materials into the body for single plane display of images developed from the capture of radioactive emissions

Body Part Character 4	Radionuclide Character 5	Qualifier Character 6	Qualifier Character 7
Ø Abdomen 1 Abdomen and Pelvis 4 Chest and Abdomen 6 Chest and Neck B Head and Neck D Lower Extremity J Pelvic Region M Upper Extremity N Whole Body	1 Technetium 99m (Tc-99m) D Indium 111 (In-111) F Iodine 123 (I-123) G Iodine 131 (I-131) L Gallium 67 (Ga-67) S Thallium 201 (Tl-201) Y Other Radionuclide	Z None	Z None
3 Chest	1 Technetium 99m (Tc-99m) D Indium 111 (In-111) F Iodine 123 (I-123) G Iodine 131 (I-131) K Fluorine 18 (F-18) L Gallium 67 (Ga-67) S Thallium 201 (Tl-201) Y Other Radionuclide	Z None	Z None
Y Anatomical Regions, Multiple	Y Other Radionuclide	Z None	Z None
Z Anatomical Region, Other	Z None	Z None	Z None

C   **Nuclear Medicine**
W   **Anatomical Regions**
2   **Tomographic (Tomo) Nuclear Medicine Imaging**   Definition: Introduction of radioactive materials into the body for three dimensional display of images developed from the capture of radioactive emissions

Body Part Character 4	Radionuclide Character 5	Qualifier Character 6	Qualifier Character 7
Ø Abdomen 1 Abdomen and Pelvis 3 Chest 4 Chest and Abdomen 6 Chest and Neck B Head and Neck D Lower Extremity J Pelvic Region M Upper Extremity	1 Technetium 99m (Tc-99m) D Indium 111 (In-111) F Iodine 123 (I-123) G Iodine 131 (I-131) K Fluorine 18 (F-18) L Gallium 67 (Ga-67) S Thallium 201 (Tl-201) Y Other Radionuclide	Z None	Z None
Y Anatomical Regions, Multiple	Y Other Radionuclide	Z None	Z None

C   **Nuclear Medicine**
W   **Anatomical Regions**
3   **Positron Emission Tomographic (PET) Imaging**   Definition: Introduction of radioactive materials into the body for three dimensional display of images developed from the simultaneous capture, 180 degrees apart, of radioactive emissions

Body Part Character 4	Radionuclide Character 5	Qualifier Character 6	Qualifier Character 7
N Whole Body	Y Other Radionuclide	Z None	Z None

C   Nuclear Medicine
W   Anatomical Regions
5   Nonimaging Nuclear Medicine Probe   Definition: Introduction of radioactive materials into the body for the study of distribution and fate of certain substances by the detection of radioactive emissions; or, alternatively, measurement of absorption of radioactive emissions from an external source

Body Part Character 4	Radionuclide Character 5	Qualifier Character 6	Qualifier Character 7
Ø Abdomen 1 Abdomen and Pelvis 3 Chest 4 Chest and Abdomen 6 Chest and Neck B Head and Neck D Lower Extremity J Pelvic Region M Upper Extremity	1 Technetium 99m (Tc-99m) D Indium 111 (In-111) Y Other Radionuclide	Z None	Z None

C   Nuclear Medicine
W   Anatomical Regions
7   Systemic Nuclear Medicine Therapy   Definition: Introduction of unsealed radioactive materials into the body for treatment

Body Part Character 4	Radionuclide Character 5	Qualifier Character 6	Qualifier Character 7
Ø Abdomen 3 Chest	N Phosphorus 32 (P-32) Y Other Radionuclide	Z None	Z None
G Thyroid	G Iodine 131 (I-131) Y Other Radionuclide	Z None	Z None
N Whole Body	8 Samarium 153 (Sm-153) G Iodine 131 (I-131) N Phosphorus 32 (P-32) P Strontium 89 (Sr-89) Y Other Radionuclide	Z None	Z None
Y Anatomical Regions, Multiple	Y Other Radionuclide	Z None	Z None

Radiation Therapy D00–DWY

AHA Coding Clinic for table D01
2020, 4Q, 43-44	Insertion of radioactive element
2020, 4Q, 69-70	Cesium 131 brachytherapy
2019, 4Q, 42-44	Unidirectional source brachytherapy

AHA Coding Clinic for table D0Y
2020, 4Q, 70	Intraoperative radiation therapy

AHA Coding Clinic for table D71
2020, 4Q, 43-44	Insertion of radioactive element
2020, 4Q, 69-70	Cesium 131 brachytherapy
2019, 4Q, 42-44	Unidirectional source brachytherapy

AHA Coding Clinic for table D81
2020, 4Q, 43-44	Insertion of radioactive element
2020, 4Q, 69-70	Cesium 131 brachytherapy
2019, 4Q, 42-44	Unidirectional source brachytherapy

AHA Coding Clinic for table D91
2020, 4Q, 43-44	Insertion of radioactive element
2020, 4Q, 69-70	Cesium 131 brachytherapy
2019, 4Q, 42-44	Unidirectional source brachytherapy

AHA Coding Clinic for table DB1
2020, 4Q, 43-44	Insertion of radioactive element
2020, 4Q, 69-70	Cesium 131 brachytherapy
2019, 4Q, 42-44	Unidirectional source brachytherapy

AHA Coding Clinic for table DD1
2020, 4Q, 43-44	Insertion of radioactive element
2020, 4Q, 69-70	Cesium 131 brachytherapy
2019, 4Q, 42-44	Unidirectional source brachytherapy

AHA Coding Clinic for table DF1
2020, 4Q, 43-44	Insertion of radioactive element
2020, 4Q, 69-70	Cesium 131 brachytherapy
2019, 4Q, 42-44	Unidirectional source brachytherapy

AHA Coding Clinic for table DG1
2020, 4Q, 43-44	Insertion of radioactive element
2020, 4Q, 69-70	Cesium 131 brachytherapy
2019, 4Q, 42-44	Unidirectional source brachytherapy

AHA Coding Clinic for table DM1
2020, 4Q, 43-44	Insertion of radioactive element
2020, 4Q, 69-70	Cesium 131 brachytherapy
2019, 4Q, 42-44	Unidirectional source brachytherapy

AHA Coding Clinic for table DT1
2020, 4Q, 43-44	Insertion of radioactive element
2020, 4Q, 69-70	Cesium 131 brachytherapy
2019, 4Q, 42-44	Unidirectional source brachytherapy

AHA Coding Clinic for table DU1
2020, 4Q, 43-44	Insertion of radioactive element
2020, 4Q, 69-70	Cesium 131 brachytherapy
2019, 4Q, 42-44	Unidirectional source brachytherapy
2017, 4Q, 104	Intrauterine brachytherapy & placement of tandems & ovoids

AHA Coding Clinic for table DV1
2020, 4Q, 43-44	Insertion of radioactive element
2020, 4Q, 69-70	Cesium 131 brachytherapy
2019, 4Q, 42-44	Unidirectional source brachytherapy

AHA Coding Clinic for table DW1
2020, 4Q, 43-44	Insertion of radioactive element
2020, 4Q, 69-70	Cesium 131 brachytherapy
2019, 4Q, 42-44	Unidirectional source brachytherapy

AHA Coding Clinic for table DWY
2019, 4Q, 37	Hyperthermic antineoplastic chemotherapy

D   Radiation Therapy
0   Central and Peripheral Nervous System
0   Beam Radiation

Treatment Site Character 4	Modality Qualifier Character 5	Isotope Character 6	Qualifier Character 7
0 Brain 1 Brain Stem 6 Spinal Cord 7 Peripheral Nerve	0 Photons <1 MeV 1 Photons 1- 10 MeV 2 Photons >10 MeV 4 Heavy Particles (Protons, Ions) 5 Neutrons 6 Neutron Capture	Z None	Z None
0 Brain 1 Brain Stem 6 Spinal Cord 7 Peripheral Nerve	3 Electrons	Z None	0 Intraoperative Z None

D   Radiation Therapy
0   Central and Peripheral Nervous System
1   Brachytherapy

Treatment Site Character 4	Modality Qualifier Character 5	Isotope Character 6	Qualifier Character 7
0 Brain 1 Brain Stem 6 Spinal Cord 7 Peripheral Nerve	9 High Dose Rate (HDR)	7 Cesium 137 (Cs-137) 8 Iridium 192 (Ir-192) 9 Iodine 125 (I-125) B Palladium 103 (Pd-103) C Californium 252 (Cf-252) Y Other Isotope	Z None
0 Brain 1 Brain Stem 6 Spinal Cord 7 Peripheral Nerve	B Low Dose Rate (LDR)	6 Cesium 131 (Cs-131) 7 Cesium 137 (Cs-137) 8 Iridium 192 (Ir-192) 9 Iodine 125 (I-125) C Californium 252 (Cf-252) Y Other Isotope	Z None
0 Brain 1 Brain Stem 6 Spinal Cord 7 Peripheral Nerve	B Low Dose Rate (LDR)	B Palladium 103 (Pd-103)	1 Unidirectional Source Z None

NC Noncovered Procedure   LC Limited Coverage   QA Questionable OB Admit   NT New Tech Add-on   ⊞ Combination Member   ♂ Male   ♀ Female

Radiation Therapy

D   Radiation Therapy
0   Central and Peripheral Nervous System
2   Stereotactic Radiosurgery

Treatment Site Character 4	Modality Qualifier Character 5	Isotope Character 6	Qualifier Character 7

0   Brain
1   Brain Stem
6   Spinal Cord
7   Peripheral Nerve
	D Stereotactic Other Photon
	     Radiosurgery
	H Stereotactic Particulate
	     Radiosurgery
	J Stereotactic Gamma Beam
	     Radiosurgery
		Z None	Z None

DRG Non-OR   All treatment site, modality, isotope, and qualifier values

D   Radiation Therapy
0   Central and Peripheral Nervous System
Y   Other Radiation

Treatment Site Character 4	Modality Qualifier Character 5	Isotope Character 6	Qualifier Character 7
0 Brain 1 Brain Stem 6 Spinal Cord 7 Peripheral Nerve	7 Contact Radiation 8 Hyperthermia C Intraoperative Radiation Therapy (IORT) F Plaque Radiation K Laser Interstitial Thermal Therapy	Z None	Z None

Valid OR   D0Y[0,1,6,7]KZZ

D   Radiation Therapy
7   Lymphatic and Hematologic System
0   Beam Radiation

Treatment Site Character 4	Modality Qualifier Character 5	Isotope Character 6	Qualifier Character 7
0 Bone Marrow 1 Thymus 2 Spleen 3 Lymphatics, Neck 4 Lymphatics, Axillary 5 Lymphatics, Thorax 6 Lymphatics, Abdomen 7 Lymphatics, Pelvis 8 Lymphatics, Inguinal	0 Photons <1 MeV 1 Photons 1- 10 MeV 2 Photons >10 MeV 4 Heavy Particles (Protons, Ions) 5 Neutrons 6 Neutron Capture	Z None	Z None
0 Bone Marrow 1 Thymus 2 Spleen 3 Lymphatics, Neck 4 Lymphatics, Axillary 5 Lymphatics, Thorax 6 Lymphatics, Abdomen 7 Lymphatics, Pelvis 8 Lymphatics, Inguinal	3 Electrons	Z None	0 Intraoperative Z None

D   Radiation Therapy
7   Lymphatic and Hematologic System
1   Brachytherapy

Treatment Site Character 4	Modality Qualifier Character 5	Isotope Character 6	Qualifier Character 7
0 Bone Marrow 1 Thymus 2 Spleen 3 Lymphatics, Neck 4 Lymphatics, Axillary 5 Lymphatics, Thorax 6 Lymphatics, Abdomen 7 Lymphatics, Pelvis 8 Lymphatics, Inguinal	9 High Dose Rate (HDR)	7 Cesium 137 (Cs-137) 8 Iridium 192 (Ir-192) 9 Iodine 125 (I-125) B Palladium 103 (Pd-103) C Californium 252 (Cf-252) Y Other Isotope	Z None
0 Bone Marrow 1 Thymus 2 Spleen 3 Lymphatics, Neck 4 Lymphatics, Axillary 5 Lymphatics, Thorax 6 Lymphatics, Abdomen 7 Lymphatics, Pelvis 8 Lymphatics, Inguinal	B Low Dose Rate (LDR)	6 Cesium 131 (Cs-131) 7 Cesium 137 (Cs-137) 8 Iridium 192 (Ir-192) 9 Iodine 125 (I-125) C Californium 252 (Cf-252) Y Other Isotope	Z None
0 Bone Marrow 1 Thymus 2 Spleen 3 Lymphatics, Neck 4 Lymphatics, Axillary 5 Lymphatics, Thorax 6 Lymphatics, Abdomen 7 Lymphatics, Pelvis 8 Lymphatics, Inguinal	B Low Dose Rate (LDR)	B Palladium 103 (Pd-103)	1 Unidirectional Source Z None

D   Radiation Therapy
7   Lymphatic and Hematologic System
2   Stereotactic Radiosurgery

Treatment Site Character 4	Modality Qualifier Character 5	Isotope Character 6	Qualifier Character 7

0   Bone Marrow
1   Thymus
2   Spleen
3   Lymphatics, Neck
4   Lymphatics, Axillary
5   Lymphatics, Thorax
6   Lymphatics, Abdomen
7   Lymphatics, Pelvis
8   Lymphatics, Inguinal
	D Stereotactic Other Photon
	     Radiosurgery
	H Stereotactic Particulate
	     Radiosurgery
	J Stereotactic Gamma Beam
	     Radiosurgery
		Z None	Z None

DRG Non-OR   All treatment site, modality, isotope, and qualifier values

D   Radiation Therapy
7   Lymphatic and Hematologic System
Y   Other Radiation

Treatment Site Character 4	Modality Qualifier Character 5	Isotope Character 6	Qualifier Character 7
0 Bone Marrow 1 Thymus 2 Spleen 3 Lymphatics, Neck 4 Lymphatics, Axillary 5 Lymphatics, Thorax 6 Lymphatics, Abdomen 7 Lymphatics, Pelvis 8 Lymphatics, Inguinal	8 Hyperthermia F Plaque Radiation	Z None	Z None

NC Noncovered Procedure   **LC** Limited Coverage   **QA** Questionable OB Admit   **NT** New Tech Add-on   ✛ Combination Member   ♂ Male   ♀ Female

ICD-10-PCS 2022   783

Radiation Therapy

D Radiation Therapy
8 Eye
Ø Beam Radiation

Treatment Site Character 4	Modality Qualifier Character 5	Isotope Character 6	Qualifier Character 7
Ø Eye	Ø Photons <1 MeV 1 Photons 1- 10 MeV 2 Photons >10 MeV 4 Heavy Particles (Protons, Ions) 5 Neutrons 6 Neutron Capture	Z None	Z None
Ø Eye	3 Electrons	Z None	Ø Intraoperative Z None

D Radiation Therapy
8 Eye
1 Brachytherapy

Treatment Site Character 4	Modality Qualifier Character 5	Isotope Character 6	Qualifier Character 7
Ø Eye	9 High Dose Rate (HDR)	7 Cesium 137 (Cs-137) 8 Iridium 192 (Ir-192) 9 Iodine 125 (I-125) B Palladium 103 (Pd-103) C Californium 252 (Cf-252) Y Other Isotope	Z None
Ø Eye	B Low Dose Rate (LDR)	6 Cesium 131 (Cs-131) 7 Cesium 137 (Cs-137) 8 Iridium 192 (Ir-192) 9 Iodine 125 (I-125) C Californium 252 (Cf-252) Y Other Isotope	Z None
Ø Eye	B Low Dose Rate (LDR)	B Palladium 103 (Pd-103)	1 Unidirectional Source Z None

D Radiation Therapy
8 Eye
2 Stereotactic Radiosurgery

Treatment Site Character 4	Modality Qualifier Character 5	Isotope Character 6	Qualifier Character 7
Ø Eye	D Stereotactic Other Photon Radiosurgery H Stereotactic Particulate Radiosurgery J Stereotactic Gamma Beam Radiosurgery	Z None	Z None

DRG Non-OR All treatment site, modality, isotope, and qualifier values

D Radiation Therapy
8 Eye
Y Other Radiation

Treatment Site Character 4	Modality Qualifier Character 5	Isotope Character 6	Qualifier Character 7
Ø Eye	7 Contact Radiation 8 Hyperthermia F Plaque Radiation	Z None	Z None

D   **Radiation Therapy**
9   **Ear, Nose, Mouth and Throat**
0   **Beam Radiation**

Treatment Site Character 4	Modality Qualifier Character 5	Isotope Character 6	Qualifier Character 7
0 Ear 1 Nose 3 Hypopharynx 4 Mouth 5 Tongue 6 Salivary Glands 7 Sinuses 8 Hard Palate 9 Soft Palate B Larynx D Nasopharynx F Oropharynx	0 Photons <1 MeV 1 Photons 1- 10 MeV 2 Photons >10 MeV 4 Heavy Particles (Protons, Ions) 5 Neutrons 6 Neutron Capture	Z None	Z None
0 Ear 1 Nose 3 Hypopharynx 4 Mouth 5 Tongue 6 Salivary Glands 7 Sinuses 8 Hard Palate 9 Soft Palate B Larynx D Nasopharynx F Oropharynx	3 Electrons	Z None	0 Intraoperative Z None

D   **Radiation Therapy**
9   **Ear, Nose, Mouth and Throat**
1   **Brachytherapy**

Treatment Site Character 4	Modality Qualifier Character 5	Isotope Character 6	Qualifier Character 7
0 Ear 1 Nose 3 Hypopharynx 4 Mouth 5 Tongue 6 Salivary Glands 7 Sinuses 8 Hard Palate 9 Soft Palate B Larynx D Nasopharynx F Oropharynx	9 High Dose Rate (HDR)	7 Cesium 137 (Cs-137) 8 Iridium 192 (Ir-192) 9 Iodine 125 (I-125) B Palladium 103 (Pd-103) C Californium 252 (Cf-252) Y Other Isotope	Z None
0 Ear 1 Nose 3 Hypopharynx 4 Mouth 5 Tongue 6 Salivary Glands 7 Sinuses 8 Hard Palate 9 Soft Palate B Larynx D Nasopharynx F Oropharynx	B Low Dose Rate (LDR)	6 Cesium 131 (Cs-131) 7 Cesium 137 (Cs-137) 8 Iridium 192 (Ir-192) 9 Iodine 125 (I-125) C Californium 252 (Cf-252) Y Other Isotope	Z None
0 Ear 1 Nose 3 Hypopharynx 4 Mouth 5 Tongue 6 Salivary Glands 7 Sinuses 8 Hard Palate 9 Soft Palate B Larynx D Nasopharynx F Oropharynx	B Low Dose Rate (LDR)	B Palladium 103 (Pd-103)	1 Unidirectional Source Z None

NC Noncovered Procedure   LC Limited Coverage   QA Questionable OB Admit   NT New Tech Add-on   ⊞ Combination Member   ♂ Male   ♀ Female

ICD-10-PCS 2022   785

Radiation Therapy

D Radiation Therapy
9 Ear, Nose, Mouth and Throat
2 Stereotactic Radiosurgery

Treatment Site Character 4	Modality Qualifier Character 5	Isotope Character 6	Qualifier Character 7

Ø Ear
1 Nose
4 Mouth
5 Tongue
6 Salivary Glands
7 Sinuses
8 Hard Palate
9 Soft Palate
B Larynx
C Pharynx
D Nasopharynx
	D Stereotactic Other Photon
	   Radiosurgery
	H Stereotactic Particulate
	   Radiosurgery
	J Stereotactic Gamma Beam
	   Radiosurgery
		Z None	Z None

DRG Non-OR   All treatment site, modality, isotope, and qualifier values

D Radiation Therapy
9 Ear, Nose, Mouth and Throat
Y Other Radiation

Treatment Site Character 4	Modality Qualifier Character 5	Isotope Character 6	Qualifier Character 7
Ø Ear 1 Nose 5 Tongue 6 Salivary Glands 7 Sinuses 8 Hard Palate 9 Soft Palate	7 Contact Radiation 8 Hyperthermia F Plaque Radiation	Z None	Z None
3 Hypopharynx F Oropharynx	7 Contact Radiation 8 Hyperthermia	Z None	Z None
4 Mouth B Larynx D Nasopharynx	7 Contact Radiation 8 Hyperthermia C Intraoperative Radiation Therapy (IORT) F Plaque Radiation	Z None	Z None
C Pharynx	C Intraoperative Radiation Therapy (IORT) F Plaque Radiation	Z None	Z None

D Radiation Therapy
B Respiratory System
Ø Beam Radiation

Treatment Site Character 4	Modality Qualifier Character 5	Isotope Character 6	Qualifier Character 7
Ø Trachea 1 Bronchus 2 Lung 5 Pleura 6 Mediastinum 7 Chest Wall 8 Diaphragm	Ø Photons <1 MeV 1 Photons 1- 10 MeV 2 Photons >10 MeV 4 Heavy Particles (Protons, Ions) 5 Neutrons 6 Neutron Capture	Z None	Z None
Ø Trachea 1 Bronchus 2 Lung 5 Pleura 6 Mediastinum 7 Chest Wall 8 Diaphragm	3 Electrons	Z None	Ø Intraoperative Z None

D Radiation Therapy
B Respiratory System
1 Brachytherapy

Treatment Site Character 4	Modality Qualifier Character 5	Isotope Character 6	Qualifier Character 7
Ø Trachea 1 Bronchus 2 Lung 5 Pleura 6 Mediastinum 7 Chest Wall 8 Diaphragm	9 High Dose Rate (HDR)	7 Cesium 137 (Cs-137) 8 Iridium 192 (Ir-192) 9 Iodine 125 (I-125) B Palladium 103 (Pd-103) C Californium 252 (Cf-252) Y Other Isotope	Z None
Ø Trachea 1 Bronchus 2 Lung 5 Pleura 6 Mediastinum 7 Chest Wall 8 Diaphragm	B Low Dose Rate (LDR)	6 Cesium 131 (Cs-131) 7 Cesium 137 (Cs-137) 8 Iridium 192 (Ir-192) 9 Iodine 125 (I-125) C Californium 252 (Cf-252) Y Other Isotope	Z None
Ø Trachea 1 Bronchus 2 Lung 5 Pleura 6 Mediastinum 7 Chest Wall 8 Diaphragm	B Low Dose Rate (LDR)	B Palladium 103 (Pd-103)	1 Unidirectional Source Z None

D Radiation Therapy
B Respiratory System
2 Stereotactic Radiosurgery

Treatment Site Character 4	Modality Qualifier Character 5	Isotope Character 6	Qualifier Character 7

Ø Trachea
1 Bronchus
2 Lung
5 Pleura
6 Mediastinum
7 Chest Wall
8 Diaphragm
	D Stereotactic Other Photon
	   Radiosurgery
	H Stereotactic Particulate
	   Radiosurgery
	J Stereotactic Gamma Beam
	   Radiosurgery
		Z None	Z None

DRG Non-OR All treatment site, modality, isotope, and qualifier values

D Radiation Therapy
B Respiratory System
Y Other Radiation

Treatment Site Character 4	Modality Qualifier Character 5	Isotope Character 6	Qualifier Character 7
Ø Trachea 1 Bronchus 2 Lung 5 Pleura 6 Mediastinum 7 Chest Wall 8 Diaphragm	7 Contact Radiation 8 Hyperthermia F Plaque Radiation K Laser Interstitial Thermal Therapy	Z None	Z None

Valid OR DBY[Ø,1,2,5,6,7,8]KZZ

Radiation Therapy

D   **Radiation Therapy**
D   **Gastrointestinal System**
Ø   **Beam Radiation**

Treatment Site Character 4	Modality Qualifier Character 5	Isotope Character 6	Qualifier Character 7
Ø Esophagus 1 Stomach 2 Duodenum 3 Jejunum 4 Ileum 5 Colon 7 Rectum	Ø Photons <1 MeV 1 Photons 1- 10 MeV 2 Photons >10 MeV 4 Heavy Particles (Protons, Ions) 5 Neutrons 6 Neutron Capture	Z None	Z None
Ø Esophagus 1 Stomach 2 Duodenum 3 Jejunum 4 Ileum 5 Colon 7 Rectum	3 Electrons	Z None	Ø Intraoperative Z None

D   **Radiation Therapy**
D   **Gastrointestinal System**
1   **Brachytherapy**

Treatment Site Character 4	Modality Qualifier Character 5	Isotope Character 6	Qualifier Character 7
Ø Esophagus 1 Stomach 2 Duodenum 3 Jejunum 4 Ileum 5 Colon 7 Rectum	9 High Dose Rate (HDR)	7 Cesium 137 (Cs-137) 8 Iridium 192 (Ir-192) 9 Iodine 125 (I-125) B Palladium 103 (Pd-103) C Californium 252 (Cf-252) Y Other Isotope	Z None
Ø Esophagus 1 Stomach 2 Duodenum 3 Jejunum 4 Ileum 5 Colon 7 Rectum	B Low Dose Rate (LDR)	6 Cesium 131 (Cs-131) 7 Cesium 137 (Cs-137) 8 Iridium 192 (Ir-192) 9 Iodine 125 (I-125) C Californium 252 (Cf-252) Y Other Isotope	Z None
Ø Esophagus 1 Stomach 2 Duodenum 3 Jejunum 4 Ileum 5 Colon 7 Rectum	B Low Dose Rate (LDR)	B Palladium 103 (Pd-103)	1 Unidirectional Source Z None

D   **Radiation Therapy**
D   **Gastrointestinal System**
2   **Stereotactic Radiosurgery**

Treatment Site Character 4	Modality Qualifier Character 5	Isotope Character 6	Qualifier Character 7
Ø Esophagus 1 Stomach 2 Duodenum 3 Jejunum 4 Ileum 5 Colon 7 Rectum	D Stereotactic Other Photon Radiosurgery H Stereotactic Particulate Radiosurgery J Stereotactic Gamma Beam Radiosurgery	Z None	Z None

DRG Non-OR   All treatment site, modality, isotope, and qualifier values

D   **Radiation therapy**
D   **Gastrointestinal System**
Y   **Other Radiation**

Treatment Site Character 4	Modality Qualifier Character 5	Isotope Character 6	Qualifier Character 7
Ø Esophagus	7 Contact Radiation 8 Hyperthermia F Plaque Radiation K Laser Interstitial Thermal Therapy	Z None	Z None
1 Stomach 2 Duodenum 3 Jejunum 4 Ileum 5 Colon 7 Rectum	7 Contact Radiation 8 Hyperthermia C Intraoperative Radiation Therapy (IORT) F Plaque Radiation K Laser Interstitial Thermal Therapy	Z None	Z None
8 Anus	C Intraoperative Radiation Therapy (IORT) F Plaque Radiation K Laser Interstitial Thermal Therapy	Z None	Z None

Valid OR   DDYØKZZ
Valid OR   DDY[1,2,3,4,5,7]KZZ
Valid OR   DDY8KZZ

D   **Radiation Therapy**
F   **Hepatobiliary System and Pancreas**
Ø   **Beam Radiation**

Treatment Site Character 4	Modality Qualifier Character 5	Isotope Character 6	Qualifier Character 7
Ø Liver 1 Gallbladder 2 Bile Ducts 3 Pancreas	Ø Photons <1 MeV 1 Photons 1- 10 MeV 2 Photons >10 MeV 4 Heavy Particles (Protons, Ions) 5 Neutrons 6 Neutron Capture	Z None	Z None
Ø Liver 1 Gallbladder 2 Bile Ducts 3 Pancreas	3 Electrons	Z None	Ø Intraoperative Z None

D   **Radiation Therapy**
F   **Hepatobiliary System and Pancreas**
1   **Brachytherapy**

Treatment Site Character 4	Modality Qualifier Character 5	Isotope Character 6	Qualifier Character 7
Ø Liver 1 Gallbladder 2 Bile Ducts 3 Pancreas	9 High Dose Rate (HDR)	7 Cesium 137 (Cs-137) 8 Iridium 192 (Ir-192) 9 Iodine 125 (I-125) B Palladium 103 (Pd-103) C Californium 252 (Cf-252) Y Other Isotope	Z None
Ø Liver 1 Gallbladder 2 Bile Ducts 3 Pancreas	B Low Dose Rate (LDR)	6 Cesium 131 (Cs-131) 7 Cesium 137 (Cs-137) 8 Iridium 192 (Ir-192) 9 Iodine 125 (I-125) C Californium 252 (Cf-252) Y Other Isotope	Z None
Ø Liver 1 Gallbladder 2 Bile Ducts 3 Pancreas	B Low Dose Rate (LDR)	B Palladium 103 (Pd-103)	1 Unidirectional Source Z None

NC Noncovered Procedure   **LC** Limited Coverage   **QA** Questionable OB Admit   **NT** New Tech Add-on   ⊞ Combination Member   ♂ Male   ♀ Female

ICD-10-PCS 2022   **789**

Radiation Therapy

D   **Radiation Therapy**
F   **Hepatobiliary System and Pancreas**
2   **Stereotactic Radiosurgery**

Treatment Site Character 4	Modality Qualifier Character 5	Isotope Character 6	Qualifier Character 7
Ø Liver 1 Gallbladder 2 Bile Ducts 3 Pancreas	D Stereotactic Other Photon Radiosurgery H Stereotactic Particulate Radiosurgery J Stereotactic Gamma Beam Radiosurgery	Z None	Z None

DRG Non-OR   All treatment site, modality, isotope, and qualifier values

D   **Radiation Therapy**
F   **Hepatobiliary System and Pancreas**
Y   **Other Radiation**

Treatment Site Character 4	Modality Qualifier Character 5	Isotope Character 6	Qualifier Character 7
Ø Liver 1 Gallbladder 2 Bile Ducts 3 Pancreas	7 Contact Radiation 8 Hyperthermia C Intraoperative Radiation Therapy (IORT) F Plaque Radiation K Laser Interstitial Thermal Therapy	Z None	Z None

Valid OR   DFY[Ø,1,2,3]KZZ

D   **Radiation Therapy**
G   **Endocrine System**
Ø   **Beam Radiation**

Treatment Site Character 4	Modality Qualifier Character 5	Isotope Character 6	Qualifier Character 7
Ø Pituitary Gland 1 Pineal Body 2 Adrenal Glands 4 Parathyroid Glands 5 Thyroid	Ø Photons <1 MeV 1 Photons 1- 10 MeV 2 Photons >10 MeV 5 Neutrons 6 Neutron Capture	Z None	Z None
Ø Pituitary Gland 1 Pineal Body 2 Adrenal Glands 4 Parathyroid Glands 5 Thyroid	3 Electrons	Z None	Ø Intraoperative Z None

D   **Radiation Therapy**
G   **Endocrine System**
1   **Brachytherapy**

Treatment Site Character 4	Modality Qualifier Character 5	Isotope Character 6	Qualifier Character 7
Ø Pituitary Gland 1 Pineal Body 2 Adrenal Glands 4 Parathyroid Glands 5 Thyroid	9 High Dose Rate (HDR)	7 Cesium 137 (Cs-137) 8 Iridium 192 (Ir-192) 9 Iodine 125 (I-125) B Palladium 103 (Pd-103) C Californium 252 (Cf-252) Y Other Isotope	Z None
Ø Pituitary Gland 1 Pineal Body 2 Adrenal Glands 4 Parathyroid Glands 5 Thyroid	B Low Dose Rate (LDR)	6 Cesium 131 (Cs-131) 7 Cesium 137 (Cs-137) 8 Iridium 192 (Ir-192) 9 Iodine 125 (I-125) C Californium 252 (Cf-252) Y Other Isotope	Z None
Ø Pituitary Gland 1 Pineal Body 2 Adrenal Glands 4 Parathyroid Glands 5 Thyroid	B Low Dose Rate (LDR)	B Palladium 103 (Pd-103)	1 Unidirectional Source Z None

Non-OR Procedure   DRG Non-OR Procedure   Valid OR Procedure   HAC Associated Procedure   Combination Only   New/Revised GREEN

D Radiation Therapy
G Endocrine System
2 Stereotactic Radiosurgery

Treatment Site Character 4	Modality Qualifier Character 5	Isotope Character 6	Qualifier Character 7

Ø Pituitary Gland
1 Pineal Body
2 Adrenal Glands
4 Parathyroid Glands
5 Thyroid
	D Stereotactic Other Photon
	   Radiosurgery
	H Stereotactic Particulate
	   Radiosurgery
	J Stereotactic Gamma Beam
	   Radiosurgery
		Z None	Z None

DRG Non-OR All treatment site, modality, isotope, and qualifier values

D Radiation therapy
G Endocrine System
Y Other Radiation

Treatment Site Character 4	Modality Qualifier Character 5	Isotope Character 6	Qualifier Character 7
Ø Pituitary Gland 1 Pineal Body 2 Adrenal Glands 4 Parathyroid Glands 5 Thyroid	7 Contact Radiation 8 Hyperthermia F Plaque Radiation K Laser Interstitial Thermal Therapy	Z None	Z None

Valid OR DGY[Ø,1,2,4,5]KZZ

D Radiation Therapy
H Skin
Ø Beam Radiation

Treatment Site Character 4	Modality Qualifier Character 5	Isotope Character 6	Qualifier Character 7
2 Skin, Face 3 Skin, Neck 4 Skin, Arm 6 Skin, Chest 7 Skin, Back 8 Skin, Abdomen 9 Skin, Buttock B Skin, Leg	Ø Photons <1 MeV 1 Photons 1- 10 MeV 2 Photons >10 MeV 4 Heavy Particles (Protons, Ions) 5 Neutrons 6 Neutron Capture	Z None	Z None
2 Skin, Face 3 Skin, Neck 4 Skin, Arm 6 Skin, Chest 7 Skin, Back 8 Skin, Abdomen 9 Skin, Buttock B Skin, Leg	3 Electrons	Z None	Ø Intraoperative Z None

D Radiation Therapy
H Skin
Y Other Radiation

Treatment Site Character 4	Modality Qualifier Character 5	Isotope Character 6	Qualifier Character 7
2 Skin, Face 3 Skin, Neck 4 Skin, Arm 6 Skin, Chest 7 Skin, Back 8 Skin, Abdomen 9 Skin, Buttock B Skin, Leg	7 Contact Radiation 8 Hyperthermia F Plaque Radiation	Z None	Z None
5 Skin, Hand C Skin, Foot	F Plaque Radiation	Z None	Z None

Radiation Therapy

D Radiation Therapy
M Breast
Ø Beam Radiation

Treatment Site Character 4	Modality Qualifier Character 5	Isotope Character 6	Qualifier Character 7
Ø Breast, Left 1 Breast, Right	Ø Photons <1 MeV 1 Photons 1- 10 MeV 2 Photons >10 MeV 4 Heavy Particles (Protons, Ions) 5 Neutrons 6 Neutron Capture	Z None	Z None
Ø Breast, Left 1 Breast, Right	3 Electrons	Z None	Ø Intraoperative Z None

D Radiation Therapy
M Breast
1 Brachytherapy

Treatment Site Character 4	Modality Qualifier Character 5	Isotope Character 6	Qualifier Character 7
Ø Breast, Left 1 Breast, Right	9 High Dose Rate (HDR)	7 Cesium 137 (Cs-137) 8 Iridium 192 (Ir-192) 9 Iodine 125 (I-125) B Palladium 103 (Pd-103) C Californium 252 (Cf-252) Y Other Isotope	Z None
Ø Breast, Left 1 Breast, Right	B Low Dose Rate (LDR)	6 Cesium 131 (Cs-131) 7 Cesium 137 (Cs-137) 8 Iridium 192 (Ir-192) 9 Iodine 125 (I-125) C Californium 252 (Cf-252) Y Other Isotope	Z None
Ø Breast, Left 1 Breast, Right	B Low Dose Rate (LDR)	B Palladium 103 (Pd-103)	1 Unidirectional Source Z None

D Radiation Therapy
M Breast
2 Stereotactic Radiosurgery

Treatment Site Character 4	Modality Qualifier Character 5	Isotope Character 6	Qualifier Character 7
Ø Breast, Left 1 Breast, Right	D Stereotactic Other Photon Radiosurgery H Stereotactic Particulate Radiosurgery J Stereotactic Gamma Beam Radiosurgery	Z None	Z None

DRG Non-OR All treatment site, modality, isotope, and qualifier values

D Radiation Therapy
M Breast
Y Other Radiation

Treatment Site Character 4	Modality Qualifier Character 5	Isotope Character 6	Qualifier Character 7
Ø Breast, Left 1 Breast, Right	7 Contact Radiation 8 Hyperthermia F Plaque Radiation K Laser Interstitial Thermal Therapy	Z None	Z None

Valid OR DMY[Ø,1]KZZ

D   **Radiation Therapy**
P   **Musculoskeletal System**
Ø   **Beam Radiation**

Treatment Site Character 4	Modality Qualifier Character 5	Isotope Character 6	Qualifier Character 7
Ø Skull 2 Maxilla 3 Mandible 4 Sternum 5 Rib(s) 6 Humerus 7 Radius/Ulna 8 Pelvic Bones 9 Femur B Tibia/Fibula C Other Bone	Ø Photons <1 MeV 1 Photons 1- 10 MeV 2 Photons >10 MeV 4 Heavy Particles (Protons, Ions) 5 Neutrons 6 Neutron Capture	Z None	Z None
Ø Skull 2 Maxilla 3 Mandible 4 Sternum 5 Rib(s) 6 Humerus 7 Radius/Ulna 8 Pelvic Bones 9 Femur B Tibia/Fibula C Other Bone	3 Electrons	Z None	Ø Intraoperative Z None

D   **Radiation Therapy**
P   **Musculoskeletal System**
Y   **Other Radiation**

Treatment Site Character 4	Modality Qualifier Character 5	Isotope Character 6	Qualifier Character 7
Ø Skull 2 Maxilla 3 Mandible 4 Sternum 5 Rib(s) 6 Humerus 7 Radius/Ulna 8 Pelvic Bones 9 Femur B Tibia/Fibula C Other Bone	7 Contact Radiation 8 Hyperthermia F Plaque Radiation	Z None	Z None

D   **Radiation Therapy**
T   **Urinary System**
Ø   **Beam Radiation**

Treatment Site Character 4	Modality Qualifier Character 5	Isotope Character 6	Qualifier Character 7
Ø Kidney 1 Ureter 2 Bladder 3 Urethra	Ø Photons <1 MeV 1 Photons 1- 10 MeV 2 Photons >10 MeV 4 Heavy Particles (Protons, Ions) 5 Neutrons 6 Neutron Capture	Z None	Z None
Ø Kidney 1 Ureter 2 Bladder 3 Urethra	3 Electrons	Z None	Ø Intraoperative Z None

NC Noncovered Procedure   LC Limited Coverage   QA Questionable OB Admit   NT New Tech Add-on   ⊞ Combination Member   ♂ Male   ♀ Female

ICD-10-PCS 2022   793

Radiation Therapy

D   Radiation Therapy
T   Urinary System
1   Brachytherapy

Treatment Site Character 4	Modality Qualifier Character 5	Isotope Character 6	Qualifier Character 7
Ø Kidney 1 Ureter 2 Bladder 3 Urethra	9 High Dose Rate (HDR)	7 Cesium 137 (Cs-137) 8 Iridium 192 (Ir-192) 9 Iodine 125 (I-125) B Palladium 103 (Pd-103) C Californium 252 (Cf-252) Y Other Isotope	Z None
Ø Kidney 1 Ureter 2 Bladder 3 Urethra	B Low Dose Rate (LDR)	6 Cesium 131 (Cs-131) 7 Cesium 137 (Cs-137) 8 Iridium 192 (Ir-192) 9 Iodine 125 (I-125) C Californium 252 (Cf-252) Y Other Isotope	Z None
Ø Kidney 1 Ureter 2 Bladder 3 Urethra	B Low Dose Rate (LDR)	B Palladium 103 (Pd-103)	1 Unidirectional Source Z None

D   Radiation Therapy
T   Urinary System
2   Stereotactic Radiosurgery

Treatment Site Character 4	Modality Qualifier Character 5	Isotope Character 6	Qualifier Character 7

Ø Kidney
1 Ureter
2 Bladder
3 Urethra
	D Stereotactic Other Photon
	    Radiosurgery
	H Stereotactic Particulate
	    Radiosurgery
	J Stereotactic Gamma Beam
	    Radiosurgery
		Z None	Z None

DRG Non-OR   All treatment site, modality, isotope, and qualifier values

D   Radiation Therapy
T   Urinary System
Y   Other Radiation

Treatment Site Character 4	Modality Qualifier Character 5	Isotope Character 6	Qualifier Character 7
Ø Kidney 1 Ureter 2 Bladder 3 Urethra	7 Contact Radiation 8 Hyperthermia C Intraoperative Radiation Therapy (IORT) F Plaque Radiation	Z None	Z None

D   Radiation Therapy
U   Female Reproductive System
Ø   Beam Radiation

Treatment Site Character 4	Modality Qualifier Character 5	Isotope Character 6	Qualifier Character 7
Ø Ovary ♀ 1 Cervix ♀ 2 Uterus ♀	Ø Photons <1 MeV 1 Photons 1- 10 MeV 2 Photons >10 MeV 4 Heavy Particles (Protons, Ions) 5 Neutrons 6 Neutron Capture	Z None	Z None
Ø Ovary ♀ 1 Cervix ♀ 2 Uterus ♀	3 Electrons	Z None	Ø Intraoperative Z None

♀   All treatment site, modality, isotope, and qualifier values

Radiation Therapy

D   Radiation Therapy
U   Female Reproductive System
1   Brachytherapy

Treatment Site Character 4	Modality Qualifier Character 5	Isotope Character 6	Qualifier Character 7
Ø Ovary ♀ 1 Cervix 2 Uterus ♀	9 High Dose Rate (HDR)	7 Cesium 137 (Cs-137) 8 Iridium 192 (Ir-192) 9 Iodine 125 (I-125) B Palladium 103 (Pd-103) C Californium 252 (Cf-252) Y Other Isotope	Z None
Ø Ovary ♀ 1 Cervix ♀ 2 Uterus ♀	B Low Dose Rate (LDR)	6 Cesium 131 (Cs-131) 7 Cesium 137 (Cs-137) 8 Iridium 192 (Ir-192) 9 Iodine 125 (I-125) C Californium 252 (Cf-252) Y Other Isotope	Z None
Ø Ovary ♀ 1 Cervix ♀ 2 Uterus ♀	B Low Dose Rate (LDR)	B Palladium 103 (Pd-103)	1 Unidirectional Source Z None

♀   All treatment site, modality, isotope, and qualifier values

D   Radiation Therapy
U   Female Reproductive System
2   Stereotactic Radiosurgery

Treatment Site Character 4	Modality Qualifier Character 5	Isotope Character 6	Qualifier Character 7

Ø Ovary ♀
1 Cervix ♀
2 Uterus ♀
	D Stereotactic Other Photon
	   Radiosurgery
	H Stereotactic Particulate
	   Radiosurgery
	J Stereotactic Gamma Beam
	   Radiosurgery
		Z None	Z None

DRG Non-OR   All treatment site, modality, isotope, and qualifier values
♀   All treatment site, modality, isotope, and qualifier values

D   Radiation Therapy
U   Female Reproductive System
Y   Other Radiation

Treatment Site Character 4	Modality Qualifier Character 5	Isotope Character 6	Qualifier Character 7
Ø Ovary ♀ 1 Cervix ♀ 2 Uterus ♀	7 Contact Radiation 8 Hyperthermia C Intraoperative Radiation Therapy (IORT) F Plaque Radiation	Z None	Z None

♀   All treatment site, modality, isotope, and qualifier values

D   Radiation Therapy
V   Male Reproductive System
Ø   Beam Radiation

Treatment Site Character 4	Modality Qualifier Character 5	Isotope Character 6	Qualifier Character 7
Ø Prostate ♂ 1 Testis ♂	Ø Photons <1 MeV 1 Photons 1- 10 MeV 2 Photons >10 MeV 4 Heavy Particles (Protons, Ions) 5 Neutrons 6 Neutron Capture	Z None	Z None
Ø Prostate ♂ 1 Testis ♂	3 Electrons	Z None	Ø Intraoperative Z None

♂   All treatment site, modality, isotope, and qualifier values

NC Noncovered Procedure   LC Limited Coverage   QA Questionable OB Admit   NT New Tech Add-on   ⊞ Combination Member   ♂ Male   ♀ Female

ICD-10-PCS 2022   795

Radiation Therapy

D   Radiation Therapy
V   Male Reproductive System
1   Brachytherapy

Treatment Site Character 4	Modality Qualifier Character 5	Isotope Character 6	Qualifier Character 7
Ø Prostate ♂ 1 Testis ♂	9 High Dose Rate (HDR)	7 Cesium 137 (Cs-137) 8 Iridium 192 (Ir-192) 9 Iodine 125 (I-125) B Palladium 103 (Pd-103) C Californium 252 (Cf-252) Y Other Isotope	Z None
Ø Prostate ♂ 1 Testis ♂	B Low Dose Rate (LDR)	6 Cesium 131 (Cs-131) 7 Cesium 137 (Cs-137) 8 Iridium 192 (Ir-192) 9 Iodine 125 (I-125) C Californium 252 (Cf-252) Y Other Isotope	Z None
Ø Prostate ♂ 1 Testis ♂	B Low Dose Rate (LDR)	B Palladium 103 (Pd-103)	1 Unidirectional Source Z None

♂   All treatment site, modality, isotope, and qualifier values

D   Radiation Therapy
V   Male Reproductive System
2   Stereotactic Radiosurgery

Treatment Site Character 4	Modality Qualifier Character 5	Isotope Character 6	Qualifier Character 7

Ø   Prostate   ♂
1   Testis   ♂
	D Stereotactic Other Photon
	     Radiosurgery
	H Stereotactic Particulate
	     Radiosurgery
	J Stereotactic Gamma Beam
	     Radiosurgery
		Z None	Z None

DRG Non-OR   All treatment site, modality, isotope, and qualifier values
♂   All treatment site, modality, isotope, and qualifier values

D   Radiation Therapy
V   Male Reproductive System
Y   Other Radiation

Treatment Site Character 4	Modality Qualifier Character 5	Isotope Character 6	Qualifier Character 7
Ø Prostate ♂	7 Contact Radiation 8 Hyperthermia C Intraoperative Radiation Therapy (IORT) F Plaque Radiation K Laser Interstitial Thermal Therapy	Z None	Z None
1 Testis ♂	7 Contact Radiation 8 Hyperthermia F Plaque Radiation	Z None	Z None

Valid OR   DVYØKZZ
♂   All treatment site, modality, isotope, and qualifier values

D   Radiation Therapy
W   Anatomical Regions
Ø   Beam Radiation

Treatment Site Character 4	Modality Qualifier Character 5	Isotope Character 6	Qualifier Character 7
1 Head and Neck 2 Chest 3 Abdomen 4 Hemibody 5 Whole Body 6 Pelvic Region	Ø Photons <1 MeV 1 Photons 1- 10 MeV 2 Photons >10 MeV 4 Heavy Particles (Protons, Ions) 5 Neutrons 6 Neutron Capture	Z None	Z None
1 Head and Neck 2 Chest 3 Abdomen 4 Hemibody 5 Whole Body 6 Pelvic Region	3 Electrons	Z None	Ø Intraoperative Z None

Non-OR Procedure   DRG Non-OR Procedure   Valid OR Procedure   HAC Associated Procedure   Combination Only   New/Revised GREEN

D   **Radiation Therapy**
W   **Anatomical Regions**
1   **Brachytherapy**

Treatment Site Character 4	Modality Qualifier Character 5	Isotope Character 6	Qualifier Character 7
Ø Cranial Cavity K Upper Back L Lower Back P Gastrointestinal Tract Q Respiratory Tract R Genitourinary Tract X Upper Extremity Y Lower Extremity	B Low Dose Rate (LDR)	B Palladium 103 (Pd-103)	1 Unidirectional Source Z None
1 Head and Neck 2 Chest 3 Abdomen 6 Pelvic Region	9 High Dose Rate (HDR)	7 Cesium 137 (Cs-137) 8 Iridium 192 (Ir-192) 9 Iodine 125 (I-125) B Palladium 103 (Pd-103) C Californium 252 (Cf-252) Y Other Isotope	Z None
1 Head and Neck 2 Chest 3 Abdomen 6 Pelvic Region	B Low Dose Rate (LDR)	6 Cesium 131 (Cs-131) 7 Cesium 137 (Cs-137) 8 Iridium 192 (Ir-192) 9 Iodine 125 (I-125) C Californium 252 (Cf-252) Y Other Isotope	Z None
1 Head and Neck 2 Chest 3 Abdomen 6 Pelvic Region	B Low Dose Rate (LDR)	B Palladium 103 (Pd-103)	1 Unidirectional Source Z None

D   **Radiation Therapy**
W   **Anatomical Regions**
2   **Stereotactic Radiosurgery**

Treatment Site Character 4	Modality Qualifier Character 5	Isotope Character 6	Qualifier Character 7

1 Head and Neck
2 Chest
3 Abdomen
6 Pelvic Region
	D Stereotactic Other Photon
	   Radiosurgery
	H Stereotactic Particulate
	   Radiosurgery
	J Stereotactic Gamma Beam
	   Radiosurgery
		Z None	Z None

DRG Non-OR All treatment site, modality, isotope, and qualifier values

D   **Radiation Therapy**
W   **Anatomical Regions**
Y   **Other Radiation**

Treatment Site Character 4	Modality Qualifier Character 5	Isotope Character 6	Qualifier Character 7
1 Head and Neck 2 Chest 3 Abdomen 4 Hemibody 6 Pelvic Region	7 Contact Radiation 8 Hyperthermia F Plaque Radiation	Z None	Z None
5 Whole Body	7 Contact Radiation 8 Hyperthermia F Plaque Radiation	Z None	Z None
5 Whole Body	G Isotope Administration	D Iodine 131 (I-131) F Phosphorus 32 (P-32) G Strontium 89 (Sr-89) H Strontium 90 (Sr-90) Y Other Isotope	Z None

Radiation Therapy

NC Noncovered Procedure   LC Limited Coverage   OA Questionable OB Admit   NT New Tech Add-on   ⊞ Combination Member   ♂ Male   ♀ Female

ICD-10-PCS 2022   797

Physical Rehabilitation and Diagnostic Audiology F00–F15

F   **Physical Rehabilitation and Diagnostic Audiology**
0   **Rehabilitation**
0   **Speech Assessment**   Definition: Measurement of speech and related functions

Body System/Region Character 4	Type Qualifier Character 5	Equipment Character 6	Qualifier Character 7
3 Neurological System - Whole Body	**G** Communicative/Cognitive Integration Skills	**K** Audiovisual **M** Augmentative / Alternative Communication **P** Computer **Y** Other Equipment **Z** None	**Z** None
Z None	**0** Filtered Speech **3** Staggered Spondaic Word **Q** Performance Intensity Phonetically Balanced Speech Discrimination **R** Brief Tone Stimuli **S** Distorted Speech **T** Dichotic Stimuli **V** Temporal Ordering of Stimuli **W** Masking Patterns	**1** Audiometer **2** Sound Field / Booth **K** Audiovisual **Z** None	**Z** None
Z None	**1** Speech Threshold **2** Speech/Word Recognition	**1** Audiometer **2** Sound Field / Booth **9** Cochlear Implant **K** Audiovisual **Z** None	**Z** None
Z None	**4** Sensorineural Acuity Level	**1** Audiometer **2** Sound Field / Booth **Z** None	**Z** None
Z None	**5** Synthetic Sentence Identification	**1** Audiometer **2** Sound Field / Booth **9** Cochlear Implant **K** Audiovisual	**Z** None
Z None	**6** Speech and/or Language Screening **7** Nonspoken Language **8** Receptive/Expressive Language **C** Aphasia **G** Communicative/Cognitive Integration Skills **L** Augmentative/Alternative Communication System	**K** Audiovisual **M** Augmentative / Alternative Communication **P** Computer **Y** Other Equipment **Z** None	**Z** None
Z None	**9** Articulation/Phonology	**K** Audiovisual **P** Computer **Q** Speech Analysis **Y** Other Equipment **Z** None	**Z** None
Z None	**B** Motor Speech	**K** Audiovisual **N** Biosensory Feedback **P** Computer **Q** Speech Analysis **T** Aerodynamic Function **Y** Other Equipment **Z** None	**Z** None
Z None	**D** Fluency	**K** Audiovisual **N** Biosensory Feedback **P** Computer **Q** Speech Analysis **S** Voice Analysis **T** Aerodynamic Function **Y** Other Equipment **Z** None	**Z** None
Z None	**F** Voice	**K** Audiovisual **N** Biosensory Feedback **P** Computer **S** Voice Analysis **T** Aerodynamic Function **Y** Other Equipment **Z** None	**Z** None

DRG Non-OR   All body system/region, type qualifier, equipment, and qualifier values

F00 Continued on next page

NC Noncovered Procedure   **LC** Limited Coverage   **QA** Questionable OB Admit   **NT** New Tech Add-on   ⊞ Combination Member   ♂ Male   ♀ Female

F   Physical Rehabilitation and Diagnostic Audiology
Ø   Rehabilitation
Ø   Speech Assessment   Definition: Measurement of speech and related functions

Body System/Region Character 4	Type Qualifier Character 5	Equipment Character 6	Qualifier Character 7
Z None	H Bedside Swallowing and Oral Function P Oral Peripheral Mechanism	Y Other Equipment Z None	Z None
Z None	J Instrumental Swallowing and Oral Function	T Aerodynamic Function W Swallowing Y Other Equipment	Z None
Z None	K Orofacial Myofunctional	K Audiovisual P Computer Y Other Equipment Z None	Z None
Z None	M Voice Prosthetic	K Audiovisual P Computer S Voice Analysis V Speech Prosthesis Y Other Equipment Z None	Z None
Z None	N Non-invasive Instrumental Status	N Biosensory Feedback P Computer Q Speech Analysis S Voice Analysis T Aerodynamic Function Y Other Equipment	Z None
Z None	X Other Specified Central Auditory Processing	Z None	Z None

DRG Non-OR   All body system/region, type qualifier, equipment, and qualifier values

F   Physical Rehabilitation and Diagnostic Audiology
Ø   Rehabilitation
1   Motor and/or Nerve Function Assessment   Definition: Measurement of motor, nerve, and related functions

Body System/Region Character 4	Type Qualifier Character 5	Equipment Character 6	Qualifier Character 7
Ø Neurological System - Head and Neck 1 Neurological System - Upper Back/ Upper Extremity 2 Neurological System - Lower Back/ Lower Extremity 3 Neurological System - Whole Body	Ø Muscle Performance	E Orthosis F Assistive, Adaptive, Supportive or Protective U Prosthesis Y Other Equipment Z None	Z None
Ø Neurological System - Head and Neck 1 Neurological System - Upper Back/ Upper Extremity 2 Neurological System - Lower Back/ Lower Extremity 3 Neurological System - Whole Body	1 Integumentary Integrity 3 Coordination/Dexterity 4 Motor Function G Reflex Integrity	Z None	Z None
Ø Neurological System - Head and Neck 1 Neurological System - Upper Back/ Upper Extremity 2 Neurological System - Lower Back/ Lower Extremity 3 Neurological System - Whole Body	5 Range of Motion and Joint Integrity 6 Sensory Awareness/Processing/ Integrity	Y Other Equipment Z None	Z None
D Integumentary System - Head and Neck F Integumentary System - Upper Back/ Upper Extremity G Integumentary System - Lower Back/ Lower Extremity H Integumentary System - Whole Body J Musculoskeletal System - Head and Neck K Musculoskeletal System - Upper Back/ Upper Extremity L Musculoskeletal System - Lower Back/ Lower Extremity M Musculoskeletal System - Whole Body	Ø Muscle Performance	E Orthosis F Assistive, Adaptive, Supportive or Protective U Prosthesis Y Other Equipment Z None	Z None

DRG Non-OR   All body system/region, type qualifier, equipment, and qualifier values

F01 Continued on next page

Non-OR Procedure   DRG Non-OR Procedure   Valid OR Procedure   HAC Associated Procedure   Combination Only   New/Revised GREEN

F   **Physical Rehabilitation and Diagnostic Audiology**
Ø   **Rehabilitation**
1   **Motor and/or Nerve Function Assessment**   Definition: Measurement of motor, nerve, and related functions

Body System/Region Character 4	Type Qualifier Character 5	Equipment Character 6	Qualifier Character 7
D Integumentary System - Head and Neck **F** Integumentary System - Upper Back/ Upper Extremity **G** Integumentary System - Lower Back/ Lower Extremity **H** Integumentary System - Whole Body **J** Musculoskeletal System - Head and Neck **K** Musculoskeletal System - Upper Back/ Upper Extremity **L** Musculoskeletal System - Lower Back/ Lower Extremity **M** Musculoskeletal System - Whole Body	**1** Integumentary Integrity	**Z** None	**Z** None
D Integumentary System - Head and Neck **F** Integumentary System - Upper Back/ Upper Extremity **G** Integumentary System - Lower Back/ Lower Extremity **H** Integumentary System - Whole Body **J** Musculoskeletal System - Head and Neck **K** Musculoskeletal System - Upper Back/ Upper Extremity **L** Musculoskeletal System - Lower Back/ Lower Extremity **M** Musculoskeletal System - Whole Body	**5** Range of Motion and Joint Integrity **6** Sensory Awareness/Processing/ Integrity	**Y** Other Equipment **Z** None	**Z** None
N Genitourinary System	**Ø** Muscle Performance	**E** Orthosis **F** Assistive, Adaptive, Supportive or Protective **U** Prosthesis **Y** Other Equipment **Z** None	**Z** None
Z None	**2** Visual Motor Integration	**K** Audiovisual **M** Augmentative / Alternative Communication **N** Biosensory Feedback **P** Computer **Q** Speech Analysis **S** Voice Analysis **Y** Other Equipment **Z** None	**Z** None
Z None	**7** Facial Nerve Function	**7** Electrophysiologic	**Z** None
Z None	**9** Somatosensory Evoked Potentials	**J** Somatosensory	**Z** None
Z None	**B** Bed Mobility **C** Transfer **F** Wheelchair Mobility	**E** Orthosis **F** Assistive, Adaptive, Supportive or Protective **U** Prosthesis **Z** None	**Z** None
Z None	**D** Gait and/or Balance	**E** Orthosis **F** Assistive, Adaptive, Supportive or Protective **U** Prosthesis **Y** Other Equipment **Z** None	**Z** None

DRG Non-OR   All body system/region, type qualifier, equipment, and qualifier values

NC Noncovered Procedure   **LC** Limited Coverage   **QA** Questionable OB Admit   **NT** New Tech Add-on   ⊞ Combination Member   ♂ Male   ♀ Female

ICD-10-PCS 2022   801

Physical Rehabilitation and Diagnostic Audiology

F   **Physical Rehabilitation and Diagnostic Audiology**
Ø   **Rehabilitation**
2   **Activities of Daily Living Assessment**   Definition: Measurement of functional level for activities of daily living

Body System/Region Character 4	Type Qualifier Character 5	Equipment Character 6	Qualifier Character 7
Ø Neurological System - Head and Neck	9 Cranial Nerve Integrity D Neuromotor Development	Y Other Equipment Z None	Z None
1 Neurological System - Upper Back/Upper Extremity 2 Neurological System - Lower Back/Lower Extremity 3 Neurological System - Whole Body	D Neuromotor Development	Y Other Equipment Z None	Z None
4 Circulatory System - Head and Neck 5 Circulatory System - Upper Back/Upper Extremity 6 Circulatory System - Lower Back/Lower Extremity 8 Respiratory System - Head and Neck 9 Respiratory System - Upper Back/Upper Extremity B Respiratory System - Lower Back/Lower Extremity	G Ventilation, Respiration and Circulation	C Mechanical G Aerobic Endurance and Conditioning Y Other Equipment Z None	Z None
7 Circulatory System - Whole Body C Respiratory System - Whole Body	7 Aerobic Capacity and Endurance	E Orthosis G Aerobic Endurance and Conditioning U Prosthesis Y Other Equipment Z None	Z None
7 Circulatory System - Whole Body C Respiratory System - Whole Body	G Ventilation, Respiration and Circulation	C Mechanical G Aerobic Endurance and Conditioning Y Other Equipment Z None	Z None
Z None	Ø Bathing/Showering 1 Dressing 3 Grooming/Personal Hygiene 4 Home Management	E Orthosis F Assistive, Adaptive, Supportive or Protective U Prosthesis Z None	Z None
Z None	2 Feeding/Eating 8 Anthropometric Characteristics F Pain	Y Other Equipment Z None	Z None
Z None	5 Perceptual Processing	K Audiovisual M Augmentative / Alternative Communication N Biosensory Feedback P Computer Q Speech Analysis S Voice Analysis Y Other Equipment Z None	Z None
Z None	6 Psychosocial Skills	Z None	Z None
Z None	B Environmental, Home and Work Barriers C Ergonomics and Body Mechanics	E Orthosis F Assistive, Adaptive, Supportive or Protective U Prosthesis Y Other Equipment Z None	Z None
Z None	H Vocational Activities and Functional Community or Work Reintegration Skills	E Orthosis F Assistive, Adaptive, Supportive or Protective G Aerobic Endurance and Conditioning U Prosthesis Y Other Equipment Z None	Z None

DRG Non-OR All body system/region, type qualifier, equipment, and qualifier values

Non-OR Procedure   DRG Non-OR Procedure   Valid OR Procedure   HAC Associated Procedure   Combination Only   New/Revised GREEN

F   **Physical Rehabilitation and Diagnostic Audiology**
Ø   **Rehabilitation**
6   **Speech Treatment**   Definition: Application of techniques to improve, augment, or compensate for speech and related functional impairment

Body System/Region Character 4	Type Qualifier Character 5	Equipment Character 6	Qualifier Character 7
3 Neurological System - Whole Body	6 Communicative/Cognitive Integration Skills	K Audiovisual M Augmentative / Alternative Communication P Computer Y Other Equipment Z None	Z None

Z None	0 Nonspoken Language
	3 Aphasia
	6 Communicative/Cognitive
	     Integration Skills
		K Audiovisual
		M Augmentative / Alternative
		     Communication
		P Computer
		Y Other Equipment
		Z None
			Z None

Z None	1 Speech-Language Pathology and
	     Related Disorders Counseling
	2 Speech-Language Pathology and
	     Related Disorders Prevention
		K Audiovisual
		Z None
			Z None

Z None	4 Articulation/Phonology	K Audiovisual P Computer Q Speech Analysis T Aerodynamic Function Y Other Equipment Z None	Z None
Z None	5 Aural Rehabilitation	K Audiovisual L Assistive Listening M Augmentative / Alternative Communication N Biosensory Feedback P Computer Q Speech Analysis S Voice Analysis Y Other Equipment Z None	Z None
Z None	7 Fluency	4 Electroacoustic Immitance / Acoustic Reflex K Audiovisual N Biosensory Feedback Q Speech Analysis S Voice Analysis T Aerodynamic Function Y Other Equipment Z None	Z None
Z None	8 Motor Speech	K Audiovisual N Biosensory Feedback P Computer Q Speech Analysis S Voice Analysis T Aerodynamic Function Y Other Equipment Z None	Z None
Z None	9 Orofacial Myofunctional	K Audiovisual P Computer Y Other Equipment Z None	Z None
Z None	B Receptive/Expressive Language	K Audiovisual L Assistive Listening M Augmentative / Alternative Communication P Computer Y Other Equipment Z None	Z None

DRG Non-OR   All body system/region, type qualifier, equipment, and qualifier values

F06 Continued on next page

NC Noncovered Procedure   **LC** Limited Coverage   **QA** Questionable OB Admit   **NT** New Tech Add-on   ⊞ Combination Member   ♂ Male   ♀ Female

ICD-10-PCS 2022   **803**

F06 Continued

F   **Physical Rehabilitation and Diagnostic Audiology**
Ø   **Rehabilitation**
6   **Speech Treatment**   Definition: Application of techniques to improve, augment, or compensate for speech and related functional impairment

Body System/Region Character 4	Type Qualifier Character 5	Equipment Character 6	Qualifier Character 7
Z None	C Voice	K Audiovisual N Biosensory Feedback P Computer S Voice Analysis T Aerodynamic Function V Speech Prosthesis Y Other Equipment Z None	Z None
Z None	D Swallowing Dysfunction	M Augmentative / Alternative Communication T Aerodynamic Function V Speech Prosthesis Y Other Equipment Z None	Z None

DRG Non-OR   All body system/region, type qualifier, equipment, and qualifier values

F   **Physical Rehabilitation and Diagnostic Audiology**
Ø   **Rehabilitation**
7   **Motor Treatment**   Definition: Exercise or activities to increase or facilitate motor function

Body System/Region Character 4	Type Qualifier Character 5	Equipment Character 6	Qualifier Character 7
Ø Neurological System - Head and Neck 1 Neurological System - Upper Back/Upper Extremity 2 Neurological System - Lower Back/Lower Extremity 3 Neurological System - Whole Body D Integumentary System - Head and Neck F Integumentary System - Upper Back/Upper Extremity G Integumentary System - Lower Back/Lower Extremity H Integumentary System - Whole Body J Musculoskeletal System - Head and Neck K Musculoskeletal System - Upper Back/Upper Extremity L Musculoskeletal System - Lower Back/Lower Extremity M Musculoskeletal System - Whole Body	Ø Range of Motion and Joint Mobility 1 Muscle Performance 2 Coordination/Dexterity 3 Motor Function	E Orthosis F Assistive, Adaptive, Supportive or Protective U Prosthesis Y Other Equipment Z None	Z None
Ø Neurological System - Head and Neck 1 Neurological System - Upper Back/Upper Extremity 2 Neurological System - Lower Back/Lower Extremity 3 Neurological System - Whole Body D Integumentary System - Head and Neck F Integumentary System - Upper Back/Upper Extremity G Integumentary System - Lower Back/Lower Extremity H Integumentary System - Whole Body J Musculoskeletal System - Head and Neck K Musculoskeletal System - Upper Back/Upper Extremity L Musculoskeletal System - Lower Back/Lower Extremity M Musculoskeletal System - Whole Body	6 Therapeutic Exercise	B Physical Agents C Mechanical D Electrotherapeutic E Orthosis F Assistive, Adaptive, Supportive or Protective G Aerobic Endurance and Conditioning H Mechanical or Electromechanical U Prosthesis Y Other Equipment Z None	Z None

DRG Non-OR   All body system/region, type qualifier, equipment, and qualifier values

F07 Continued on next page

F Physical Rehabilitation and Diagnostic Audiology
Ø Rehabilitation
7 Motor Treatment Definition: Exercise or activities to increase or facilitate motor function

Body System/Region Character 4	Type Qualifier Character 5	Equipment Character 6	Qualifier Character 7

Ø Neurological System - Head and Neck
1 Neurological System - Upper Back/
   Upper Extremity
2 Neurological System - Lower Back/
   Lower Extremity
3 Neurological System - Whole Body
D Integumentary System - Head and
   Neck
F Integumentary System - Upper Back/
   Upper Extremity
G Integumentary System - Lower Back/
   Lower Extremity
H Integumentary System - Whole Body
J Musculoskeletal System - Head and
   Neck
K Musculoskeletal System - Upper Back/
   Upper Extremity
L Musculoskeletal System - Lower Back/
   Lower Extremity
M Musculoskeletal System - Whole Body
	7 Manual Therapy Techniques	Z None	Z None

4 Circulatory System - Head and Neck
5 Circulatory System - Upper Back /
   Upper Extremity
6 Circulatory System - Lower Back /
   Lower Extremity
7 Circulatory System - Whole Body
8 Respiratory System - Head and Neck
9 Respiratory System - Upper Back /
   Upper Extremity
B Respiratory System - Lower Back /
   Lower Extremity
C Respiratory System - Whole Body
	6 Therapeutic Exercise	B Physical Agents
		C Mechanical
		D Electrotherapeutic
		E Orthosis
		F Assistive, Adaptive, Supportive or
		   Protective
		G Aerobic Endurance and
		   Conditioning
		H Mechanical or Electromechanical
		U Prosthesis
		Y Other Equipment
		Z None
			Z None

N Genitourinary System	1 Muscle Performance	E Orthosis F Assistive, Adaptive, Supportive or Protective U Prosthesis Y Other Equipment Z None	Z None

N Genitourinary System	6 Therapeutic Exercise	B Physical Agents
		C Mechanical
		D Electrotherapeutic
		E Orthosis
		F Assistive, Adaptive, Supportive or
		   Protective
		G Aerobic Endurance and
		   Conditioning
		H Mechanical or Electromechanical
		U Prosthesis
		Y Other Equipment
		Z None
			Z None

Z None	4 Wheelchair Mobility	D Electrotherapeutic E Orthosis F Assistive, Adaptive, Supportive or Protective U Prosthesis Y Other Equipment Z None	Z None
Z None	5 Bed Mobility	C Mechanical E Orthosis F Assistive, Adaptive, Supportive or Protective U Prosthesis Y Other Equipment Z None	Z None
Z None	8 Transfer Training	C Mechanical D Electrotherapeutic E Orthosis F Assistive, Adaptive, Supportive or Protective U Prosthesis Y Other Equipment Z None	Z None

DRG Non-OR All body system/region, type qualifier, equipment, and qualifier values

F07 Continued on next page

NC Noncovered Procedure   **LC** Limited Coverage   **QA** Questionable OB Admit   **NT** New Tech Add-on   **⊞** Combination Member   ♂ Male   ♀ Female

F   Physical Rehabilitation and Diagnostic Audiology
Ø   Rehabilitation
7   Motor Treatment   Definition: Exercise or activities to increase or facilitate motor function

Body System/Region Character 4	Type Qualifier Character 5	Equipment Character 6	Qualifier Character 7

Z None	9 Gait Training/Functional
	    Ambulation
		C Mechanical
		D Electrotherapeutic
		E Orthosis
		F Assistive, Adaptive, Supportive or
		    Protective
		G Aerobic Endurance and
		    Conditioning
		U Prosthesis
		Y Other Equipment
		Z None
			Z None

DRG Non-OR   All body system/region, type qualifier, equipment, and qualifier values

F   Physical Rehabilitation and Diagnostic Audiology
Ø   Rehabilitation
8   Activities of Daily Living Treatment   Definition: Exercise or activities to facilitate functional competence for activities of daily living

Body System/Region Character 4	Type Qualifier Character 5	Equipment Character 6	Qualifier Character 7

D   Integumentary System - Head and
    Neck
F   Integumentary System - Upper Back/
    Upper Extremity
G   Integumentary System - Lower Back/
    Lower Extremity
H   Integumentary System - Whole Body
J   Musculoskeletal System - Head and
    Neck
K   Musculoskeletal System - Upper Back/
    Upper Extremity
L   Musculoskeletal System - Lower Back/
    Lower Extremity
M   Musculoskeletal System - Whole Body
	5 Wound Management	B Physical Agents
		C Mechanical
		D Electrotherapeutic
		E Orthosis
		F Assistive, Adaptive, Supportive or
		    Protective
		U Prosthesis
		Y Other Equipment
		Z None
			Z None

Z None	Ø Bathing/Showering Techniques 1 Dressing Techniques 2 Grooming/Personal Hygiene	E Orthosis F Assistive, Adaptive, Supportive or Protective U Prosthesis Y Other Equipment Z None	Z None
Z None	3 Feeding/Eating	C Mechanical D Electrotherapeutic E Orthosis F Assistive, Adaptive, Supportive or Protective U Prosthesis Y Other Equipment Z None	Z None
Z None	4 Home Management	D Electrotherapeutic E Orthosis F Assistive, Adaptive, Supportive or Protective U Prosthesis Y Other Equipment Z None	Z None
Z None	6 Psychosocial Skills	Z None	Z None

Z None	7 Vocational Activities and
	    Functional Community or Work
	    Reintegration Skills
		B Physical Agents
		C Mechanical
		D Electrotherapeutic
		E Orthosis
		F Assistive, Adaptive, Supportive or
		    Protective
		G Aerobic Endurance and
		    Conditioning
		U Prosthesis
		Y Other Equipment
		Z None
			Z None

DRG Non-OR   All body system/region, type qualifier, equipment, and qualifier values

Non-OR Procedure   DRG Non-OR Procedure   Valid OR Procedure   HAC Associated Procedure   Combination Only   New/Revised GREEN

F   **Physical Rehabilitation and Diagnostic Audiology**
0   **Rehabilitation**
9   **Hearing Treatment**   Definition: Application of techniques to improve, augment, or compensate for hearing and related functional impairment

Body System/Region Character 4	Type Qualifier Character 5	Equipment Character 6	Qualifier Character 7
Z None	0 Hearing and Related Disorders Counseling 1 Hearing and Related Disorders Prevention	K Audiovisual Z None	Z None
Z None	2 Auditory Processing	K Audiovisual L Assistive Listening P Computer Y Other Equipment Z None	Z None
Z None	3 Cerumen Management	X Cerumen Management Z None	Z None

DRG Non-OR   All body system/region, type qualifier, equipment, and qualifier values

F   **Physical Rehabilitation and Diagnostic Audiology**
0   **Rehabilitation**
B   **Cochlear Implant Treatment**   Definition: Application of techniques to improve the communication abilities of individuals with cochlear implant

Body System/Region Character 4	Type Qualifier Character 5	Equipment Character 6	Qualifier Character 7
Z None	0 Cochlear Implant Rehabilitation	1 Audiometer 2 Sound Field / Booth 9 Cochlear Implant K Audiovisual P Computer Y Other Equipment	Z None

DRG Non-OR   All body system/region, type qualifier, equipment, and qualifier values

F   **Physical Rehabilitation and Diagnostic Audiology**
0   **Rehabilitation**
C   **Vestibular Treatment**   Definition: Application of techniques to improve, augment, or compensate for vestibular and related functional impairment

Body System/Region Character 4	Type Qualifier Character 5	Equipment Character 6	Qualifier Character 7
3 Neurological System - Whole Body H Integumentary System - Whole Body M Musculoskeletal System - Whole Body	3 Postural Control	E Orthosis F Assistive, Adaptive, Supportive or Protective U Prosthesis Y Other Equipment Z None	Z None
Z None	0 Vestibular	8 Vestibular / Balance Z None	Z None
Z None	1 Perceptual Processing 2 Visual Motor Integration	K Audiovisual L Assistive Listening N Biosensory Feedback P Computer Q Speech Analysis S Voice Analysis T Aerodynamic Function Y Other Equipment Z None	Z None

DRG Non-OR   All body system/region, type qualifier, equipment, and qualifier values

NC Noncovered Procedure   **LC** Limited Coverage   **QA** Questionable OB Admit   **NT** New Tech Add-on   ⊞ Combination Member   ♂ Male   ♀ Female

ICD-10-PCS 2022   807

F   **Physical Rehabilitation and Diagnostic Audiology**
0   **Rehabilitation**
D   **Device Fitting**   Definition: Fitting of a device designed to facilitate or support achievement of a higher level of function

Body System/Region Character 4	Type Qualifier Character 5	Equipment Character 6	Qualifier Character 7
Z None	0 Tinnitus Masker	5 Hearing Aid Selection / Fitting / Test Z None	Z None
Z None	1 Monaural Hearing Aid 2 Binaural Hearing Aid 5 Assistive Listening Device	1 Audiometer 2 Sound Field / Booth 5 Hearing Aid Selection / Fitting / Test K Audiovisual L Assistive Listening Z None	Z None
Z None	3 Augmentative/Alternative Communication System	M Augmentative / Alternative Communication	Z None
Z None	4 Voice Prosthetic	S Voice Analysis V Speech Prosthesis	Z None
Z None	6 Dynamic Orthosis 7 Static Orthosis 8 Prosthesis 9 Assistive, Adaptive, Supportive or Protective Devices	E Orthosis F Assistive, Adaptive, Supportive or Protective U Prosthesis Z None	Z None

DRG Non-OR	F0DZ0[5,Z]Z
DRG Non-OR	F0DZ[1, 2,5][1,2,5, K,L,Z]Z
DRG Non-OR	F0DZ3MZ
DRG Non-OR	F0DZ4[S,V]Z
DRG Non-OR	F0DZ[6,7][E,F,U,Z]Z
DRG Non-OR	F0DZ8[E,F,U]Z

F   **Physical Rehabilitation and Diagnostic Audiology**
0   **Rehabilitation**
F   **Caregiver Training**   Definition: Training in activities to support patient's optimal level of function

Body System/Region Character 4	Type Qualifier Character 5	Equipment Character 6	Qualifier Character 7
Z None	0 Bathing/Showering Technique 1 Dressing 2 Feeding and Eating 3 Grooming/Personal Hygiene 4 Bed Mobility 5 Transfer 6 Wheelchair Mobility 7 Therapeutic Exercise 8 Airway Clearance Techniques 9 Wound Management B Vocational Activities and Functional Community or Work Reintegration Skills C Gait Training/Functional Ambulation D Application, Proper Use and Care of Devices F Application, Proper Use and Care of Orthoses G Application, Proper Use and Care of Prosthesis H Home Management	E Orthosis F Assistive, Adaptive, Supportive or Protective U Prosthesis Z None	Z None
Z None	J Communication Skills	K Audiovisual L Assistive Listening M Augmentative / Alternative Communication P Computer Z None	Z None

DRG Non-OR	All body system/region, type qualifier, equipment, and qualifier values

F   Physical Rehabilitation and Diagnostic Audiology
1   Diagnostic Audiology
3   Hearing Assessment   Definition: Measurement of hearing and related functions

Body System/Region Character 4	Type Qualifier Character 5	Equipment Character 6	Qualifier Character 7
Z None	**0** Hearing Screening	**0** Occupational Hearing **1** Audiometer **2** Sound Field / Booth **3** Tympanometer **8** Vestibular / Balance **9** Cochlear Implant **Z** None	**Z** None
Z None	**1** Pure Tone Audiometry, Air **2** Pure Tone Audiometry, Air and Bone	**0** Occupational Hearing **1** Audiometer **2** Sound Field / Booth **Z** None	**Z** None
Z None	**3** Bekesy Audiometry **6** Visual Reinforcement Audiometry **9** Short Increment Sensitivity Index **B** Stenger **C** Pure Tone Stenger	**1** Audiometer **2** Sound Field / Booth **Z** None	**Z** None
Z None	**4** Conditioned Play Audiometry **5** Select Picture Audiometry	**1** Audiometer **2** Sound Field / Booth **K** Audiovisual **Z** None	**Z** None
Z None	**7** Alternate Binaural or Monaural Loudness Balance	**1** Audiometer **K** Audiovisual **Z** None	**Z** None
Z None	**8** Tone Decay **D** Tympanometry **F** Eustachian Tube Function **G** Acoustic Reflex Patterns **H** Acoustic Reflex Threshold **J** Acoustic Reflex Decay	**3** Tympanometer **4** Electroacoustic Immitance / Acoustic Reflex **Z** None	**Z** None
Z None	**K** Electrocochleography **L** Auditory Evoked Potentials	**7** Electrophysiologic **Z** None	**Z** None
Z None	**M** Evoked Otoacoustic Emissions, Screening **N** Evoked Otoacoustic Emissions, Diagnostic	**6** Otoacoustic Emission (OAE) **Z** None	**Z** None
Z None	**P** Aural Rehabilitation Status	**1** Audiometer **2** Sound Field / Booth **4** Electroacoustic Immitance / Acoustic Reflex **9** Cochlear Implant **K** Audiovisual **L** Assistive Listening **P** Computer **Z** None	**Z** None
Z None	**Q** Auditory Processing	**K** Audiovisual **P** Computer **Y** Other Equipment **Z** None	**Z** None

NC Noncovered Procedure   **LC** Limited Coverage   **QA** Questionable OB Admit   **NT** New Tech Add-on   ⊞ Combination Member   ♂ Male   ♀ Female

ICD-10-PCS 2022   809

F **Physical Rehabilitation and Diagnostic Audiology**
1 **Diagnostic Audiology**
4 **Hearing Aid Assessment**   Definition: Measurement of the appropriateness and/or effectiveness of a hearing device

Body System/Region Character 4	Type Qualifier Character 5	Equipment Character 6	Qualifier Character 7
Z None	Ø Cochlear Implant	1 Audiometer 2 Sound Field / Booth 3 Tympanometer 4 Electroacoustic Immitance / Acoustic Reflex 5 Hearing Aid Selection / Fitting / Test 7 Electrophysiologic 9 Cochlear Implant K Audiovisual L Assistive Listening P Computer Y Other Equipment Z None	Z None

Z None	1 Ear Canal Probe Microphone
	6 Binaural Electroacoustic Hearing
	   Aid Check
	8 Monaural Electroacoustic Hearing
	   Aid Check
		5 Hearing Aid Selection / Fitting / Test
		Z None
			Z None

Z None	2 Monaural Hearing Aid 3 Binaural Hearing Aid	1 Audiometer 2 Sound Field / Booth 3 Tympanometer 4 Electroacoustic Immitance / Acoustic Reflex 5 Hearing Aid Selection / Fitting / Test K Audiovisual L Assistive Listening P Computer Z None	Z None

Z None	4 Assistive Listening System/Device
	   Selection
		1 Audiometer
		2 Sound Field / Booth
		3 Tympanometer
		4 Electroacoustic Immitance /
		   Acoustic Reflex
		K Audiovisual
		L Assistive Listening
		Z None
			Z None

Z None	5 Sensory Aids	1 Audiometer 2 Sound Field / Booth 3 Tympanometer 4 Electroacoustic Immitance / Acoustic Reflex 5 Hearing Aid Selection / Fitting / Test K Audiovisual L Assistive Listening Z None	Z None
Z None	7 Ear Protector Attentuation	Ø Occupational Hearing Z None	Z None

F **Physical Rehabilitation and Diagnostic Audiology**
1 **Diagnostic Audiology**
5 **Vestibular Assessment**   Definition: Measurement of the vestibular system and related functions

Body System/Region Character 4	Type Qualifier Character 5	Equipment Character 6	Qualifier Character 7

Z None	Ø Bithermal, Binaural Caloric
	   Irrigation
	1 Bithermal, Monaural Caloric
	   Irrigation
	2 Unithermal Binaural Screen
	3 Oscillating Tracking
	4 Sinusoidal Vertical Axis Rotational
	5 Dix-Hallpike Dynamic
	6 Computerized Dynamic
	   Posturography
		8 Vestibular / Balance
		Z None
			Z None

Z None	7 Tinnitus Masker	5 Hearing Aid Selection / Fitting / Test Z None	Z None

Non-OR Procedure   DRG Non-OR Procedure   Valid OR Procedure   HAC Associated Procedure   Combination Only   New/Revised GREEN

Mental Health GZ1–GZJ

G **Mental Health**
Z **None**
1 **Psychological Tests**　Definition: The administration and interpretation of standardized psychological tests and measurement instruments for the assessment of psychological function

Qualifier Character 4	Qualifier Character 5	Qualifier Character 6	Qualifier Character 7
Ø Developmental 1 Personality and Behavioral 2 Intellectual and Psychoeducational 3 Neuropsychological 4 Neurobehavioral and Cognitive Status	Z None	Z None	Z None

G **Mental Health**
Z **None**
2 **Crisis Intervention**　Definition: Treatment of a traumatized, acutely disturbed or distressed individual for the purpose of short-term stabilization

Qualifier Character 4	Qualifier Character 5	Qualifier Character 6	Qualifier Character 7
Z None	Z None	Z None	Z None

G **Mental Health**
Z **None**
3 **Medication Management**　Definition: Monitoring and adjusting the use of medications for the treatment of a mental health disorder

Qualifier Character 4	Qualifier Character 5	Qualifier Character 6	Qualifier Character 7
Z None	Z None	Z None	Z None

G **Mental Health**
Z **None**
5 **Individual Psychotherapy**　Definition: Treatment of an individual with a mental health disorder by behavioral, cognitive, psychoanalytic, psychodynamic or psychophysiological means to improve functioning or well-being

Qualifier Character 4	Qualifier Character 5	Qualifier Character 6	Qualifier Character 7
Ø Interactive 1 Behavioral 2 Cognitive 3 Interpersonal 4 Psychoanalysis 5 Psychodynamic 6 Supportive 8 Cognitive-Behavioral 9 Psychophysiological	Z None	Z None	Z None

G **Mental Health**
Z **None**
6 **Counseling**　Definition: The application of psychological methods to treat an individual with normal developmental issues and psychological problems in order to increase function, improve well-being, alleviate distress, maladjustment or resolve crises

Qualifier Character 4	Qualifier Character 5	Qualifier Character 6	Qualifier Character 7
Ø Educational 1 Vocational 3 Other Counseling	Z None	Z None	Z None

G **Mental Health**
Z **None**
7 **Family Psychotherapy**　Definition: Treatment that includes one or more family members of an individual with a mental health disorder by behavioral, cognitive, psychoanalytic, psychodynamic or psychophysiological means to improve functioning or well-being
　　Explanation: Remediation of emotional or behavioral problems presented by one or more family members in cases where psychotherapy with more than one family member is indicated

Qualifier Character 4	Qualifier Character 5	Qualifier Character 6	Qualifier Character 7
2 Other Family Psychotherapy	Z None	Z None	Z None

NC Noncovered Procedure　**LC** Limited Coverage　**QA** Questionable OB Admit　**NT** New Tech Add-on　⊞ Combination Member　♂ Male　♀ Female

ICD-10-PCS 2022　　811

G   **Mental Health**
Z   **None**
B   **Electroconvulsive Therapy**   Definition: The application of controlled electrical voltages to treat a mental health disorder

Qualifier Character 4	Qualifier Character 5	Qualifier Character 6	Qualifier Character 7
Ø Unilateral-Single Seizure 1 Unilateral-Multiple Seizure 2 Bilateral-Single Seizure 3 Bilateral-Multiple Seizure 4 Other Electroconvulsive Therapy	Z None	Z None	Z None

G   **Mental Health**
Z   **None**
C   **Biofeedback**   Definition: Provision of information from the monitoring and regulating of physiological processes in conjunction with cognitive-behavioral techniques to improve patient functioning or well-being

Qualifier Character 4	Qualifier Character 5	Qualifier Character 6	Qualifier Character 7
9 Other Biofeedback	Z None	Z None	Z None

G   **Mental Health**
Z   **None**
F   **Hypnosis**   Definition: Induction of a state of heightened suggestibility by auditory, visual and tactile techniques to elicit an emotional or behavioral response

Qualifier Character 4	Qualifier Character 5	Qualifier Character 6	Qualifier Character 7
Z None	Z None	Z None	Z None

G   **Mental Health**
Z   **None**
G   **Narcosynthesis**   Definition: Administration of intravenous barbiturates in order to release suppressed or repressed thoughts

Qualifier Character 4	Qualifier Character 5	Qualifier Character 6	Qualifier Character 7
Z None	Z None	Z None	Z None

G   **Mental Health**
Z   **None**
H   **Group Psychotherapy**   Definition: Treatment of two or more individuals with a mental health disorder by behavioral, cognitive, psychoanalytic, psychodynamic or psychophysiological means to improve functioning or well-being

Qualifier Character 4	Qualifier Character 5	Qualifier Character 6	Qualifier Character 7
Z None	Z None	Z None	Z None

G   **Mental Health**
Z   **None**
J   **Light Therapy**   Definition: Application of specialized light treatments to improve functioning or well-being

Qualifier Character 4	Qualifier Character 5	Qualifier Character 6	Qualifier Character 7
Z None	Z None	Z None	Z None

Substance Abuse Treatment HZ2–HZ9

AHA Coding Clinic for table HZ2
2020, 1Q, 21   Inpatient detoxification services

AHA Coding Clinic for table HZ9
2020, 1Q, 21   Inpatient detoxification services

H   **Substance Abuse Treatment**
Z   **None**
2   **Detoxification Services**   Definition: Detoxification from alcohol and/or drugs

Explanation: Not a treatment modality, but helps the patient stabilize physically and psychologically until the body becomes free of drugs and the effects of alcohol

Qualifier Character 4	Qualifier Character 5	Qualifier Character 6	Qualifier Character 7
Z None	Z None	Z None	Z None

H   **Substance Abuse Treatment**
Z   **None**
3   **Individual Counseling**   Definition: The application of psychological methods to treat an individual with addictive behavior

Explanation: Comprised of several different techniques, which apply various strategies to address drug addiction

Qualifier Character 4	Qualifier Character 5	Qualifier Character 6	Qualifier Character 7
Ø Cognitive	Z None	Z None	Z None
1 Behavioral			
2 Cognitive-Behavioral			
3 12-Step			
4 Interpersonal			
5 Vocational			
6 Psychoeducation			
7 Motivational Enhancement			
8 Confrontational			
9 Continuing Care			
B Spiritual			
C Pre/Post-Test Infectious Disease			

DRG Non-OR   HZ3[Ø,1,2,3,4,5,6,7,8,9,B]ZZZ

H   **Substance Abuse Treatment**
Z   **None**
4   **Group Counseling**   Definition: The application of psychological methods to treat two or more individuals with addictive behavior

Explanation: Provides structured group counseling sessions and healing power through the connection with others

Qualifier Character 4	Qualifier Character 5	Qualifier Character 6	Qualifier Character 7
Ø Cognitive	Z None	Z None	Z None
1 Behavioral			
2 Cognitive-Behavioral			
3 12-Step			
4 Interpersonal			
5 Vocational			
6 Psychoeducation			
7 Motivational Enhancement			
8 Confrontational			
9 Continuing Care			
B Spiritual			
C Pre/Post-Test Infectious Disease			

DRG Non-OR   HZ4[Ø,1,2,3,4,5,6,7,8,9,B]ZZZ

NC Noncovered Procedure   LC Limited Coverage   QA Questionable OB Admit   NT New Tech Add-on   ✚ Combination Member   ♂ Male   ♀ Female

ICD-10-PCS 2022   813

HZ2–HZ4

H   **Substance Abuse Treatment**
Z   **None**
5   **Individual Psychotherapy**   Definition: Treatment of an individual with addictive behavior by behavioral, cognitive, psychoanalytic, psychodynamic or psychophysiological means

Qualifier Character 4	Qualifier Character 5	Qualifier Character 6	Qualifier Character 7
Ø Cognitive	Z None	Z None	Z None
1 Behavioral			
2 Cognitive-Behavioral			
3 12-Step			
4 Interpersonal			
5 Interactive			
6 Psychoeducation			
7 Motivational Enhancement			
8 Confrontational			
9 Supportive			
B Psychoanalysis			
C Psychodynamic			
D Psychophysiological			

DRG Non-OR   For all qualifier values

H   **Substance Abuse Treatment**
Z   **None**
6   **Family Counseling**   Definition: The application of psychological methods that includes one or more family members to treat an individual with addictive behavior

     Explanation: Provides support and education for family members of addicted individuals. Family member participation is seen as a critical area of substance abuse treatment

Qualifier Character 4	Qualifier Character 5	Qualifier Character 6	Qualifier Character 7
3 Other Family Counseling	Z None	Z None	Z None

H   **Substance Abuse Treatment**
Z   **None**
8   **Medication Management**   Definition: Monitoring or adjusting the use of replacement medications for the treatment of addiction

Qualifier Character 4	Qualifier Character 5	Qualifier Character 6	Qualifier Character 7
Ø Nicotine Replacement	Z None	Z None	Z None
1 Methadone Maintenance			
2 Levo-alpha-acetyl-methadol (LAAM)			
3 Antabuse			
4 Naltrexone			
5 Naloxone			
6 Clonidine			
7 Bupropion			
8 Psychiatric Medication			
9 Other Replacement Medication			

H   **Substance Abuse Treatment**
Z   **None**
9   **Pharmacotherapy**   Definition: The use of replacement medications for the treatment of addiction

Qualifier Character 4	Qualifier Character 5	Qualifier Character 6	Qualifier Character 7
Ø Nicotine Replacement	Z None	Z None	Z None
1 Methadone Maintenance			
2 Levo-alpha-acetyl-methadol (LAAM)			
3 Antabuse			
4 Naltrexone			
5 Naloxone			
6 Clonidine			
7 Bupropion			
8 Psychiatric Medication			
9 Other Replacement Medication			

Non-OR Procedure   DRG Non-OR Procedure   Valid OR Procedure   HAC Associated Procedure   Combination Only   New/Revised GREEN

New Technology X27–XYØ

AHA Coding Clinic for all tables in the New Technology Section
2015, 4Q, 8-11 New Section X codes - New Technology procedures

AHA Coding Clinic for table X27
2019, 4Q, 45-46 Sustained released drug-eluting stent

AHA Coding Clinic for table X2A
2021, 1Q, 16 Placement of Sentinel™ embolic protection device with deployment of single filter
2020, 4Q, 70-71 Cerebral embolic filtration extracorporeal flow reversal circuit
2019, 4Q, 46 Cerebral embolic filtration
2016, 4Q, 115-116 Cerebral embolic filtration

AHA Coding Clinic for table X2C
2016, 4Q, 82-83 Coronary artery, number of arteries
2015, 4Q, 8-14 New Section X codes—New Technology procedures

AHA Coding Clinic for table X2R
2016, 4Q, 116 Aortic valve rapid deployment
2015, 4Q, 8-12 New Section X codes—New Technology procedures

AHA Coding Clinic for table XHR
2016, 4Q, 116 Application of wound matrix

AHA Coding Clinic for table XKØ
2017, 4Q, 74 Intramuscular autologous bone marrow cell therapy

AHA Coding Clinic for table XNS
2017, 4Q, 74-75 Magnetic growth rods
2016, 4Q, 117 Placement of magnetic growth rods

AHA Coding Clinic for table XNU
2020, 4Q, 72 Implantation of vertebral mechanically expandable device

AHA Coding Clinic for table XRG
2017, 4Q, 76 Radiolucent porous interbody fusion device

AHA Coding Clinic for table XT2
2019, 4Q, 46-47 Renal function monitoring

AHA Coding Clinic for table XV5
2018, 4Q, 55 Robotic waterjet ablation

AHA Coding Clinic for table XWØ
2021, 1Q, 49 Frequently asked questions regarding ICD-10-CM and ICD-10-PCS coding for COVID-19
2020, 4Q, 72-76 Introduction of new therapeutic substances
2020, 4Q, 95 Frequently Asked Questions Regarding ICD-10-PCS Coding for COVID-19
2020, 3Q, 17-21 New procedure codes for introduction or infusion of therapeutics
2019, 4Q, 47-50 New therapeutic substances
2018, 4Q, 56 New therapeutic substances
2015, 4Q, 8-15 New Section X codes—New Technology procedures

AHA Coding Clinic for table XW1
2020, 3Q, 17-21 New procedure codes for introduction or infusion of therapeutics

AHA Coding Clinic for table XW2
2020, 4Q, 77-78 Transfusion of chimeric antigen receptor (CAR) T cell immunotherapy

AHA Coding Clinic for table XXE
2020, 4Q, 78-79 Measurement of infection
2020, 4Q, 78-79 Positive blood culture fluorescence hybridization
2020, 4Q, 79 Nucleic acid-base microbial detection
2019, 4Q, 50-51 Whole blood nucleic acid-base microbial detection

AHA Coding Clinic for table XYØ
2017, 4Q, 78 Intraoperative treatment of vascular grafts

X **New Technology**
2 **Cardiovascular System**
7 **Dilation**   Definition: Expanding an orifice or the lumen of a tubular body part

Explanation: The orifice can be a natural orifice or an artificially created orifice. Accomplished by stretching a tubular body part using intraluminal pressure or by cutting part of the orifice or wall of the tubular body part.

Body Part Character 4	Approach Character 5	Device/Substance/Technology Character 6	Qualifier Character 7
H Femoral Artery, Right	3 Percutaneous	8 Intraluminal Device, Sustained **NT** Release Drug-eluting	5 New Technology Group 5
J Femoral Artery, Left		9 Intraluminal Device, Sustained **NT** Release Drug-eluting, Two	
K Popliteal Artery, Proximal Right			
L Popliteal Artery, Proximal Left		B Intraluminal Device, Sustained **NT** Release Drug-eluting, Three	
M Popliteal Artery, Distal Right		C Intraluminal Device, Sustained **NT** Release Drug-eluting, Four or More	
N Popliteal Artery, Distal Left			
P Anterior Tibial Artery, Right			
Q Anterior Tibial Artery, Left			
R Posterior Tibial Artery, Right			
S Posterior Tibial Artery, Left			
T Peroneal Artery, Right			
U Peroneal Artery, Left			

Valid OR All body part, approach, device/substance/technology, and qualifier values
NT X27[H,J,K,L]3[8,9,B,C]5 *See* Appendix H for applicable device trade name

X **New Technology**
2 **Cardiovascular System**
A **Assistance**   Definition: Taking over a portion of a physiological function by extracorporeal means

Explanation: None

Body Part Character 4	Approach Character 5	Device/Substance/Technology Character 6	Qualifier Character 7
5 Innominate Artery and Left Common Carotid Artery	3 Percutaneous	1 Cerebral Embolic Filtration, Dual Filter	2 New Technology Group 2
6 Aortic Arch	3 Percutaneous	2 Cerebral Embolic Filtration, Single Deflection Filter	5 New Technology Group 5
H Common Carotid Artery, Right	3 Percutaneous	3 Cerebral Embolic Filtration, Extracorporeal Flow Reversal Circuit	6 New Technology Group 6
J Common Carotid Artery, Left			

X New Technology
2 Cardiovascular System
C Extirpation

Definition: Taking or cutting out solid matter from a body part

Explanation: The solid matter may be an abnormal byproduct of a biological function or a foreign body; it may be imbedded in a body part or in the lumen of a tubular body part. The solid matter may or may not have been previously broken into pieces.

Body Part Character 4	Approach Character 5	Device/Substance/Technology Character 6	Qualifier Character 7
P Abdominal Aorta **Q** Upper Extremity Vein, Right **R** Upper Extremity Vein, Left **S** Lower Extremity Artery, Right **T** Lower Extremity Artery, Left **U** Lower Extremity Vein, Right **V** Lower Extremity Vein, Left **Y** Great Vessel	**3** Percutaneous	**T** Computer-aided Mechanical Aspiration	**7** New Technology Group 7

X New Technology
2 Cardiovascular System
J Inspection

Definition: Visually and/or manually exploring a body part

Explanation: None

Body Part Character 4	Approach Character 5	Device/Substance/Technology Character 6	Qualifier Character 7
A Heart	**X** External	**4** Transthoracic Echocardiography, Computer-aided Guidance	**7** New Technology Group 7

X New Technology
2 Cardiovascular System
K Bypass

Definition: Altering the route of passage of the contents of a tubular body part

Explanation: None

Body Part Character 4	Approach Character 5	Device/Substance/Technology Character 6	Qualifier Character 7
B Radial Artery, Right **C** Radial Artery, Left	**3** Percutaneous	**1** Thermal Resistance Energy	**7** New Technology Group 7

X New Technology
2 Cardiovascular System
R Replacement

Definition: Putting in or on biological or synthetic material that physically takes the place and/or function of all or a portion of a body part

Explanation: The body part may have been taken out or replaced, or may be taken out, physically eradicated, or rendered nonfunctional during the REPLACEMENT procedure. A REMOVAL procedure is coded for taking out the device used in a previous replacement procedure

Body Part Character 4	Approach Character 5	Device/Substance/Technology Character 6	Qualifier Character 7
F Aortic Valve	**Ø** Open **3** Percutaneous **4** Percutaneous Endoscopic	**3** Zooplastic Tissue, Rapid Deployment Technique	**2** New Technology Group 2
X Thoracic Aorta, Arch	**Ø** Open	**N** Branched Synthetic Substitute with Intraluminal Device	**7** New Technology Group 7

Valid OR X2RF[Ø,3,4]32

X New Technology
2 Cardiovascular System
V Restriction

Definition: Partially closing an orifice or the lumen of a tubular body part

Explanation: None

Body Part Character 4	Approach Character 5	Device/Substance/Technology Character 6	Qualifier Character 7
7 Coronary Sinus	**3** Percutaneous	**Q** Reduction Device	**7** New Technology Group 7
W Thoracic Aorta, Descending	**Ø** Open	**N** Branched Synthetic Substitute with Intraluminal Device	**7** New Technology Group 7

Valid OR X2V73Q7

X New Technology
D Gastrointestinal System
2 Monitoring

Definition: Determining the level of a physiological or physical function repetitively over a period of time

Explanation: None

Body Part Character 4	Approach Character 5	Device/Substance/Technology Character 6	Qualifier Character 7
G Upper GI **H** Lower GI	**4** Percutaneous Endoscopic **8** Via Natural or Artificial Opening Endoscopic	**V** Oxygen Saturation	**7** New Technology Group 7

X New Technology
D Gastrointestinal System
P Irrigation Definition: Putting in or on a cleansing substance
Explanation: None

Body Part Character 4	Approach Character 5	Device/Substance/Technology Character 6	Qualifier Character 7
H Lower GI	8 Via Natural or Artificial Opening Endoscopic	K Intraoperative Single-use Oversleeve	7 New Technology Group 7

X New Technology
F Hepatobiliary System and Pancreas
J Inspection Definition: Visually and/or manually exploring a body part
Explanation: None

Body Part Character 4	Approach Character 5	Device/Substance/Technology Character 6	Qualifier Character 7
B Hepatobiliary Duct D Pancreatic Duct	8 Via Natural or Artificial Opening Endoscopic	A Single-use Duodenoscope	7 New Technology Group 7

X New Technology
H Skin, Subcutaneous Tissue, Fascia and Breast
R Replacement Definition: Putting in or on biological or synthetic material that physically takes the place and/or function of all or a portion of a body part
Explanation: The body part may have been taken out or replaced, or may be taken out, physically eradicated, or rendered nonfunctional during the REPLACEMENT procedure. A REMOVAL procedure is coded for taking out the device used in a previous replacement procedure

Body Part Character 4	Approach Character 5	Device/Substance/Technology Character 6	Qualifier Character 7
P Skin	X External	F Bioengineered Allogeneic Construct	7 New Technology Group 7
P Skin	X External	L Skin Substitute, Porcine Liver Derived	2 New Technology Group 2

Valid OR XHRPXL2

X New Technology
K Muscles, Tendons, Bursae and Ligaments
Ø Introduction Definition: Putting in or on a therapeutic, diagnostic, nutritional, physiological, or prophylactic substance except blood or blood products
Explanation: None

Body Part Character 4	Approach Character 5	Device/Substance/Technology Character 6	Qualifier Character 7
2 Muscle	3 Percutaneous	Ø Concentrated Bone Marrow Aspirate	3 New Technology Group 3

NC Noncovered Procedure **LC** Limited Coverage **QA** Questionable OB Admit **NT** New Tech Add-on ✚ Combination Member ♂ Male ♀ Female

New Technology

X New Technology
N Bones
S Reposition

Definition: Moving to its normal location, or other suitable location, all or a portion of a body part

Explanation: The body part is moved to a new location from an abnormal location, or from a normal location where it is not functioning correctly. The body part may or may not be cut out or off to be moved to the new location.

Body Part Character 4	Approach Character 5	Device/Substance/Technology Character 6	Qualifier Character 7
Ø Lumbar Vertebra	Ø Open	3 Magnetically Controlled Growth Rod(s)	2 New Technology Group 2
Ø Lumbar Vertebra	Ø Open	C Posterior (Dynamic) Distraction Device	7 New Technology Group 7
Ø Lumbar Vertebra	3 Percutaneous	3 Magnetically Controlled Growth Rod(s)	2 New Technology Group 2
Ø Lumbar Vertebra	3 Percutaneous	C Posterior (Dynamic) Distraction Device	7 New Technology Group 7
3 Cervical Vertebra	Ø Open 3 Percutaneous	3 Magnetically Controlled Growth Rod(s)	2 New Technology Group 2
4 Thoracic Vertebra	Ø Open	3 Magnetically Controlled Growth Rod(s)	2 New Technology Group 2
4 Thoracic Vertebra	Ø Open	C Posterior (Dynamic) Distraction Device	7 New Technology Group 7
4 Thoracic Vertebra	3 Percutaneous	3 Magnetically Controlled Growth Rod(s)	2 New Technology Group 2
4 Thoracic Vertebra	3 Percutaneous	C Posterior (Dynamic) Distraction Device	7 New Technology Group 7

Valid OR XNSØØ32
Valid OR XNSØ332
Valid OR XNS3[Ø,3]32
Valid OR XNS4Ø32
Valid OR XNS4332

X New Technology
N Bones
U Supplement

Definition: Putting in or on biological or synthetic material that physically reinforces and/or augments the function of a portion of a body part

Explanation: None

Body Part Character 4	Approach Character 5	Device/Substance/Technology Character 6	Qualifier Character 7
Ø Lumbar Vertebra 4 Thoracic Vertebra	3 Percutaneous	5 Synthetic Substitute, Mechanically Expandable (Paired) **NT**	6 New Technology Group 6

Valid OR XNU[Ø,4]356
NT XNU[Ø,4]356 *See* Appendix H for applicable device trade name

X   New Technology
R   Joints
G   Fusion   Definition: Joining together portions of an articular body part rendering the articular body part immobile
                 Explanation: The body part is joined together by fixation device, bone graft, or other means

Body Part Character 4	Approach Character 5	Device/Substance/Technology Character 6	Qualifier Character 7
Ø Occipital-cervical Joint	Ø Open	9 Interbody Fusion Device, Nanotextured Surface	2 New Technology Group 2
Ø Occipital-cervical Joint	Ø Open	F Interbody Fusion Device, Radiolucent Porous	3 New Technology Group 3
1 Cervical Vertebral Joint	Ø Open	9 Interbody Fusion Device, Nanotextured Surface	2 New Technology Group 2
1 Cervical Vertebral Joint	Ø Open	F Interbody Fusion Device, Radiolucent Porous	3 New Technology Group 3
2 Cervical Vertebral Joints, 2 or more	Ø Open	9 Interbody Fusion Device, Nanotextured Surface	2 New Technology Group 2
2 Cervical Vertebral Joints, 2 or more	Ø Open	F Interbody Fusion Device, Radiolucent Porous	3 New Technology Group 3
4 Cervicothoracic Vertebral Joint	Ø Open	9 Interbody Fusion Device, Nanotextured Surface	2 New Technology Group 2
4 Cervicothoracic Vertebral Joint	Ø Open	F Interbody Fusion Device, Radiolucent Porous	3 New Technology Group 3
6 Thoracic Vertebral Joint	Ø Open	9 Interbody Fusion Device, Nanotextured Surface	2 New Technology Group 2
6 Thoracic Vertebral Joint	Ø Open	F Interbody Fusion Device, Radiolucent Porous	3 New Technology Group 3
7 Thoracic Vertebral Joints, 2 to 7 ⊞	Ø Open	9 Interbody Fusion Device, Nanotextured Surface	2 New Technology Group 2
7 Thoracic Vertebral Joints, 2 to 7 ⊞	Ø Open	F Interbody Fusion Device, Radiolucent Porous	3 New Technology Group 3
8 Thoracic Vertebral Joints, 8 or more	Ø Open	9 Interbody Fusion Device, Nanotextured Surface	2 New Technology Group 2
8 Thoracic Vertebral Joints, 8 or more	Ø Open	F Interbody Fusion Device, Radiolucent Porous	3 New Technology Group 3
A Thoracolumbar Vertebral Joint	Ø Open	9 Interbody Fusion Device, Nanotextured Surface	2 New Technology Group 2
A Thoracolumbar Vertebral Joint	Ø Open	F Interbody Fusion Device, Radiolucent Porous	3 New Technology Group 3
A Thoracolumbar Vertebral Joint	Ø Open 3 Percutaneous 4 Percutaneous Endoscopic	R Interbody Fusion Device, Customizable	7 New Technology Group 7
B Lumbar Vertebral Joint	Ø Open	9 Interbody Fusion Device, Nanotextured Surface	2 New Technology Group 2
B Lumbar Vertebral Joint	Ø Open	F Interbody Fusion Device, Radiolucent Porous	3 New Technology Group 3
B Lumbar Vertebral Joint	Ø Open 3 Percutaneous 4 Percutaneous Endoscopic	R Interbody Fusion Device, Customizable	7 New Technology Group 7
C Lumbar Vertebral Joints, 2 or more ⊞	Ø Open	9 Interbody Fusion Device, Nanotextured Surface	2 New Technology Group 2
C Lumbar Vertebral Joints, 2 or more ⊞	Ø Open	F Interbody Fusion Device, Radiolucent Porous	3 New Technology Group 3
C Lumbar Vertebral Joints, 2 or more	Ø Open 3 Percutaneous 4 Percutaneous Endoscopic	R Interbody Fusion Device, Customizable	7 New Technology Group 7
D Lumbosacral Joint	Ø Open	9 Interbody Fusion Device, Nanotextured Surface	2 New Technology Group 2
D Lumbosacral Joint	Ø Open	F Interbody Fusion Device, Radiolucent Porous	3 New Technology Group 3
D Lumbosacral Joint	Ø Open 3 Percutaneous 4 Percutaneous Endoscopic	R Interbody Fusion Device, Customizable	7 New Technology Group 7

Valid OR   All body part, approach, device/substance/technology, and qualifier values
HAC   XRG[Ø,1,2,4,6,7,8,A,B,C,D]Ø92 when reported with SDx K68.11 or T81.40–T81.49, T84.60-T84.619, T84.63-T84.7 with 7th character A
HAC   XRG[Ø,1,2,4,6,7,8,A,B,C,D]ØF3 when reported with SDx K68.11 or T81.40–T81.49, T84.60-T84.619, T84.63-T84.7 with 7th character A

See Appendix L for Procedure Combinations
⊞ XRG7Ø92
⊞ XRG7ØF3
⊞ XRGCØ92
⊞ XRGCØF3

X   New Technology
T   Urinary System
2   Monitoring   Definition: Determining the level of a physiological or physical function repetitively over a period of time
                 Explanation: None

Body Part Character 4	Approach Character 5	Device/Substance/Technology Character 6	Qualifier Character 7
5 Kidney	X External	E Fluorescent Pyrazine	5 New Technology Group 5

 Noncovered Procedure   Limited Coverage   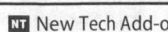 Questionable OB Admit   **NT** New Tech Add-on   ⊞ Combination Member   ♂ Male   ♀ Female

New Technology

X   **New Technology**
V   **Male Reproductive System**
5   **Destruction**   Definition: Physical eradication of all or a portion of a body part by the direct use of energy, force, or a destructive agent
                     Explanation: None of the body part is physically taken out

Body Part Character 4	Approach Character 5	Device/Substance/Technology Character 6	Qualifier Character 7
0 Prostate	8 Via Natural or Artificial Opening Endoscopic	A Robotic Waterjet Ablation	4 New Technology Group 4

Valid OR   All body part, approach, device/substance/technology, and qualifier values

X   **New Technology**
W   **Anatomical Regions**
0   **Introduction**   Definition: Putting in or on a therapeutic, diagnostic, nutritional, physiological, or prophylactic substance except blood or blood products
                     Explanation: None

Body Part Character 4	Approach Character 5	Device/Substance/Technology Character 6	Qualifier Character 7
0 Skin	X External	2 Bromelain-enriched Proteolytic Enzyme	7 New Technology Group 7
1 Subcutaneous Tissue	3 Percutaneous	9 Satralizumab-mwge	7 New Technology Group 7
1 Subcutaneous Tissue	3 Percutaneous	F Other New Technology Therapeutic Substance	5 New Technology Group 5
1 Subcutaneous Tissue	3 Percutaneous	H Other New Technology Monoclonal Antibody K Leronlimab Monoclonal Antibody S COVID-19 Vaccine Dose 1 T COVID-19 Vaccine Dose 2 U COVID-19 Vaccine	6 New Technology Group 6
1 Subcutaneous Tissue	3 Percutaneous	W Caplacizumab **NT**	5 New Technology Group 5
1 Subcutaneous Tissue	X External	2 Bromelain-enriched Proteolytic Enzyme	7 New Technology Group 7
2 Muscle	3 Percutaneous	S COVID-19 Vaccine Dose 1 T COVID-19 Vaccine Dose 2 U COVID-19 Vaccine	6 New Technology Group 6
3 Peripheral Vein	3 Percutaneous	0 Brexanolone 2 Nerinitide 3 Durvalumab Antineoplastic **NT**	6 New Technology Group 6
3 Peripheral Vein	3 Percutaneous	5 Narsoplimab Monoclonal Antibody	7 New Technology Group 7
3 Peripheral Vein	3 Percutaneous	6 Lefamulin Anti-infective **NT**	6 New Technology Group 6
3 Peripheral Vein	3 Percutaneous	6 Terlipressin	7 New Technology Group 7
3 Peripheral Vein	3 Percutaneous	7 Coagulation Factor Xa, Inactivated **NT**	2 New Technology Group 2
3 Peripheral Vein	3 Percutaneous	7 Trilaciclib 8 Lurbinectedin	7 New Technology Group 7
3 Peripheral Vein	3 Percutaneous	9 Defibrotide Sodium Anticoagulant	2 New Technology Group 2
3 Peripheral Vein	3 Percutaneous	9 Ceftolozane/Tazobactam Anti-infective **NT**	6 New Technology Group 6
3 Peripheral Vein	3 Percutaneous	A Bezlotoxumab Monoclonal Antibody	3 New Technology Group 3
3 Peripheral Vein	3 Percutaneous	A Cefiderocol Anti-infective **NT**	6 New Technology Group 6
3 Peripheral Vein	3 Percutaneous	A Ciltacabtagene Autoleucel	7 New Technology Group 7
3 Peripheral Vein	3 Percutaneous	B Cytarabine and Daunorubicin Liposome Antineoplastic	3 New Technology Group 3
3 Peripheral Vein	3 Percutaneous	B Omadacycline Anti-infective **NT**	6 New Technology Group 6
3 Peripheral Vein	3 Percutaneous	B Amivantamab Monoclonal Antibody	7 New Technology Group 7
3 Peripheral Vein	3 Percutaneous	C Eculizumab **NT**	6 New Technology Group 6
3 Peripheral Vein	3 Percutaneous	C Engineered Chimeric Antigen Receptor T-cell Immunotherapy, Autologous	7 New Technology Group 7
3 Peripheral Vein	3 Percutaneous	D Atezolizumab Antineoplastic **NT**	6 New Technology Group 6
3 Peripheral Vein	3 Percutaneous	E Remdesivir Anti-infective **NT**	5 New Technology Group 5
3 Peripheral Vein	3 Percutaneous	E Etesevimab Monoclonal Antibody	6 New Technology Group 6
3 Peripheral Vein	3 Percutaneous	F Other New Technology Therapeutic Substance	3 New Technology Group 3
3 Peripheral Vein	3 Percutaneous	F Other New Technology Therapeutic Substance	5 New Technology Group 5
3 Peripheral Vein	3 Percutaneous	F Bamlanivimab Monoclonal Antibody	6 New Technology Group 6
3 Peripheral Vein	3 Percutaneous	G Plazomicin Anti-infective **NT**	4 New Technology Group 4
3 Peripheral Vein	3 Percutaneous	G Sarilumab	5 New Technology Group 5

DRG Non-OR	XW033C7	**NT**	XW03366	**NT**	XW033A6	**NT**	XW033D6
NT	XW013W5	**NT**	XW03372	**NT**	XW033B6	**NT**	XW033E5
NT	XW03336	**NT**	XW03396	**NT**	XW033C6	**NT**	XW033G4

* For all codes with NT icon *see* Appendix I for registered or trade name of substance

XW0 Continued on next page

Non-OR Procedure   DRG Non-OR Procedure   Valid OR Procedure   HAC Associated Procedure   Combination Only   New/Revised GREEN

X New Technology
W Anatomical Regions
Ø Introduction

XWØ Continued

Definition: Putting in or on a therapeutic, diagnostic, nutritional, physiological, or prophylactic substance except blood or blood products
Explanation: None

Body Part Character 4	Approach Character 5	Device/Substance/Technology Character 6	Qualifier Character 7
3 Peripheral Vein	3 Percutaneous	G REGN-COV2 Monoclonal Antibody	6 New Technology Group 6
3 Peripheral Vein	3 Percutaneous	G Engineered Chimeric Antigen Receptor T-cell Immunotherapy, Allogeneic	7 New Technology Group 7
3 Peripheral Vein	3 Percutaneous	H Synthetic Human Angiotensin II	4 New Technology Group 4
3 Peripheral Vein	3 Percutaneous	H Tocilizumab	5 New Technology Group 5
3 Peripheral Vein	3 Percutaneous	H Other New Technology Monoclonal Antibody	6 New Technology Group 6
3 Peripheral Vein	3 Percutaneous	H Axicabtagene Ciloleucel Immunotherapy J Tisagenlecleucel Immunotherapy	7 New Technology Group 7
3 Peripheral Vein	3 Percutaneous	K Fosfomycin Anti-infective	5 New Technology Group 5
3 Peripheral Vein	3 Percutaneous	K Idecabtagene Vicleucel Immunotherapy	7 New Technology Group 7
3 Peripheral Vein	3 Percutaneous	L CD24Fc Immunomodulator	6 New Technology Group 6
3 Peripheral Vein	3 Percutaneous	L Lifileucel Immunotherapy M Brexucabtagene Autoleucel Immunotherapy	7 New Technology Group 7
3 Peripheral Vein	3 Percutaneous	N Meropenem-vaborbactam Anti-infective	5 New Technology Group 5
3 Peripheral Vein	3 Percutaneous	N Lisocabtagene Maraleucel Immunotherapy	7 New Technology Group 7
3 Peripheral Vein	3 Percutaneous	Q Tagraxofusp-erzs Antineoplastic **NT** S Iobenguane I-131 Antineoplastic **NT** U Imipenem-cilastatin-relebactam Anti-infective **NT** W Caplacizumab **NT**	5 New Technology Group 5
4 Central Vein	3 Percutaneous	Ø Brexanolone 2 Nerinitide 3 Durvalumab Antineoplastic **NT**	6 New Technology Group 6
4 Central Vein	3 Percutaneous	5 Narsoplimab Monoclonal Antibody	7 New Technology Group 7
4 Central Vein	3 Percutaneous	6 Lefamulin Anti-infective **NT**	6 New Technology Group 6
4 Central Vein	3 Percutaneous	6 Terlipressin	7 New Technology Group 7
4 Central Vein	3 Percutaneous	7 Coagulation Factor Xa, Inactivated **NT**	2 New Technology Group 2
4 Central Vein	3 Percutaneous	7 Trilaciclib 8 Lurbinectedin	7 New Technology Group 7
4 Central Vein	3 Percutaneous	9 Defibrotide Sodium Anticoagulant	2 New Technology Group 2
4 Central Vein	3 Percutaneous	9 Ceftolozane/Tazobactam Anti-infective **NT**	6 New Technology Group 6
4 Central Vein	3 Percutaneous	A Bezlotoxumab Monoclonal Antibody	3 New Technology Group 3
4 Central Vein	3 Percutaneous	A Cefiderocol Anti-infective **NT**	6 New Technology Group 6
4 Central Vein	3 Percutaneous	A Ciltacabtagene Autoleucel	7 New Technology Group 7
4 Central Vein	3 Percutaneous	B Cytarabine and Daunorubicin Liposome Antineoplastic	3 New Technology Group 3
4 Central Vein	3 Percutaneous	B Omadacycline Anti-infective **NT**	6 New Technology Group 6
4 Central Vein	3 Percutaneous	B Amivantamab Monoclonal Antibody	7 New Technology Group 7
4 Central Vein	3 Percutaneous	C Eculizumab **NT**	6 New Technology Group 6
4 Central Vein	3 Percutaneous	C Engineered Chimeric Antigen Receptor T-cell Immunotherapy, Autologous	7 New Technology Group 7
4 Central Vein	3 Percutaneous	D Atezolizumab Antineoplastic **NT**	6 New Technology Group 6
4 Central Vein	3 Percutaneous	E Remdesivir Anti-infective **NT**	5 New Technology Group 5
4 Central Vein	3 Percutaneous	E Etesevimab Monoclonal Antibody	6 New Technology Group 6
4 Central Vein	3 Percutaneous	F Other New Technology Therapeutic Substance	3 New Technology Group 3
4 Central Vein	3 Percutaneous	F Other New Technology Therapeutic Substance	5 New Technology Group 5
4 Central Vein	3 Percutaneous	F Bamlanivimab Monoclonal Antibody	6 New Technology Group 6
4 Central Vein	3 Percutaneous	G Plazomicin Anti-infective **NT**	4 New Technology Group 4

DRG Non-OR	XWØ33G7	**NT**	XWØ33[Q,S,U,W]5	**NT**	XWØ4396	**NT**	XWØ43D6
DRG Non-OR	XWØ33[H,J]7	**NT**	XWØ4336	**NT**	XWØ43A6	**NT**	XWØ43E5
DRG Non-OR	XWØ33K7	**NT**	XWØ4366	**NT**	XWØ43B6	**NT**	XWØ43G4
DRG Non-OR	XWØ33[L,M]7	**NT**	XWØ4372	**NT**	XWØ43C6		
DRG Non-OR	XWØ33N7						
DRG Non-OR	XWØ43C7						

* For all codes with NT icon *see* Appendix I for registered or trade name of substance

XWØ Continued on next page

NC Noncovered Procedure   **LC** Limited Coverage   **QA** Questionable OB Admit   **NT** New Tech Add-on   ⊞ Combination Member   ♂ Male   ♀ Female

New Technology

X New Technology
W Anatomical Regions
Ø Introduction

XWØ Continued

Definition: Putting in or on a therapeutic, diagnostic, nutritional, physiological, or prophylactic substance except blood or blood products
Explanation: None

Body Part Character 4	Approach Character 5	Device/Substance/Technology Character 6	Qualifier Character 7
4 Central Vein	3 Percutaneous	G Sarilumab	5 New Technology Group 5
4 Central Vein	3 Percutaneous	G REGN-COV2 Monoclonal Antibody	6 New Technology Group 6
4 Central Vein	3 Percutaneous	G Engineered Chimeric Antigen Receptor T-cell Immunotherapy, Allogeneic	7 New Technology Group 7
4 Central Vein	3 Percutaneous	H Synthetic Human Angiotensin II	4 New Technology Group 4
4 Central Vein	3 Percutaneous	H Tocilizumab	5 New Technology Group 5
4 Central Vein	3 Percutaneous	H Other New Technology Monoclonal Antibody	6 New Technology Group 6
4 Central Vein	3 Percutaneous	H Axicabtagene Ciloleucel Immunotherapy J Tisagenlecleucel Immunotherapy	7 New Technology Group 7
4 Central Vein	3 Percutaneous	K Fosfomycin Anti-infective	5 New Technology Group 5
4 Central Vein	3 Percutaneous	K Idecabtagene Vicleucel Immunotherapy	7 New Technology Group 7
4 Central Vein	3 Percutaneous	L CD24Fc Immunomodulator	6 New Technology Group 6
4 Central Vein	3 Percutaneous	L Lifileucel Immunotherapy M Brexucabtagene Autoleucel Immunotherapy	7 New Technology Group 7
4 Central Vein	3 Percutaneous	N Meropenem-vaborbactam Anti-infective	5 New Technology Group 5
4 Central Vein	3 Percutaneous	N Lisocabtagene Maraleucel Immunotherapy	7 New Technology Group 7
4 Central Vein	3 Percutaneous	Q Tagraxofusp-erzs Antineoplastic NT S Iobenguane I-131 Antineoplastic NT U Imipenem-cilastatin-relebactam Anti-infective NT W Caplacizumab NT	5 New Technology Group 5
9 Nose	7 Via Natural or Artificial Opening	M Esketamine Hydrochloride NT	5 New Technology Group 5
D Mouth and Pharynx	X External	6 Lefamulin Anti-infective NT	6 New Technology Group 6
D Mouth and Pharynx	X External	8 Uridine Triacetate	2 New Technology Group 2
D Mouth and Pharynx	X External	F Other New Technology Therapeutic Substance J Apalutamide Antineoplastic L Erdafitinib Antineoplastic NT	5 New Technology Group 5
D Mouth and Pharynx	X External	M Baricitinib NT	6 New Technology Group 6
D Mouth and Pharynx	X External	R Venetoclax Antineoplastic T Ruxolitinib NT V Gilteritinib Antineoplastic NT	5 New Technology Group 5
G Upper GI H Lower GI	7 Via Natural or Artificial Opening	M Baricitinib NT	6 New Technology Group 6
G Upper GI H Lower GI	8 Via Natural or Artificial Opening Endoscopic	8 Mineral-based Topical Hemostatic Agent NT	6 New Technology Group 6
Q Cranial Cavity and Brain	3 Percutaneous	1 Eladocagene exuparvovec	6 New Technology Group 6
V Bones	Ø Open	P Antibiotic-eluting Bone Void Filler	7 New Technology Group 7

DRG Non-OR	XWØ43G7	NT	XWØ43[Q,S,U,W]5	NT	XWØDXL5	NT	XWØ[G,H]7M6
DRG Non-OR	XWØ43[H,J]7	NT	XWØ97M5	NT	XWØDXM6	NT	XWØ[G,H]886
DRG Non-OR	XWØ43K7	NT	XWØDX66	NT	XWØDX[T,V]5		
DRG Non-OR	XWØ43[L,M]7						
DRG Non-OR	XWØ43N7						

* For all codes with NT icon *see* Appendix I for registered or trade name of substance

X New Technology
W Anatomical Regions
1 Transfusion   Definition: Putting in blood or blood products
        Explanation: None

Body Part Character 4	Approach Character 5	Device/Substance/Technology Character 6	Qualifier Character 7
3 Peripheral Vein	3 Percutaneous	2 Plasma, Convalescent (Nonautologous) **NT**	5 New Technology Group 5
3 Peripheral Vein	3 Percutaneous	D High-Dose Intravenous Immune Globulin E Hyperimmune Globulin	7 New Technology Group 7
4 Central Vein	3 Percutaneous	2 Plasma, Convalescent (Nonautologous) **NT**	5 New Technology Group 5
4 Central Vein	3 Percutaneous	D High-Dose Intravenous Immune Globulin E Hyperimmune Globulin	7 New Technology Group 7

NT XW13325
NT XW14325

X New Technology
W Anatomical Regions
H Insertion   Definition: Putting in a nonbiological appliance that monitors, assists, performs, or prevents a physiological function but does not physically take the place of a body part
        Explanation: None

Body Part Character 4	Approach Character 5	Device/Substance/Technology Character 6	Qualifier Character 7
D Mouth and Pharynx	7 Via Natural or Artificial Opening	Q Neurostimulator Lead	7 New Technology Group 7

X New Technology
X Physiological Systems
E Measurement   Definition: Determining the level of a physiological or physical function at a point in time
        Explanation: None

Body Part Character 4	Approach Character 5	Device/Substance/Technology Character 6	Qualifier Character 7
Ø Central Nervous	X External	Ø Intracranial Vascular Activity, Computer-aided Assessment	7 New Technology Group 7
3 Arterial	X External	2 Pulmonary Artery Flow, Computer-aided Triage and Notification	7 New Technology Group 7
5 Circulatory	X External	M Infection, Whole Blood Nucleic Acid-base Microbial Detection **NT**	5 New Technology Group 5
5 Circulatory	X External	N Infection, Positive Blood Culture Fluorescence Hybridization for Organism Identification, Concentration and Susceptibility	6 New Technology Group 6
5 Circulatory	X External	R Infection, Mechanical Initial Specimen Diversion Technique Using Active Negative Pressure T Intracranial Arterial Flow, Whole Blood mRNA V Infection, Serum/Plasma Nanoparticle Fluorescence SARS-CoV-2 Antibody Detection	7 New Technology Group 7
9 Nose	7 Via Natural or Artificial Opening	U Infection, Nasopharyngeal Fluid SARS-CoV-2 Polymerase Chain Reaction	7 New Technology Group 7
B Respiratory	X External	Q Infection, Lower Respiratory Fluid Nucleic Acid-base Microbial Detection	6 New Technology Group 6

NT XXE5XM5 for T2 Bacteria Test Panel

X New Technology
Y Extracorporeal
Ø Introduction   Definition: Putting in or on a therapeutic, diagnostic, nutritional, physiological, or prophylactic substance except blood or blood products
        Explanation: None

Body Part Character 4	Approach Character 5	Device/Substance/Technology Character 6	Qualifier Character 7
V Vein Graft	X External	8 Endothelial Damage Inhibitor	3 New Technology Group 3
Y Extracorporeal	X External	3 Nafamostat Anticoagulant	7 New Technology Group 7

NC Noncovered Procedure   **LC** Limited Coverage   **QA** Questionable OB Admit   **NT** New Tech Add-on   ⊞ Combination Member   ♂ Male   ♀ Female

ICD-10-PCS 2022   823

XW1–XYØ

Appendixes

Appendix A: Components of the Medical and Surgical Approach Definitions

ICD-10-PCS Value	Definition	Access Location	Method	Type of Instrumentation	Example
Open (Ø)	Cutting through the skin or mucous membrane and any other body layers necessary to expose the site of the procedure	Skin or mucous membrane, any other body layers	Cutting	None	Abdominal hysterectomy
Percutaneous (3)	Entry, by puncture or minor incision, of instrumentation through the skin or mucous membrane and any other body layers necessary to reach the site of the procedure	Skin or mucous membrane, any other body layers	Puncture or minor incision	Without visualization	Needle biopsy of liver, Liposuction
Percutaneous endoscopic (4)	Entry, by puncture or minor incision, of instrumentation through the skin or mucous membrane and any other body layers necessary to reach and visualize the site of the procedure	Skin or mucous membrane, any other body layers	Puncture or minor incision	With visualization	Arthroscopy, Laparoscopic cholecystectomy
Via natural or artificial opening (7)	Entry of instrumentation through a natural or artificial external opening to reach the site of the procedure	Natural or artificial external opening	Direct entry	Without visualization	Endotracheal tube insertion, Foley catheter placement
Via natural or artificial opening endoscopic (8)	Entry of instrumentation through a natural or artificial external opening to reach and visualize the site of the procedure	Natural or artificial external opening	Direct entry	With visualization	Sigmoidoscopy, EGD, ERCP
Via natural or artificial opening with percutaneous endoscopic assistance (F)	Entry of instrumentation through a natural or artificial external opening and entry, by puncture or minor incision, of instrumentation through the skin or mucous membrane and any other body layers necessary to aid in the performance of the procedure	Skin or mucous membrane, any other body layers	Direct entry with puncture or minor incision for instrumentation only	With visualization	Laparoscopic-assisted vaginal hysterectomy
External (X)	Procedures performed directly on the skin or mucous membrane and procedures performed indirectly by the application of external force through the skin or mucous membrane	Skin or mucous membrane	Direct or indirect application	None	Closed fracture reduction, Resection of tonsils

Open (Ø)

Percutaneous (3)

Percutaneous Endoscopic (4)

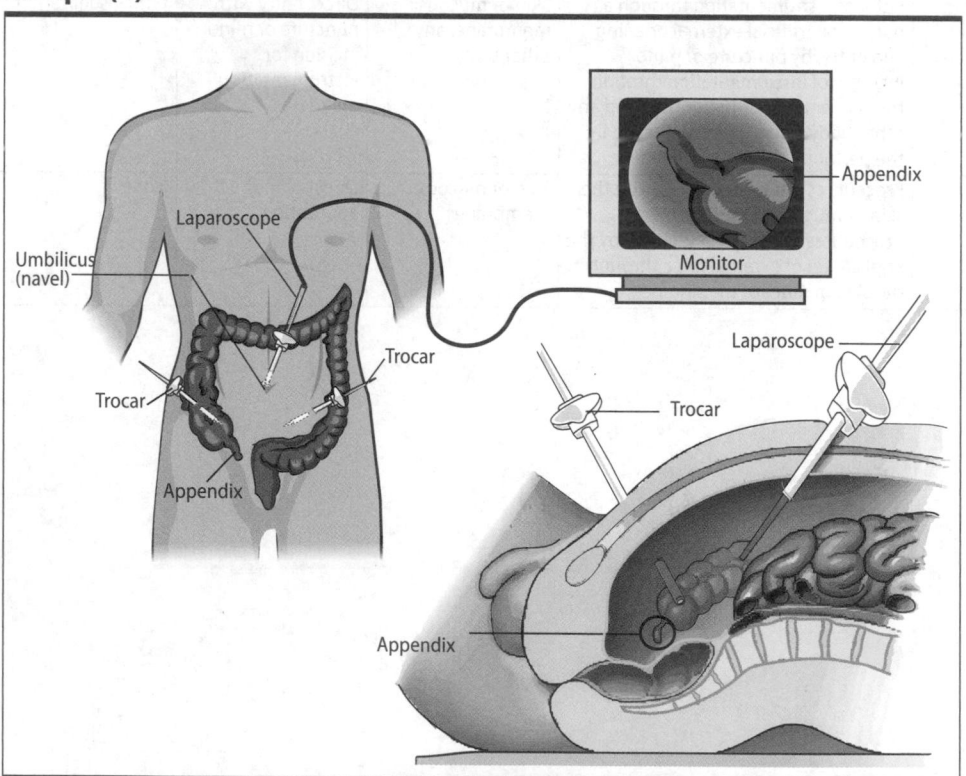

Via Natural or Artificial Opening (7)

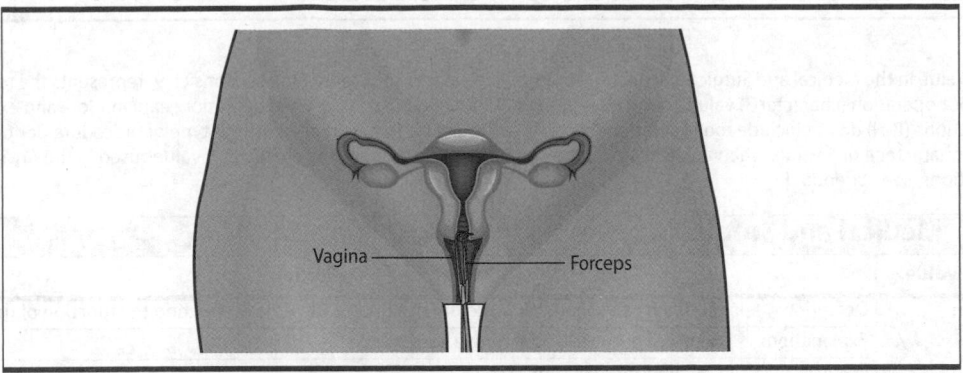

Via Natural or Artificial Opening, Endoscopic (8)

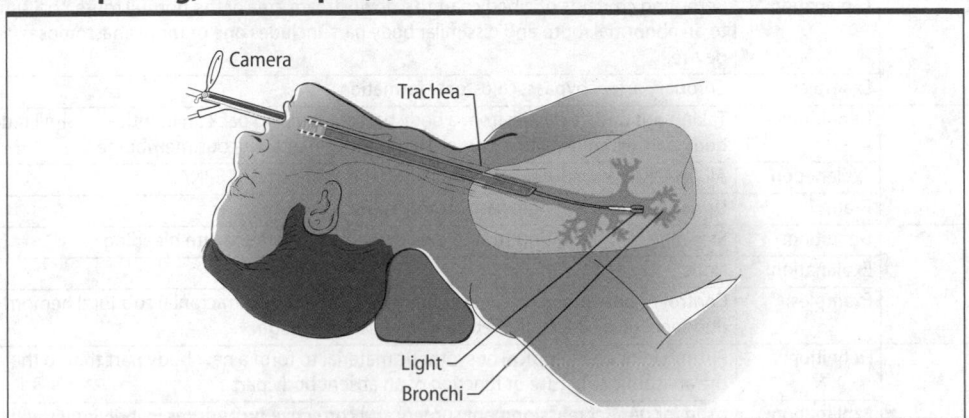

Via Natural or Artificial Opening with Percutaneous Endoscopic Assistance (F)

External (X)

Appendix B: Root Operation Definitions

The character 3 value in the Medical and Surgical section (Ø) and the Medical and Surgical-related sections (1-9) represents the root operation. This resource provides each root operation (character 3) value, found in sections Ø-9, as well as their associated definition, explanation, and examples, where applicable. The Ancillary sections (B-H) do not include root operations; instead the character 3 value represents the type of procedure performed with additional detail provided by the character 4 or 5 value, when applicable. For the character 3, character 4, and character 5 values used in the Ancillary sections of B-H, along with their definitions, see appendix J.

Ø	Medical and Surgical		
ICD-1Ø-PCS Value			**Definition**
Ø	Alteration	Definition:	Modifying the anatomic structure of a body part without affecting the function of the body part
		Explanation:	Principal purpose is to improve appearance
		Examples:	Face lift, breast augmentation
1	Bypass	Definition:	Altering the route of passage of the contents of a tubular body part
		Explanation:	Rerouting contents of a body part to a downstream area of the normal route, to a similar route and body part, or to an abnormal route and dissimilar body part. Includes one or more anastomoses, with or without the use of a device.
		Examples:	Coronary artery bypass, colostomy formation
2	Change	Definition:	Taking out or off a device from a body part and putting back an identical or similar device in or on the same body part without cutting or puncturing the skin or a mucous membrane
		Explanation:	All CHANGE procedures are coded using the approach EXTERNAL
		Example:	Urinary catheter change, gastrostomy tube change
3	Control	Definition:	Stopping, or attempting to stop, postprocedural or other acute bleeding
		Explanation:	None
		Examples:	Control of post-prostatectomy hemorrhage, control of intracranial subdural hemorrhage, control of bleeding duodenal ulcer, control of retroperitoneal hemorrhage
4	Creation	Definition:	Putting in or on biological or synthetic material to form a new body part that to the extent possible replicates the anatomic structure or function of an absent body part
		Explanation:	Used for gender reassignment surgery and corrective procedures in individuals with congenital anomalies
		Examples:	Creation of vagina in a male, creation of right and left atrioventricular valve from common atrioventricular valve
5	Destruction	Definition:	Physical eradication of all or a portion of a body part by the direct use of energy, force, or a destructive agent
		Explanation:	None of the body part is physically taken out
		Examples:	Fulguration of rectal polyp, cautery of skin lesion
6	Detachment	Definition:	Cutting off all or a portion of the upper or lower extremities
		Explanation:	The body part value is the site of the detachment, with a qualifier if applicable to further specify the level where the extremity was detached
		Examples:	Below knee amputation, disarticulation of shoulder
7	Dilation	Definition:	Expanding an orifice or the lumen of a tubular body part
		Explanation:	The orifice can be a natural orifice or an artificially created orifice. Accomplished by stretching a tubular body part using intraluminal pressure or by cutting part of the orifice or wall of the tubular body part.
		Examples:	Percutaneous transluminal angioplasty, internal urethrotomy
8	Division	Definition:	Cutting into a body part, without draining fluids and/or gases from the body part, in order to separate or transect a body part
		Explanation:	All or a portion of the body part is separated into two or more portions
		Examples:	Spinal cordotomy, osteotomy
9	Drainage	Definition:	Taking or letting out fluids and/or gases from a body part
		Explanation:	The qualifier DIAGNOSTIC is used to identify drainage procedures that are biopsies
		Examples:	Thoracentesis, incision and drainage
B	Excision	Definition:	Cutting out or off, without replacement, a portion of a body part
		Explanation:	The qualifier DIAGNOSTIC is used to identify excision procedures that are biopsies
		Examples:	Partial nephrectomy, liver biopsy
C	Extirpation	Definition:	Taking or cutting out solid matter from a body part
		Explanation:	The solid matter may be an abnormal byproduct of a biological function or a foreign body; it may be imbedded in a body part or in the lumen of a tubular body part. The solid matter may or may not have been previously broken into pieces.
		Examples:	Thrombectomy, choledocholithotomy

Continued on next page

Ø	**Medical and Surgical**		*Continued from previous page*
ICD-1Ø-PCS Value			**Definition**
D	Extraction	Definition:	Pulling or stripping out or off all or a portion of a body part by the use of force
		Explanation:	The qualifier DIAGNOSTIC is used to identify extractions that are biopsies
		Examples:	Dilation and curettage, vein stripping
F	Fragmentation	Definition:	Breaking solid matter in a body part into pieces
		Explanation:	Physical force (e.g., manual, ultrasonic) applied directly or indirectly is used to break the solid matter into pieces. The solid matter may be an abnormal byproduct of a biological function or a foreign body. The pieces of solid matter are not taken out.
		Examples:	Extracorporeal shockwave lithotripsy, transurethral lithotripsy
G	Fusion	Definition:	Joining together portions of an articular body part rendering the articular body part immobile
		Explanation:	The body part is joined together by fixation device, bone graft, or other means
		Examples:	Spinal fusion, ankle arthrodesis
H	Insertion	Definition:	Putting in a nonbiological appliance that monitors, assists, performs, or prevents a physiological function but does not physically take the place of a body part
		Explanation:	None
		Examples:	Insertion of radioactive implant, insertion of central venous catheter
J	Inspection	Definition:	Visually and/or manually exploring a body part
		Explanation:	Visual exploration may be performed with or without optical instrumentation. Manual exploration may be performed directly or through intervening body layers.
		Examples:	Diagnostic arthroscopy, exploratory laparotomy
K	Map	Definition:	Locating the route of passage of electrical impulses and/or locating functional areas in a body part
		Explanation:	Applicable only to the cardiac conduction mechanism and the central nervous system
		Examples:	Cardiac mapping, cortical mapping
L	Occlusion	Definition:	Completely closing an orifice or a lumen of a tubular body part
		Explanation:	The orifice can be a natural orifice or an artificially created orifice
		Examples:	Fallopian tube ligation, ligation of inferior vena cava
M	Reattachment	Definition:	Putting back in or on all or a portion of a separated body part to its normal location or other suitable location
		Explanation:	Vascular circulation and nervous pathways may or may not be reestablished
		Examples:	Reattachment of hand, reattachment of avulsed kidney
N	Release	Definition:	Freeing a body part from an abnormal physical constraint by cutting or by use of force
		Explanation:	Some of the restraining tissue may be taken out but none of the body part is taken out
		Examples:	Adhesiolysis, carpal tunnel release
P	Removal	Definition:	Taking out or off a device from a body part
		Explanation:	If a device is taken out and a similar device put in without cutting or puncturing the skin or mucous membrane, the procedure is coded to the root operation CHANGE. Otherwise, the procedure for taking out a device is coded to the root operation REMOVAL.
		Examples:	Drainage tube removal, cardiac pacemaker removal
Q	Repair	Definition:	Restoring, to the extent possible, a body part to its normal anatomic structure and function
		Explanation:	Used only when the method to accomplish the repair is not one of the other root operations
		Examples:	Colostomy takedown, suture of laceration
R	Replacement	Definition:	Putting in or on biological or synthetic material that physically takes the place and/or function of all or a portion of a body part
		Explanation:	The body part may have been taken out or replaced, or may be taken out, physically eradicated, or rendered nonfunctional during the REPLACEMENT procedure. A REMOVAL procedure is coded for taking out the device used in a previous replacement procedure.
		Examples:	Total hip replacement, bone graft, free skin graft
S	Reposition	Definition:	Moving to its normal location, or other suitable location, all or a portion of a body part
		Explanation:	The body part is moved to a new location from an abnormal location, or from a normal location where it is not functioning correctly. The body part may or may not be cut out or off to be moved to the new location.
		Examples:	Reposition of undescended testicle, fracture reduction
T	Resection	Definition:	Cutting out or off, without replacement, all of a body part
		Explanation:	None
		Examples:	Total nephrectomy, total lobectomy of lung
V	Restriction	Definition:	Partially closing an orifice or the lumen of a tubular body part
		Explanation:	The orifice can be a natural orifice or an artificially created orifice
		Examples:	Esophagogastric fundoplication, cervical cerclage

Continued on next page

Ø	Medical and Surgical			*Continued from previous page*

ICD-10-PCS Value			Definition
W	Revision	Definition:	Correcting, to the extent possible, a portion of a malfunctioning device or the position of a displaced device
		Explanation:	Revision can include correcting a malfunctioning or displaced device by taking out or putting in components of the device such as a screw or pin
		Examples:	Adjustment of position of pacemaker lead, recementing of hip prosthesis
U	Supplement	Definition:	Putting in or on biological or synthetic material that physically reinforces and/or augments the function of a portion of a body part
		Explanation:	The biological material is non-living, or is living and from the same individual. The body part may have been previously replaced, and the SUPPLEMENT procedure is performed to physically reinforce and/or augment the function of the replaced body part.
		Examples:	Herniorrhaphy using mesh, mitral valve ring annuloplasty, put a new acetabular liner in a previous hip replacement
X	Transfer	Definition:	Moving, without taking out, all or a portion of a body part to another location to take over the function of all or a portion of a body part
		Explanation:	The body part transferred remains connected to its vascular and nervous supply
		Examples:	Tendon transfer, skin pedicle flap transfer
Y	Transplantation	Definition:	Putting in or on all or a portion of a living body part taken from another individual or animal to physically take the place and/or function of all or a portion of a similar body part
		Explanation:	The native body part may or may not be taken out, and the transplanted body part may take over all or a portion of its function
		Examples:	Kidney transplant, heart transplant

Root Operation Definitions for Other Sections

1	Obstetrics		

ICD-10-PCS Value			Definition
2	Change	Definition:	Taking out or off a device from a body part and putting back an identical or similar device in or on the same body part without cutting or puncturing the skin or a mucous membrane
		Explanation:	None
		Examples:	Replacement of fetal scalp electrode
9	Drainage	Definition:	Taking or letting out fluids and/or gases from a body part
		Explanation:	None
		Examples:	Biopsy of amniotic fluid
A	Abortion	Definition:	Artificially terminating a pregnancy
		Explanation:	None
		Examples:	Transvaginal abortion using vacuum aspiration technique
D	Extraction	Definition:	Pulling or stripping out or off all or a portion of a body part by the use of force
		Explanation:	None
		Examples:	Low-transverse C-section
E	Delivery	Definition:	Assisting the passage of the products of conception from the genital canal
		Explanation:	None
		Examples:	Manually-assisted delivery
H	Insertion	Definition:	Putting in a nonbiological appliance that monitors, assists, performs, or prevents a physiological function but does not physically take the place of a body part
		Explanation:	None
		Examples:	Placement of fetal scalp electrode
J	Inspection	Definition:	Visually and/or manually exploring a body part
		Explanation:	Visual exploration may be performed with or without optical instrumentation. Manual exploration may be performed directly or through intervening body layers.
		Examples:	Bimanual pregnancy exam
P	Removal	Definition:	Taking out or off a device from a body part, region or orifice
		Explanation:	If a device is taken out and a similar device put in without cutting or puncturing the skin or mucous membrane, the procedure is coded to the root operation CHANGE. Otherwise, the procedure for taking out a device is coded to the root operation REMOVAL.
		Examples:	Removal of fetal monitoring electrode

Continued on next page

1   Obstetrics

Continued from previous page

ICD-10-PCS Value			Definition
Q	Repair	Definition:	Restoring, to the extent possible, a body part to its normal anatomic structure and function
		Explanation:	Used only when the method to accomplish the repair is not one of the other root operations
		Examples:	In utero repair of congenital diaphragmatic hernia
S	Reposition	Definition:	Moving to its normal location, or other suitable location, all or a portion of a body part
		Explanation:	The body part is moved to a new location from an abnormal location, or from a normal location where it is not functioning correctly. The body part may or may not be cut out or off to be moved to the new location.
		Examples:	External version of fetus
T	Resection	Definition:	Cutting out or off, without replacement, all of a body part
		Explanation:	None
		Examples:	Total excision of tubal pregnancy
Y	Transplantation	Definition:	Putting in or on all or a portion of a living body part taken from another individual or animal to physically take the place and/or function of all or a portion of a similar body part
		Explanation:	The native body part may or may not be taken out, and the transplanted body part may take over all or a portion of its function
		Examples:	In utero fetal kidney transplant

2   Placement

ICD-10-PCS Value			Definition
Ø	Change	Definition:	Taking out or off a device from a body part and putting back an identical or similar device in or on the same body part without cutting or puncturing the skin or a mucous membrane
		Examples:	Change of vaginal packing
1	Compression	Definition:	Putting pressure on a body region
		Examples:	Placement of pressure dressing on abdominal wall
2	Dressing	Definition:	Putting material on a body region for protection
		Examples:	Application of sterile dressing to head wound
3	Immobilization	Definition:	Limiting or preventing motion of a body region
		Examples:	Placement of splint on left finger
4	Packing	Definition:	Putting material in a body region or orifice
		Examples:	Placement of nasal packing
5	Removal	Definition:	Taking out or off a device from a body part
		Examples:	Removal of stereotactic head frame
6	Traction	Definition:	Exerting a pulling force on a body region in a distal direction
		Examples:	Lumbar traction using motorized split-traction table

3   Administration

ICD-10-PCS Value			Definition
Ø	Introduction	Definition:	Putting in or on a therapeutic, diagnostic, nutritional, physiological, or prophylactic substance except blood or blood products
		Examples:	Nerve block injection to median nerve
1	Irrigation	Definition:	Putting in or on a cleansing substance
		Examples:	Flushing of eye
2	Transfusion	Definition:	Putting in blood or blood products
		Examples:	Transfusion of cell saver red cells into central venous line

4   Measurement and Monitoring

ICD-10-PCS Value			Definition
Ø	Measurement	Definition:	Determining the level of a physiological or physical function at a point in time
		Examples:	External electrocardiogram(EKG), single reading
1	Monitoring	Definition:	Determining the level of a physiological or physical function repetitively over a period of time
		Examples:	Urinary pressure monitoring

5   Extracorporeal or Systemic Assistance and Performance

ICD-10-PCS Value			Definition
Ø	Assistance	Definition:	Taking over a portion of a physiological function by extracorporeal means
		Examples:	Hyperbaric oxygenation of wound
1	Performance	Definition:	Completely taking over a physiological function by extracorporeal means
		Examples:	Cardiopulmonary bypass in conjunction with CABG
2	Restoration	Definition:	Returning, or attempting to return, a physiological function to its original state by extracorporeal means
		Examples:	Attempted cardiac defibrillation, unsuccessful

6   Extracorporeal or Systemic Therapies

ICD-10-PCS Value			Definition
Ø	Atmospheric Control	Definition:	Extracorporeal control of atmospheric pressure and composition
		Examples:	Antigen-free air conditioning, series treatment
1	Decompression	Definition:	Extracorporeal elimination of undissolved gas from body fluids
		Examples:	Hyperbaric decompression treatment, single
2	Electromagnetic Therapy	Definition:	Extracorporeal treatment by electromagnetic rays
		Examples:	TMS (transcranial magnetic stimulation), series treatment
3	Hyperthermia	Definition:	Extracorporeal raising of body temperature
		Examples:	None
4	Hypothermia	Definition:	Extracorporeal lowering of body temperature
		Examples:	Whole body hypothermia treatment for temperature imbalances, series
5	Pheresis	Definition:	Extracorporeal separation of blood products
		Examples:	Therapeutic leukopheresis, single treatment
6	Phototherapy	Definition:	Extracorporeal treatment by light rays
		Examples:	Phototherapy of circulatory system, series treatment
7	Ultrasound Therapy	Definition:	Extracorporeal treatment by ultrasound
		Examples:	Therapeutic ultrasound of peripheral vessels, single treatment
8	Ultraviolet Light Therapy	Definition:	Extracorporeal treatment by ultraviolet light
		Examples:	Ultraviolet light phototherapy, series treatment
9	Shock Wave Therapy	Definition:	Extracorporeal treatment by shock waves
		Examples:	Shockwave therapy of plantar fascia, single treatment
B	Perfusion	Definition:	Extracorporeal treatment by diffusion of therapeutic fluid
		Examples:	Perfusion of donor liver while preparing transplant patient

7   Osteopathic

ICD-10-PCS Value			Definition
Ø	Treatment	Definition:	Manual treatment to eliminate or alleviate somatic dysfunction and related disorders
		Examples:	Fascial release of abdomen, osteopathic treatment

8   Other Procedures

ICD-10-PCS Value			Definition
Ø	Other Procedures	Definition:	Methodologies which attempt to remediate or cure a disorder or disease
		Examples:	Acupuncture, yoga therapy

9   Chiropractic

ICD-10-PCS Value			Definition
B	Manipulation	Definition:	Manual procedure that involves a directed thrust to move a joint past the physiological range of motion, without exceeding the anatomical limit
		Examples:	Chiropractic treatment of cervical spine, short lever specific contact

Appendix C: Comparison of Medical and Surgical Root Operations

Note: the character associated with each operation appears in parentheses after its title.

Procedures That Take Out Some or All of a Body Part

Root Operation	Objective of Procedure	Site of Procedure	Example
Destruction (5)	Eradicating without taking out or replacement	Some/all of a body part	Fulguration of endometrium
Detachment (6)	Cutting out/off without replacement	Extremity only, any level	Amputation above elbow
Excision (B)	Cutting out/off without replacement	Some of a body part	Breast lumpectomy
Extraction (D)	Pulling out or off without replacement	Some/all of a body part	Suction D&C
Resection (T)	Cutting out/off without replacement	All of a body part	Total mastectomy

Procedures That Put in/Put Back or Move Some/All of a Body Part

Root Operation	Objective of Procedure	Site of Procedure	Example
Reattachment (M)	Putting back a detached body part	Some/all of a body part	Reattach finger
Reposition (S)	Moving a body part to normal or other suitable location	Some/all of a body part	Move undescended testicle
Transfer (X)	Moving a body part to function for a similar body part	Some/all of a body part	Skin pedicle transfer flap
Transplantation (Y)	Putting in a living body part from a person/animal	Some/all of a body part	Kidney transplant

Procedures That Take Out or Eliminate Solid Matter, Fluids, or Gases From a Body Part

Root Operation	Objective of Procedure	Site of Procedure	Example
Drainage (9)	Taking or letting out	Fluids and/or gases from a body part	Incision and drainage
Extirpation (C)	Taking or cutting out	Solid matter in a body part	Thrombectomy
Fragmentation (F)	Breaking into pieces	Solid matter within a body part	Lithotripsy

Procedures That Involve Only Examination of Body Parts and Regions

Root Operation	Objective of Procedure	Site of Procedure	Example
Inspection (J)	Visual/manual exploration	Some/all of a body part	Diagnostic cystoscopy Exploratory laparoscopy
Map (K)	Locating electrical impulse route/functional areas	Brain/cardiac conduction mechanism	Cardiac mapping

Procedures That Alter the Diameter/Route of a Tubular Body Part

Root Operation	Objective of Procedure	Site of Procedure	Example
Bypass (1)	Altering route of passage of contents	Tubular body part	Coronary artery bypass graft (CABG)
Dilation (7)	Expanding natural or artificially created orifice/lumen	Tubular body part	Percutaneous transluminal coronary angioplasty (PTCA)
Occlusion (L)	Completely closing natural or artificially created orifice/lumen	Tubular body part	Fallopian tube ligation
Restriction (V)	Partially closing natural or artificially created orifice/lumen	Tubular body part	Gastroesophageal fundoplication

Procedures That Always Involve Devices

Root Operation		Objective of Procedure	Site of Procedure	Example
Change (2)	DVC	Exchanging device w/out cutting/puncturing	In/on a body part	Gastrostomy tube change
Insertion (H)	DVC	Putting in nonbiological device	In/on a body part	Central line insertion
Removal (P)	DVC	Taking out device	In/on a body part	Central line removal
Replacement (R)	DVC	Putting in device that replaces a body part	Some/all of a body part	Total hip replacement
Revision (W)	DVC	Correcting a malfunctioning/displaced device	In/on a body part	Revision of pacemaker
Supplement (U)	DVC	Putting in device that reinforces or augments a body part	In/on a body part	Abdominal wall herniorrhaphy using mesh

DVC = Device involved in root operation

Procedures Involving Cutting or Separation Only

Root Operation	Objective of Procedure	Site of Procedure	Example
Division (8)	Cutting into/separating	A body part	Neurotomy
Release (N)	Freeing a body part from constraint	Around a body part	Adhesiolysis

Procedures That Define Other Repairs

Root Operation	Objective of Procedure	Site of Procedure	Example
Control (3)	Stopping/attempting to stop postprocedural or other acute bleeding	Anatomical region or nasal mucosa/soft tissue	Post-prostatectomy bleeding control, control subdural hemorrhage, bleeding ulcer, retroperitoneal hemorrhage
Repair (Q)	Restoring body part to its normal structure/function	Some/all of a body part	Suture laceration

Procedures That Define Other Objectives

Root Operation	Objective of Procedure	Site of Procedure	Example
Alteration (Ø)	Modifying body part for cosmetic purposes without affecting function	Some/all of a body part	Face lift
Creation (4)	Using biological or synthetic material to form a new body part that replicates the anatomic structure or function of a missing body part	Perineum, valve	Sex change/artificial vagina/penis, atrioventricular valve creation
Fusion (G)	Unification or immobilization	Joint or articular body part	Spinal fusion

Appendix D: Body Part Key

Term	ICD-10-PCS Value
Abdominal aortic plexus	Abdominal Sympathetic Nerve
Abdominal esophagus	Esophagus, Lower
Abductor hallucis muscle	Foot Muscle, Right
	Foot Muscle, Left
Accessory cephalic vein	Cephalic Vein, Right
	Cephalic Vein, Left
Accessory obturator nerve	Lumbar Plexus
Accessory phrenic nerve	Phrenic nerve
Accessory spleen	Spleen
Acetabulofemoral joint	Hip Joint, Right
	Hip Joint, Left
Achilles tendon	Lower Leg Tendon, Right
	Lower Leg Tendon, Left
Acromioclavicular ligament	Shoulder Bursa and Ligament, Right
	Shoulder Bursa and Ligament, Left
Acromion (process)	Scapula, Right
	Scapula, Left
Adductor brevis muscle	Upper Leg Muscle, Right
	Upper Leg Muscle, Left
Adductor hallucis muscle	Foot Muscle, Right
	Foot Muscle, Left
Adductor longus muscle	Upper Leg Muscle, Right
	Upper Leg Muscle, Left
Adductor magnus muscle	Upper Leg Muscle, Right
	Upper Leg Muscle, Left
Adenohypophysis	Pituitary Gland
Alar ligament of axis	Head and Neck Bursa and Ligament
Alveolar process of mandible	Mandible, Right
	Mandible, Left
Alveolar process of maxilla	Maxilla
Anal orifice	Anus
Anatomical snuffbox	Lower Arm and Wrist Muscle, Right
	Lower Arm and Wrist Muscle, Left
Angular artery	Face Artery
Angular vein	Face Vein, Right
	Face Vein, Left
Annular ligament	Elbow Bursa and Ligament, Right
	Elbow Bursa and Ligament, Left
Anorectal junction	Rectum
Ansa cervicalis	Cervical Plexus
Antebrachial fascia	Subcutaneous Tissue and Fascia, Right Lower Arm
	Subcutaneous Tissue and Fascia, Left Lower Arm
Anterior (pectoral) lymph node	Lymphatic, Right Axillary
	Lymphatic, Left Axillary
Anterior cerebral artery	Intracranial Artery
Anterior cerebral vein	Intracranial Vein
Anterior choroidal artery	Intracranial Artery
Anterior circumflex humeral artery	Axillary Artery, Right
	Axillary Artery, Left
Anterior communicating artery	Intracranial Artery
Anterior cruciate ligament (ACL)	Knee Bursa and Ligament, Right
	Knee Bursa and Ligament, Left

Term	ICD-10-PCS Value
Anterior crural nerve	Femoral Nerve
Anterior facial vein	Face Vein, Right
	Face Vein, Left
Anterior intercostal artery	Internal Mammary Artery, Right
	Internal Mammary Artery, Left
Anterior interosseous nerve	Median Nerve
Anterior lateral malleolar artery	Anterior Tibial Artery, Right
	Anterior Tibial Artery, Left
Anterior lingual gland	Minor Salivary Gland
Anterior medial malleolar artery	Anterior Tibial Artery, Right
	Anterior Tibial Artery, Left
Anterior spinal artery	Vertebral Artery, Right
	Vertebral Artery, Left
Anterior tibial recurrent artery	Anterior Tibial Artery, Right
	Anterior Tibial Artery, Left
Anterior ulnar recurrent artery	Ulnar Artery, Right
	Ulnar Artery, Left
Anterior vagal trunk	Vagus Nerve
Anterior vertebral muscle	Neck Muscle, Right
	Neck Muscle, Left
Antihelix	External Ear, Right
	External Ear, Left
	External Ear, Bilateral
Antitragus	External Ear, Right
	External Ear, Left
	External Ear, Bilateral
Antrum of Highmore	Maxillary Sinus, Right
	Maxillary Sinus, Left
Aortic annulus	Aortic Valve
Aortic arch	Thoracic Aorta, Ascending/Arch
Aortic intercostal artery	Upper Artery
Apical (subclavicular) lymph node	Lymphatic, Right Axillary
	Lymphatic, Left Axillary
Apneustic center	Pons
Aqueduct of Sylvius	Cerebral Ventricle
Aqueous humour	Anterior Chamber, Right
	Anterior Chamber, Left
Arachnoid mater, intracranial	Cerebral Meninges
Arachnoid mater, spinal	Spinal Meninges
Arcuate artery	Foot Artery, Right
	Foot Artery, Left
Areola	Nipple, Right
	Nipple, Left
Arterial canal (duct)	Pulmonary Artery, Left
Aryepiglottic fold	Larynx
Arytenoid cartilage	Larynx
Arytenoid muscle	Neck Muscle, Right
	Neck Muscle, Left
Ascending aorta	Thoracic Aorta, Ascending/Arch
Ascending palatine artery	Face Artery
Ascending pharyngeal artery	External Carotid Artery, Right
	External Carotid Artery, Left
Atlantoaxial joint	Cervical Vertebral Joint

Term	ICD-10-PCS Value
Atrioventricular node	Conduction Mechanism
Atrium dextrum cordis	Atrium, Right
Atrium pulmonale	Atrium, Left
Auditory tube	Eustachian Tube, Right
	Eustachian Tube, Left
Auerbach's (myenteric)plexus	Abdominal Sympathetic Nerve
Auricle	External Ear, Right
	External Ear, Left
	External Ear, Bilateral
Auricularis muscle	Head Muscle
Axillary fascia	Subcutaneous Tissue and Fascia, Right Upper Arm
	Subcutaneous Tissue and Fascia, Left Upper Arm
Axillary nerve	Brachial Plexus
Bartholin's (greater vestibular) gland	Vestibular Gland
Basal (internal) cerebral vein	Intracranial Vein
Basal nuclei	Basal Ganglia
Base of tongue	Pharynx
Basilar artery	Intracranial Artery
Basis pontis	Pons
Biceps brachii muscle	Upper Arm Muscle, Right
	Upper Arm Muscle, Left
Biceps femoris muscle	Upper Leg Muscle, Right
	Upper Leg Muscle, Left
Bicipital aponeurosis	Subcutaneous Tissue and Fascia, Right Lower Arm
	Subcutaneous Tissue and Fascia, Left Lower Arm
Bicuspid valve	Mitral Valve
Body of femur	Femoral Shaft, Right
	Femoral Shaft, Left
Body of fibula	Fibula, Right
	Fibula, Left
Bony labyrinth	Inner Ear, Right
	Inner Ear, Left
Bony orbit	Orbit, Right
	Orbit, Left
Bony vestibule	Inner Ear, Right
	Inner Ear, Left
Botallo's duct	Pulmonary Artery, Left
Brachial (lateral) lymph node	Lymphatic, Right Axillary
	Lymphatic, Left Axillary
Brachialis muscle	Upper Arm Muscle, Right
	Upper Arm Muscle, Left
Brachiocephalic artery	Innominate Artery
Brachiocephalic trunk	Innominate Artery
Brachiocephalic vein	Innominate Vein, Right
	Innominate Vein, Left
Brachioradialis muscle	Lower Arm and Wrist Muscle, Right
	Lower Arm and Wrist Muscle, Left
Breast procedures, skin only	Skin, Chest
Broad ligament	Uterine Supporting Structure
Bronchial artery	Upper Artery
Bronchus intermedius	Main Bronchus, Right
Buccal gland	Buccal Mucosa

Term	ICD-10-PCS Value
Buccinator lymph node	Lymphatic, Head
Buccinator muscle	Facial Muscle
Bulbospongiosus muscle	Perineum Muscle
Bulbourethral (Cowper's) gland	Urethra
Bundle of His	Conduction Mechanism
Bundle of Kent	Conduction Mechanism
Calcaneocuboid joint	Tarsal Joint, Right
	Tarsal Joint, Left
Calcaneocuboid ligament	Foot Bursa and Ligament, Right
	Foot Bursa and Ligament, Left
Calcaneofibular ligament	Ankle Bursa and Ligament, Right
	Ankle Bursa and Ligament, Left
Calcaneus	Tarsal, Right
	Tarsal, Left
Capitate bone	Carpal, Right
	Carpal, Left
Cardia	Esophagogastric Junction
Cardiac plexus	Thoracic Sympathetic Nerve
Cardioesophageal junction	Esophagogastric Junction
Caroticotympanic artery	Internal Carotid Artery, Right
	Internal Carotid Artery, Left
Carotid glomus	Carotid Body, Right
	Carotid Body, Left
	Carotid Bodies, Bilateral
Carotid sinus	Internal Carotid Artery, Right
	Internal Carotid Artery, Left
Carotid sinus nerve	Glossopharyngeal Nerve
Carpometacarpal ligament	Hand Bursa and Ligament, Right
	Hand Bursa and Ligament, Left
Cauda equina	Lumbar Spinal Cord
Cavernous plexus	Head and Neck Sympathetic Nerve
Celiac ganglion	Abdominal Sympathetic Nerve
Celiac (solar) plexus	Abdominal Sympathetic Nerve
Celiac lymph node	Lymphatic, Aortic
Celiac trunk	Celiac Artery
Central axillary lymph node	Lymphatic, Right Axillary
	Lymphatic, Left Axillary
Cerebral aqueduct (Sylvius)	Cerebral Ventricle
Cerebrum	Brain
Cervical esophagus	Esophagus, Upper
Cervical facet joint	Cervical Vertebral Joint
	Cervical Vertebral Joints, 2 or more
Cervical ganglion	Head and Neck Sympathetic Nerve
Cervical interspinous ligament	Head and Neck Bursa and Ligament
Cervical intertransverse ligament	Head and Neck Bursa and Ligament
Cervical ligamentum flavum	Head and Neck Bursa and Ligament
Cervical lymph node	Lymphatic, Right Neck
	Lymphatic, Left Neck
Cervicothoracic facet joint	Cervicothoracic Vertebral Joint
Choana	Nasopharynx
Chondroglossus muscle	Tongue, Palate, Pharynx Muscle
Chorda tympani	Facial Nerve
Choroid plexus	Cerebral Ventricle
Ciliary body	Eye, Right
	Eye, Left

Term	ICD-10-PCS Value
Ciliary ganglion	Head and Neck Sympathetic Nerve
Circle of Willis	Intracranial Artery
Circumflex illiac artery	Femoral Artery, Right
	Femoral Artery, Left
Claustrum	Basal Ganglia
Coccygeal body	Coccygeal Glomus
Coccygeus muscle	Trunk Muscle, Right
	Trunk Muscle, Left
Cochlea	Inner Ear, Right
	Inner Ear, Left
Cochlear nerve	Acoustic Nerve
Columella	Nasal Mucosa and Soft Tissue
Common digital vein	Foot Vein, Right
	Foot Vein, Left
Common facial vein	Face Vein, Right
	Face Vein, Left
Common fibular nerve	Peroneal Nerve
Common hepatic artery	Hepatic Artery
Common iliac (subaortic) lymph node	Lymphatic, Pelvis
Common interosseous artery	Ulnar Artery, Right
	Ulnar Artery, Left
Common peroneal nerve	Peroneal Nerve
Condyloid process	Mandible, Right
	Mandible, Left
Conus arteriosus	Ventricle, Right
Conus medullaris	Lumbar Spinal Cord
Coracoacromial ligament	Shoulder Bursa and Ligament, Right
	Shoulder Bursa and Ligament, Left
Coracobrachialis muscle	Upper Arm Muscle, Right
	Upper Arm Muscle, Left
Coracoclavicular ligament	Shoulder Bursa and Ligament, Right
	Shoulder Bursa and Ligament, Left
Coracohumeral ligament	Shoulder Bursa and Ligament, Right
	Shoulder Bursa and Ligament, Left
Coracoid process	Scapula, Right
	Scapula, Left
Corniculate cartilage	Larynx
Corpus callosum	Brain
Corpus cavernosum	Penis
Corpus spongiosum	Penis
Corpus striatum	Basal Ganglia
Corrugator supercilii muscle	Facial Muscle
Costocervical trunk	Subclavian Artery, Right
	Subclavian Artery, Left
Costoclavicular ligament	Shoulder Bursa and Ligament, Right
	Shoulder Bursa and Ligament, Left
Costotransverse joint	Thoracic Vertebral Joint
Costotransverse ligament	Rib(s) Bursa and Ligament
Costovertebral joint	Thoracic Vertebral Joint
Costoxiphoid ligament	Sternum Bursa and Ligament
Cowper's (bulbourethral) gland	Urethra
Cremaster muscle	Perineum Muscle
Cribriform plate	Ethmoid Bone, Right
	Ethmoid Bone, Left
Cricoid cartilage	Trachea

Term	ICD-10-PCS Value
Cricothyroid artery	Thyroid Artery, Right
	Thyroid Artery, Left
Cricothyroid muscle	Neck Muscle, Right
	Neck Muscle, Left
Crural fascia	Subcutaneous Tissue and Fascia, Right Upper Leg
	Subcutaneous Tissue and Fascia, Left Upper Leg
Cubital lymph node	Lymphatic, Right Upper Extremity
	Lymphatic, Left Upper Extremity
Cubital nerve	Ulnar Nerve
Cuboid bone	Tarsal, Right
	Tarsal, Left
Cuboideonavicular joint	Tarsal Joint, Right
	Tarsal Joint, Left
Culmen	Cerebellum
Cuneiform cartilage	Larynx
Cuneonavicular joint	Tarsal Joint, Right
	Tarsal Joint, Left
Cuneonavicular ligament	Foot Bursa and Ligament, Right
	Foot Bursa and Ligament, Left
Cutaneous (transverse) cervical nerve	Cervical Plexus
Deep cervical fascia	Subcutaneous Tissue and Fascia, Right Neck
	Subcutaneous Tissue and Fascia, Left Neck
Deep cervical vein	Vertebral Vein, Right
	Vertebral Vein, Left
Deep circumflex iliac artery	External Iliac Artery, Right
	External Iliac Artery, Left
Deep facial vein	Face Vein, Right
	Face Vein, Left
Deep femoral artery	Femoral Artery, Right
	Femoral Artery, Left
Deep femoral (profunda femoris) vein	Femoral Vein, Right
	Femoral Vein, Left
Deep palmar arch	Hand Artery, Right
	Hand Artery, Left
Deep transverse perineal muscle	Perineum Muscle
Deferential artery	Internal Iliac Artery, Right
	Internal Iliac Artery, Left
Deltoid fascia	Subcutaneous Tissue and Fascia, Right Upper Arm
	Subcutaneous Tissue and Fascia, Left Upper Arm
Deltoid ligament	Ankle Bursa and Ligament, Right
	Ankle Bursa and Ligament, Left
Deltoid muscle	Shoulder Muscle, Right
	Shoulder Muscle, Left
Deltopectoral (infraclavicular) lymph node	Lymphatic, Right Upper Extremity
	Lymphatic, Left Upper Extremity
Dens	Cervical Vertebra
Denticulate (dentate) ligament	Spinal Meninges
Depressor anguli oris muscle	Facial Muscle
Depressor labii inferioris muscle	Facial Muscle

Term	ICD-10-PCS Value
Depressor septi nasi muscle	Facial Muscle
Depressor supercilii muscle	Facial Muscle
Dermis	Skin
Descending genicular artery	Femoral Artery, Right
	Femoral Artery, Left
Diaphragma sellae	Dura Mater
Distal humerus	Humeral Shaft, Right
	Humeral Shaft, Left
Distal humerus, involving joint	Elbow Joint, Right
	Elbow Joint, Left
Distal radioulnar joint	Wrist Joint, Right
	Wrist Joint, Left
Dorsal digital nerve	Radial Nerve
Dorsal metacarpal vein	Hand Vein, Right
	Hand Vein, Left
Dorsal metatarsal artery	Foot Artery, Right
	Foot Artery, Left
Dorsal metatarsal vein	Foot Vein, Right
	Foot Vein, Left
Dorsal root ganglion	Cervical Spinal Cord
	Lumbar Spinal Cord
	Spinal Cord
	Thoracic Spinal Cord
Dorsal scapular artery	Subclavian Artery, Right
	Subclavian Artery, Left
Dorsal scapular nerve	Brachial Plexus
Dorsal venous arch	Foot Vein, Right
	Foot Vein, Left
Dorsalis pedis artery	Anterior Tibial Artery, Right
	Anterior Tibial Artery, Left
Duct of Santorini	Pancreatic Duct, Accessory
Duct of Wirsung	Pancreatic Duct
Ductus deferens	Vas Deferens, Right
	Vas Deferens, Left
	Vas Deferens, Bilateral
	Vas Deferens
Duodenal ampulla	Ampulla of Vater
Duodenojejunal flexure	Jejunum
Dura mater, intracranial	Dura Mater
Dura mater, spinal	Spinal Meninges
Dural venous sinus	Intracranial Vein
Earlobe	External Ear, Right
	External Ear, Left
	External Ear, Bilateral
Eighth cranial nerve	Acoustic Nerve
Ejaculatory duct	Vas Deferens, Right
	Vas Deferens, Left
	Vas Deferens, Bilateral
	Vas Deferens
Eleventh cranial nerve	Accessory Nerve
Encephalon	Brain
Ependyma	Cerebral Ventricle
Epidermis	Skin
Epidural space, spinal	Spinal Canal
Epiploic foramen	Peritoneum
Epithalamus	Thalamus

Term	ICD-10-PCS Value
Epitroclear lymph node	Lymphatic, Right Upper Extremity
	Lymphatic, Left Upper Extremity
Erector spinae muscle	Trunk Muscle, Right
	Trunk Muscle, Left
Esophageal artery	Upper Artery
Esophageal plexus	Thoracic Sympathetic Nerve
Ethmoidal air cell	Ethmoid Sinus, Right
	Ethmoid Sinus, Left
Extensor carpi radialis muscle	Lower Arm and Wrist Muscle, Right
	Lower Arm and Wrist Muscle, Left
Extensor carpi ulnaris muscle	Lower Arm and Wrist Muscle, Right
	Lower Arm and Wrist Muscle, Left
Extensor digitorum brevis muscle	Foot Muscle, Right
	Foot Muscle, Left
Extensor digitorum longus muscle	Lower Leg Muscle, Right
	Lower Leg Muscle, Left
Extensor hallucis brevis muscle	Foot Muscle, Right
	Foot Muscle, Left
Extensor hallucis longus muscle	Lower Leg Muscle, Right
	Lower Leg Muscle, Left
External anal sphincter	Anal Sphincter
External auditory meatus	External Auditory Canal, Right
	External Auditory Canal, Left
External maxillary artery	Face Artery
External naris	Nasal Mucosa and Soft Tissue
External oblique aponeurosis	Subcutaneous Tissue and Fascia, Trunk
External oblique muscle	Abdomen Muscle, Right
	Abdomen Muscle, Left
External popliteal nerve	Peroneal Nerve
External pudendal artery	Femoral Artery, Right
	Femoral Artery, Left
External pudenal vein	Saphenous Vein, Right
	Saphenous Vein, Left
External urethral sphincter	Urethra
Extradural space, intracranial	Epidural Space, Intracranial
Extradural space, spinal	Spinal Canal
Facial artery	Face Artery
False vocal cord	Larynx
Falx cerebri	Dura Mater
Fascia lata	Subcutaneous Tissue and Fascia, Right Upper Leg
	Subcutaneous Tissue and Fascia, Left Upper Leg
Femoral head	Upper Femur, Right
	Upper Femur, Left
Femoral lymph node	Lymphatic, Right Lower Extremity
	Lymphatic, Left Lower Extremity
Femoropatellar joint	Knee Joint, Right
	Knee Joint, Left
	Knee Joint, Femoral Surface, Right
	Knee Joint, Femoral Surface, Left
Femorotibial joint	Knee Joint, Right
	Knee Joint, Left
	Knee Joint, Tibial Surface, Right
	Knee Joint, Tibial Surface, Left
Fibular artery	Peroneal Artery, Right
	Peroneal Artery, Left

Term	ICD-10-PCS Value
Fibular sesamoid	Metatarsal, Right
	Metatarsal, Left
Fibularis brevis muscle	Lower Leg Muscle, Right
	Lower Leg Muscle, Left
Fibularis longus muscle	Lower Leg Muscle, Right
	Lower Leg Muscle, Left
Fifth cranial nerve	Trigeminal Nerve
Filum terminale	Spinal Meninges
First cranial nerve	Olfactory Nerve
First intercostal nerve	Brachial Plexus
Flexor carpi radialis muscle	Lower Arm and Wrist Muscle, Right
	Lower Arm and Wrist Muscle, Left
Flexor carpi ulnaris muscle	Lower Arm and Wrist Muscle, Right
	Lower Arm and Wrist Muscle, Left
Flexor digitorum brevis muscle	Foot Muscle, Right
	Foot Muscle, Left
Flexor digitorum longus muscle	Lower Leg Muscle, Right
	Lower Leg Muscle, Left
Flexor hallucis brevis muscle	Foot Muscle, Right
	Foot Muscle, Left
Flexor hallucis longus muscle	Lower Leg Muscle, Right
	Lower Leg Muscle, Left
Flexor pollicis longus muscle	Lower Arm and Wrist Muscle, Right
	Lower Arm and Wrist Muscle, Left
Foramen magnum	Occipital Bone
Foramen of Monro (intraventricular)	Cerebral Ventricle
Foreskin	Prepuce
Fossa of Rosenmuller	Nasopharynx
Fourth cranial nerve	Trochlear Nerve
Fourth ventricle	Cerebral Ventricle
Fovea	Retina, Right
	Retina, Left
Frenulum labii inferioris	Lower Lip
Frenulum labii superioris	Upper Lip
Frenulum linguae	Tongue
Frontal lobe	Cerebral Hemisphere
Frontal vein	Face Vein, Right
	Face Vein, Left
Fundus uteri	Uterus
Galea aponeurotica	Subcutaneous Tissue and Fascia, Scalp
Ganglion impar (ganglion of Walther)	Sacral Sympathetic Nerve
Gasserian ganglion	Trigeminal Nerve
Gastric lymph node	Lymphatic, Aortic
Gastric plexus	Abdominal Sympathetic Nerve
Gastrocnemius muscle	Lower Leg Muscle, Right
	Lower Leg Muscle, Left
Gastrocolic ligament	Omentum
Gastrocolic omentum	Omentum
Gastroduodenal artery	Hepatic Artery
Gastroesophageal (GE) junction	Esophagogastric Junction
Gastrohepatic omentum	Omentum
Gastrophrenic ligament	Omentum
Gastrosplenic ligament	Omentum
Gemellus muscle	Hip Muscle, Right
	Hip Muscle, Left
Geniculate ganglion	Facial Nerve

Term	ICD-10-PCS Value
Geniculate nucleus	Thalamus
Genioglossus muscle	Tongue, Palate, Pharynx Muscle
Genitofemoral nerve	Lumbar Plexus
Glans penis	Prepuce
Glenohumeral joint	Shoulder Joint, Right
	Shoulder Joint, Left
Glenohumeral ligament	Shoulder Bursa and Ligament, Right
	Shoulder Bursa and Ligament, Left
Glenoid fossa (of scapula)	Glenoid Cavity, Right
	Glenoid Cavity, Left
Glenoid ligament (labrum)	Shoulder Joint, Right
	Shoulder Joint, Left
Globus pallidus	Basal Ganglia
Glossoepiglottic fold	Epiglottis
Glottis	Larynx
Gluteal lymph node	Lymphatic, Pelvis
Gluteal vein	Hypogastric Vein, Right
	Hypogastric Vein, Left
Gluteus maximus muscle	Hip Muscle, Right
	Hip Muscle, Left
Gluteus medius muscle	Hip Muscle, Right
	Hip Muscle, Left
Gluteus minimus muscle	Hip Muscle, Right
	Hip Muscle, Left
Gracilis muscle	Upper Leg Muscle, Right
	Upper Leg Muscle, Left
Great auricular nerve	Cervical Plexus
Great cerebral vein	Intracranial Vein
Great(er) saphenous vein	Saphenous Vein, Right
	Saphenous Vein, Left
Greater alar cartilage	Nasal Mucosa and Soft Tissue
Greater occipital nerve	Cervical Nerve
Greater omentum	Omentum
Greater splanchnic nerve	Thoracic Sympathetic Nerve
Greater superficial petrosal nerve	Facial Nerve
Greater trochanter	Upper Femur, Right
	Upper Femur, Left
Greater tuberosity	Humeral Head, Right
	Humeral Head, Left
Greater vestibular (Bartholin's) gland	Vestibular Gland
Greater wing	Sphenoid Bone
Hallux	1st Toe, Right
	1st Toe, Left
Hamate bone	Carpal, Right
	Carpal, Left
Head of fibula	Fibula, Right
	Fibula, Left
Helix	External Ear, Right
	External Ear, Left
	External Ear, Bilateral
Hepatic artery proper	Hepatic Artery
Hepatic flexure	Transverse Colon
Hepatic lymph node	Lymphatic, Aortic
Hepatic plexus	Abdominal Sympathetic Nerve
Hepatic portal vein	Portal Vein
Hepatogastric ligament	Omentum

Term	ICD-10-PCS Value
Hepatopancreatic ampulla	Ampulla of Vater
Humeroradial joint	Elbow Joint, Right
	Elbow Joint, Left
Humeroulnar joint	Elbow Joint, Right
	Elbow Joint, Left
Humerus, distal	Humeral Shaft, Right
	Humeral Shaft, Left
Hyoglossus muscle	Tongue, Palate, Pharynx Muscle
Hyoid artery	Thyroid Artery, Right
	Thyroid Artery, Left
Hypogastric artery	Internal Iliac Artery, Right
	Internal Iliac Artery, Left
Hypopharynx	Pharynx
Hypophysis	Pituitary Gland
Hypothenar muscle	Hand Muscle, Right
	Hand Muscle, Left
Ileal artery	Superior Mesenteric Artery
Ileocolic artery	Superior Mesenteric Artery
Ileocolic vein	Colic Vein
Iliac crest	Pelvic Bone, Right
	Pelvic Bone, Left
Iliac fascia	Subcutaneous Tissue and Fascia, Right Upper Leg
	Subcutaneous Tissue and Fascia, Left Upper Leg
Iliac lymph node	Lymphatic, Pelvis
Iliacus muscle	Hip Muscle, Right
	Hip Muscle, Left
Iliofemoral ligament	Hip Bursa and Ligament, Right
	Hip Bursa and Ligament, Left
Iliohypogastric nerve	Lumbar Plexus
Ilioinguinal nerve	Lumbar Plexus
Iliolumbar artery	Internal Iliac Artery, Right
	Internal Iliac Artery, Left
Iliolumbar ligament	Lower Spine Bursa and Ligament
Iliotibial tract (band)	Subcutaneous Tissue and Fascia, Right Upper Leg
	Subcutaneous Tissue and Fascia, Left Upper Leg
Ilium	Pelvic Bone, Right
	Pelvic Bone, Left
Incus	Auditory Ossicle, Right
	Auditory Ossicle, Left
Inferior cardiac nerve	Thoracic Sympathetic Nerve
Inferior cerebellar vein	Intracranial Vein
Inferior cerebral vein	Intracranial Vein
Inferior epigastric artery	External Iliac Artery, Right
	External Iliac Artery, Left
Inferior epigastric lymph node	Lymphatic, Pelvis
Inferior genicular artery	Popliteal Artery, Right
	Popliteal Artery, Left
Inferior gluteal artery	Internal Iliac Artery, Right
	Internal Iliac Artery, Left
Inferior gluteal nerve	Sacral Plexus
Inferior hypogastric plexus	Abdominal Sympathetic Nerve
Inferior labial artery	Face Artery
Inferior longitudinal muscle	Tongue, Palate, Pharynx Muscle

Term	ICD-10-PCS Value
Inferior mesenteric ganglion	Abdominal Sympathetic Nerve
Inferior mesenteric lymph node	Lymphatic, Mesenteric
Inferior mesenteric plexus	Abdominal Sympathetic Nerve
Inferior oblique muscle	Extraocular Muscle, Right
	Extraocular Muscle, Left
Inferior pancreaticoduo-denal artery	Superior Mesenteric Artery
Inferior phrenic artery	Abdominal Aorta
Inferior rectus muscle	Extraocular Muscle, Right
	Extraocular Muscle, Left
Inferior suprarenal artery	Renal Artery, Right
	Renal Artery, Left
Inferior tarsal plate	Lower Eyelid, Right
	Lower Eyelid, Left
Inferior thyroid vein	Innominate Vein, Right
	Innominate Vein, Left
Inferior tibiofibular joint	Ankle Joint, Right
	Ankle Joint, Left
Inferior turbinate	Nasal Turbinate
Inferior ulnar collateral artery	Brachial Artery, Right
	Brachial Artery, Left
Inferior vesical artery	Internal Iliac Artery, Right
	Internal Iliac Artery, Left
Infraauricular lymph node	Lymphatic, Head
Infraclavicular (deltopectoral) lymph node	Lymphatic, Right Upper Extremity
	Lymphatic, Left Upper Extremity
Infrahyoid muscle	Neck Muscle, Right
	Neck Muscle, Left
Infraparotid lymph node	Lymphatic, Head
Infraspinatus fascia	Subcutaneous Tissue and Fascia, Right Upper Arm
	Subcutaneous Tissue and Fascia, Left Upper Arm
Infraspinatus muscle	Shoulder Muscle, Right
	Shoulder Muscle, Left
Infundibulopelvic ligament	Uterine Supporting Structure
Inguinal canal	Inguinal Region, Right
	Inguinal Region, Left
	Inguinal Region, Bilateral
Inguinal triangle	Inguinal Region, Right
	Inguinal Region, Left
	Inguinal Region, Bilateral
Interatrial septum	Atrial Septum
Intercarpal joint	Carpal Joint, Right
	Carpal Joint, Left
Intercarpal ligament	Hand Bursa and Ligament, Right
	Hand Bursa and Ligament, Left
Interclavicular ligament	Shoulder Bursa and Ligament, Right
	Shoulder Bursa and Ligament, Left
Intercostal lymph node	Lymphatic, Thorax
Intercostal muscle	Thorax Muscle, Right
	Thorax Muscle, Left
Intercostal nerve	Thoracic Nerve
Intercostobrachial nerve	Thoracic Nerve
Intercuneiform joint	Tarsal Joint, Right
	Tarsal Joint, Left

Term	ICD-10-PCS Value
Intercuneiform ligament	Foot Bursa and Ligament, Right
	Foot Bursa and Ligament, Left
Intermediate bronchus	Main Bronchus, Right
Intermediate cuneiform bone	Tarsal, Right
	Tarsal, Left
Internal anal sphincter	Anal Sphincter
Internal (basal) cerebral vein	Intracranial Vein
Internal carotid artery, intracranial portion	Intracranial Artery
Internal carotid plexus	Head and Neck Sympathetic Nerve
Internal iliac vein	Hypogastric Vein, Right
	Hypogastric Vein, Left
Internal maxillary artery	External Carotid Artery, Right
	External Carotid Artery, Left
Internal naris	Nasal Mucosa and Soft Tissue
Internal oblique muscle	Abdomen Muscle, Right
	Abdomen Muscle, Left
Internal pudendal artery	Internal Iliac Artery, Right
	Internal Iliac Artery, Left
Internal pudendal vein	Hypogastric Vein, Right
	Hypogastric Vein, Left
Internal thoracic artery	Internal Mammary Artery, Right
	Internal Mammary Artery, Left
	Subclavian Artery, Right
	Subclavian Artery, Left
Internal urethral sphincter	Urethra
Interphalangeal (IP) joint	Finger Phalangeal Joint, Right
	Finger Phalangeal Joint, Left
	Toe Phalangeal Joint, Right
	Toe Phalangeal Joint, Left
Interphalangeal ligament	Foot Bursa and Ligament, Right
	Foot Bursa and Ligament, Left
	Hand Bursa and Ligament, Right
	Hand Bursa and Ligament, Left
Interspinalis muscle	Trunk Muscle, Right
	Trunk Muscle, Left
Interspinous ligament, cervical	Head and Neck Bursa and Ligament
Interspinous ligament, lumbar	Lower Spine Bursa and Ligament
Interspinous ligament, thoracic	Upper Spine Bursa and Ligament
Intertransversarius muscle	Trunk Muscle, Right
	Trunk Muscle, Left
Intertransverse ligament, cervical	Head and Neck Bursa and Ligament
Intertransverse ligament, lumbar	Lower Spine Bursa and Ligament
Intertransverse ligament, thoracic	Upper Spine Bursa and Ligament
Interventricular foramen (Monro)	Cerebral Ventricle
Interventricular septum	Ventricular Septum
Intestinal lymphatic trunk	Cisterna Chyli
Ischiatic nerve	Sciatic Nerve
Ischiocavernosus muscle	Perineum Muscle
Ischiofemoral ligament	Hip Bursa and Ligament, Right
	Hip Bursa and Ligament, Left

Term	ICD-10-PCS Value
Ischium	Pelvic Bone, Right
	Pelvic Bone, Left
Jejunal artery	Superior Mesenteric Artery
Jugular body	Glomus Jugulare
Jugular lymph node	Lymphatic, Right Neck
	Lymphatic, Left Neck
Labia majora	Vulva
Labia minora	Vulva
Labial gland	Upper Lip
	Lower Lip
Lacrimal canaliculus	Lacrimal Duct, Right
	Lacrimal Duct, Left
Lacrimal punctum	Lacrimal Duct, Right
	Lacrimal Duct, Left
Lacrimal sac	Lacrimal Duct, Right
	Lacrimal Duct, Left
Laryngopharynx	Pharynx
Lateral (brachial) lymph node	Lymphatic, Right Axillary
	Lymphatic, Left Axillary
Lateral canthus	Upper Eyelid, Right
	Upper Eyelid, Left
Lateral collateral ligament (LCL)	Knee Bursa and Ligament, Right
	Knee Bursa and Ligament, Left
Lateral condyle of femur	Lower Femur, Right
	Lower Femur, Left
Lateral condyle of tibia	Tibia, Right
	Tibia, Left
Lateral cuneiform bone	Tarsal, Right
	Tarsal, Left
Lateral epicondyle of femur	Lower Femur, Right
	Lower Femur, Left
Lateral epicondyle of humerus	Humeral Shaft, Right
	Humeral Shaft, Left
Lateral femoral cutaneous nerve	Lumbar Plexus
Lateral malleolus	Fibula, Right
	Fibula, Left
Lateral meniscus	Knee Joint, Right
	Knee Joint, Left
Lateral nasal cartilage	Nasal Mucosa and Soft Tissue
Lateral plantar artery	Foot Artery, Right
	Foot Artery, Left
Lateral plantar nerve	Tibial Nerve
Lateral rectus muscle	Extraocular Muscle, Right
	Extraocular Muscle, Left
Lateral sacral artery	Internal Iliac Artery, Right
	Internal Iliac Artery, Left
Lateral sacral vein	Hypogastric Vein, Right
	Hypogastric Vein, Left
Lateral sural cutaneous nerve	Peroneal Nerve
Lateral tarsal artery	Foot Artery, Right
	Foot Artery, Left
Lateral temporo-mandibular ligament	Head and Neck Bursa and Ligament
Lateral thoracic artery	Axillary Artery, Right
	Axillary Artery, Left
Latissimus dorsi muscle	Trunk Muscle, Right
	Trunk Muscle, Left

Term	ICD-10-PCS Value
Least splanchnic nerve	Thoracic Sympathetic Nerve
Left ascending lumbar vein	Hemiazygos Vein
Left atrioventricular valve	Mitral Valve
Left auricular appendix	Atrium, Left
Left colic vein	Colic Vein
Left coronary sulcus	Heart, Left
Left gastric artery	Gastric Artery
Left gastroepiploic artery	Splenic Artery
Left gastroepiploic vein	Splenic Vein
Left inferior phrenic vein	Renal Vein, Left
Left inferior pulmonary vein	Pulmonary Vein, Left
Left jugular trunk	Thoracic Duct
Left lateral ventricle	Cerebral Ventricle
Left ovarian vein	Renal Vein, Left
Left second lumbar vein	Renal Vein, Left
Left subclavian trunk	Thoracic Duct
Left subcostal vein	Hemiazygos Vein
Left superior pulmonary vein	Pulmonary Vein, Left
Left suprarenal vein	Renal Vein, Left
Left testicular vein	Renal Vein, Left
Leptomeninges, intracranial	Cerebral Meninges
Leptomeninges, spinal	Spinal Meninges
Lesser alar cartilage	Nasal Mucosa and Soft Tissue
Lesser occipital nerve	Cervical Plexus
Lesser omentum	Omentum
Lesser saphenous vein	Saphenous Vein, Right
	Saphenous Vein, Left
Lesser splanchnic nerve	Thoracic Sympathetic Nerve
Lesser trochanter	Upper Femur, Right
	Upper Femur, Left
Lesser tuberosity	Humeral Head, Right
	Humeral Head, Left
Lesser wing	Sphenoid Bone
Levator anguli oris muscle	Facial Muscle
Levator ani muscle	Perineum Muscle
Levator labii superioris alaeque nasi muscle	Facial Muscle
Levator labii superioris muscle	Facial Muscle
Levator palpebrae superioris muscle	Upper Eyelid, Right
	Upper Eyelid, Left
Levator scapulae muscle	Neck Muscle, Right
	Neck Muscle, Left
Levator veli palatini muscle	Tongue, Palate, Pharynx Muscle
Levatores costarum muscle	Thorax Muscle, Right
	Thorax Muscle, Left
Ligament of head of fibula	Knee Bursa and Ligament, Right
	Knee Bursa and Ligament, Left
Ligament of the lateral malleolus	Ankle Bursa and Ligament, Right
	Ankle Bursa and Ligament, Left
Ligamentum flavum, cervical	Head and Neck Bursa and Ligament
Ligamentum flavum, lumbar	Lower Spine Bursa and Ligament
Ligamentum flavum, thoracic	Upper Spine Bursa and Ligament

Term	ICD-10-PCS Value
Lingual artery	External Carotid Artery, Right
	External Carotid Artery, Left
Lingual tonsil	Pharynx
Locus ceruleus	Pons
Long thoracic nerve	Brachial Plexus
Lumbar artery	Abdominal Aorta
Lumbar facet joint	Lumbar Vertebral Joint
Lumbar ganglion	Lumbar Sympathetic Nerve
Lumbar lymph node	Lymphatic, Aortic
Lumbar lymphatic trunk	Cisterna Chyli
Lumbar splanchnic nerve	Lumbar Sympathetic Nerve
Lumbosacral facet joint	Lumbosacral Joint
Lumbosacral trunk	Lumbar Nerve
Lunate bone	Carpal, Right
	Carpal, Left
Lunotriquetral ligament	Hand Bursa and Ligament, Right
	Hand Bursa and Ligament, Left
Macula	Retina, Right
	Retina, Left
Malleus	Auditory Ossicle, Right
	Auditory Ossicle, Left
Mammary duct	Breast, Right
	Breast, Left
	Breast, Bilateral
Mammary gland	Breast, Right
	Breast, Left
	Breast, Bilateral
Mammillary body	Hypothalamus
Mandibular nerve	Trigeminal Nerve
Mandibular notch	Mandible, Right
	Mandible, Left
Manubrium	Sternum
Masseter muscle	Head Muscle
Masseteric fascia	Subcutaneous Tissue and Fascia, Face
Mastoid (postauricular) lymph node	Lymphatic, Right Neck
	Lymphatic, Left Neck
Mastoid air cells	Mastoid Sinus, Right
	Mastoid Sinus, Left
Mastoid process	Temporal Bone, Right
	Temporal Bone, Left
Maxillary artery	External Carotid Artery, Right
	External Carotid Artery, Left
Maxillary nerve	Trigeminal Nerve
Medial canthus	Lower Eyelid, Right
	Lower Eyelid, Left
Medial collateral ligament (MCL)	Knee Bursa and Ligament, Right
	Knee Bursa and Ligament, Left
Medial condyle of femur	Lower Femur, Right
	Lower Femur, Left
Medial condyle of tibia	Tibia, Right
	Tibia, Left
Medial cuneiform bone	Tarsal, Right
	Tarsal, Left
Medial epicondyle of femur	Lower Femur, Right
	Lower Femur, Left
Medial epicondyle of humerus	Humeral Shaft, Right
	Humeral Shaft, Left

Term	ICD-10-PCS Value
Medial malleolus	Tibia, Right
	Tibia, Left
Medial meniscus	Knee Joint, Right
	Knee Joint, Left
Medial plantar artery	Foot Artery, Right
	Foot Artery, Left
Medial plantar nerve	Tibial Nerve
Medial popliteal nerve	Tibial Nerve
Medial rectus muscle	Extraocular Muscle, Right
	Extraocular Muscle, Left
Medial sural cutaneous nerve	Tibial Nerve
Median antebrachial vein	Basilic Vein, Right
	Basilic Vein, Left
Median cubital vein	Basilic Vein, Right
	Basilic Vein, Left
Median sacral artery	Abdominal Aorta
Mediastinal cavity	Mediastinum
Mediastinal lymph node	Lymphatic, Thorax
Mediastinal space	Mediastinum
Meissner's (submucous) plexus	Abdominal Sympathetic Nerve
Membranous urethra	Urethra
Mental foramen	Mandible, Right
	Mandible, Left
Mentalis muscle	Facial Muscle
Mesoappendix	Mesentery
Mesocolon	Mesentery
Metacarpal ligament	Hand Bursa and Ligament, Right
	Hand Bursa and Ligament, Left
Metacarpophalangeal ligament	Hand Bursa and Ligament, Right
	Hand Bursa and Ligament, Left
Metatarsal ligament	Foot Bursa and Ligament, Right
	Foot Bursa and Ligament, Left
Metatarsophalangeal ligament	Foot Bursa and Ligament, Right
	Foot Bursa and Ligament, Left
Metatarsophalangeal (MTP) joint	Metatarsal-Phalangeal Joint, Right
	Metatarsal-Phalangeal Joint, Left
Metathalamus	Thalamus
Midcarpal joint	Carpal Joint, Right
	Carpal Joint, Left
Middle cardiac nerve	Thoracic Sympathetic Nerve
Middle cerebral artery	Intracranial Artery
Middle cerebral vein	Intracranial Vein
Middle colic vein	Colic Vein
Middle genicular artery	Popliteal Artery, Right
	Popliteal Artery, Left
Middle hemorrhoidal vein	Hypogastric Vein, Right
	Hypogastric Vein, Left
Middle rectal artery	Internal Iliac Artery, Right
	Internal Iliac Artery, Left
Middle suprarenal artery	Abdominal Aorta
Middle temporal artery	Temporal Artery, Right
	Temporal Artery, Left
Middle turbinate	Nasal Turbinate
Mitral annulus	Mitral Valve
Molar gland	Buccal Mucosa
Musculocutaneous nerve	Brachial Plexus

Term	ICD-10-PCS Value
Musculophrenic artery	Internal Mammary Artery, Right
	Internal Mammary Artery, Left
Musculospiral nerve	Radial Nerve
Myelencephalon	Medulla Oblongata
Myenteric (Auerbach's) plexus	Abdominal Sympathetic Nerve
Myometrium	Uterus
Nail bed	Finger Nail
	Toe Nail
Nail plate	Finger Nail
	Toe Nail
Nasal cavity	Nasal Mucosa and Soft Tissue
Nasal concha	Nasal Turbinate
Nasalis muscle	Facial Muscle
Nasolacrimal duct	Lacrimal Duct, Right
	Lacrimal Duct, Left
Navicular bone	Tarsal, Right
	Tarsal, Left
Neck of femur	Upper Femur, Right
	Upper Femur, Left
Neck of humerus (anatomical) (surgical)	Humeral Head, Right
	Humeral Head, Left
Nerve to the stapedius	Facial Nerve
Neurohypophysis	Pituitary Gland
Ninth cranial nerve	Glossopharyngeal Nerve
Nostril	Nasal Mucosa and Soft Tissue
Obturator artery	Internal Iliac Artery, Right
	Internal Iliac Artery, Left
Obturator lymph node	Lymphatic, Pelvis
Obturator muscle	Hip Muscle, Right
	Hip Muscle, Left
Obturator nerve	Lumbar Plexus
Obturator vein	Hypogastric Vein, Right
	Hypogastric Vein, Left
Obtuse margin	Heart, Left
Occipital artery	External Carotid Artery, Right
	External Carotid Artery, Left
Occipital lobe	Cerebral Hemisphere
Occipital lymph node	Lymphatic, Right Neck
	Lymphatic, Left Neck
Occipitofrontalis muscle	Facial Muscle
Odontoid process	Cervical Vertebra
Olecranon bursa	Elbow Bursa and Ligament, Right
	Elbow Bursa and Ligament, Left
Olecranon process	Ulna, Right
	Ulna, Left
Olfactory bulb	Olfactory Nerve
Ophthalmic artery	Intracranial Artery
Ophthalmic nerve	Trigeminal Nerve
Ophthalmic vein	Intracranial Vein
Optic chiasma	Optic Nerve
Optic disc	Retina, Right
	Retina, Left
Optic foramen	Sphenoid Bone
Orbicularis oculi muscle	Upper Eyelid, Right
	Upper Eyelid, Left
Orbicularis oris muscle	Facial Muscle
Orbital fascia	Subcutaneous Tissue and Fascia, Face

Term	ICD-10-PCS Value
Orbital portion of ethmoid bone	Orbit, Right
	Orbit, Left
Orbital portion of frontal bone	Orbit, Right
	Orbit, Left
Orbital portion of lacrimal bone	Orbit, Right
	Orbit, Left
Orbital portion of maxilla	Orbit, Right
	Orbit, Left
Orbital portion of palatine bone	Orbit, Right
	Orbit, Left
Orbital portion of sphenoid bone	Orbit, Right
	Orbit, Left
Orbital portion of zygomatic bone	Orbit, Right
	Orbit, Left
Oropharynx	Pharynx
Otic ganglion	Head and Neck Sympathetic Nerve
Oval window	Middle Ear, Right
	Middle Ear, Left
Ovarian artery	Abdominal Aorta
Ovarian ligament	Uterine Supporting Structure
Oviduct	Fallopian Tube, Right
	Fallopian Tube, Left
Palatine gland	Buccal Mucosa
Palatine tonsil	Tonsils
Palatine uvula	Uvula
Palatoglossal muscle	Tongue, Palate, Pharynx Muscle
Palatopharyngeal muscle	Tongue, Palate, Pharynx Muscle
Palmar (volar) digital vein	Hand Vein, Right
	Hand Vein, Left
Palmar (volar) metacarpal vein	Hand Vein, Right
	Hand Vein, Left
Palmar cutaneous nerve	Median Nerve
	Radial Nerve
Palmar fascia (aponeurosis)	Subcutaneous Tissue and Fascia, Right Hand
	Subcutaneous Tissue and Fascia, Left Hand
Palmar interosseous muscle	Hand Muscle, Right
	Hand Muscle, Left
Palmar ulnocarpal ligament	Wrist Bursa and Ligament, Right
	Wrist Bursa and Ligament, Left
Palmaris longus muscle	Lower Arm and Wrist Muscle, Right
	Lower Arm and Wrist Muscle, Left
Pancreatic artery	Splenic Artery
Pancreatic plexus	Abdominal Sympathetic Nerve
Pancreatic vein	Splenic Vein
Pancreaticosplenic lymph node	Lymphatic, Aortic
Paraaortic lymph node	Lymphatic, Aortic
Parapharyngeal space	Neck
Pararectal lymph node	Lymphatic, Mesenteric
Parasternal lymph node	Lymphatic, Thorax
Paratracheal lymph node	Lymphatic, Thorax
Paraurethral (Skene's) gland	Vestibular Gland
Parietal lobe	Cerebral Hemisphere
Parotid lymph node	Lymphatic, Head
Parotid plexus	Facial Nerve

Term	ICD-10-PCS Value
Pars flaccida	Tympanic Membrane, Right
	Tympanic Membrane, Left
Patellar ligament	Knee Bursa and Ligament, Right
	Knee Bursa and Ligament, Left
Patellar tendon	Knee Tendon, Right
	Knee Tendon, Left
Patellofemoral joint	Knee Joint, Right
	Knee Joint, Left
	Knee Joint, Femoral Surface, Right
	Knee Joint, Femoral Surface, Left
Pectineus muscle	Upper Leg Muscle, Right
	Upper Leg Muscle, Left
Pectoral (anterior) lymph node	Lymphatic, Right Axillary
	Lymphatic, Left Axillary
Pectoral fascia	Subcutaneous Tissue and Fascia, Chest
Pectoralis major muscle	Thorax Muscle, Right
	Thorax Muscle, Left
Pectoralis minor muscle	Thorax Muscle, Right
	Thorax Muscle, Left
Pelvic splanchnic nerve	Abdominal Sympathetic Nerve
	Sacral Sympathetic Nerve
Penile urethra	Urethra
Pericardiophrenic artery	Internal Mammary Artery, Right
	Internal Mammary Artery, Left
Perimetrium	Uterus
Peroneus brevis muscle	Lower Leg Muscle, Right
	Lower Leg Muscle, Left
Peroneus longus muscle	Lower Leg Muscle, Right
	Lower Leg Muscle, Left
Petrous part of temporal bone	Temporal Bone, Right
	Temporal Bone, Left
Pharyngeal constrictor muscle	Tongue, Palate, Pharynx Muscle
Pharyngeal plexus	Vagus Nerve
Pharyngeal recess	Nasopharynx
Pharyngeal tonsil	Adenoids
Pharyngotympanic tube	Eustachian Tube, Right
	Eustachian Tube, Left
Pia mater, intracranial	Cerebral Meninges
Pia mater, spinal	Spinal Meninges
Pinna	External Ear, Right
	External Ear, Left
	External Ear, Bilateral
Piriform recess (sinus)	Pharynx
Piriformis muscle	Hip Muscle, Right
	Hip Muscle, Left
Pisiform bone	Carpal, Right
	Carpal, Left
Pisohamate ligament	Hand Bursa and Ligament, Right
	Hand Bursa and Ligament, Left
Pisometacarpal ligament	Hand Bursa and Ligament, Right
	Hand Bursa and Ligament, Left
Plantar digital vein	Foot Vein, Right
	Foot Vein, Left
Plantar fascia (aponeurosis)	Subcutaneous Tissue and Fascia, Right Foot
	Subcutaneous Tissue and Fascia, Left Foot

Term	ICD-10-PCS Value
Plantar metatarsal vein	Foot Vein, Right
	Foot Vein, Left
Plantar venous arch	Foot Vein, Right
	Foot Vein, Left
Platysma muscle	Neck Muscle, Right
	Neck Muscle, Left
Plica semilunaris	Conjunctiva, Right
	Conjunctiva, Left
Pneumogastric nerve	Vagus Nerve
Pneumotaxic center	Pons
Pontine tegmentum	Pons
Popliteal ligament	Knee Bursa and Ligament, Right
	Knee Bursa and Ligament, Left
Popliteal lymph node	Lymphatic, Left Lower Extremity
	Lymphatic, Right Lower Extremity
Popliteal vein	Femoral Vein, Right
	Femoral Vein, Left
Popliteus muscle	Lower Leg Muscle, Right
	Lower Leg Muscle, Left
Postauricular (mastoid) lymph node	Lymphatic, Right Neck
	Lymphatic, Left Neck
Postcava	Inferior Vena Cava
Posterior (subscapular) lymph node	Lymphatic, Right Axillary
	Lymphatic, Left Axillary
Posterior auricular artery	External Carotid Artery, Right
	External Carotid Artery, Left
Posterior auricular nerve	Facial Nerve
Posterior auricular vein	External Jugular Vein, Right
	External Jugular Vein, Left
Posterior cerebral artery	Intracranial Artery
Posterior chamber	Eye, Right
	Eye, Left
Posterior circumflex humeral artery	Axillary Artery, Right
	Axillary Artery, Left
Posterior communicating artery	Intracranial Artery
Posterior cruciate ligament (PCL)	Knee Bursa and Ligament, Right
	Knee Bursa and Ligament, Left
Posterior facial (retromandibular) vein	Face Vein, Right
	Face Vein, Left
Posterior femoral cutaneous nerve	Sacral Plexus
Posterior inferior cerebellar artery (PICA)	Intracranial Artery
Posterior interosseous nerve	Radial Nerve
Posterior labial nerve	Pudendal Nerve
Posterior scrotal nerve	Pudendal Nerve
Posterior spinal artery	Vertebral Artery, Right
	Vertebral Artery, Left
Posterior tibial recurrent artery	Anterior Tibial Artery, Right
	Anterior Tibial Artery, Left
Posterior ulnar recurrent artery	Ulnar Artery, Right
	Ulnar Artery, Left
Posterior vagal trunk	Vagus Nerve
Preauricular lymph node	Lymphatic, Head
Precava	Superior Vena Cava
Prepatellar bursa	Knee Bursa and Ligament, Right
	Knee Bursa and Ligament, Left

Term	ICD-10-PCS Value
Pretracheal fascia	Subcutaneous Tissue and Fascia, Right Neck
	Subcutaneous Tissue and Fascia, Left Neck
Prevertebral fascia	Subcutaneous Tissue and Fascia, Right Neck
	Subcutaneous Tissue and Fascia, Left Neck
Princeps pollicis artery	Hand Artery, Right
	Hand Artery, Left
Procerus muscle	Facial Muscle
Profunda brachii	Brachial Artery, Right
	Brachial Artery, Left
Profunda femoris (deep femoral) vein	Femoral Vein, Right
	Femoral Vein, Left
Pronator quadratus muscle	Lower Arm and Wrist Muscle, Right
	Lower Arm and Wrist Muscle, Left
Pronator teres muscle	Lower Arm and Wrist Muscle, Right
	Lower Arm and Wrist Muscle, Left
Prostatic urethra	Urethra
Proximal radioulnar joint	Elbow Joint, Right
	Elbow Joint, Left
Psoas muscle	Hip Muscle, Right
	Hip Muscle, Left
Pterygoid muscle	Head Muscle
Pterygoid process	Sphenoid Bone
Pterygopalatine (sphenopalatine) ganglion	Head and Neck Sympathetic Nerve
Pubis	Pelvic Bone, Right
	Pelvic Bone, Left
Pubofemoral ligament	Hip Bursa and Ligament, Right
	Hip Bursa and Ligament, Left
Pudendal nerve	Sacral Plexus
Pulmoaortic canal	Pulmonary Artery, Left
Pulmonary annulus	Pulmonary Valve
Pulmonary plexus	Thoracic Sympathetic Nerve
	Vagus Nerve
Pulmonic valve	Pulmonary Valve
Pulvinar	Thalamus
Pyloric antrum	Stomach, Pylorus
Pyloric canal	Stomach, Pylorus
Pyloric sphincter	Stomach, Pylorus
Pyramidalis muscle	Abdomen Muscle, Right
	Abdomen Muscle, Left
Quadrangular cartilage	Nasal Septum
Quadrate lobe	Liver
Quadratus femoris muscle	Hip Muscle, Right
	Hip Muscle, Left
Quadratus lumborum muscle	Trunk Muscle, Right
	Trunk Muscle, Left
Quadratus plantae muscle	Foot Muscle, Right
	Foot Muscle, Left
Quadriceps (femoris)	Upper Leg Muscle, Right
	Upper Leg Muscle, Left
Radial collateral carpal ligament	Wrist Bursa and Ligament, Right
	Wrist Bursa and Ligament, Left
Radial collateral ligament	Elbow Bursa and Ligament, Right
	Elbow Bursa and Ligament, Left
Radial notch	Ulna, Right
	Ulna, Left

Term	ICD-10-PCS Value
Radial recurrent artery	Radial Artery, Right
	Radial Artery, Left
Radial vein	Brachial Vein, Right
	Brachial Vein, Left
Radialis indicis	Hand Artery, Right
	Hand Artery, Left
Radiocarpal joint	Wrist Joint, Right
	Wrist Joint, Left
Radiocarpal ligament	Wrist Bursa and Ligament, Right
	Wrist Bursa and Ligament, Left
Radioulnar ligament	Wrist Bursa and Ligament, Right
	Wrist Bursa and Ligament, Left
Rectosigmoid junction	Sigmoid Colon
Rectus abdominis muscle	Abdomen Muscle, Right
	Abdomen Muscle, Left
Rectus femoris muscle	Upper Leg Muscle, Right
	Upper Leg Muscle, Left
Recurrent laryngeal nerve	Vagus Nerve
Renal calyx	Kidney, Right
	Kidney, Left
	Kidneys, Bilateral
	Kidney
Renal capsule	Kidney, Right
	Kidney, Left
	Kidneys, Bilateral
	Kidney
Renal cortex	Kidney, Right
	Kidney, Left
	Kidneys, Bilateral
	Kidney
Renal nerve	Abdominal sympathetic Nerve
Renal plexus	Abdominal Sympathetic Nerve
Renal segment	Kidney, Right
	Kidney, Left
	Kidneys, Bilateral
	Kidney
Renal segmental artery	Renal Artery, Right
	Renal Artery, Left
Retroperitoneal cavity	Retroperitoneum
Retroperitoneal lymph node	Lymphatic, Aortic
Retroperitoneal space	Retroperitoneum
Retropharyngeal lymph node	Lymphatic, Right Neck
	Lymphatic, Left Neck
Retropharyngeal space	Neck
Retropubic space	Pelvic Cavity
Rhinopharynx	Nasopharynx
Rhomboid major muscle	Trunk Muscle, Right
	Trunk Muscle, Left
Rhomboid minor muscle	Trunk Muscle, Right
	Trunk Muscle, Left
Right ascending lumbar vein	Azygos Vein
Right atrioventricular valve	Tricuspid Valve
Right auricular appendix	Atrium, Right
Right colic vein	Colic Vein
Right coronary sulcus	Heart, Right
Right gastric artery	Gastric Artery

Term	ICD-10-PCS Value
Right gastroepiploic vein	Superior Mesenteric Vein
Right inferior phrenic vein	Inferior Vena Cava
Right inferior pulmonary vein	Pulmonary Vein, Right
Right jugular trunk	Lymphatic, Right Neck
Right lateral ventricle	Cerebral Ventricle
Right lymphatic duct	Lymphatic, Right Neck
Right ovarian vein	Inferior Vena Cava
Right second lumbar vein	Inferior Vena Cava
Right subclavian trunk	Lymphatic, Right Neck
Right subcostal vein	Azygos Vein
Right superior pulmonary vein	Pulmonary Vein, Right
Right suprarenal vein	Inferior Vena Cava
Right testicular vein	Inferior Vena Cava
Rima glottidis	Larynx
Risorius muscle	Facial Muscle
Round ligament of uterus	Uterine Supporting Structure
Round window	Inner Ear, Right
	Inner Ear, Left
Sacral ganglion	Sacral Sympathetic Nerve
Sacral lymph node	Lymphatic, Pelvis
Sacral splanchnic nerve	Sacral Sympathetic Nerve
Sacrococcygeal ligament	Lower Spine Bursa and Ligament
Sacrococcygeal symphysis	Sacrococcygeal Joint
Sacroiliac ligament	Lower Spine Bursa and Ligament
Sacrospinous ligament	Lower Spine Bursa and Ligament
Sacrotuberous ligament	Lower Spine Bursa and Ligament
Salpingopharyngeus muscle	Tongue, Palate, Pharynx Muscle
Salpinx	Fallopian Tube, Right
	Fallopian Tube, Left
Saphenous nerve	Femoral Nerve
Sartorius muscle	Upper Leg Muscle, Right
	Upper Leg Muscle, Left
Scalene muscle	Neck Muscle, Right
	Neck Muscle, Left
Scaphoid bone	Carpal, Right
	Carpal, Left
Scapholunate ligament	Wrist Bursa and Ligament, Right
	Wrist Bursa and Ligament, Left
Scaphotrapezium ligament	Hand Bursa and Ligament, Right
	Hand Bursa and Ligament, Left
Scarpa's (vestibular) ganglion	Acoustic Nerve
Sebaceous gland	Skin
Second cranial nerve	Optic Nerve
Sella turcica	Sphenoid Bone
Semicircular canal	Inner Ear, Right
	Inner Ear, Left
Semimembranosus muscle	Upper Leg Muscle, Right
	Upper Leg Muscle, Left
Semitendinosus muscle	Upper Leg Muscle, Right
	Upper Leg Muscle, Left
Septal cartilage	Nasal Septum
Serratus anterior muscle	Thorax Muscle, Right
	Thorax Muscle, Left
Serratus posterior muscle	Trunk Muscle, Right
	Trunk Muscle, Left

Term	ICD-10-PCS Value
Seventh cranial nerve	Facial Nerve
Short gastric artery	Splenic Artery
Sigmoid artery	Inferior Mesenteric Artery
Sigmoid flexure	Sigmoid Colon
Sigmoid vein	Inferior Mesenteric Vein
Sinoatrial node	Conduction Mechanism
Sinus venosus	Atrium, Right
Sixth cranial nerve	Abducens Nerve
Skene's (paraurethral) gland	Vestibular Gland
Small saphenous vein	Saphenous Vein, Right
	Saphenous Vein, Left
Solar (celiac) plexus	Abdominal Sympathetic Nerve
Soleus muscle	Lower Leg Muscle, Right
	Lower Leg Muscle, Left
Sphenomandibular ligament	Head and Neck Bursa and Ligament
Sphenopalatine (pterygopalatine) ganglion	Head and Neck Sympathetic Nerve
Spinal nerve, cervical	Cervical Nerve
Spinal nerve, lumbar	Lumbar Nerve
Spinal nerve, sacral	Sacral Nerve
Spinal nerve, thoracic	Thoracic Nerve
Spinous process	Cervical Vertebra
	Lumbar Vertebra
	Thoracic Vertebra
Spiral ganglion	Acoustic Nerve
Splenic flexure	Transverse Colon
Splenic plexus	Abdominal Sympathetic Nerve
Splenius capitis muscle	Head Muscle
Splenius cervicis muscle	Neck Muscle, Right
	Neck Muscle, Left
Stapes	Auditory Ossicle, Right
	Auditory Ossicle, Left
Stellate ganglion	Head and Neck Sympathetic Nerve
Stensen's duct	Parotid Duct, Right
	Parotid Duct, Left
Sternoclavicular ligament	Shoulder Bursa and Ligament, Right
	Shoulder Bursa and Ligament, Left
Sternocleidomastoid artery	Thyroid Artery, Right
	Thyroid Artery, Left
Sternocleidomastoid muscle	Neck Muscle, Right
	Neck Muscle, Left
Sternocostal ligament	Sternum Bursa and Ligament
Styloglossus muscle	Tongue, Palate, Pharynx Muscle
Stylomandibular ligament	Head and Neck Bursa and Ligament
Stylopharyngeus muscle	Tongue, Palate, Pharynx Muscle
Subacromial bursa	Shoulder Bursa and Ligament, Right
	Shoulder Bursa and Ligament, Left
Subaortic (common iliac) lymph node	Lymphatic, Pelvis
Subarachnoid space, spinal	Spinal Canal
Subclavicular (apical) lymph node	Lymphatic, Right Axillary
	Lymphatic, Left Axillary
Subclavius muscle	Thorax Muscle, Right
	Thorax Muscle, Left
Subclavius nerve	Brachial Plexus
Subcostal artery	Upper Artery

Term	ICD-10-PCS Value
Subcostal muscle	Thorax Muscle, Right
	Thorax Muscle, Left
Subcostal nerve	Thoracic Nerve
Subdural space, spinal	Spinal Canal
Submandibular ganglion	Facial Nerve
	Head and Neck Sympathetic Nerve
Submandibular gland	Submaxillary Gland, Right
	Submaxillary Gland, Left
Submandibular lymph node	Lymphatic, Head
Submandibular space	Subcutaneous Tissue and Fascia, Face
Submaxillary ganglion	Head and Neck Sympathetic Nerve
Submaxillary lymph node	Lymphatic, Head
Submental artery	Face Artery
Submental lymph node	Lymphatic, Head
Submucous (Meissner's) plexus	Abdominal Sympathetic Nerve
Suboccipital nerve	Cervical Nerve
Suboccipital venous plexus	Vertebral Vein, Right
	Vertebral Vein, Left
Subparotid lymph node	Lymphatic, Head
Subscapular aponeurosis	Subcutaneous Tissue and Fascia, Right Upper Arm
	Subcutaneous Tissue and Fascia, Left Upper Arm
Subscapular artery	Axillary Artery, Right
	Axillary Artery, Left
Subscapular (posterior) lymph node	Lymphatic, Right Axillary
	Lymphatic, Left Axillary
Subscapularis muscle	Shoulder Muscle, Right
	Shoulder Muscle, Left
Substantia nigra	Basal Ganglia
Subtalar (talocalcaneal) joint	Tarsal Joint, Right
	Tarsal Joint, Left
Subtalar ligament	Foot Bursa and Ligament, Right
	Foot Bursa and Ligament, Left
Subthalamic nucleus	Basal Ganglia
Superficial circumflex iliac vein	Saphenous Vein, Right
	Saphenous Vein, Left
Superficial epigastric artery	Femoral Artery, Right
	Femoral Artery, Left
Superficial epigastric vein	Saphenous Vein, Right
	Saphenous Vein, Left
Superficial palmar arch	Hand Artery, Right
	Hand Artery, Left
Superficial palmar venous arch	Hand Vein, Right
	Hand Vein, Left
Superficial temporal artery	Temporal Artery, Right
	Temporal Artery, Left
Superficial transverse perineal muscle	Perineum Muscle
Superior cardiac nerve	Thoracic Sympathetic Nerve
Superior cerebellar vein	Intracranial Vein
Superior cerebral vein	Intracranial Vein
Superior clunic (cluneal) nerve	Lumbar Nerve
Superior epigastric artery	Internal Mammary Artery, Right
	Internal Mammary Artery, Left

Term	ICD-10-PCS Value
Superior genicular artery	Popliteal Artery, Right
	Popliteal Artery, Left
Superior gluteal artery	Internal Iliac Artery, Right
	Internal Iliac Artery, Left
Superior gluteal nerve	Lumbar Plexus
Superior hypogastric plexus	Abdominal Sympathetic Nerve
Superior labial artery	Face Artery
Superior laryngeal artery	Thyroid Artery, Right
	Thyroid Artery, Left
Superior laryngeal nerve	Vagus Nerve
Superior longitudinal muscle	Tongue, Palate, Pharynx Muscle
Superior mesenteric ganglion	Abdominal Sympathetic Nerve
Superior mesenteric lymph node	Lymphatic, Mesenteric
Superior mesenteric plexus	Abdominal Sympathetic Nerve
Superior oblique muscle	Extraocular Muscle, Right
	Extraocular Muscle, Left
Superior olivary nucleus	Pons
Superior rectal artery	Inferior Mesenteric Artery
Superior rectal vein	Inferior Mesenteric Vein
Superior rectus muscle	Extraocular Muscle, Right
	Extraocular Muscle, Left
Superior tarsal plate	Upper Eyelid, Right
	Upper Eyelid, Left
Superior thoracic artery	Axillary Artery, Right
	Axillary Artery, Left
Superior thyroid artery	External Carotid Artery, Right
	External Carotid Artery, Left
	Thyroid Artery, Right
	Thyroid Artery, Left
Superior turbinate	Nasal Turbinate
Superior ulnar collateral artery	Brachial Artery, Right
	Brachial Artery, Left
Supraclavicular nerve	Cervical Plexus
Supraclavicular (Virchow's) lymph node	Lymphatic, Right Neck
	Lymphatic, Left Neck
Suprahyoid lymph node	Lymphatic, Head
Suprahyoid muscle	Neck Muscle, Right
	Neck Muscle, Left
Suprainguinal lymph node	Lymphatic, Pelvis
Supraorbital vein	Face Vein, Right
	Face Vein, Left
Suprarenal gland	Adrenal Gland, Right
	Adrenal Gland, Left
	Adrenal Glands, Bilateral
	Adrenal Gland
Suprarenal plexus	Abdominal Sympathetic Nerve
Suprascapular nerve	Brachial Plexus
Supraspinatus fascia	Subcutaneous Tissue and Fascia, Right Upper Arm
	Subcutaneous Tissue and Fascia, Left Upper Arm
Supraspinatus muscle	Shoulder Muscle, Right
	Shoulder Muscle, Left
Supraspinous ligament	Upper Spine Bursa and Ligament
	Lower Spine Bursa and Ligament

Term	ICD-10-PCS Value
Suprasternal notch	Sternum
Supratrochlear lymph node	Lymphatic, Right Upper Extremity
	Lymphatic, Left Upper Extremity
Sural artery	Popliteal Artery, Right
	Popliteal Artery, Left
Sweat gland	Skin
Talocalcaneal ligament	Foot Bursa and Ligament, Right
	Foot Bursa and Ligament, Left
Talocalcaneal (subtalar) joint	Tarsal Joint, Right
	Tarsal Joint, Left
Talocalcaneonavicular joint	Tarsal Joint, Right
	Tarsal Joint, Left
Talocalcaneonavicular ligament	Foot Bursa and Ligament, Right
	Foot Bursa and Ligament, Left
Talocrural joint	Ankle Joint, Right
	Ankle Joint, Left
Talofibular ligament	Ankle Bursa and Ligament, Right
	Ankle Bursa and Ligament, Left
Talus bone	Tarsal, Right
	Tarsal, Left
Tarsometatarsal ligament	Foot Bursa and Ligament, Right
	Foot Bursa and Ligament, Left
Temporal lobe	Cerebral Hemisphere
Temporalis muscle	Head Muscle
Temporoparietalis muscle	Head Muscle
Tensor fasciae latae muscle	Hip Muscle, Right
	Hip Muscle, Left
Tensor veli palatini muscle	Tongue, Palate, Pharynx Muscle
Tenth cranial nerve	Vagus Nerve
Tentorium cerebelli	Dura Mater
Teres major muscle	Shoulder Muscle, Right
	Shoulder Muscle, Left
Teres minor muscle	Shoulder Muscle, Right
	Shoulder Muscle, Left
Testicular artery	Abdominal Aorta
Thenar muscle	Hand Muscle, Right
	Hand Muscle, Left
Third cranial nerve	Oculomotor Nerve
Third occipital nerve	Cervical Nerve
Third ventricle	Cerebral Ventricle
Thoracic aortic plexus	Thoracic Sympathetic Nerve
Thoracic esophagus	Esophagus, Middle
Thoracic facet joint	Thoracic Vertebral Joint
Thoracic ganglion	Thoracic Sympathetic Nerve
Thoracoacromial artery	Axillary Artery, Right
	Axillary Artery, Left
Thoracolumbar facet joint	Thoracolumbar Vertebral Joint
Thymus gland	Thymus
Thyroarytenoid muscle	Neck Muscle, Right
	Neck Muscle, Left
Thyrocervical trunk	Thyroid Artery, Right
	Thyroid Artery, Left
Thyroid cartilage	Larynx
Tibial sesamoid	Metatarsal, Right
	Metatarsal, Left
Tibialis anterior muscle	Lower Leg Muscle, Right
	Lower Leg Muscle, Left

Term	ICD-10-PCS Value
Tibialis posterior muscle	Lower Leg Muscle, Right
	Lower Leg Muscle, Left
Tibiofemoral joint	Knee Joint, Right
	Knee Joint, Left
	Knee Joint, Tibial Surface, Right
	Knee Joint, Tibial Surface, Left
Tibioperoneal trunk	Popliteal Artery, Right
	Popliteal Artery, Left
Tongue, base of	Pharynx
Tracheobronchial lymph node	Lymphatic, Thorax
Tragus	External Ear, Right
	External Ear, Left
	External Ear, Bilateral
Transversalis fascia	Subcutaneous Tissue and Fascia, Trunk
Transverse acetabular ligament	Hip Bursa and Ligament, Right
	Hip Bursa and Ligament, Left
Transverse (cutaneous) cervical nerve	Cervical Plexus
Transverse facial artery	Temporal Artery, Right
	Temporal Artery, Left
Transverse foramen	Cervical Vertebra
Transverse humeral ligament	Shoulder Bursa and Ligament, Right
	Shoulder Bursa and Ligament, Left
Transverse ligament of atlas	Head and Neck Bursa and Ligament
Transverse process	Cervical Vertebra
	Thoracic Vertebra
	Lumbar Vertebra
Transverse scapular ligament	Shoulder Bursa and Ligament, Right
	Shoulder Bursa and Ligament, Left
Transverse thoracis muscle	Thorax Muscle, Right
	Thorax Muscle, Left
Transversospinalis muscle	Trunk Muscle, Right
	Trunk Muscle, Left
Transversus abdominis muscle	Abdomen Muscle, Right
	Abdomen Muscle, Left
Trapezium bone	Carpal, Right
	Carpal, Left
Trapezius muscle	Trunk Muscle, Right
	Trunk Muscle, Left
Trapezoid bone	Carpal, Right
	Carpal, Left
Triceps brachii muscle	Upper Arm Muscle, Right
	Upper Arm Muscle, Left
Tricuspid annulus	Tricuspid Valve
Trifacial nerve	Trigeminal Nerve
Trigone of bladder	Bladder
Triquetral bone	Carpal, Right
	Carpal, Left
Trochantericbursa	Hip Bursa and Ligament, Right
	Hip Bursa and Ligament, Left
Twelfth cranial nerve	Hypoglossal Nerve
Tympanic cavity	Middle Ear, Right
	Middle Ear, Left
Tympanic nerve	Glossopharyngeal Nerve
Tympanic part of temoporal bone	Temporal Bone, Right
	Temporal Bone, Left

Term	ICD-10-PCS Value
Ulnar collateral carpal ligament	Wrist Bursa and Ligament, Right
	Wrist Bursa and Ligament, Left
Ulnar collateral ligament	Elbow Bursa and Ligament, Right
	Elbow Bursa and Ligament, Left
Ulnar notch	Radius, Right
	Radius, Left
Ulnar vein	Brachial Vein, Right
	Brachial Vein, Left
Umbilical artery	Internal Iliac Artery, Right
	Internal Iliac Artery, Left
	Lower Artery
Ureteral orifice	Ureter, Right
	Ureter, Left
	Ureters, Bilateral
	Ureter
Ureteropelvic junction (UPJ)	Kidney Pelvis, Right
	Kidney Pelvis, Left
Ureterovesical orifice	Ureter, Right
	Ureter, Left
	Ureters, Bilateral
	Ureter
Uterine artery	Internal Iliac Artery, Right
	Internal Iliac Artery, Left
Uterine cornu	Uterus
Uterine tube	Fallopian Tube, Right
	Fallopian Tube, Left
Uterine vein	Hypogastric Vein, Right
	Hypogastric Vein, Left
Vaginal artery	Internal Iliac Artery, Right
	Internal Iliac Artery, Left
Vaginal vein	Hypogastric Vein, Right
	Hypogastric Vein, Left
Vastus intermedius muscle	Upper Leg Muscle, Right
	Upper Leg Muscle, Left
Vastus lateralis muscle	Upper Leg Muscle, Right
	Upper Leg Muscle, Left
Vastus medialis muscle	Upper Leg Muscle, Right
	Upper Leg Muscle, Left
Ventricular fold	Larynx
Vermiform appendix	Appendix
Vermilion border	Upper Lip
	Lower Lip
Vertebral arch	Cervical Vertebra
	Lumbar Vertebra
	Thoracic Vertebra
Vertebral body	Cervical Vertebra
	Lumbar Vertebra
	Thoracic Vertebra
Vertebral canal	Spinal Canal
Vertebral foramen	Cervical Vertebra
	Lumbar Vertebra
	Thoracic Vertebra
Vertebral lamina	Cervical Vertebra
	Lumbar Vertebra
	Thoracic Vertebra
Vertebral pedicle	Cervical Vertebra
	Lumbar Vertebra
	Thoracic Vertebra

Appendix D: Body Part Key

Term	ICD-10-PCS Value
Vesical vein	Hypogastric Vein, Right
	Hypogastric Vein, Left
Vestibular (Scarpa's) ganglion	Acoustic Nerve
Vestibular nerve	Acoustic Nerve
Vestibulocochlear nerve	Acoustic Nerve
Virchow's (supraclavicular) lymph node	Lymphatic, Right Neck
	Lymphatic, Left Neck
Vitreous body	Vitreous, Right
	Vitreous, Left
Vocal fold	Vocal Cord, Right
	Vocal Cord, Left
Volar (palmar) digital vein	Hand Vein, Right
	Hand Vein, Left
Volar (palmar) metacarpal vein	Hand Vein, Right
	Hand Vein, Left
Vomer bone	Nasal Septum
Vomer of nasal septum	Nasal Bone
Xiphoid process	Sternum
Zonule of Zinn	Lens, Right
	Lens, Left
Zygomatic process of frontal bone	Frontal Bone
Zygomatic process of temporal bone	Temporal Bone, Right
	Temporal Bone, Left
Zygomaticus muscle	Facial Muscle

Appendix E: Body Part Definitions

ICD-10-PCS Value	Definition
1st Toe, Left 1st Toe, Right	**Includes:** Hallux
Abdomen Muscle, Left Abdomen Muscle, Right	**Includes:** External oblique muscle Internal oblique muscle Pyramidalis muscle Rectus abdominis muscle Transversus abdominis muscle
Abdominal Aorta	**Includes:** Inferior phrenic artery Lumbar artery Median sacral artery Middle suprarenal artery Ovarian artery Testicular artery
Abdominal Sympathetic Nerve	**Includes:** Abdominal aortic plexus Auerbach's (myenteric) plexus Celiac (solar) plexus Celiac ganglion Gastric plexus Hepatic plexus Inferior hypogastric plexus Inferior mesenteric ganglion Inferior mesenteric plexus Meissner's (submucous) plexus Myenteric (Auerbach's) plexus Pancreatic plexus Pelvic splanchnic nerve Renal nerve Renal plexus Solar (celiac) plexus Splenic plexus Submucous (Meissner's) plexus Superior hypogastric plexus Superior mesenteric ganglion Superior mesenteric plexus Suprarenal plexus
Abducens Nerve	**Includes:** Sixth cranial nerve
Accessory Nerve	**Includes:** Eleventh cranial nerve
Acoustic Nerve	**Includes:** Cochlear nerve Eighth cranial nerve Scarpa's (vestibular) ganglion Spiral ganglion Vestibular (Scarpa's) ganglion Vestibular nerve Vestibulocochlear nerve
Adenoids	**Includes:** Pharyngeal tonsil
Adrenal Gland Adrenal Gland, Left Adrenal Gland, Right Adrenal Glands, Bilateral	**Includes:** Suprarenal gland
Ampulla of Vater	**Includes:** Duodenal ampulla Hepatopancreatic ampulla
Anal Sphincter	**Includes:** External anal sphincter Internal anal sphincter

ICD-10-PCS Value	Definition
Ankle Bursa and Ligament, Left Ankle Bursa and Ligament, Right	**Includes:** Calcaneofibular ligament Deltoid ligament Ligament of the lateral malleolus Talofibular ligament
Ankle Joint, Left Ankle Joint, Right	**Includes:** Inferior tibiofibular joint Talocrural joint
Anterior Chamber, Left Anterior Chamber, Right	**Includes:** Aqueous humour
Anterior Tibial Artery, Left Anterior Tibial Artery, Right	**Includes:** Anterior lateral malleolar artery Anterior medial malleolar artery Anterior tibial recurrent artery Dorsalis pedis artery Posterior tibial recurrent artery
Anus	**Includes:** Anal orifice
Aortic Valve	**Includes:** Aortic annulus
Appendix	**Includes:** Vermiform appendix
Atrial Septum	**Includes:** Interatrial septum
Atrium, Left	**Includes:** Atrium pulmonale Left auricular appendix
Atrium, Right	**Includes:** Atrium dextrum cordis Right auricular appendix Sinus venosus
Auditory Ossicle, Left Auditory Ossicle, Right	**Includes:** Incus Malleus Stapes
Axillary Artery, Left Axillary Artery, Right	**Includes:** Anterior circumflex humeral artery Lateral thoracic artery Posterior circumflex humeral artery Subscapular artery Superior thoracic artery Thoracoacromial artery
Azygos Vein	**Includes:** Right ascending lumbar vein Right subcostal vein
Basal Ganglia	**Includes:** Basal nuclei Claustrum Corpus striatum Globus pallidus Substantia nigra Subthalamic nucleus
Basilic Vein, Left Basilic Vein, Right	**Includes:** Median antebrachial vein Median cubital vein
Bladder	**Includes:** Trigone of bladder
Brachial Artery, Left Brachial Artery, Right	**Includes:** Inferior ulnar collateral artery Profunda brachii Superior ulnar collateral artery

ICD-10-PCS Value	Definition
Brachial Plexus	**Includes:** Axillary nerve Dorsal scapular nerve First intercostal nerve Long thoracic nerve Musculocutaneous nerve Subclavius nerve Suprascapular nerve
Brachial Vein, Left **Brachial Vein, Right**	**Includes:** Radial vein Ulnar vein
Brain	**Includes:** Cerebrum Corpus callosum Encephalon
Breast, Bilateral **Breast, Left** **Breast, Right**	**Includes:** Mammary duct Mammary gland
Buccal Mucosa	**Includes:** Buccal gland Molar gland Palatine gland
Carotid Bodies, Bilateral **Carotid Body, Left** **Carotid Body, Right**	**Includes:** Carotid glomus
Carpal Joint, Left **Carpal Joint, Right**	**Includes:** Intercarpal joint Midcarpal joint
Carpal, Left **Carpal, Right**	**Includes:** Capitate bone Hamate bone Lunate bone Pisiform bone Scaphoid bone Trapezium bone Trapezoid bone Triquetral bone
Celiac Artery	**Includes:** Celiac trunk
Cephalic Vein, Left **Cephalic Vein, Right**	**Includes:** Accessory cephalic vein
Cerebellum	**Includes:** Culmen
Cerebral Hemisphere	**Includes:** Frontal lobe Occipital lobe Parietal lobe Temporal lobe
Cerebral Meninges	**Includes:** Arachnoid mater, intracranial Leptomeninges, intracranial Pia mater, intracranial
Cerebral Ventricle	**Includes:** Aqueduct of Sylvius Cerebral aqueduct (Sylvius) Choroid plexus Ependyma Foramen of Monro (intraventricular) Fourth ventricle Interventricular foramen (Monro) Left lateral ventricle Right lateral ventricle Third ventricle

ICD-10-PCS Value	Definition
Cervical Nerve	**Includes:** Greater occipital nerve Spinal nerve, cervical Suboccipital nerve Third occipital nerve
Cervical Plexus	**Includes:** Ansa cervicalis Cutaneous (transverse) cervical nerve Great auricular nerve Lesser occipital nerve Supraclavicular nerve Transverse (cutaneous) cervical nerve
Cervical Spinal Cord	**Includes:** Dorsal root ganglion
Cervical Vertebra	**Includes:** Dens Odontoid process Spinous process Transverse foramen Transverse process Vertebral arch Vertebral body Vertebral foramen Vertebral lamina Vertebral pedicle
Cervical Vertebral Joint	**Includes:** Atlantoaxial joint Cervical facet joint
Cervical Vertebral Joints, 2 or more	**Includes:** Cervical facet joint
Cervicothoracic Vertebral Joint	**Includes:** Cervicothoracic facet joint
Cisterna Chyli	**Includes:** Intestinal lymphatic trunk Lumbar lymphatic trunk
Coccygeal Glomus	**Includes:** Coccygeal body
Colic Vein	**Includes:** Ileocolic vein Left colic vein Middle colic vein Right colic vein
Conduction Mechanism	**Includes:** Atrioventricular node Bundle of His Bundle of Kent Sinoatrial node
Conjunctiva, Left **Conjunctiva, Right**	**Includes:** Plica semilunaris
Dura Mater	**Includes:** Diaphragma sellae Dura mater, intracranial Falx cerebri Tentorium cerebelli
Elbow Bursa and Ligament, Left **Elbow Bursa and Ligament, Right**	**Includes:** Annular ligament Olecranon bursa Radial collateral ligament Ulnar collateral ligament
Elbow Joint, Left **Elbow Joint, Right**	**Includes:** Distal humerus, involving joint Humeroradial joint Humeroulnar joint Proximal radioulnar joint
Epidural Space, Intracranial	**Includes:** Extradural space, intracranial

ICD-10-PCS Value	Definition
Epiglottis	**Includes:** Glossoepiglottic fold
Esophagogastric Junction	**Includes:** Cardia Cardioesophageal junction Gastroesophageal (GE) junction
Esophagus, Lower	**Includes:** Abdominal esophagus
Esophagus, Middle	**Includes:** Thoracic esophagus
Esophagus, Upper	**Includes:** Cervical esophagus
Ethmoid Bone, Left **Ethmoid Bone, Right**	**Includes:** Cribriform plate
Ethmoid Sinus, Left **Ethmoid Sinus, Right**	**Includes:** Ethmoidal air cell
Eustachian Tube, Left **Eustachian Tube, Right**	**Includes:** Auditory tube Pharyngotympanic tube
External Auditory Canal, Left **External Auditory Canal, Right**	**Includes:** External auditory meatus
External Carotid Artery, Left **External Carotid Artery, Right**	**Includes:** Ascending pharyngeal artery Internal maxillary artery Lingual artery Maxillary artery Occipital artery Posterior auricular artery Superior thyroid artery
External Ear, Bilateral **External Ear, Left** **External Ear, Right**	**Includes:** Antihelix Antitragus Auricle Earlobe Helix Pinna Tragus
External Iliac Artery, Left **External Iliac Artery, Right**	**Includes:** Deep circumflex iliac artery Inferior epigastric artery
External Jugular Vein, Left **External Jugular Vein, Right**	**Includes:** Posterior auricular vein
Extraocular Muscle, Left **Extraocular Muscle, Right**	**Includes:** Inferior oblique muscle Inferior rectus muscle Lateral rectus muscle Medial rectus muscle Superior oblique muscle Superior rectus muscle
Eye, Left **Eye, Right**	**Includes:** Ciliary body Posterior chamber
Face Artery	**Includes:** Angular artery Ascending palatine artery External maxillary artery Facial artery Inferior labial artery Submental artery Superior labial artery

ICD-10-PCS Value	Definition
Face Vein, Left **Face Vein, Right**	**Includes:** Angular vein Anterior facial vein Common facial vein Deep facial vein Frontal vein Posterior facial (retromandibular) vein Supraorbital vein
Facial Muscle	**Includes:** Buccinator muscle Corrugator supercilii muscle Depressor anguli oris muscle Depressor labii inferioris muscle Depressor septi nasi muscle Depressor supercilii muscle Levator anguli oris muscle Levator labii superioris alaeque nasi muscle Levator labii superioris muscle Mentalis muscle Nasalis muscle Occipitofrontalis muscle Orbicularis oris muscle Procerus muscle Risorius muscle Zygomaticus muscle
Facial Nerve	**Includes:** Chorda tympani Geniculate ganglion Greater superficial petrosal nerve Nerve to the stapedius Parotid plexus Posterior auricular nerve Seventh cranial nerve Submandibular ganglion
Fallopian Tube, Left **Fallopian Tube, Right**	**Includes:** Oviduct Salpinx Uterine tube
Femoral Artery, Left **Femoral Artery, Right**	**Includes:** Circumflex iliac artery Deep femoral artery Descending genicular artery External pudendal artery Superficial epigastric artery
Femoral Nerve	**Includes:** Anterior crural nerve Saphenous nerve
Femoral Shaft, Left **Femoral Shaft, Right**	**Includes:** Body of femur
Femoral Vein, Left **Femoral Vein, Right**	**Includes:** Deep femoral (profunda femoris) vein Popliteal vein Profunda femoris (deep femoral) vein
Fibula, Left **Fibula, Right**	**Includes:** Body of fibula Head of fibula Lateral malleolus
Finger Nail	**Includes:** Nail bed Nail plate
Finger Phalangeal Joint, Left **Finger Phalangeal Joint, Right**	**Includes:** Interphalangeal (IP) joint

ICD-10-PCS Value	Definition
Foot Artery, Left Foot Artery, Right	**Includes:** Arcuate artery Dorsal metatarsal artery Lateral plantar artery Lateral tarsal artery Medial plantar artery
Foot Bursa and Ligament, Left Foot Bursa and Ligament, Right	**Includes:** Calcaneocuboid ligament Cuneonavicular ligament Intercuneiform ligament Interphalangeal ligament Metatarsal ligament Metatarsophalangeal ligament Subtalar ligament Talocalcaneal ligament Talocalcaneonavicular ligament Tarsometatarsal ligament
Foot Muscle, Left Foot Muscle, Right	**Includes:** Abductor hallucis muscle Adductor hallucis muscle Extensor digitorum brevis muscle Extensor hallucis brevis muscle Flexor digitorum brevis muscle Flexor hallucis brevis muscle Quadratus plantae muscle
Foot Vein, Left Foot Vein, Right	**Includes:** Common digital vein Dorsal metatarsal vein Dorsal venous arch Plantar digital vein Plantar metatarsal vein Plantar venous arch
Frontal Bone	**Includes:** Zygomatic process of frontal bone
Gastric Artery	**Includes:** Left gastric artery Right gastric artery
Glenoid Cavity, Left Glenoid Cavity, Right	**Includes:** Glenoid fossa (of scapula)
Glomus Jugulare	**Includes:** Jugular body
Glossopharyngeal Nerve	**Includes:** Carotid sinus nerve Ninth cranial nerve Tympanic nerve
Hand Artery, Left Hand Artery, Right	**Includes:** Deep palmar arch Princeps pollicis artery Radialis indicis Superficial palmar arch
Hand Bursa and Ligament, Left Hand Bursa and Ligament, Right	**Includes:** Carpometacarpal ligament Intercarpal ligament Interphalangeal ligament Lunotriquetral ligament Metacarpal ligament Metacarpophalangeal ligament Pisohamate ligament Pisometacarpal ligament Scaphotrapezium ligament
Hand Muscle, Left Hand Muscle, Right	**Includes:** Hypothenar muscle Palmar interosseous muscle Thenar muscle

ICD-10-PCS Value	Definition
Hand Vein, Left Hand Vein, Right	**Includes:** Dorsal metacarpal vein Palmar (volar) digital vein Palmar (volar) metacarpal vein Superficial palmar venous arch Volar (palmar) digital vein Volar (palmar) metacarpal vein
Head and Neck Bursa and Ligament	**Includes:** Alar ligament of axis Cervical interspinous ligament Cervical intertransverse ligament Cervical ligamentum flavum Interspinous ligament, cervical Intertransverse ligament, cervical Lateral temporomandibular ligament Ligamentum flavum, cervical Sphenomandibular ligament Stylomandibular ligament Transverse ligament of atlas
Head and Neck Sympathetic Nerve	**Includes:** Cavernous plexus Cervical ganglion Ciliary ganglion Internal carotid plexus Otic ganglion Pterygopalatine (sphenopalatine) ganglion Sphenopalatine (pterygopalatine) ganglion Stellate ganglion Submandibular ganglion Submaxillary ganglion
Head Muscle	**Includes:** Auricularis muscle Masseter muscle Pterygoid muscle Splenius capitis muscle Temporalis muscle Temporoparietalis muscle
Heart, Left	**Includes:** Left coronary sulcus Obtuse margin
Heart, Right	**includes:** Right coronary sulcus
Hemiazygos Vein	**Includes:** Left ascending lumbar vein Left subcostal vein
Hepatic Artery	**Includes:** Common hepatic artery Gastroduodenal artery Hepatic artery proper
Hip Bursa and Ligament, Left Hip Bursa and Ligament, Right	**Includes:** Iliofemoral ligament Ischiofemoral ligament Pubofemoral ligament Transverse acetabular ligament Trochanteric bursa
Hip Joint, Left Hip Joint, Right	**Includes:** Acetabulofemoral joint
Hip Muscle, Left Hip Muscle, Right	**Includes:** Gemellus muscle Gluteus maximus muscle Gluteus medius muscle Gluteus minimus muscle Iliacus muscle Obturator muscle Piriformis muscle Psoas muscle Quadratus femoris muscle Tensor fasciae latae muscle

ICD-10-PCS Value	Definition
Humeral Head, Left **Humeral Head, Right**	**Includes:** Greater tuberosity Lesser tuberosity Neck of humerus (anatomical)(surgical)
Humeral Shaft, Left **Humeral Shaft, Right**	**Includes:** Distal humerus Humerus, distal Lateral epicondyle of humerus Medial epicondyle of humerus
Hypogastric Vein, Left **Hypogastric Vein, Right**	**Includes:** Gluteal vein Internal iliac vein Internal pudendal vein Lateral sacral vein Middle hemorrhoidal vein Obturator vein Uterine vein Vaginal vein Vesical vein
Hypoglossal Nerve	**Includes:** Twelfth cranial nerve
Hypothalamus	**Includes:** Mammillary body
Inferior Mesenteric Artery	**Includes:** Sigmoid artery Superior rectal artery
Inferior Mesenteric Vein	**Includes:** Sigmoid vein Superior rectal vein
Inferior Vena Cava	**Includes:** Postcava Right inferior phrenic vein Right ovarian vein Right second lumbar vein Right suprarenal vein Right testicular vein
Inguinal Region, Bilateral **Inguinal Region, Left** **Inguinal Region, Right**	**Includes:** Inguinal canal Inguinal triangle
Inner Ear, Left **Inner Ear, Right**	**Includes:** Bony labyrinth Bony vestibule Cochlea Round window Semicircular canal
Innominate Artery	**Includes:** Brachiocephalic artery Brachiocephalic trunk
Innominate Vein, Left **Innominate Vein, Right**	**Includes:** Brachiocephalic vein Inferior thyroid vein
Internal Carotid Artery, Left **Internal Carotid Artery, Right**	**Includes:** Caroticotympanic artery Carotid sinus

ICD-10-PCS Value	Definition
Internal Iliac Artery, Left **Internal Iliac Artery, Right**	**Includes:** Deferential artery Hypogastric artery Iliolumbar artery Inferior gluteal artery Inferior vesical artery Internal pudendal artery Lateral sacral artery Middle rectal artery Obturator artery Superior gluteal artery Umbilical artery Uterine artery Vaginal artery
Internal Mammary Artery, Left **Internal Mammary Artery, Right**	**Includes:** Anterior intercostal artery Internal thoracic artery Musculophrenic artery Pericardiophrenic artery Superior epigastric artery
Intracranial Artery	**Includes:** Anterior cerebral artery Anterior choroidal artery Anterior communicating artery Basilar artery Circle of Willis Internal carotid artery, intracranial portion Middle cerebral artery Ophthalmic artery Posterior cerebral artery Posterior communicating artery Posterior inferior cerebellar artery (PICA)
Intracranial Vein	**Includes:** Anterior cerebral vein Basal (internal) cerebral vein Dural venous sinus Great cerebral vein Inferior cerebellar vein Inferior cerebral vein Internal (basal) cerebral vein Middle cerebral vein Ophthalmic vein Superior cerebellar vein Superior cerebral vein
Jejunum	**Includes:** Duodenojejunal flexure
Kidney	**Includes:** Renal calyx Renal capsule Renal cortex Renal segment
Kidney Pelvis, Left **Kidney Pelvis, Right**	**Includes:** Ureteropelvic junction (UPJ)
Kidney, Left **Kidney, Right** **Kidneys, Bilateral**	**Includes:** Renal calyx Renal capsule Renal cortex Renal segment
Knee Bursa and Ligament, Left **Knee Bursa and Ligament, Right**	**Includes:** Anterlor cruciate ligament (ACL) Lateral collateral ligament (LCL) Ligament of head of fibula Medial collateral ligament (MCL) Patellar ligament Popliteal ligament Posterior cruciate ligament (PCL) Prepatellar bursa

Appendix E: Body Part Definitions

ICD-10-PCS Value	Definition
Knee Joint, Femoral Surface, Left Knee Joint, Femoral Surface, Right	**Includes:** Femoropatellar joint Patellofemoral joint
Knee Joint, Left Knee Joint, Right	**Includes:** Femoropatellar joint Femorotibial joint Lateral meniscus Medial meniscus Patellofemoral joint Tibiofemoral joint
Knee Joint, Tibial Surface, Left Knee Joint, Tibial Surface, Right	**Includes:** Femorotibial joint Tibiofemoral joint
Knee Tendon, Left Knee Tendon, Right	**Includes:** Patellar tendon
Lacrimal Duct, Left Lacrimal Duct, Right	**Includes:** Lacrimal canaliculus Lacrimal punctum Lacrimal sac Nasolacrimal duct
Larynx	**Includes:** Aryepiglottic fold Arytenoid cartilage Corniculate cartilage Cuneiform cartilage False vocal cord Glottis Rima glottidis Thyroid cartilage Ventricular fold
Lens, Left Lens, Right	**Includes:** Zonule of Zinn
Liver	**Includes:** Quadrate lobe
Lower Arm and Wrist Muscle, Left Lower Arm and Wrist Muscle, Right	**Includes:** Anatomical snuffbox Brachioradialis muscle Extensor carpi radialis muscle Extensor carpi ulnaris muscle Flexor carpi radialis muscle Flexor carpi ulnaris muscle Flexor pollicis longus muscle Palmaris longus muscle Pronator quadratus muscle Pronator teres muscle
Lower Artery	**Includes:** Umbilical artery
Lower Eyelid, Left Lower Eyelid, Right	**Includes:** Inferior tarsal plate Medial canthus
Lower Femur, Left Lower Femur, Right	**Includes:** Lateral condyle of femur Lateral epicondyle of femur Medial condyle of femur Medial epicondyle of femur

ICD-10-PCS Value	Definition
Lower Leg Muscle, Left Lower Leg Muscle, Right	**Includes:** Extensor digitorum longus muscle Extensor hallucis longus muscle Fibularis brevis muscle Fibularis longus muscle Flexor digitorum longus muscle Flexor hallucis longus muscle Gastrocnemius muscle Peroneus brevis muscle Peroneus longus muscle Popliteus muscle Soleus muscle Tibialis anterior muscle Tibialis posterior muscle
Lower Leg Tendon, Left Lower Leg Tendon, Right	**Includes:** Achilles tendon
Lower Lip	**Includes:** Frenulum labii inferioris Labial gland Vermilion border
Lower Spine Bursa and Ligament	**Includes:** Iliolumbar ligament Interspinous ligament, lumbar Intertransverse ligament, lumbar Ligamentum flavum, lumbar Sacrococcygeal ligament Sacroiliac ligament Sacrospinous ligament Sacrotuberous ligament Supraspinous ligament
Lumbar Nerve	**Includes:** Lumbosacral trunk Spinal nerve, lumbar Superior clunic (cluneal) nerve
Lumbar Plexus	**Includes:** Accessory obturator nerve Genitofemoral nerve Iliohypogastric nerve Ilioinguinal nerve Lateral femoral cutaneous nerve Obturator nerve Superior gluteal nerve
Lumbar Spinal Cord	**Includes:** Cauda equina Conus medullaris Dorsal root ganglion
Lumbar Sympathetic Nerve	**Includes:** Lumbar ganglion Lumbar splanchnic nerve
Lumbar Vertebra	**Includes:** Spinous process Transverse process Vertebral arch Vertebral body Vertebral foramen Vertebral lamina Vertebral pedicle
Lumbar Vertebral Joint	**Includes:** Lumbar facet joint
Lumbosacral Joint	**Includes:** Lumbosacral facet joint

ICD-10-PCS Value	Definition
Lymphatic, Aortic	**Includes:** Celiac lymph node Gastric lymph node Hepatic lymph node Lumbar lymph node Pancreaticosplenic lymph node Paraaortic lymph node Retroperitoneal lymph node
Lymphatic, Head	**Includes:** Buccinator lymph node Infraauricular lymph node Infraparotid lymph node Parotid lymph node Preauricular lymph node Submandibular lymph node Submaxillary lymph node Submental lymph node Subparotid lymph node Suprahyoid lymph node
Lymphatic, Left Axillary	**Includes:** Anterior (pectoral) lymph node Apical (subclavicular) lymph node Brachial (lateral) lymph node Central axillary lymph node Lateral (brachial) lymph node Pectoral (anterior) lymph node Posterior (subscapular) lymph node Subclavicular (apical) lymph node Subscapular (posterior) lymph node
Lymphatic, Left Lower Extremity	**Includes:** Femoral lymph node Popliteal lymph node
Lymphatic, Left Neck	**Includes:** Cervical lymph node Jugular lymph node Mastoid (postauricular) lymph node Occipital lymph node Postauricular (mastoid) lymph node Retropharyngeal lymph node Supraclavicular (Virchow's) lymph node Virchow's (supraclavicular) lymph node
Lymphatic, Left Upper Extremity	**Includes:** Cubital lymph node Deltopectoral (infraclavicular) lymph node Epitrochlear lymph node Infraclavicular (deltopectoral) lymph node Supratrochlear lymph node
Lymphatic, Mesenteric	**Includes:** Inferior mesenteric lymph node Pararectal lymph node Superior mesenteric lymph node
Lymphatic, Pelvis	**Includes:** Common iliac (subaortic) lymph node Gluteal lymph node Iliac lymph node Inferior epigastric lymph node Obturator lymph node Sacral lymph node Subaortic (common iliac) lymph node Suprainguinal lymph node

ICD-10-PCS Value	Definition
Lymphatic, Right Axillary	**Includes:** Anterior (pectoral) lymph node Apical (subclavicular) lymph node Brachial (lateral) lymph node Central axillary lymph node Lateral (brachial) lymph node Pectoral (anterior) lymph node Posterior (subscapular) lymph node Subclavicular (apical) lymph node Subscapular (posterior) lymph node
Lymphatic, Right Lower Extremity	**Includes:** Femoral lymph node Popliteal lymph node
Lymphatic, Right Neck	**Includes:** Cervical lymph node Jugular lymph node Mastoid (postauricular) lymph node Occipital lymph node Postauricular (mastoid) lymph node Retropharyngeal lymph node Right jugular trunk Right lymphatic duct Right subclavian trunk Supraclavicular (Virchow's) lymph node Virchow's (supraclavicular) lymph node
Lymphatic, Right Upper Extremity	**Includes:** Cubital lymph node Deltopectoral (infraclavicular) lymph node Epitrochlear lymph node Infraclavicular (deltopectoral) lymph node Supratrochlear lymph node
Lymphatic, Thorax	**Includes:** Intercostal lymph node Mediastinal lymph node Parasternal lymph node Paratracheal lymph node Tracheobronchial lymph node
Main Bronchus, Right	**Includes:** Bronchus intermedius Intermediate bronchus
Mandible, Left **Mandible, Right**	**Includes:** Alveolar process of mandible Condyloid process Mandibular notch Mental foramen
Mastoid Sinus, Left **Mastoid Sinus, Right**	**Includes:** Mastoid air cells
Metatarsal, Left **Metatarsal, Right**	**Includes:** Fibular sesamoid Tibial sesamoid
Maxilla	**Includes:** Alveolar process of maxilla
Maxillary Sinus, Left **Maxillary Sinus, Right**	**Includes:** Antrum of Highmore
Median Nerve	**Includes:** Anterior interosseous nerve Palmar cutaneous nerve
Mediastinum	**Includes:** Mediastinal cavity Mediastinal space
Medulla Oblongata	**Includes:** Myelencephalon
Mesentery	**Includes:** Mesoappendix Mesocolon

ICD-10-PCS Value	Definition
Metatarsal, Right Metatarsal, Left	Includes: Fibular sesamoid Tibial sesamoid
Metatarsal-Phalangeal Joint, Left Metatarsal-Phalangeal Joint, Right	Includes: Metatarsophalangeal (MTP) joint
Middle Ear, Left Middle Ear, Right	Includes: Oval window Tympanic cavity
Minor Salivary Gland	Includes: Anterior lingual gland
Mitral Valve	Includes: Bicuspid valve Left atrioventricular valve Mitral annulus
Nasal Bone	Includes: Vomer of nasal septum
Nasal Mucosa and Soft Tissue	Includes: Columella External naris Greater alar cartilage Internal naris Lateral nasal cartilage Lesser alar cartilage Nasal cavity Nostril
Nasal Septum	Includes: Quadrangular cartilage Septal cartilage Vomer bone
Nasal Turbinate	Includes: Inferior turbinate Middle turbinate Nasal concha Superior turbinate
Nasopharynx	Includes: Choana Fossa of Rosenmuller Pharyngeal recess Rhinopharynx
Neck	Includes: Parapharyngeal space Retropharyngeal space
Neck Muscle, Left Neck Muscle, Right	Includes: Anterior vertebral muscle Arytenoid muscle Cricothyroid muscle Infrahyoid muscle Levator scapulae muscle Platysma muscle Scalene muscle Splenius cervicis muscle Sternocleidomastoid muscle Suprahyoid muscle Thyroarytenoid muscle
Nipple, Left Nipple, Right	Includes: Areola
Occipital Bone	Includes: Foramen magnum
Oculomotor Nerve	Includes: Third cranial nerve
Olfactory Nerve	Includes: First cranial nerve Olfactory bulb

ICD-10-PCS Value	Definition
Omentum	Includes: Gastrocolic ligament Gastrocolic omentum Gastrohepatic omentum Gastrophrenic ligament Gastrosplenic ligament Greater Omentum Hepatogastric ligament Lesser Omentum
Optic Nerve	Includes: Optic chiasma Second cranial nerve
Orbit, Left Orbit, Right	Includes: Bony orbit Orbital portion of ethmoid bone Orbital portion of frontal bone Orbital portion of lacrimal bone Orbital portion of maxilla Orbital portion of palatine bone Orbital portion of sphenoid bone Orbital portion of zygomatic bone
Pancreatic Duct	Includes: Duct of Wirsung
Pancreatic Duct, Accessory	Includes: Duct of Santorini
Parotid Duct, Left Parotid Duct, Right	Includes: Stensen's duct
Pelvic Bone, Left Pelvic Bone, Right	Includes: Iliac crest Ilium Ischium Pubis
Pelvic Cavity	Includes: Retropubic space
Penis	Includes: Corpus cavernosum Corpus spongiosum
Perineum Muscle	Includes: Bulbospongiosus muscle Cremaster muscle Deep transverse perineal muscle Ischiocavernosus muscle Levator ani muscle Superficial transverse perineal muscle
Peritoneum	Includes: Epiploic foramen
Peroneal Artery, Left Peroneal Artery, Right	Includes: Fibular artery
Peroneal Nerve	Includes: Common fibular nerve Common peroneal nerve External popliteal nerve Lateral sural cutaneous nerve
Pharynx	Includes: Base of Tongue Hypopharynx Laryngopharynx Lingual tonsil Oropharynx Piriform recess (sinus) Tongue, base of
Phrenic Nerve	Includes: Accessory phrenic nerve
Pituitary Gland	Includes: Adenohypophysis Hypophysis Neurohypophysis

ICD-10-PCS Value	Definition
Pons	**Includes:** Apneustic center Basis pontis Locus ceruleus Pneumotaxic center Pontine tegmentum Superior olivary nucleus
Popliteal Artery, Left Popliteal Artery, Right	**Includes:** Inferior genicular artery Middle genicular artery Superior genicular artery Sural artery Tibioperoneal trunk
Portal Vein	**Includes:** Hepatic portal vein
Prepuce	**Includes:** Foreskin Glans penis
Pudendal Nerve	**Includes:** Posterior labial nerve Posterior scrotal nerve
Pulmonary Artery, Left	**Includes:** Arterial canal (duct) Botallo's duct Pulmoaortic canal
Pulmonary Valve	**Includes:** Pulmonary annulus Pulmonic valve
Pulmonary Vein, Left	**Includes:** Left inferior pulmonary vein Left superior pulmonary vein
Pulmonary Vein, Right	**Includes:** Right inferior pulmonary vein Right superior pulmonary vein
Radial Artery, Left Radial Artery, Right	**Includes:** Radial recurrent artery
Radial Nerve	**Includes:** Dorsal digital nerve Musculospiral nerve Palmar cutaneous nerve Posterior interosseous nerve
Radius, Left Radius, Right	**Includes:** Ulnar notch
Rectum	**Includes:** Anorectal junction
Renal Artery, Left Renal Artery, Right	**Includes:** Inferior suprarenal artery Renal segmental artery
Renal Vein, Left	**Includes:** Left inferior phrenic vein Left ovarian vein Left second lumbar vein Left suprarenal vein Left testicular vein
Retina, Left Retina, Right	**Includes:** Fovea Macula Optic disc
Retroperitoneum	**Includes:** Retroperitoneal cavity Retroperitoneal space
Rib(s) Bursa and Ligament	**Includes:** Costotransverse ligament
Sacral Nerve	**Includes:** Spinal nerve, sacral

ICD-10-PCS Value	Definition
Sacral Plexus	**Includes:** Inferior gluteal nerve Posterior femoral cutaneous nerve Pudendal nerve
Sacral Sympathetic Nerve	**Includes:** Ganglion impar (ganglion of Walther) Pelvic splanchnic nerve Sacral ganglion Sacral splanchnic nerve
Sacrococcygeal Joint	**Includes:** Sacrococcygeal symphysis
Saphenous Vein, Left Saphenous Vein, Right	**Includes:** External pudendal vein Great(er) saphenous vein Lesser saphenous vein Small saphenous vein Superficial circumflex iliac vein Superficial epigastric vein
Scapula, Left Scapula, Right	**Includes:** Acromion (process) Coracoid process
Sciatic Nerve	**Includes:** Ischiatic nerve
Shoulder Bursa and Ligament, Left Shoulder Bursa and Ligament, Right	**Includes:** Acromioclavicular ligament Coracoacromial ligament Coracoclavicular ligament Coracohumeral ligament Costoclavicular ligament Glenohumeral ligament Interclavicular ligament Sternoclavicular ligament Subacromial bursa Transverse humeral ligament Transverse scapular ligament
Shoulder Joint, Left Shoulder Joint, Right	**Includes:** Glenohumeral joint Glenoid ligament (labrum)
Shoulder Muscle, Left Shoulder Muscle, Right	**Includes:** Deltoid muscle Infraspinatus muscle Subscapularis muscle Supraspinatus muscle Teres major muscle Teres minor muscle
Sigmoid Colon	**Includes:** Rectosigmoid junction Sigmoid flexure
Skin	**Includes:** Dermis Epidermis Sebaceous gland Sweat gland
Skin, Chest	**Includes:** Breast procedures, skin only
Sphenoid Bone	**Includes:** Greater wing Lesser wing Optic foramen Pterygoid process Sella turcica
Spinal Canal	**Includes:** Epidural space, spinal Extradural space, spinal Subarachnoid space, spinal Subdural space, spinal Vertebral canal

ICD-10-PCS Value	Definition
Spinal Cord	**Includes:** Dorsal root ganglion
Spinal Meninges	**Includes:** Arachnoid mater, spinal Denticulate (dentate) ligament Dura mater, spinal Filum terminale Leptomeninges, spinal Pia mater, spinal
Spleen	**Includes:** Accessory spleen
Splenic Artery	**Includes:** Left gastroepiploic artery Pancreatic artery Short gastric artery
Splenic Vein	**Includes:** Left gastroepiploic vein Pancreatic vein
Sternum	**Includes:** Manubrium Suprasternal notch Xiphoid process
Sternum Bursa and Ligament	**Includes:** Costoxiphoid ligament Sternocostal ligament
Stomach, Pylorus	**Includes:** Pyloric antrum Pyloric canal Pyloric sphincter
Subclavian Artery, Left Subclavian Artery, Right	**Includes:** Costocervical trunk Dorsal scapular artery Internal thoracic artery
Subcutaneous Tissue and Fascia, Chest	**Includes:** Pectoral fascia
Subcutaneous Tissue and Fascia, Face	**Includes:** Masseteric fascia Orbital fascia Submandibular space
Subcutaneous Tissue and Fascia, Left Foot	**Includes:** Plantar fascia (aponeurosis)
Subcutaneous Tissue and Fascia, Left Hand	**Includes:** Palmar fascia (aponeurosis)
Subcutaneous Tissue and Fascia, Left Lower Arm	**Includes:** Antebrachial fascia Bicipital aponeurosis
Subcutaneous Tissue and Fascia, Left Neck	**Includes:** Deep cervical fascia Pretracheal fascia Prevertebral fascia
Subcutaneous Tissue and Fascia, Left Upper Arm	**Includes:** Axillary fascia Deltoid fascia Infraspinatus fascia Subscapular aponeurosis Supraspinatus fascia
Subcutaneous Tissue and Fascia, Left Upper Leg	**Includes:** Crural fascia Fascia lata Iliac fascia Iliotibial tract (band)
Subcutaneous Tissue and Fascia, Right Foot	**Includes:** Plantar fascia (aponeurosis)
Subcutaneous Tissue and Fascia, Right Hand	**Includes:** Palmar fascia (aponeurosis)

ICD-10-PCS Value	Definition
Subcutaneous Tissue and Fascia, Right Lower Arm	**Includes:** Antebrachial fascia Bicipital aponeurosis
Subcutaneous Tissue and Fascia, Right Neck	**Includes:** Deep cervical fascia Pretracheal fascia Prevertebral fascia
Subcutaneous Tissue and Fascia, Right Upper Arm	**Includes:** Axillary fascia Deltoid fascia Infraspinatus fascia Subscapular aponeurosis Supraspinatus fascia
Subcutaneous Tissue and Fascia, Right Upper Leg	**Includes:** Crural fascia Fascia lata Iliac fascia Iliotibial tract (band)
Subcutaneous Tissue and Fascia, Scalp	**Includes:** Galea aponeurotica
Subcutaneous Tissue and Fascia, Trunk	**Includes:** External oblique aponeurosis Transversalis fascia
Submaxillary Gland, Left Submaxillary Gland, Right	**Includes:** Submandibular gland
Superior Mesenteric Artery	**Includes:** Ileal artery Ileocolic artery Inferior pancreaticoduodenal artery Jejunal artery
Superior Mesenteric Vein	**Includes:** Right gastroepiploic vein
Superior Vena Cava	**Includes:** Precava
Tarsal Joint, Left Tarsal Joint, Right	**Includes:** Calcaneocuboid joint Cuboideonavicular joint Cuneonavicular joint Intercuneiform joint Subtalar (talocalcaneal) joint Talocalcaneal (subtalar) joint Talocalcaneonavicular joint
Tarsal, Left Tarsal, Right	**Includes:** Calcaneus Cuboid bone Intermediate cuneiform bone Lateral cuneiform bone Medial cuneiform bone Navicular bone Talus bone
Temporal Artery, Left Temporal Artery, Right	**Includes:** Middle temporal artery Superficial temporal artery Transverse facial artery
Temporal Bone, Left Temporal Bone, Right	**Includes:** Mastoid process Petrous part of temporal bone Tympanic part of temporal bone Zygomatic process of temporal bone
Thalamus	**Includes:** Epithalamus Geniculate nucleus Metathalamus Pulvinar
Thoracic Aorta, Ascending/Arch	**Includes:** Aortic arch Ascending aorta

ICD-10-PCS Value	Definition
Thoracic Duct	**Includes:** Left jugular trunk Left subclavian trunk
Thoracic Nerve	**Includes:** Intercostal nerve Intercostobrachial nerve Spinal nerve, thoracic Subcostal nerve
Thoracic Spinal Cord	**Includes:** Dorsal root ganglion
Thoracic Sympathetic Nerve	**Includes:** Cardiac plexus Esophageal plexus Greater splanchnic nerve Inferior cardiac nerve Least splanchnic nerve Lesser splanchnic nerve Middle cardiac nerve Pulmonary plexus Superior cardiac nerve Thoracic aortic plexus Thoracic ganglion
Thoracic Vertebra	**Includes:** Spinous process Transverse process Vertebral arch Vertebral body Vertebral foramen Vertebral lamina Vertebral pedicle
Thoracic Vertebral Joint	**Includes:** Costotransverse joint Costovertebral joint Thoracic facet joint
Thoracolumbar Vertebral Joint	**Includes:** Thoracolumbar facet joint
Thorax Muscle, Left **Thorax Muscle, Right**	**Includes:** Intercostal muscle Levatores costarum muscle Pectoralis major muscle Pectoralis minor muscle Serratus anterior muscle Subclavius muscle Subcostal muscle Transverse thoracis muscle
Thymus	**Includes:** Thymus gland
Thyroid Artery, Left **Thyroid Artery, Right**	**Includes:** Cricothyroid artery Hyoid artery Sternocleidomastoid artery Superior laryngeal artery Superior thyroid artery Thyrocervical trunk
Tibia, Left **Tibia, Right**	**Includes:** Lateral condyle of tibia Medial condyle of tibia Medial malleolus
Tibial Nerve	**Includes:** Lateral plantar nerve Medial plantar nerve Medial popliteal nerve Medial sural cutaneous nerve
Toe Nail	**Includes:** Nail bed Nail plate

ICD-10-PCS Value	Definition
Toe Phalangeal Joint, Left **Toe Phalangeal Joint, Right**	**Includes:** Interphalangeal (IP) joint
Tongue	**Includes:** Frenulum linguae
Tongue, Palate, Pharynx Muscle	**Includes:** Chondroglossus muscle Genioglossus muscle Hyoglossus muscle Inferior longitudinal muscle Levator veli palatini muscle Palatoglossal muscle Palatopharyngeal muscle Pharyngeal constrictor muscle Salpingopharyngeus muscle Styloglossus muscle Stylopharyngeus muscle Superior longitudinal muscle Tensor veli palatini muscle
Tonsils	**Includes:** Palatine tonsil
Trachea	**Includes:** Cricoid cartilage
Transverse Colon	**Includes:** Hepatic flexure Splenic flexure
Tricuspid Valve	**Includes:** Right atrioventricular valve Tricuspid annulus
Trigeminal Nerve	**Includes:** Fifth cranial nerve Gasserian ganglion Mandibular nerve Maxillary nerve Ophthalmic nerve Trifacial nerve
Trochlear Nerve	**Includes:** Fourth cranial nerve
Trunk Muscle, Left **Trunk Muscle, Right**	**Includes:** Coccygeus muscle Erector spinae muscle Interspinalis muscle Intertransversarius muscle Latissimus dorsi muscle Quadratus lumborum muscle Rhomboid major muscle Rhomboid minor muscle Serratus posterior muscle Transversospinalis muscle Trapezius muscle
Tympanic Membrane, Left **Tympanic Membrane, Right**	**Includes:** Pars flaccida
Ulna, Left **Ulna, Right**	**Includes:** Olecranon process Radial notch
Ulnar Artery, Left **Ulnar Artery, Right**	**Includes:** Anterior ulnar recurrent artery Common interosseous artery Posterior ulnar recurrent artery
Ulnar Nerve	**Includes:** Cubital nerve
Upper Arm Muscle, Left **Upper Arm Muscle, Right**	**Includes:** Biceps brachii muscle Brachialis muscle Coracobrachialis muscle Triceps brachii muscle

Appendix E: Body Part Definitions

ICD-10-PCS Value	Definition
Upper Artery	**Includes:** Aortic intercostal artery Bronchial artery Esophageal artery Subcostal artery
Upper Eyelid, Left Upper Eyelid, Right	**Includes:** Lateral canthus Levator palpebrae superioris muscle Orbicularis oculi muscle Superior tarsal plate
Upper Femur, Left Upper Femur, Right	**Includes:** Femoral head Greater trochanter Lesser trochanter Neck of femur
Upper Leg Muscle, Left Upper Leg Muscle, Right	**Includes:** Adductor brevis muscle Adductor longus muscle Adductor magnus muscle Biceps femoris muscle Gracilis muscle Pectineus muscle Quadriceps (femoris) Rectus femoris muscle Sartorius muscle Semimembranosus muscle Semitendinosus muscle Vastus intermedius muscle Vastus lateralis muscle Vastus medialis muscle
Upper Lip	**Includes:** Frenulum labii superioris Labial gland Vermilion border
Upper Spine Bursa and Ligament	**Includes:** Interspinous ligament, thoracic Intertransverse ligament, thoracic Ligamentum flavum, thoracic Supraspinous ligament
Ureter Ureter, Left Ureter, Right Ureters, Bilateral	**Includes:** Ureteral orifice Ureterovesical orifice
Urethra	**Includes:** Bulbourethral (Cowper's) gland Cowper's (bulbourethral) gland External urethral sphincter Internal urethral sphincter Membranous urethra Penile urethra Prostatic urethra
Uterine Supporting Structure	**Includes:** Broad ligament Infundibulopelvic ligament Ovarian ligament Round ligament of uterus
Uterus	**Includes:** Fundus uteri Myometrium Perimetrium Uterine cornu
Uvula	**Includes:** Palatine uvula

ICD-10-PCS Value	Definition
Vagus Nerve	**Includes:** Anterior vagal trunk Pharyngeal plexus Pneumogastric nerve Posterior vagal trunk Pulmonary plexus Recurrent laryngeal nerve Superior laryngeal nerve Tenth cranial nerve
Vas Deferens Vas Deferens, Bilateral Vas Deferens, Left Vas Deferens, Right	**Includes:** Ductus deferens Ejaculatory duct
Ventricle, Right	**Includes:** Conus arteriosus
Ventricular Septum	**Includes:** Interventricular septum
Vertebral Artery, Left Vertebral Artery, Right	**Includes:** Anterior spinal artery Posterior spinal artery
Vertebral Vein, Left Vertebral Vein, Right	**Includes:** Deep cervical vein Suboccipital venous plexus
Vestibular Gland	**Includes:** Bartholin's (greater vestibular) gland Greater vestibular (Bartholin's) gland Paraurethral (Skene's) gland Skene's (paraurethral) gland
Vitreous, Left Vitreous, Right	**Includes:** Vitreous body
Vocal Cord, Left Vocal Cord, Right	**Includes:** Vocal fold
Vulva	**Includes:** Labia majora Labia minora
Wrist Bursa and Ligament, Left Wrist Bursa and Ligament, Right	**Includes:** Palmar ulnocarpal ligament Radial collateral carpal ligament Radiocarpal ligament Radioulnar ligament Scapholunate ligament Ulnar collateral carpal ligament
Wrist Joint, Left Wrist Joint, Right	**Includes:** Distal radioulnar joint Radiocarpal joint

Appendix F: Device Classification

In most PCS codes, the sixth character of the code classifies the device. The sixth character device value "defines the material or appliance used to accomplish the objective of the procedure that remains in or on the procedure site at the end of the procedure." If the device is the means by which the procedural objective is accomplished, then a specific device value is coded in the sixth character. If no device is used to accomplish the objective of the procedure, the device value No Device is coded in the sixth character. In limited root operations, the classification provides the qualifier values Temporary and Intraoperative, for specific procedures involving clinically significant devices whose purpose is brief use during the procedure or current inpatient stay.

Material that is classified as a PCS device is distinguished from material classified as a PCS substance by its having a specific location. A device is intended to maintain a fixed location at the procedure site where it was put, whereas a substance is intended to disperse or be absorbed in the body. There are circumstances in which a device does not stay where it was put and may need to be "revised" in a subsequent procedure to move the device back to its intended location.

Material classified as a PCS device is also distinguishable by the fact that it is removable. Although it may not be practical to remove some types of devices once they become established at the site, it is physically possible to remove a device for some time after the procedure. A skin graft, for example, once it "takes," may be nearly indistinguishable from the surrounding skin and so is no longer clearly identifiable as a device. Nevertheless, procedures that involve material coded as a device can for the most part be "reversed" by removing the device from the procedure site.

General Device Types

Device Type	Definition	Examples
Grafts	Biological or synthetic material that **takes the place of all or a portion of a body part.**	Full- or partial-thickness skin grafts: • Autologous • Nonautologous • Synthetic • Zooplastic Other tissue grafts: • Bone • Tendon • Vascular
Prosthesis	Biological or synthetic material that **takes the place of all or a portion of a body part.**	Joint prosthesis: • Autologous • Nonautologous • Synthetic
Implants	**Therapeutic** material that is not absorbed by, eliminated by, or incorporated into a body part.	External fixation device Internal fixation device: • Orthopaedic pins • Intramedullary rods Radioactive element implant Mesh
Simple or mechanical appliances	Biological or synthetic material that **assists or prevents a physiological function.**	Drainage device Extraluminal device Endobrachial device Fusion device Intraluminal device (can be temporary) Tracheostomy device IUD
Electronic appliances	Electronic appliances used to **assist, monitor, take the pace of, or prevent a physiological function.**	Cardiac leads Diaphragmatic pacemaker External heart assist system Short-term external heart assist system (Intraoperative) Fetal monitoring Hearing device Monitoring device Neurostimulator
External appliances	Performed without making an incision or a puncture, external appliances are used for the purpose of **protection, immobilization, stretching, compression, or packing.**	Bandage Cast Packing material Pressure dressing Traction apparatus

Transplant/Grafting Tissue Type Terminology

Tissue Type	Terminology
Tissue or organ transferred into a new position in **the body of the same individual**	Autograft Autologous Autoplastic
Having to do with individuals or tissues that have **identical genes**, such as identical twins	Isograft Isologous Syngeneic Syngraft
Tissue or organ taken from **different individuals** of the same species	Allogeneic Allograft Homologous Homograft
Tissue or organ from a **cadaver**	Nonautologous
Tissue or organ from individuals of **different species**	Heterogeneic Heterologous Xenogeneic Xenograft Zooplastic

Appendix G: Device Key and Aggregation Table

This **NT** symbol next to a device in the Term column identifies that the device has been approved for NTAP (new technology add-on payment). CMS provides incremental payment, in addition to the DRG payment, for technologies that have received an NTAP designation.

Device Key

Term	ICD-10-PCS Value
3f (Aortic) Bioprosthesis valve	Zooplastic Tissue in Heart and Great Vessels
AbioCor® Total Replacement Heart	Synthetic Substitute
Absolute Pro Vascular (OTW) Self-Expanding Stent System	Intraluminal Device
Acculink (RX) Carotid Stent System	Intraluminal Device
Acellular Hydrated Dermis	Nonautologous Tissue Substitute
Acetabular cup	Liner in Lower Joints
Activa PC neurostimulator	Stimulator Generator, Multiple Array for Insertion in Subcutaneous Tissue and Fascia
Activa RC neurostimulator	Stimulator Generator, Multiple Array Rechargeable for Insertion in Subcutaneous Tissue and Fascia
Activa SC neurostimulator	Stimulator Generator, Single Array for Insertion in Subcutaneous Tissue and Fascia
ACUITY™ Steerable Lead	Cardiac Lead, Pacemaker for Insertion in Heart and Great Vessels Cardiac Lead, Defibrillator for Insertion in Heart and Great Vessels
Advisa (MRI)	Pacemaker, Dual Chamber for Insertion in Subcutaneous Tissue and Fascia
AFX® Endovascular AAA System	Intraluminal Device
Alfapump® system	Other Device
AMPLATZER® Muscular VSD Occluder	Synthetic Substitute
AMS 800® Urinary Control System	Artificial Sphincter in Urinary System
AneuRx® AAA Advantage®	Intraluminal Device
Annuloplasty ring	Synthetic Substitute
ApiFix® Minimally Invasive Deformity Correction (MID-C) System (C)	Posterior (Dynamic) Distraction Device in New Technology
Aprevo™	Interbody Fusion Device, Customizable in New Technology
Articulating Spacer (Antibiotic)	Articulating Spacer in Lower Joints
Artificial anal sphincter (AAS)	Artificial Sphincter in Gastrointestinal System
Artificial bowel sphincter (neosphincter)	Artificial Sphincter in Gastrointestinal System
Artificial urinary sphincter (AUS)	Artificial Sphincter in Urinary System
Ascenda Intrathecal Catheter	Infusion Device
Assurant (Cobalt) stent	Intraluminal Device
AtriClip LAA Exclusion System	Extraluminal Device
Attain Ability® Lead	Cardiac Lead, Pacemaker for Insertion in Heart and Great Vessels Cardiac Lead, Defibrillator for Insertion in Heart and Great Vessels

Term	ICD-10-PCS Value
Attain StarFix® (OTW) Lead	Cardiac Lead, Pacemaker for Insertion in Heart and Great Vessels Cardiac Lead, Defibrillator for Insertion in Heart and Great Vessels
Autograft	Autologous Tissue Substitute
Autologous artery graft	Autologous Arterial Tissue in Heart and Great Vessels Autologous Arterial Tissue in Upper Arteries Autologous Arterial Tissue in Lower Arteries Autologous Arterial Tissue in Upper Veins Autologous Arterial Tissue in Lower Veins
Autologous vein graft	Autologous Venous Tissue in Heart and Great Vessels Autologous Venous Tissue in Upper Arteries Autologous Venous Tissue in Lower Arteries Autologous Venous Tissue in Upper Veins Autologous Venous Tissue in Lower Veins
Axial Lumbar Interbody Fusion System	Interbody Fusion Device in Lower Joints
AxiaLIF® System	Interbody Fusion Device in Lower Joints
BAK/C® Interbody Cervical Fusion System	Interbody Fusion Device in Upper Joints
Bard® Composix® (E/X)(LP) mesh	Synthetic Substitute
Bard® Composix® Kugel® patch	Synthetic Substitute
Bard® Dulex™ mesh	Synthetic Substitute
Bard® Ventralex™ hernia patch	Synthetic Substitute
Baroreflex Activation Therapy® (BAT®) **NT**	Stimulator Lead in Upper Arteries Stimulator Generator in Subcutaneous Tissue and Fascia
Barricaid® Annular Closure Device (ACD)	Synthetic Substitute
Berlin Heart Ventricular Assist Device	Implantable Heart Assist System in Heart and Great Vessels
Bioactive embolization coil(s)	Intraluminal Device, Bioactive in Upper Arteries
Biventricular external heart assist system	Short-term External Heart Assist System in Heart and Great Vessels
Blood glucose monitoring system	Monitoring Device
Bone anchored hearing device	Hearing Device, Bone Conduction for Insertion in Ear, Nose, Sinus Hearing Device, in Head and Facial Bones
Bone bank bone graft	Nonautologous Tissue Substitute
Bone screw (interlocking)(lag)(pedicle)(recessed)	Internal Fixation Device in Head and Facial Bones Internal Fixation Device in Upper Bones Internal Fixation Device in Lower Bones
Bovine pericardial valve	Zooplastic Tissue in Heart and Great Vessels
Bovine pericardium graft	Zooplastic Tissue in Heart and Great Vessels
Brachytherapy seeds	Radioactive Element

Term	ICD-10-PCS Value
BRYAN® Cervical Disc System	Synthetic Substitute
BVS 5000 Ventricular Assist Device	Short-term External Heart Assist System in Heart and Great Vessels
Cardiac contractility modulation lead **NT**	Cardiac Lead in Heart and Great Vessels
Cardiac event recorder	Monitoring Device
Cardiac resynchronization therapy (CRT) lead	Cardiac Lead, Pacemaker for Insertion in Heart and Great Vessels Cardiac Lead, Defibrillator for Insertion in Heart and Great Vessels
CardioMEMS® pressure sensor	Monitoring Device, Pressure Sensor for Insertion in Heart and Great Vessels
Carmat total artificial heart (TAH)	Biologic with Synthetic Substitute, Autoregulated Electrohydraulic for Replacement in Heart and Great Vessels
Carotid (artery) sinus (baroreceptor) lead	Stimulator Lead in Upper Arteries
Carotid WALLSTENT® Monorail® Endoprosthesis	Intraluminal Device
Centrimag® Blood Pump	Short-term External Heart Assist System in Heart and Great Vessels
Ceramic on ceramic bearing surface	Synthetic Substitute, Ceramic for Replacement in Lower Joints
Cesium-131 Collagen Implant	Radioactive Element, Cesium-131 Collagen Implant for Insertion in Central Nervous System and Cranial Nerves
CivaSheet®	Radioactive Element
Clamp and rod internal fixation system (CRIF)	Internal Fixation Device in Upper Bones Internal Fixation Device in Lower Bones
COALESCE® radiolucent interbody fusion device	Interbody Fusion Device, Radiolucent Porous in New Technology
CoAxia NeuroFlo catheter	Intraluminal Device
Cobalt/chromium head and polyethylene socket	Synthetic Substitute, Metal on Polyethylene for Replacement in Lower Joints
Cobalt/chromium head and socket	Synthetic Substitute, Metal for Replacement in Lower Joints
Cochlear implant (CI), multiple channel (electrode)	Hearing Device, Multiple Channel Cochlear Prosthesis for Insertion in Ear, Nose, Sinus
Cochlear implant (CI), single channel (electrode)	Hearing Device, Single Channel Cochlear Prosthesis for Insertion in Ear, Nose, Sinus
COGNIS® CRT-D	Cardiac Resynchronization Defibrillator Pulse Generator for Insertion in Subcutaneous Tissue and Fascia
COHERE® radiolucent interbody fusion device	Interbody Fusion Device, Radiolucent Porous in New Technology
Colonic Z-Stent®	Intraluminal Device
Complete (SE) stent	Intraluminal Device
Concerto II CRT-D	Cardiac Resynchronization Defibrillator Pulse Generator for Insertion in Subcutaneous Tissue and Fascia
CONSERVE® PLUS Total Resurfacing Hip System	Resurfacing Device in Lower Joints
Consulta CRT-D	Cardiac Resynchronization Defibrillator Pulse Generator for Insertion in Subcutaneous Tissue and Fascia
Consulta CRT-P	Cardiac Resynchronization Pacemaker Pulse Generator for Insertion in Subcutaneous Tissue and Fascia

Term	ICD-10-PCS Value
CONTAK RENEWAL® 3 RF (HE) CRT-D	Cardiac Resynchronization Defibrillator Pulse Generator for Insertion in Subcutaneous Tissue and Fascia
Contegra Pulmonary Valved Conduit	Zooplastic Tissue in Heart and Great Vessels
Continuous Glucose Monitoring (CGM) device	Monitoring Device
Cook Biodesign® Fistula Plug(s)	Nonautologous Tissue Substitute
Cook Biodesign® Hernia Graft(s)	Nonautologous Tissue Substitute
Cook Biodesign® Layered Graft(s)	Nonautologous Tissue Substitute
Cook Zenapro™ Layered Graft(s)	Nonautologous Tissue Substitute
Cook Zenith AAA Endovascular Graft	Intraluminal Device
Cook Zenith® Fenestrated AAA Endovascular Graft	Intraluminal Device, Branched or Fenestrated, One or Two Arteries for Restriction in Lower Arteries Intraluminal Device, Branched or Fenestrated, Three or More Arteries for Restriction in Lower Arteries
CoreValve transcatheter aortic valve	Zooplastic Tissue in Heart and Great Vessels
Cormet Hip Resurfacing System	Resurfacing Device in Lower Joints
CoRoent® XL	Interbody Fusion Device in Lower Joints
Corox (OTW) Bipolar Lead	Cardiac Lead, Pacemaker for Insertion in Heart and Great Vessels Cardiac Lead, Defibrillator for Insertion in Heart and Great Vessels
Cortical strip neurostimulator lead	Neurostimulator Lead in Central Nervous System and Cranial Nerves
Corvia IASD®	Synthetic Substitute
Cultured epidermal cell autograft	Autologous Tissue Substitute
CYPHER® Stent	Intraluminal Device, Drug-eluting in Heart and Great Vessels
Cystostomy tube	Drainage Device
DBS lead	Neurostimulator Lead in Central Nervous System and Cranial Nerves
DeBakey Left Ventricular Assist Device	Implantable Heart Assist System in Heart and Great Vessels
Deep brain neurostimulator lead	Neurostimulator Lead in Central Nervous System and Cranial Nerves
Delta frame external fixator	External Fixation Device, Hybrid for Insertion in Upper Bones External Fixation Device, Hybrid for Reposition in Upper Bones External Fixation Device, Hybrid for Insertion in Lower Bones External Fixation Device, Hybrid for Reposition in Lower Bones
Delta III Reverse shoulder prosthesis	Synthetic Substitute, Reverse Ball and Socket for Replacement in Upper Joints
Diaphragmatic pacemaker generator	Stimulator Generator in Subcutaneous Tissue and Fascia
Direct Lateral Interbody Fusion (DLIF) device	Interbody Fusion Device in Lower Joints
Driver stent (RX) (OTW)	Intraluminal Device
DuraHeart Left Ventricular Assist System	Implantable Heart Assist System in Heart and Great Vessels

Term	ICD-10-PCS Value
Durata® Defibrillation Lead	Cardiac Lead, Defibrillator for Insertion in Heart and Great Vessels
DynaNail®	Internal Fixation Device, Sustained Compression for Fusion in Lower Joints Internal Fixation Device, Sustained Compression for Fusion in Upper Joints
DynaNail Mini®	Internal Fixation Device, Sustained Compression for Fusion in Lower Joints Internal Fixation Device, Sustained Compression for Fusion in Upper Joints
Dynesys® Dynamic Stabilization System	Spinal Stabilization Device, Pedicle-Based for Insertion in Upper Joints Spinal Stabilization Device, Pedicle-Based for Insertion in Lower Joints
E-Luminexx™ (Biliary)(Vascular) Stent	Intraluminal Device
EDWARDS INTUITY Elite valve system	Zooplastic Tissue, Rapid Deployment Technique in New Technology
Electrical bone growth stimulator (EBGS)	Bone Growth Stimulator in Head and Facial Bones Bone Growth Stimulator in Upper Bones Bone Growth Stimulator in Lower Bones
Electrical muscle stimulation (EMS) lead	Stimulator Lead in Muscles
Electronic muscle stimulator lead	Stimulator Lead in Muscles
Eluvia™ Drug-eluting **NT** Vascular Stent System	Intraluminal Device, Sustained Release Drug-eluting In New Technology Intraluminal Device, Sustained Release Drug-eluting, Two in New Technology Intraluminal Device, Sustained Release Drug-eluting, Three in New Technology Intraluminal Device, Sustained Release Drug-eluting, Four or More in New Technology
Embolization coil(s)	Intraluminal Device
Endeavor® (III)(IV) (Sprint) Zotarolimus-eluting Coronary Stent System	Intraluminal Device, Drug-eluting in Heart and Great Vessels
Endologix AFX® Endovascular AAA System	Intraluminal Device
EndoSure® sensor	Monitoring Device, Pressure Sensor for Insertion in Heart and Great Vessels
ENDOTAK RELIANCE® (G) Defibrillation Lead	Cardiac Lead, Defibrillator for Insertion in Heart and Great Vessels
Endotracheal tube (cuffed)(double-lumen)	Intraluminal Device, Endotracheal Airway in Respiratory System
Endurant® Endovascular Stent Graft	Intraluminal Device
Endurant® II AAA stent graft system	Intraluminal Device
EnRhythm	Pacemaker, Dual Chamber for Insertion in Subcutaneous Tissue and Fascia
Enterra gastric neurostimulator	Stimulator Generator, Multiple Array for Insertion in Subcutaneous Tissue and Fascia
Epic™ Stented Tissue Valve (aortic)	Zooplastic Tissue in Heart and Great Vessels
Epicel® cultured epidermal autograft	Autologous Tissue Substitute

Term	ICD-10-PCS Value
Esophageal obturator airway (EOA)	Intraluminal Device, Airway in Gastrointestinal System
Esteem® implantable hearing system	Hearing Device in Ear, Nose, Sinus
Evera (XT)(S)(DR/VR)	Defibrillator Generator for Insertion in Subcutaneous Tissue and Fascia
Everolimus-eluting coronary stent	Intraluminal Device, Drug-eluting in Heart and Great Vessels
Ex-PRESS™ mini glaucoma shunt	Synthetic Substitute
EXCLUDER® AAA Endoprosthesis	Intraluminal Device Intraluminal Device, Branched or Fenestrated, One or Two Arteries for Restriction in Lower Arteries Intraluminal Device, Branched or Fenestrated, Three or More Arteries for Restriction in Lower Arteries
EXCLUDER® IBE Endoprosthesis	Intraluminal Device, Branched or Fenestrated, One or Two Arteries for Restriction in Lower Arteries
Express® (LD) Premounted Stent System	Intraluminal Device
Express® Biliary SD Monorail® Premounted Stent System	Intraluminal Device
Express® SD Renal Monorail® Premounted Stent System	Intraluminal Device
External fixator	External Fixation Device in Head and Facial Bones External Fixation Device in Upper Bones External Fixation Device in Lower Bones External Fixation Device in Upper Joints External Fixation Device in Lower Joints
EXtreme Lateral Interbody Fusion (XLIF) device	Interbody Fusion Device in Lower Joints
Facet replacement spinal stabilization device	Spinal Stabilization Device, Facet Replacement for Insertion in Upper Joints Spinal Stabilization Device, Facet Replacement for Insertion in Lower Joints
FLAIR® Endovascular Stent Graft	Intraluminal Device
Flexible Composite Mesh	Synthetic Substitute
Flow Diverter embolization device	Intraluminal Device, Flow Diverter for Restriction in Upper Arteries
Foley catheter	Drainage Device
Formula™ Balloon-Expandable Renal Stent System	Intraluminal Device
Freestyle (Stentless) Aortic Root Bioprosthesis	Zooplastic Tissue in Heart and Great Vessels
Fusion screw (compression)(lag)(locking)	Internal Fixation Device in Upper Joints Internal Fixation Device in Lower Joints
GammaTile™	Radioactive Element, Cesium-131 Collagen Implant for Insertion in Central Nervous System and Cranial Nerves
Gastric electrical stimulation (GES) lead	Stimulator Lead in Gastrointestinal System
Gastric pacemaker lead	Stimulator Lead in Gastrointestinal System

Term	ICD-10-PCS Value
GORE EXCLUDER® AAA Endoprosthesis	Intraluminal Device Intraluminal Device, Branched or Fenestrated, One or Two Arteries for Restriction in Lower Arteries Intraluminal Device, Branched or Fenestrated, Three or More Arteries for Restriction in Lower Arteries
GORE EXCLUDER® IBE Endoprosthesis	Intraluminal Device, Branched or Fenestrated, One or Two Arteries for Restriction in Lower Arteries
GORE TAG® Thoracic Endoprosthesis	Intraluminal Device
GORE® DUALMESH®	Synthetic Substitute
Guedel airway	Intraluminal Device, Airway in Mouth and Throat
Hancock Bioprosthesis (aortic)(mitral) valve	Zooplastic Tissue in Heart and Great Vessels
Hancock Bioprosthetic Valved Conduit	Zooplastic Tissue in Heart and Great Vessels
HeartMate 3™ LVAS	Implantable Heart Assist System in Heart and Great Vessels
HeartMate II® Left Ventricular Assist Device (LVAD)	Implantable Heart Assist System in Heart and Great Vessels
HeartMate XVE® Left Ventricular Assist Device (LVAD)	Implantable Heart Assist System in Heart and Great Vessels
Herculink (RX) Elite Renal Stent System	Intraluminal Device
Hip (joint) liner	Liner in Lower Joints
Holter valve ventricular shunt	Synthetic Substitute
IASD® (InterAtrial Shunt Device), Corvia	Synthetic Substitute
Ilizarov external fixator	External Fixation Device, Ring for Insertion in Upper Bones External Fixation Device, Ring for Reposition in Upper Bones External Fixation Device, Ring for Insertion in Lower Bones External Fixation Device, Ring for Reposition in Lower Bones
Ilizarov-Vecklich device	External Fixation Device, Limb Lengthening for Insertion in Upper Bones External Fixation Device, Limb Lengthening for Insertion in Lower Bones
Impella® heart pump	Short-term External Heart Assist System in Heart and Great Vessels
Implantable cardioverter-defibrillator (ICD)	Defibrillator Generator for Insertion in Subcutaneous Tissue and Fascia
Implantable drug infusion pump (anti-spasmodic) (chemotherapy)(pain)	Infusion Device, Pump in Subcutaneous Tissue and Fascia
Implantable glucose monitoring device	Monitoring Device
Implantable hemodynamic monitor (IHM)	Monitoring Device, Hemodynamic for Insertion in Subcutaneous Tissue and Fascia
Implantable hemodynamic monitoring system (IHMS)	Monitoring Device, Hemodynamic for Insertion in Subcutaneous Tissue and Fascia
Implantable Miniature Telescope™ (IMT)	Synthetic Substitute, Intraocular Telescope for Replacement in Eye

Term	ICD-10-PCS Value
Implanted (venous)(access) port	Vascular Access Device, Totally Implantable in Subcutaneous Tissue and Fascia
InDura, intrathecal catheter (1P) (spinal)	Infusion Device
Injection reservoir, port	Vascular Access Device, Totally Implantable in Subcutaneous Tissue and Fascia
Injection reservoir, pump	Infusion Device, Pump in Subcutaneous Tissue and Fascia
InterAtrial Shunt Device IASD®, Corvia	Synthetic Substitute
Interbody fusion (spine) cage	Interbody Fusion Device in Upper Joints Interbody Fusion Device in Lower Joints
Interspinous process spinal stabilization device	Spinal Stabilization Device, Interspinous Process for Insertion in Upper Joints Spinal Stabilization Device, Interspinous Process for Insertion in Lower Joints
InterStim™ Micro Therapy neurostimulator	Stimulator Generator, Single Array Rechargeable for Insertion in Subcutaneous Tissue and Fascia
InterStim® Therapy lead	Neurostimulator Lead in Peripheral Nervous System
InterStim™ II Therapy neurostimulator	Stimulator Generator, Single Array for Insertion in Subcutaneous Tissue and Fascia
Intramedullary (IM) rod (nail)	Internal Fixation Device, Intramedullary in Upper Bones Internal Fixation Device, Intramedullary in Lower Bones
Intramedullary skeletal kinetic distractor (ISKD)	Internal Fixation Device, Intramedullary in Upper Bones Internal Fixation Device, Intramedullary in Lower Bones
Intrauterine Device (IUD)	Contraceptive Device in Female Reproductive System
INTUITY Elite valve system, EDWARDS	Zooplastic Tissue, Rapid Deployment Technique in New Technology
Itrel (3)(4) neurostimulator	Stimulator Generator, Single Array for Insertion in Subcutaneous Tissue and Fascia
Joint fixation plate	Internal Fixation Device in Upper Joints Internal Fixation Device in Lower Joints
Joint liner (insert)	Liner in Lower Joints
Joint spacer (antibiotic)	Spacer in Upper Joints Spacer in Lower Joints
Kappa	Pacemaker, Dual Chamber for Insertion in Subcutaneous Tissue and Fascia
Kirschner wire (K-wire)	Internal Fixation Device in Head and Facial Bones Internal Fixation Device in Upper Bones Internal Fixation Device in Lower Bones Internal Fixation Device in Upper Joints Internal Fixation Device in Lower Joints
Knee (implant) insert	Liner in Lower Joints
Kuntscher nail	Internal Fixation Device, Intramedullary in Upper Bones Internal Fixation Device, Intramedullary in Lower Bones
LAP-BAND® adjustable gastric banding system	Extraluminal Device
LifeStent® (Flexstar)(XL) Vascular Stent System	Intraluminal Device

Term	ICD-10-PCS Value
LIVIAN™ CRT-D	Cardiac Resynchronization Defibrillator Pulse Generator for Insertion in Subcutaneous Tissue and Fascia
Loop recorder, implantable	Monitoring Device
MAGEC® Spinal Bracing and Distraction System	Magnetically Controlled Growth Rod(s) in New Technology
Mark IV Breathing Pacemaker System	Stimulator Generator in Subcutaneous Tissue and Fascia
Maximo II DR (VR)	Defibrillator Generator for Insertion in Subcutaneous Tissue and Fascia
Maximo II DR CRT-D	Cardiac Resynchronization Defibrillator Pulse Generator for Insertion in Subcutaneous Tissue and Fascia
Medtronic Endurant® II AAA stent graft system	Intraluminal Device
Melody® transcatheter pulmonary valve	Zooplastic Tissue in Heart and Great Vessels
Metal on metal bearing surface	Synthetic Substitute, Metal for Replacement in Lower Joints
Micro-Driver stent (RX) (OTW)	Intraluminal Device
MicroMed HeartAssist	Implantable Heart Assist System in Heart and Great Vessels
Micrus CERECYTE microcoil	Intraluminal Device, Bioactive in Upper Arteries
MIRODERM™ Biologic Wound Matrix	Skin Substitute, Porcine Liver Derived in New Technology
MitraClip valve repair system	Synthetic Substitute
Mitroflow® Aortic Pericardial Heart Valve	Zooplastic Tissue in Heart and Great Vessels
Mosaic Bioprosthesis (aortic) (mitral) valve	Zooplastic Tissue in Heart and Great Vessels
MULTI-LINK (VISION)(MINI-VISION)(ULTRA) Coronary Stent System	Intraluminal Device
nanoLOCK™ interbody fusion device	Interbody Fusion Device, Nanotextured Surface in New Technology
Nasopharyngeal airway (NPA)	Intraluminal Device, Airway in Ear, Nose, Sinus
Neovasc Reducer™	Reduction Device in New Technology
Neuromuscular electrical stimulation (NEMS) lead	Stimulator Lead in Muscles
Neurostimulator generator, multiple channel	Stimulator Generator, Multiple Array for Insertion in Subcutaneous Tissue and Fascia
Neurostimulator generator, multiple channel rechargeable	Stimulator Generator, Multiple Array Rechargeable for Insertion in Subcutaneous Tissue and Fascia
Neurostimulator generator, single channel	Stimulator Generator, Single Array for Insertion in Subcutaneous Tissue and Fascia
Neurostimulator generator, single channel rechargeable	Stimulator Generator, Single Array Rechargeable for Insertion in Subcutaneous Tissue and Fascia
Neutralization plate	Internal Fixation Device in Head and Facial Bones Internal Fixation Device in Upper Bones Internal Fixation Device in Lower Bones
Nitinol framed polymer mesh	Synthetic Substitute
Non-tunneled central venous catheter	Infusion Device
Novacor Left Ventricular Assist Device	Implantable Heart Assist System in Heart and Great Vessels

Term	ICD-10-PCS Value
Novation® Ceramic AHS® (Articulation Hip System)	Synthetic Substitute, Ceramic for Replacement in Lower Joints
Omnilink Elite Vascular Balloon Expandable Stent System	Intraluminal Device
Open Pivot Aortic Valve Graft (AVG)	Synthetic Substitute
Open Pivot (mechanical) Valve	Synthetic Substitute
Optimizer™ III implantable NT pulse generator	Contractility Modulation Device for Insertion in Subcutaneous Tissue and Fascia
Oropharyngeal airway (OPA)	Intraluminal Device, Airway in Mouth and Throat
Ovatio™ CRT-D	Cardiac Resynchronization Defibrillator Pulse Generator for Insertion in Subcutaneous Tissue and Fascia
OXINIUM	Synthetic Substitute, Oxidized Zirconium on Polyethylene for Replacement in Lower Joints
Paclitaxel-eluting coronary stent	Intraluminal Device, Drug-eluting in Heart and Great Vessels
Paclitaxel-eluting peripheral stent	Intraluminal Device, Drug-eluting in Upper Arteries Intraluminal Device, Drug-eluting in Lower Arteries
Partially absorbable mesh	Synthetic Substitute
Pedicle-based dynamic stabilization device	Spinal Stabilization Device, Pedicle-Based for Insertion in Upper Joints Spinal Stabilization Device, Pedicle-Based for Insertion in Lower Joints
PERCEPT™ PC neurostimulator	Stimulator Generator, Multiple Array for Insertion in Subcutaneous Tissue and Fascia
Perceval sutureless valve	Zooplastic Tissue, Rapid Deployment Technique in New Technology
Percutaneous endoscopic gastrojejunostomy (PEG/J) tube	Feeding Device in Gastrointestinal System
Percutaneous endoscopic gastrostomy (PEG) tube	Feeding Device in Gastrointestinal System
Percutaneous nephrostomy catheter	Drainage Device
Peripherally inserted central catheter (PICC)	Infusion Device
Pessary ring	Intraluminal Device, Pessary in Female Reproductive System
Phrenic nerve stimulator generator	Stimulator Generator in Subcutaneous Tissue and Fascia
Phrenic nerve stimulator lead	Diaphragmatic Pacemaker Lead in Respiratory System
PHYSIOMESH™ Flexible Composite Mesh	Synthetic Substitute
Pipeline™ (Flex) embolization device	Intraluminal Device, Flow Diverter for Restriction in Upper Arteries
Polyethylene socket	Synthetic Substitute, Polyethylene for Replacement in Lower Joints
Polymethylmethacrylate (PMMA)	Synthetic Substitute
Polypropylene mesh	Synthetic Substitute
Porcine (bioprosthetic) valve	Zooplastic Tissue in Heart and Great Vessels

Appendix G: Device Key and Aggregation Table

Term	ICD-10-PCS Value
PRECICE intramedullary limb lengthening system	Internal Fixation Device, Intramedullary Limb Lengthening for Insertion in Upper Bones Internal Fixation Device, Intramedullary Limb Lengthening for Insertion in Lower Bones
PRESTIGE® Cervical Disc	Synthetic Substitute
PrimeAdvanced neurostimulator (SureScan)(MRI Safe)	Stimulator Generator, Multiple Array for Insertion in Subcutaneous Tissue and Fascia
PROCEED™ Ventral Patch	Synthetic Substitute
Prodisc-C	Synthetic Substitute
Prodisc-L	Synthetic Substitute
PROLENE Polypropylene Hernia System (PHS)	Synthetic Substitute
Protecta XT CRT-D	Cardiac Resynchronization Defibrillator Pulse Generator for Insertion in Subcutaneous Tissue and Fascia
Protecta XT DR (XT VR)	Defibrillator Generator for Insertion in Subcutaneous Tissue and Fascia
Protégé® RX Carotid Stent System	Intraluminal Device
Pump reservoir	Infusion Device, Pump in Subcutaneous Tissue and Fascia
REALIZE® Adjustable Gastric Band	Extraluminal Device
Rebound HRD® (Hernia Repair Device)	Synthetic Substitute
Reducer™ System	Reduction Device in New Technology
RestoreAdvanced neurostimulator (SureScan)(MRI Safe)	Stimulator Generator, Multiple Array Rechargeable for Insertion in Subcutaneous Tissue and Fascia
RestoreSensor neurostimulator (SureScan)(MRI Safe)	Stimulator Generator, Multiple Array Rechargeable for Insertion in Subcutaneous Tissue and Fascia
RestoreUltra neurostimulator (SureScan)(MRI Safe)	Stimulator Generator, Multiple Array Rechargeable for Insertion in Subcutaneous Tissue and Fascia
Reveal (LINQ)(DX)(XT)	Monitoring Device
Reverse® Shoulder Prosthesis	Synthetic Substitute, Reverse Ball and Socket for Replacement in Upper Joints
Revo MRI™ SureScan® pacemaker	Pacemaker, Dual Chamber for Insertion in Subcutaneous Tissue and Fascia
Rheos® System device	Stimulator Generator in Subcutaneous Tissue and Fascia
Rheos® System lead	Stimulator Lead in Upper Arteries
RNS System lead	Neurostimulator Lead in Central Nervous System and Cranial Nerves
RNS system neurostimulator generator	Neurostimulator Generator in Head and Facial Bones
S-ICD™ lead	Subcutaneous Defibrillator Lead in Subcutaneous Tissue and Fascia
Sacral nerve modulation (SNM) lead	Stimulator Lead in Urinary System
Sacral neuromodulation lead	Stimulator Lead in Urinary System
SAPIEN transcatheter aortic valve	Zooplastic Tissue in Heart and Great Vessels

Term	ICD-10-PCS Value
SAVAL below-the-knee (BTK) drug-eluting stent system	Intraluminal Device, Sustained Release Drug-eluting in New Technology Intraluminal Device, Sustained Release Drug-eluting, Two in New Technology Intraluminal Device, Sustained Release Drug-eluting, Three in New Technology Intraluminal Device, Sustained Release Drug-eluting, Four or More in New Technology
Secura (DR) (VR)	Defibrillator Generator for Insertion in Subcutaneous Tissue and Fascia
Sheffield hybrid external fixator	External Fixation Device, Hybrid for Insertion in Upper Bones External Fixation Device, Hybrid for Reposition in Upper Bones External Fixation Device, Hybrid for Insertion in Lower Bones External Fixation Device, Hybrid for Reposition in Lower Bones
Sheffield ring external fixator	External Fixation Device, Ring for Insertion in Upper Bones External Fixation Device, Ring for Reposition in Upper Bones External Fixation Device, Ring for Insertion in Lower Bones External Fixation Device, Ring for Reposition in Lower Bones
Single lead pacemaker (atrium)(ventricle)	Pacemaker, Single Chamber for Insertion in Subcutaneous Tissue and Fascia
Single lead rate responsive pacemaker (atrium)(ventricle)	Pacemaker, Single Chamber Rate Responsive for Insertion in Subcutaneous Tissue and Fascia
Sirolimus-eluting coronary stent	Intraluminal Device, Drug-eluting in Heart and Great Vessels
SJM Biocor® Stented Valve System	Zooplastic Tissue in Heart and Great Vessels
Spacer, Articulating (Antibiotic)	Articulating Spacer in Lower Joints
Spacer, Static (Antibiotic)	Spacer in Lower Joints
Spinal cord neurostimulator lead	Neurostimulator Lead in Central Nervous System and Cranial Nerves
Spinal growth rods, magnetically controlled	Magnetically Controlled Growth Rod(s) in New Technology
SpineJack® system **NT**	Synthetic Substitute, Mechanically Expandable (Paired) in New Technology
Spiration IBV™ Valve System	Intraluminal Device, Endobronchial Valve in Respiratory System
Static Spacer (Antibiotic)	Spacer in Lower Joints
Stent, intraluminal (cardiovascular) (gastrointestinal) (hepatobiliary)(urinary)	Intraluminal Device
Stented tissue valve	Zooplastic Tissue in Heart and Great Vessels
Stratos LV	Cardiac Resynchronization Pacemaker Pulse Generator for Insertion in Subcutaneous Tissue and Fascia
Subcutaneous injection reservoir, port	Vascular Access Device, Totally Implantable in Subcutaneous Tissue and Fascia
Subcutaneous injection reservoir, pump	Infusion Device, Pump in Subcutaneous Tissue and Fascia

Term	ICD-10-PCS Value
Subdermal progesterone implant	Contraceptive Device in Subcutaneous Tissue and Fascia
Surpass Streamline™ Flow Diverter	Intraluminal Device, Flow Diverter for Restriction in Upper Arteries
Sutureless valve, Perceval	Zooplastic Tissue, Rapid Deployment Technique in New Technology
SynCardia (temporary) Total Artificial Heart (TAH)	Synthetic Substitute, Pneumatic for Replacement in Heart and Great Vessels
SynCardia Total Artificial Heart	Synthetic Substitute
Synchra CRT-P	Cardiac Resynchronization Pacemaker Pulse Generator for Insertion in Subcutaneous Tissue and Fascia
SyncroMed Pump	Infusion Device, Pump in Subcutaneous Tissue and Fascia
Talent® Converter	Intraluminal Device
Talent® Occluder	Intraluminal Device
Talent® Stent Graft (abdominal)(thoracic)	Intraluminal Device
TandemHeart® System	Short-term External Heart Assist System in Heart and Great Vessels
TAXUS® Liberté® Paclitaxel-eluting Coronary Stent System	Intraluminal Device, Drug-eluting in Heart and Great Vessels
Therapeutic occlusion coil(s)	Intraluminal Device
Thoracostomy tube	Drainage Device
Thoraflex™ Hybrid device	Branched Synthetic Substitute with Intraluminal Device in New Technology
Thoratec IVAD (Implantable Ventricular Assist Device)	Implantable Heart Assist System in Heart and Great Vessels
Thoratec Paracorporeal Ventricular Assist Device	Short-term External Heart Assist System in Heart and Great Vessels
Tibial insert	Liner in Lower Joints
Tissue bank graft	Nonautologous Tissue Substitute
Tissue expander (inflatable)(injectable)	Tissue Expander in Skin and Breast Tissue Expander in Subcutaneous Tissue and Fascia
Titanium Sternal Fixation System (TSFS)	Internal Fixation Device, Rigid Plate for Insertion in Upper Bones Internal Fixation Device, Rigid Plate for Reposition in Upper Bones
Total artificial (replacement) heart	Synthetic Substitute
Tracheostomy tube	Tracheostomy Device in Respiratory System
Trifecta™ Valve (aortic)	Zooplastic Tissue in Heart and Great Vessels
Tunneled central venous catheter	Vascular Access Device, Tunneled in Subcutaneous Tissue and Fascia
Tunneled spinal (intrathecal) catheter	Infusion Device
Two lead pacemaker	Pacemaker, Dual Chamber for Insertion in Subcutaneous Tissue and Fascia
Ultraflex™ Precision Colonic Stent System	Intraluminal Device
ULTRAPRO Hernia System (UHS)	Synthetic Substitute
ULTRAPRO Partially Absorbable Lightweight Mesh	Synthetic Substitute
ULTRAPRO Plug	Synthetic Substitute

Term	ICD-10-PCS Value
Ultrasonic osteogenic stimulator	Bone Growth Stimulator in Head and Facial Bones Bone Growth Stimulator in Upper Bones Bone Growth Stimulator in Lower Bones
Ultrasound bone healing system	Bone Growth Stimulator in Head and Facial Bones Bone Growth Stimulator in Upper Bones Bone Growth Stimulator in Lower Bones
Uniplanar external fixator	External Fixation Device, Monoplanar for Insertion in Upper Bones External Fixation Device, Monoplanar for Reposition in Upper Bones External Fixation Device, Monoplanar for Insertion in Lower Bones External Fixation Device, Monoplanar for Reposition in Lower Bones
Urinary incontinence stimulator lead	Stimulator Lead in Urinary System
V-Wave Interatrial Shunt System	Synthetic Substitute
Vaginal pessary	Intraluminal Device, Pessary in Female Reproductive System
Valiant Thoracic Stent Graft	Intraluminal Device
Vectra® Vascular Access Graft	Vascular Access Device, Tunneled in Subcutaneous Tissue and Fascia
Ventrio™ Hernia Patch	Synthetic Substitute
Versa	Pacemaker, Dual Chamber for Insertion in Subcutaneous Tissue and Fascia
Virtuoso (II) (DR) (VR)	Defibrillator Generator for Insertion in Subcutaneous Tissue and Fascia
Viva(XT)(S)	Cardiac Resynchronization Defibrillator Pulse Generator for Insertion in Subcutaneous Tissue and Fascia
WALLSTENT® Endoprosthesis	Intraluminal Device
X-STOP® Spacer	Spinal Stabilization Device, Interspinous Process for Insertion in Upper Joints Spinal Stabilization Device, Interspinous Process for Insertion in Lower Joints
Xact Carotid Stent System	Intraluminal Device
Xenograft	Zooplastic Tissue in Heart and Great Vessels
XIENCE Everolimus Eluting Coronary Stent System	Intraluminal Device, Drug-eluting in Heart and Great Vessels
XLIF® System	Interbody Fusion Device in Lower Joints
Zenith® Fenestrated AAA Endovascular Graft	Intraluminal Device, Branched or Fenestrated, One or Two Arteries for Restriction in Lower Arteries Intraluminal Device, Branched or Fenestrated, Three or More Arteries for Restriction in Lower Arteries Intraluminal Device
Zenith Flex® AAA Endovascular Graft	Intraluminal Device
Zenith TX2® TAA Endovascular Graft	Intraluminal Device
Zenith® Renu™ AAA Ancillary Graft	Intraluminal Device
Zilver® PTX® (paclitaxel) Drug-Eluting Peripheral Stent	Intraluminal Device, Drug-eluting in Upper Arteries Intraluminal Device, Drug-eluting in Lower Arteries
Zimmer® NexGen® LPS Mobile Bearing Knee	Synthetic Substitute

Term	ICD-10-PCS Value
Zimmer® NexGen® LPS-Flex Mobile Knee	Synthetic Substitute
Zotarolimus-eluting coronary stent	Intraluminal Device, Drug-eluting in Heart and Great Vessels

Device Aggregation Table

This table crosswalks specific device character value definitions for specific root operations in a specific body system to the more general device character value to be used when the root operation covers a wide range of body parts and the device character represents an entire family of devices.

Specific Device	for Operation	in Body System	General Device	
Autologous Arterial Tissue (A)	All applicable	Heart and Great Vessels Lower Arteries Lower Veins Upper Arteries Upper Veins	7	Autologous Tissue Substitute
Autologous Venous Tissue (9)	All applicable	Heart and Great Vessels Lower Arteries Lower Veins Upper Arteries Upper Veins	7	Autologous Tissue Substitute
Cardiac Lead, Defibrillator (K)	Insertion	Heart and Great Vessels	M	Cardiac Lead
Cardiac Lead, Pacemaker (J)	Insertion	Heart and Great Vessels	M	Cardiac Lead
Cardiac Resynchronization Defibrillator Pulse Generator (9)	Insertion	Subcutaneous Tissue and Fascia	P	Cardiac Rhythm Related Device
Cardiac Resynchronization Pacemaker Pulse Generator (7)	Insertion	Subcutaneous Tissue and Fascia	P	Cardiac Rhythm Related Device
Contractility Modulation Device (A)	Insertion	Subcutaneous Tissue and Fascia	P	Cardiac Rhythm Related Device
Defibrillator Generator (8)	Insertion	Subcutaneous Tissue and Fascia	P	Cardiac Rhythm Related Device
Epiretinal Visual Prosthesis (5)	All applicable	Eye	J	Synthetic Substitute
External Fixation Device, Hybrid (D)	Insertion	Lower Bones Upper Bones	5	External Fixation Device
External Fixation Device, Hybrid (D)	Reposition	Lower Bones Upper Bones	5	External Fixation Device
External Fixation Device, Limb Lengthening (8)	Insertion	Lower Bones Upper Bones	5	External Fixation Device
External Fixation Device, Monoplanar (B)	Insertion	Lower Bones Upper Bones	5	External Fixation Device
External Fixation Device, Monoplanar (B)	Reposition	Lower Bones Upper Bones	5	External Fixation Device
External Fixation Device, Ring (C)	Insertion	Lower Bones Upper Bones	5	External Fixation Device
External Fixation Device, Ring (C)	Reposition	Lower Bones Upper Bones	5	External Fixation Device
Hearing Device, Bone Conduction (4)	Insertion	Ear, Nose, Sinus	S	Hearing Device
Hearing Device, Multiple Channel Cochlear Prosthesis (6)	Insertion	Ear, Nose, Sinus	S	Hearing Device
Hearing Device, Single Channel Cochlear Prosthesis (5)	Insertion	Ear, Nose, Sinus	S	Hearing Device
Internal Fixation Device, Intramedullary (6)	All applicable	Lower Bones Upper Bones	4	Internal Fixation Device
Internal Fixation Device, Intramedullary Limb Lengthening (7)	Insertion	Lower Bones Upper Bones	6	Internal Fixation Device, Intramedullary
Internal Fixation Device, Rigid Plate (Ø)	Insertion	Upper Bones	4	Internal Fixation Device
Internal Fixation Device, Rigid Plate (Ø)	Reposition	Upper Bones	4	Internal Fixation Device
Intraluminal Device, Airway (B)	All applicable	Ear, Nose, Sinus Gastrointestinal System Mouth and Throat	D	Intraluminal Device
Intraluminal Device, Bioactive (B)	All applicable	Upper Arteries	D	Intraluminal Device
Intraluminal Device, Branched or Fenestrated, One or Two Arteries (E)	Restriction	Heart and Great Vessels Lower Arteries	D	Intraluminal Device

Specific Device	for Operation	in Body System	General Device	
Intraluminal Device, Branched or Fenestrated, Three or More Arteries (F)	Restriction	Heart and Great Vessels Lower Arteries	D	Intraluminal Device
Intraluminal Device, Drug-eluting (4)	All applicable	Heart and Great Vessels Lower Arteries Upper Arteries	D	Intraluminal Device
Intraluminal Device, Drug-eluting, Four or More (7)	All applicable	Heart and Great Vessels Lower Arteries Upper Arteries	D	Intraluminal Device
Intraluminal Device, Drug-eluting, Three (6)	All applicable	Heart and Great Vessels Lower Arteries Upper Arteries	D	Intraluminal Device
Intraluminal Device, Drug-eluting, Two (5)	All applicable	Heart and Great Vessels Lower Arteries Upper Arteries	D	Intraluminal Device
Intraluminal Device, Endobronchial Valve (G)	All applicable	Respiratory System	D	Intraluminal Device
Intraluminal Device, Endotracheal Airway (E)	All applicable	Respiratory System	D	Intraluminal Device
Intraluminal Device, Flow Diverter (H)	Restriction	Upper Arteries	D	Intraluminal Device
Intraluminal Device, Four or More (G)	All applicable	Heart and Great Vessels Lower Arteries Upper Arteries	D	Intraluminal Device
Intraluminal Device, Pessary (G)	All applicable	Female Reproductive System	D	Intraluminal Device
Intraluminal Device, Radioactive (T)	All applicable	Heart and Great Vessels	D	Intraluminal Device
Intraluminal Device, Three (F)	All applicable	Heart and Great Vessels Lower Arteries Upper Arteries	D	Intraluminal Device
Intraluminal Device, Two (E)	All applicable	Heart and Great Vessels Lower Arteries Upper Arteries	D	Intraluminal Device
Monitoring Device, Hemodynamic (Ø)	Insertion	Subcutaneous Tissue and Fascia	2	Monitoring Device
Monitoring Device, Pressure Sensor (Ø)	Insertion	Heart and Great Vessels	2	Monitoring Device
Pacemaker, Dual Chamber (6)	Insertion	Subcutaneous Tissue and Fascia	P	Cardiac Rhythm Related Device
Pacemaker, Single Chamber (4)	Insertion	Subcutaneous Tissue and Fascia	P	Cardiac Rhythm Related Device
Pacemaker, Single Chamber Rate Responsive (5)	Insertion	Subcutaneous Tissue and Fascia	P	Cardiac Rhythm Related Device
Spinal Stabilization Device, Facet Replacement (D)	Insertion	Lower Joints Upper Joints	4	Internal Fixation Device
Spinal Stabilization Device, Interspinous Process (B)	Insertion	Lower Joints Upper Joints	4	Internal Fixation Device
Spinal Stabilization Device, Pedicle-Based (C)	Insertion	Lower Joints Upper Joints	4	Internal Fixation Device
Spinal Stabilization Device, Vertebral Body Tether (3)	Reposition	Lower Bones Upper Bones	4	Internal Fixation Device
Stimulator Generator, Multiple Array (D)	Insertion	Subcutaneous Tissue and Fascia	M	Stimulator Generator
Stimulator Generator, Multiple Array Rechargeable (E)	Insertion	Subcutaneous Tissue and Fascia	M	Stimulator Generator
Stimulator Generator, Single Array (B)	Insertion	Subcutaneous Tissue and Fascia	M	Stimulator Generator
Stimulator Generator, Single Array Rechargeable (C)	Insertion	Subcutaneous Tissue and Fascia	M	Stimulator Generator
Synthetic Substitute, Ceramic (3)	Replacement	Lower Joints	J	Synthetic Substitute
Synthetic Substitute, Ceramic on Polyethylene (4)	Replacement	Lower Joints	J	Synthetic Substitute
Synthetic Substitute, Intraocular Telescope (Ø)	Replacement	Eye	J	Synthetic Substitute
Synthetic Substitute, Metal (1)	Replacement	Lower Joints	J	Synthetic Substitute
Synthetic Substitute, Metal on Polyethylene (2)	Replacement	Lower Joints	J	Synthetic Substitute
Synthetic Substitute, Oxidized Zirconium on Polyethylene (6)	Replacement	Lower Joints	J	Synthetic Substitute
Synthetic Substitute, Polyethylene (Ø)	Replacement	Lower Joints	J	Synthetic Substitute
Synthetic Substitute, Reverse Ball and Socket (Ø)	Replacement	Upper Joints	J	Synthetic Substitute

Appendix H: Device Definitions

This **NT** symbol next to a device in the Definition column identifies that the device has been approved for NTAP (new technology add-on payment). CMS provides incremental payment, in addition to the DRG payment, for technologies that have received an NTAP designation.

ICD-10-PCS Value	Definition
Articulating Spacer in Lower Joints	**Includes:** Articulating Spacer (Antibiotic) Spacer, Articulating (Antibiotic)
Artificial Sphincter in Gastrointestinal System	**Includes:** Artificial anal sphincter (AAS) Artificial bowel sphincter (neosphincter)
Artificial Sphincter in Urinary System	**Includes:** AMS 800® Urinary Control System Artificial urinary sphincter (AUS)
Autologous Arterial Tissue in Heart and Great Vessels	**Includes:** Autologous artery graft
Autologous Arterial Tissue in Lower Arteries	**Includes:** Autologous artery graft
Autologous Arterial Tissue in Lower Veins	**Includes:** Autologous artery graft
Autologous Arterial Tissue in Upper Arteries	**Includes:** Autologous artery graft
Autologous Arterial Tissue in Upper Veins	**Includes:** Autologous artery graft
Autologous Tissue Substitute	**Includes:** Autograft Cultured epidermal cell autograft Epicel® cultured epidermal autograft
Autologous Venous Tissue in Heart and Great Vessels	**Includes:** Autologous vein graft
Autologous Venous Tissue in Lower Arteries	**Includes:** Autologous vein graft
Autologous Venous Tissue in Lower Veins	**Includes:** Autologous vein graft
Autologous Venous Tissue in Upper Arteries	**Includes:** Autologous vein graft
Autologous Venous Tissue in Upper Veins	**Includes:** Autologous vein graft
Biologic with Synthetic Substitute, Autoregulated Electrohydraulic for Replacement in Heart and Great Vessels	**Includes:** Carmat total artificial heart (TAH)
Bone Growth Stimulator in Head and Facial Bones	**Includes:** Electrical bone growth stimulator (EBGS) Ultrasonic osteogenic stimulator Ultrasound bone healing system
Bone Growth Stimulator in Lower Bones	**Includes:** Electrical bone growth stimulator (EBGS) Ultrasonic osteogenic stimulator Ultrasound bone healing system
Bone Growth Stimulator in Upper Bones	**Includes:** Electrical bone growth stimulator (EBGS) Ultrasonic osteogenic stimulator Ultrasound bone healing system
Branched Synthetic Substitute with Intraluminal Device in New Technology	**Includes:** Thoraflex™ Hybrid device

ICD-10-PCS Value	Definition
Cardiac Lead in Heart and Great Vessels	**Includes:** Cardiac contractility modulation lead **NT**
Cardiac Lead, Defibrillator for Insertion in Heart and Great Vessels	**Includes:** ACUITY™ Steerable Lead Attain Ability® lead Attain StarFix® (OTW) lead Cardiac resynchronization therapy (CRT) lead Corox (OTW) Bipolar Lead Durata® Defibrillation Lead ENDOTAK RELIANCE® (G) Defibrillation Lead
Cardiac Lead, Pacemaker for Insertion in Heart and Great Vessels	**Includes:** ACUITY™ Steerable Lead Attain Ability® lead Attain StarFix® (OTW) lead Cardiac resynchronization therapy (CRT) lead Corox (OTW) Bipolar Lead
Cardiac Resynchronization Defibrillator Pulse Generator for Insertion in Subcutaneous Tissue and Fascia	**Includes:** COGNIS® CRT-D Concerto II CRT-D Consulta CRT-D CONTAK RENEWA® 3 RF (HE) CRT-D LIVIAN™ CRT-D Maximo II DR CRT-D Ovatio™ CRT-D Protecta XT CRT-D Viva (XT)(S)
Cardiac Resynchronization Pacemaker Pulse Generator for Insertion in Subcutaneous Tissue and Fascia	**Includes:** Consulta CRT-P Stratos LV Synchra CRT-P
Contraceptive Device in Female Reproductive System	**Includes:** Intrauterine device (IUD)
Contraceptive Device in Subcutaneous Tissue and Fascia	**Includes:** Subdermal progesterone implant
Contractility Modulation Device for Insertion in Subcutaneous Tissue and Fascia	**Includes:** Optimizer™ III implantable pulse generator **NT**
Defibrillator Generator for Insertion in Subcutaneous Tissue and Fascia	**Includes:** Evera (XT)(S)(DR/VR) Implantable cardioverter-defibrillator (ICD) Maximo II DR (VR) Protecta XT DR (XT VR) Secura (DR) (VR) Virtuoso (II) (DR) (VR)
Diaphragmatic Pacemaker Lead in Respiratory System	**Includes:** Phrenic nerve stimulator lead
Drainage Device	**Includes:** Cystostomy tube Foley catheter Percutaneous nephrostomy catheter Thoracostomy tube

ICD-10-PCS Value	Definition	ICD-10-PCS Value	Definition
External Fixation Device in Head and Facial Bones	Includes: External fixator	**Hearing Device in Ear, Nose, Sinus**	Includes: Esteem® implantable hearing system
External Fixation Device in Lower Bones	Includes: External fixator	**Hearing Device in Head and Facial Bones**	Includes: Bone anchored hearing device
External Fixation Device in Lower Joints	Includes: External fixator	**Hearing Device, Bone Conduction for Insertion in Ear, Nose, Sinus**	Includes: Bone anchored hearing device
External Fixation Device in Upper Bones	Includes: External fixator	**Hearing Device, Multiple Channel Cochlear Prosthesis for Insertion in Ear, Nose, Sinus**	Includes: Cochlear implant (CI), multiple channel (electrode)
External Fixation Device in Upper Joints	Includes: External fixator	**Hearing Device, Single Channel Cochlear Prosthesis for Insertion in Ear, Nose, Sinus**	Includes: Cochlear implant (CI), single channel (electrode)
External Fixation Device, Hybrid for Insertion in Lower Bones	Includes: Delta frame external fixator Sheffield hybrid external fixator	**Implantable Heart Assist System in Heart and Great Vessels**	Includes: Berlin Heart Ventricular Assist Device DeBakey Left Ventricular Assist Device DuraHeart Left Ventricular Assist System HeartMate 3™ LVAS HeartMate II® Left Ventricular Assist Device (LVAD) HeartMate XVE® Left Ventricular Assist Device (LVAD) MicroMed HeartAssist Novacor Left Ventricular Assist Device Thoratec IVAD (Implantable Ventricular Assist Device)
External Fixation Device, Hybrid for Insertion in Upper Bones	Includes: Delta frame external fixator Sheffield hybrid external fixator		
External Fixation Device, Hybrid for Reposition in Lower Bones	Includes: Delta frame external fixator Sheffield hybrid external fixator		
External Fixation Device, Hybrid for Reposition in Upper Bones	Includes: Delta frame external fixator Sheffield hybrid external fixator		
External Fixation Device, Limb Lengthening for Insertion in Lower Bones	Includes: Ilizarov-Vecklich device	**Infusion Device**	Includes: Ascenda Intrathecal Catheter InDura, intrathecal catheter (1P) (spinal) Non-tunneled central venous catheter Peripherally inserted central catheter (PICC) Tunneled spinal (intrathecal) catheter
External Fixation Device, Limb Lengthening for Insertion in Upper Bones	Includes: Ilizarov-Vecklich device		
External Fixation Device, Monoplanar for Insertion in Lower Bones	Includes: Uniplanar external fixator	**Infusion Device, Pump in Subcutaneous Tissue and Fascia**	Includes: Implantable drug infusion pump (anti-spasmodic)(chemotherapy) (pain) Injection reservoir, pump Pump reservoir Subcutaneous injection reservoir, pump SynchroMed pump
External Fixation Device, Monoplanar for Insertion in Upper Bones	Includes: Uniplanar external fixator		
External Fixation Device, Monoplanar for Reposition in Lower Bones	Includes: Uniplanar external fixator		
External Fixation Device, Monoplanar for Reposition in Upper Bones	Includes: Uniplanar external fixator	**Interbody Fusion Device, Customizable in New Technology**	Includes: aprevo™
External Fixation Device, Ring for Insertion in Lower Bones	Includes: Ilizarov external fixator Sheffield ring external fixator	**Interbody Fusion Device in Lower Joints**	Includes: Axial Lumbar Interbody Fusion System AxiaLIF® System CoRoent® XL Direct Lateral Interbody Fusion (DLIF) device EXtreme Lateral Interbody Fusion (XLIF) device Interbody fusion (spine) cage XLIF® System
External Fixation Device, Ring for Insertion in Upper Bones	Includes: Ilizarov external fixator Sheffield ring external fixator		
External Fixation Device, Ring for Reposition in Lower Bones	Includes: Ilizarov external fixator Sheffield ring external fixator		
External Fixation Device, Ring for Reposition in Upper Bones	Includes: Ilizarov external fixator Sheffield ring external fixator	**Interbody Fusion Device in Upper Joints**	Includes: BAK/C® Interbody Cervical Fusion System Interbody fusion (spine) cage
Extraluminal Device	Includes: AtriClip LAA Exclusion System LAP-BAND® adjustable gastric banding system REALIZE® Adjustable Gastric Band	**Interbody Fusion Device, Customizable in New Technology**	Includes: aprevo™
Feeding Device in Gastrointestinal System	Includes: Percutaneous endoscopic gastrojejunostomy (PEG/J) tube Percutaneous endoscopic gastrostomy (PEG) tube	**Interbody Fusion Device, Nanotextured Surface in New Technology**	Includes: nanoLOCK™ interbody fusion device

ICD-10-PCS Value	Definition
Interbody Fusion Device, Radiolucent Porous in New Technology	Includes: COALESCE® radiolucent interbody fusion device COHERE® radiolucent interbody fusion device
Internal Fixation Device in Head and Facial Bones	Includes: Bone screw (interlocking)(lag)(pedicle) (recessed) Kirschner wire (K-wire) Neutralization plate
Internal Fixation Device in Lower Bones	Includes: Bone screw (interlocking)(lag)(pedicle) (recessed) Clamp and rod internal fixation system (CRIF) Kirschner wire (K-wire) Neutralization plate
Internal Fixation Device in Lower Joints	Includes: Fusion screw (compression)(lag)(locking) Joint fixation plate Kirschner wire (K-wire)
Internal Fixation Device in Upper Bones	Includes: Bone screw (interlocking)(lag)(pedicle) (recessed) Clamp and rod internal fixation system (CRIF) Kirschner wire (K-wire) Neutralization plate
Internal Fixation Device in Upper Joints	Includes: Fusion screw (compression)(lag)(locking) Joint fixation plate Kirschner wire (K-wire)
Internal Fixation Device, Intramedullary in Lower Bones	Includes: Intramedullary (IM) rod (nail) Intramedullary skeletal kinetic distractor (ISKD) Kuntscher nail
Internal Fixation Device, Intramedullary in Upper Bones	Includes: Intramedullary (IM) rod (nail) Intramedullary skeletal kinetic distractor (ISKD) Kuntscher nail
Internal Fixation Device Intramedullary Limb Lengthening for Insertion in Lower Bones	Includes: PRECICE intramedullary limb lengthening system
Internal Fixation Device Intramedullary Limb Lengthening for Insertion in Upper Bones	Includes: PRECICE intramedullary limb lengthening system
Internal Fixation Device, Rigid Plate for Insertion in Upper Bones	Includes: Titanium Sternal Fixation System (TSFS)
Internal Fixation Device, Rigid Plate for Reposition in Upper Bones	Includes: Titanium Sternal Fixation System (TSFS)
Internal Fixation Device, Sustained Compression for Fusion in Lower Joints	Includes: DynaNail® DynaNail Mini®
Internal Fixation Device, Sustained Compression for Fusion in Upper Joints	Includes: DynaNail® DynaNail Mini®

ICD-10-PCS Value	Definition
Intraluminal Device	Includes: Absolute Pro Vascular (OTW) Self-Expanding Stent System Acculink (RX) Carotid Stent System AFX® Endovascular AAA System AneuRx® AAA Advantage® Assurant (Cobalt) stent Carotid WALLSTENT® Monorail® Endoprosthesis CoAxia NeuroFlo catheter Colonic Z-Stent® Complete (SE) stent Cook Zenith AAA Endovascular Graft Driver stent (RX) (OTW) E-Luminexx™ (Biliary)(Vascular) Stent Embolization coil(s) Endologix AFX® Endovascular AAA System Endurant® Endovascular Stent Graft Endurant® II AAA stent graft system EXCLUDER® AAA Endoprosthesis Express® (LD) Premounted Stent System Express® Biliary SD Monorail® Premounted Stent System Express® SD Renal Monorail® Premounted Stent System FLAIR® Endovascular Stent Graft Formula™ Balloon-Expandable Renal Stent System GORE EXCLUDER® AAA Endoprosthesis GORE TAG® Thoracic Endoprosthesis Herculink (RX) Elite Renal Stent System LifeStent® (Flexstar)(XL) Vascular Stent System Medtronic Endurant® II AAA stent graft system Micro-Driver stent (RX) (OTW) MULTI-LINK (VISION)(MINI-VISION)(ULTRA) Coronary Stent System Omnilink Elite Vascular Balloon Expandable Stent System Protege® RX Carotid Stent System Stent, intraluminal (cardiovascular) (gastrointestinal)(hepatobiliary) (urinary) Talent® Converter Talent® Occluder Talent® Stent Graft (abdominal)(thoracic) Therapeutic occlusion coil(s) Ultraflex™ Precision Colonic Stent System Valiant Thoracic Stent Graft WALLSTENT® Endoprosthesis Xact Carotid Stent System Zenith AAA Endovascular Graft Zenith Flex® AAA Endovascular Graft Zenith TX2® TAA Endovascular Graft Zenith® Renu™ AAA Ancillary Graft
Intraluminal Device, Airway in Ear, Nose, Sinus	Includes: Nasopharyngeal airway (NPA)
Intraluminal Device, Airway in Gastrointestinal System	Includes: Esophageal obturator airway (EOA)
Intraluminal Device, Airway in Mouth and Throat	Includes: Guedel airway Oropharyngeal airway (OPA)
Intraluminal Device, Bioactive in Upper Arteries	Includes: Bioactive embolization coil(s) Micrus CERECYTE microcoil

ICD-10-PCS Value	Definition
Intraluminal Device, Branched or Fenestrated, One or Two Arteries for Restriction in Lower Arteries	**Includes:** Cook Zenith® Fenestrated AAA Endovascular Graft EXCLUDER® AAA Endoprosthesis EXCLUDER® IBE Endoprosthesis GORE EXCLUDER® AAA Endoprosthesis GORE EXCLUDER®IBE Endoprosthesis Zenith® Fenestrated AAA Endovascular Graft
Intraluminal Device, Branched or Fenestrated, Three or More Arteries for Restriction in Lower Arteries	**Includes:** Cook Zenith® Fenestrated AAA Endovascular Graft EXCLUDER® AAA Endoprosthesis GORE EXCLUDER® AAA Endoprosthesis Zenith® Fenestrated AAA Endovascular Graft
Intraluminal Device, Drug-eluting in Heart and Great Vessels	**Includes:** CYPHER® Stent Endeavor® (III)(IV) (Sprint) Zotarolimus-eluting Coronary Stent System Everolimus-eluting coronary stent Paclitaxel-eluting coronary stent Sirolimus-eluting coronary stent TAXUS® Liberte® Paclitaxel-eluting Coronary Stent System XIENCE Everolimus Eluting Coronary Stent System Zotarolimus-eluting coronary stent
Intraluminal Device, Drug-eluting in Lower Arteries	**Includes:** Paclitaxel-eluting peripheral stent Zilver® PTX® (paclitaxel) Drug-Eluting Peripheral Stent
Intraluminal Device, Drug-eluting in Upper Arteries	**Includes:** Paclitaxel-eluting peripheral stent Zilver® PTX® (paclitaxel) Drug-Eluting Peripheral Stent
Intraluminal Device, Endobronchial Valve in Respiratory System	**Includes:** Spiration IBV™ Valve System
Intraluminal Device, Endotracheal Airway in Respiratory System	**Includes:** Endotracheal tube (cuffed)(double-lumen)
Intraluminal Device, Flow Diverter for Restriction in Upper Arteries	**Includes:** Flow Diverter embolization device Pipeline™ (Flex) embolization device Surpass Streamline™ Flow Diverter
Intraluminal Device, Pessary in Female Reproductive System	**Includes:** Pessary ring Vaginal pessary
Intraluminal Device, Sustained Release Drug-eluting in New Technology	**Includes:** Eluvia™ Drug-eluting Vascular Stent System **NT** SAVAL below-the-knee (BTK) drug-eluting stent system
Intraluminal Device, Sustained Release Drug-eluting, Four or More in New Technology	**Includes:** Eluvia™ Drug-eluting Vascular Stent System **NT** SAVAL below-the-knee (BTK) drug-eluting stent system
Intraluminal Device, Sustained Release Drug-eluting, Three in New Technology	**Includes:** Eluvia™ Drug-eluting Vascular Stent System **NT** SAVAL below-the-knee (BTK) drug-eluting stent system

ICD-10-PCS Value	Definition
Intraluminal Device, Sustained Release Drug-eluting, Two in New Technology	**Includes:** Eluvia™ Drug-eluting Vascular Stent System **NT** SAVAL below-the-knee (BTK) drug-eluting stent system
Liner in Lower Joints	**Includes:** Acetabular cup Hip (joint) liner Joint liner (insert) Knee (implant) insert Tibial insert
Magnetically Controlled Growth Rod(s) in New Technology	**Includes:** MAGEC® Spinal Bracing and Distraction System Spinal growth rods, magnetically controlled
Monitoring Device	**Includes:** Blood glucose monitoring system Cardiac event recorder Continuous Glucose Monitoring (CGM) device Implantable glucose monitoring device Loop recorder, implantable Reveal (LINQ)(DX)(XT)
Monitoring Device, Hemodynamic for Insertion in Subcutaneous Tissue and Fascia	**Includes:** Implantable hemodynamic monitor (IHM) Implantable hemodynamic monitoring system (IHMS)
Monitoring Device, Pressure Sensor for Insertion in Heart and Great Vessels	**Includes:** CardioMEMS® pressure sensor EndoSure® sensor
Neurostimulator Generator in Head and Facial Bones	**Includes:** RNS system neurostimulator generator
Neurostimulator Lead in Central Nervous System and Cranial Nerves	**Includes:** Cortical strip neurostimulator lead DBS lead Deep brain neurostimulator lead RNS System lead Spinal cord neurostimulator lead
Neurostimulator Lead in Peripheral Nervous System	**Includes:** InterStim® Therapy lead
Nonautologous Tissue Substitute	**Includes:** Acellular Hydrated Dermis Bone bank bone graft Cook Biodesign® Fistula Plug(s) Cook Biodesign® Hernia Graft(s) Cook Biodesign® Layered Graft(s) Cook Zenapro™ Layered Graft(s) Tissue bank graft
Other Device	**Includes:** Alfapump® system
Pacemaker, Dual Chamber for Insertion in Subcutaneous Tissue and Fascia	**Includes:** Advisa (MRI) EnRhythm Kappa Revo MRI™ SureScan® pacemaker Two lead pacemaker Versa
Pacemaker, Single Chamber for Insertion in Subcutaneous Tissue and Fascia	**Includes:** Single lead pacemaker (atrium)(ventricle)

Appendix H: Device Definitions

ICD-10-PCS Value	Definition	ICD-10-PCS Value	Definition
Pacemaker, Single Chamber Rate Responsive for Insertion in Subcutaneous Tissue and Fascia	Includes: Single lead rate responsive pacemaker (atrium)(ventricle)	**Stimulator Generator in Subcutaneous Tissue and Fascia**	Includes: Baroreflex Activation Therapy® (BAT®) [NT] Diaphragmatic pacemaker generator Mark IV Breathing Pacemaker System Phrenic nerve stimulator generator Rheos® System device
Posterior (Dynamic) Distraction Device in New Technology	Includes: ApiFix® Minimally Invasive Deformity Correction (MID-C) System	**Stimulator Generator, Multiple Array for Insertion in Subcutaneous Tissue and Fascia**	Includes: Activa PC neurostimulator Enterra gastric neurostimulator Neurostimulator generator, multiple channel PERCEPT™ PC neurostimulator PrimeAdvanced neurostimulator (SureScan)(MRI Safe)
Radioactive Element	Includes: Brachytherapy seeds CivaSheet®		
Radioactive Element, Cesium-131 Collagen Implant for Insertion in Central Nervous System and Cranial Nerves	Includes: Cesium-131 Collagen Implant GammaTile™	**Stimulator Generator, Multiple Array Rechargeable for Insertion in Subcutaneous Tissue and Fascia**	Includes: Activa RC neurostimulator Neurostimulator generator, multiple channel rechargeable RestoreAdvanced neurostimulator (SureScan)(MRI Safe) RestoreSensor neurostimulator (SureScan)(MRI Safe) RestoreUltra neurostimulator (SureScan)(MRI Safe)
Reduction Device in New Technology	Includes: Neovasc Reducer™ Reducer™ System		
Resurfacing Device in Lower Joints	Includes: CONSERVE® PLUS Total Resurfacing Hip System Cormet Hip Resurfacing System		
Short-term External Heart Assist System in Heart and Great Vessels	Includes: Biventricular external heart assist system BVS 5000 Ventricular Assist Device Centrimag® Blood Pump Impella® heart pump TandemHeart® System Thoratec Paracorporeal Ventricular Assist Device	**Stimulator Generator, Single Array for Insertion in Subcutaneous Tissue and Fascia**	Includes: Activa SC neurostimulator InterStim™ II Therapy neurostimulator Itrel (3)(4) neurostimulator Neurostimulator generator, single channel
		Stimulator Generator, Single Array Rechargeable for Insertion in Subcutaneous Tissue and Fascia	Includes: InterStim™ Micro Therapy neurostimulator Neurostimulator generator, single channel rechargeable
Skin Substitute, Porcine Liver Derived in New Technology	Includes: MIRODERM™ Biologic Wound Matrix		
Spacer in Lower Joints	Includes: Joint spacer (antibiotic) Spacer, Static (Antibiotic) Static Spacer (Antibiotic)	**Stimulator Lead in Gastrointestinal System**	Includes: Gastric electrical stimulation (GES) lead Gastric pacemaker lead
Spacer in Upper Joints	Includes: Joint spacer (antibiotic)	**Stimulator Lead in Muscles**	Includes: Electrical muscle stimulation (EMS) lead Electronic muscle stimulator lead Neuromuscular electrical stimulation (NEMS) lead
Spinal Stabilization Device, Facet Replacement for Insertion in Lower Joints	Includes: Facet replacement spinal stabilization device		
Spinal Stabilization Device, Facet Replacement for Insertion in Upper Joints	Includes: Facet replacement spinal stabilization device	**Stimulator Lead in Upper Arteries**	Includes: Baroreflex Activation Therapy® (BAT®) [NT] Carotid (artery) sinus (baroreceptor) lead Rheos® System lead
Spinal Stabilization Device, Interspinous Process for Insertion in Lower Joints	Includes: Interspinous process spinal stabilization device X-STOP® Spacer	**Stimulator Lead in Urinary System**	Includes: Sacral nerve modulation (SNM) lead Sacral neuromodulation lead Urinary incontinence stimulator lead
Spinal Stabilization Device, Interspinous Process for Insertion in Upper Joints	Includes: Interspinous process spinal stabilization device X-STOP® Spacer	**Subcutaneous Defibrillator Lead in Subcutaneous Tissue and Fascia**	Includes: S-ICD™ lead
Spinal Stabilization Device, Pedicle-Based for Insertion in Lower Joints	Includes: Dynesys® Dynamic Stabilization System Pedicle-based dynamic stabilization device		
Spinal Stabilization Device, Pedicle-Based for Insertion in Upper Joints	Includes: Dynesys® Dynamic Stabilization System Pedicle-based dynamic stabilization device		

ICD-10-PCS Value	Definition
Synthetic Substitute	**Includes:** AbioCor® Total Replacement Heart AMPLATZER® Muscular VSD Occluder Annuloplasty ring Bard® Composix® (E/X) (LP) mesh Bard® Composix® Kugel® patch Bard® Dulex™ mesh Bard® Ventralex™ hernia patch Barricaid® Annular Closure Device (ACD) BRYAN® Cervical Disc System Corvia IASD® Ex-PRESS™ mini glaucoma shunt Flexible Composite Mesh GORE® DUALMESH® Holter valve ventricular shunt IASD® (InterAtrial Shunt Device), Corvia InterAtrial Shunt Device IASD®, Corvia MitraClip valve repair system Nitinol framed polymer mesh Open Pivot (mechanical) valve Open Pivot Aortic Valve Graft (AVG) Partially absorbable mesh PHYSIOMESH™ Flexible Composite Mesh Polymethylmethacrylate (PMMA) Polypropylene mesh PRESTIGE® Cervical Disc PROCEED™ Ventral Patch Prodisc-C Prodisc-L PROLENE Polypropylene Hernia System (PHS) Rebound HRD® (Hernia Repair Device) SynCardia Total Artificial Heart Total artificial (replacement) heart ULTRAPRO Hernia System (UHS) ULTRAPRO Partially Absorbable Lightweight Mesh ULTRAPRO Plug V-Wave Interatrial Shunt System Ventrio™ Hernia Patch Zimmer® NexGen® LPS Mobile Bearing Knee Zimmer® NexGen® LPS-Flex Mobile Knee
Synthetic Substitute, Ceramic for Replacement in Lower Joints	**Includes:** Ceramic on ceramic bearing surface Novation® Ceramic AHS® (Articulation Hip System)
Synthetic Substitute, Intraocular Telescope for Replacement in Eye	**Includes:** Implantable Miniature Telescope™ (IMT)
Synthetic Substitute, Mechanically Expandable (Paired) in New Technology	**Includes:** SpineJack® system **NT**
Synthetic Substitute, Metal for Replacement in Lower Joints	**Includes:** Cobalt/chromium head and socket Metal on metal bearing surface
Synthetic Substitute, Metal on Polyethylene for Replacement in Lower Joints	**Includes:** Cobalt/chromium head and polyethylene socket
Synthetic Substitute, Oxidized Zirconium on Polyethylene for Replacement in Lower Joints	**Includes:** OXINIUM
Synthetic Substitute, Pneumatic for Replacement in Heart and Great Vessels	**Includes:** SynCardia (temporary) total artificial heart (TAH)

ICD-10-PCS Value	Definition
Synthetic Substitute, Polyethylene for Replacement in Lower Joints	**Includes:** Polyethylene socket
Synthetic Substitute, Reverse Ball and Socket for Replacement in Upper Joints	**Includes:** Delta III Reverse shoulder prosthesis Reverse® Shoulder Prosthesis
Tissue Expander in Skin and Breast	**Includes:** Tissue expander (inflatable) (injectable)
Tissue Expander in Subcutaneous Tissue and Fascia	**Includes:** Tissue expander (inflatable) (injectable)
Tracheostomy Device in Respiratory System	**Includes:** Tracheostomy tube
Vascular Access Device, Totally Implantable in Subcutaneous Tissue and Fascia	**Includes:** Implanted (venous)(access) port Injection reservoir, port Subcutaneous injection reservoir, port
Vascular Access Device, Tunneled in Subcutaneous Tissue and Fascia	**Includes:** Tunneled central venous catheter Vectra® Vascular Access Graft
Zooplastic Tissue in Heart and Great Vessels	**Includes:** 3f (Aortic) Bioprosthesis valve Bovine pericardial valve Bovine pericardium graft Contegra Pulmonary Valved Conduit CoreValve transcatheter aortic valve Epic™ Stented Tissue Valve (aortic) Freestyle (Stentless) Aortic Root Bioprosthesis Hancock Bioprosthesis (aortic) (mitral) valve Hancock Bioprosthetic Valved Conduit Melody® transcatheter pulmonary valve Mitroflow® Aortic Pericardial Heart Valve Mosaic Bioprosthesis (aortic) (mitral) valve Porcine (bioprosthetic) valve SAPIEN transcatheter aortic valve SJM Biocor® Stented Valve System Stented tissue valve Trifecta™ Valve (aortic) Xenograft
Zooplastic Tissue, Rapid Deployment Technique in New Technology	**Includes:** EDWARDS INTUITY Elite valve system INTUITY Elite valve system, EDWARDS Perceval sutureless valve Sutureless valve, Perceval

Appendix I: Substance Key/Substance Definitions

Substance Key

This table crosswalks a specific substance, listed by trade name or synonym, to the PCS value that would be used to represent that substance in either the Administration or New Technology section. The ICD-10-PCS value may be located in either the 6th-character Substance column or the 7th-character Qualifier column depending on the section/table to which it is classified. The most specific character is listed in the table.

This **NT** symbol next to a substance/technology in the Trade Name or Synonym column identifies that the substance/technology has been approved for NTAP (new technology add-on payment). CMS provides incremental payment, in addition to the DRG payment, for technologies that have received an NTAP designation.

Substances denoted by an asterisk (*) in the Trade Name or Synonym column, although not included in the official ICD-10-PCS classification, were added based on information provided in the FY 2022 IPPS proposed rule.

Trade Name or Synonym	ICD-10-PCS Value	PCS Section
ABECMA®	Idecabtagene Vicleucel Immunotherapy (K)	New Technology (X)
ACTEMRA®	Tocilizumab (H)	New Technology (X)
AIGISRx Antibacterial Envelope	Anti-Infective Envelope (A)	Administration (3)
Andexanet Alfa, Factor Xa Inhibitor Reversal Agent	Coagulation Factor Xa, Inactivated (7)	New Technology (X)
Andexxa **NT**	Coagulation Factor Xa, Inactivated (7)	New Technology (X)
Angiotensin II	Synthetic Human Angiotensin II (H)	New Technology (X)
Antibacterial Envelope (TYRX) (AIGISRx)	Anti-Infective Envelope (A)	Administration (3)
Antimicrobial envelope	Anti-Infective Envelope (A)	Administration (3)
Anti-SARS-CoV-2 hyperimmune globulin	Hyperimmune Globulin (E)	New Technology (X)
AVYCAZ® (ceftazidime-avibactam)	Other Anti-infective (9)	Administration (3)
Axicabtagene Ciloeucel	Axicabtagene Ciloleucel Immunotherapy (H)	New Technology (X)
AZEDRA® **NT**	Iobenguane I-131 Antineoplastic (S)	New Technology (X)
*Balversa™ **NT**	Erdafitinib Antineoplastic (L)	New Technology (X)
Blinatumomab	Other Antineoplastic (5)	Administration (3)
BLINCYTO® (blinatumomab)	Other Antineoplastic (5)	Administration (3)
Bone morphogenetic protein 2 (BMP 2)	Recombinant Bone Morphogenetic Protein (B)	Administration (3)
Brexucabtagene Autoleucel	Brexucabtagene Autoleucel Immunotherapy (4)	New Technology (X)
*CABLIVI® **NT**	Caplacizumab (W)	New Technology (X)
Casirivimab (REGN10933) and Imdevimab (REGN10987)	REGN-COV2 Monoclonal Antibody (G)	New Technology (X)
CBMA (Concentrated Bone Marrow Aspirate)	Concentrated Bone Marrow Aspirate (Ø)	New Technology (X)
Ceftazidime-avibactam	Other Anti-infective (9)	Administration (3)
CERAMENT® G	Antibiotic-eluting Bone Void Filler (P)	New Technology (X)
cilta-cel	Ciltacabtagene Autoleucel (A)	New Technology (X)
Clolar	Clofarabine (P)	Administration (3)
Coagulation Factor Xa, (Recombinant) Inactivated	Coagulation Factor Xa, Inactivated (7)	New Technology (X)
CONTEPO™	Fosfomycin Anti-infective (K)	New Technology (X)
COSELA™	Trilaciclib (7)	New Technology (X)
CRESEMBA® (isavuconazonium sulfate)	Other Anti-infective (9)	Administration (3)
Defitelio	Defibrotide Sodium Anticoagulant (9)	New Technology (X)
DuraGraft® Endothelial Damage Inhibitor	Endothelial Damage Inhibitor (8)	New Technology (X)
ELZONRIS™ **NT**	Tagraxofusp-erzs Antineoplastic (Q)	New Technology (X)
ENSPRYNG™	Satralizumab-mwge (9)	New Technology (X)
ERLEADA™	Apalutamide Antineoplastic (J)	New Technology (X)
Factor Xa Inhibitor Reversal Agent, Andexanet Alfa	Coagulation Factor Xa, Inactivated (7)	New Technology (X)
FETROJA® **NT**	Cefiderocol Anti-infective (A)	New Technology (X)
Fosfomycin injection	Fosfomycin Anti-infective (K)	New Technology (X)
Gammaglobulin	Globulin (S)	Administration (3)
GAMUNEX-C, for COVID-19 treatment	High-Dose Intravenous Immune Globulin (D)	New Technology (X)
GIAPREZA™	Synthetic Human Angiotensin II (H)	New Technology (X)
GS-5734	Remdesivir Anti-infective (E)	New Technology (X)
hdIVIG (high-dose intravenous immunoglobulin), for COVID-19 treatment	High-Dose Intravenous Immune Globulin (D)	New Technology (X)
Hemospray® Endoscopic Hemostat **NT**	Mineral-based Topical Hemostatic Agent (8)	New Technology (X)
HIG (hyperimmune globulin), for COVID-19 treatment	Hyperimmune Globulin (E)	New Technology (X)

Trade Name or Synonym	ICD-10-PCS Value	PCS Section
High-dose intravenous immunoglobulin (hdIVIG), for COVID-19 treatment	Hyperimmune Globulin (E)	New Technology (X)
hIVIG (hyperimmune intravenous immunoglobulin), for COVID-19 treatment	Hyperimmune Globulin (E)	New Technology (X)
Human angiotensin II, synthetic	Synthetic Human Angiotensin II (H)	New Technology (X)
Hyperimmune globulin	Globulin (S)	Administration (3)
Hyperimmune intravenous immunoglobulin (hIVIG), for COVID-19 treatment	Hyperimmune Globulin (E)	New Technology (X)
Idarucizumab, Pradaxa® (dabigatran) reversal agent	Other Therapeutic Substance (G)	Administration (3)
Idecabtagene Vicleucel	Idecabtagene Vicleucel Immunotherapy (K)	New Technology (X)
Ide-cel	Idecabtagene Vicleucel Immunotherapy (K)	New Technology (X)
IGIV-C, for COVID-19 treatment	Hyperimmune Globulin (E)	New Technology (X)
Imdevimab (REGN10987) and Casirivimab (REGN10933)	REGN-COV2 Monoclonal Antibody (G)	New Technology (X)
IMFINZI® **NT**	Durvalumab Antineoplastic (3)	New Technology (X)
IMI/REL	Imipenem-cilastatin-relebactam Anti-infective (U)	New Technology (X)
Immunoglobulin	Globulin (S)	Administration (3)
INTERCEPT Blood System for Plasma Pathogen Reduced Cryoprecipitated Fibrinogen Complex	Pathogen Reduced Cryoprecipitated Fibrinogen Complex (D)	Administration (3)
INTERCEPT Fibrinogen Complex	Pathogen Reduced Cryoprecipitated Fibrinogen Complex (D)	Administration (3)
Iobenguane I-131, High Specific Activity (HSA)	Iobenguane I-131 Antineoplastic (S)	New Technology (X)
Isavuconazole (isavuconazonium sulfate)	Other Anti-infective (9)	Administration (3)
Jakafi® **NT**	Ruxolitinib (T)	New Technology (X)
Kcentra	4-Factor Prothrombin Complex Concentrate (B)	Administration (3)
KEVZARA®	Sarilumab (G)	New Technology (X)
KYMRIAH	Tisagenlecleucel Immunotherapy (J)	New Technology (X)
Lifileucel	Lifileucel Immunotherapy (L)	New Technology (X)
Lisocabtagene Maraleucel	Lisocabtagene Maraleucel Immunotherapy (7)	New Technology (X)
LTX Regional Anticoagulant	Nafamostat Anticoagulant (3)	New Technology (X)
NA-1 (Nerinitide)	Nerinitide (2)	New Technology (X)
Nesiritide	Human B-type Natriuretic Peptide (H)	Administration (3)
NexoBrid™	Bromelain-enriched Proteolytic Enzyme (2)	New Technology (X)
Niyad™	Nafamostat Anticoagulant (3)	New Technology (X)
NUZYRA™ **NT**	Omadacycline Anti-infective (B)	New Technology (X)
Octagam 10%, for COVID-19 treatment	High-Dose Intravenous Immune Globulin (D)	New Technology (X)
Olumiant® **NT**	Baricitinib (M)	New Technology (X)
OTL-101	Hematopoietic Stem/Progenitor Cells, Genetically Modified (C)	Administration (3)
OTL-103	Hematopoietic Stem/Progenitor Cells, Genetically Modified (C)	Administration (3)
OTL-200	Hematopoietic Stem/Progenitor Cells, Genetically Modified (C)	Administration (3)
Polyclonal hyperimmune globulin	Globulin (S)	Administration (3)
Praxbind® (idarucizumab), Pradaxa® (dabigatran) reversal agent	Other Therapeutic Substance (G)	Administration (3)
*RECARBRIO™ **NT**	Imipenem-cilastatin-relebactam Anti-infective (U)	New Technology (X)
rhBMP-2	Recombinant Bone Morphogenetic Protein (B)	Administration (3)
Seprafilm	Adhesion Barrier (5)	Administration (3)
Soliris® **NT**	Eculizumab (C)	New Technology (X)
SPRAVATO™ **NT**	Esketamine Hydrochloride (M)	New Technology (X)
STELARA®	Other New Technology Therapeutic Substance (F)	New Technology (X)
StrataGraft®	Bioengineered Allogeneic Construct (F)	New Technology (X)
Tecartus™	Brexucabtagene Autoleucel Immunotherapy (M)	New Technology (X)
TECENTRIQ® **NT**	Atezolizumab Antineoplastic (D)	New Technology (X)
TERLIVAZ®	Terlipressin (6)	New Technology (X)
Tisagenlecleucel	Tisagenlecleucel Immunotherapy (J)	New Technology (X)
Tissue Plasminogen Activator (tPA)(r- tPA)	Other Thrombolytic (7)	Administration (3)
TYRX Antibacterial Envelope	Anti-Infective Envelope (A)	Administration (3)
Ustekinumab	Other New Technology Therapeutic Substance (F)	New Technology (X)
Vabomere™	Meropenem-vaborbactam Anti-infective (N)	New Technology (X)
Veklury **NT**	Remdesivir Anti-infective (E)	New Technology (X)
Venclexta®	Ventoclax Antineoplastic (R)	New Technology (X)

Trade Name or Synonym		ICD-10-PCS Value	PCS Section
Vistogard®		Uridine Triacetate (8)	New Technology (X)
Voraxaze		Glucarpidase (Q)	Administration (3)
VYXEOS™		Cytarabine and Daunorubicin Liposome Antineoplastic (B)	New Technology (X)
XENLETA™	**NT**	Lefamulin Anti-infective (6)	New Technology (X)
XOSPATA®	**NT**	Gilteritinib Antineoplastic (V)	New Technology (X)
*ZEMDRI™	**NT**	Plazomicin Anti-infective (6)	New Technology (X)
ZEPZELCA™		Lurbinectedin (8)	New Technology (X)
ZERBAXA®	**NT**	Ceftolozane/Tazobactam Anti-infective (9)	New Technology (X)
ZINPLAVA™		Bezlotoxumab Monoclonal Antibody (A)	New Technology (X)
ZULRESSO™		Brexanolone (Ø)	New Technology (X)
Zyvox		Oxazolidinones (8)	Administration (3)

Substance Definitions

This table crosswalks a PCS value, used in the Administration or New Technology section, to a specific substance. The specific substances are listed by trade name or synonym. The ICD-10-PCS value may be located in either the 6th-character Substance column or the 7th-character Qualifier column depending on the section/table to which it is classified.

This **NT** symbol next to a substance/technology in the Trade Name or Synonym column identifies that the substance/technology has been approved for NTAP (new technology add-on payment). CMS provides incremental payment, in addition to the DRG payment, for technologies that have received an NTAP designation.

Substances denoted by an asterisk (*) in the Trade Name or Synonym column, although not included in the official ICD-10-PCS classification, were added based on information provided in the FY 2022 IPPS proposed rule.

ICD-10-PCS Value	Trade Name or Synonym		PCS Section
4-Factor Prothrombin Complex Concentrate (B)	**Includes:** Kcentra		Administration (3)
Adhesion Barrier (5)	**Includes:** Seprafilm		Administration (3)
Antibiotic-eluting Bone Void Filler (P)	**Includes:** CERAMENT® G		New Technology (X)
Anti-Infective Envelope (A)	**Includes:** AIGISRx Antibacterial Envelope Antimicrobial envelope Antibacterial Envelope (TYRX) (AIGISRx) TYRX Antibacterial Envelope		Administration (3)
Apalutamide Antineoplastic (J)	**Includes:** ERLEADA™		New Technology (X)
Atezolizumab Antineoplastic (D)	**Includes:** TECENTRIQ®	**NT**	New Technology (X)
Axicabtagene Ciloleucel Immunotherapy (H)	**Includes:** Axicabtagene Ciloleucel Yescarta®		New Technology (X)
Baricitinib (M)	**Includes:** Olumiant®	**NT**	New Technology (X)
Bezlotoxumab Monoclonal Antibody (A)	**Includes:** ZINPLAVA™		New Technology (X)
Bioengineered Allogeneic Construct (F)	**Includes:** StrataGraft®		New Technology (X)
Brexanolone (Ø)	**Includes:** ZULRESSO™		New Technology (X)
Brexucabtagene Autoleucel Immunotherapy (M)	**Includes:** Tecartus™		New Technology (X)
Bromelain-enriched Proteolytic Enzyme (2)	**Includes:** NexoBrid™		New Technology (X)
Caplacizumab (W)	**Includes:** *CABLIVI®	**NT**	New Technology (X)
Cefiderocol Anti-infective (A)	**Includes:** FETROJA®	**NT**	New Technology (X)
Ceftolozane/Tazobactam Anti- infective (9)	**Includes:** ZERBAXA®	**NT**	New Technology (X)
Ciltacabtagene Autoleucel (A)	**Includes:** cilta-cel		New Technology (X)
Clofarabine (P)	**Includes:** Clolar		Administration (3)
Coagulation Factor Xa, Inactivated (7)	**Includes:** Andexanet Alfa, Factor Xa Inhibitor Reversal Agent Andexxa **NT** Coagulation Factor Xa, (Recombinant) Inactivated Factor Xa Inhibitor Reversal Agent, Andexanet Alfa		New Technology (X)
Concentrated Bone Marrow Aspirate (Ø)	**Includes:** CBMA (Concentrated Bone Marrow Aspirate)		New Technology (X)
Cytarabine and Daunorubicin Liposome Antineoplastic (B)	**Includes:** VYXEOS™		New Technology (X)
Defibrotide Sodium Anticoagulant (9)	**Includes:** Defitelio		New Technology (X)
Durvalumab Antineoplastic (3)	**Includes:** IMFINZI®	**NT**	New Technology (X)
Eculizumab (C)	**Includes:** Soliris®	**NT**	New Technology (X)
Endothelial Damage Inhibitor (8)	**Includes:** DuraGraft® Endothelial Damage Inhibitor		New Technology (X)
Erdafitinib Antineoplastic (L)	**Includes:** *Balversa™	**NT**	New Technology (X)
Esketamine Hydrochloride (M)	**Includes:** SPRAVATO™	**NT**	New Technology (X)

ICD-10-PCS Value	Trade Name or Synonym		PCS Section
Fosfomycin Anti-infective (K)	**Includes:**	CONTEPO™ Fosfomycin injection	New Technology (X)
Gilteritinib Antineoplastic (V)	**Includes:**	XOSPATA® **NT**	New Technology (X)
Globulin (S)	**Includes:**	Gammaglobulin Hyperimmune globulin Immunoglobulin Polyclonal hyperimmune globulin	Administration (3)
Glucarpidase (Q)	**Includes:**	Voraxaze	Administration (3)
Hematopoietic Stem/Progenitor Cells, Genetically Modified (C)	**Includes:**	OTL-101 OTL-103 OTL-200	Administration (3)
High-Dose Intravenous Immune Globulin (D)	**Includes:**	GAMUNEX-C, for COVID-19 treatment hdIVIG (high-dose intravenous immunoglobulin), for COVID-19 treatment High-dose intravenous immunoglobulin (hdIVIG), for COVID-19 treatment Octagam 10%, for COVID-19 treatment	New Technology (X)
Human B-type Natriuretic Peptide (H)	**Includes:**	Nesiritide	Administration (3)
Hyperimmune Globulin (E)	**Includes:**	Anti-SARS-CoV-2 hyperimmune globulin HIG (hyperimmune globulin), for COVID-19 treatment hIVIG (hyperimmune intravenous immunoglobulin), for COVID-19 treatment Hyperimmune intravenous immunoglobulin (hIVIG), for COVID-19 treatment IGIV-C, for COVID-19 treatment	New Technology (X)
Idecabtagene Vicleucel Immunotherapy (K)	**Includes:**	ABECMA® Idecabtagene Vicleucel Ide-cel	New Technology (X)
Imipenem-cilastatin-relebactam Anti-infective (U)	**Includes:**	IMI/REL *RECARBRIO™ **NT**	New Technology (X)
Iobenguane I-131 Antineoplastic (S)	**Includes:**	AZEDRA® **NT** Iobenguane I-131, High Specific Activity (HSA)	New Technology (X)
Lefamulin Anti-infective (6)	**Includes:**	XENLETA™ **NT**	New Technology (X)
Lifileucel Immunotherapy (L)	**Includes:**	Lifileucel	New Technology (X)
Lisocabtagene Maraleucel Immunotherapy (7)	**Includes:**	Lisocabtagene Maraleucel	New Technology (X)
Lurbinectedin (8)	**Includes:**	ZEPZELCA™	New Technology (X)
Meropenem-vaborbactam Anti-infective (N)	**Includes:**	Vabomere™	New Technology (X)
Mineral-based Topical Hemostatic Agent (8)	**Includes:**	Hemospray® Endoscopic Hemostat **NT**	New Technology (X)
Nafamostat Anticoagulant (3)	**Includes:**	LTX Regional Anticoagulant Niyad™	New Technology (X)
Nerinitide (2)	**Includes:**	NA-1 (Nerinitide)	New Technology (X)
Omadacycline Anti-infective (B)	**Includes:**	NUZYRA™ **NT**	New Technology (X)
Other Anti-infective (9)	**Includes:**	AVYCAZ® (ceftazidime-avibactam) Ceftazidime-avibactam CRESEMBA® (isavuconazonium sulfate) Isavuconazole (isavuconazonium sulfate)	Administration (3)
Other Antineoplastic (5)	**Includes:**	Blinatumomab BLINCYTO® (blinatumomab)	Administration (3)
Other New Technology Therapeutic Substance (F)	**Includes:**	STELARA® Ustekinumab	New Technology (X)
Other Therapeutic Substance (G)	**Includes:**	Idarucizumab, Pradaxa® (dabigatran) reversal agent Praxbind® (idarucizumab), Pradaxa® (dabigatran) reversal agent	Administration (3)
Other Thrombolytic (7)	**Includes:**	Tissue Plasminogen Activator (tPA)(r-tPA)	Administration (3)
Oxazolidinones (8)	**Includes:**	Zyvox	Administration (3)
Pathogen Reduced Cryoprecipitated Fibrinogen Complex (D)	**Includes:**	INTERCEPT Blood System for Plasma Pathogen Reduced Cryoprecipitated Fibrinogen Complex INTERCEPT Fibrinogen Complex	Administration (3)
Plazomicin Anti-infective (G)	**Includes:**	*ZEMDRI™ **NT**	New Technology (X)
Recombinant Bone Morphogenetic Protein (B)	**Includes:**	Bone morphogenetic protein 2 (BMP 2) rhBMP-2	Administration (3)
REGN-COV2 Monoclonal Antibody (G)	**Includes:**	Casirivimab (REGN10933) and Imdevimab (REGN10987) Imdevimab (REGN10987) and Casirivimab (REGN10933)	New Technology (X)

ICD-10-PCS Value	Trade Name or Synonym		PCS Section
Remdesivir Anti-infective (E)	**Includes:**	GS-5734 Veklury ⬛NT	New Technology (X)
Ruxolitinib (T)	**Includes:**	Jakafi® ⬛NT	New Technology (X)
Sarilumab (G)	**Includes:**	KEVZARA®	New Technology (X)
Satralizumab-mwge (9)	**Includes:**	ENSPRYNG™	New Technology (X)
Synthetic Human Angiotensin II (H)	**Includes:**	Angiotensin II GIAPREZA™ Human angiotensin II, synthetic	New Technology (X)
Tagraxofusp-erzs Antineoplastic (Q)	**Includes:**	ELZONRIS™ ⬛NT	New Technology (X)
Terlipressin (6)	**Includes:**	TERLIVAZ®	New Technology (X)
Tisagenlecleucel Immunotherapy (J)	**Includes:**	KYMRIAH® Tisagenlecleucel	New Technology (X)
Tocilizumab (H)	**Includes:**	ACTEMRA®	New Technology (X)
Trilaciclib (7)	**Includes:**	COSELA™	New Technology (X)
Uridine Triacetate (8)	**Includes:**	Vistogard®	New Technology (X)
Venetoclax Antineoplastic (R)	**Includes:**	Venclexta®	New Technology (X)

Appendix J: Sections B–H Character Definitions

Sections B–H (Imaging through Substance Abuse Treatment) do not include root operations. Instead, the character 3 value represents the type of procedure performed with additional details about that procedure provided by the character 4 or 5 value, when appropriate. This resource provides the specific ICD-10-PCS value and its associated definition for the character 3, character 4, and character 5 values in the ancillary sections of B–H.

Section B–Imaging

ICD-10-PCS Value (Character 3)	Definition
Computerized Tomography (CT Scan) (2)	Computer reformatted digital display of multiplanar images developed from the capture of multiple exposures of external ionizing radiation
Fluoroscopy (1)	Single plane or bi-plane real time display of an image developed from the capture of external ionizing radiation on a fluorescent screen. The image may also be stored by either digital or analog means.
Magnetic Resonance Imaging (MRI) (3)	Computer reformatted digital display of multiplanar images developed from the capture of radiofrequency signals emitted by nuclei in a body site excited within a magnetic field
Other Imaging (5)	Other specified modality for visualizing a body part
Plain Radiography (Ø)	Planar display of an image developed from the capture of external ionizing radiation on photographic or photoconductive plate
Ultrasonography (4)	Real time display of images of anatomy or flow information developed from the capture of reflected and attenuated high frequency sound waves

Section C–Nuclear Medicine

ICD-10-PCS Value (Character 3)	Definition
Nonimaging Nuclear Medicine Assay (6)	Introduction of radioactive materials into the body for the study of body fluids and blood elements, by the detection of radioactive emissions
Nonimaging Nuclear Medicine Probe (5)	Introduction of radioactive materials into the body for the study of distribution and fate of certain substances by the detection of radioactive emissions; or, alternatively, measurement of absorption of radioactive emissions from an external source
Nonimaging Nuclear Medicine Uptake (4)	Introduction of radioactive materials into the body for measurements of organ function, from the detection of radioactive emissions
Planar Nuclear Medicine Imaging (1)	Introduction of radioactive materials into the body for single plane display of images developed from the capture of radioactive emissions
Positron Emission Tomographic (PET) Imaging (3)	Introduction of radioactive materials into the body for three dimensional display of images developed from the simultaneous capture, 18Ø degrees apart, of radioactive emissions
Systemic Nuclear Medicine Therapy (7)	Introduction of unsealed radioactive materials into the body for treatment
Tomographic (Tomo) Nuclear Medicine Imaging (2)	Introduction of radioactive materials into the body for three dimensional display of images developed from the capture of radioactive emissions

Section F–Physical Rehabilitation and Diagnostic Audiology

ICD-10-PCS Value (Character 3)	Definition
Activities of Daily Living Assessment (2)	Measurement of functional level for activities of daily living
Activities of Daily Living Treatment (8)	Exercise or activities to facilitate functional competence for activities of daily living
Caregiver Training (F)	Training in activities to support patient's optimal level of function
Cochlear Implant Treatment (B)	Application of techniques to improve the communication abilities of individuals with cochlear implant
Device Fitting (D)	Fitting of a device designed to facilitate or support achievement of a higher level of function
Hearing Aid Assessment (4)	Measurement of the appropriateness and/or effectiveness of a hearing device
Hearing Assessment (3)	Measurement of hearing and related functions
Hearing Treatment (9)	Application of techniques to improve, augment, or compensate for hearing and related functional impairment
Motor and/or Nerve Function Assessment (1)	Measurement of motor, nerve, and related functions

Continued on next page

Section F–Physical Rehabilitation and Diagnostic Audiology

Continued from previous page

ICD-10-PCS Value (Character 3)	Definition
Motor Treatment (7)	Exercise or activities to increase or facilitate motor function
Speech Assessment (Ø)	Measurement of speech and related functions
Speech Treatment (6)	Application of techniques to improve, augment, or compensate for speech and related functional impairment
Vestibular Assessment (5)	Measurement of the vestibular system and related functions
Vestibular Treatment (C)	Application of techniques to improve, augment, or compensate for vestibular and related functional impairment

Section F–Physical Rehabilitation and Diagnostic Audiology

ICD-10-PCS Value Qualifier (Character 5)	Definition
Acoustic Reflex Decay (J)	Measures reduction in size/strength of acoustic reflex over time Includes/Examples: Includes site of lesion test
Acoustic Reflex Patterns (G)	Defines site of lesion based upon presence/absence of acoustic reflexes with ipsilateral vs. contralateral stimulation
Acoustic Reflex Threshold (H)	Determines minimal intensity that acoustic reflex occurs with ipsilateral and/or contralateral stimulation
Aerobic Capacity and Endurance (7)	Measures autonomic responses to positional changes; perceived exertion, dyspnea or angina during activity; performance during exercise protocols; standard vital signs; and blood gas analysis or oxygen consumption
Alternate Binaural or Monaural Loudness Balance (7)	Determines auditory stimulus parameter that yields the same objective sensation Includes/Examples: Sound intensities that yield same loudness perception
Anthropometric Characteristics (B)	Measures edema, body fat composition, height, weight, length and girth
Aphasia (Assessment) (C)	Measures expressive and receptive speech and language function including reading and writing
Aphasia (Treatment) (3)	Applying techniques to improve, augment, or compensate for receptive/ expressive language impairments
Articulation/Phonology (Assessment) (9)	Measures speech production
Articulation/Phonology (Treatment) (4)	Applying techniques to correct, improve, or compensate for speech productive impairment
Assistive Listening Device (5)	Assists in use of effective and appropriate assistive listening device/system
Assistive Listening System/Device Selection (4)	Measures the effectiveness and appropriateness of assistive listening systems/devices
Assistive, Adaptive, Supportive or Protective Devices (9)	Explanation: Devices to facilitate or support achievement of a higher level of function in wheelchair mobility; bed mobility; transfer or ambulation ability; bath and showering ability; dressing; grooming; personal hygiene; play or leisure
Auditory Evoked Potentials (L)	Measures electric responses produced by the VIIIth cranial nerve and brainstem following auditory stimulation
Auditory Processing (Assessment) (Q)	Evaluates ability to receive and process auditory information and comprehension of spoken language
Auditory Processing (Treatment) (2)	Applying techniques to improve the receiving and processing of auditory information and comprehension of spoken language
Augmentative/Alternative Communication System (Assessment) (L)	Determines the appropriateness of aids, techniques, symbols, and/or strategies to augment or replace speech and enhance communication Includes/Examples: Includes the use of telephones, writing equipment, emergency equipment, and TDD
Augmentative/Alternative Communication System (Treatment) (3)	Includes/Examples: Includes augmentative communication devices and aids
Aural Rehabilitation (5)	Applying techniques to improve the communication abilities associated with hearing loss
Aural Rehabilitation Status (P)	Measures impact of a hearing loss including evaluation of receptive and expressive communication skills
Bathing/Showering (Ø)	Includes/Examples: Includes obtaining and using supplies; soaping, rinsing, and drying body parts; maintaining bathing position; and transferring to and from bathing positions

Continued on next page

Section F–Physical Rehabilitation and Diagnostic Audiology
Continued from previous page

ICD-10-PCS Value Qualifier (Character 5)	Definition
Bathing/Showering Techniques (Ø)	Activities to facilitate obtaining and using supplies, soaping, rinsing and drying body parts, maintaining bathing position, and transferring to and from bathing positions
Bed Mobility (Assessment) (B)	Transitional movement within bed
Bed Mobility (Treatment) (5)	Exercise or activities to facilitate transitional movements within bed
Bedside Swallowing and Oral Function (H)	Includes/Examples: Bedside swallowing includes assessment of sucking, masticating, coughing, and swallowing. Oral function includes assessment of musculature for controlled movements, structures, and functions to determine coordination and phonation.
Bekesy Audiometry (3)	Uses an instrument that provides a choice of discrete or continuously varying pure tones; choice of pulsed or continuous signal
Binaural Electroacoustic Hearing Aid Check (6)	Determines mechanical and electroacoustic function of bilateral hearing aids using hearing aid test box
Binaural Hearing Aid (Assessment) (3)	Measures the candidacy, effectiveness, and appropriateness of a hearing aid Explanation: Measures bilateral fit
Binaural Hearing Aid (Treatment) (2)	Explanation: Assists in achieving maximum understanding and performance
Bithermal, Binaural Caloric Irrigation (Ø)	Measures the rhythmic eye movements stimulated by changing the temperature of the vestibular system
Bithermal, Monaural Caloric Irrigation (1)	Measures the rhythmic eye movements stimulated by changing the temperature of the vestibular system in one ear
Brief Tone Stimuli (R)	Measures specific central auditory process
Cerumen Management (3)	Includes examination of external auditory canal and tympanic membrane and removal of cerumen from external ear canal
Cochlear Implant (Ø)	Measures candidacy for cochlear implant
Cochlear Implant Rehabilitation (Ø)	Applying techniques to improve the communication abilities of individuals with cochlear implant; includes programming the device, providing patients/families with information
Communicative/Cognitive Integration Skills (Assessment) (G)	Measures ability to use higher cortical functions Includes/Examples: Includes orientation, recognition, attention span, initiation and termination of activity, memory, sequencing, categorizing, concept formation, spatial operations, judgment, problem solving, generalization and pragmatic communication
Communicative/Cognitive Integration Skills (Treatment) (6)	Activities to facilitate the use of higher cortical functions Includes/Examples: Includes level of arousal, orientation, recognition, attention span, initiation and termination of activity, memory sequencing, judgment and problem solving, learning and generalization, and pragmatic communication
Computerized Dynamic Posturography (6)	Measures the status of the peripheral and central vestibular system and the sensory/motor component of balance; evaluates the efficacy of vestibular rehabilitation
Conditioned Play Audiometry (4)	Behavioral measures using nonspeech and speech stimuli to obtain frequency-specific and ear-specific information on auditory status from the patient Explanation: Obtains speech reception threshold by having patient point to pictures of spondaic words
Coordination/Dexterity (Assessment) (3)	Measures large and small muscle groups for controlled goal-directed movements Explanation: Dexterity includes object manipulation
Coordination/Dexterity (Treatment) (2)	Exercise or activities to facilitate gross coordination and fine coordination
Cranial Nerve Integrity (9)	Measures cranial nerve sensory and motor functions, including tastes, smell and facial expression
Dichotic Stimuli (T)	Measures specific central auditory process
Distorted Speech (S)	Measures specific central auditory process
Dix-Hallpike Dynamic (5)	Measures nystagmus following Dix-Hallpike maneuver
Dressing (1)	Includes/Examples: Includes selecting clothing and accessories, obtaining clothing from storage, dressing, fastening and adjusting clothing and shoes, and applying and removing personal devices, prosthesis or orthosis
Dressing Techniques (1)	Activities to facilitate selecting clothing and accessories, dressing and undressing, adjusting clothing and shoes, applying and removing devices, prostheses or orthoses
Dynamic Orthosis (6)	Includes/Examples: Includes customized and prefabricated splints, inhibitory casts, spinal and other braces, and protective devices; allows motion through transfer of movement from other body parts or by use of outside forces

Continued on next page

Section F–Physical Rehabilitation and Diagnostic Audiology

Continued from previous page

ICD-10-PCS Value Qualifier (Character 5)	Definition
Ear Canal Probe Microphone (1)	Real ear measures
Ear Protector Attentuation (7)	Measures ear protector fit and effectiveness
Electrocochleography (K)	Measures the VIIIth cranial nerve action potential
Environmental, Home, Work Barriers (B)	Measures current and potential barriers to optimal function, including safety hazards, access problems and home or office design
Ergonomics and Body Mechanics (C)	Ergonomic measurement of job tasks, work hardening or work conditioning needs; functional capacity; and body mechanics
Eustachian Tube Function (F)	Measures eustachian tube function and patency of eustachian tube
Evoked Otoacoustic Emissions, Diagnostic (N)	Measures auditory evoked potentials in a diagnostic format
Evoked Otoacoustic Emissions, Screening (M)	Measures auditory evoked potentials in a screening format
Facial Nerve Function (7)	Measures electrical activity of the VIIth cranial nerve (facial nerve)
Feeding/Eating (Assessment) (2)	Includes/Examples: Includes setting up food, selecting and using utensils and tableware, bringing food or drink to mouth, cleaning face, hands, and clothing, and management of alternative methods of nourishment
Feeding/Eating (Treatment) (3)	Exercise or activities to facilitate setting up food, selecting and using utensils and tableware, bringing food or drink to mouth, cleaning face, hands, and clothing, and management of alternative methods of nourishment
Filtered Speech (Ø)	Uses high or low pass filtered speech stimuli to assess central auditory processing disorders, site of lesion testing
Fluency (Assessment) (D)	Measures speech fluency or stuttering
Fluency (Treatment) (7)	Applying techniques to improve and augment fluent speech
Gait and/or Balance (D)	Measures biomechanical, arthrokinematic and other spatial and temporal characteristics of gait and balance
Gait Training/Functional Ambulation (9)	Exercise or activities to facilitate ambulation on a variety of surfaces and in a variety of environments
Grooming/Personal Hygiene (Assessment) (3)	Includes/Examples: Includes ability to obtain and use supplies in a sequential fashion, general grooming, oral hygiene, toilet hygiene, personal care devices, including care for artificial airways
Grooming/Personal Hygiene (Treatment) (2)	Activities to facilitate obtaining and using supplies in a sequential fashion: general grooming, oral hygiene, toilet hygiene, cleaning body, and personal care devices, including artificial airways
Hearing and Related Disorders Counseling (Ø)	Provides patients/families/caregivers with information, support, referrals to facilitate recovery from a communication disorder Includes/Examples: Includes strategies for psychosocial adjustment to hearing loss for clients and families/caregivers
Hearing and Related Disorders Prevention (1)	Provides patients/families/caregivers with information and support to prevent communication disorders
Hearing Screening (Ø)	Pass/refer measures designed to identify need for further audiologic assessment
Home Management (Assessment) (4)	Obtaining and maintaining personal and household possessions and environment Includes/Examples: Includes clothing care, cleaning, meal preparation and cleanup, shopping, money management, household maintenance, safety procedures, and childcare/parenting
Home Management (Treatment) (4)	Activities to facilitate obtaining and maintaining personal household possessions and environment Includes/Examples: Includes clothing care, cleaning, meal preparation and clean-up, shopping, money management, household maintenance, safety procedures, childcare/parenting
Instrumental Swallowing and Oral Function (J)	Measures swallowing function using instrumental diagnostic procedures Explanation: Methods include videofluoroscopy, ultrasound, manometry, endoscopy
Integumentary Integrity (1)	Includes/Examples: Includes burns, skin conditions, ecchymosis, bleeding, blisters, scar tissue, wounds and other traumas, tissue mobility, turgor and texture
Manual Therapy Techniques (7)	Techniques in which the therapist uses his/her hands to administer skilled movements Includes/Examples: Includes connective tissue massage, joint mobilization and manipulation, manual lymph drainage, manual traction, soft tissue mobilization and manipulation
Masking Patterns (W)	Measures central auditory processing status

Continued on next page

Section F–Physical Rehabilitation and Diagnostic Audiology

Continued from previous page

ICD-10-PCS Value Qualifier (Character 5)	Definition
Monaural Electroacoustic Hearing Aid Check (8)	Determines mechanical and electroacoustic function of one hearing aid using hearing aid test box
Monaural Hearing Aid (Assessment) (2)	Measures the candidacy, effectiveness, and appropriateness of a hearing aid Explanation: Measures unilateral fit
Monaural Hearing Aid (Treatment) (1)	Explanation: Assists in achieving maximum understanding and performance
Motor Function (Assessment) (4)	Measures the body's functional and versatile movement patterns Includes/Examples: Includes motor assessment scales, analysis of head, trunk and limb movement, and assessment of motor learning
Motor Function (Treatment) (3)	Exercise or activities to facilitate crossing midline, laterality, bilateral integration, praxis, neuromuscular relaxation, inhibition, facilitation, motor function and motor learning
Motor Speech (Assessment) (B)	Measures neurological motor aspects of speech production
Motor Speech (Treatment) (8)	Applying techniques to improve and augment the impaired neurological motor aspects of speech production
Muscle Performance (Assessment) (Ø)	Measures muscle strength, power and endurance using manual testing, dynamometry or computer-assisted electromechanical muscle test; functional muscle strength, power and endurance; muscle pain, tone, or soreness; or pelvic-floor musculature Explanation: Muscle endurance refers to the ability to contract a muscle repeatedly over time
Muscle Performance (Treatment) (1)	Exercise or activities to increase the capacity of a muscle to do work in terms of strength, power, and/or endurance Explanation: Muscle strength is the force exerted to overcome resistance in one maximal effort. Muscle power is work produced per unit of time, or the product of strength and speed. Muscle endurance is the ability to contract a muscle repeatedly over time.
Neuromotor Development (D)	Measures motor development, righting and equilibrium reactions, and reflex and equilibrium reactions
Non-invasive Instrumental Status (N)	Instrumental measures of oral, nasal, vocal, and velopharyngeal functions as they pertain to speech production
Nonspoken Language (Assessment) (7)	Measures nonspoken language (print, sign, symbols) for communication
Nonspoken Language (Treatment) (Ø)	Applying techniques that improve, augment, or compensate spoken communication
Oral Peripheral Mechanism (P)	Structural measures of face, jaw, lips, tongue, teeth, hard and soft palate, pharynx as related to speech production
Orofacial Myofunctional (Assessment) (K)	Measures orofacial myofunctional patterns for speech and related functions
Orofacial Myofunctional (Treatment) (9)	Applying techniques to improve, alter, or augment impaired orofacial myofunctional patterns and related speech production errors
Oscillating Tracking (3)	Measures ability to visually track
Pain (F)	Measures muscle soreness, pain and soreness with joint movement, and pain perception Includes/Examples: Includes questionnaires, graphs, symptom magnification scales or visual analog scales
Perceptual Processing (Assessment) (5)	Measures stereognosis, kinesthesia, body schema, right-left discrimination, form constancy, position in space, visual closure, figure-ground, depth perception, spatial relations and topographical orientation
Perceptual Processing (Treatment) (1)	Exercise and activities to facilitate perceptual processing Explanation: Includes stereognosis, kinesthesia, body schema, right-left discrimination, form constancy, position in space, visual closure, figure-ground, depth perception, spatial relations, and topographical orientation Includes/Examples: Includes stereognosis, kinesthesia, body schema, right-left discrimination, form constancy, position in space, visual closure, figure-ground, depth perception, spatial relations, and topographical orientation
Performance Intensity Phonetically Balanced Speech Discrimination (Q)	Measures word recognition over varying intensity levels
Postural Control (3)	Exercise or activities to increase postural alignment and control
Prosthesis (8)	Explanation: Artificial substitutes for missing body parts that augment performance or function Includes/Examples: Limb prosthesis, ocular prosthesis

Continued on next page

Section F–Physical Rehabilitation and Diagnostic Audiology
Continued from previous page

ICD-10-PCS Value Qualifier (Character 5)	Definition
Psychosocial Skills (Assessment) (6)	The ability to interact in society and to process emotions Includes/Examples: Includes psychological (values, interests, self-concept); social (role performance, social conduct, interpersonal skills, self expression); self-management (coping skills, time management, self-control)
Psychosocial Skills (Treatment) (6)	The ability to interact in society and to process emotions Includes/Examples: Includes psychological (values, interests, self-concept); social (role performance, social conduct, interpersonal skills, self expression); self-management (coping skills, time management, self-control)
Pure Tone Audiometry, Air (1)	Air-conduction pure tone threshold measures with appropriate masking
Pure Tone Audiometry, Air and Bone (2)	Air-conduction and bone-conduction pure tone threshold measures with appropriate masking
Pure Tone Stenger (C)	Measures unilateral nonorganic hearing loss based on simultaneous presentation of pure tones of differing volume
Range of Motion and Joint Integrity (5)	Measures quantity, quality, grade, and classification of joint movement and/or mobility Explanation: Range of Motion is the space, distance or angle through which movement occurs at a joint or series of joints. Joint integrity is the conformance of joints to expected anatomic, biomechanical and kinematic norms.
Range of Motion and Joint Mobility (Ø)	Exercise or activities to increase muscle length and joint mobility
Receptive/Expressive Language (Assessment) (8)	Measures receptive and expressive language
Receptive/Expressive Language (Treatment) (B)	Applying techniques to improve and augment receptive/expressive language
Reflex Integrity (G)	Measures the presence, absence, or exaggeration of developmentally appropriate, pathologic or normal reflexes
Select Picture Audiometry (5)	Establishes hearing threshold levels for speech using pictures
Sensorineural Acuity Level (4)	Measures sensorineural acuity masking presented via bone conduction
Sensory Aids (5)	Determines the appropriateness of a sensory prosthetic device, other than a hearing aid or assistive listening system/device
Sensory Awareness/ Processing/ Integrity (6)	Includes/Examples: Includes light touch, pressure, temperature, pain, sharp/dull, proprioception, vestibular, visual, auditory, gustatory, and olfactory
Short Increment Sensitivity Index (9)	Measures the ear's ability to detect small intensity changes; site of lesion test requiring a behavioral response
Sinusoidal Vertical Axis Rotational (4)	Measures nystagmus following rotation
Somatosensory Evoked Potentials (9)	Measures neural activity from sites throughout the body
Speech/Language Screening (6)	Identifies need for further speech and/or language evaluation
Speech Threshold (1)	Measures minimal intensity needed to repeat spondaic words
Speech-Language Pathology and Related Disorders Counseling (1)	Provides patients/families with information, support, referrals to facilitate recovery from a communication disorder
Speech-Language Pathology and Related Disorders Prevention (2)	Applying techniques to avoid or minimize onset and/or development of a communication disorder
Speech/Word Recognition (2)	Measures ability to repeat/identify single syllable words; scores given as a percentage; includes word recognition/speech discrimination
Staggered Spondaic Word (3)	Measures central auditory processing site of lesion based upon dichotic presentation of spondaic words
Static Orthosis (7)	Includes/Examples: Includes customized and prefabricated splints, inhibitory casts, spinal and other braces, and protective devices; has no moving parts, maintains joint(s) in desired position
Stenger (B)	Measures unilateral nonorganic hearing loss based on simultaneous presentation of signals of differing volume
Swallowing Dysfunction (D)	Activities to improve swallowing function in coordination with respiratory function Includes/Examples: Includes function and coordination of sucking, mastication, coughing, swallowing
Synthetic Sentence Identification (5)	Measures central auditory dysfunction using identification of third order approximations of sentences and competing messages

Continued on next page

Section F–Physical Rehabilitation and Diagnostic Audiology

Continued from previous page

ICD-10-PCS Value Qualifier (Character 5)	Definition
Temporal Ordering of Stimuli (V)	Measures specific central auditory process
Therapeutic Exercise (6)	Exercise or activities to facilitate sensory awareness, sensory processing, sensory integration, balance training, conditioning, reconditioning Includes/Examples: Includes developmental activities, breathing exercises, aerobic endurance activities, aquatic exercises, stretching and ventilatory muscle training
Tinnitus Masker (Assessment) (7)	Determines candidacy for tinnitus masker
Tinnitus Masker (Treatment) (Ø)	Explanation: Used to verify physical fit, acoustic appropriateness, and benefit; assists in achieving maximum benefit
Tone Decay (8)	Measures decrease in hearing sensitivity to a tone; site of lesion test requiring a behavioral response
Transfer (C)	Transitional movement from one surface to another
Transfer Training (8)	Exercise or activities to facilitate movement from one surface to another
Tympanometry (D)	Measures the integrity of the middle ear; measures ease at which sound flows through the tympanic membrane while air pressure against the membrane is varied
Unithermal Binaural Screen (2)	Measures the rhythmic eye movements stimulated by changing the temperature of the vestibular system in both ears using warm water, screening format
Ventilation/Respiration/Circulation (G)	Measures ventilatory muscle strength, power and endurance, pulmonary function and ventilatory mechanics Includes/Examples: Includes ability to clear airway, activities that aggravate or relieve edema, pain, dyspnea or other symptoms, chest wall mobility, cardiopulmonary response to performance of ADL and IAD, cough and sputum, standard vital signs
Vestibular (Ø)	Applying techniques to compensate for balance disorders; includes habituation, exercise therapy, and balance retraining
Visual Motor Integration (Assessment) (2)	Coordinating the interaction of information from the eyes with body movement during activity
Visual Motor Integration (Treatment) (2)	Exercise or activities to facilitate coordinating the interaction of information from eyes with body movement during activity
Visual Reinforcement Audiometry (6)	Behavioral measures using nonspeech and speech stimuli to obtain frequency/ear-specific information on auditory status Includes/Examples: Includes a conditioned response of looking toward a visual reinforcer (e.g., lights, animated toy) every time auditory stimuli are heard
Vocational Activities and Functional Community or Work Reintegration Skills (Assessment) (H)	Measures environmental, home, work (job/school/play) barriers that keep patients from functioning optimally in their environment Includes/Examples: Includes assessment of vocational skills and interests, environment of work (job/school/play), injury potential and injury prevention or reduction, ergonomic stressors, transportation skills, and ability to access and use community resources
Vocational Activities and Functional Community or Work Reintegration Skills (Treatment) (7)	Activities to facilitate vocational exploration, body mechanics training, job acquisition, and environmental or work (job/school/play) task adaptation Includes/Examples: Includes injury prevention and reduction, ergonomic stressor reduction, job coaching and simulation, work hardening and conditioning, driving training, transportation skills, and use of community resources
Voice (Assessment) (F)	Measures vocal structure, function and production
Voice (Treatment) (C)	Applying techniques to improve voice and vocal function
Voice Prosthetic (Assessment) (M)	Determines the appropriateness of voice prosthetic/adaptive device to enhance or facilitate communication
Voice Prosthetic (Treatment) (4)	Includes/Examples: Includes electrolarynx, and other assistive, adaptive, supportive devices
Wheelchair Mobility (Assessment) (F)	Measures fit and functional abilities within wheelchair in a variety of environments
Wheelchair Mobility (Treatment) (4)	Management, maintenance and controlled operation of a wheelchair, scooter or other device, in and on a variety of surfaces and environments
Wound Management (5)	Includes/Examples: Includes non-selective and selective debridement (enzymes, autolysis, sharp debridement), dressings (wound coverings, hydrogel, vacuum-assisted closure), topical agents, etc.

Section G–Mental Health

ICD-10-PCS Value (Character 3)	Definition
Biofeedback (C)	Provision of information from the monitoring and regulating of physiological processes in conjunction with cognitive-behavioral techniques to improve patient functioning or well-being Includes/Examples: Includes EEG, blood pressure, skin temperature or peripheral blood flow, ECG, electrooculogram, EMG, respirometry or capnometry, GSR/EDR, perineometry to monitor/regulate bowel/bladder activity, electrogastrogram to monitor/regulate gastric motility
Counseling (6)	The application of psychological methods to treat an individual with normal developmental issues and psychological problems in order to increase function, improve well-being, alleviate distress, maladjustment or resolve crises
Crisis Intervention (2)	Treatment of a traumatized, acutely disturbed or distressed individual for the purpose of short-term stabilization Includes/Examples: Includes defusing, debriefing, counseling, psychotherapy and/or coordination of care with other providers or agencies
Electroconvulsive Therapy (B)	The application of controlled electrical voltages to treat a mental health disorder Includes/Examples: Includes appropriate sedation and other preparation of the individual
Family Psychotherapy (7)	Treatment that includes one or more family members of an individual with a mental health disorder by behavioral, cognitive, psychoanalytic, psychodynamic or psychophysiological means to improve functioning or well-being Explanation: Remediation of emotional or behavioral problems presented by one or more family members in cases where psychotherapy with more than one family member is indicated
Group Psychotherapy (H)	Treatment of two or more individuals with a mental health disorder by behavioral, cognitive, psychoanalytic, psychodynamic or psychophysiological means to improve functioning or well-being
Hypnosis (F)	Induction of a state of heightened suggestibility by auditory, visual and tactile techniques to elicit an emotional or behavioral response
Individual Psychotherapy (5)	Treatment of an individual with a mental health disorder by behavioral, cognitive, psychoanalytic, psychodynamic or psychophysiological means to improve functioning or well-being
Light Therapy (J)	Application of specialized light treatments to improve functioning or well-being
Medication Management (3)	Monitoring and adjusting the use of medications for the treatment of a mental health disorder
Narcosynthesis (G)	Administration of intravenous barbiturates in order to release suppressed or repressed thoughts
Psychological Tests (1)	The administration and interpretation of standardized psychological tests and measurement instruments for the assessment of psychological function
Behavioral (1)	Primarily to modify behavior Includes/Examples: Includes modeling and role playing, positive reinforcement of target behaviors, response cost, and training of self-management skills
Cognitive (2)	Primarily to correct cognitive distortions and errors
Cognitive-Behavioral (8)	Combining cognitive and behavioral treatment strategies to improve functioning Explanation: Maladaptive responses are examined to determine how cognitions relate to behavior patterns in response to an event. Uses learning principles and information-processing models.
Developmental (Ø)	Age-normed developmental status of cognitive, social and adaptive behavior skills
Intellectual and Psychoeducational (2)	Intellectual abilities, academic achievement and learning capabilities (including behaviors and emotional factors affecting learning)
Interactive (Ø)	Uses primarily physical aids and other forms of non-oral interaction with a patient who is physically, psychologically or developmentally unable to use ordinary language for communication Includes/Examples: Includes the use of toys in symbolic play
Interpersonal (3)	Helps an individual make changes in interpersonal behaviors to reduce psychological dysfunction Includes/Examples: Includes exploratory techniques, encouragement of affective expression, clarification of patient statements, analysis of communication patterns, use of therapy relationship and behavior change techniques
Neurobehavioral and Cognitive Status (4)	Includes neurobehavioral status exam, interview(s), and observation for the clinical assessment of thinking, reasoning and judgment, acquired knowledge, attention, memory, visual spatial abilities, language functions, and planning
Neuropsychological (3)	Thinking, reasoning and judgment, acquired knowledge, attention, memory, visual spatial abilities, language functions, planning
Personality and Behavioral (1)	Mood, emotion, behavior, social functioning, psychopathological conditions, personality traits and characteristics

Continued on next page

Section G–Mental Health

Continued from previous page

ICD-10-PCS Value (Character 3)	Definition
Psychoanalysis (4)	Methods of obtaining a detailed account of past and present mental and emotional experiences to determine the source and eliminate or diminish the undesirable effects of unconscious conflicts Explanation: Accomplished by making the individual aware of their existence, origin, and inappropriate expression in emotions and behavior
Psychodynamic (5)	Exploration of past and present emotional experiences to understand motives and drives using insight-oriented techniques to reduce the undesirable effects of internal conflicts on emotions and behavior Explanation: Techniques include empathetic listening, clarifying self-defeating behavior patterns, and exploring adaptive alternatives
Psychophysiological (9)	Monitoring and alteration of physiological processes to help the individual associate physiological reactions combined with cognitive and behavioral strategies to gain improved control of these processes to help the individual cope more effectively
Supportive (6)	Formation of therapeutic relationship primarily for providing emotional support to prevent further deterioration in functioning during periods of particular stress Explanation: Often used in conjunction with other therapeutic approaches
Vocational (1)	Exploration of vocational interests, aptitudes and required adaptive behavior skills to develop and carry out a plan for achieving a successful vocational placement Includes/Examples: Includes enhancing work related adjustment and/or pursuing viable options in training education or preparation

Section H–Substance Abuse Treatment

ICD-10-PCS Value (Character 3)	Definition
Detoxification Services (2)	Detoxification from alcohol and/or drugs Explanation: Not a treatment modality, but helps the patient stabilize physically and psychologically until the body becomes free of drugs and the effects of alcohol
Family Counseling (6)	The application of psychological methods that includes one or more family members to treat an individual with addictive behavior Explanation: Provides support and education for family members of addicted individuals. Family member participation is seen as a critical area of substance abuse treatment.
Group Counseling (4)	The application of psychological methods to treat two or more individuals with addictive behavior Explanation: Provides structured group counseling sessions and healing power through the connection with others
Individual Counseling (3)	The application of psychological methods to treat an individual with addictive behavior Explanation: Comprised of several different techniques, which apply various strategies to address drug addiction
Individual Psychotherapy (5)	Treatment of an individual with addictive behavior by behavioral, cognitive, psychoanalytic, psychodynamic or psychophysiological means
Medication Management (8)	Monitoring and adjusting the use of replacement medications for the treatment of addiction
Pharmacotherapy (9)	The use of replacement medications for the treatment of addiction

Appendix K: Hospital Acquired Conditions

Hospital acquired conditions (HACs) are conditions considered reasonably preventable through the application of evidence-based guidelines. Although it is the ICD-10-CM diagnosis code that drives a HAC designation, in some cases a specific ICD-10-PCS procedure code must also be present before that diagnosis code can be considered a HAC. This resource provides only those HAC categories that require both an ICD-10-PCS code and an ICD-10-CM diagnosis code. The official descriptions for each code are also provided. To see all 14 HAC categories and their corresponding codes, refer to Optum360's *ICD-10-CM Expert for Hospitals*.

Note: The resource used to compile this list is the proposed, version 39, MS-DRG Grouper software and Definitions Manual files published with the fiscal 2022 IPPS proposed rule. For the final, version 39, MS-DRG Grouper software and Definitions Manual files, refer to the following: https://www.cms.gov/Medicare/Medicare-Fee-for-Service-Payment/AcuteInpatientPPS/MS-DRG-Classifications-and-Software.

HAC 08: Surgical Site Infection of Mediastinitis After Coronary Bypass Graft (CABG) Procedures

Secondary diagnosis not POA:

J98.51	Mediastinitis
J98.59	Other diseases of mediastinum, not elsewhere classified

AND

Any of the following procedures:

0210083	Bypass Coronary Artery, One Artery from Coronary Artery with Zooplastic Tissue, Open Approach
0210088	Bypass Coronary Artery, One Artery from Right Internal Mammary with Zooplastic Tissue, Open Approach
0210089	Bypass Coronary Artery, One Artery from Left Internal Mammary with Zooplastic Tissue, Open Approach
021008C	Bypass Coronary Artery, One Artery from Thoracic Artery with Zooplastic Tissue, Open Approach
021008F	Bypass Coronary Artery, One Artery from Abdominal Artery with Zooplastic Tissue, Open Approach
021008W	Bypass Coronary Artery, One Artery from Aorta with Zooplastic Tissue, Open Approach
0210093	Bypass Coronary Artery, One Artery from Coronary Artery with Autologous Venous Tissue, Open Approach
0210098	Bypass Coronary Artery, One Artery from Right Internal Mammary with Autologous Venous Tissue, Open Approach
0210099	Bypass Coronary Artery, One Artery from Left Internal Mammary with Autologous Venous Tissue, Open Approach
021009C	Bypass Coronary Artery, One Artery from Thoracic Artery with Autologous Venous Tissue, Open Approach
021009F	Bypass Coronary Artery, One Artery from Abdominal Artery with Autologous Venous Tissue, Open Approach
021009W	Bypass Coronary Artery, One Artery from Aorta with Autologous Venous Tissue, Open Approach
02100A3	Bypass Coronary Artery, One Artery from Coronary Artery with Autologous Arterial Tissue, Open Approach
02100A8	Bypass Coronary Artery, One Artery from Right Internal Mammary with Autologous Arterial Tissue, Open Approach
02100A9	Bypass Coronary Artery, One Artery from Left Internal Mammary with Autologous Arterial Tissue, Open Approach
02100AC	Bypass Coronary Artery, One Artery from Thoracic Artery with Autologous Arterial Tissue, Open Approach
02100AF	Bypass Coronary Artery, One Artery from Abdominal Artery with Autologous Arterial Tissue, Open Approach
02100AW	Bypass Coronary Artery, One Artery from Aorta with Autologous Arterial Tissue, Open Approach

02100J3	Bypass Coronary Artery, One Artery from Coronary Artery with Synthetic Substitute, Open Approach
02100J8	Bypass Coronary Artery, One Artery from Right Internal Mammary with Synthetic Substitute, Open Approach
02100J9	Bypass Coronary Artery, One Artery from Left Internal Mammary with Synthetic Substitute, Open Approach
02100JC	Bypass Coronary Artery, One Artery from Thoracic Artery with Synthetic Substitute, Open Approach
02100JF	Bypass Coronary Artery, One Artery from Abdominal Artery with Synthetic Substitute, Open Approach
02100JW	Bypass Coronary Artery, One Artery from Aorta with Synthetic Substitute, Open Approach
02100K3	Bypass Coronary Artery, One Artery from Coronary Artery with Nonautologous Tissue Substitute, Open Approach
02100K8	Bypass Coronary Artery, One Artery from Right Internal Mammary with Nonautologous Tissue Substitute, Open Approach
02100K9	Bypass Coronary Artery, One Artery from Left Internal Mammary with Nonautologous Tissue Substitute, Open Approach
02100KC	Bypass Coronary Artery, One Artery from Thoracic Artery with Nonautologous Tissue Substitute, Open Approach
02100KF	Bypass Coronary Artery, One Artery from Abdominal Artery with Nonautologous Tissue Substitute, Open Approach
02100KW	Bypass Coronary Artery, One Artery from Aorta with Nonautologous Tissue Substitute, Open Approach
02100Z3	Bypass Coronary Artery, One Artery from Coronary Artery, Open Approach
02100Z8	Bypass Coronary Artery, One Artery from Right Internal Mammary, Open Approach
02100Z9	Bypass Coronary Artery, One Artery from Left Internal Mammary, Open Approach
02100ZC	Bypass Coronary Artery, One Artery from Thoracic Artery, Open Approach
02100ZF	Bypass Coronary Artery, One Artery from Abdominal Artery, Open Approach
0210483	Bypass Coronary Artery, One Artery from Coronary Artery with Zooplastic Tissue, Percutaneous Endoscopic Approach
0210488	Bypass Coronary Artery, One Artery from Right Internal Mammary with Zooplastic Tissue, Percutaneous Endoscopic Approach
0210489	Bypass Coronary Artery, One Artery from Left Internal Mammary with Zooplastic Tissue, Percutaneous Endoscopic Approach

021048C	Bypass Coronary Artery, One Artery from Thoracic Artery with Zooplastic Tissue, Percutaneous Endoscopic Approach
021048F	Bypass Coronary Artery, One Artery from Abdominal Artery with Zooplastic Tissue, Percutaneous Endoscopic Approach
021048W	Bypass Coronary Artery, One Artery from Aorta with Zooplastic Tissue, Percutaneous Endoscopic Approach
0210493	Bypass Coronary Artery, One Artery from Coronary Artery with Autologous Venous Tissue, Percutaneous Endoscopic Approach
0210498	Bypass Coronary Artery, One Artery from Right Internal Mammary with Autologous Venous Tissue, Percutaneous Endoscopic Approach
0210499	Bypass Coronary Artery, One Artery from Left Internal Mammary with Autologous Venous Tissue, Percutaneous Endoscopic Approach
021049C	Bypass Coronary Artery, One Artery from Thoracic Artery with Autologous Venous Tissue, Percutaneous Endoscopic Approach
021049F	Bypass Coronary Artery, One Artery from Abdominal Artery with Autologous Venous Tissue, Percutaneous Endoscopic Approach
021049W	Bypass Coronary Artery, One Artery from Aorta with Autologous Venous Tissue, Percutaneous Endoscopic Approach
02104A3	Bypass Coronary Artery, One Artery from Coronary Artery with Autologous Arterial Tissue, Percutaneous Endoscopic Approach
02104A8	Bypass Coronary Artery, One Artery from Right Internal Mammary with Autologous Arterial Tissue, Percutaneous Endoscopic Approach
02104A9	Bypass Coronary Artery, One Artery from Left Internal Mammary with Autologous Arterial Tissue, Percutaneous Endoscopic Approach
02104AC	Bypass Coronary Artery, One Artery from Thoracic Artery with Autologous Arterial Tissue, Percutaneous Endoscopic Approach
02104AF	Bypass Coronary Artery, One Artery from Abdominal Artery with Autologous Arterial Tissue, Percutaneous Endoscopic Approach
02104AW	Bypass Coronary Artery, One Artery from Aorta with Autologous Arterial Tissue, Percutaneous Endoscopic Approach
02104J3	Bypass Coronary Artery, One Artery from Coronary Artery with Synthetic Substitute, Percutaneous Endoscopic Approach

HAC 08: Surgical Site Infection of Mediastinitis After Coronary Bypass Graft (CABG) Procedures (continued)

Ø2104J8   Bypass Coronary Artery, One Artery from Right Internal Mammary with Synthetic Substitute, Percutaneous Endoscopic Approach

Ø2104J9   Bypass Coronary Artery, One Artery from Left Internal Mammary with Synthetic Substitute, Percutaneous Endoscopic Approach

Ø2104JC   Bypass Coronary Artery, One Artery from Thoracic Artery with Synthetic Substitute, Percutaneous Endoscopic Approach

Ø2104JF   Bypass Coronary Artery, One Artery from Abdominal Artery with Synthetic Substitute, Percutaneous Endoscopic Approach

Ø2104JW   Bypass Coronary Artery, One Artery from Aorta with Synthetic Substitute, Percutaneous Endoscopic Approach

Ø2104K3   Bypass Coronary Artery, One Artery from Coronary Artery with Nonautologous Tissue Substitute, Percutaneous Endoscopic Approach

Ø2104K8   Bypass Coronary Artery, One Artery from Right Internal Mammary with Nonautologous Tissue Substitute, Percutaneous Endoscopic Approach

Ø2104K9   Bypass Coronary Artery, One Artery from Left Internal Mammary with Nonautologous Tissue Substitute, Percutaneous Endoscopic Approach

Ø2104KC   Bypass Coronary Artery, One Artery from Thoracic Artery with Nonautologous Tissue Substitute, Percutaneous Endoscopic Approach

Ø2104KF   Bypass Coronary Artery, One Artery from Abdominal Artery with Nonautologous Tissue Substitute, Percutaneous Endoscopic Approach

Ø2104KW   Bypass Coronary Artery, One Artery from Aorta with Nonautologous Tissue Substitute, Percutaneous Endoscopic Approach

Ø2104Z3   Bypass Coronary Artery, One Artery from Coronary Artery, Percutaneous Endoscopic Approach

Ø2104Z8   Bypass Coronary Artery, One Artery from Right Internal Mammary, Percutaneous Endoscopic Approach

Ø2104Z9   Bypass Coronary Artery, One Artery from Left Internal Mammary, Percutaneous Endoscopic Approach

Ø2104ZC   Bypass Coronary Artery, One Artery from Thoracic Artery, Percutaneous Endoscopic Approach

Ø2104ZF   Bypass Coronary Artery, One Artery from Abdominal Artery, Percutaneous Endoscopic Approach

Ø211Ø83   Bypass Coronary Artery, Two Arteries from Coronary Artery with Zooplastic Tissue, Open Approach

Ø211Ø88   Bypass Coronary Artery, Two Arteries from Right Internal Mammary with Zooplastic Tissue, Open Approach

Ø211Ø89   Bypass Coronary Artery, Two Arteries from Left Internal Mammary with Zooplastic Tissue, Open Approach

Ø211Ø8C   Bypass Coronary Artery, Two Arteries from Thoracic Artery with Zooplastic Tissue, Open Approach

Ø211Ø8F   Bypass Coronary Artery, Two Arteries from Abdominal Artery with Zooplastic Tissue, Open Approach

Ø211Ø8W   Bypass Coronary Artery, Two Arteries from Aorta with Zooplastic Tissue, Open Approach

Ø211Ø93   Bypass Coronary Artery, Two Arteries from Coronary Artery with Autologous Venous Tissue, Open Approach

Ø211Ø98   Bypass Coronary Artery, Two Arteries from Right Internal Mammary with Autologous Venous Tissue, Open Approach

Ø211Ø99   Bypass Coronary Artery, Two Arteries from Left Internal Mammary with Autologous Venous Tissue, Open Approach

Ø211Ø9C   Bypass Coronary Artery, Two Arteries from Thoracic Artery with Autologous Venous Tissue, Open Approach

Ø211Ø9F   Bypass Coronary Artery, Two Arteries from Abdominal Artery with Autologous Venous Tissue, Open Approach

Ø211Ø9W   Bypass Coronary Artery, Two Arteries from Aorta with Autologous Venous Tissue, Open Approach

Ø211ØA3   Bypass Coronary Artery, Two Arteries from Coronary Artery with Autologous Arterial Tissue, Open Approach

Ø211ØA8   Bypass Coronary Artery, Two Arteries from Right Internal Mammary with Autologous Arterial Tissue, Open Approach

Ø211ØA9   Bypass Coronary Artery, Two Arteries from Left Internal Mammary with Autologous Arterial Tissue, Open Approach

Ø211ØAC   Bypass Coronary Artery, Two Arteries from Thoracic Artery with Autologous Arterial Tissue, Open Approach

Ø211ØAF   Bypass Coronary Artery, Two Arteries from Abdominal Artery with Autologous Arterial Tissue, Open Approach

Ø211ØAW   Bypass Coronary Artery, Two Arteries from Aorta with Autologous Arterial Tissue, Open Approach

Ø211ØJ3   Bypass Coronary Artery, Two Arteries from Coronary Artery with Synthetic Substitute, Open Approach

Ø211ØJ8   Bypass Coronary Artery, Two Arteries from Right Internal Mammary with Synthetic Substitute, Open Approach

Ø211ØJ9   Bypass Coronary Artery, Two Arteries from Left Internal Mammary with Synthetic Substitute, Open Approach

Ø211ØJC   Bypass Coronary Artery, Two Arteries from Thoracic Artery with Synthetic Substitute, Open Approach

Ø211ØJF   Bypass Coronary Artery, Two Arteries from Abdominal Artery with Synthetic Substitute, Open Approach

Ø211ØJW   Bypass Coronary Artery, Two Arteries from Aorta with Synthetic Substitute, Open Approach

Ø211ØK3   Bypass Coronary Artery, Two Arteries from Coronary Artery with Nonautologous Tissue Substitute, Open Approach

Ø211ØK8   Bypass Coronary Artery, Two Arteries from Right Internal Mammary with Nonautologous Tissue Substitute, Open Approach

Ø211ØK9   Bypass Coronary Artery, Two Arteries from Left Internal Mammary with Nonautologous Tissue Substitute, Open Approach

Ø211ØKC   Bypass Coronary Artery, Two Arteries from Thoracic Artery with Nonautologous Tissue Substitute, Open Approach

Ø211ØKF   Bypass Coronary Artery, Two Arteries from Abdominal Artery with Nonautologous Tissue Substitute, Open Approach

Ø211ØKW   Bypass Coronary Artery, Two Arteries from Aorta with Nonautologous Tissue Substitute, Open Approach

Ø211ØZ3   Bypass Coronary Artery, Two Arteries from Coronary Artery, Open Approach

Ø211ØZ8   Bypass Coronary Artery, Two Arteries from Right Internal Mammary, Open Approach

Ø211ØZ9   Bypass Coronary Artery, Two Arteries from Left Internal Mammary, Open Approach

Ø211ØZC   Bypass Coronary Artery, Two Arteries from Thoracic Artery, Open Approach

Ø211ØZF   Bypass Coronary Artery, Two Arteries from Abdominal Artery, Open Approach

Ø211483   Bypass Coronary Artery, Two Arteries from Coronary Artery with Zooplastic Tissue, Percutaneous Endoscopic Approach

Ø211488   Bypass Coronary Artery, Two Arteries from Right Internal Mammary with Zooplastic Tissue, Percutaneous Endoscopic Approach

Ø211489   Bypass Coronary Artery, Two Arteries from Left Internal Mammary with Zooplastic Tissue, Percutaneous Endoscopic Approach

Ø21148C   Bypass Coronary Artery, Two Arteries from Thoracic Artery with Zooplastic Tissue, Percutaneous Endoscopic Approach

Ø21148F   Bypass Coronary Artery, Two Arteries from Abdominal Artery with Zooplastic Tissue, Percutaneous Endoscopic Approach

Ø21148W   Bypass Coronary Artery, Two Arteries from Aorta with Zooplastic Tissue, Percutaneous Endoscopic Approach

Ø211493   Bypass Coronary Artery, Two Arteries from Coronary Artery with Autologous Venous Tissue, Percutaneous Endoscopic Approach

Ø211498   Bypass Coronary Artery, Two Arteries from Right Internal Mammary with Autologous Venous Tissue, Percutaneous Endoscopic Approach

Ø211499   Bypass Coronary Artery, Two Arteries from Left Internal Mammary with Autologous Venous Tissue, Percutaneous Endoscopic Approach

Ø21149C   Bypass Coronary Artery, Two Arteries from Thoracic Artery with Autologous Venous Tissue, Percutaneous Endoscopic Approach

Ø21149F   Bypass Coronary Artery, Two Arteries from Abdominal Artery with Autologous Venous Tissue, Percutaneous Endoscopic Approach

Ø21149W   Bypass Coronary Artery, Two Arteries from Aorta with Autologous Venous Tissue, Percutaneous Endoscopic Approach

Ø2114A3   Bypass Coronary Artery, Two Arteries from Coronary Artery with Autologous Arterial Tissue, Percutaneous Endoscopic Approach

Ø2114A8   Bypass Coronary Artery, Two Arteries from Right Internal Mammary with Autologous Arterial Tissue, Percutaneous Endoscopic Approach

Ø2114A9   Bypass Coronary Artery, Two Arteries from Left Internal Mammary with Autologous Arterial Tissue, Percutaneous Endoscopic Approach

Ø2114AC   Bypass Coronary Artery, Two Arteries from Thoracic Artery with Autologous Arterial Tissue, Percutaneous Endoscopic Approach

Ø2114AF   Bypass Coronary Artery, Two Arteries from Abdominal Artery with Autologous Arterial Tissue, Percutaneous Endoscopic Approach

Appendix K: Hospital Acquired Conditions

HAC 08: Surgical Site Infection of Mediastinitis After Coronary Bypass Graft (CABG) Procedures (continued)

Ø2114AW Bypass Coronary Artery, Two Arteries from Aorta with Autologous Arterial Tissue, Percutaneous Endoscopic Approach

Ø2114J3 Bypass Coronary Artery, Two Arteries from Coronary Artery with Synthetic Substitute, Percutaneous Endoscopic Approach

Ø2114J8 Bypass Coronary Artery, Two Arteries from Right Internal Mammary with Synthetic Substitute, Percutaneous Endoscopic Approach

Ø2114J9 Bypass Coronary Artery, Two Arteries from Left Internal Mammary with Synthetic Substitute, Percutaneous Endoscopic Approach

Ø2114JC Bypass Coronary Artery, Two Arteries from Thoracic Artery with Synthetic Substitute, Percutaneous Endoscopic Approach

Ø2114JF Bypass Coronary Artery, Two Arteries from Abdominal Artery with Synthetic Substitute, Percutaneous Endoscopic Approach

Ø2114JW Bypass Coronary Artery, Two Arteries from Aorta with Synthetic Substitute, Percutaneous Endoscopic Approach

Ø2114K3 Bypass Coronary Artery, Two Arteries from Coronary Artery with Nonautologous Tissue Substitute, Percutaneous Endoscopic Approach

Ø2114K8 Bypass Coronary Artery, Two Arteries from Right Internal Mammary with Nonautologous Tissue Substitute, Percutaneous Endoscopic Approach

Ø2114K9 Bypass Coronary Artery, Two Arteries from Left Internal Mammary with Nonautologous Tissue Substitute, Percutaneous Endoscopic Approach

Ø2114KC Bypass Coronary Artery, Two Arteries from Thoracic Artery with Nonautologous Tissue Substitute, Percutaneous Endoscopic Approach

Ø2114KF Bypass Coronary Artery, Two Arteries from Abdominal Artery with Nonautologous Tissue Substitute, Percutaneous Endoscopic Approach

Ø2114KW Bypass Coronary Artery, Two Arteries from Aorta with Nonautologous Tissue Substitute, Percutaneous Endoscopic Approach

Ø2114Z3 Bypass Coronary Artery, Two Arteries from Coronary Artery, Percutaneous Endoscopic Approach

Ø2114Z8 Bypass Coronary Artery, Two Arteries from Right Internal Mammary, Percutaneous Endoscopic Approach

Ø2114Z9 Bypass Coronary Artery, Two Arteries from Left Internal Mammary, Percutaneous Endoscopic Approach

Ø2114ZC Bypass Coronary Artery, Two Arteries from Thoracic Artery, Percutaneous Endoscopic Approach

Ø2114ZF Bypass Coronary Artery, Two Arteries from Abdominal Artery, Percutaneous Endoscopic Approach

Ø212Ø83 Bypass Coronary Artery, Three Arteries from Coronary Artery with Zooplastic Tissue, Open Approach

Ø212Ø88 Bypass Coronary Artery, Three Arteries from Right Internal Mammary with Zooplastic Tissue, Open Approach

Ø212Ø89 Bypass Coronary Artery, Three Arteries from Left Internal Mammary with Zooplastic Tissue, Open Approach

Ø212Ø8C Bypass Coronary Artery, Three Arteries from Thoracic Artery with Zooplastic Tissue, Open Approach

Ø212Ø8F Bypass Coronary Artery, Three Arteries from Abdominal Artery with Zooplastic Tissue, Open Approach

Ø212Ø8W Bypass Coronary Artery, Three Arteries from Aorta with Zooplastic Tissue, Open Approach

Ø212Ø93 Bypass Coronary Artery, Three Arteries from Coronary Artery with Autologous Venous Tissue, Open Approach

Ø212Ø98 Bypass Coronary Artery, Three Arteries from Right Internal Mammary with Autologous Venous Tissue, Open Approach

Ø212Ø99 Bypass Coronary Artery, Three Arteries from Left Internal Mammary with Autologous Venous Tissue, Open Approach

Ø212Ø9C Bypass Coronary Artery, Three Arteries from Thoracic Artery with Autologous Venous Tissue, Open Approach

Ø212Ø9F Bypass Coronary Artery, Three Arteries from Abdominal Artery with Autologous Venous Tissue, Open Approach

Ø212Ø9W Bypass Coronary Artery, Three Arteries from Aorta with Autologous Venous Tissue, Open Approach

Ø212ØA3 Bypass Coronary Artery, Three Arteries from Coronary Artery with Autologous Arterial Tissue, Open Approach

Ø212ØA8 Bypass Coronary Artery, Three Arteries from Right Internal Mammary with Autologous Arterial Tissue, Open Approach

Ø212ØA9 Bypass Coronary Artery, Three Arteries from Left Internal Mammary with Autologous Arterial Tissue, Open Approach

Ø212ØAC Bypass Coronary Artery, Three Arteries from Thoracic Artery with Autologous Arterial Tissue, Open Approach

Ø212ØAF Bypass Coronary Artery, Three Arteries from Abdominal Artery with Autologous Arterial Tissue, Open Approach

Ø212ØAW Bypass Coronary Artery, Three Arteries from Aorta with Autologous Arterial Tissue, Open Approach

Ø212ØJ3 Bypass Coronary Artery, Three Arteries from Coronary Artery with Synthetic Substitute, Open Approach

Ø212ØJ8 Bypass Coronary Artery, Three Arteries from Right Internal Mammary with Synthetic Substitute, Open Approach

Ø212ØJ9 Bypass Coronary Artery, Three Arteries from Left Internal Mammary with Synthetic Substitute, Open Approach

Ø212ØJC Bypass Coronary Artery, Three Arteries from Thoracic Artery with Synthetic Substitute, Open Approach

Ø212ØJF Bypass Coronary Artery, Three Arteries from Abdominal Artery with Synthetic Substitute, Open Approach

Ø212ØJW Bypass Coronary Artery, Three Arteries from Aorta with Synthetic Substitute, Open Approach

Ø212ØK3 Bypass Coronary Artery, Three Arteries from Coronary Artery with Nonautologous Tissue Substitute, Open Approach

Ø212ØK8 Bypass Coronary Artery, Three Arteries from Right Internal Mammary with Nonautologous Tissue Substitute, Open Approach

Ø212ØK9 Bypass Coronary Artery, Three Arteries from Left Internal Mammary with Nonautologous Tissue Substitute, Open Approach

Ø212ØKC Bypass Coronary Artery, Three Arteries from Thoracic Artery with Nonautologous Tissue Substitute, Open Approach

Ø212ØKF Bypass Coronary Artery, Three Arteries from Abdominal Artery with Nonautologous Tissue Substitute, Open Approach

Ø212ØKW Bypass Coronary Artery, Three Arteries from Aorta with Nonautologous Tissue Substitute, Open Approach

Ø212ØZ3 Bypass Coronary Artery, Three Arteries from Coronary Artery, Open Approach

Ø212ØZ8 Bypass Coronary Artery, Three Arteries from Right Internal Mammary, Open Approach

Ø212ØZ9 Bypass Coronary Artery, Three Arteries from Left Internal Mammary, Open Approach

Ø212ØZC Bypass Coronary Artery, Three Arteries from Thoracic Artery, Open Approach

Ø212ØZF Bypass Coronary Artery, Three Arteries from Abdominal Artery, Open Approach

Ø21248 3 Bypass Coronary Artery, Three Arteries from Coronary Artery with Zooplastic Tissue, Percutaneous Endoscopic Approach

Ø21248 8 Bypass Coronary Artery, Three Arteries from Right Internal Mammary with Zooplastic Tissue, Percutaneous Endoscopic Approach

Ø21248 9 Bypass Coronary Artery, Three Arteries from Left Internal Mammary with Zooplastic Tissue, Percutaneous Endoscopic Approach

Ø21248C Bypass Coronary Artery, Three Arteries from Thoracic Artery with Zooplastic Tissue, Percutaneous Endoscopic Approach

Ø21248F Bypass Coronary Artery, Three Arteries from Abdominal Artery with Zooplastic Tissue, Percutaneous Endoscopic Approach

Ø21248W Bypass Coronary Artery, Three Arteries from Aorta with Zooplastic Tissue, Percutaneous Endoscopic Approach

Ø21249 3 Bypass Coronary Artery, Three Arteries from Coronary Artery with Autologous Venous Tissue, Percutaneous Endoscopic Approach

Ø21249 8 Bypass Coronary Artery, Three Arteries from Right Internal Mammary with Autologous Venous Tissue, Percutaneous Endoscopic Approach

Ø21249 9 Bypass Coronary Artery, Three Arteries from Left Internal Mammary with Autologous Venous Tissue, Percutaneous Endoscopic Approach

Ø21249C Bypass Coronary Artery, Three Arteries from Thoracic Artery with Autologous Venous Tissue, Percutaneous Endoscopic Approach

Ø21249F Bypass Coronary Artery, Three Arteries from Abdominal Artery with Autologous Venous Tissue, Percutaneous Endoscopic Approach

Ø21249W Bypass Coronary Artery, Three Arteries from Aorta with Autologous Venous Tissue, Percutaneous Endoscopic Approach

HAC 08: Surgical Site Infection of Mediastinitis After Coronary Bypass Graft (CABG) Procedures (continued)

02124A3 Bypass Coronary Artery, Three Arteries from Coronary Artery with Autologous Arterial Tissue, Percutaneous Endoscopic Approach

02124A8 Bypass Coronary Artery, Three Arteries from Right Internal Mammary with Autologous Arterial Tissue, Percutaneous Endoscopic Approach

02124A9 Bypass Coronary Artery, Three Arteries from Left Internal Mammary with Autologous Arterial Tissue, Percutaneous Endoscopic Approach

02124AC Bypass Coronary Artery, Three Arteries from Thoracic Artery with Autologous Arterial Tissue, Percutaneous Endoscopic Approach

02124AF Bypass Coronary Artery, Three Arteries from Abdominal Artery with Autologous Arterial Tissue, Percutaneous Endoscopic Approach

02124AW Bypass Coronary Artery, Three Arteries from Aorta with Autologous Arterial Tissue, Percutaneous Endoscopic Approach

02124J3 Bypass Coronary Artery, Three Arteries from Coronary Artery with Synthetic Substitute, Percutaneous Endoscopic Approach

02124J8 Bypass Coronary Artery, Three Arteries from Right Internal Mammary with Synthetic Substitute, Percutaneous Endoscopic Approach

02124J9 Bypass Coronary Artery, Three Arteries from Left Internal Mammary with Synthetic Substitute, Percutaneous Endoscopic Approach

02124JC Bypass Coronary Artery, Three Arteries from Thoracic Artery with Synthetic Substitute, Percutaneous Endoscopic Approach

02124JF Bypass Coronary Artery, Three Arteries from Abdominal Artery with Synthetic Substitute, Percutaneous Endoscopic Approach

02124JW Bypass Coronary Artery, Three Arteries from Aorta with Synthetic Substitute, Percutaneous Endoscopic Approach

02124K3 Bypass Coronary Artery, Three Arteries from Coronary Artery with Nonautologous Tissue Substitute, Percutaneous Endoscopic Approach

02124K8 Bypass Coronary Artery, Three Arteries from Right Internal Mammary with Nonautologous Tissue Substitute, Percutaneous Endoscopic Approach

02124K9 Bypass Coronary Artery, Three Arteries from Left Internal Mammary with Nonautologous Tissue Substitute, Percutaneous Endoscopic Approach

02124KC Bypass Coronary Artery, Three Arteries from Thoracic Artery with Nonautologous Tissue Substitute, Percutaneous Endoscopic Approach

02124KF Bypass Coronary Artery, Three Arteries from Abdominal Artery with Nonautologous Tissue Substitute, Percutaneous Endoscopic Approach

02124KW Bypass Coronary Artery, Three Arteries from Aorta with Nonautologous Tissue Substitute, Percutaneous Endoscopic Approach

02124Z3 Bypass Coronary Artery, Three Arteries from Coronary Artery, Percutaneous Endoscopic Approach

02124Z8 Bypass Coronary Artery, Three Arteries from Right Internal Mammary, Percutaneous Endoscopic Approach

02124Z9 Bypass Coronary Artery, Three Arteries from Left Internal Mammary, Percutaneous Endoscopic Approach

02124ZC Bypass Coronary Artery, Three Arteries from Thoracic Artery, Percutaneous Endoscopic Approach

02124ZF Bypass Coronary Artery, Three Arteries from Abdominal Artery, Percutaneous Endoscopic Approach

0213083 Bypass Coronary Artery, Four or More Arteries from Coronary Artery with Zooplastic Tissue, Open Approach

0213088 Bypass Coronary Artery, Four or More Arteries from Right Internal Mammary with Zooplastic Tissue, Open Approach

0213089 Bypass Coronary Artery, Four or More Arteries from Left Internal Mammary with Zooplastic Tissue, Open Approach

021308C Bypass Coronary Artery, Four or More Arteries from Thoracic Artery with Zooplastic Tissue, Open Approach

021308F Bypass Coronary Artery, Four or More Arteries from Abdominal Artery with Zooplastic Tissue, Open Approach

021308W Bypass Coronary Artery, Four or More Arteries from Aorta with Zooplastic Tissue, Open Approach

0213093 Bypass Coronary Artery, Four or More Arteries from Coronary Artery with Autologous Venous Tissue, Open Approach

0213098 Bypass Coronary Artery, Four or More Arteries from Right Internal Mammary with Autologous Venous Tissue, Open Approach

0213099 Bypass Coronary Artery, Four or More Arteries from Left Internal Mammary with Autologous Venous Tissue, Open Approach

021309C Bypass Coronary Artery, Four or More Arteries from Thoracic Artery with Autologous Venous Tissue, Open Approach

021309F Bypass Coronary Artery, Four or More Arteries from Abdominal Artery with Autologous Venous Tissue, Open Approach

021309W Bypass Coronary Artery, Four or More Arteries from Aorta with Autologous Venous Tissue, Open Approach

02130A3 Bypass Coronary Artery, Four or More Arteries from Coronary Artery with Autologous Arterial Tissue, Open Approach

02130A8 Bypass Coronary Artery, Four or More Arteries from Right Internal Mammary with Autologous Arterial Tissue, Open Approach

02130A9 Bypass Coronary Artery, Four or More Arteries from Left Internal Mammary with Autologous Arterial Tissue, Open Approach

02130AC Bypass Coronary Artery, Four or More Arteries from Thoracic Artery with Autologous Arterial Tissue, Open Approach

02130AF Bypass Coronary Artery, Four or More Arteries from Abdominal Artery with Autologous Arterial Tissue, Open Approach

02130AW Bypass Coronary Artery, Four or More Arteries from Aorta with Autologous Arterial Tissue, Open Approach

02130J3 Bypass Coronary Artery, Four or More Arteries from Coronary Artery with Synthetic Substitute, Open Approach

02130J8 Bypass Coronary Artery, Four or More Arteries from Right Internal Mammary with Synthetic Substitute, Open Approach

02130J9 Bypass Coronary Artery, Four or More Arteries from Left Internal Mammary with Synthetic Substitute, Open Approach

02130JC Bypass Coronary Artery, Four or More Arteries from Thoracic Artery with Synthetic Substitute, Open Approach

02130JF Bypass Coronary Artery, Four or More Arteries from Abdominal Artery with Synthetic Substitute, Open Approach

02130JW Bypass Coronary Artery, Four or More Arteries from Aorta with Synthetic Substitute, Open Approach

02130K3 Bypass Coronary Artery, Four or More Arteries from Coronary Artery with Nonautologous Tissue Substitute, Open Approach

02130K8 Bypass Coronary Artery, Four or More Arteries from Right Internal Mammary with Nonautologous Tissue Substitute, Open Approach

02130K9 Bypass Coronary Artery, Four or More Arteries from Left Internal Mammary with Nonautologous Tissue Substitute, Open Approach

02130KC Bypass Coronary Artery, Four or More Arteries from Thoracic Artery with Nonautologous Tissue Substitute, Open Approach

02130KF Bypass Coronary Artery, Four or More Arteries from Abdominal Artery with Nonautologous Tissue Substitute, Open Approach

02130KW Bypass Coronary Artery, Four or More Arteries from Aorta with Nonautologous Tissue Substitute, Open Approach

02130Z3 Bypass Coronary Artery, Four or More Arteries from Coronary Artery, Open Approach

02130Z8 Bypass Coronary Artery, Four or More Arteries from Right Internal Mammary, Open Approach

02130Z9 Bypass Coronary Artery, Four or More Arteries from Left Internal Mammary, Open Approach

02130ZC Bypass Coronary Artery, Four or More Arteries from Thoracic Artery, Open Approach

02130ZF Bypass Coronary Artery, Four or More Arteries from Abdominal Artery, Open Approach

0213483 Bypass Coronary Artery, Four or More Arteries from Coronary Artery with Zooplastic Tissue, Percutaneous Endoscopic Approach

0213488 Bypass Coronary Artery, Four or More Arteries from Right Internal Mammary with Zooplastic Tissue, Percutaneous Endoscopic Approach

0213489 Bypass Coronary Artery, Four or More Arteries from Left Internal Mammary with Zooplastic Tissue, Percutaneous Endoscopic Approach

021348C Bypass Coronary Artery, Four or More Arteries from Thoracic Artery with Zooplastic Tissue, Percutaneous Endoscopic Approach

HAC 08: Surgical Site Infection of Mediastinitis After Coronary Bypass Graft (CABG) Procedures (continued)

021348F Bypass Coronary Artery, Four or More Arteries from Abdominal Artery with Zooplastic Tissue, Percutaneous Endoscopic Approach

021348W Bypass Coronary Artery, Four or More Arteries from Aorta with Zooplastic Tissue, Percutaneous Endoscopic Approach

0213493 Bypass Coronary Artery, Four or More Arteries from Coronary Artery with Autologous Venous Tissue, Percutaneous Endoscopic Approach

0213498 Bypass Coronary Artery, Four or More Arteries from Right Internal Mammary with Autologous Venous Tissue, Percutaneous Endoscopic Approach

0213499 Bypass Coronary Artery, Four or More Arteries from Left Internal Mammary with Autologous Venous Tissue, Percutaneous Endoscopic Approach

021349C Bypass Coronary Artery, Four or More Arteries from Thoracic Artery with Autologous Venous Tissue, Percutaneous Endoscopic Approach

021349F Bypass Coronary Artery, Four or More Arteries from Abdominal Artery with Autologous Venous Tissue, Percutaneous Endoscopic Approach

021349W Bypass Coronary Artery, Four or More Arteries from Aorta with Autologous Venous Tissue, Percutaneous Endoscopic Approach

02134A3 Bypass Coronary Artery, Four or More Arteries from Coronary Artery with Autologous Arterial Tissue, Percutaneous Endoscopic Approach

02134A8 Bypass Coronary Artery, Four or More Arteries from Right Internal Mammary with Autologous Arterial Tissue, Percutaneous Endoscopic Approach

02134A9 Bypass Coronary Artery, Four or More Arteries from Left Internal Mammary with Autologous Arterial Tissue, Percutaneous Endoscopic Approach

02134AC Bypass Coronary Artery, Four or More Arteries from Thoracic Artery with Autologous Arterial Tissue, Percutaneous Endoscopic Approach

02134AF Bypass Coronary Artery, Four or More Arteries from Abdominal Artery with Autologous Arterial Tissue, Percutaneous Endoscopic Approach

02134AW Bypass Coronary Artery, Four or More Arteries from Aorta with Autologous Arterial Tissue, Percutaneous Endoscopic Approach

02134J3 Bypass Coronary Artery, Four or More Arteries from Coronary Artery with Synthetic Substitute, Percutaneous Endoscopic Approach

02134J8 Bypass Coronary Artery, Four or More Arteries from Right Internal Mammary with Synthetic Substitute, Percutaneous Endoscopic Approach

02134J9 Bypass Coronary Artery, Four or More Arteries from Left Internal Mammary with Synthetic Substitute, Percutaneous Endoscopic Approach

02134JC Bypass Coronary Artery, Four or More Arteries from Thoracic Artery with Synthetic Substitute, Percutaneous Endoscopic Approach

02134JF Bypass Coronary Artery, Four or More Arteries from Abdominal Artery with Synthetic Substitute, Percutaneous Endoscopic Approach

02134JW Bypass Coronary Artery, Four or More Arteries from Aorta with Synthetic Substitute, Percutaneous Endoscopic Approach

02134K3 Bypass Coronary Artery, Four or More Arteries from Coronary Artery with Nonautologous Tissue Substitute, Percutaneous Endoscopic Approach

02134K8 Bypass Coronary Artery, Four or More Arteries from Right Internal Mammary with Nonautologous Tissue Substitute, Percutaneous Endoscopic Approach

02134K9 Bypass Coronary Artery, Four or More Arteries from Left Internal Mammary with Nonautologous Tissue Substitute, Percutaneous Endoscopic Approach

02134KC Bypass Coronary Artery, Four or More Arteries from Thoracic Artery with Nonautologous Tissue Substitute, Percutaneous Endoscopic Approach

02134KF Bypass Coronary Artery, Four or More Arteries from Abdominal Artery with Nonautologous Tissue Substitute, Percutaneous Endoscopic Approach

02134KW Bypass Coronary Artery, Four or More Arteries from Aorta with Nonautologous Tissue Substitute, Percutaneous Endoscopic Approach

02134Z3 Bypass Coronary Artery, Four or More Arteries from Coronary Artery, Percutaneous Endoscopic Approach

02134Z8 Bypass Coronary Artery, Four or More Arteries from Right Internal Mammary, Percutaneous Endoscopic Approach

02134Z9 Bypass Coronary Artery, Four or More Arteries from Left Internal Mammary, Percutaneous Endoscopic Approach

02134ZC Bypass Coronary Artery, Four or More Arteries from Thoracic Artery, Percutaneous Endoscopic Approach

02134ZF Bypass Coronary Artery, Four or More Arteries from Abdominal Artery, Percutaneous Endoscopic Approach

HAC 10: Deep Vein Thrombosis (DVT) or Pulmonary Embolism (PE) with Total Knee or Hip Replacement

Secondary diagnosis not POA:

I26.02 Saddle embolus of pulmonary artery with acute cor pulmonale

I26.09 Other pulmonary embolism with acute cor pulmonale

I26.92 Saddle embolus of pulmonary artery without acute cor pulmonale

I26.93 Single subsegmental pulmonary embolism without acute cor pulmonale

I26.94 Multiple subsegmental pulmonary emboli without acute cor pulmonale

I26.99 Other pulmonary embolism without acute cor pulmonale

I82.401 Acute embolism and thrombosis of unspecified deep veins of right lower extremity

I82.402 Acute embolism and thrombosis of unspecified deep veins of left lower extremity

I82.403 Acute embolism and thrombosis of unspecified deep veins of lower extremity, bilateral

I82.409 Acute embolism and thrombosis of unspecified deep veins of unspecified lower extremity

I82.411 Acute embolism and thrombosis of right femoral vein

I82.412 Acute embolism and thrombosis of left femoral vein

I82.413 Acute embolism and thrombosis of femoral vein, bilateral

I82.419 Acute embolism and thrombosis of unspecified femoral vein

I82.421 Acute embolism and thrombosis of right iliac vein

I82.422 Acute embolism and thrombosis of left iliac vein

I82.423 Acute embolism and thrombosis of iliac vein, bilateral

I82.429 Acute embolism and thrombosis of unspecified iliac vein

I82.431 Acute embolism and thrombosis of right popliteal vein

I82.432 Acute embolism and thrombosis of left popliteal vein

I82.433 Acute embolism and thrombosis of popliteal vein, bilateral

I82.439 Acute embolism and thrombosis of unspecified popliteal vein

I82.441 Acute embolism and thrombosis of right tibial vein

I82.442 Acute embolism and thrombosis of left tibial vein

I82.443 Acute embolism and thrombosis of tibial vein, bilateral

I82.449 Acute embolism and thrombosis of unspecified tibial vein

I82.451 Acute embolism and thrombosis of right peroneal vein

I82.452 Acute embolism and thrombosis of left peroneal vein

I82.453 Acute embolism and thrombosis of peroneal vein, bilateral

I82.459 Acute embolism and thrombosis of unspecified peroneal vein

I82.491 Acute embolism and thrombosis of other specified deep vein of right lower extremity

I82.492 Acute embolism and thrombosis of other specified deep vein of left lower extremity

I82.493 Acute embolism and thrombosis of other specified deep vein of lower extremity, bilateral

I82.499 Acute embolism and thrombosis of other specified deep vein of unspecified lower extremity

I82.4Y1 Acute embolism and thrombosis of unspecified deep veins of right proximal lower extremity

I82.4Y2 Acute embolism and thrombosis of unspecified deep veins of left proximal lower extremity

I82.4Y3 Acute embolism and thrombosis of unspecified deep veins of proximal lower extremity, bilateral

I82.4Y9 Acute embolism and thrombosis of unspecified deep veins of unspecified proximal lower extremity

I82.4Z1 Acute embolism and thrombosis of unspecified deep veins of right distal lower extremity

I82.4Z2 Acute embolism and thrombosis of unspecified deep veins of left distal lower extremity

I82.4Z3 Acute embolism and thrombosis of unspecified deep veins of distal lower extremity, bilateral

I82.4Z9 Acute embolism and thrombosis of unspecified deep veins of unspecified distal lower extremity

HAC 10: Deep Vein Thrombosis (DVT) or Pulmonary Embolism (PE) with Total Knee or Hip Replacement (continued)

AND

Any of the following procedures:

ØSR9019 Replacement of Right Hip Joint with Metal Synthetic Substitute, Cemented, Open Approach

ØSR901A Replacement of Right Hip Joint with Metal Synthetic Substitute, Uncemented, Open Approach

ØSR901Z Replacement of Right Hip Joint with Metal Synthetic Substitute, Open Approach

ØSR9029 Replacement of Right Hip Joint with Metal on Polyethylene Synthetic Substitute, Cemented, Open Approach

ØSR902A Replacement of Right Hip Joint with Metal on Polyethylene Synthetic Substitute, Uncemented, Open Approach

ØSR902Z Replacement of Right Hip Joint with Metal on Polyethylene Synthetic Substitute, Open Approach

ØSR9039 Replacement of Right Hip Joint with Ceramic Synthetic Substitute, Cemented, Open Approach

ØSR903A Replacement of Right Hip Joint with Ceramic Synthetic Substitute, Uncemented, Open Approach

ØSR903Z Replacement of Right Hip Joint with Ceramic Synthetic Substitute, Open Approach

ØSR9049 Replacement of Right Hip Joint with Ceramic on Polyethylene Synthetic Substitute, Cemented, Open Approach

ØSR904A Replacement of Right Hip Joint with Ceramic on Polyethylene Synthetic Substitute, Uncemented, Open Approach

ØSR904Z Replacement of Right Hip Joint with Ceramic on Polyethylene Synthetic Substitute, Open Approach

ØSR9069 Replacement of Right Hip Joint with Oxidized Zirconium on Polyethylene Synthetic Substitute, Cemented, Open Approach

ØSR906A Replacement of Right Hip Joint with Oxidized Zirconium on Polyethylene Synthetic Substitute, Uncemented, Open Approach

ØSR906Z Replacement of Right Hip Joint with Oxidized Zirconium on Polyethylene Synthetic Substitute, Open Approach

ØSR907Z Replacement of Right Hip Joint with Autologous Tissue Substitute, Open Approach

ØSR90EZ Replacement of Right Hip Joint with Articulating Spacer, Open Approach

ØSR90J9 Replacement of Right Hip Joint with Synthetic Substitute, Cemented, Open Approach

ØSR90JA Replacement of Right Hip Joint with Synthetic Substitute, Uncemented, Open Approach

ØSR90JZ Replacement of Right Hip Joint with Synthetic Substitute, Open Approach

ØSR90KZ Replacement of Right Hip Joint with Nonautologous Tissue Substitute, Open Approach

ØSRAØØ9 Replacement of Right Hip Joint, Acetabular Surface with Polyethylene Synthetic Substitute, Cemented, Open Approach

ØSRAØØA Replacement of Right Hip Joint, Acetabular Surface with Polyethylene Synthetic Substitute, Uncemented, Open Approach

ØSRAØØZ Replacement of Right Hip Joint, Acetabular Surface with Polyethylene Synthetic Substitute, Open Approach

ØSRAØ19 Replacement of Right Hip Joint, Acetabular Surface with Metal Synthetic Substitute, Cemented, Open Approach

ØSRAØ1A Replacement of Right Hip Joint, Acetabular Surface with Metal Synthetic Substitute, Uncemented, Open Approach

ØSRAØ1Z Replacement of Right Hip Joint, Acetabular Surface with Metal Synthetic Substitute, Open Approach

ØSRAØ39 Replacement of Right Hip Joint, Acetabular Surface with Ceramic Synthetic Substitute, Cemented, Open Approach

ØSRAØ3A Replacement of Right Hip Joint, Acetabular Surface with Ceramic Synthetic Substitute, Uncemented, Open Approach

ØSRAØ3Z Replacement of Right Hip Joint, Acetabular Surface with Ceramic Synthetic Substitute, Open Approach

ØSRAØ7Z Replacement of Right Hip Joint, Acetabular Surface with Autologous Tissue Substitute, Open Approach

ØSRAØJ9 Replacement of Right Hip Joint, Acetabular Surface with Synthetic Substitute, Cemented, Open Approach

ØSRAØJA Replacement of Right Hip Joint, Acetabular Surface with Synthetic Substitute, Uncemented, Open Approach

ØSRAØJZ Replacement of Right Hip Joint, Acetabular Surface with Synthetic Substitute, Open Approach

ØSRAØKZ Replacement of Right Hip Joint, Acetabular Surface with Nonautologous Tissue Substitute, Open Approach

ØSRBØ19 Replacement of Left Hip Joint with Metal Synthetic Substitute, Cemented, Open Approach

ØSRBØ1A Replacement of Left Hip Joint with Metal Synthetic Substitute, Uncemented, Open Approach

ØSRBØ1Z Replacement of Left Hip Joint with Metal Synthetic Substitute, Open Approach

ØSRBØ29 Replacement of Left Hip Joint with Metal on Polyethylene Synthetic Substitute, Cemented, Open Approach

ØSRBØ2A Replacement of Left Hip Joint with Metal on Polyethylene Synthetic Substitute, Uncemented, Open Approach

ØSRBØ2Z Replacement of Left Hip Joint with Metal on Polyethylene Synthetic Substitute, Open Approach

ØSRBØ39 Replacement of Left Hip Joint with Ceramic Synthetic Substitute, Cemented, Open Approach

ØSRBØ3A Replacement of Left Hip Joint with Ceramic Synthetic Substitute, Uncemented, Open Approach

ØSRBØ3Z Replacement of Left Hip Joint with Ceramic Synthetic Substitute, Open Approach

ØSRBØ49 Replacement of Left Hip Joint with Ceramic on Polyethylene Synthetic Substitute, Cemented, Open Approach

ØSRBØ4A Replacement of Left Hip Joint with Ceramic on Polyethylene Synthetic Substitute, Uncemented, Open Approach

ØSRBØ4Z Replacement of Left Hip Joint with Ceramic on Polyethylene Synthetic Substitute, Open Approach

ØSRBØ69 Replacement of Left Hip Joint with Oxidized Zirconium on Polyethylene Synthetic Substitute, Cemented, Open Approach

ØSRBØ6A Replacement of Left Hip Joint with Oxidized Zirconium on Polyethylene Synthetic Substitute, Uncemented, Open Approach

ØSRBØ6Z Replacement of Left Hip Joint with Oxidized Zirconium on Polyethylene Synthetic Substitute, Open Approach

ØSRBØ7Z Replacement of Left Hip Joint with Autologous Tissue Substitute, Open Approach

ØSRBØEZ Replacement of Left Hip Joint with Articulating Spacer, Open Approach

ØSRBØJ9 Replacement of Left Hip Joint with Synthetic Substitute, Cemented, Open Approach

ØSRBØJA Replacement of Left Hip Joint with Synthetic Substitute, Uncemented, Open Approach

ØSRBØJZ Replacement of Left Hip Joint with Synthetic Substitute, Open Approach

ØSRBØKZ Replacement of Left Hip Joint with Nonautologous Tissue Substitute, Open Approach

ØSRC069 Replacement of Right Knee Joint with Oxidized Zirconium on Polyethylene Synthetic Substitute, Cemented, Open Approach

ØSRC06A Replacement of Right Knee Joint with Oxidized Zirconium on Polyethylene Synthetic Substitute, Uncemented, Open Approach

ØSRC06Z Replacement of Right Knee Joint with Oxidized Zirconium on Polyethylene Synthetic Substitute, Open Approach

ØSRC07Z Replacement of Right Knee Joint with Autologous Tissue Substitute, Open Approach

ØSRC0EZ Replacement of Right Knee Joint with Articulating Spacer, Open Approach

ØSRC0J9 Replacement of Right Knee Joint with Synthetic Substitute, Cemented, Open Approach

ØSRC0JA Replacement of Right Knee Joint with Synthetic Substitute, Uncemented, Open Approach

ØSRC0JZ Replacement of Right Knee Joint with Synthetic Substitute, Open Approach

ØSRC0KZ Replacement of Right Knee Joint with Nonautologous Tissue Substitute, Open Approach

ØSRC0L9 Replacement of Right Knee Joint with Medial Unicondylar Synthetic Substitute, Cemented, Open Approach

ØSRC0LA Replacement of Right Knee Joint with Medial Unicondylar Synthetic Substitute, Uncemented, Open Approach

ØSRC0LZ Replacement of Right Knee Joint with Medial Unicondylar Synthetic Substitute, Open Approach

ØSRC0M9 Replacement of Right Knee Joint with Lateral Unicondylar Synthetic Substitute, Cemented, Open Approach

ØSRC0MA Replacement of Right Knee Joint with Lateral Unicondylar Synthetic Substitute, Uncemented, Open Approach

ØSRC0MZ Replacement of Right Knee Joint with Lateral Unicondylar Synthetic Substitute, Open Approach

ØSRC0N9 Replacement of Right Knee Joint with Patellofemoral Synthetic Substitute, Cemented, Open Approach

ØSRC0NA Replacement of Right Knee Joint with Patellofemoral Synthetic Substitute, Uncemented, Open Approach

HAC 10: Deep Vein Thrombosis (DVT) or Pulmonary Embolism (PE) with Total Knee or Hip Replacement (continued)

ØSRCØNZ Replacement of Right Knee Joint with Patellofemoral Synthetic Substitute, Open Approach

ØSRDØ69 Replacement of Left Knee Joint with Oxidized Zirconium on Polyethylene Synthetic Substitute, Cemented, Open Approach

ØSRDØ6A Replacement of Left Knee Joint with Oxidized Zirconium on Polyethylene Synthetic Substitute, Uncemented, Open Approach

ØSRDØ6Z Replacement of Left Knee Joint with Oxidized Zirconium on Polyethylene Synthetic Substitute, Open Approach

ØSRDØ7Z Replacement of Left Knee Joint with Autologous Tissue Substitute, Open Approach

ØSRDØEZ Replacement of Left Knee Joint with Articulating Spacer, Open Approach

ØSRDØJ9 Replacement of Left Knee Joint with Synthetic Substitute, Cemented, Open Approach

ØSRDØJA Replacement of Left Knee Joint with Synthetic Substitute, Uncemented, Open Approach

ØSRDØJZ Replacement of Left Knee Joint with Synthetic Substitute, Open Approach

ØSRDØKZ Replacement of Left Knee Joint with Nonautologous Tissue Substitute, Open Approach

ØSRDØL9 Replacement of Left Knee Joint with Medial Unicondylar Synthetic Substitute, Cemented, Open Approach

ØSRDØLA Replacement of Left Knee Joint with Medial Unicondylar Synthetic Substitute, Uncemented, Open Approach

ØSRDØLZ Replacement of Left Knee Joint with Medial Unicondylar Synthetic Substitute, Open Approach

ØSRDØM9 Replacement of Left Knee Joint with Lateral Unicondylar Synthetic Substitute, Cemented, Open Approach

ØSRDØMA Replacement of Left Knee Joint with Lateral Unicondylar Synthetic Substitute, Uncemented, Open Approach

ØSRDØMZ Replacement of Left Knee Joint with Lateral Unicondylar Synthetic Substitute, Open Approach

ØSRDØN9 Replacement of Left Knee Joint with Patellofemoral Synthetic Substitute, Cemented, Open Approach

ØSRDØNA Replacement of Left Knee Joint with Patellofemoral Synthetic Substitute, Uncemented, Open Approach

ØSRDØNZ Replacement of Left Knee Joint with Patellofemoral Synthetic Substitute, Open Approach

ØSREØØ9 Replacement of Left Hip Joint, Acetabular Surface with Polyethylene Synthetic Substitute, Cemented, Open Approach

ØSREØØA Replacement of Left Hip Joint, Acetabular Surface with Polyethylene Synthetic Substitute, Uncemented, Open Approach

ØSREØØZ Replacement of Left Hip Joint, Acetabular Surface with Polyethylene Synthetic Substitute, Open Approach

ØSREØ19 Replacement of Left Hip Joint, Acetabular Surface with Metal Synthetic Substitute, Cemented, Open Approach

ØSREØ1A Replacement of Left Hip Joint, Acetabular Surface with Metal Synthetic Substitute, Uncemented, Open Approach

ØSREØ1Z Replacement of Left Hip Joint, Acetabular Surface with Metal Synthetic Substitute, Open Approach

ØSREØ39 Replacement of Left Hip Joint, Acetabular Surface with Ceramic Synthetic Substitute, Cemented, Open Approach

ØSREØ3A Replacement of Left Hip Joint, Acetabular Surface with Ceramic Synthetic Substitute, Uncemented, Open Approach

ØSREØ3Z Replacement of Left Hip Joint, Acetabular Surface with Ceramic Synthetic Substitute, Open Approach

ØSREØ7Z Replacement of Left Hip Joint, Acetabular Surface with Autologous Tissue Substitute, Open Approach

ØSREØJ9 Replacement of Left Hip Joint, Acetabular Surface with Synthetic Substitute, Cemented, Open Approach

ØSREØJA Replacement of Left Hip Joint, Acetabular Surface with Synthetic Substitute, Uncemented, Open Approach

ØSREØJZ Replacement of Left Hip Joint, Acetabular Surface with Synthetic Substitute, Open Approach

ØSREØKZ Replacement of Left Hip Joint, Acetabular Surface with Nonautologous Tissue Substitute, Open Approach

ØSRRØ19 Replacement of Right Hip Joint, Femoral Surface with Metal Synthetic Substitute, Cemented, Open Approach

ØSRRØ1A Replacement of Right Hip Joint, Femoral Surface with Metal Synthetic Substitute, Uncemented, Open Approach

ØSRRØ1Z Replacement of Right Hip Joint, Femoral Surface with Metal Synthetic Substitute, Open Approach

ØSRRØ39 Replacement of Right Hip Joint, Femoral Surface with Ceramic Synthetic Substitute, Cemented, Open Approach

ØSRRØ3A Replacement of Right Hip Joint, Femoral Surface with Ceramic Synthetic Substitute, Uncemented, Open Approach

ØSRRØ3Z Replacement of Right Hip Joint, Femoral Surface with Ceramic Synthetic Substitute, Open Approach

ØSRRØ7Z Replacement of Right Hip Joint, Femoral Surface with Autologous Tissue Substitute, Open Approach

ØSRRØJ9 Replacement of Right Hip Joint, Femoral Surface with Synthetic Substitute, Cemented, Open Approach

ØSRRØJA Replacement of Right Hip Joint, Femoral Surface with Synthetic Substitute, Uncemented, Open Approach

ØSRRØJZ Replacement of Right Hip Joint, Femoral Surface with Synthetic Substitute, Open Approach

ØSRRØKZ Replacement of Right Hip Joint, Femoral Surface with Nonautologous Tissue Substitute, Open Approach

ØSRSØ19 Replacement of Left Hip Joint, Femoral Surface with Metal Synthetic Substitute, Cemented, Open Approach

ØSRSØ1A Replacement of Left Hip Joint, Femoral Surface with Metal Synthetic Substitute, Uncemented, Open Approach

ØSRSØ1Z Replacement of Left Hip Joint, Femoral Surface with Metal Synthetic Substitute, Open Approach

ØSRSØ39 Replacement of Left Hip Joint, Femoral Surface with Ceramic Synthetic Substitute, Cemented, Open Approach

ØSRSØ3A Replacement of Left Hip Joint, Femoral Surface with Ceramic Synthetic Substitute, Uncemented, Open Approach

ØSRSØ3Z Replacement of Left Hip Joint, Femoral Surface with Ceramic Synthetic Substitute, Open Approach

ØSRSØ7Z Replacement of Left Hip Joint, Femoral Surface with Autologous Tissue Substitute, Open Approach

ØSRSØJ9 Replacement of Left Hip Joint, Femoral Surface with Synthetic Substitute, Cemented, Open Approach

ØSRSØJA Replacement of Left Hip Joint, Femoral Surface with Synthetic Substitute, Uncemented, Open Approach

ØSRSØJZ Replacement of Left Hip Joint, Femoral Surface with Synthetic Substitute, Open Approach

ØSRSØKZ Replacement of Left Hip Joint, Femoral Surface with Nonautologous Tissue Substitute, Open Approach

ØSRTØ7Z Replacement of Right Knee Joint, Femoral Surface with Autologous Tissue Substitute, Open Approach

ØSRTØJ9 Replacement of Right Knee Joint, Femoral Surface with Synthetic Substitute, Cemented, Open Approach

ØSRTØJA Replacement of Right Knee Joint, Femoral Surface with Synthetic Substitute, Uncemented, Open Approach

ØSRTØJZ Replacement of Right Knee Joint, Femoral Surface with Synthetic Substitute, Open Approach

ØSRTØKZ Replacement of Right Knee Joint, Femoral Surface with Nonautologous Tissue Substitute, Open Approach

ØSRUØ7Z Replacement of Left Knee Joint, Femoral Surface with Autologous Tissue Substitute, Open Approach

ØSRUØJ9 Replacement of Left Knee Joint, Femoral Surface with Synthetic Substitute, Cemented, Open Approach

ØSRUØJA Replacement of Left Knee Joint, Femoral Surface with Synthetic Substitute, Uncemented, Open Approach

ØSRUØJZ Replacement of Left Knee Joint, Femoral Surface with Synthetic Substitute, Open Approach

ØSRUØKZ Replacement of Left Knee Joint, Femoral Surface with Nonautologous Tissue Substitute, Open Approach

ØSRVØ7Z Replacement of Right Knee Joint, Tibial Surface with Autologous Tissue Substitute, Open Approach

ØSRVØJ9 Replacement of Right Knee Joint, Tibial Surface with Synthetic Substitute, Cemented, Open Approach

ØSRVØJA Replacement of Right Knee Joint, Tibial Surface with Synthetic Substitute, Uncemented, Open Approach

ØSRVØJZ Replacement of Right Knee Joint, Tibial Surface with Synthetic Substitute, Open Approach

ØSRVØKZ Replacement of Right Knee Joint, Tibial Surface with Nonautologous Tissue Substitute, Open Approach

ØSRWØ7Z Replacement of Left Knee Joint, Tibial Surface with Autologous Tissue Substitute, Open Approach

ØSRWØJ9 Replacement of Left Knee Joint, Tibial Surface with Synthetic Substitute, Cemented, Open Approach

ØSRWØJA Replacement of Left Knee Joint, Tibial Surface with Synthetic Substitute, Uncemented, Open Approach

ØSRWØJZ Replacement of Left Knee Joint, Tibial Surface with Synthetic Substitute, Open Approach

HAC 10: Deep Vein Thrombosis (DVT) or Pulmonary Embolism (PE) with Total Knee or Hip Replacement (continued)

ØSRWØKZ Replacement of Left Knee Joint, Tibial Surface with Nonautologous Tissue Substitute, Open Approach
ØSU9ØBZ Supplement Right Hip Joint with Resurfacing Device, Open Approach
ØSUAØBZ Supplement Right Hip Joint, Acetabular Surface with Resurfacing Device, Open Approach
ØSUBØBZ Supplement Left Hip Joint with Resurfacing Device, Open Approach
ØSUEØBZ Supplement Left Hip Joint, Acetabular Surface with Resurfacing Device, Open Approach
ØSURØBZ Supplement Right Hip Joint, Femoral Surface with Resurfacing Device, Open Approach
ØSUSØBZ Supplement Left Hip Joint, Femoral Surface with Resurfacing Device, Open Approach

HAC 11: Surgical Site Infection-Bariatric Surgery

Principal diagnosis of:
E66.Ø1 Morbid (severe) obesity due to excess calories

AND

Secondary diagnosis not POA:
K68.11 Postprocedural retroperitoneal abscess
K95.Ø1 Infection due to gastric band procedure
K95.81 Infection due to other bariatric procedure
T81.4ØXA Infection following a procedure, unspecified, initial encounter
T81.41XA Infection following a procedure, superficial incisional surgical site, initial encounter
T81.42XA Infection following a procedure, deep incisional surgical site, initial encounter
T81.43XA Infection following a procedure, organ and space surgical site, initial encounter
T81.44XA Sepsis following a procedure, initial encounter
T81.49XA Infection following a procedure, other surgical site, initial encounter

AND

Any of the following procedures:
ØD16Ø79 Bypass Stomach to Duodenum with Autologous Tissue Substitute, Open Approach
ØD16Ø7A Bypass Stomach to Jejunum with Autologous Tissue Substitute, Open Approach
ØD16Ø7B Bypass Stomach to Ileum with Autologous Tissue Substitute, Open Approach
ØD16Ø7L Bypass Stomach to Transverse Colon with Autologous Tissue Substitute, Open Approach
ØD16ØJ9 Bypass Stomach to Duodenum with Synthetic Substitute, Open Approach
ØD16ØJA Bypass Stomach to Jejunum with Synthetic Substitute, Open Approach
ØD16ØJB Bypass Stomach to Ileum with Synthetic Substitute, Open Approach
ØD16ØJL Bypass Stomach to Transverse Colon with Synthetic Substitute, Open Approach
ØD16ØK9 Bypass Stomach to Duodenum with Nonautologous Tissue Substitute, Open Approach
ØD16ØKA Bypass Stomach to Jejunum with Nonautologous Tissue Substitute, Open Approach
ØD16ØKB Bypass Stomach to Ileum with Nonautologous Tissue Substitute, Open Approach

ØD16ØKL Bypass Stomach to Transverse Colon with Nonautologous Tissue Substitute, Open Approach
ØD16ØZ9 Bypass Stomach to Duodenum, Open Approach
ØD16ØZA Bypass Stomach to Jejunum, Open Approach
ØD16ØZB Bypass Stomach to Ileum, Open Approach
ØD16ØZL Bypass Stomach to Transverse Colon, Open Approach
ØD16479 Bypass Stomach to Duodenum with Autologous Tissue Substitute, Percutaneous Endoscopic Approach
ØD1647A Bypass Stomach to Jejunum with Autologous Tissue Substitute, Percutaneous Endoscopic Approach
ØD1647B Bypass Stomach to Ileum with Autologous Tissue Substitute, Percutaneous Endoscopic Approach
ØD1647L Bypass Stomach to Transverse Colon with Autologous Tissue Substitute, Percutaneous Endoscopic Approach
ØD164J9 Bypass Stomach to Duodenum with Synthetic Substitute, Percutaneous Endoscopic Approach
ØD164JA Bypass Stomach to Jejunum with Synthetic Substitute, Percutaneous Endoscopic Approach
ØD164JB Bypass Stomach to Ileum with Synthetic Substitute, Percutaneous Endoscopic Approach
ØD164JL Bypass Stomach to Transverse Colon with Synthetic Substitute, Percutaneous Endoscopic Approach
ØD164K9 Bypass Stomach to Duodenum with Nonautologous Tissue Substitute, Percutaneous Endoscopic Approach
ØD164KA Bypass Stomach to Jejunum with Nonautologous Tissue Substitute, Percutaneous Endoscopic Approach
ØD164KB Bypass Stomach to Ileum with Nonautologous Tissue Substitute, Percutaneous Endoscopic Approach
ØD164KL Bypass Stomach to Transverse Colon with Nonautologous Tissue Substitute, Percutaneous Endoscopic Approach
ØD164Z9 Bypass Stomach to Duodenum, Percutaneous Endoscopic Approach
ØD164ZA Bypass Stomach to Jejunum, Percutaneous Endoscopic Approach
ØD164ZB Bypass Stomach to Ileum, Percutaneous Endoscopic Approach
ØD164ZL Bypass Stomach to Transverse Colon, Percutaneous Endoscopic Approach
ØD16879 Bypass Stomach to Duodenum with Autologous Tissue Substitute, Via Natural or Artificial Opening Endoscopic
ØD1687A Bypass Stomach to Jejunum with Autologous Tissue Substitute, Via Natural or Artificial Opening Endoscopic
ØD1687B Bypass Stomach to Ileum with Autologous Tissue Substitute, Via Natural or Artificial Opening Endoscopic
ØD1687L Bypass Stomach to Transverse Colon with Autologous Tissue Substitute, Via Natural or Artificial Opening Endoscopic
ØD168J9 Bypass Stomach to Duodenum with Synthetic Substitute, Via Natural or Artificial Opening Endoscopic
ØD168JA Bypass Stomach to Jejunum with Synthetic Substitute, Via Natural or Artificial Opening Endoscopic
ØD168JB Bypass Stomach to Ileum with Synthetic Substitute, Via Natural or Artificial Opening Endoscopic

ØD168JL Bypass Stomach to Transverse Colon with Synthetic Substitute, Via Natural or Artificial Opening Endoscopic
ØD168K9 Bypass Stomach to Duodenum with Nonautologous Tissue Substitute, Via Natural or Artificial Opening Endoscopic
ØD168KA Bypass Stomach to Jejunum with Nonautologous Tissue Substitute, Via Natural or Artificial Opening Endoscopic
ØD168KB Bypass Stomach to Ileum with Nonautologous Tissue Substitute, Via Natural or Artificial Opening Endoscopic
ØD168KL Bypass Stomach to Transverse Colon with Nonautologous Tissue Substitute, Via Natural or Artificial Opening Endoscopic
ØD168Z9 Bypass Stomach to Duodenum, Via Natural or Artificial Opening Endoscopic
ØD168ZA Bypass Stomach to Jejunum, Via Natural or Artificial Opening Endoscopic
ØD168ZB Bypass Stomach to Ileum, Via Natural or Artificial Opening Endoscopic
ØD168ZL Bypass Stomach to Transverse Colon, Via Natural or Artificial Opening Endoscopic
ØDV64CZ Restriction of Stomach with Extraluminal Device, Percutaneous Endoscopic Approach

HAC 12: Surgical Site Infection-Certain Orthopedic Procedures of the Spine, Shoulder, and Elbow

Secondary diagnosis not POA:
K68.11 Postprocedural retroperitoneal abscess
T81.4ØXA Infection following a procedure, unspecified, initial encounter
T81.41XA Infection following a procedure, superficial incisional surgical site, initial encounter
T81.42XA Infection following a procedure, deep incisional surgical site, initial encounter
T81.43XA Infection following a procedure, organ and space surgical site, initial encounter
T81.44XA Sepsis following a procedure, initial encounter
T81.49XA Infection following a procedure, other surgical site, initial encounter
T84.6ØXA Infection and inflammatory reaction due to internal fixation device of unspecified site, initial encounter
T84.61ØA Infection and inflammatory reaction due to internal fixation device of right humerus, initial encounter
T84.611A Infection and inflammatory reaction due to internal fixation device of left humerus, initial encounter
T84.612A Infection and inflammatory reaction due to internal fixation device of right radius, initial encounter
T84.613A Infection and inflammatory reaction due to internal fixation device of left radius, initial encounter
T84.614A Infection and inflammatory reaction due to internal fixation device of right ulna, initial encounter
T84.615A Infection and inflammatory reaction due to internal fixation device of left ulna, initial encounter
T84.619A Infection and inflammatory reaction due to internal fixation device of unspecified bone of arm, initial encounter
T84.63XA Infection and inflammatory reaction due to internal fixation device of spine, initial encounter
T84.69XA Infection and inflammatory reaction due to internal fixation device of other site, initial encounter

HAC 12: Surgical Site Infection-Certain Orthopedic Procedures of the Spine, Shoulder, and Elbow (continued)

T84.7XXA Infection and inflammatory reaction due to other internal orthopedic prosthetic devices, implants and grafts, initial encounter

AND

Any of the following procedures:

ØRG0070 Fusion of Occipital-cervical Joint with Autologous Tissue Substitute, Anterior Approach, Anterior Column, Open Approach

ØRG0071 Fusion of Occipital-cervical Joint with Autologous Tissue Substitute, Posterior Approach, Posterior Column, Open Approach

ØRG007J Fusion of Occipital-cervical Joint with Autologous Tissue Substitute, Posterior Approach, Anterior Column, Open Approach

ØRG00A0 Fusion of Occipital-cervical Joint with Interbody Fusion Device, Anterior Approach, Anterior Column, Open Approach

ØRG00AJ Fusion of Occipital-cervical Joint with Interbody Fusion Device, Posterior Approach, Anterior Column, Open Approach

ØRG00J0 Fusion of Occipital-cervical Joint with Synthetic Substitute, Anterior Approach, Anterior Column, Open Approach

ØRG00J1 Fusion of Occipital-cervical Joint with Synthetic Substitute, Posterior Approach, Posterior Column, Open Approach

ØRG00JJ Fusion of Occipital-cervical Joint with Synthetic Substitute, Posterior Approach, Anterior Column, Open Approach

ØRG00K0 Fusion of Occipital-cervical Joint with Nonautologous Tissue Substitute, Anterior Approach, Anterior Column, Open Approach

ØRG00K1 Fusion of Occipital-cervical Joint with Nonautologous Tissue Substitute, Posterior Approach, Posterior Column, Open Approach

ØRG00KJ Fusion of Occipital-cervical Joint with Nonautologous Tissue Substitute, Posterior Approach, Anterior Column, Open Approach

ØRG0370 Fusion of Occipital-cervical Joint with Autologous Tissue Substitute, Anterior Approach, Anterior Column, Percutaneous Approach

ØRG0371 Fusion of Occipital-cervical Joint with Autologous Tissue Substitute, Posterior Approach, Posterior Column, Percutaneous Approach

ØRG037J Fusion of Occipital-cervical Joint with Autologous Tissue Substitute, Posterior Approach, Anterior Column, Percutaneous Approach

ØRG03A0 Fusion of Occipital-cervical Joint with Interbody Fusion Device, Anterior Approach, Anterior Column, Percutaneous Approach

ØRG03AJ Fusion of Occipital-cervical Joint with Interbody Fusion Device, Posterior Approach, Anterior Column, Percutaneous Approach

ØRG03J0 Fusion of Occipital-cervical Joint with Synthetic Substitute, Anterior Approach, Anterior Column, Percutaneous Approach

ØRG03J1 Fusion of Occipital-cervical Joint with Synthetic Substitute, Posterior Approach, Posterior Column, Percutaneous Approach

ØRG03JJ Fusion of Occipital-cervical Joint with Synthetic Substitute, Posterior Approach, Anterior Column, Percutaneous Approach

ØRG03K0 Fusion of Occipital-cervical Joint with Nonautologous Tissue Substitute, Anterior Approach, Anterior Column, Percutaneous Approach

ØRG03K1 Fusion of Occipital-cervical Joint with Nonautologous Tissue Substitute, Posterior Approach, Posterior Column, Percutaneous Approach

ØRG03KJ Fusion of Occipital-cervical Joint with Nonautologous Tissue Substitute, Posterior Approach, Anterior Column, Percutaneous Approach

ØRG0470 Fusion of Occipital-cervical Joint with Autologous Tissue Substitute, Anterior Approach, Anterior Column, Percutaneous Endoscopic Approach

ØRG0471 Fusion of Occipital-cervical Joint with Autologous Tissue Substitute, Posterior Approach, Posterior Column, Percutaneous Endoscopic Approach

ØRG047J Fusion of Occipital-cervical Joint with Autologous Tissue Substitute, Posterior Approach, Anterior Column, Percutaneous Endoscopic Approach

ØRG04A0 Fusion of Occipital-cervical Joint with Interbody Fusion Device, Anterior Approach, Anterior Column, Percutaneous Endoscopic Approach

ØRG04AJ Fusion of Occipital-cervical Joint with Interbody Fusion Device, Posterior Approach, Anterior Column, Percutaneous Endoscopic Approach

ØRG04J0 Fusion of Occipital-cervical Joint with Synthetic Substitute, Anterior Approach, Anterior Column, Percutaneous Endoscopic Approach

ØRG04J1 Fusion of Occipital-cervical Joint with Synthetic Substitute, Posterior Approach, Posterior Column, Percutaneous Endoscopic Approach

ØRG04JJ Fusion of Occipital-cervical Joint with Synthetic Substitute, Posterior Approach, Anterior Column, Percutaneous Endoscopic Approach

ØRG04K0 Fusion of Occipital-cervical Joint with Nonautologous Tissue Substitute, Anterior Approach, Anterior Column, Percutaneous Endoscopic Approach

ØRG04K1 Fusion of Occipital-cervical Joint with Nonautologous Tissue Substitute, Posterior Approach, Posterior Column, Percutaneous Endoscopic Approach

ØRG04KJ Fusion of Occipital-cervical Joint with Nonautologous Tissue Substitute, Posterior Approach, Anterior Column, Percutaneous Endoscopic Approach

ØRG1070 Fusion of Cervical Vertebral Joint with Autologous Tissue Substitute, Anterior Approach, Anterior Column, Open Approach

ØRG1071 Fusion of Cervical Vertebral Joint with Autologous Tissue Substitute, Posterior Approach, Posterior Column, Open Approach

ØRG107J Fusion of Cervical Vertebral Joint with Autologous Tissue Substitute, Posterior Approach, Anterior Column, Open Approach

ØRG10A0 Fusion of Cervical Vertebral Joint with Interbody Fusion Device, Anterior Approach, Anterior Column, Open Approach

ØRG10AJ Fusion of Cervical Vertebral Joint with Interbody Fusion Device, Posterior Approach, Anterior Column, Open Approach

ØRG10J0 Fusion of Cervical Vertebral Joint with Synthetic Substitute, Anterior Approach, Anterior Column, Open Approach

ØRG10J1 Fusion of Cervical Vertebral Joint with Synthetic Substitute, Posterior Approach, Posterior Column, Open Approach

ØRG10JJ Fusion of Cervical Vertebral Joint with Synthetic Substitute, Posterior Approach, Anterior Column, Open Approach

ØRG10K0 Fusion of Cervical Vertebral Joint with Nonautologous Tissue Substitute, Anterior Approach, Anterior Column, Open Approach

ØRG10K1 Fusion of Cervical Vertebral Joint with Nonautologous Tissue Substitute, Posterior Approach, Posterior Column, Open Approach

ØRG10KJ Fusion of Cervical Vertebral Joint with Nonautologous Tissue Substitute, Posterior Approach, Anterior Column, Open Approach

ØRG1370 Fusion of Cervical Vertebral Joint with Autologous Tissue Substitute, Anterior Approach, Anterior Column, Percutaneous Approach

ØRG1371 Fusion of Cervical Vertebral Joint with Autologous Tissue Substitute, Posterior Approach, Posterior Column, Percutaneous Approach

ØRG137J Fusion of Cervical Vertebral Joint with Autologous Tissue Substitute, Posterior Approach, Anterior Column, Percutaneous Approach

ØRG13A0 Fusion of Cervical Vertebral Joint with Interbody Fusion Device, Anterior Approach, Anterior Column, Percutaneous Approach

ØRG13AJ Fusion of Cervical Vertebral Joint with Interbody Fusion Device, Posterior Approach, Anterior Column, Percutaneous Approach

ØRG13J0 Fusion of Cervical Vertebral Joint with Synthetic Substitute, Anterior Approach, Anterior Column, Percutaneous Approach

ØRG13J1 Fusion of Cervical Vertebral Joint with Synthetic Substitute, Posterior Approach, Posterior Column, Percutaneous Approach

ØRG13JJ Fusion of Cervical Vertebral Joint with Synthetic Substitute, Posterior Approach, Anterior Column, Percutaneous Approach

ØRG13K0 Fusion of Cervical Vertebral Joint with Nonautologous Tissue Substitute, Anterior Approach, Anterior Column, Percutaneous Approach

ØRG13K1 Fusion of Cervical Vertebral Joint with Nonautologous Tissue Substitute, Posterior Approach, Posterior Column, Percutaneous Approach

ØRG13KJ Fusion of Cervical Vertebral Joint with Nonautologous Tissue Substitute, Posterior Approach, Anterior Column, Percutaneous Approach

ØRG1470 Fusion of Cervical Vertebral Joint with Autologous Tissue Substitute, Anterior Approach, Anterior Column, Percutaneous Endoscopic Approach

HAC 12: Surgical Site Infection-Certain Orthopedic Procedures of the Spine, Shoulder, and Elbow (continued)

ØRG1471 Fusion of Cervical Vertebral Joint with Autologous Tissue Substitute, Posterior Approach, Posterior Column, Percutaneous Endoscopic Approach

ØRG147J Fusion of Cervical Vertebral Joint with Autologous Tissue Substitute, Posterior Approach, Anterior Column, Percutaneous Endoscopic Approach

ØRG14A0 Fusion of Cervical Vertebral Joint with Interbody Fusion Device, Anterior Approach, Anterior Column, Percutaneous Endoscopic Approach

ØRG14AJ Fusion of Cervical Vertebral Joint with Interbody Fusion Device, Posterior Approach, Anterior Column, Percutaneous Endoscopic Approach

ØRG14J0 Fusion of Cervical Vertebral Joint with Synthetic Substitute, Anterior Approach, Anterior Column, Percutaneous Endoscopic Approach

ØRG14J1 Fusion of Cervical Vertebral Joint with Synthetic Substitute, Posterior Approach, Posterior Column, Percutaneous Endoscopic Approach

ØRG14JJ Fusion of Cervical Vertebral Joint with Synthetic Substitute, Posterior Approach, Anterior Column, Percutaneous Endoscopic Approach

ØRG14K0 Fusion of Cervical Vertebral Joint with Nonautologous Tissue Substitute, Anterior Approach, Anterior Column, Percutaneous Endoscopic Approach

ØRG14K1 Fusion of Cervical Vertebral Joint with Nonautologous Tissue Substitute, Posterior Approach, Posterior Column, Percutaneous Endoscopic Approach

ØRG14KJ Fusion of Cervical Vertebral Joint with Nonautologous Tissue Substitute, Posterior Approach, Anterior Column, Percutaneous Endoscopic Approach

ØRG2070 Fusion of 2 or more Cervical Vertebral Joints with Autologous Tissue Substitute, Anterior Approach, Anterior Column, Open Approach

ØRG2071 Fusion of 2 or more Cervical Vertebral Joints with Autologous Tissue Substitute, Posterior Approach, Posterior Column, Open Approach

ØRG207J Fusion of 2 or more Cervical Vertebral Joints with Autologous Tissue Substitute, Posterior Approach, Anterior Column, Open Approach

ØRG20A0 Fusion of 2 or more Cervical Vertebral Joints with Interbody Fusion Device, Anterior Approach, Anterior Column, Open Approach

ØRG20AJ Fusion of 2 or more Cervical Vertebral Joints with Interbody Fusion Device, Posterior Approach, Anterior Column, Open Approach

ØRG20J0 Fusion of 2 or more Cervical Vertebral Joints with Synthetic Substitute, Anterior Approach, Anterior Column, Open Approach

ØRG20J1 Fusion of 2 or more Cervical Vertebral Joints with Synthetic Substitute, Posterior Approach, Posterior Column, Open Approach

ØRG20JJ Fusion of 2 or more Cervical Vertebral Joints with Synthetic Substitute, Posterior Approach, Anterior Column, Open Approach

ØRG20K0 Fusion of 2 or more Cervical Vertebral Joints with Nonautologous Tissue Substitute, Anterior Approach, Anterior Column, Open Approach

ØRG20K1 Fusion of 2 or more Cervical Vertebral Joints with Nonautologous Tissue Substitute, Posterior Approach, Posterior Column, Open Approach

ØRG20KJ Fusion of 2 or more Cervical Vertebral Joints with Nonautologous Tissue Substitute, Posterior Approach, Anterior Column, Open Approach

ØRG2370 Fusion of 2 or more Cervical Vertebral Joints with Autologous Tissue Substitute, Anterior Approach, Anterior Column, Percutaneous Approach

ØRG2371 Fusion of 2 or more Cervical Vertebral Joints with Autologous Tissue Substitute, Posterior Approach, Posterior Column, Percutaneous Approach

ØRG237J Fusion of 2 or more Cervical Vertebral Joints with Autologous Tissue Substitute, Posterior Approach, Anterior Column, Percutaneous Approach

ØRG23A0 Fusion of 2 or more Cervical Vertebral Joints with Interbody Fusion Device, Anterior Approach, Anterior Column, Percutaneous Approach

ØRG23AJ Fusion of 2 or more Cervical Vertebral Joints with Interbody Fusion Device, Posterior Approach, Anterior Column, Percutaneous Approach

ØRG23J0 Fusion of 2 or more Cervical Vertebral Joints with Synthetic Substitute, Anterior Approach, Anterior Column, Percutaneous Approach

ØRG23J1 Fusion of 2 or more Cervical Vertebral Joints with Synthetic Substitute, Posterior Approach, Posterior Column, Percutaneous Approach

ØRG23JJ Fusion of 2 or more Cervical Vertebral Joints with Synthetic Substitute, Posterior Approach, Anterior Column, Percutaneous Approach

ØRG23K0 Fusion of 2 or more Cervical Vertebral Joints with Nonautologous Tissue Substitute, Anterior Approach, Anterior Column, Percutaneous Approach

ØRG23K1 Fusion of 2 or more Cervical Vertebral Joints with Nonautologous Tissue Substitute, Posterior Approach, Posterior Column, Percutaneous Approach

ØRG23KJ Fusion of 2 or more Cervical Vertebral Joints with Nonautologous Tissue Substitute, Posterior Approach, Anterior Column, Percutaneous Approach

ØRG2470 Fusion of 2 or more Cervical Vertebral Joints with Autologous Tissue Substitute, Anterior Approach, Anterior Column, Percutaneous Endoscopic Approach

ØRG2471 Fusion of 2 or more Cervical Vertebral Joints with Autologous Tissue Substitute, Posterior Approach, Posterior Column, Percutaneous Endoscopic Approach

ØRG247J Fusion of 2 or more Cervical Vertebral Joints with Autologous Tissue Substitute, Posterior Approach, Anterior Column, Percutaneous Endoscopic Approach

ØRG24A0 Fusion of 2 or more Cervical Vertebral Joints with Interbody Fusion Device, Anterior Approach, Anterior Column, Percutaneous Endoscopic Approach

ØRG24AJ Fusion of 2 or more Cervical Vertebral Joints with Interbody Fusion Device, Posterior Approach, Anterior Column, Percutaneous Endoscopic Approach

ØRG24J0 Fusion of 2 or more Cervical Vertebral Joints with Synthetic Substitute, Anterior Approach, Anterior Column, Percutaneous Endoscopic Approach

ØRG24J1 Fusion of 2 or more Cervical Vertebral Joints with Synthetic Substitute, Posterior Approach, Posterior Column, Percutaneous Endoscopic Approach

ØRG24JJ Fusion of 2 or more Cervical Vertebral Joints with Synthetic Substitute, Posterior Approach, Anterior Column, Percutaneous Endoscopic Approach

ØRG24K0 Fusion of 2 or more Cervical Vertebral Joints with Nonautologous Tissue Substitute, Anterior Approach, Anterior Column, Percutaneous Endoscopic Approach

ØRG24K1 Fusion of 2 or more Cervical Vertebral Joints with Nonautologous Tissue Substitute, Posterior Approach, Posterior Column, Percutaneous Endoscopic Approach

ØRG24KJ Fusion of 2 or more Cervical Vertebral Joints with Nonautologous Tissue Substitute, Posterior Approach, Anterior Column, Percutaneous Endoscopic Approach

ØRG4070 Fusion of Cervicothoracic Vertebral Joint with Autologous Tissue Substitute, Anterior Approach, Anterior Column, Open Approach

ØRG4071 Fusion of Cervicothoracic Vertebral Joint with Autologous Tissue Substitute, Posterior Approach, Posterior Column, Open Approach

ØRG407J Fusion of Cervicothoracic Vertebral Joint with Autologous Tissue Substitute, Posterior Approach, Anterior Column, Open Approach

ØRG40A0 Fusion of Cervicothoracic Vertebral Joint with Interbody Fusion Device, Anterior Approach, Anterior Column, Open Approach

ØRG40AJ Fusion of Cervicothoracic Vertebral Joint with Interbody Fusion Device, Posterior Approach, Anterior Column, Open Approach

ØRG40J0 Fusion of Cervicothoracic Vertebral Joint with Synthetic Substitute, Anterior Approach, Anterior Column, Open Approach

ØRG40J1 Fusion of Cervicothoracic Vertebral Joint with Synthetic Substitute, Posterior Approach, Posterior Column, Open Approach

ØRG40JJ Fusion of Cervicothoracic Vertebral Joint with Synthetic Substitute, Posterior Approach, Anterior Column, Open Approach

ØRG40K0 Fusion of Cervicothoracic Vertebral Joint with Nonautologous Tissue Substitute, Anterior Approach, Anterior Column, Open Approach

ØRG40K1 Fusion of Cervicothoracic Vertebral Joint with Nonautologous Tissue Substitute, Posterior Approach, Posterior Column, Open Approach

ØRG40KJ Fusion of Cervicothoracic Vertebral Joint with Nonautologous Tissue Substitute, Posterior Approach, Anterior Column, Open Approach

ØRG4370 Fusion of Cervicothoracic Vertebral Joint with Autologous Tissue Substitute, Anterior Approach, Anterior Column, Percutaneous Approach

Appendix K: Hospital Acquired Conditions

HAC 12: Surgical Site Infection-Certain Orthopedic Procedures of the Spine, Shoulder, and Elbow (continued)

ØRG4371 Fusion of Cervicothoracic Vertebral Joint with Autologous Tissue Substitute, Posterior Approach, Posterior Column, Percutaneous Approach

ØRG437J Fusion of Cervicothoracic Vertebral Joint with Autologous Tissue Substitute, Posterior Approach, Anterior Column, Percutaneous Approach

ØRG43AØ Fusion of Cervicothoracic Vertebral Joint with Interbody Fusion Device, Anterior Approach, Anterior Column, Percutaneous Approach

ØRG43AJ Fusion of Cervicothoracic Vertebral Joint with Interbody Fusion Device, Posterior Approach, Anterior Column, Percutaneous Approach

ØRG43JØ Fusion of Cervicothoracic Vertebral Joint with Synthetic Substitute, Anterior Approach, Anterior Column, Percutaneous Approach

ØRG43J1 Fusion of Cervicothoracic Vertebral Joint with Synthetic Substitute, Posterior Approach, Posterior Column, Percutaneous Approach

ØRG43JJ Fusion of Cervicothoracic Vertebral Joint with Synthetic Substitute, Posterior Approach, Anterior Column, Percutaneous Approach

ØRG43KØ Fusion of Cervicothoracic Vertebral Joint with Nonautologous Tissue Substitute, Anterior Approach, Anterior Column, Percutaneous Approach

ØRG43K1 Fusion of Cervicothoracic Vertebral Joint with Nonautologous Tissue Substitute, Posterior Approach, Posterior Column, Percutaneous Approach

ØRG43KJ Fusion of Cervicothoracic Vertebral Joint with Nonautologous Tissue Substitute, Posterior Approach, Anterior Column, Percutaneous Approach

ØRG447Ø Fusion of Cervicothoracic Vertebral Joint with Autologous Tissue Substitute, Anterior Approach, Anterior Column, Percutaneous Endoscopic Approach

ØRG4471 Fusion of Cervicothoracic Vertebral Joint with Autologous Tissue Substitute, Posterior Approach, Posterior Column, Percutaneous Endoscopic Approach

ØRG447J Fusion of Cervicothoracic Vertebral Joint with Autologous Tissue Substitute, Posterior Approach, Anterior Column, Percutaneous Endoscopic Approach

ØRG44AØ Fusion of Cervicothoracic Vertebral Joint with Interbody Fusion Device, Anterior Approach, Anterior Column, Percutaneous Endoscopic Approach

ØRG44AJ Fusion of Cervicothoracic Vertebral Joint with Interbody Fusion Device, Posterior Approach, Anterior Column, Percutaneous Endoscopic Approach

ØRG44JØ Fusion of Cervicothoracic Vertebral Joint with Synthetic Substitute, Anterior Approach, Anterior Column, Percutaneous Endoscopic Approach

ØRG44J1 Fusion of Cervicothoracic Vertebral Joint with Synthetic Substitute, Posterior Approach, Posterior Column, Percutaneous Endoscopic Approach

ØRG44JJ Fusion of Cervicothoracic Vertebral Joint with Synthetic Substitute, Posterior Approach, Anterior Column, Percutaneous Endoscopic Approach

ØRG44KØ Fusion of Cervicothoracic Vertebral Joint with Nonautologous Tissue Substitute, Anterior Approach, Anterior Column, Percutaneous Endoscopic Approach

ØRG44K1 Fusion of Cervicothoracic Vertebral Joint with Nonautologous Tissue Substitute, Posterior Approach, Posterior Column, Percutaneous Endoscopic Approach

ØRG44KJ Fusion of Cervicothoracic Vertebral Joint with Nonautologous Tissue Substitute, Posterior Approach, Anterior Column, Percutaneous Endoscopic Approach

ØRG6Ø7Ø Fusion of Thoracic Vertebral Joint with Autologous Tissue Substitute, Anterior Approach, Anterior Column, Open Approach

ØRG6Ø71 Fusion of Thoracic Vertebral Joint with Autologous Tissue Substitute, Posterior Approach, Posterior Column, Open Approach

ØRG6Ø7J Fusion of Thoracic Vertebral Joint with Autologous Tissue Substitute, Posterior Approach, Anterior Column, Open Approach

ØRG6ØAØ Fusion of Thoracic Vertebral Joint with Interbody Fusion Device, Anterior Approach, Anterior Column, Open Approach

ØRG6ØAJ Fusion of Thoracic Vertebral Joint with Interbody Fusion Device, Posterior Approach, Anterior Column, Open Approach

ØRG6ØJØ Fusion of Thoracic Vertebral Joint with Synthetic Substitute, Anterior Approach, Anterior Column, Open Approach

ØRG6ØJ1 Fusion of Thoracic Vertebral Joint with Synthetic Substitute, Posterior Approach, Posterior Column, Open Approach

ØRG6ØJJ Fusion of Thoracic Vertebral Joint with Synthetic Substitute, Posterior Approach, Anterior Column, Open Approach

ØRG6ØKØ Fusion of Thoracic Vertebral Joint with Nonautologous Tissue Substitute, Anterior Approach, Anterior Column, Open Approach

ØRG6ØK1 Fusion of Thoracic Vertebral Joint with Nonautologous Tissue Substitute, Posterior Approach, Posterior Column, Open Approach

ØRG6ØKJ Fusion of Thoracic Vertebral Joint with Nonautologous Tissue Substitute, Posterior Approach, Anterior Column, Open Approach

ØRG637Ø Fusion of Thoracic Vertebral Joint with Autologous Tissue Substitute, Anterior Approach, Anterior Column, Percutaneous Approach

ØRG6371 Fusion of Thoracic Vertebral Joint with Autologous Tissue Substitute, Posterior Approach, Posterior Column, Percutaneous Approach

ØRG637J Fusion of Thoracic Vertebral Joint with Autologous Tissue Substitute, Posterior Approach, Anterior Column, Percutaneous Approach

ØRG63AØ Fusion of Thoracic Vertebral Joint with Interbody Fusion Device, Anterior Approach, Anterior Column, Percutaneous Approach

ØRG63AJ Fusion of Thoracic Vertebral Joint with Interbody Fusion Device, Posterior Approach, Anterior Column, Percutaneous Approach

ØRG63JØ Fusion of Thoracic Vertebral Joint with Synthetic Substitute, Anterior Approach, Anterior Column, Percutaneous Approach

ØRG63J1 Fusion of Thoracic Vertebral Joint with Synthetic Substitute, Posterior Approach, Posterior Column, Percutaneous Approach

ØRG63JJ Fusion of Thoracic Vertebral Joint with Synthetic Substitute, Posterior Approach, Anterior Column, Percutaneous Approach

ØRG63KØ Fusion of Thoracic Vertebral Joint with Nonautologous Tissue Substitute, Anterior Approach, Anterior Column, Percutaneous Approach

ØRG63K1 Fusion of Thoracic Vertebral Joint with Nonautologous Tissue Substitute, Posterior Approach, Posterior Column, Percutaneous Approach

ØRG63KJ Fusion of Thoracic Vertebral Joint with Nonautologous Tissue Substitute, Posterior Approach, Anterior Column, Percutaneous Approach

ØRG647Ø Fusion of Thoracic Vertebral Joint with Autologous Tissue Substitute, Anterior Approach, Anterior Column, Percutaneous Endoscopic Approach

ØRG6471 Fusion of Thoracic Vertebral Joint with Autologous Tissue Substitute, Posterior Approach, Posterior Column, Percutaneous Endoscopic Approach

ØRG647J Fusion of Thoracic Vertebral Joint with Autologous Tissue Substitute, Posterior Approach, Anterior Column, Percutaneous Endoscopic Approach

ØRG64AØ Fusion of Thoracic Vertebral Joint with Interbody Fusion Device, Anterior Approach, Anterior Column, Percutaneous Endoscopic Approach

ØRG64AJ Fusion of Thoracic Vertebral Joint with Interbody Fusion Device, Posterior Approach, Anterior Column, Percutaneous Endoscopic Approach

ØRG64JØ Fusion of Thoracic Vertebral Joint with Synthetic Substitute, Anterior Approach, Anterior Column, Percutaneous Endoscopic Approach

ØRG64J1 Fusion of Thoracic Vertebral Joint with Synthetic Substitute, Posterior Approach, Posterior Column, Percutaneous Endoscopic Approach

ØRG64JJ Fusion of Thoracic Vertebral Joint with Synthetic Substitute, Posterior Approach, Anterior Column, Percutaneous Endoscopic Approach

ØRG64KØ Fusion of Thoracic Vertebral Joint with Nonautologous Tissue Substitute, Anterior Approach, Anterior Column, Percutaneous Endoscopic Approach

ØRG64K1 Fusion of Thoracic Vertebral Joint with Nonautologous Tissue Substitute, Posterior Approach, Posterior Column, Percutaneous Endoscopic Approach

ØRG64KJ Fusion of Thoracic Vertebral Joint with Nonautologous Tissue Substitute, Posterior Approach, Anterior Column, Percutaneous Endoscopic Approach

ØRG7Ø7Ø Fusion of 2 to 7 Thoracic Vertebral Joints with Autologous Tissue Substitute, Anterior Approach, Anterior Column, Open Approach

ØRG7Ø71 Fusion of 2 to 7 Thoracic Vertebral Joints with Autologous Tissue Substitute, Posterior Approach, Posterior Column, Open Approach

ØRG7Ø7J Fusion of 2 to 7 Thoracic Vertebral Joints with Autologous Tissue Substitute, Posterior Approach, Anterior Column, Open Approach

HAC 12: Surgical Site Infection-Certain Orthopedic Procedures of the Spine, Shoulder, and Elbow (continued)

ØRG70AØ   Fusion of 2 to 7 Thoracic Vertebral Joints with Interbody Fusion Device, Anterior Approach, Anterior Column, Open Approach

ØRG70AJ   Fusion of 2 to 7 Thoracic Vertebral Joints with Interbody Fusion Device, Posterior Approach, Anterior Column, Open Approach

ØRG70JØ   Fusion of 2 to 7 Thoracic Vertebral Joints with Synthetic Substitute, Anterior Approach, Anterior Column, Open Approach

ØRG70J1   Fusion of 2 to 7 Thoracic Vertebral Joints with Synthetic Substitute, Posterior Approach, Posterior Column, Open Approach

ØRG70JJ   Fusion of 2 to 7 Thoracic Vertebral Joints with Synthetic Substitute, Posterior Approach, Anterior Column, Open Approach

ØRG70KØ   Fusion of 2 to 7 Thoracic Vertebral Joints with Nonautologous Tissue Substitute, Anterior Approach, Anterior Column, Open Approach

ØRG70K1   Fusion of 2 to 7 Thoracic Vertebral Joints with Nonautologous Tissue Substitute, Posterior Approach, Posterior Column, Open Approach

ØRG70KJ   Fusion of 2 to 7 Thoracic Vertebral Joints with Nonautologous Tissue Substitute, Posterior Approach, Anterior Column, Open Approach

ØRG737Ø   Fusion of 2 to 7 Thoracic Vertebral Joints with Autologous Tissue Substitute, Anterior Approach, Anterior Column, Percutaneous Approach

ØRG7371   Fusion of 2 to 7 Thoracic Vertebral Joints with Autologous Tissue Substitute, Posterior Approach, Posterior Column, Percutaneous Approach

ØRG737J   Fusion of 2 to 7 Thoracic Vertebral Joints with Autologous Tissue Substitute, Posterior Approach, Anterior Column, Percutaneous Approach

ØRG73AØ   Fusion of 2 to 7 Thoracic Vertebral Joints with Interbody Fusion Device, Anterior Approach, Anterior Column, Percutaneous Approach

ØRG73AJ   Fusion of 2 to 7 Thoracic Vertebral Joints with Interbody Fusion Device, Posterior Approach, Anterior Column, Percutaneous Approach

ØRG73JØ   Fusion of 2 to 7 Thoracic Vertebral Joints with Synthetic Substitute, Anterior Approach, Anterior Column, Percutaneous Approach

ØRG73J1   Fusion of 2 to 7 Thoracic Vertebral Joints with Synthetic Substitute, Posterior Approach, Posterior Column, Percutaneous Approach

ØRG73JJ   Fusion of 2 to 7 Thoracic Vertebral Joints with Synthetic Substitute, Posterior Approach, Anterior Column, Percutaneous Approach

ØRG73KØ   Fusion of 2 to 7 Thoracic Vertebral Joints with Nonautologous Tissue Substitute, Anterior Approach, Anterior Column, Percutaneous Approach

ØRG73K1   Fusion of 2 to 7 Thoracic Vertebral Joints with Nonautologous Tissue Substitute, Posterior Approach, Posterior Column, Percutaneous Approach

ØRG73KJ   Fusion of 2 to 7 Thoracic Vertebral Joints with Nonautologous Tissue Substitute, Posterior Approach, Anterior Column, Percutaneous Approach

ØRG747Ø   Fusion of 2 to 7 Thoracic Vertebral Joints with Autologous Tissue Substitute, Anterior Approach, Anterior Column, Percutaneous Endoscopic Approach

ØRG7471   Fusion of 2 to 7 Thoracic Vertebral Joints with Autologous Tissue Substitute, Posterior Approach, Posterior Column, Percutaneous Endoscopic Approach

ØRG747J   Fusion of 2 to 7 Thoracic Vertebral Joints with Autologous Tissue Substitute, Posterior Approach, Anterior Column, Percutaneous Endoscopic Approach

ØRG74AØ   Fusion of 2 to 7 Thoracic Vertebral Joints with Interbody Fusion Device, Anterior Approach, Anterior Column, Percutaneous Endoscopic Approach

ØRG74AJ   Fusion of 2 to 7 Thoracic Vertebral Joints with Interbody Fusion Device, Posterior Approach, Anterior Column, Percutaneous Endoscopic Approach

ØRG74JØ   Fusion of 2 to 7 Thoracic Vertebral Joints with Synthetic Substitute, Anterior Approach, Anterior Column, Percutaneous Endoscopic Approach

ØRG74J1   Fusion of 2 to 7 Thoracic Vertebral Joints with Synthetic Substitute, Posterior Approach, Posterior Column, Percutaneous Endoscopic Approach

ØRG74JJ   Fusion of 2 to 7 Thoracic Vertebral Joints with Synthetic Substitute, Posterior Approach, Anterior Column, Percutaneous Endoscopic Approach

ØRG74KØ   Fusion of 2 to 7 Thoracic Vertebral Joints with Nonautologous Tissue Substitute, Anterior Approach, Anterior Column, Percutaneous Endoscopic Approach

ØRG74K1   Fusion of 2 to 7 Thoracic Vertebral Joints with Nonautologous Tissue Substitute, Posterior Approach, Posterior Column, Percutaneous Endoscopic Approach

ØRG74KJ   Fusion of 2 to 7 Thoracic Vertebral Joints with Nonautologous Tissue Substitute, Posterior Approach, Anterior Column, Percutaneous Endoscopic Approach

ØRG807Ø   Fusion of 8 or More Thoracic Vertebral Joints with Autologous Tissue Substitute, Anterior Approach, Anterior Column, Open Approach

ØRG8071   Fusion of 8 or More Thoracic Vertebral Joints with Autologous Tissue Substitute, Posterior Approach, Posterior Column, Open Approach

ØRG807J   Fusion of 8 or More Thoracic Vertebral Joints with Autologous Tissue Substitute, Posterior Approach, Anterior Column, Open Approach

ØRG80AØ   Fusion of 8 or More Thoracic Vertebral Joints with Interbody Fusion Device, Anterior Approach, Anterior Column, Open Approach

ØRG80AJ   Fusion of 8 or More Thoracic Vertebral Joints with Interbody Fusion Device, Posterior Approach, Anterior Column, Open Approach

ØRG80JØ   Fusion of 8 or More Thoracic Vertebral Joints with Synthetic Substitute, Anterior Approach, Anterior Column, Open Approach

ØRG80J1   Fusion of 8 or More Thoracic Vertebral Joints with Synthetic Substitute, Posterior Approach, Posterior Column, Open Approach

ØRG80JJ   Fusion of 8 or More Thoracic Vertebral Joints with Synthetic Substitute, Posterior Approach, Anterior Column, Open Approach

ØRG80KØ   Fusion of 8 or More Thoracic Vertebral Joints with Nonautologous Tissue Substitute, Anterior Approach, Anterior Column, Open Approach

ØRG80K1   Fusion of 8 or More Thoracic Vertebral Joints with Nonautologous Tissue Substitute, Posterior Approach, Posterior Column, Open Approach

ØRG80KJ   Fusion of 8 or More Thoracic Vertebral Joints with Nonautologous Tissue Substitute, Posterior Approach, Anterior Column, Open Approach

ØRG837Ø   Fusion of 8 or More Thoracic Vertebral Joints with Autologous Tissue Substitute, Anterior Approach, Anterior Column, Percutaneous Approach

ØRG8371   Fusion of 8 or More Thoracic Vertebral Joints with Autologous Tissue Substitute, Posterior Approach, Posterior Column, Percutaneous Approach

ØRG837J   Fusion of 8 or More Thoracic Vertebral Joints with Autologous Tissue Substitute, Posterior Approach, Anterior Column, Percutaneous Approach

ØRG83AØ   Fusion of 8 or More Thoracic Vertebral Joints with Interbody Fusion Device, Anterior Approach, Anterior Column, Percutaneous Approach

ØRG83AJ   Fusion of 8 or More Thoracic Vertebral Joints with Interbody Fusion Device, Posterior Approach, Anterior Column, Percutaneous Approach

ØRG83JØ   Fusion of 8 or More Thoracic Vertebral Joints with Synthetic Substitute, Anterior Approach, Anterior Column, Percutaneous Approach

ØRG83J1   Fusion of 8 or More Thoracic Vertebral Joints with Synthetic Substitute, Posterior Approach, Posterior Column, Percutaneous Approach

ØRG83JJ   Fusion of 8 or More Thoracic Vertebral Joints with Synthetic Substitute, Posterior Approach, Anterior Column, Percutaneous Approach

ØRG83KØ   Fusion of 8 or More Thoracic Vertebral Joints with Nonautologous Tissue Substitute, Anterior Approach, Anterior Column, Percutaneous Approach

ØRG83K1   Fusion of 8 or More Thoracic Vertebral Joints with Nonautologous Tissue Substitute, Posterior Approach, Posterior Column, Percutaneous Approach

ØRG83KJ   Fusion of 8 or More Thoracic Vertebral Joints with Nonautologous Tissue Substitute, Posterior Approach, Anterior Column, Percutaneous Approach

ØRG847Ø   Fusion of 8 or More Thoracic Vertebral Joints with Autologous Tissue Substitute, Anterior Approach, Anterior Column, Percutaneous Endoscopic Approach

ØRG8471   Fusion of 8 or More Thoracic Vertebral Joints with Autologous Tissue Substitute, Posterior Approach, Posterior Column, Percutaneous Endoscopic Approach

ØRG847J   Fusion of 8 or More Thoracic Vertebral Joints with Autologous Tissue Substitute, Posterior Approach, Anterior Column, Percutaneous Endoscopic Approach

ØRG84AØ   Fusion of 8 or More Thoracic Vertebral Joints with Interbody Fusion Device, Anterior Approach, Anterior Column, Percutaneous Endoscopic Approach

HAC 12: Surgical Site Infection-Certain Orthopedic Procedures of the Spine, Shoulder, and Elbow (continued)

ØRG84AJ Fusion of 8 or More Thoracic Vertebral Joints with Interbody Fusion Device, Posterior Approach, Anterior Column, Percutaneous Endoscopic Approach

ØRG84J0 Fusion of 8 or More Thoracic Vertebral Joints with Synthetic Substitute, Anterior Approach, Anterior Column, Percutaneous Endoscopic Approach

ØRG84J1 Fusion of 8 or More Thoracic Vertebral Joints with Synthetic Substitute, Posterior Approach, Posterior Column, Percutaneous Endoscopic Approach

ØRG84JJ Fusion of 8 or More Thoracic Vertebral Joints with Synthetic Substitute, Posterior Approach, Anterior Column, Percutaneous Endoscopic Approach

ØRG84KØ Fusion of 8 or More Thoracic Vertebral Joints with Nonautologous Tissue Substitute, Anterior Approach, Anterior Column, Percutaneous Endoscopic Approach

ØRG84K1 Fusion of 8 or More Thoracic Vertebral Joints with Nonautologous Tissue Substitute, Posterior Approach, Posterior Column, Percutaneous Endoscopic Approach

ØRG84KJ Fusion of 8 or More Thoracic Vertebral Joints with Nonautologous Tissue Substitute, Posterior Approach, Anterior Column, Percutaneous Endoscopic Approach

ØRGAØ7Ø Fusion of Thoracolumbar Vertebral Joint with Autologous Tissue Substitute, Anterior Approach, Anterior Column, Open Approach

ØRGAØ71 Fusion of Thoracolumbar Vertebral Joint with Autologous Tissue Substitute, Posterior Approach, Posterior Column, Open Approach

ØRGAØ7J Fusion of Thoracolumbar Vertebral Joint with Autologous Tissue Substitute, Posterior Approach, Anterior Column, Open Approach

ØRGAØAØ Fusion of Thoracolumbar Vertebral Joint with Interbody Fusion Device, Anterior Approach, Anterior Column, Open Approach

ØRGAØAJ Fusion of Thoracolumbar Vertebral Joint with Interbody Fusion Device, Posterior Approach, Anterior Column, Open Approach

ØRGAØJØ Fusion of Thoracolumbar Vertebral Joint with Synthetic Substitute, Anterior Approach, Anterior Column, Open Approach

ØRGAØJ1 Fusion of Thoracolumbar Vertebral Joint with Synthetic Substitute, Posterior Approach, Posterior Column, Open Approach

ØRGAØJJ Fusion of Thoracolumbar Vertebral Joint with Synthetic Substitute, Posterior Approach, Anterior Column, Open Approach

ØRGAØKØ Fusion of Thoracolumbar Vertebral Joint with Nonautologous Tissue Substitute, Anterior Approach, Anterior Column, Open Approach

ØRGAØK1 Fusion of Thoracolumbar Vertebral Joint with Nonautologous Tissue Substitute, Posterior Approach, Posterior Column, Open Approach

ØRGAØKJ Fusion of Thoracolumbar Vertebral Joint with Nonautologous Tissue Substitute, Posterior Approach, Anterior Column, Open Approach

ØRGA37Ø Fusion of Thoracolumbar Vertebral Joint with Autologous Tissue Substitute, Anterior Approach, Anterior Column, Percutaneous Approach

ØRGA371 Fusion of Thoracolumbar Vertebral Joint with Autologous Tissue Substitute, Posterior Approach, Posterior Column, Percutaneous Approach

ØRGA37J Fusion of Thoracolumbar Vertebral Joint with Autologous Tissue Substitute, Posterior Approach, Anterior Column, Percutaneous Approach

ØRGA3AØ Fusion of Thoracolumbar Vertebral Joint with Interbody Fusion Device, Anterior Approach, Anterior Column, Percutaneous Approach

ØRGA3AJ Fusion of Thoracolumbar Vertebral Joint with Interbody Fusion Device, Posterior Approach, Anterior Column, Percutaneous Approach

ØRGA3JØ Fusion of Thoracolumbar Vertebral Joint with Synthetic Substitute, Anterior Approach, Anterior Column, Percutaneous Approach

ØRGA3J1 Fusion of Thoracolumbar Vertebral Joint with Synthetic Substitute, Posterior Approach, Posterior Column, Percutaneous Approach

ØRGA3JJ Fusion of Thoracolumbar Vertebral Joint with Synthetic Substitute, Posterior Approach, Anterior Column, Percutaneous Approach

ØRGA3KØ Fusion of Thoracolumbar Vertebral Joint with Nonautologous Tissue Substitute, Anterior Approach, Anterior Column, Percutaneous Approach

ØRGA3K1 Fusion of Thoracolumbar Vertebral Joint with Nonautologous Tissue Substitute, Posterior Approach, Posterior Column, Percutaneous Approach

ØRGA3KJ Fusion of Thoracolumbar Vertebral Joint with Nonautologous Tissue Substitute, Posterior Approach, Anterior Column, Percutaneous Approach

ØRGA47Ø Fusion of Thoracolumbar Vertebral Joint with Autologous Tissue Substitute, Anterior Approach, Anterior Column, Percutaneous Endoscopic Approach

ØRGA471 Fusion of Thoracolumbar Vertebral Joint with Autologous Tissue Substitute, Posterior Approach, Posterior Column, Percutaneous Endoscopic Approach

ØRGA47J Fusion of Thoracolumbar Vertebral Joint with Autologous Tissue Substitute, Posterior Approach, Anterior Column, Percutaneous Endoscopic Approach

ØRGA4AØ Fusion of Thoracolumbar Vertebral Joint with Interbody Fusion Device, Anterior Approach, Anterior Column, Percutaneous Endoscopic Approach

ØRGA4AJ Fusion of Thoracolumbar Vertebral Joint with Interbody Fusion Device, Posterior Approach, Anterior Column, Percutaneous Endoscopic Approach

ØRGA4JØ Fusion of Thoracolumbar Vertebral Joint with Synthetic Substitute, Anterior Approach, Anterior Column, Percutaneous Endoscopic Approach

ØRGA4J1 Fusion of Thoracolumbar Vertebral Joint with Synthetic Substitute, Posterior Approach, Posterior Column, Percutaneous Endoscopic Approach

ØRGA4JJ Fusion of Thoracolumbar Vertebral Joint with Synthetic Substitute, Posterior Approach, Anterior Column, Percutaneous Endoscopic Approach

ØRGA4KØ Fusion of Thoracolumbar Vertebral Joint with Nonautologous Tissue Substitute, Anterior Approach, Anterior Column, Percutaneous Endoscopic Approach

ØRGA4K1 Fusion of Thoracolumbar Vertebral Joint with Nonautologous Tissue Substitute, Posterior Approach, Posterior Column, Percutaneous Endoscopic Approach

ØRGA4KJ Fusion of Thoracolumbar Vertebral Joint with Nonautologous Tissue Substitute, Posterior Approach, Anterior Column, Percutaneous Endoscopic Approach

ØRGEØ4Z Fusion of Right Sternoclavicular Joint with Internal Fixation Device, Open Approach

ØRGEØ7Z Fusion of Right Sternoclavicular Joint with Autologous Tissue Substitute, Open Approach

ØRGEØJZ Fusion of Right Sternoclavicular Joint with Synthetic Substitute, Open Approach

ØRGEØKZ Fusion of Right Sternoclavicular Joint with Nonautologous Tissue Substitute, Open Approach

ØRGE34Z Fusion of Right Sternoclavicular Joint with Internal Fixation Device, Percutaneous Approach

ØRGE37Z Fusion of Right Sternoclavicular Joint with Autologous Tissue Substitute, Percutaneous Approach

ØRGE3JZ Fusion of Right Sternoclavicular Joint with Synthetic Substitute, Percutaneous Approach

ØRGE3KZ Fusion of Right Sternoclavicular Joint with Nonautologous Tissue Substitute, Percutaneous Approach

ØRGE44Z Fusion of Right Sternoclavicular Joint with Internal Fixation Device, Percutaneous Endoscopic Approach

ØRGE47Z Fusion of Right Sternoclavicular Joint with Autologous Tissue Substitute, Percutaneous Endoscopic Approach

ØRGE4JZ Fusion of Right Sternoclavicular Joint with Synthetic Substitute, Percutaneous Endoscopic Approach

ØRGE4KZ Fusion of Right Sternoclavicular Joint with Nonautologous Tissue Substitute, Percutaneous Endoscopic Approach

ØRGFØ4Z Fusion of Left Sternoclavicular Joint with Internal Fixation Device, Open Approach

ØRGFØ7Z Fusion of Left Sternoclavicular Joint with Autologous Tissue Substitute, Open Approach

ØRGFØJZ Fusion of Left Sternoclavicular Joint with Synthetic Substitute, Open Approach

ØRGFØKZ Fusion of Left Sternoclavicular Joint with Nonautologous Tissue Substitute, Open Approach

ØRGF34Z Fusion of Left Sternoclavicular Joint with Internal Fixation Device, Percutaneous Approach

ØRGF37Z Fusion of Left Sternoclavicular Joint with Autologous Tissue Substitute, Percutaneous Approach

ØRGF3JZ Fusion of Left Sternoclavicular Joint with Synthetic Substitute, Percutaneous Approach

ØRGF3KZ Fusion of Left Sternoclavicular Joint with Nonautologous Tissue Substitute, Percutaneous Approach

ØRGF44Z Fusion of Left Sternoclavicular Joint with Internal Fixation Device, Percutaneous Endoscopic Approach

HAC 12: Surgical Site Infection-Certain Orthopedic Procedures of the Spine, Shoulder, and Elbow (continued)

ØRGF47Z Fusion of Left Sternoclavicular Joint with Autologous Tissue Substitute, Percutaneous Endoscopic Approach

ØRGF4JZ Fusion of Left Sternoclavicular Joint with Synthetic Substitute, Percutaneous Endoscopic Approach

ØRGF4KZ Fusion of Left Sternoclavicular Joint with Nonautologous Tissue Substitute, Percutaneous Endoscopic Approach

ØRGGØ4Z Fusion of Right Acromioclavicular Joint with Internal Fixation Device, Open Approach

ØRGGØ7Z Fusion of Right Acromioclavicular Joint with Autologous Tissue Substitute, Open Approach

ØRGGØJZ Fusion of Right Acromioclavicular Joint with Synthetic Substitute, Open Approach

ØRGGØKZ Fusion of Right Acromioclavicular Joint with Nonautologous Tissue Substitute, Open Approach

ØRGG34Z Fusion of Right Acromioclavicular Joint with Internal Fixation Device, Percutaneous Approach

ØRGG37Z Fusion of Right Acromioclavicular Joint with Autologous Tissue Substitute, Percutaneous Approach

ØRGG3JZ Fusion of Right Acromioclavicular Joint with Synthetic Substitute, Percutaneous Approach

ØRGG3KZ Fusion of Right Acromioclavicular Joint with Nonautologous Tissue Substitute, Percutaneous Approach

ØRGG44Z Fusion of Right Acromioclavicular Joint with Internal Fixation Device, Percutaneous Endoscopic Approach

ØRGG47Z Fusion of Right Acromioclavicular Joint with Autologous Tissue Substitute, Percutaneous Endoscopic Approach

ØRGG4JZ Fusion of Right Acromioclavicular Joint with Synthetic Substitute, Percutaneous Endoscopic Approach

ØRGG4KZ Fusion of Right Acromioclavicular Joint with Nonautologous Tissue Substitute, Percutaneous Endoscopic Approach

ØRGHØ4Z Fusion of Left Acromioclavicular Joint with Internal Fixation Device, Open Approach

ØRGHØ7Z Fusion of Left Acromioclavicular Joint with Autologous Tissue Substitute, Open Approach

ØRGHØJZ Fusion of Left Acromioclavicular Joint with Synthetic Substitute, Open Approach

ØRGHØKZ Fusion of Left Acromioclavicular Joint with Nonautologous Tissue Substitute, Open Approach

ØRGH34Z Fusion of Left Acromioclavicular Joint with Internal Fixation Device, Percutaneous Approach

ØRGH37Z Fusion of Left Acromioclavicular Joint with Autologous Tissue Substitute, Percutaneous Approach

ØRGH3JZ Fusion of Left Acromioclavicular Joint with Synthetic Substitute, Percutaneous Approach

ØRGH3KZ Fusion of Left Acromioclavicular Joint with Nonautologous Tissue Substitute, Percutaneous Approach

ØRGH44Z Fusion of Left Acromioclavicular Joint with Internal Fixation Device, Percutaneous Endoscopic Approach

ØRGH47Z Fusion of Left Acromioclavicular Joint with Autologous Tissue Substitute, Percutaneous Endoscopic Approach

ØRGH4JZ Fusion of Left Acromioclavicular Joint with Synthetic Substitute, Percutaneous Endoscopic Approach

ØRGH4KZ Fusion of Left Acromioclavicular Joint with Nonautologous Tissue Substitute, Percutaneous Endoscopic Approach

ØRGJØ4Z Fusion of Right Shoulder Joint with Internal Fixation Device, Open Approach

ØRGJØ7Z Fusion of Right Shoulder Joint with Autologous Tissue Substitute, Open Approach

ØRGJØJZ Fusion of Right Shoulder Joint with Synthetic Substitute, Open Approach

ØRGJØKZ Fusion of Right Shoulder Joint with Nonautologous Tissue Substitute, Open Approach

ØRGJ34Z Fusion of Right Shoulder Joint with Internal Fixation Device, Percutaneous Approach

ØRGJ37Z Fusion of Right Shoulder Joint with Autologous Tissue Substitute, Percutaneous Approach

ØRGJ3JZ Fusion of Right Shoulder Joint with Synthetic Substitute, Percutaneous Approach

ØRGJ3KZ Fusion of Right Shoulder Joint with Nonautologous Tissue Substitute, Percutaneous Approach

ØRGJ44Z Fusion of Right Shoulder Joint with Internal Fixation Device, Percutaneous Endoscopic Approach

ØRGJ47Z Fusion of Right Shoulder Joint with Autologous Tissue Substitute, Percutaneous Endoscopic Approach

ØRGJ4JZ Fusion of Right Shoulder Joint with Synthetic Substitute, Percutaneous Endoscopic Approach

ØRGJ4KZ Fusion of Right Shoulder Joint with Nonautologous Tissue Substitute, Percutaneous Endoscopic Approach

ØRGKØ4Z Fusion of Left Shoulder Joint with Internal Fixation Device, Open Approach

ØRGKØ7Z Fusion of Left Shoulder Joint with Autologous Tissue Substitute, Open Approach

ØRGKØJZ Fusion of Left Shoulder Joint with Synthetic Substitute, Open Approach

ØRGKØKZ Fusion of Left Shoulder Joint with Nonautologous Tissue Substitute, Open Approach

ØRGK34Z Fusion of Left Shoulder Joint with Internal Fixation Device, Percutaneous Approach

ØRGK37Z Fusion of Left Shoulder Joint with Autologous Tissue Substitute, Percutaneous Approach

ØRGK3JZ Fusion of Left Shoulder Joint with Synthetic Substitute, Percutaneous Approach

ØRGK3KZ Fusion of Left Shoulder Joint with Nonautologous Tissue Substitute, Percutaneous Approach

ØRGK44Z Fusion of Left Shoulder Joint with Internal Fixation Device, Percutaneous Endoscopic Approach

ØRGK47Z Fusion of Left Shoulder Joint with Autologous Tissue Substitute, Percutaneous Endoscopic Approach

ØRGK4JZ Fusion of Left Shoulder Joint with Synthetic Substitute, Percutaneous Endoscopic Approach

ØRGK4KZ Fusion of Left Shoulder Joint with Nonautologous Tissue Substitute, Percutaneous Endoscopic Approach

ØRGLØ3Z Fusion of Right Elbow Joint with Sustained Compression Internal Fixation Device, Open Approach

ØRGLØ4Z Fusion of Right Elbow Joint with Internal Fixation Device, Open Approach

ØRGLØ5Z Fusion of Right Elbow Joint with External Fixation Device, Open Approach

ØRGLØ7Z Fusion of Right Elbow Joint with Autologous Tissue Substitute, Open Approach

ØRGLØJZ Fusion of Right Elbow Joint with Synthetic Substitute, Open Approach

ØRGLØKZ Fusion of Right Elbow Joint with Nonautologous Tissue Substitute, Open Approach

ØRGL33Z Fusion of Right Elbow Joint with Sustained Compression Internal Fixation Device, Percutaneous Approach

ØRGL34Z Fusion of Right Elbow Joint with Internal Fixation Device, Percutaneous Approach

ØRGL35Z Fusion of Right Elbow Joint with External Fixation Device, Percutaneous Approach

ØRGL37Z Fusion of Right Elbow Joint with Autologous Tissue Substitute, Percutaneous Approach

ØRGL3JZ Fusion of Right Elbow Joint with Synthetic Substitute, Percutaneous Approach

ØRGL3KZ Fusion of Right Elbow Joint with Nonautologous Tissue Substitute, Percutaneous Approach

ØRGL43Z Fusion of Right Elbow Joint with Sustained Compression Internal Fixation Device, Percutaneous Endoscopic Approach

ØRGL44Z Fusion of Right Elbow Joint with Internal Fixation Device, Percutaneous Endoscopic Approach

ØRGL45Z Fusion of Right Elbow Joint with External Fixation Device, Percutaneous Endoscopic Approach

ØRGL47Z Fusion of Right Elbow Joint with Autologous Tissue Substitute, Percutaneous Endoscopic Approach

ØRGL4JZ Fusion of Right Elbow Joint with Synthetic Substitute, Percutaneous Endoscopic Approach

ØRGL4KZ Fusion of Right Elbow Joint with Nonautologous Tissue Substitute, Percutaneous Endoscopic Approach

ØRGMØ3Z Fusion of Left Elbow Joint with Sustained Compression Internal Fixation Device, Open Approach

ØRGMØ4Z Fusion of Left Elbow Joint with Internal Fixation Device, Open Approach

ØRGMØ5Z Fusion of Left Elbow Joint with External Fixation Device, Open Approach

ØRGMØ7Z Fusion of Left Elbow Joint with Autologous Tissue Substitute, Open Approach

ØRGMØJZ Fusion of Left Elbow Joint with Synthetic Substitute, Open Approach

ØRGMØKZ Fusion of Left Elbow Joint with Nonautologous Tissue Substitute, Open Approach

ØRGM33Z Fusion of Left Elbow Joint with Sustained Compression Internal Fixation Device, Percutaneous Approach

ØRGM34Z Fusion of Left Elbow Joint with Internal Fixation Device, Percutaneous Approach

ØRGM35Z Fusion of Left Elbow Joint with External Fixation Device, Percutaneous Approach

ØRGM37Z Fusion of Left Elbow Joint with Autologous Tissue Substitute, Percutaneous Approach

ØRGM3JZ Fusion of Left Elbow Joint with Synthetic Substitute, Percutaneous Approach

ØRGM3KZ Fusion of Left Elbow Joint with Nonautologous Tissue Substitute, Percutaneous Approach

ØRGM43Z Fusion of Left Elbow Joint with Sustained Compression Internal Fixation Device, Percutaneous Endoscopic Approach

HAC 12: Surgical Site Infection-Certain Orthopedic Procedures of the Spine, Shoulder, and Elbow (continued)

ØRGM44Z Fusion of Left Elbow Joint with Internal Fixation Device, Percutaneous Endoscopic Approach

ØRGM45Z Fusion of Left Elbow Joint with External Fixation Device, Percutaneous Endoscopic Approach

ØRGM47Z Fusion of Left Elbow Joint with Autologous Tissue Substitute, Percutaneous Endoscopic Approach

ØRGM4JZ Fusion of Left Elbow Joint with Synthetic Substitute, Percutaneous Endoscopic Approach

ØRGM4KZ Fusion of Left Elbow Joint with Nonautologous Tissue Substitute, Percutaneous Endoscopic Approach

ØRQEØZZ Repair Right Sternoclavicular Joint, Open Approach

ØRQE3ZZ Repair Right Sternoclavicular Joint, Percutaneous Approach

ØRQE4ZZ Repair Right Sternoclavicular Joint, Percutaneous Endoscopic Approach

ØRQEXZZ Repair Right Sternoclavicular Joint, External Approach

ØRQFØZZ Repair Left Sternoclavicular Joint, Open Approach

ØRQF3ZZ Repair Left Sternoclavicular Joint, Percutaneous Approach

ØRQF4ZZ Repair Left Sternoclavicular Joint, Percutaneous Endoscopic Approach

ØRQFXZZ Repair Left Sternoclavicular Joint, External Approach

ØRQGØZZ Repair Right Acromioclavicular Joint, Open Approach

ØRQG3ZZ Repair Right Acromioclavicular Joint, Percutaneous Approach

ØRQG4ZZ Repair Right Acromioclavicular Joint, Percutaneous Endoscopic Approach

ØRQGXZZ Repair Right Acromioclavicular Joint, External Approach

ØRQHØZZ Repair Left Acromioclavicular Joint, Open Approach

ØRQH3ZZ Repair Left Acromioclavicular Joint, Percutaneous Approach

ØRQH4ZZ Repair Left Acromioclavicular Joint, Percutaneous Endoscopic Approach

ØRQHXZZ Repair Left Acromioclavicular Joint, External Approach

ØRQJØZZ Repair Right Shoulder Joint, Open Approach

ØRQJ3ZZ Repair Right Shoulder Joint, Percutaneous Approach

ØRQJ4ZZ Repair Right Shoulder Joint, Percutaneous Endoscopic Approach

ØRQJXZZ Repair Right Shoulder Joint, External Approach

ØRQKØZZ Repair Left Shoulder Joint, Open Approach

ØRQK3ZZ Repair Left Shoulder Joint, Percutaneous Approach

ØRQK4ZZ Repair Left Shoulder Joint, Percutaneous Endoscopic Approach

ØRQKXZZ Repair Left Shoulder Joint, External Approach

ØRQLØZZ Repair Right Elbow Joint, Open Approach

ØRQL3ZZ Repair Right Elbow Joint, Percutaneous Approach

ØRQL4ZZ Repair Right Elbow Joint, Percutaneous Endoscopic Approach

ØRQLXZZ Repair Right Elbow Joint, External Approach

ØRQMØZZ Repair Left Elbow Joint, Open Approach

ØRQM3ZZ Repair Left Elbow Joint, Percutaneous Approach

ØRQM4ZZ Repair Left Elbow Joint, Percutaneous Endoscopic Approach

ØRQMXZZ Repair Left Elbow Joint, External Approach

ØRUEØ7Z Supplement Right Sternoclavicular Joint with Autologous Tissue Substitute, Open Approach

ØRUEØJZ Supplement Right Sternoclavicular Joint with Synthetic Substitute, Open Approach

ØRUEØKZ Supplement Right Sternoclavicular Joint with Nonautologous Tissue Substitute, Open Approach

ØRUE37Z Supplement Right Sternoclavicular Joint with Autologous Tissue Substitute, Percutaneous Approach

ØRUE3JZ Supplement Right Sternoclavicular Joint with Synthetic Substitute, Percutaneous Approach

ØRUE3KZ Supplement Right Sternoclavicular Joint with Nonautologous Tissue Substitute, Percutaneous Approach

ØRUE47Z Supplement Right Sternoclavicular Joint with Autologous Tissue Substitute, Percutaneous Endoscopic Approach

ØRUE4JZ Supplement Right Sternoclavicular Joint with Synthetic Substitute, Percutaneous Endoscopic Approach

ØRUE4KZ Supplement Right Sternoclavicular Joint with Nonautologous Tissue Substitute, Percutaneous Endoscopic Approach

ØRUFØ7Z Supplement Left Sternoclavicular Joint with Autologous Tissue Substitute, Open Approach

ØRUFØJZ Supplement Left Sternoclavicular Joint with Synthetic Substitute, Open Approach

ØRUFØKZ Supplement Left Sternoclavicular Joint with Nonautologous Tissue Substitute, Open Approach

ØRUF37Z Supplement Left Sternoclavicular Joint with Autologous Tissue Substitute, Percutaneous Approach

ØRUF3JZ Supplement Left Sternoclavicular Joint with Synthetic Substitute, Percutaneous Approach

ØRUF3KZ Supplement Left Sternoclavicular Joint with Nonautologous Tissue Substitute, Percutaneous Approach

ØRUF47Z Supplement Left Sternoclavicular Joint with Autologous Tissue Substitute, Percutaneous Endoscopic Approach

ØRUF4JZ Supplement Left Sternoclavicular Joint with Synthetic Substitute, Percutaneous Endoscopic Approach

ØRUF4KZ Supplement Left Sternoclavicular Joint with Nonautologous Tissue Substitute, Percutaneous Endoscopic Approach

ØRUGØ7Z Supplement Right Acromioclavicular Joint with Autologous Tissue Substitute, Open Approach

ØRUGØJZ Supplement Right Acromioclavicular Joint with Synthetic Substitute, Open Approach

ØRUGØKZ Supplement Right Acromioclavicular Joint with Nonautologous Tissue Substitute, Open Approach

ØRUG37Z Supplement Right Acromioclavicular Joint with Autologous Tissue Substitute, Percutaneous Approach

ØRUG3JZ Supplement Right Acromioclavicular Joint with Synthetic Substitute, Percutaneous Approach

ØRUG3KZ Supplement Right Acromioclavicular Joint with Nonautologous Tissue Substitute, Percutaneous Approach

ØRUG47Z Supplement Right Acromioclavicular Joint with Autologous Tissue Substitute, Percutaneous Endoscopic Approach

ØRUG4JZ Supplement Right Acromioclavicular Joint with Synthetic Substitute, Percutaneous Endoscopic Approach

ØRUG4KZ Supplement Right Acromioclavicular Joint with Nonautologous Tissue Substitute, Percutaneous Endoscopic Approach

ØRUHØ7Z Supplement Left Acromioclavicular Joint with Autologous Tissue Substitute, Open Approach

ØRUHØJZ Supplement Left Acromioclavicular Joint with Synthetic Substitute, Open Approach

ØRUHØKZ Supplement Left Acromioclavicular Joint with Nonautologous Tissue Substitute, Open Approach

ØRUH37Z Supplement Left Acromioclavicular Joint with Autologous Tissue Substitute, Percutaneous Approach

ØRUH3JZ Supplement Left Acromioclavicular Joint with Synthetic Substitute, Percutaneous Approach

ØRUH3KZ Supplement Left Acromioclavicular Joint with Nonautologous Tissue Substitute, Percutaneous Approach

ØRUH47Z Supplement Left Acromioclavicular Joint with Autologous Tissue Substitute, Percutaneous Endoscopic Approach

ØRUH4JZ Supplement Left Acromioclavicular Joint with Synthetic Substitute, Percutaneous Endoscopic Approach

ØRUH4KZ Supplement Left Acromioclavicular Joint with Nonautologous Tissue Substitute, Percutaneous Endoscopic Approach

ØRUJØ7Z Supplement Right Shoulder Joint with Autologous Tissue Substitute, Open Approach

ØRUJØJZ Supplement Right Shoulder Joint with Synthetic Substitute, Open Approach

ØRUJØKZ Supplement Right Shoulder Joint with Nonautologous Tissue Substitute, Open Approach

ØRUJ37Z Supplement Right Shoulder Joint with Autologous Tissue Substitute, Percutaneous Approach

ØRUJ3JZ Supplement Right Shoulder Joint with Synthetic Substitute, Percutaneous Approach

ØRUJ3KZ Supplement Right Shoulder Joint with Nonautologous Tissue Substitute, Percutaneous Approach

ØRUJ47Z Supplement Right Shoulder Joint with Autologous Tissue Substitute, Percutaneous Endoscopic Approach

ØRUJ4JZ Supplement Right Shoulder Joint with Synthetic Substitute, Percutaneous Endoscopic Approach

ØRUJ4KZ Supplement Right Shoulder Joint with Nonautologous Tissue Substitute, Percutaneous Endoscopic Approach

ØRUKØ7Z Supplement Left Shoulder Joint with Autologous Tissue Substitute, Open Approach

ØRUKØJZ Supplement Left Shoulder Joint with Synthetic Substitute, Open Approach

ØRUKØKZ Supplement Left Shoulder Joint with Nonautologous Tissue Substitute, Open Approach

ØRUK37Z Supplement Left Shoulder Joint with Autologous Tissue Substitute, Percutaneous Approach

ØRUK3JZ Supplement Left Shoulder Joint with Synthetic Substitute, Percutaneous Approach

ØRUK3KZ Supplement Left Shoulder Joint with Nonautologous Tissue Substitute, Percutaneous Approach

HAC 12: Surgical Site Infection-Certain Orthopedic Procedures of the Spine, Shoulder, and Elbow (continued)

ØRUK47Z Supplement Left Shoulder Joint with Autologous Tissue Substitute, Percutaneous Endoscopic Approach

ØRUK4JZ Supplement Left Shoulder Joint with Synthetic Substitute, Percutaneous Endoscopic Approach

ØRUK4KZ Supplement Left Shoulder Joint with Nonautologous Tissue Substitute, Percutaneous Endoscopic Approach

ØRULØ7Z Supplement Right Elbow Joint with Autologous Tissue Substitute, Open Approach

ØRULØJZ Supplement Right Elbow Joint with Synthetic Substitute, Open Approach

ØRULØKZ Supplement Right Elbow Joint with Nonautologous Tissue Substitute, Open Approach

ØRUL37Z Supplement Right Elbow Joint with Autologous Tissue Substitute, Percutaneous Approach

ØRUL3JZ Supplement Right Elbow Joint with Synthetic Substitute, Percutaneous Approach

ØRUL3KZ Supplement Right Elbow Joint with Nonautologous Tissue Substitute, Percutaneous Approach

ØRUL47Z Supplement Right Elbow Joint with Autologous Tissue Substitute, Percutaneous Endoscopic Approach

ØRUL4JZ Supplement Right Elbow Joint with Synthetic Substitute, Percutaneous Endoscopic Approach

ØRUL4KZ Supplement Right Elbow Joint with Nonautologous Tissue Substitute, Percutaneous Endoscopic Approach

ØRUMØ7Z Supplement Left Elbow Joint with Autologous Tissue Substitute, Open Approach

ØRUMØJZ Supplement Left Elbow Joint with Synthetic Substitute, Open Approach

ØRUMØKZ Supplement Left Elbow Joint with Nonautologous Tissue Substitute, Open Approach

ØRUM37Z Supplement Left Elbow Joint with Autologous Tissue Substitute, Percutaneous Approach

ØRUM3JZ Supplement Left Elbow Joint with Synthetic Substitute, Percutaneous Approach

ØRUM3KZ Supplement Left Elbow Joint with Nonautologous Tissue Substitute, Percutaneous Approach

ØRUM47Z Supplement Left Elbow Joint with Autologous Tissue Substitute, Percutaneous Endoscopic Approach

ØRUM4JZ Supplement Left Elbow Joint with Synthetic Substitute, Percutaneous Endoscopic Approach

ØRUM4KZ Supplement Left Elbow Joint with Nonautologous Tissue Substitute, Percutaneous Endoscopic Approach

ØSGØØ7Ø Fusion of Lumbar Vertebral Joint with Autologous Tissue Substitute, Anterior Approach, Anterior Column, Open Approach

ØSGØØ71 Fusion of Lumbar Vertebral Joint with Autologous Tissue Substitute, Posterior Approach, Posterior Column, Open Approach

ØSGØØ7J Fusion of Lumbar Vertebral Joint with Autologous Tissue Substitute, Posterior Approach, Anterior Column, Open Approach

ØSGØØAØ Fusion of Lumbar Vertebral Joint with Interbody Fusion Device, Anterior Approach, Anterior Column, Open Approach

ØSGØØAJ Fusion of Lumbar Vertebral Joint with Interbody Fusion Device, Posterior Approach, Anterior Column, Open Approach

ØSGØØJØ Fusion of Lumbar Vertebral Joint with Synthetic Substitute, Anterior Approach, Anterior Column, Open Approach

ØSGØØJ1 Fusion of Lumbar Vertebral Joint with Synthetic Substitute, Posterior Approach, Posterior Column, Open Approach

ØSGØØJJ Fusion of Lumbar Vertebral Joint with Synthetic Substitute, Posterior Approach, Anterior Column, Open Approach

ØSGØØKØ Fusion of Lumbar Vertebral Joint with Nonautologous Tissue Substitute, Anterior Approach, Anterior Column, Open Approach

ØSGØØK1 Fusion of Lumbar Vertebral Joint with Nonautologous Tissue Substitute, Posterior Approach, Posterior Column, Open Approach

ØSGØØKJ Fusion of Lumbar Vertebral Joint with Nonautologous Tissue Substitute, Posterior Approach, Anterior Column, Open Approach

ØSGØ37Ø Fusion of Lumbar Vertebral Joint with Autologous Tissue Substitute, Anterior Approach, Anterior Column, Percutaneous Approach

ØSGØ371 Fusion of Lumbar Vertebral Joint with Autologous Tissue Substitute, Posterior Approach, Posterior Column, Percutaneous Approach

ØSGØ37J Fusion of Lumbar Vertebral Joint with Autologous Tissue Substitute, Posterior Approach, Anterior Column, Percutaneous Approach

ØSGØ3AØ Fusion of Lumbar Vertebral Joint with Interbody Fusion Device, Anterior Approach, Anterior Column, Percutaneous Approach

ØSGØ3AJ Fusion of Lumbar Vertebral Joint with Interbody Fusion Device, Posterior Approach, Anterior Column, Percutaneous Approach

ØSGØ3JØ Fusion of Lumbar Vertebral Joint with Synthetic Substitute, Anterior Approach, Anterior Column, Percutaneous Approach

ØSGØ3J1 Fusion of Lumbar Vertebral Joint with Synthetic Substitute, Posterior Approach, Posterior Column, Percutaneous Approach

ØSGØ3JJ Fusion of Lumbar Vertebral Joint with Synthetic Substitute, Posterior Approach, Anterior Column, Percutaneous Approach

ØSGØ3KØ Fusion of Lumbar Vertebral Joint with Nonautologous Tissue Substitute, Anterior Approach, Anterior Column, Percutaneous Approach

ØSGØ3K1 Fusion of Lumbar Vertebral Joint with Nonautologous Tissue Substitute, Posterior Approach, Posterior Column, Percutaneous Approach

ØSGØ3KJ Fusion of Lumbar Vertebral Joint with Nonautologous Tissue Substitute, Posterior Approach, Anterior Column, Percutaneous Approach

ØSGØ47Ø Fusion of Lumbar Vertebral Joint with Autologous Tissue Substitute, Anterior Approach, Anterior Column, Percutaneous Endoscopic Approach

ØSGØ471 Fusion of Lumbar Vertebral Joint with Autologous Tissue Substitute, Posterior Approach, Posterior Column, Percutaneous Endoscopic Approach

ØSGØ47J Fusion of Lumbar Vertebral Joint with Autologous Tissue Substitute, Posterior Approach, Anterior Column, Percutaneous Endoscopic Approach

ØSGØ4AØ Fusion of Lumbar Vertebral Joint with Interbody Fusion Device, Anterior Approach, Anterior Column, Percutaneous Endoscopic Approach

ØSGØ4AJ Fusion of Lumbar Vertebral Joint with Interbody Fusion Device, Posterior Approach, Anterior Column, Percutaneous Endoscopic Approach

ØSGØ4JØ Fusion of Lumbar Vertebral Joint with Synthetic Substitute, Anterior Approach, Anterior Column, Percutaneous Endoscopic Approach

ØSGØ4J1 Fusion of Lumbar Vertebral Joint with Synthetic Substitute, Posterior Approach, Posterior Column, Percutaneous Endoscopic Approach

ØSGØ4JJ Fusion of Lumbar Vertebral Joint with Synthetic Substitute, Posterior Approach, Anterior Column, Percutaneous Endoscopic Approach

ØSGØ4KØ Fusion of Lumbar Vertebral Joint with Nonautologous Tissue Substitute, Anterior Approach, Anterior Column, Percutaneous Endoscopic Approach

ØSGØ4K1 Fusion of Lumbar Vertebral Joint with Nonautologous Tissue Substitute, Posterior Approach, Posterior Column, Percutaneous Endoscopic Approach

ØSGØ4KJ Fusion of Lumbar Vertebral Joint with Nonautologous Tissue Substitute, Posterior Approach, Anterior Column, Percutaneous Endoscopic Approach

ØSG1Ø7Ø Fusion of 2 or More Lumbar Vertebral Joints with Autologous Tissue Substitute, Anterior Approach, Anterior Column, Open Approach

ØSG1Ø71 Fusion of 2 or More Lumbar Vertebral Joints with Autologous Tissue Substitute, Posterior Approach, Posterior Column, Open Approach

ØSG1Ø7J Fusion of 2 or More Lumbar Vertebral Joints with Autologous Tissue Substitute, Posterior Approach, Anterior Column, Open Approach

ØSG1ØAØ Fusion of 2 or More Lumbar Vertebral Joints with Interbody Fusion Device, Anterior Approach, Anterior Column, Open Approach

ØSG1ØAJ Fusion of 2 or More Lumbar Vertebral Joints with Interbody Fusion Device, Posterior Approach, Anterior Column, Open Approach

ØSG1ØJØ Fusion of 2 or More Lumbar Vertebral Joints with Synthetic Substitute, Anterior Approach, Anterior Column, Open Approach

ØSG1ØJ1 Fusion of 2 or More Lumbar Vertebral Joints with Synthetic Substitute, Posterior Approach, Posterior Column, Open Approach

ØSG1ØJJ Fusion of 2 or More Lumbar Vertebral Joints with Synthetic Substitute, Posterior Approach, Anterior Column, Open Approach

ØSG1ØKØ Fusion of 2 or More Lumbar Vertebral Joints with Nonautologous Tissue Substitute, Anterior Approach, Anterior Column, Open Approach

HAC 12: Surgical Site Infection-Certain Orthopedic Procedures of the Spine, Shoulder, and Elbow (continued)

ØSG10K1   Fusion of 2 or More Lumbar Vertebral Joints with Nonautologous Tissue Substitute, Posterior Approach, Posterior Column, Open Approach

ØSG10KJ   Fusion of 2 or More Lumbar Vertebral Joints with Nonautologous Tissue Substitute, Posterior Approach, Anterior Column, Open Approach

ØSG137Ø   Fusion of 2 or More Lumbar Vertebral Joints with Autologous Tissue Substitute, Anterior Approach, Anterior Column, Percutaneous Approach

ØSG1371   Fusion of 2 or More Lumbar Vertebral Joints with Autologous Tissue Substitute, Posterior Approach, Posterior Column, Percutaneous Approach

ØSG137J   Fusion of 2 or More Lumbar Vertebral Joints with Autologous Tissue Substitute, Posterior Approach, Anterior Column, Percutaneous Approach

ØSG13AØ   Fusion of 2 or More Lumbar Vertebral Joints with Interbody Fusion Device, Anterior Approach, Anterior Column, Percutaneous Approach

ØSG13AJ   Fusion of 2 or More Lumbar Vertebral Joints with Interbody Fusion Device, Posterior Approach, Anterior Column, Percutaneous Approach

ØSG13JØ   Fusion of 2 or More Lumbar Vertebral Joints with Synthetic Substitute, Anterior Approach, Anterior Column, Percutaneous Approach

ØSG13J1   Fusion of 2 or More Lumbar Vertebral Joints with Synthetic Substitute, Posterior Approach, Posterior Column, Percutaneous Approach

ØSG13JJ   Fusion of 2 or More Lumbar Vertebral Joints with Synthetic Substitute, Posterior Approach, Anterior Column, Percutaneous Approach

ØSG13KØ   Fusion of 2 or More Lumbar Vertebral Joints with Nonautologous Tissue Substitute, Anterior Approach, Anterior Column, Percutaneous Approach

ØSG13K1   Fusion of 2 or More Lumbar Vertebral Joints with Nonautologous Tissue Substitute, Posterior Approach, Posterior Column, Percutaneous Approach

ØSG13KJ   Fusion of 2 or More Lumbar Vertebral Joints with Nonautologous Tissue Substitute, Posterior Approach, Anterior Column, Percutaneous Approach

ØSG147Ø   Fusion of 2 or More Lumbar Vertebral Joints with Autologous Tissue Substitute, Anterior Approach, Anterior Column, Percutaneous Endoscopic Approach

ØSG1471   Fusion of 2 or More Lumbar Vertebral Joints with Autologous Tissue Substitute, Posterior Approach, Posterior Column, Percutaneous Endoscopic Approach

ØSG147J   Fusion of 2 or More Lumbar Vertebral Joints with Autologous Tissue Substitute, Posterior Approach, Anterior Column, Percutaneous Endoscopic Approach

ØSG14AØ   Fusion of 2 or More Lumbar Vertebral Joints with Interbody Fusion Device, Anterior Approach, Anterior Column, Percutaneous Endoscopic Approach

ØSG14AJ   Fusion of 2 or More Lumbar Vertebral Joints with Interbody Fusion Device, Posterior Approach, Anterior Column, Percutaneous Endoscopic Approach

ØSG14JØ   Fusion of 2 or More Lumbar Vertebral Joints with Synthetic Substitute, Anterior Approach, Anterior Column, Percutaneous Endoscopic Approach

ØSG14J1   Fusion of 2 or More Lumbar Vertebral Joints with Synthetic Substitute, Posterior Approach, Posterior Column, Percutaneous Endoscopic Approach

ØSG14JJ   Fusion of 2 or More Lumbar Vertebral Joints with Synthetic Substitute, Posterior Approach, Anterior Column, Percutaneous Endoscopic Approach

ØSG14KØ   Fusion of 2 or More Lumbar Vertebral Joints with Nonautologous Tissue Substitute, Anterior Approach, Anterior Column, Percutaneous Endoscopic Approach

ØSG14K1   Fusion of 2 or More Lumbar Vertebral Joints with Nonautologous Tissue Substitute, Posterior Approach, Posterior Column, Percutaneous Endoscopic Approach

ØSG14KJ   Fusion of 2 or More Lumbar Vertebral Joints with Nonautologous Tissue Substitute, Posterior Approach, Anterior Column, Percutaneous Endoscopic Approach

ØSG3Ø7Ø   Fusion of Lumbosacral Joint with Autologous Tissue Substitute, Anterior Approach, Anterior Column, Open Approach

ØSG3Ø71   Fusion of Lumbosacral Joint with Autologous Tissue Substitute, Posterior Approach, Posterior Column, Open Approach

ØSG3Ø7J   Fusion of Lumbosacral Joint with Autologous Tissue Substitute, Posterior Approach, Anterior Column, Open Approach

ØSG3ØAØ   Fusion of Lumbosacral Joint with Interbody Fusion Device, Anterior Approach, Anterior Column, Open Approach

ØSG3ØAJ   Fusion of Lumbosacral Joint with Interbody Fusion Device, Posterior Approach, Anterior Column, Open Approach

ØSG3ØJØ   Fusion of Lumbosacral Joint with Synthetic Substitute, Anterior Approach, Anterior Column, Open Approach

ØSG3ØJ1   Fusion of Lumbosacral Joint with Synthetic Substitute, Posterior Approach, Posterior Column, Open Approach

ØSG3ØJJ   Fusion of Lumbosacral Joint with Synthetic Substitute, Posterior Approach, Anterior Column, Open Approach

ØSG3ØKØ   Fusion of Lumbosacral Joint with Nonautologous Tissue Substitute, Anterior Approach, Anterior Column, Open Approach

ØSG3ØK1   Fusion of Lumbosacral Joint with Nonautologous Tissue Substitute, Posterior Approach, Posterior Column, Open Approach

ØSG3ØKJ   Fusion of Lumbosacral Joint with Nonautologous Tissue Substitute, Posterior Approach, Anterior Column, Open Approach

ØSG337Ø   Fusion of Lumbosacral Joint with Autologous Tissue Substitute, Anterior Approach, Anterior Column, Percutaneous Approach

ØSG3371   Fusion of Lumbosacral Joint with Autologous Tissue Substitute, Posterior Approach, Posterior Column, Percutaneous Approach

ØSG337J   Fusion of Lumbosacral Joint with Autologous Tissue Substitute, Posterior Approach, Anterior Column, Percutaneous Approach

ØSG33AØ   Fusion of Lumbosacral Joint with Interbody Fusion Device, Anterior Approach, Anterior Column, Percutaneous Approach

ØSG33AJ   Fusion of Lumbosacral Joint with Interbody Fusion Device, Posterior Approach, Anterior Column, Percutaneous Approach

ØSG33JØ   Fusion of Lumbosacral Joint with Synthetic Substitute, Anterior Approach, Anterior Column, Percutaneous Approach

ØSG33J1   Fusion of Lumbosacral Joint with Synthetic Substitute, Posterior Approach, Posterior Column, Percutaneous Approach

ØSG33JJ   Fusion of Lumbosacral Joint with Synthetic Substitute, Posterior Approach, Anterior Column, Percutaneous Approach

ØSG33KØ   Fusion of Lumbosacral Joint with Nonautologous Tissue Substitute, Anterior Approach, Anterior Column, Percutaneous Approach

ØSG33K1   Fusion of Lumbosacral Joint with Nonautologous Tissue Substitute, Posterior Approach, Posterior Column, Percutaneous Approach

ØSG33KJ   Fusion of Lumbosacral Joint with Nonautologous Tissue Substitute, Posterior Approach, Anterior Column, Percutaneous Approach

ØSG347Ø   Fusion of Lumbosacral Joint with Autologous Tissue Substitute, Anterior Approach, Anterior Column, Percutaneous Endoscopic Approach

ØSG3471   Fusion of Lumbosacral Joint with Autologous Tissue Substitute, Posterior Approach, Posterior Column, Percutaneous Endoscopic Approach

ØSG347J   Fusion of Lumbosacral Joint with Autologous Tissue Substitute, Posterior Approach, Anterior Column, Percutaneous Endoscopic Approach

ØSG34AØ   Fusion of Lumbosacral Joint with Interbody Fusion Device, Anterior Approach, Anterior Column, Percutaneous Endoscopic Approach

ØSG34AJ   Fusion of Lumbosacral Joint with Interbody Fusion Device, Posterior Approach, Anterior Column, Percutaneous Endoscopic Approach

ØSG34JØ   Fusion of Lumbosacral Joint with Synthetic Substitute, Anterior Approach, Anterior Column, Percutaneous Endoscopic Approach

ØSG34J1   Fusion of Lumbosacral Joint with Synthetic Substitute, Posterior Approach, Posterior Column, Percutaneous Endoscopic Approach

ØSG34JJ   Fusion of Lumbosacral Joint with Synthetic Substitute, Posterior Approach, Anterior Column, Percutaneous Endoscopic Approach

ØSG34KØ   Fusion of Lumbosacral Joint with Nonautologous Tissue Substitute, Anterior Approach, Anterior Column, Percutaneous Endoscopic Approach

ØSG34K1   Fusion of Lumbosacral Joint with Nonautologous Tissue Substitute, Posterior Approach, Posterior Column, Percutaneous Endoscopic Approach

HAC 12: Surgical Site Infection-Certain Orthopedic Procedures of the Spine, Shoulder, and Elbow (continued)

0SG34KJ Fusion of Lumbosacral Joint with Nonautologous Tissue Substitute, Posterior Approach, Anterior Column, Percutaneous Endoscopic Approach

0SG704Z Fusion of Right Sacroiliac Joint with Internal Fixation Device, Open Approach

0SG707Z Fusion of Right Sacroiliac Joint with Autologous Tissue Substitute, Open Approach

0SG70JZ Fusion of Right Sacroiliac Joint with Synthetic Substitute, Open Approach

0SG70KZ Fusion of Right Sacroiliac Joint with Nonautologous Tissue Substitute, Open Approach

0SG734Z Fusion of Right Sacroiliac Joint with Internal Fixation Device, Percutaneous Approach

0SG737Z Fusion of Right Sacroiliac Joint with Autologous Tissue Substitute, Percutaneous Approach

0SG73JZ Fusion of Right Sacroiliac Joint with Synthetic Substitute, Percutaneous Approach

0SG73KZ Fusion of Right Sacroiliac Joint with Nonautologous Tissue Substitute, Percutaneous Approach

0SG744Z Fusion of Right Sacroiliac Joint with Internal Fixation Device, Percutaneous Endoscopic Approach

0SG747Z Fusion of Right Sacroiliac Joint with Autologous Tissue Substitute, Percutaneous Endoscopic Approach

0SG74JZ Fusion of Right Sacroiliac Joint with Synthetic Substitute, Percutaneous Endoscopic Approach

0SG74KZ Fusion of Right Sacroiliac Joint with Nonautologous Tissue Substitute, Percutaneous Endoscopic Approach

0SG804Z Fusion of Left Sacroiliac Joint with Internal Fixation Device, Open Approach

0SG807Z Fusion of Left Sacroiliac Joint with Autologous Tissue Substitute, Open Approach

0SG80JZ Fusion of Left Sacroiliac Joint with Synthetic Substitute, Open Approach

0SG80KZ Fusion of Left Sacroiliac Joint with Nonautologous Tissue Substitute, Open Approach

0SG834Z Fusion of Left Sacroiliac Joint with Internal Fixation Device, Percutaneous Approach

0SG837Z Fusion of Left Sacroiliac Joint with Autologous Tissue Substitute, Percutaneous Approach

0SG83JZ Fusion of Left Sacroiliac Joint with Synthetic Substitute, Percutaneous Approach

0SG83KZ Fusion of Left Sacroiliac Joint with Nonautologous Tissue Substitute, Percutaneous Approach

0SG844Z Fusion of Left Sacroiliac Joint with Internal Fixation Device, Percutaneous Endoscopic Approach

0SG847Z Fusion of Left Sacroiliac Joint with Autologous Tissue Substitute, Percutaneous Endoscopic Approach

0SG84JZ Fusion of Left Sacroiliac Joint with Synthetic Substitute, Percutaneous Endoscopic Approach

0SG84KZ Fusion of Left Sacroiliac Joint with Nonautologous Tissue Substitute, Percutaneous Endoscopic Approach

XRG0092 Fusion of Occipital-cervical Joint using Nanotextured Surface Interbody Fusion Device, Open Approach, New Technology Group 2

XRG00F3 Fusion of Occipital-cervical Joint using Radiolucent Porous Interbody Fusion Device, Open Approach, New Technology Group 3

XRG1092 Fusion of Cervical Vertebral Joint using Nanotextured Surface Interbody Fusion Device, Open Approach, New Technology Group 2

XRG10F3 Fusion of Cervical Vertebral Joint using Radiolucent Porous Interbody Fusion Device, Open Approach, New Technology Group 3

XRG2092 Fusion of 2 or more Cervical Vertebral Joints using Nanotextured Surface Interbody Fusion Device, Open Approach, New Technology Group 2

XRG20F3 Fusion of 2 or more Cervical Vertebral Joints using Radiolucent Porous Interbody Fusion Device, Open Approach, New Technology Group 3

XRG4092 Fusion of Cervicothoracic Vertebral Joint using Nanotextured Surface Interbody Fusion Device, Open Approach, New Technology Group 2

XRG40F3 Fusion of Cervicothoracic Vertebral Joint using Radiolucent Porous Interbody Fusion Device, Open Approach, New Technology Group 3

XRG6092 Fusion of Thoracic Vertebral Joint using Nanotextured Surface Interbody Fusion Device, Open Approach, New Technology Group 2

XRG60F3 Fusion of Thoracic Vertebral Joint using Radiolucent Porous Interbody Fusion Device, Open Approach, New Technology Group 3

XRG7092 Fusion of 2 to 7 Thoracic Vertebral Joints using Nanotextured Surface Interbody Fusion Device, Open Approach, New Technology Group 2

XRG70F3 Fusion of 2 to 7 Thoracic Vertebral Joints using Radiolucent Porous Interbody Fusion Device, Open Approach, New Technology Group 3

XRG8092 Fusion of 8 or more Thoracic Vertebral Joints using Nanotextured Surface Interbody Fusion Device, Open Approach, New Technology Group 2

XRG80F3 Fusion of 8 or more Thoracic Vertebral Joints using Radiolucent Porous Interbody Fusion Device, Open Approach, New Technology Group 3

XRGA092 Fusion of Thoracolumbar Vertebral Joint using Nanotextured Surface Interbody Fusion Device, Open Approach, New Technology Group 2

XRGA0F3 Fusion of Thoracolumbar Vertebral Joint using Radiolucent Porous Interbody Fusion Device, Open Approach, New Technology Group 3

XRGB092 Fusion of Lumbar Vertebral Joint using Nanotextured Surface Interbody Fusion Device, Open Approach, New Technology Group 2

XRGB0F3 Fusion of Lumbar Vertebral Joint using Radiolucent Porous Interbody Fusion Device, Open Approach, New Technology Group 3

XRGC092 Fusion of 2 or more Lumbar Vertebral Joints using Nanotextured Surface Interbody Fusion Device, Open Approach, New Technology Group 2

XRGC0F3 Fusion of 2 or more Lumbar Vertebral Joints using Radiolucent Porous Interbody Fusion Device, Open Approach, New Technology Group 3

XRGD092 Fusion of Lumbosacral Joint using Nanotextured Surface Interbody Fusion Device, Open Approach, New Technology Group 2

XRGD0F3 Fusion of Lumbosacral Joint using Radiolucent Porous Interbody Fusion Device, Open Approach, New Technology Group 3

HAC 13: Surgical Site Infection (SSI) Following Cardiac Implantable Electronic Device (CIED) Procedures

Secondary diagnosis not POA:

K68.11 Postprocedural retroperitoneal abscess

T81.40XA Infection following a procedure, unspecified, initial encounter

T81.41XA Infection following a procedure, superficial incisional surgical site, initial encounter

T81.42XA Infection following a procedure, deep incisional surgical site, initial encounter

T81.43XA Infection following a procedure, organ and space surgical site, initial encounter

T81.44XA Sepsis following a procedure, initial encounter

T81.49XA Infection following a procedure, other surgical site, initial encounter

T82.6XXA Infection and inflammatory reaction due to cardiac valve prosthesis, initial encounter

T82.7XXA Infection and inflammatory reaction due to other internal orthopedic prosthetic devices, implants and grafts, initial encounter

AND

Any of the following procedures:

02H43JZ Insertion of Pacemaker Lead into Coronary Vein, Percutaneous Approach

02H43KZ Insertion of Defibrillator Lead into Coronary Vein, Percutaneous Approach

02H43MZ Insertion of Cardiac Lead into Coronary Vein, Percutaneous Approach

02H63JZ Insertion of Pacemaker Lead Into Right Atrium, Percutaneous Approach

02H63MZ Insertion of Cardiac Lead into Right Atrium, Percutaneous Approach

02H73JZ Insertion of Pacemaker Lead into Left Atrium, Percutaneous Approach

02H73MZ Insertion of Cardiac Lead into Left Atrium, Percutaneous Approach

02HK3JZ Insertion of Pacemaker Lead into Right Ventricle, Percutaneous Approach

02HL3JZ Insertion of Pacemaker Lead into Left Ventricle, Percutaneous Approach

02HN0JZ Insertion of Pacemaker Lead into Pericardium, Open Approach

02HN0MZ Insertion of Cardiac Lead into Pericardium, Open Approach

02HN3JZ Insertion of Pacemaker Lead into Pericardium, Percutaneous Approach

02HN3MZ Insertion of Cardiac Lead into Pericardium, Percutaneous Approach

02HN4JZ Insertion of Pacemaker Lead into Pericardium, Percutaneous Endoscopic Approach

02HN4MZ Insertion of Cardiac Lead into Pericardium, Percutaneous Endoscopic Approach

02PA0MZ Removal of Cardiac Lead from Heart, Open Approach

02PA3MZ Removal of Cardiac Lead from Heart, Percutaneous Approach

02PA4MZ Removal of Cardiac Lead from Heart, Percutaneous Endoscopic Approach

HAC 13: Surgical Site Infection (SSI) Following Cardiac Implantable Electronic Device (CIED) Procedures (continued)

02PAXMZ	Removal of Cardiac Lead from Heart, External Approach
02WA0MZ	Revision of Cardiac Lead in Heart, Open Approach
02WA3MZ	Revision of Cardiac Lead in Heart, Percutaneous Approach
02WA4MZ	Revision of Cardiac Lead in Heart, Percutaneous Endoscopic Approach
0JH604Z	Insertion of Pacemaker, Single Chamber into Chest Subcutaneous Tissue and Fascia, Open Approach
0JH605Z	Insertion of Pacemaker, Single Chamber Rate Responsive into Chest Subcutaneous Tissue and Fascia, Open Approach
0JH606Z	Insertion of Pacemaker, Dual Chamber into Chest Subcutaneous Tissue and Fascia, Open Approach
0JH607Z	Insertion of Cardiac Resynchronization Pacemaker Pulse Generator into Chest Subcutaneous Tissue and Fascia, Open Approach
0JH608Z	Insertion of Defibrillator Generator into Chest Subcutaneous Tissue and Fascia, Open Approach
0JH609Z	Insertion of Cardiac Resynchronization Defibrillator Pulse Generator into Chest Subcutaneous Tissue and Fascia, Open Approach
0JH60PZ	Insertion of Cardiac Rhythm Related Device into Chest Subcutaneous Tissue and Fascia, Open Approach
0JH634Z	Insertion of Pacemaker, Single Chamber into Chest Subcutaneous Tissue and Fascia, Percutaneous Approach
0JH635Z	Insertion of Pacemaker, Single Chamber Rate Responsive into Chest Subcutaneous Tissue and Fascia, Percutaneous Approach
0JH636Z	Insertion of Pacemaker, Dual Chamber into Chest Subcutaneous Tissue and Fascia, Percutaneous Approach
0JH637Z	Insertion of Cardiac Resynchronization Pacemaker Pulse Generator into Chest Subcutaneous Tissue and Fascia, Percutaneous Approach
0JH638Z	Insertion of Defibrillator Generator into Chest Subcutaneous Tissue and Fascia, Percutaneous Approach
0JH639Z	Insertion of Cardiac Resynchronization Defibrillator Pulse Generator into Chest Subcutaneous Tissue and Fascia, Percutaneous Approach
0JH63PZ	Insertion of Cardiac Rhythm Related Device into Chest Subcutaneous Tissue and Fascia, Percutaneous Approach
0JH804Z	Insertion of Pacemaker, Single Chamber into Abdomen Subcutaneous Tissue and Fascia, Open Approach
0JH805Z	Insertion of Pacemaker, Single Chamber Rate Responsive into Abdomen Subcutaneous Tissue and Fascia, Open Approach
0JH806Z	Insertion of Pacemaker, Dual Chamber into Abdomen Subcutaneous Tissue and Fascia, Open Approach
0JH807Z	Insertion of Cardiac Resynchronization Pacemaker Pulse Generator into Abdomen Subcutaneous Tissue and Fascia, Open Approach
0JH808Z	Insertion of Defibrillator Generator into Abdomen Subcutaneous Tissue and Fascia, Open Approach
0JH809Z	Insertion of Cardiac Resynchronization Defibrillator Pulse Generator into Abdomen Subcutaneous Tissue and Fascia, Open Approach
0JH80PZ	Insertion of Cardiac Rhythm Related Device into Abdomen Subcutaneous Tissue and Fascia, Open Approach
0JH834Z	Insertion of Pacemaker, Single Chamber into Abdomen Subcutaneous Tissue and Fascia, Percutaneous Approach
0JH835Z	Insertion of Pacemaker, Single Chamber Rate Responsive into Abdomen Subcutaneous Tissue and Fascia, Percutaneous Approach
0JH836Z	Insertion of Pacemaker, Dual Chamber into Abdomen Subcutaneous Tissue and Fascia, Percutaneous Approach
0JH837Z	Insertion of Cardiac Resynchronization Pacemaker Pulse Generator into Abdomen Subcutaneous Tissue and Fascia, Percutaneous Approach
0JH838Z	Insertion of Defibrillator Generator into Abdomen Subcutaneous Tissue and Fascia, Percutaneous Approach
0JH839Z	Insertion of Cardiac Resynchronization Defibrillator Pulse Generator into Abdomen Subcutaneous Tissue and Fascia, Percutaneous Approach
0JH83PZ	Insertion of Cardiac Rhythm Related Device into Abdomen Subcutaneous Tissue and Fascia, Percutaneous Approach
0JPT0FZ	Removal of Subcutaneous Defibrillator Lead from Trunk Subcutaneous Tissue and Fascia, Open Approach
0JPT0PZ	Removal of Cardiac Rhythm Related Device from Trunk Subcutaneous Tissue and Fascia, Open Approach
0JPT3FZ	Removal of Subcutaneous Defibrillator Lead from Trunk Subcutaneous Tissue and Fascia, Percutaneous Approach
0JPT3PZ	Removal of Cardiac Rhythm Related Device from Trunk Subcutaneous Tissue and Fascia, Percutaneous Approach
0JWT0FZ	Revision of Subcutaneous Defibrillator Lead in Trunk Subcutaneous Tissue and Fascia, Open Approach
0JWT0PZ	Revision of Cardiac Rhythm Related Device in Trunk Subcutaneous Tissue and Fascia, Open Approach
0JWT3FZ	Revision of Subcutaneous Defibrillator Lead in Trunk Subcutaneous Tissue and Fascia, Percutaneous Approach
0JWT3PZ	Revision of Cardiac Rhythm Related Device in Trunk Subcutaneous Tissue and Fascia, Percutaneous Approach

HAC 14: Iatrogenic Pneumothorax with Venous Catheterization

Secondary diagnosis not POA:

J95.811	Postprocedural pneumothorax

AND

Any of the following procedures:

02H633Z	Insertion of Infusion Device into Right Atrium, Percutaneous Approach
02HK33Z	Insertion of Infusion Device into Right Ventricle, Percutaneous Approach
02HS33Z	Insertion of Infusion Device into Right Pulmonary Vein, Percutaneous Approach
02HS43Z	Insertion of Infusion Device into Right Pulmonary Vein, Percutaneous Endoscopic Approach
02HT33Z	Insertion of Infusion Device into Left Pulmonary Vein, Percutaneous Approach
02HT43Z	Insertion of Infusion Device into Left Pulmonary Vein, Percutaneous Endoscopic Approach
02HV33Z	Insertion of Infusion Device into Superior Vena Cava, Percutaneous Approach
02HV43Z	Insertion of Infusion Device into Superior Vena Cava, Percutaneous Endoscopic Approach
05H033Z	Insertion of Infusion Device into Azygos Vein, Percutaneous Approach
05H043Z	Insertion of Infusion Device into Azygos Vein, Percutaneous Endoscopic Approach
05H133Z	Insertion of Infusion Device into Hemiazygos Vein, Percutaneous Approach
05H143Z	Insertion of Infusion Device into Hemiazygos Vein, Percutaneous Endoscopic Approach
05H333Z	Insertion of Infusion Device into Right Innominate Vein, Percutaneous Approach
05H343Z	Insertion of Infusion Device into Right Innominate Vein, Percutaneous Endoscopic Approach
05H433Z	Insertion of Infusion Device into Left Innominate Vein, Percutaneous Approach
05H443Z	Insertion of Infusion Device into Left Innominate Vein, Percutaneous Endoscopic Approach
05H533Z	Insertion of Infusion Device into Right Subclavian Vein, Percutaneous Approach
05H543Z	Insertion of Infusion Device into Right Subclavian Vein, Percutaneous Endoscopic Approach
05H633Z	Insertion of Infusion Device into Left Subclavian Vein, Percutaneous Approach
05H643Z	Insertion of Infusion Device into Left Subclavian Vein, Percutaneous Endoscopic Approach
05HM33Z	Insertion of Infusion Device into Right Internal Jugular Vein, Percutaneous Approach
05HN33Z	Insertion of Infusion Device into Left Internal Jugular Vein, Percutaneous Approach
05HP33Z	Insertion of Infusion Device into Right External Jugular Vein, Percutaneous Approach
05HQ33Z	Insertion of Infusion Device into Left External Jugular Vein, Percutaneous Approach
0JH63XZ	Insertion of Vascular Access Device into Chest Subcutaneous Tissue and Fascia, Percutaneous Approach

Appendix L: Procedure Combination Tables

The tables below were developed to help simplify the relationship between ICD-10-PCS coding and MS-DRG assignment. The Centers for Medicare & Medicaid Services (CMS) has identified in the MS-DRG Definitions Manual certain procedure combinations that must occur in order to assign a specific MS-DRG. There are many factors influencing MS-DRG assignment, including principal and secondary diagnoses, MCC or CC use, sex of the patient, and discharge status. These tables should be used only as a guide. These tables were created based on the proposed, version 39, MS-DRG Grouper software and Definitions Manual files published with the fiscal 2022 IPPS proposed rule. To view the final, version 39, MS-DRG Grouper software and Definitions Manual files, refer to the following: https://www.cms.gov/Medicare/Medicare-Fee-for-Service-Payment/AcuteInpatientPPS/MS-DRG-Classifications-and-Software.

DRG 001-002 Heart Transplant or Implant of Heart Assist System

Heart Transplant
Replacement of Right and Left Ventricle   02RK0JZ and 02RL0JZ

Insertion With Removal of Heart Assist System

Type of Heart Assist System	Code as appropriate Insertion by approach	Code also as appropriate Removal of Heart Assist System by approach
Biventricular External	02HA[0,3,4]RS	02PA[0,3,4]RZ
External	02HA[0,4]RZ	02PA[0,3,4]RZ

Revision With Removal of Heart Assist System

Type of Heart Assist System	Code as appropriate Revision by approach	Code also as appropriate Removal of Heart Assist System by approach
Implantable	02WA[0,3,4]QZ	02PA[0,3,4]RZ
External	02WA[0,3,4]RZ	02PA[0,3,4]RZ

DRG 008 Simultaneous Pancreas/Kidney Transplant

Transplanted Body Part	Code Transplant as appropriate by tissue type			Code also Pancreas Transplant as appropriate by tissue type		
	Allogeneic	Syngeneic	Zooplastic	Allogeneic	Syngeneic	Zooplastic
Kidney, Right	0TY00Z0	0TY00Z1	0TY00Z2	0FYG0Z0	0FYG0Z1	0FYG0Z2
Kidney, Left	0TY10Z0	0TY10Z1	0TY10Z2			

DRG 019 Simultaneous Pancreas/Kidney Transplant with Hemodialysis

Transplanted Body Part	Code Transplant as appropriate by tissue type			Code also Pancreas Transplant as appropriate by tissue type			Code also Hemodialysis		
	Allogeneic	Syngeneic	Zooplastic	Allogeneic	Syngeneic	Zooplastic	< 6 Hours	6-18 Hours	> 18 Hours
Kidney, Right	0TY00Z0	0TY00Z1	0TY00Z2	0FYG0Z0	0FYG0Z1	0FYG0Z2	5A1D07Z	5A1D80Z	5A1D90Z
Kidney, Left	0TY10Z0	0TY10Z1	0TY10Z2						

DRG 023-027 Craniotomy

Site of Neurostimulator Lead	Code as appropriate Insertion of Lead by approach	Code also as appropriate Insertion of Device by type and subcutaneous site						
		Neuro-stimulator Generator	Stimulator Multiple Array Code as appropriate by approach			Stimulator Multiple Array, Rechargeable Code as appropriate by approach		
		Skull	Chest	Back	Abdomen	Chest	Back	Abdomen
Brain	00H0[0,3,4]MZ	0NH00NZ	0JH6[0,3]DZ	0JH7[0,3]DZ	0JH8[0,3]DZ	0JH6[0,3]EZ	0JH7[0,3]EZ	0JH8[0,3]EZ
Cerebral Ventricle	00H6[0,3,4]MZ	0NH00NZ	0JH6[0,3]DZ	0JH7[0,3]DZ	0JH8[0,3]DZ	0JH6[0,3]EZ	0JH7[0,3]EZ	0JH8[0,3]EZ

DRG 028-030 Spinal Procedures

Generator Type	Insertion of Generator by Site			Code also as appropriate Insertion of Neurostimulator Lead by approach	
	Chest	Abdomen	Back	Spinal Canal	Spinal Cord
Single Array	ØJH6[Ø,3]BZ	ØJH8[Ø,3]BZ	ØJH7[Ø,3]BZ	ØØHU[Ø,3,4]MZ	ØØHV[Ø,3,4]MZ
Single Array, Rechargeable	ØJH6[Ø,3]CZ	ØJH8[Ø,3]CZ	ØJH7[Ø,3]CZ	ØØHU[Ø,3,4]MZ	ØØHV[Ø,3,4]MZ
Multiple Array	ØJH6[Ø,3]DZ	ØJH8[Ø,3]DZ	ØJH7[Ø,3]DZ	ØØHU[Ø,3,4]MZ	ØØHV[Ø,3,4]MZ
Multiple Array, Rechargable	ØJH6[Ø,3]EZ	—	ØJH7[Ø,3]EZ	ØØHU[Ø,3,4]MZ	ØØHV[Ø,3,4]MZ
Multiple Array, Rechargable	—	ØJH8[Ø,3]EZ	—	ØØHU[Ø,3,4]MZ	ØØHV[Ø,3,4]MZ

DRG 040-042 Peripheral and Cranial Nerve and Other Nervous System Procedures

Insertion of Neurostimulator Lead With Device

Site of Neurostimulator Lead	Code as appropriate Insertion by approach	Code also as appropriate Insertion of Device by type and subcutaneous site					
		Stimulator Single Array Code as appropriate by approach			Stimulator Single Array, Rechargeable Code as appropriate by approach		
		Chest	Back	Abdomen	Chest	Back	Abdomen
Cranial Nerve	ØØHE[Ø,3,4]MZ	ØJH6[Ø,3]BZ	ØJH7[Ø,3]BZ	ØJH8[Ø,3]BZ	ØJH6[Ø,3]CZ	ØJH7[Ø,3]CZ	ØJH8[Ø,3]CZ
Peripheral Nerve	Ø1HY[Ø,3,4]MZ	ØJH6[Ø,3]BZ	ØJH7[Ø,3]BZ	ØJH8[Ø,3]BZ	ØJH6[Ø,3]CZ	ØJH7[Ø,3]CZ	ØJH8[Ø,3]CZ
Stomach	ØDH6[Ø,3,4]MZ	ØJH6[Ø,3]BZ	ØJH7[Ø,3]BZ	ØJH8[Ø,3]BZ	ØJH6[Ø,3]CZ	ØJH7[Ø,3]CZ	ØJH8[Ø,3]CZ
Azygos vein	Ø5HØ[Ø,3,4]MZ	ØJH6[Ø,3]BZ	ØJH7[Ø,S]BZ	ØJH8[Ø,3]BZ	ØJH6[Ø,3]CZ	ØJH7[Ø,S]CZ	ØJH8[Ø,3]CZ
Innominate Vein, Right	Ø5H3[Ø,3,4]MZ	ØJH6[Ø,3]BZ	ØJH7[Ø,S]BZ	ØJH8[Ø,3]BZ	ØJH6[Ø,3]CZ	ØJH7[Ø,S]CZ	ØJH8[Ø,3]CZ
Innominate Vein, Left	Ø5H4[Ø,3,4]MZ	ØJH6[Ø,3]BZ	ØJH7[Ø,S]BZ	ØJH8[Ø,3]BZ	ØJH6[Ø,3]CZ	ØJH7[Ø,S]CZ	ØJH8[Ø,3]CZ
		Stimulator Multiple Array Code as appropriate by approach			Stimulator Multiple Array, Rechargeable Code as appropriate by approach		
		Chest	Back	Abdomen	Chest	Back	Abdomen
Cranial Nerve	ØØHE[Ø,3,4]MZ	ØJH6[Ø,3]DZ	ØJH7[Ø,3]DZ	ØJH8[Ø,3]DZ	ØJH6[Ø,3]EZ	ØJH7[Ø,3]EZ	ØJH8[Ø,3]EZ
Peripheral Nerve	Ø1HY[Ø,3,4]MZ	ØJH6[Ø,3]DZ	ØJH7[Ø,3]DZ	ØJH8[Ø,3]DZ	ØJH6[Ø,3]EZ	ØJH7[Ø,3]EZ	ØJH8[Ø,3]EZ
Stomach	ØDH6[Ø,3,4]MZ	ØJH6[Ø,3]DZ	ØJH7[Ø,3]DZ	ØJH8[Ø,3]DZ	ØJH6[Ø,3]EZ	ØJH7[Ø,3]EZ	ØJH8[Ø,3]EZ
Azygos vein	Ø5HØ[Ø,3,4]MZ	ØJH6[Ø,3]DZ	ØJH7[Ø,S]DZ	ØJH8[Ø,3]DZ	ØJH6[Ø,3]EZ	ØJH7[Ø,S]EZ	ØJH8[Ø,3]EZ
Innominate Vein, Right	Ø5H3[Ø,3,4]MZ	ØJH6[Ø,3]DZ	ØJH7[Ø,S]DZ	ØJH8[Ø,3]DZ	ØJH6[Ø,3]EZ	ØJH7[Ø,S]EZ	ØJH8[Ø,3]EZ
Innominate Vein, Left	Ø5H4[Ø,3,4]MZ	ØJH6[Ø,3]DZ	ØJH7[Ø,S]DZ	ØJH8[Ø,3]DZ	ØJH6[Ø,3]EZ	ØJH7[Ø,S]EZ	ØJH8[Ø,3]EZ

DRG 222-227 Cardiac Defibrillator Implant

Insertion of Generator With Insertion of Lead(s) into Coronary Vein, Atrium or Ventricle

Generator Type	Insertion of Generator by Site		Code also as appropriate Insertion of Leads by site				
	Chest	Abdomen	Coronary Vein	Atrium		Ventricle	
				Right	Left	Right	Left
Defibrillator	ØJH6[Ø,3]8Z	ØJH8[Ø,3]8Z	Ø2H4[Ø,4]KZ	Ø2H6[Ø,3,4]KZ	Ø2H7[Ø,3,4]KZ	Ø2HK[Ø,3,4]KZ	Ø2HL[Ø,3,4]KZ
Cardiac Resynch Defibrillator Pulse Generator	ØJH6[Ø,3]9Z	ØJH8[Ø,3]9Z	Ø2H4[Ø,3,4]KZ or Ø2H43[J,M]Z	Ø2H6[Ø,3,4]KZ	Ø2H7[Ø,3,4]KZ	Ø2HK[Ø,3,4]KZ	Ø2HL[Ø,3,4]KZ
Contractility Modulation Device	ØJH6[Ø,3]AZ	ØJH8[Ø,3]AZ	—	Ø2H6[Ø,3,4]MZ	—	Ø2HK[Ø,3,4]MZ	—

Insertion of Generator with Insertion of Lead(s) into Pericardium or Chest

Generator Type	Insertion of Generator by Site		Code also as appropriate Insertion of Leads by Site and Type			
	Chest	Abdomen	Pericardium			Chest
			Pacemaker	Defibrillator	Cardiac	Subcutaneous
Defibrillator	ØJH6[Ø,3]8Z	ØJH8[Ø,3]8Z	Ø2HN[Ø,3,4]JZ	Ø2HN[Ø,3,4]KZ	Ø2HN[Ø,3,4]MZ	ØJH6[Ø,3]FZ
Cardiac Resynch Defibrillator Pulse Generator	ØJH6[Ø,3]9Z	ØJH8[Ø,3]9Z	Ø2HN[Ø,3,4]JZ	Ø2HN[Ø,3,4]KZ	Ø2HN[Ø,3,4]MZ	ØJH6[Ø,3]FZ

Appendix L: Procedure Combination Tables

DRG 242-244 Permanent Cardiac Pacemaker Implant

Insertion of Generator and Lead(s) Only

Generator Type	Insertion of Generator by Site		Code also as appropriate Insertion of Leads by site					
	Chest	Abdomen	Coronary Vein	Atrium		Ventricle		Pericardium
				Right	Left	Right	Left	
Single Chamber	ØJH6[Ø,3]4Z	ØJH8[Ø,3]4Z	02H4[Ø,3,4][J,M]Z	02H6[Ø,3,4][J,M]Z	02H7[Ø,3,4][J,M]Z	02HK[Ø,3,4][J,M]Z	02HL[Ø,3,4][J,M]Z	02HN[Ø,3,4][J,M]Z
Single Chamber RR	ØJH6[Ø,3]5Z	ØJH8[Ø,3]5Z	02H4[Ø,3,4][J,M]Z	02H6[Ø,3,4][J,M]Z	02H7[Ø,3,4][J,M]Z	02HK[Ø,3,4][J,M]Z	02HL[Ø,3,4][J,M]Z	02HN[Ø,3,4][J,M]Z
Dual Chamber	ØJH6[Ø,3]6Z	ØJH8[Ø,3]6Z	02H4[Ø,3,4][J,M]Z	02H6[Ø,3,4][J,M]Z	02H7[Ø,3,4][J,M]Z	02HK[Ø,3,4][J,M]Z	02HL[Ø,3,4][J,M]Z	02HN[Ø,3,4][J,M]Z
Cardiac Resynch Pulse Generator	ØJH6[Ø,3]7Z	ØJH8[Ø,3]7Z	02H4[Ø,3,4][J,M]Z	02H6[Ø,3,4][J,M]Z	02H7[Ø,3,4][J,M]Z	02HK[Ø,3,4][J,M]Z	02HL[Ø,3,4][J,M]Z	02HN[Ø,3,4][J,M]Z
Cardiac Rhythm Related	ØJH6[Ø,3]PZ	ØJH8[Ø,3]PZ	02H4[Ø,3,4][J,M]Z	02H6[Ø,3,4][J,M]Z	02H7[Ø,3,4][J,M]Z	02HK[Ø,3,4][J,M]Z	02HL[Ø,3,4][J,M]Z	02HN[Ø,3,4][J,M]Z

DRG 326-328 Stomach, Esophageal and Duodenal Procedures

Site	Resection by Open Approach	Code also as appropriate Resection of Pancreas by Open Approach
Duodenum	ØDT9ØZZ	ØFTGØZZ

DRG 344-346 Minor Small and Large Bowel Procedures

Site	Repair by Open Approach	Code also as appropriate Repair by external approach of Abdominal Wall Stoma
Small Intestine	ØDQ8ØZZ	ØWQFXZ2
Duodenum	ØDQ9ØZZ	ØWQFXZ2
Jejunum	ØDQAØZZ	ØWQFXZ2
Ileum	ØDQBØZZ	ØWQFXZ2
Large Intestine	ØDQEØZZ	ØWQFXZ2
Large Intestine, Right	ØDQFØZZ	ØWQFXZ2
Large Intestine, Left	ØDQGØZZ	ØWQFXZ2
Cecum	ØDQHØZZ	ØWQFXZ2
Ascending Colon	ØDQKØZZ	ØWQFXZ2
Transverse Colon	ØDQLØZZ	ØWQFXZ2
Descending Colon	ØDQMØZZ	ØWQFXZ2
Sigmoid Colon	ØDQNØZZ	ØWQFXZ2

DRG 456-458 Spinal Fusion Except Cervical with Spinal Curvature/Malignancy/Infection or Extensive Fusions

Fusion of Thoracic and Lumbar Vertebra, Anterior Column

2 to 7 Thoracic Vertebra		Code also 2 or more Lumbar Vertebra	
ØRG[Ø,3,4][7,A,J,K]Ø	XRG7ØF3	ØSG1[Ø,3,4][7,A,J,K]Ø	XRGCØF3

Fusion of Thoracic and Lumbar Vertebra, Posterior Column

2 to 7 Thoracic Vertebra			Code also 2 or more Lumbar Vertebra		
Posterior Approach	Anterior Approach	New Technology	Posterior Approach	Anterior Approach	New Technology
ØRG7[Ø,3,4][7,J,K]1	ØRG7[Ø,3,4][7,A,J,K]J	XRG7092 XRG7ØF3	ØSG1[Ø,3,4][7,J,K]1	ØSG1[Ø,3,4][7,A,J,K]J	XRGC092 XRGCØF3

DRG 461-462 Bilateral or Multiple Major Joint Procedures of Lower Extremity

For procedures to qualify as bilateral or multiple joint procedures, at least one replacement code or combination removal and replacement code from two different lower extremity sites from the following table(s) must be reported.

Examples: Left hip and right hip codes (bilateral); left hip and left knee codes (multiple); left hip and right ankle codes (multiple); left knee and right knee codes (bilateral); right hip removal and replacement, with right knee replacement

Hip, RT	Hip, LT	Knee, RT	Knee, LT	Ankle, RT	Ankle, LT
ØSR9Ø19	ØSRBØ19	ØSRCØ69	ØSRDØ69	ØSRFØ7Z	ØSRGØ7Z
ØSR9Ø1A	ØSRBØ1A	ØSRCØ6A	ØSRDØ6A	ØSRFØJ9	ØSRGØJ9
ØSR9Ø1Z	ØSRBØ1Z	ØSRCØ6Z	ØSRDØ6Z	ØSRFØJA	ØSRGØJA
ØSR9Ø29	ØSRBØ29	ØSRCØ7Z	ØSRDØ7Z	ØSRFØJZ	ØSRGØJZ
ØSR9Ø2A	ØSRBØ2A	ØSRCØJ9	ØSRDØJ9	ØSRFØKZ	ØSRGØKZ
ØSR9Ø2Z	ØSRBØ2Z	ØSRCØJA	ØSRDØJA		
ØSR9Ø39	ØSRBØ39	ØSRCØJZ	ØSRDØJZ		
ØSR9Ø3A	ØSRBØ3A	ØSRCØKZ	ØSRDØKZ		
ØSR9Ø3Z	ØSRBØ3Z	ØSRCØL9	ØSRDØL9		
ØSR9Ø49	ØSRBØ49	ØSRCØLA	ØSRDØLA		
ØSR9Ø4A	ØSRBØ4A	ØSRCØLZ	ØSRDØLZ		
ØSR9Ø4Z	ØSRBØ4Z	ØSRCØM9	ØSRDØM9		
ØSR9Ø69	ØSRBØ69	ØSRCØMA	ØSRDØMA		
ØSR9Ø6A	ØSRBØ6A	ØSRCØMZ	ØSRDØMZ		
ØSR9Ø6Z	ØSRBØ6Z	ØSRCØN9	ØSRDØN9		
ØSR9Ø7Z	ØSRBØ7Z	ØSRCØNA	ØSRDØNA		
ØSR9ØJ9	ØSRBØJ9	ØSRCØNZ	ØSRDØNZ		
ØSR9ØJA	ØSRBØJA	ØSRTØ7Z	ØSRUØ7Z		
ØSR9ØJZ	ØSRBØJZ	ØSRTØJ9	ØSRUØJ9		
ØSR9ØKZ	ØSRBØKZ	ØSRTØJA	ØSRUØJA		
ØSRAØØ9	ØSREØØ9	ØSRTØJZ	ØSRUØJZ		
ØSRAØØA	ØSREØØA	ØSRTØKZ	ØSRUØKZ		
ØSRAØØZ	ØSREØØZ	ØSRVØ7Z	ØSRWØ7Z		
ØSRAØ19	ØSREØ19	ØSRVØJ9	ØSRWØJ9		
ØSRAØ1A	ØSREØ1A	ØSRVØJA	ØSRWØJA		
ØSRAØ1Z	ØSREØ1Z	ØSRVØJZ	ØSRWØJZ		
ØSRAØ39	ØSREØ39	ØSRVØKZ	ØSRWØKZ		
ØSRAØ3A	ØSREØ3A	ØSPCØJZ	ØSPDØJZ		
ØSRAØ3Z	ØSREØ3Z				
ØSRAØ7Z	ØSREØ7Z				
ØSRAØJ9	ØSREØJ9				
ØSRAØJA	ØSREØJA				
ØSRAØJZ	ØSREØJZ				
ØSRAØKZ	ØSREØKZ				
ØSRRØ19	ØSRSØ19				
ØSRRØ1A	ØSRSØ1A				
ØSRRØ1Z	ØSRSØ1Z				
ØSRRØ39	ØSRSØ39				
ØSRRØ3A	ØSRSØ3A				
ØSRRØ3Z	ØSRSØ3Z				
ØSRRØ7Z	ØSRSØ7Z				
ØSRRØJ9	ØSRSØJ9				
ØSRRØJA	ØSRSØJA				
ØSRRØJZ	ØSRSØJZ				
ØSRRØKZ	ØSRSØKZ				
ØSU9ØBZ	ØSUBØBZ				
ØSUAØBZ	ØSUEØBZ				
ØSURØBZ	ØSUSØBZ				
ØSP9ØJZ	ØSPBØJZ				

Hip Procedure Combinations

Open Removal of Hip Spacer with Replacement

Removal of Spacer		Code also as appropriate Replacement by Device Type					
		Metal	Metal on Poly	Ceramic	Ceramic on Poly	Oxidized Zirc on Poly	Synth Subst
Hip, RT	ØSP9Ø8Z	ØSR9Ø1[9,A,Z]	ØSR9Ø2[9,A,Z]	ØSR9Ø3[9,A,Z]	ØSR9Ø4[9,A,Z]	ØSR9Ø6[9,A,Z]	ØSR9ØJ[9,A,Z]
Hip, LT	ØSPBØ8Z	ØSRBØ1[9,A,Z]	ØSRBØ2[9,A,Z]	ØSRBØ3[9,A,Z]	ØSRBØ4[9,A,Z]	ØSRBØ6[9,A,Z]	ØSRBØJ[9,A,Z]

Open Removal of Hip Spacer with Replacement

Removal of Spacer		Code also as appropriate Replacement by Device Type						
		Acetabular Surface				Femoral Surface		
		Poly	Metal	Ceramic	Synthetic	Metal	Ceramic	Synth
Hip, RT	ØSP9Ø8Z	ØSRAØØ[9,A,Z]	ØSRAØ1[9,A,Z]	ØSRAØ3[9,A,Z]	ØSRAØJ[9,A,Z]	ØSRRØ1[9,A,Z]	ØSRRØ3[9,A,Z]	ØSRRØJ[9,A,Z]
Hip, LT	ØSPBØ8Z	ØSREØØ[9,A,Z]	ØSREØ1[9,A,Z]	ØSREØ3[9,A,Z]	ØSREØJ[9,A,Z]	ØSRSØ1[9,A,Z]	ØSRSØ3[9,A,Z]	ØSRSØJ[9,A,Z]

Open Removal of Hip Liner with Replacement

Removal of Liner		Code also as appropriate Replacement by Device Type					
		Metal	Metal on Poly	Ceramic	Ceramic on Poly	Oxidized Zirc on Poly	Synth Subst
Hip, RT	ØSP9Ø9Z	ØSR9Ø1[9,A,Z]	ØSR9Ø2[9,A,Z]	ØSR9Ø3[9,A,Z]	ØSR9Ø4[9,A,Z]	ØSR9Ø6[9,A,Z]	ØSR9ØJ[9,A,Z]
Hip, LT	ØSPBØ9Z	ØSRBØ1[9,A,Z]	ØSRBØ2[9,A,Z]	ØSRBØ3[9,A,Z]	ØSRBØ4[9,A,Z]	ØSRBØ6[9,A,Z]	ØSRBØJ[9,A,Z]

Open Removal of Hip Liner with Replacement

Removal of Liner		Code also as appropriate Replacement by Device Type						
		Acetabular Surface				Femoral Surface		
		Poly	Metal	Ceramic	Synthetic	Metal	Ceramic	Synth
Hip, RT	ØSP9Ø9Z	ØSRAØØ[9,A,Z]	ØSRAØ1[9,A,Z]	ØSRAØ3[9,A,Z]	ØSRAØJ[9,A,Z]	ØSRRØ1[9,A,Z]	ØSRRØ3[9,A,Z]	ØSRRØJ[9,A,Z]
Hip, LT	ØSPBØ9Z	ØSREØØ[9,A,Z]	ØSREØ1[9,A,Z]	ØSREØ3[9,A,Z]	ØSREØJ[9,A,Z]	ØSRSØ1[9,A,Z]	ØSRSØ3[9,A,Z]	ØSRSØJ[9,A,Z]

Open Removal of Hip Resurfacing Device with Replacement

Removal of Resurfacing Device		Code also as appropriate Replacement by Device Type					
		Metal	Metal on Poly	Ceramic	Ceramic on Poly	Oxidized Zirc on Poly	Synth Subst
Hip, RT	ØSP9ØBZ	ØSR9Ø1[9,A,Z]	ØSR9Ø2[9,A,Z]	ØSR9Ø3[9,A,Z]	ØSR9Ø4[9,A,Z]	ØSR9Ø6[9,A,Z]	ØSR9ØJ[9,A,Z]
Hip, LT	ØSPBØBZ	ØSRBØ1[9,A,Z]	ØSRBØ2[9,A,Z]	ØSRBØ3[9,A,Z]	ØSRBØ4[9,A,Z]	ØSRBØ6[9,A,Z]	ØSRBØJ[9,A,Z]

Open Removal of Hip Resurfacing Device with Replacement

Removal of Resurfacing Device		Code also as appropriate Replacement by Device Type						
		Acetabular Surface				Femoral Surface		
		Poly	Metal	Ceramic	Synthetic	Metal	Ceramic	Synth
Hip, RT	ØSP9ØBZ	ØSRAØØ[9,A,Z]	ØSRAØ1[9,A,Z]	ØSRAØ3[9,A,Z]	ØSRAØJ[9,A,Z]	ØSRRØ1[9,A,Z]	ØSRRØ3[9,A,Z]	ØSRRØJ[9,A,Z]
Hip, LT	ØSPBØBZ	ØSREØØ[9,A,Z]	ØSREØ1[9,A,Z]	ØSREØ3[9,A,Z]	ØSREØJ[9,A,Z]	ØSRSØ1[9,A,Z]	ØSRSØ3[9,A,Z]	ØSRSØJ[9,A,Z]

Open Removal of Hip Articulating Spacer with Replacement

Removal of Articulating Spacer		Code also as appropriate Replacement by Device Type					
		Metal	Metal on Poly	Ceramic	Ceramic on Poly	Oxidized Zirc on Poly	Synth Subst
Hip, RT	ØSP9ØEZ	ØSR9Ø1[9,A,Z]	ØSR9Ø2[9,A,Z]	ØSR9Ø3[9,A,Z]	ØSR9Ø4[9,A,Z]	ØSR9Ø6[9,A,Z]	ØSR9ØJ[9,A,Z]
Hip, LT	ØSPBØEZ	ØSRBØ1[9,A,Z]	ØSRBØ2[9,A,Z]	ØSRBØ3[9,A,Z]	ØSRBØ4[9,A,Z]	ØSRBØ6[9,A,Z]	ØSRBØJ[9,A,Z]

Open Removal of Hip Articulating Spacer with Replacement

Removal of Articulating Spacer		Code also as appropriate Replacement by Device Type						
		Acetabular Surface				Femoral Surface		
		Poly	Metal	Ceramic	Synthetic	Metal	Ceramic	Synth
Hip, RT	ØSP90EZ	ØSRAØØ[9,A,Z]	ØSRAØ1[9,A,Z]	ØSRAØ3[9,A,Z]	ØSRAØJ[9,A,Z]	ØSRRØ1[9,A,Z]	ØSRRØ3[9,A,Z]	ØSRRØJ[9,A,Z]
Hip, LT	ØSPBØEZ	ØSREØØ[9,A,Z]	ØSREØ1[9,A,Z]	ØSREØ3[9,A,Z]	ØSREØJ[9,A,Z]	ØSRSØ1[9,A,Z]	ØSRSØ3[9,A,Z]	ØSRSØJ[9,A,Z]

Open Removal of Hip Synthetic Substitute with Replacement

Removal of Synthetic Substitute		Code also as appropriate Replacement by Device Type					
		Metal	Metal on Poly	Ceramic	Ceramic on Poly	Oxidized Zirc on Poly	Synth Subst
Hip, RT	ØSP[9,A,R]ØJZ	ØSR9Ø1[9,A,Z]	ØSR9Ø2[9,A,Z]	ØSR9Ø3[9,A,Z]	ØSR9Ø4[9,A,Z]	ØSR9Ø6[9,A,Z]	ØSR9ØJ[9,A,Z]
Hip, LT	ØSP[B,E,S]ØJZ	ØSRBØ1[9,A,Z]	ØSRBØ2[9,A,Z]	ØSRBØ3[9,A,Z]	ØSRBØ4[9,A,Z]	ØSRBØ6[9,A,Z]	ØSRBØJ[9,A,Z]

Open Removal of Hip Synthetic Substitute with Replacement

Removal of Synthetic Substitute		Code also as appropriate Replacement by Device Type						
		Acetabular Surface				Femoral Surface		
		Poly	Metal	Ceramic	Synthetic	Metal	Ceramic	Synth
Hip, RT	ØSP[9,A,R]ØJZ	ØSRAØØ[9,A,Z]	ØSRAØ1[9,A,Z]	ØSRAØ3[9,A,Z]	ØSRAØJ[9,A,Z]	ØSRRØ1[9,A,Z]	ØSRRØ3[9,A,Z]	ØSRRØJ[9,A,Z]
Hip, LT	ØSP[B,E,S]ØJZ	ØSREØØ[9,A,Z]	ØSREØ1[9,A,Z]	ØSREØ3[9,A,Z]	ØSREØJ[9,A,Z]	ØSRSØ1[9,A,Z]	ØSRSØ3[9,A,Z]	ØSRSØJ[9,A,Z]

Percutaneous Endoscopic Removal of Hip Spacer with Open Replacement

Removal of Spacer		Code also as appropriate Replacement by Device Type					
		Metal	Metal on Poly	Ceramic	Ceramic on Poly	Oxidized Zirc on Poly	Synth Subst
Hip, RT	ØSP948Z	ØSR9Ø1[9,A,Z]	ØSR9Ø2[9,A,Z]	ØSR9Ø3[9,A,Z]	ØSR9Ø4[9,A,Z]	ØSR9Ø6[9,A,Z]	ØSR9ØJ[9,A,Z]
Hip, LT	ØSPB48Z	ØSRBØ1[9,A,Z]	ØSRBØ2[9,A,Z]	ØSRBØ3[9,A,Z]	ØSRBØ4[9,A,Z]	ØSRBØ6[9,A,Z]	ØSRBØJ[9,A,Z]

Percutaneous Endoscopic Removal of Hip Spacer with Open Replacement

Removal of Spacer		Code also as appropriate Replacement by Device Type						
		Acetabular Surface				Femoral Surface		
		Poly	Metal	Ceramic	Synthetic	Metal	Ceramic	Synth
Hip, RT	ØSP948Z	ØSRAØØ[9,A,Z]	ØSRAØ1[9,A,Z]	ØSRAØ3[9,A,Z]	ØSRAØJ[9,A,Z]	ØSRRØ1[9,A,Z]	ØSRRØ3[9,A,Z]	ØSRRØJ[9,A,Z]
Hip, LT	ØSPB48Z	ØSREØØ[9,A,Z]	ØSREØ1[9,A,Z]	ØSREØ3[9,A,Z]	ØSREØJ[9,A,Z]	ØSRSØ1[9,A,Z]	ØSRSØ3[9,A,Z]	ØSRSØJ[9,A,Z]

Percutaneous Endoscopic Removal of Hip Synthetic Substitute with Open Replacement

Removal of Synthetic Substitute		Code also as appropriate Replacement by Device Type					
		Metal	Metal on Poly	Ceramic	Ceramic on Poly	Oxidized Zirc on Poly	Synth Subst
Hip, RT	ØSP[9,A,R]4JZ	ØSR9Ø1[9,A,Z]	ØSR9Ø2[9,A,Z]	ØSR9Ø3[9,A,Z]	ØSR9Ø4[9,A,Z]	ØSR9Ø6[9,A,Z]	ØSR9ØJ[9,A,Z]
Hip, LT	ØSP[B,E,S]4JZ	ØSRBØ1[9,A,Z]	ØSRBØ2[9,A,Z]	ØSRBØ3[9,A,Z]	ØSRBØ4[9,A,Z]	ØSRBØ6[9,A,Z]	ØSRBØJ[9,A,Z]

Percutaneous Endoscopic Removal of Hip Synthetic Substitute with Open Replacement

Removal of Synthetic Substitute		Code also as appropriate Replacement by Device Type						
		Acetabular Surface				Femoral Surface		
		Poly	Metal	Ceramic	Synthetic	Metal	Ceramic	Synth
Hip, RT	ØSP[9,A,R]4JZ	ØSRAØØ[9,A,Z]	ØSRAØ1[9,A,Z]	ØSRAØ3[9,A,Z]	ØSRAØJ[9,A,Z]	ØSRRØ1[9,A,Z]	ØSRRØ3[9,A,Z]	ØSRRØJ[9,A,Z]
Hip, LT	ØSP[B,E,S]4JZ	ØSREØØ[9,A,Z]	ØSREØ1[9,A,Z]	ØSREØ3[9,A,Z]	ØSREØJ[9,A,Z]	ØSRSØ1[9,A,Z]	ØSRSØ3[9,A,Z]	ØSRSØJ[9,A,Z]

Knee Procedure Combinations

Open Removal of Knee Spacer with Synthetic Substitute Replacement

Removal of Spacer		Code also as appropriate Replacement by Type of Synthetic Substitute				
		Oxidized Zircon on Poly	Synth Subst	Patello-femoral	Femoral Surface	Tibial Surface
Knee, RT	ØSPCØ8Z	ØSRCØ6[9,A,Z]	ØSRCØJ[9,A,Z]	ØSRCØN[9,A,Z]	ØSRTØJ[9,A,Z]	ØSRVØJ[9,A,Z]
Knee, LT	ØSPDØ8Z	ØSRDØ6[9,A,Z]	ØSRDØJ[9,A,Z]	ØSRDØN[9,A,Z]	ØSRUØJ[9,A,Z]	ØSRWØJ[9,A,Z]

Open Removal of Knee Liner with Synthetic Substitute Replacement

Removal of Liner		Code also as appropriate Replacement by Type of Synthetic Substitute						
		Oxidized Zircon on Poly	Synth Subst	Medial Unicondylar	Lateral Unicondylar	Patello-femoral	Femoral Surface	Tibial Surface
Knee, RT	ØSPCØ9Z	ØSRCØ6[9,A,Z]	ØSRCØJ[9,A,Z]	ØSRCØL[9,A,Z]	ØSRCØM[9,A,Z]	ØSRCØN[9,A,Z]	ØSRTØJ[9,A,Z]	ØSRVØJ[9,A,Z]
Knee, LT	ØSPDØ9Z	ØSRDØ6[9,A,Z]	ØSRDØJ[9,A,Z]	ØSRDØL[9,A,Z]	ØSRDØM[9,A,Z]	ØSRDØN[9,A,Z]	ØSRUØJ[9,A,Z]	ØSRWØJ[9,A,Z]

Open Removal of Knee Articulating Spacer with Synthetic Substitute Replacement

Removal of Articulating Spacer		Code also as appropriate Replacement by Type of Synthetic Substitute			
		Oxidized Zircon on Poly	Synth Subst	Femoral Surface	Tibial Surface
Knee, RT	ØSPCØEZ	ØSRCØ6[9,A,Z]	ØSRCØJ[9,A,Z]	ØSRTØJ[9,A,Z]	ØSRVØJ[9,A,Z]
Knee, LT	ØSPDØEZ	ØSRDØ6[9,A,Z]	ØSRDØJ[9,A,Z]	ØSRUØJ[9,A,Z]	ØSRWØJ[9,A,Z]

Open Removal of Patellar Surface of Knee with Synthetic Substitute Replacement

Removal of Patellar Surface		Code also as appropriate Replacement by Type of Synthetic Substitute				
		Oxidized Zircon on Poly	Synth Subst	Patello-femoral	Femoral Surface	Tibial Surface
Knee, RT	ØSPCØJC	ØSRCØ6[9,A,Z]	ØSRCØJ[9,A,Z]	ØSRCØN[9,A,Z]	ØSRTØJ[9,A,Z]	ØSRVØJ[9,A,Z]
Knee, LT	ØSPDØJC	ØSRDØ6[9,A,Z]	ØSRDØJ[9,A,Z]	ØSRDØN[9,A,Z]	ØSRUØJ[9,A,Z]	ØSRWØJ[9,A,Z]

Open Removal of Knee Synthetic Substitute with Synthetic Substitute Replacement

Removal of Synthetic Substitute		Code also as appropriate Replacement by Type of Synthetic Substitute						
		Oxidized Zircon on Poly	Synth Subst	Medial Unicondylar	Lateral Unicondylar	Patello-femoral	Femoral Surface	Tibial Surface
Knee, RT	ØSPCØJZ	ØSRCØ6[9,A,Z]	ØSRCØJ[9,A,Z]	ØSRCØL[9,A,Z]	ØSRCØM[9,A,Z]	ØSRCØN[9,A,Z]	ØSRTØJ[9,A,Z]	ØSRVØJ[9,A,Z]
Knee, LT	ØSPDØJZ	ØSRDØ6[9,A,Z]	ØSRDØJ[9,A,Z]	ØSRDØL[9,A,Z]	ØSRDØM[9,A,Z]	ØSRDØN[9,A,Z]	ØSRUØJ[9,A,Z]	ØSRWØJ[9,A,Z]

Open Removal of Medial or Lateral Unicondylar Knee with Synthetic Substitute Replacement

Removal of Medial/Lateral Unicondylar Knee		Code also as appropriate Replacement by Type of Synthetic Substitute				
		Oxidized Zircon on Poly	Synth Subst	Medial Unicondylar	Femoral Surface	Tibial Surface
Knee, RT	ØSPCØ[L,M]Z	ØSRCØ6[9,A,Z]	ØSRCØJ[9,A,Z]	ØSRCØL[9,A,Z]	ØSRTØJ[9,A,Z]	ØSRVØJ[9,A,Z]
Knee, LT	ØSPDØ[L,M]Z	ØSRDØ6[9,A,Z]	ØSRDØJ[9,A,Z]	ØSRDØL[9,A,Z]	ØSRUØJ[9,A,Z]	ØSRWØJ[9,A,Z]

Open Removal of Patellofemoral Knee with Synthetic Substitute Replacement

Removal of Patellofemoral Knee		Code also as appropriate Replacement by Type of Synthetic Substitute				
		Oxidized Zircon on Poly	Synth Subst	Medial Unicondylar	Femoral Surface	Tibial Surface
Knee, RT	ØSPCØNZ	ØSRCØ6[9,A,Z]	ØSRCØJ[9,A,Z]	ØSRCØL[9,A,Z]	ØSRTØJ[9,A,Z]	ØSRVØJ[9,A,Z]
Knee, LT	ØSPDØNZ	ØSRDØ6[9,A,Z]	ØSRDØJ[9,A,Z]	ØSRDØL[9,A,Z]	ØSRUØJ[9,A,Z]	ØSRWØJ[9,A,Z]

Open Removal of Femoral/Tibial Surface of Knee with Synthetic Substitute Replacement

Removal of Femoral/Tibial Surface of Knee		Code also as appropriate Replacement by Type of Synthetic Substitute					
		Oxidized Zircon on Poly	Synth Subst	Articulating Spacer	Patello-femoral	Femoral Surface	Tibial Surface
Knee, RT	ØSP[T,V]ØJZ	ØSRCØ6[9,A,Z]	ØSRCØJ[9,A,Z]	ØSRCØEZ	ØSRCØN[9,A,Z]	ØSRTØJ[9,A,Z]	ØSRVØJ[9,A,Z]
Knee, LT	ØSP[U,W]ØJZ	ØSRDØ6[9,A,Z]	ØSRDØJ[9,A,Z]	ØSRDØEZ	ØSRDØN[9,A,Z]	ØSRUØJ[9,A,Z]	ØSRWØJ[9,A,Z]

Percutaneous/Percutaneous Endoscopic Removal of Knee Spacer with Open Synthetic Substitute Replacement

Removal of Spacer		Code also as appropriate Replacement by Type of Synthetic Substitute				
		Oxidized Zircon on Poly	Synth Subst	Patello-femoral	Femoral Surface	Tibial Surface
Knee, RT	ØSPC[3,4]8Z	ØSRCØ6[9,A,Z]	ØSRCØJ[9,A,Z]	ØSRCØN[9,A,Z]	ØSRTØJ[9,A,Z]	ØSRVØJ[9,A,Z]
Knee, LT	ØSPD[3,4]8Z	ØSRDØ6[9,A,Z]	ØSRDØJ[9,A,Z]	ØSRDØN[9,A,Z]	ØSRUØJ[9,A,Z]	ØSRWØJ[9,A,Z]

Percutaneous Endoscopic Removal of Patellar Surface of Knee with Synthetic Substitute Replacement

Removal of Patellar Surface		Code also as appropriate Replacement by Type of Synthetic Substitute				
		Oxidized Zircon on Poly	Synth Subst	Patello-femoral	Femoral Surface	Tibial Surface
Knee, RT	ØSPC4JC	ØSRCØ6[9,A,Z]	ØSRCØJ[9,A,Z]	ØSRCØN[9,A,Z]	ØSRTØJ[9,A,Z]	ØSRVØJ[9,A,Z]
Knee, LT	ØSPD4JC	ØSRDØ6[9,A,Z]	ØSRDØJ[9,A,Z]	ØSRDØN[9,A,Z]	ØSRUØJ[9,A]	ØSRWØJ[9,A,Z]

Percutaneous Endoscopic Removal of Knee Synthetic Substitute with Synthetic Substitute Replacement

Removal of Synthetic Substitute		Code also as appropriate Replacement by Type of Synthetic Substitute						
		Oxidized Zircon on Poly	Synth Subst	Medial Unicondylar	Lateral Unicondylar	Patello-femoral	Femoral Surface	Tibial Surface
Knee, RT	ØSPC4JZ	ØSRCØ6[9,A,Z]	ØSRCØJ[9,A,Z]	ØSRCØL[9,A,Z]	ØSRCØM[9,A,Z]	ØSRCØN[9,A,Z]	ØSRTØJ[9,A,Z]	ØSRVØJ[9,A,Z]
Knee, LT	ØSPD4JZ	ØSRDØ6[9,A,Z]	ØSRDØJ[9,A,Z]	ØSRDØL[9,A,Z]	ØSRDØM[9,A,Z]	ØSRDØN[9,A,Z]	ØSRUØJ[9,A,Z]	ØSRWØJ[9,A,Z]

Percutaneous Endoscopic Removal of Medial or Lateral Unicondylar Knee with Synthetic Substitute Replacement

Removal of Medial/Lateral Unicondylar Knee		Code also as appropriate Replacement by Type of Synthetic Substitute				
		Oxidized Zircon on Poly	Synth Subst	Medial Unicondylar	Femoral Surface	Tibial Surface
Knee, RT	ØSPC4[L,M]Z	ØSRCØ6[9,A,Z]	ØSRCØJ[9,A,Z]	ØSRCØL[9,A,Z]	ØSRTØJ[9,A,Z]	ØSRVØJ[9,A,Z]
Knee, LT	ØSPD4[L,M]Z	ØSRDØ6[9,A,Z]	ØSRDØJ[9,A,Z]	ØSRDØL[9,A,Z]	ØSRUØJ[9,A,Z]	ØSRWØJ[9,A,Z]

Percutaneous Endoscopic Removal of Patellofemoral Knee with Synthetic Substitute Replacement

Removal of Patellofemoral Knee		Code also as appropriate Replacement by Type of Synthetic Substitute				
		Oxidized Zircon on Poly	Synth Subst	Medial Unicondylar	Femoral Surface	Tibial Surface
Knee, RT	ØSPC4NZ	ØSRCØ6[9,A,Z]	ØSRCØJ[9,A,Z]	ØSRCØL[9,A,Z]	ØSRTØJ[9,A,Z]	ØSRVØJ[9,A,Z]
Knee, LT	ØSPD4NZ	ØSRDØ6[9,A,Z]	ØSRDØJ[9,A,Z]	ØSRDØL[9,A,Z]	ØSRUØJ[9,A,Z]	ØSRWØJ[9,A,Z]

Percutaneous Endoscopic Removal of Femoral/Tibial Surface of Knee with Synthetic Substitute Replacement

Removal of Femoral/Tibial Surface of Knee		Code also as appropriate Replacement by Type of Synthetic Substitute					
		Oxidized Zircon on Poly	Synth Subst	Articulating Spacer	Patello-femoral	Femoral Surface	Tibial Surface
Knee, RT	ØSP[T,V]4JZ	ØSRCØ6[9,A,Z]	ØSRCØJ[9,A,Z]	ØSRCØEZ	ØSRCØN[9,A,Z]	ØSRTØJ[9,A,Z]	ØSRVØJ[9,A,Z]
Knee, LT	ØSP[U,W]4JZ	ØSRDØ6[9,A,Z]	ØSRDØJ[9,A,Z]	ØSRDØEZ	ØSRDØN[9,A,Z]	ØSRUØJ[9,A,Z]	ØSRWØJ[9,A,Z]

466-468 Revision of Hip or Knee Replacement

Hip Procedures

Open Removal of Hip Spacer with Replacement

Removal of Spacer		Code also as appropriate Replacement by Device Type						
		Metal	Metal on Poly	Ceramic	Ceramic on Poly	Oxidized Zirc on Poly	Articulating Spacer	Synth Subst
Hip, RT	ØSP9Ø8Z	ØSR9Ø1[9,A,Z]	ØSR9Ø2[9,A,Z]	ØSR9Ø3[9,A,Z]	ØSR9Ø4[9,A,Z]	ØSR9Ø6[9,A,Z]	ØSR9ØEZ	ØSR9ØJ[9,A,Z]
Hip, LT	ØSPBØ8Z	ØSRBØ1[9,A,Z]	ØSRBØ2[9,A,Z]	ØSRBØ3[9,A,Z]	ØSRBØ4[9,A,Z]	ØSRBØ6[9,A,Z]	ØSRBØEZ	ØSRBØJ[9,A,Z]

Open Removal of Hip Spacer with Replacement

Removal of Spacer		Code also as appropriate Replacement by Device Type						
		Acetabular Surface				Femoral Surface		
		Poly	Metal	Ceramic	Synthetic	Metal	Ceramic	Synth
Hip, RT	ØSP9Ø8Z	ØSRAØØ[9,A,Z]	ØSRAØ1[9,A,Z]	ØSRAØ3[9,A,Z]	ØSRAØJ[9,A,Z]	ØSRRØ1[9,A,Z]	ØSRRØ3[9,A,Z]	ØSRRØJ[9,A,Z]
Hip, LT	ØSPBØ8Z	ØSREØØ[9,A,Z]	ØSREØ1[9,A,Z]	ØSREØ3[9,A,Z]	ØSREØJ[9,A,Z]	ØSRSØ1[9,A,Z]	ØSRSØ3[9,A,Z]	ØSRSØJ[9,A,Z]

Open Removal of Hip Spacer with Liner Insertion (supplement)

Removal of Spacer		Code also as appropriate Supplement of Body Part by Site		
		Joint	Acetabular Surface	Femoral Surface
Hip, RT	ØSP9Ø8Z	ØSU9Ø9Z	ØSUAØ9Z	ØSURØ9Z
Hip, LT	ØSPBØ8Z	ØSUBØ9Z	ØSUEØ9Z	ØSUSØ9Z

Open Removal of Hip Liner with Replacement

Removal of Liner		Code also as appropriate Replacement by Device Type						
		Metal	Metal on Poly	Ceramic	Ceramic on Poly	Oxidized Zirc on Poly	Articulating Spacer	Synth Subst
Hip, RT	ØSP9Ø9Z	ØSR9Ø1[9,A,Z]	ØSR9Ø2[9,A,Z]	ØSR9Ø3[9,A,Z]	ØSR9Ø4[9,A,Z]	ØSR9Ø6[9,A,Z]	ØSR9ØEZ	ØSR9ØJ[9,A,Z]
Hip, LT	ØSPBØ9Z	ØSRBØ1[9,A,Z]	ØSRBØ2[9,A,Z]	ØSRBØ3[9,A,Z]	ØSRBØ4[9,A,Z]	ØSRBØ6[9,A,Z]	ØSRBØEZ	ØSRBØJ[9,A,Z]

Open Removal of Hip Liner with Replacement

Removal of Liner		Code also as appropriate Replacement by Device Type						
		Acetabular Surface				Femoral Surface		
		Poly	Metal	Ceramic	Synthetic	Metal	Ceramic	Synth
Hip, RT	ØSP9Ø9Z	ØSRAØØ[9,A,Z]	ØSRAØ1[9,A,Z]	ØSRAØ3[9,A,Z]	ØSRAØJ[9,A,Z]	ØSRRØ1[9,A,Z]	ØSRRØ3[9,A,Z]	ØSRRØJ[9,A,Z]
Hip, LT	ØSPBØ9Z	ØSREØØ[9,A,Z]	ØSREØ1[9,A,Z]	ØSREØ3[9,A,Z]	ØSREØJ[9,A,Z]	ØSRSØ1[9,A,Z]	ØSRSØ3[9,A,Z]	ØSRSØJ[9,A,Z]

Open Removal of Hip Liner with Liner Insertion (supplement)

Removal of Liner		Code also as appropriate Supplement of Body Part by Site		
		Joint	Acetabular Surface	Femoral Surface
Hip, RT	ØSP9Ø9Z	ØSU9Ø9Z	ØSUAØ9Z	ØSURØ9Z
Hip, LT	ØSPBØ9Z	ØSUBØ9Z	ØSUEØ9Z	ØSUSØ9Z

Open Removal of Hip Resurfacing Device with Replacement

Removal of Resurfacing Device		Code also as appropriate Replacement by Device Type						
		Metal	Metal on Poly	Ceramic	Ceramic on Poly	Oxidized Zirc on Poly	Articulating Spacer	Synth Subst
Hip, RT	ØSP9ØBZ	ØSR9Ø1[9,A,Z]	ØSR9Ø2[9,A,Z]	ØSR9Ø3[9,A,Z]	ØSR9Ø4[9,A,Z]	ØSR9Ø6[9,A,Z]	ØSR9ØEZ	ØSR9ØJ[9,A,Z]
Hip, LT	ØSPBØBZ	ØSRBØ1[9,A,Z]	ØSRBØ2[9,A,Z]	ØSRBØ3[9,A,Z]	ØSRBØ4[9,A,Z]	ØSRBØ6[9,A,Z]	ØSRBØEZ	ØSRBØJ[9,A,Z]

Open Removal of Hip Resurfacing Device with Replacement

Removal of Resurfacing Device		Code also as appropriate Replacement by Device Type						
		Acetabular Surface				Femoral Surface		
		Poly	Metal	Ceramic	Synthetic	Metal	Ceramic	Synth
Hip, RT	ØSP9ØBZ	ØSRAØØ[9,A,Z]	ØSRAØ1[9,A,Z]	ØSRAØ3[9,A,Z]	ØSRAØJ[9,A,Z]	ØSRRØ1[9,A,Z]	ØSRRØ3[9,A,Z]	ØSRRØJ[9,A,Z]
Hip, LT	ØSPBØBZ	ØSREØØ[9,A,Z]	ØSREØ1[9,A,Z]	ØSREØ3[9,A,Z]	ØSREØJ[9,A,Z]	ØSRSØ1[9,A,Z]	ØSRSØ3[9,A,Z]	ØSRSØJ[9,A,Z]

Open Removal of Hip Resurfacing Device with Liner Insertion (supplement)

Removal of Resurfacing Device		Code also as appropriate Supplement of Body Part by Site		
		Joint	Acetabular Surface	Femoral Surface
Hip, RT	ØSP9ØBZ	ØSU9Ø9Z	ØSUAØ9Z	ØSURØ9Z
Hip, LT	ØSPBØBZ	ØSUBØ9Z	ØSUEØ9Z	ØSUSØ9Z

Open Removal of Hip Articulating Spacer with Replacement

Removal of Articulating Spacer		Code also as appropriate Replacement by Device Type					
		Metal	Metal on Poly	Ceramic	Ceramic on Poly	Oxidized Zirc on Poly	Synth Subst
Hip, RT	ØSP90EZ	ØSR901[9,A,Z]	ØSR902[9,A,Z]	ØSR903[9,A,Z]	ØSR904[9,A,Z]	ØSR906[9,A,Z]	ØSR90J[9,A,Z]
Hip, LT	ØSPBØEZ	ØSRB01[9,A,Z]	ØSRB02[9,A,Z]	ØSRB03[9,A,Z]	ØSRB04[9,A,Z]	ØSRB06[9,A,Z]	ØSRB0J[9,A,Z]

Open Removal of Hip Articulating Spacer with Replacement

Removal of Articulating Spacer		Code also as appropriate Replacement by Device Type						
		Acetabular Surface				Femoral Surface		
		Poly	Metal	Ceramic	Synthetic	Metal	Ceramic	Synth
Hip, RT	ØSP90EZ	ØSRA00[9,A,Z]	ØSRA01[9,A,Z]	ØSRA03[9,A,Z]	ØSRA0J[9,A,Z]	ØSRR01[9,A,Z]	ØSRR03[9,A,Z]	ØSRR0J[9,A,Z]
Hip, LT	ØSPBØEZ	ØSRE00[9,A,Z]	ØSRE01[9,A,Z]	ØSRE03[9,A,Z]	ØSRE0J[9,A,Z]	ØSRS01[9,A,Z]	ØSRS03[9,A,Z]	ØSRS0J[9,A,Z]

Open Removal of Hip Articulating Spacer with Liner Insertion (supplement)

Removal of Articulating Spacer		Code also as appropriate Supplement of Body Part by Site		
		Joint	Acetabular Surface	Femoral Surface
Hip, RT	ØSP90EZ	ØSU909Z	ØSUA09Z	ØSUR09Z
Hip, LT	ØSPBØEZ	ØSUB09Z	ØSUE09Z	ØSUS09Z

Open Removal of Hip Synthetic Substitute with Replacement

Removal of Synthetic Substitute		Code also as appropriate Replacement by Device Type						
		Metal	Metal on Poly	Ceramic	Ceramic on Poly	Oxidized Zirc on Poly	Articulating Spacer	Synth Subst
Hip, RT	ØSP[9,A,R]ØJZ	ØSR901[9,A,Z]	ØSR902[9,A,Z]	ØSR903[9,A,Z]	ØSR904[9,A,Z]	ØSR906[9,A,Z]	ØSR90EZ	ØSR90J[9,A,Z]
Hip, LT	ØSP[B,E,S]ØJZ	ØSRB01[9,A,Z]	ØSRB02[9,A,Z]	ØSRB03[9,A,Z]	ØSRB04[9,A,Z]	ØSRB06[9,A,Z]	ØSRBØEZ	ØSRB0J[9,A,Z]

Open Removal of Hip Synthetic Substitute with Replacement

Removal of Synthetic Substitute		Code also as appropriate Replacement by Device Type						
		Acetabular Surface				Femoral Surface		
		Poly	Metal	Ceramic	Synthetic	Metal	Ceramic	Synth
Hip, RT	ØSP[9,A,R]ØJZ	ØSRA00[9,A,Z]	ØSRA01[9,A,Z]	ØSRA03[9,A,Z]	ØSRA0J[9,A,Z]	ØSRR01[9,A,Z]	ØSRR03[9,A,Z]	ØSRR0J[9,A,Z]
Hip, LT	ØSP[B,E,S]ØJZ	ØSRE00[9,A,Z]	ØSRE01[9,A,Z]	ØSRE03[9,A,Z]	ØSRE0J[9,A,Z]	ØSRS01[9,A,Z]	ØSRS03[9,A,Z]	ØSRS0J[9,A,Z]

Percutaneous Endoscopic Removal of Hip Spacer with Open Replacement

Removal of Spacer		Code also as appropriate Replacement by Device Type						
		Metal	Metal on Poly	Ceramic	Ceramic on Poly	Oxidized Zirc on Poly	Articulating Spacer	Synth Subst
Hip, RT	ØSP948Z	ØSR901[9,A,Z]	ØSR902[9,A,Z]	ØSR903[9,A,Z]	ØSR904[9,A,Z]	ØSR906[9,A,Z]	ØSR90EZ	ØSR90J[9,A,Z]
Hip, LT	ØSPB48Z	ØSRB01[9,A,Z]	ØSRB02[9,A,Z]	ØSRB03[9,A,Z]	ØSRB04[9,A,Z]	ØSRB06[9,A,Z]	ØSRBØEZ	ØSRB0J[9,A,Z]

Percutaneous Endoscopic Removal of Hip Spacer with Open Replacement

Removal of Spacer		Code also as appropriate Replacement by Device Type						
		Acetabular Surface				Femoral Surface		
		Poly	Metal	Ceramic	Synthetic	Metal	Ceramic	Synth
Hip, RT	ØSP948Z	ØSRA00[9,A,Z]	ØSRA01[9,A,Z]	ØSRA03[9,A,Z]	ØSRA0J[9,A,Z]	ØSRR01[9,A,Z]	ØSRR03[9,A,Z]	ØSRR0J[9,A,Z]
Hip, LT	ØSPB48Z	ØSRE00[9,A,Z]	ØSRE01[9,A,Z]	ØSRE03[9,A,Z]	ØSRE0J[9,A,Z]	ØSRS01[9,A,Z]	ØSRS03[9,A,Z]	ØSRS0J[9,A,Z]

Percutaneous Endoscopic Removal of Hip Spacer with Open Liner Insertion (supplement)

Removal of Spacer		Code also as appropriate Supplement of Body Part by Site		
		Joint	Acetabular Surface	Femoral Surface
Hip, RT	ØSP948Z	ØSU909Z	ØSUA09Z	ØSUR09Z
Hip, LT	ØSPB48Z	ØSUB09Z	ØSUE09Z	ØSUS09Z

Percutaneous Endoscopic Removal of Hip Synthetic Substitute with Open Replacement

Removal of Synthetic Substitute		Code also as appropriate Replacement by Device Type						
		Metal	Metal on Poly	Ceramic	Ceramic on Poly	Oxidized Zirc on Poly	Articulating Spacer	Synth Subst
Hip, RT	ØSP[9,A,R]4JZ	ØSR9Ø1[9,A,Z]	ØSR9Ø2[9,A,Z]	ØSR9Ø3[9,A,Z]	ØSR9Ø4[9,A,Z]	ØSR9Ø6[9,A,Z]	ØSR9ØEZ	ØSR9ØJ[9,A,Z]
Hip, LT	ØSP[B,E,S]4JZ	ØSRBØ1[9,A,Z]	ØSRBØ2[9,A,Z]	ØSRBØ3[9,A,Z]	ØSRBØ4[9,A,Z]	ØSRBØ6[9,A,Z]	ØSRBØEZ	ØSRBØJ[9,A,Z]

Percutaneous Endoscopic Removal of Hip Synthetic Substitute with Open Replacement

Removal of Synthetic Substitute		Code also as appropriate Replacement by Device Type						
		Acetabular Surface				Femoral Surface		
		Poly	Metal	Ceramic	Synthetic	Metal	Ceramic	Synth
Hip, RT	ØSP[9,A,R]4JZ	ØSRAØØ[9,A,Z]	ØSRAØ1[9,A,Z]	ØSRAØ3[9,A,Z]	ØSRAØJ[9,A,Z]	ØSRRØ1[9,A,Z]	ØSRRØ3[9,A,Z]	ØSRRØJ[9,A,Z]
Hip, LT	ØSP[B,E,S]4JZ	ØSREØØ[9,A,Z]	ØSREØ1[9,A,Z]	ØSREØ3[9,A,Z]	ØSREØJ[9,A,Z]	ØSRSØ1[9,A,Z]	ØSRSØ3[9,A,Z]	ØSRSØJ[9,A,Z]

Percutaneous Endoscopic Removal of Hip Synthetic Substitute with Open Liner Insertion (supplement)

Removal of Synthetic Substitute		Code also as appropriate Supplement of Body Part by Site		
		Joint	Acetabular Surface	Femoral Surface
Hip, RT	ØSP[9,A,R]4JZ	ØSU9Ø9Z	ØSUAØ9Z	ØSURØ9Z
Hip, LT	ØSP[B,E,S]4JZ	ØSUBØ9Z	ØSUEØ9Z	ØSUSØ9Z

Knee Procedures

Open Removal of Knee Spacer with Articulating Spacer Replacement

Removal of Spacer		Code also as appropriate Replacement with Articulating Spacer
Knee, RT	ØSPCØ8Z	ØSRCØEZ
Knee, LT	ØSPDØ8Z	ØSRDØEZ

Open Removal of Knee Spacer with Synthetic Substitute Replacement

Removal of Spacer		Code also as appropriate Replacement by Type of Synthetic Substitute				
		Oxidized Zircon on Poly	Synth Subst	Patello-femoral	Femoral Surface	Tibial Surface
Knee, RT	ØSPCØ8Z	ØSRCØ6[9,A,Z]	ØSRCØJ[9,A,Z]	ØSRCØN[9,A,Z]	ØSRTØJ[9,A,Z]	ØSRVØJ[9,A,Z]
Knee, LT	ØSPDØ8Z	ØSRDØ6[9,A,Z]	ØSRDØJ[9,A,Z]	ØSRDØN[9,A,Z]	ØSRUØJ[9,A,Z]	ØSRWØJ[9,A,Z]

Open Removal of Knee Liner with Articulating Spacer Replacement

Removal of Liner		Code also as appropriate Replacement with Articulating Spacer
Knee, RT	ØSPCØ9Z	ØSRCØEZ
Knee, LT	ØSPDØ9Z	ØSRDØEZ

Open Removal of Knee Liner with Synthetic Substitute Replacement

Removal of Liner		Code also as appropriate Replacement by Type of Synthetic Substitute						
		Oxidized Zircon on Poly	Synth Subst	Medial Unicondylar	Lateral Unicondylar	Patello-femoral	Femoral Surface	Tibial Surface
Knee, RT	ØSPCØ9Z	ØSRCØ6[9,A,Z]	ØSRCØJ[9,A,Z]	ØSRCØL[9,A,Z]	ØSRCØM[9,A,Z]	ØSRCØN[9,A,Z]	ØSRTØJ[9,A,Z]	ØSRVØJ[9,A,Z]
Knee, LT	ØSPDØ9Z	ØSRDØ6[9,A,Z]	ØSRDØJ[9,A,Z]	ØSRDØL[9,A,Z]	ØSRDØM[9,A,Z]	ØSRDØN[9,A,Z]	ØSRUØJ[9,A,Z]	ØSRWØJ[9,A,Z]

Open Removal of Knee Articulating Spacer with Synthetic Substitute Replacement

Removal of Articulating Spacer		Code also as appropriate Replacement by Type of Synthetic Substitute			
		Oxidized Zircon on Poly	Synth Subst	Femoral Surface	Tibial Surface
Knee, RT	ØSPCØEZ	ØSRCØ6[9,A,Z]	ØSRCØJ[9,A,Z]	ØSRTØJ[9,A,Z]	ØSRVØJ[9,A,Z]
Knee, LT	ØSPDØEZ	ØSRDØ6[9,A,Z]	ØSRDØJ[9,A,Z]	ØSRUØJ[9,A,Z]	ØSRWØJ[9,A,Z]

Open Removal of Patellar Surface of Knee with Synthetic Substitute Replacement

Removal of Patellar Surface		Code also as appropriate Replacement by Type of Synthetic Substitute				
		Oxidized Zircon on Poly	Synth Subst	Patello-femoral	Femoral Surface	Tibial Surface
Knee, RT	ØSPCØJC	ØSRCØ6[9,A,Z]	ØSRCØJ[9,A,Z]	ØSRCØN[9,A,Z]	ØSRTØJ[9,A,Z]	ØSRVØJ[9,A,Z]
Knee, LT	ØSPDØJC	ØSRDØ6[9,A,Z]	ØSRDØJ[9,A,Z]	ØSRDØN[9,A,Z]	ØSRUØJ[9,A,Z]	ØSRWØJ[9,A,Z]

Open Removal of Patellar Surface of Knee with Articulating Spacer Replacement

Removal of Patellar Surface		Code also as appropriate Replacement with Articulating Spacer
Knee, RT	ØSPCØJC	ØSRCØEZ
Knee, LT	ØSPDØJC	ØSRDØEZ

Open Removal of Knee Synthetic Substitute with Synthetic Substitute Replacement

Removal of Synthetic Substitute		Code also as appropriate Replacement by Type of Synthetic Substitute						
		Oxidized Zircon on Poly	Synth Subst	Medial Unicondylar	Lateral Unicondylar	Patello-femoral	Femoral Surface	Tibial Surface
Knee, RT	ØSPCØJZ	ØSRCØ6[9,A,Z]	ØSRCØJ[9,A,Z]	ØSRCØL[9,A,Z]	ØSRCØM[9,A,Z]	ØSRCØN[9,A,Z]	ØSRTØJ[9,A,Z]	ØSRVØJ[9,A,Z]
Knee, LT	ØSPDØJZ	ØSRDØ6[9,A,Z]	ØSRDØJ[9,A,Z]	ØSRDØL[9,A,Z]	ØSRDØM[9,A,Z]	ØSRDØN[9,A,Z]	ØSRUØJ[9,A,Z]	ØSRWØJ[9,A,Z]

Open Removal of Knee Synthetic Substitute with Articulating Spacer Replacement

Removal of Synthetic Substitute		Code also as appropriate Replacement with Articulating Spacer
Knee, RT	ØSPCØJZ	ØSRCØEZ
Knee, LT	ØSPDØJZ	ØSRDØEZ

Open Removal of Medial or Lateral Unicondylar Knee with Synthetic Substitute Replacement

Removal of Medial/Lateral Unicondylar Knee		Code also as appropriate Replacement by Type of Synthetic Substitute				
		Oxidized Zircon on Poly	Synth Subst	Medial Unicondylar	Femoral Surface	Tibial Surface
Knee, RT	ØSPCØ[L,M]Z	ØSRCØ6[9,A,Z]	ØSRCØJ[9,A,Z]	ØSRCØL[9,A,Z]	ØSRTØJ[9,A,Z]	ØSRVØJ[9,A,Z]
Knee, LT	ØSPDØ[L,M]Z	ØSRDØ6[9,A,Z]	ØSRDØJ[9,A,Z]	ØSRDØL[9,A,Z]	ØSRUØJ[9,A,Z]	ØSRWØJ[9,A,Z]

Open Removal of Patellofemoral Knee with Synthetic Substitute Replacement

Removal of Patellofemoral Knee		Code also as appropriate Replacement by Type of Synthetic Substitute				
		Oxidized Zircon on Poly	Synth Subst	Medial Unicondylar	Femoral Surface	Tibial Surface
Knee, RT	ØSPCØNZ	ØSRCØ6[9,A,Z]	ØSRCØJ[9,A,Z]	ØSRCØL[9,A,Z]	ØSRTØJ[9,A,Z]	ØSRVØJ[9,A,Z]
Knee, LT	ØSPDØNZ	ØSRDØ6[9,A,Z]	ØSRDØJ[9,A,Z]	ØSRDØL[9,A,Z]	ØSRUØJ[9,A,Z]	ØSRWØJ[9,A,Z]

Open Removal of Femoral/Tibial Surface of Knee with Synthetic Substitute Replacement

Removal of Femoral/Tibial Surface of Knee		Code also as appropriate Replacement by Type of Synthetic Substitute					
		Oxidized Zircon on Poly	Synth Subst	Articulating Spacer	Patello-femoral	Femoral Surface	Tibial Surface
Knee, RT	ØSP[T,V]ØJZ	ØSRCØ6[9,A,Z]	ØSRCØJ[9,A,Z]	ØSRCØEZ	ØSRCØN[9,A,Z]	ØSRTØJ[9,A,Z]	ØSRVØJ[9,A,Z]
Knee, LT	ØSP[U,W]ØJZ	ØSRDØ6[9,A,Z]	ØSRDØJ[9,A,Z]	ØSRDØEZ	ØSRDØN[9,A,Z]	ØSRUØJ[9,A,Z]	ØSRWØJ[9,A,Z]

Percutaneous/Percutaneous Endoscopic Removal of Knee Spacer with Open Synthetic Substitute Replacement

Removal of Spacer		Code also as appropriate Replacement by Type of Synthetic Substitute				
		Oxidized Zircon on Poly	Synth Subst	Patello-femoral	Femoral Surface	Tibial Surface
Knee, RT	ØSPC[3,4]8Z	ØSRCØ6[9,A,Z]	ØSRCØJ[9,A,Z]	ØSRCØN[9,A,Z]	ØSRTØJ[9,A,Z]	ØSRVØJ[9,A,Z]
Knee, LT	ØSPD[3,4]8Z	ØSRDØ6[9,A,Z]	ØSRDØJ[9,A,Z]	ØSRDØN[9,A,Z]	ØSRUØJ[9,A,Z]	ØSRWØJ[9,A,Z]

Percutaneous/Percutaneous Endoscopic Removal of Knee Spacer with Open Articulating Spacer Replacement

Removal of Spacer		Code also as appropriate Replacement with Articulating Spacer
Knee, RT	ØSPC[3,4]8Z	ØSRCØEZ
Knee, LT	ØSPD[3,4]8Z	ØSRDØEZ

Appendix L: Procedure Combination Tables

Percutaneous Endoscopic Removal of Patellar Surface of Knee with Synthetic Substitute Replacement

Removal of Patellar Surface		Code also as appropriate Replacement by Type of Synthetic Substitute				
		Oxidized Zircon on Poly	Synth Subst	Patello-femoral	Femoral Surface	Tibial Surface
Knee, RT	ØSPC4JC	ØSRC06[9,A,Z]	ØSRCØJ[9,A,Z]	ØSRCØN[9,A,Z]	ØSRTØJ[9,A,Z]	ØSRVØJ[9,A,Z]
Knee, LT	ØSPD4JC	ØSRD06[9,A,Z]	ØSRDØJ[9,A,Z]	ØSRDØN[9,A,Z]	ØSRUØJ[9,A,Z]	ØSRWØJ[9,A,Z]

Percutaneous Endoscopic Removal of Patellar Surface of Knee with Articulating Spacer Replacement

Removal of Patellar Surface		Code also as appropriate Replacement with Articulating Spacer
Knee, RT	ØSPC4JC	ØSRCØEZ
Knee, LT	ØSPD4JC	ØSRDØEZ

Percutaneous Endoscopic Removal of Knee Synthetic Substitute with Synthetic Substitute Replacement

Removal of Synthetic Substitute		Code also as appropriate Replacement by Type of Synthetic Substitute						
		Oxidized Zircon on Poly	Synth Subst	Medial Unicondylar	Lateral Unicondylar	Patello-femoral	Femoral Surface	Tibial Surface
Knee, RT	ØSPC4JZ	ØSRC06[9,A,Z]	ØSRCØJ[9,A,Z]	ØSRCØL[9,A,Z]	ØSRCØM[9,A,Z]	ØSRCØN[9,A,Z]	ØSRTØJ[9,A,Z]	ØSRVØJ[9,A,Z]
Knee, LT	ØSPD4JZ	ØSRD06[9,A,Z]	ØSRDØJ[9,A,Z]	ØSRDØL[9,A,Z]	ØSRDØM[9,A,Z]	ØSRDØN[9,A,Z]	ØSRUØJ[9,A,Z]	ØSRWØJ[9,A,Z]

Percutaneous Endoscopic Removal of Knee Synthetic Substitute with Articulating Spacer Replacement

Removal of Synthetic Substitute		Code also as appropriate Replacement with Articulating Spacer
Knee, RT	ØSPC4JZ	ØSRCØEZ
Knee, LT	ØSPD4JZ	ØSRDØEZ

Percutaneous Endoscopic Removal of Medial or Lateral Unicondylar Knee with Synthetic Substitute Replacement

Removal of Medial/Lateral Unicondylar Knee		Code also as appropriate Replacement by Type of Synthetic Substitute				
		Oxidized Zircon on Poly	Synth Subst	Medial Unicondylar	Femoral Surface	Tibial Surface
Knee, RT	ØSPC4[L,M]Z	ØSRC06[9,A,Z]	ØSRCØJ[9,A,Z]	ØSRCØL[9,A,Z]	ØSRTØJ[9,A,Z]	ØSRVØJ[9,A,Z]
Knee, LT	ØSPD4[L,M]Z	ØSRD06[9,A,Z]	ØSRDØJ[9,A,Z]	ØSRDØL[9,A,Z]	ØSRUØJ[9,A,Z]	ØSRWØJ[9,A,Z]

Percutaneous Endoscopic Removal of Patellofemoral Knee with Synthetic Substitute Replacement

Removal of Patellofemoral Knee		Code also as appropriate Replacement by Type of Synthetic Substitute				
		Oxidized Zircon on Poly	Synth Subst	Medial Unicondylar	Femoral Surface	Tibial Surface
Knee, RT	ØSPC4NZ	ØSRC06[9,A,Z]	ØSRCØJ[9,A,Z]	ØSRCØL[9,A,Z]	ØSRTØJ[9,A,Z]	ØSRVØJ[9,A,Z]
Knee, LT	ØSPD4NZ	ØSRD06[9,A,Z]	ØSRDØJ[9,A,Z]	ØSRDØL[9,A,Z]	ØSRUØJ[9,A,Z]	ØSRWØJ[9,A,Z]

Percutaneous Endoscopic Removal of Femoral/Tibial Surface of Knee with Synthetic Substitute Replacement

Removal of Femoral/Tibial Surface of Knee		Code also as appropriate Replacement by Type of Synthetic Substitute					
		Oxidized Zircon on Poly	Synth Subst	Articulating Spacer	Patello-femoral	Femoral Surface	Tibial Surface
Knee, RT	ØSP[T,V]4JZ	ØSRC06[9,A,Z]	ØSRCØJ[9,A,Z]	ØSRCØEZ	ØSRCØN[9,A,Z]	ØSRTØJ[9,A,Z]	ØSRVØJ[9,A,Z]
Knee, LT	ØSP[U,W]4JZ	ØSRD06[9,A,Z]	ØSRDØJ[9,A,Z]	ØSRDØEZ	ØSRDØN[9,A,Z]	ØSRUØJ[9,A,Z]	ØSRWØJ[9,A,Z]

DRG 485-489 Knee Procedures

Joint	Removal of Liner by open approach	Code also as appropriate Supplement of Tibial Surface by Site
Knee, RT	ØSPCØ9Z	ØSUVØ9Z
Knee, LT	ØSPDØ9Z	ØSUWØ9Z

DRG 515-517 Other Musculoskeletal System and Connective Tissue Procedures

Site	Reposition of Vertebra by percutaneous approach	Code also as appropriate Supplement With Synthetic Substitute by Percutaneous Approach at site of Repositioned Vertebra
Cervical	0PS33ZZ	0PU33JZ
Coccyx	0QSS3ZZ	0QUS3JZ
Lumbar	0QS03ZZ	0QU03JZ
Sacrum	0QS13ZZ	0QU13JZ
Thoracic	0PS43ZZ	0PU43JZ

DRG 518-520 Back and Neck Procedures, Except Spinal Fusion, or Disc Devices/Neurostimulators

Generator Type	Insertion of Generator by Site			Code also as appropriate Insertion Neurostimulator Lead by approach and Site	
	Chest	Abdomen	Back	Spinal Canal	Spinal Cord
Single Array	0JH6[0,3]BZ	0JH8[0,3]BZ	0JH7[0,3]BZ	00HU[0,3,4]MZ	00HV[0,3,4]MZ
Single Array, Rechargeable	0JH6[0,3]CZ	0JH8[0,3]CZ	0JH7[0,3]CZ	00HU[0,3,4]MZ	00HV[0,3,4]MZ
Multiple Array	0JH6[0,3]DZ	0JH8[0,3]DZ	0JH7[0,3]DZ	00HU[0,3,4]MZ	00HV[0,3,4]MZ
Multiple Array, Rechargable	0JH6[0,3]EZ	—	0JH7[0,3]EZ	00HU[0,3,4]MZ	00HV[0,3,4]MZ
Multiple Array, Rechargable	—	0JH8[0,3]EZ	—	00HU[0,3,4]MZ	00HV[0,3,4]MZ

DRG 582-583 Mastectomy for Malignancy

Site	Resection by Open approach	Code also as appropriate Resection of Lymph Nodes by Open approach by site			Code also as appropriate Resection of Thorax Muscle by Open approach	
		Axillary	Internal Mammary	Thorax	Right	Left
Breast, Right	0HTT0ZZ	07T50ZZ	07T80ZZ	07T70ZZ	0KTH0ZZ	—
Breast, Left	0HTU0ZZ	07T60ZZ	07T90ZZ	07T70ZZ	—	0KTJ0ZZ
Breast, Bilateral	0HTV0ZZ	07T50ZZ and 07T60ZZ	07T80ZZ and 07T90ZZ	07T70ZZ	0KTH0ZZ	0KTJ0ZZ

DRG 584-585 Breast Biopsy, Local Excision and Other Breast Procedures

Resection of Breast With Resection of Lymph Nodes and Thorax Muscle

Site	Resection by Open approach	Code also as appropriate Resection of Lymph Nodes by Open approach by site			Code also as appropriate Resection of Thorax Muscle by Open approach	
		Axillary	Internal Mammary	Thorax	Right	Left
Breast, Right	0HTT0ZZ	07T50ZZ	07T80ZZ	07T70ZZ	0KTH0ZZ	—
Breast, Left	0HTU0ZZ	07T60ZZ	07T90ZZ	07T70ZZ	—	0KTJ0ZZ
Breast, Bilateral	0HTV0ZZ	07T50ZZ and 07T60ZZ	07T80ZZ and 07T90ZZ	07T70ZZ	0KTH0ZZ	0KTJ0ZZ

Replacement of Breast Tissue

Site	Replacement by Percutaneous approach with Autologous Tissue	Code also as appropriate Extraction of Subcutaneous Tissue by Percutaneous approach					
		Abdomen	Back	Buttock	Chest	Leg, Upper, Right	Leg, Upper, Left
Breast, Right	0HRT37Z	0JD83ZZ	0JD73ZZ	0JD93ZZ	0JD63ZZ	0JDL3ZZ	0JDM3ZZ
Breast, Left	0HRU37Z	0JD83ZZ	0JD73ZZ	0JD93ZZ	0JD63ZZ	0JDL3ZZ	0JDM3ZZ
Breast, Bilateral	0HRV37Z	0JD83ZZ	0JD73ZZ	0JD93ZZ	0JD63ZZ	0JDL3ZZ	0JDM3ZZ

DRG 628-630 Other Endocrine, Nutritional and Metabolic Procedures

Hip Procedures

Open Removal of Hip Spacer with Replacement

Removal of Spacer		Code also as appropriate Replacement by Device Type					
		Metal	Metal on Poly	Ceramic	Ceramic on Poly	Oxidized Zirc on Poly	Synthetic Substitute
Hip, RT	0SP908Z	0SR901[9,A,Z]	0SR902[9,A,Z]	0SR903[9,A,Z]	0SR904[9,A,Z]	0SR906[9,A,Z]	0SR90J[9,A,Z]
Hip, LT	0SPB08Z	0SRB01[9,A,Z]	0SRB02[9,A,Z]	0SRB03[9,A,Z]	0SRB04[9,A,Z]	0SRB06[9,A,Z]	0SRB0J[9,A,Z]

Open Removal of Hip Spacer with Replacement

Removal of Spacer		Code also as appropriate Replacement by Device Type						
		Acetabular Surface				Femoral Surface		
		Poly	Metal	Ceramic	Synthetic	Metal	Ceramic	Synthetic
Hip, RT	ØSP908Z	ØSRAØØ[9,A,Z]	ØSRAØ1[9,A,Z]	ØSRAØ3[9,A,Z]	ØSRAØJ[9,A,Z]	ØSRRØ1[9,A,Z]	ØSRRØ3[9,A,Z]	ØSRRØJ[9,A,Z]
Hip, LT	ØSPBØ8Z	ØSREØØ[9,A,Z]	ØSREØ1[9,A,Z]	ØSREØ3[9,A,Z]	ØSREØJ[9,A,Z]	ØSRSØ1[9,A,Z]	ØSRSØ3[9,A,Z]	ØSRSØJ[9,A,Z]

Open Removal of Hip Spacer with Liner Insertion (supplement)

Removal of Spacer		Code also as appropriate Supplement of Body Part by Site		
		Joint	Acetabular Surface	Femoral Surface
Hip, RT	ØSP908Z	ØSU909Z	ØSUAØ9Z	ØSURØ9Z
Hip, LT	ØSPBØ8Z	ØSUBØ9Z	ØSUEØ9Z	ØSUSØ9Z

Open Removal of Hip Liner with Replacement

Removal of Liner		Code also as appropriate Replacement by Device Type					
		Metal	Metal on Poly	Ceramic	Ceramic on Poly	Oxidized Zirc on Poly	Synthetic Substitute
Hip, RT	ØSP909Z	ØSR9Ø1[9,A,Z]	ØSR9Ø2[9,A,Z]	ØSR9Ø3[9,A,Z]	ØSR9Ø4[9,A,Z]	ØSR9Ø6[9,A,Z]	ØSR9ØJ[9,A,Z]
Hip, LT	ØSPBØ9Z	ØSRBØ1[9,A,Z]	ØSRBØ2[9,A,Z]	ØSRBØ3[9,A,Z]	ØSRBØ4[9,A,Z]	ØSRBØ6[9,A,Z]	ØSRBØJ[9,A,Z]

Open Removal of Hip Liner with Replacement

Removal of Liner		Code also as appropriate Replacement by Device Type						
		Acetabular Surface				Femoral Surface		
		Poly	Metal	Ceramic	Synthetic	Metal	Ceramic	Synthetic
Hip, RT	ØSP909Z	ØSRAØØ[9,A,Z]	ØSRAØ1[9,A,Z]	ØSRAØ3[9,A,Z]	ØSRAØJ[9,A,Z]	ØSRRØ1[9,A,Z]	ØSRRØ3[9,A,Z]	ØSRRØJ[9,A,Z]
Hip, LT	ØSPBØ9Z	ØSREØØ[9,A,Z]	ØSREØ1[9,A,Z]	ØSREØ3[9,A,Z]	ØSREØJ[9,A,Z]	ØSRSØ1[9,A,Z]	ØSRSØ3[9,A,Z]	ØSRSØJ[9,A,Z]

Open Removal of Hip Liner with Liner Insertion (supplement)

Removal of Liner		Code also as appropriate Supplement of Body Part by Site		
		Joint	Acetabular Surface	Femoral Surface
Hip, RT	ØSP909Z	ØSU909Z	ØSUAØ9Z	ØSURØ9Z
Hip, LT	ØSPBØ9Z	ØSUBØ9Z	ØSUEØ9Z	ØSUSØ9Z

Open Removal of Hip Resurfacing Device with Replacement

Removal of Resurfacing Device		Code also as appropriate Replacement by Device Type					
		Metal	Metal on Poly	Ceramic	Ceramic on Poly	Oxidized Zirc on Poly	Synthetic Substitute
Hip, RT	ØSP90BZ	ØSR9Ø1[9,A,Z]	ØSR9Ø2[9,A,Z]	ØSR9Ø3[9,A,Z]	ØSR9Ø4[9,A,Z]	ØSR9Ø6[9,A,Z]	ØSR9ØJ[9,A,Z]
Hip, LT	ØSPBØBZ	ØSRBØ1[9,A,Z]	ØSRBØ2[9,A,Z]	ØSRBØ3[9,A,Z]	ØSRBØ4[9,A,Z]	ØSRBØ6[9,A,Z]	ØSRBØJ[9,A,Z]

Open Removal of Hip Resurfacing Device with Replacement

Removal of Resurfacing Device		Code also as appropriate Replacement by Device Type						
		Acetabular Surface				Femoral Surface		
		Poly	Metal	Ceramic	Synthetic	Metal	Ceramic	Synthetic
Hip, RT	ØSP90BZ	ØSRAØØ[9,A,Z]	ØSRAØ1[9,A,Z]	ØSRAØ3[9,A,Z]	ØSRAØJ[9,A,Z]	ØSRRØ1[9,A,Z]	ØSRRØ3[9,A,Z]	ØSRRØJ[9,A,Z]
Hip, LT	ØSPBØBZ	ØSREØØ[9,A,Z]	ØSREØ1[9,A,Z]	ØSREØ3[9,A,Z]	ØSREØJ[9,A,Z]	ØSRSØ1[9,A,Z]	ØSRSØ3[9,A,Z]	ØSRSØJ[9,A,Z]

Open Removal of Hip Resurfacing Device with Liner Insertion (supplement)

Removal of Resurfacing Device		Code also as appropriate Supplement of Body Part by Site		
		Joint	Acetabular Surface	Femoral Surface
Hip, RT	ØSP90BZ	ØSU909Z	ØSUAØ9Z	ØSURØ9Z
Hip, LT	ØSPBØBZ	ØSUBØ9Z	ØSUEØ9Z	ØSUSØ9Z

Open Removal of Hip Synthetic Substitute with Replacement

Removal of Synthetic Substitute		Code also as appropriate Replacement by Device Type					
		Metal	Metal on Poly	Ceramic	Ceramic on Poly	Oxidized Zirc on Poly	Synthetic Substitute
Hip, RT	0SP90JZ	0SR901[9,A,Z]	0SR902[9,A,Z]	0SR903[9,A,Z]	0SR904[9,A,Z]	0SR906[9,A,Z]	0SR90J[9,A,Z]
Hip, LT	0SPB0JZ	0SRB01[9,A,Z]	0SRB02[9,A,Z]	0SRB03[9,A,Z]	0SRB04[9,A,Z]	0SRB06[9,A,Z]	0SRB0J[9,A,Z]

Open Removal of Hip Synthetic Substitute with Replacement

Removal of Synthetic Substitute		Code also as appropriate Replacement by Device Type						
		Acetabular Surface				Femoral Surface		
		Poly	Metal	Ceramic	Synthetic	Metal	Ceramic	Synthetic
Hip, RT	0SP90JZ	0SRA00[9,A,Z]	0SRA01[9,A,Z]	0SRA03[9,A,Z]	0SRA0J[9,A,Z]	0SRR01[9,A,Z]	0SRR03[9,A,Z]	0SRR0J[9,A,Z]
Hip, LT	0SPB0JZ	0SRE00[9,A,Z]	0SRE01[9,A,Z]	0SRE03[9,A,Z]	0SRE0J[9,A,Z]	0SRS01[9,A,Z]	0SRS03[9,A,Z]	0SRS0J[9,A,Z]

Open Removal of Hip Acetabular/Femoral Surface with Replacement

Removal of Acetabular/Femoral Surface		Code also as appropriate Replacement by Device Type					
		Metal	Metal on Poly	Ceramic	Ceramic on Poly	Oxidized Zirc on Poly	Synthetic Substitute
Hip, RT	0SP[A,R]0JZ	0SR901[9,A,Z]	0SR902[9,A,Z]	0SR903[9,A,Z]	0SR904[9,A,Z]	0SR906[9,A,Z]	0SR90J[9,A,Z]
Hip, LT	0SP[E,S]0JZ	0SRB01[9,A,Z]	0SRB02[9,A,Z]	0SRB03[9,A,Z]	0SRB04[9,A,Z]	0SRB06[9,A,Z]	0SRB0J[9,A,Z]

Open Removal of Hip Acetabular/Femoral Surface with Replacement

Removal of Acetabular/Femoral Surface		Code also as appropriate Replacement by Device Type						
		Acetabular Surface				Femoral Surface		
		Poly	Metal	Ceramic	Synthetic	Metal	Ceramic	Synthetic
Hip, RT	0SP[A,R]0JZ	0SRA00[9,A,Z]	0SRA01[9,A,Z]	0SRA03[9,A,Z]	0SRA0J[9,A,Z]	0SRR01[9,A,Z]	0SRR03[9,A,Z]	0SRR0J[9,A,Z]
Hip, LT	0SP[E,S]0JZ	0SRE00[9,A,Z]	0SRE01[9,A,Z]	0SRE03[9,A,Z]	0SRE0J[9,A,Z]	0SRS01[9,A,Z]	0SRS03[9,A,Z]	0SRS0J[9,A,Z]

Percutaneous Endoscopic Removal of Hip Spacer with Replacement

Removal of Spacer		Code also as appropriate Replacement by Device Type					
		Metal	Metal on Poly	Ceramic	Ceramic on Poly	Oxidized Zirc on Poly	Synthetic Substitute
Hip, RT	0SP948Z	0SR901[9,A,Z]	0SR902[9,A,Z]	0SR903[9,A,Z]	0SR904[9,A,Z]	0SR906[9,A,Z]	0SR90J[9,A,Z]
Hip, LT	0SPB48Z	0SRB01[9,A,Z]	0SRB02[9,A,Z]	0SRB03[9,A,Z]	0SRB04[9,A,Z]	0SRB06[9,A,Z]	0SRB0J[9,A,Z]

Percutaneous Endoscopic Removal of Hip Spacer with Replacement

Removal of Spacer		Code also as appropriate Replacement by Device Type						
		Acetabular Surface				Femoral Surface		
		Poly	Metal	Ceramic	Synthetic	Metal	Ceramic	Synthetic
Hip, RT	0SP948Z	0SRA00[9,A,Z]	0SRA01[9,A,Z]	0SRA03[9,A,Z]	0SRA0J[9,A,Z]	0SRR01[9,A,Z]	0SRR03[9,A,Z]	0SRR0J[9,A,Z]
Hip, LT	0SPB48Z	0SRE00[9,A,Z]	0SRE01[9,A,Z]	0SRE03[9,A,Z]	0SRE0J[9,A,Z]	0SRS01[9,A,Z]	0SRS03[9,A,Z]	0SRS0J[9,A,Z]

Percutaneous Endoscopic Removal of Hip Spacer with Liner Insertion (supplement)

Removal of Spacer		Code also as appropriate Supplement of Body Part by Site		
		Joint	Acetabular Surface	Femoral Surface
Hip, RT	0SP948Z	0SU909Z	0SUA09Z	0SUR09Z
Hip, LT	0SPB48Z	0SUB09Z	0SUE09Z	0SUS09Z

Percutaneous Endoscopic Removal of Hip Synthetic Substitute with Replacement

Removal of Synthetic Substitute		Code also as appropriate Replacement by Device Type					
		Metal	Metal on Poly	Ceramic	Ceramic on Poly	Oxidized Zirc on Poly	Synthetic Substitute
Hip, RT	0SP94JZ	0SR901[9,A,Z]	0SR902[9,A,Z]	0SR903[9,A,Z]	0SR904[9,A,Z]	0SR906[9,A,Z]	0SR90J[9,A,Z]
Hip, LT	0SPB4JZ	0SRB01[9,A,Z]	0SRB02[9,A,Z]	0SRB03[9,A,Z]	0SRB04[9,A,Z]	0SRB06[9,A,Z]	0SRB0J[9,A,Z]

Percutaneous Endoscopic of Hip Synthetic Substitute with Replacement

Removal of Synthetic Substitute		Code also as appropriate Replacement by Device Type						
		Acetabular Surface				Femoral Surface		
		Poly	Metal	Ceramic	Synthetic	Metal	Ceramic	Synthetic
Hip, RT	ØSP94JZ	ØSRAØØ[9,A,Z]	ØSRAØ1[9,A,Z]	ØSRAØ3[9,A,Z]	ØSRAØJ[9,A,Z]	ØSRRØ1[9,A,Z]	ØSRRØ3[9,A,Z]	ØSRRØJ[9,A,Z]
Hip, LT	ØSPB4JZ	ØSREØØ[9,A,Z]	ØSREØ1[9,A,Z]	ØSREØ3[9,A,Z]	ØSREØJ[9,A,Z]	ØSRSØ1[9,A,Z]	ØSRSØ3[9,A,Z]	ØSRSØJ[9,A,Z]

Percutaneous Endoscopic Removal of Hip Synthetic Substitute with Liner Insertion (supplement)

Removal of Synthetic Substitute		Code also as appropriate Supplement of Body Part by Site		
		Joint	Acetabular Surface	Femoral Surface
Hip, RT	ØSP94JZ	ØSU9Ø9Z	ØSUAØ9Z	ØSURØ9Z
Hip, LT	ØSPB4JZ	ØSUBØ9Z	ØSUEØ9Z	ØSUSØ9Z

Percutaneous Endoscopic Removal of Hip Acetabular/Femoral Surface with Replacement

Removal of Acetabular/Femoral Surface		Code also as appropriate Replacement by Device Type					
		Metal	Metal on Poly	Ceramic	Ceramic on Poly	Oxidized Zirc on Poly	Synthetic Substitute
Hip, RT	ØSP[A,R]4JZ	ØSR9Ø1[9,A,Z]	ØSR9Ø2[9,A,Z]	ØSR9Ø3[9,A,Z]	ØSR9Ø4[9,A,Z]	ØSR9Ø6[9,A,Z]	ØSR9ØJ[9,A,Z]
Hip, LT	ØSP[E,S]4JZ	ØSRBØ1[9,A,Z]	ØSRBØ2[9,A,Z]	ØSRBØ3[9,A,Z]	ØSRBØ4[9,A,Z]	ØSRBØ6[9,A,Z]	ØSRBØJ[9,A,Z]

Percutaneous Endoscopic of Hip Acetabular/Femoral Surface with Replacement

Removal of Acetabular/Femoral Surface		Code also as appropriate Replacement by Device Type						
		Acetabular Surface				Femoral Surface		
		Poly	Metal	Ceramic	Synthetic	Metal	Ceramic	Synthetic
Hip, RT	ØSP[A,R]4JZ	ØSRAØØ[9,A,Z]	ØSRAØ1[9,A,Z]	ØSRAØ3[9,A,Z]	ØSRAØJ[9,A,Z]	ØSRRØ1[9,A,Z]	ØSRRØ3[9,A,Z]	ØSRRØJ[9,A,Z]
Hip, LT	ØSP[E,S]4JZ	ØSREØØ[9,A,Z]	ØSREØ1[9,A,Z]	ØSREØ3[9,A,Z]	ØSREØJ[9,A,Z]	ØSRSØ1[9,A,Z]	ØSRSØ3[9,A,Z]	ØSRSØJ[9,A,Z]

Percutaneous Endoscopic Removal of Hip Acetabular/Femoral Surface with Liner Insertion (supplement)

Removal of Acetabular/Femoral Surface		Code also as appropriate Supplement of Body Part by Site		
		Joint	Acetabular Surface	Femoral Surface
Hip, RT	ØSP[A,R]4JZ	ØSU9Ø9Z	ØSUAØ9Z	ØSURØ9Z
Hip, LT	ØSP[E,S]4JZ	ØSUBØ9Z	ØSUEØ9Z	ØSUSØ9Z

Knee Procedures

Open Removal of Knee Liner with Synthetic Substitute Replacement

Removal of Liner		Code also as appropriate Replacement by Type of Synthetic Substitute						
		Oxidized Zircon on Poly	Synthetic Substitute	Medial Unicondylar	Lateral Unicondylar	Patello-femoral	Femoral Surface	Tibial Surface
Knee, RT	ØSPCØ9Z	ØSRCØ6[9,A,Z]	ØSRCØJ[9,A,Z]	ØSRCØL[9,A,Z]	ØSRCØM[9,A,Z]	ØSRCØN[9,A,Z]	ØSRTØJ[9,A,Z]	ØSRVØJ[9,A,Z]
Knee, LT	ØSPDØ9Z	ØSRDØ6[9,A,Z]	ØSRDØJ[9,A,Z]	ØSRDØL[9,A,Z]	ØSRDØM[9,A,Z]	ØSRDØN[9,A,Z]	ØSRUØJ[9,A,Z]	ØSRWØJ[9,A,Z]

Open Removal of Patellar Surface of Knee with Synthetic Substitute Replacement

Removal of Patellar Surface		Code also as appropriate Replacement by Type of Synthetic Substitute	
		Femoral Surface	Tibial Surface
Knee, RT	ØSPCØJC	ØSRTØJ[9,A]	ØSRVØJ[9,A,Z]
Knee, LT	ØSPDØJC	ØSRUØJ[9,A]	ØSRWØJ[9,A,Z]

Open Removal of Knee Synthetic Substitute with Synthetic Substitute Replacement

Removal of Synthetic Substitute		Code also as appropriate Replacement by Type of Synthetic Substitute	
		Femoral Surface	Tibial Surface
Knee, RT	ØSPCØJZ	ØSRTØJ[9,A]	ØSRVØJ[9,A]
Knee, LT	ØSPDØJZ	ØSRUØJ[9,A]	ØSRWØJ[9,A,Z]

Open Removal of Knee Medial/Lateral Unicondylar Device with Synthetic Substitute Replacement

Removal of Medial/Lateral Unicondylar Device		Code also as appropriate Replacement by Type of Synthetic Substitute	
		Femoral Surface	Tibial Surface
Knee, Medial Unicondylar, RT	ØSPCØLZ	ØSRTØJ[9,A]	ØSRVØJ[9,A]
Knee, Medial Unicondylar, LT	ØSPDØLZ	ØSRUØJ[9,A]	ØSRWØJ[9,A,Z]
Knee, Lateral Unicondylar, RT	ØSPCØMZ	ØSRTØJ[9,A]	ØSRVØJ[9,A]
Knee, Lateral Unicondylar, LT	ØSPDØMZ	ØSRUØJ[9,A]	ØSRWØJ[9,A,Z]

Open Removal of Knee Patellofemoral Device with Synthetic Substitute Replacement

Removal of Patellofemoral Device		Code also as appropriate Replacement by Type of Synthetic Substitute	
		Femoral Surface	Tibial Surface
Knee, RT	ØSPCØNZ	ØSRTØJ[9,A]	ØSRVØJ[9,A]
Knee, LT	ØSPDØNZ	ØSRUØJ[9,A]	ØSRWØJ[9,A,Z]

Open Removal of Femoral/Tibial Surface of Knee with Synthetic Substitute Replacement

Removal of Femoral/Tibial Surface		Code also as appropriate Replacement by Type of Synthetic Substitute	
		Femoral Surface	Tibial Surface
Knee, RT	ØSP[T,V]ØJZ	ØSRTØJ[9,A]	ØSRVØJ[9,A]
Knee, LT	ØSP[U,W]ØJZ	ØSRUØJ[9,A]	ØSRWØJ[9,A,Z]

Percutaneous Endoscopic Removal of Patellar Surface of Knee with Synthetic Substitute Replacement

Removal of Patellar Surface		Code also as appropriate Replacement by Type of Synthetic Substitute	
		Femoral Surface	Tibial Surface
Knee, RT	ØSPC4JC	ØSRTØJ[9,A]	ØSRVØJ[9,A]
Knee, LT	ØSPD4JC	ØSRUØJ[9,A]	ØSRWØJ[9,A,Z]

Percutaneous Endoscopic Removal of Knee Synthetic Substitute with Synthetic Substitute Replacement

Removal of Synthetic Substitute		Code also as appropriate Replacement by Type of Synthetic Substitute	
		Femoral Surface	Tibial Surface
Knee, RT	ØSPC4JZ	ØSRTØJ[9,A]	ØSRVØJ[9,A,Z]
Knee, LT	ØSPD4JZ	ØSRUØJ[9,A]	ØSRWØJ[9,A,Z]

Percutaneous Endoscopic Removal of Knee Medial/Lateral Unicondylar Device with Synthetic Substitute Replacement

Removal of Medial/Lateral Unicondylar Device		Code also as appropriate Replacement by Type of Synthetic Substitute	
		Femoral Surface	Tibial Surface
Knee, Medial Unicondylar, RT	ØSPC4LZ	ØSRTØJ[9,A]	ØSRVØJ[9,A]
Knee, Medial Unicondylar, LT	ØSPD4LZ	ØSRUØJ[9,A]	ØSRWØJ[9,A,Z]
Knee, Lateral Unicondylar, RT	ØSPC4MZ	ØSRTØJ[9,A]	ØSRVØJ[9,A]
Knee, Lateral Unicondylar, LT	ØSPD4MZ	ØSRUØJ[9,A]	ØSRWØJ[9,A,Z]

Percutaneous Endoscopic Removal of Knee Patellofemoral Device with Synthetic Substitute Replacement

Removal of Patellofemoral Device		Code also as appropriate Replacement by Type of Synthetic Substitute	
		Femoral Surface	Tibial Surface
Knee, RT	ØSPC4NZ	ØSRTØJ[9,A]	ØSRVØJ[9,A]
Knee, LT	ØSPD4NZ	ØSRUØJ[9,A]	ØSRWØJ[9,A,Z]

Percutaneous Endoscopic Removal of Femoral/Tibial Surface of Knee with Synthetic Substitute Replacement

Removal of Femoral/Tibial Surface		Code also as appropriate Replacement by Type of Synthetic Substitute	
		Femoral Surface	Tibial Surface
Knee, RT	ØSP[T,V]4JZ	ØSRTØJ[9,A]	ØSRVØJ[9,A,Z]
Knee, LT	ØSP[U,W]4JZ	ØSRUØJ[9,A]	ØSRWØJ[9,A,Z]

DRG 662-664 Minor Bladder Procedure

Repair of Bladder	Code also as appropriate Repair of Abdominal Wall	
	with Stoma	without Stoma
ØTQB[Ø,3,4]ZZ	ØWQFXZ2	ØWQFXZZ

DRG 665-667 Prostatectomy

Site	Resection by approach				Code also as appropriate Resection of Seminal Vesicles, Bilateral by approach	
	Open	Percutaneous Endoscopic	Via Natural or Artificial Opening	Via Natural or Artificial Opening Endoscopic	Open	Percutaneous Endoscopic
Prostate	ØVT00ZZ	ØVT04ZZ	ØVT07ZZ	ØVT08ZZ	ØVT30ZZ	ØVT34ZZ

DRG 7Ø7-7Ø8 Major Male Pelvic Procedures

Site	Resection by approach				Code also as appropriate Resection of Seminal Vesicles, Bilateral by approach	
	Open	Percutaneous Endoscopic	Via Natural or Artificial Opening	Via Natural or Artificial Opening Endoscopic	Open	Percutaneous Endoscopic
Prostate	ØVT00ZZ	ØVT04ZZ	ØVT07ZZ	ØVT08ZZ	ØVT30ZZ	ØVT34ZZ

DRG 734-735 Pelvic Evisceration, Radical Hysterectomy and Radical Vulvectomy

Pelvic Evisceration

Resection by Site						
Bladder	Cervix	Fallopian Tubes, Bilateral	Ovaries, Bilateral	Urethra	Uterus	Vagina
ØTTBØZZ	ØUTCØZZ	ØUT7ØZZ	ØUT2ØZZ	ØTTDØZZ	ØUT9ØZZ	ØUTGØZZ

Radical Hysterectomy

Approach	Resection by Site		
	Cervix	Uterus	Uterine Support Structure
Vaginal	ØUTC[7,8]ZZ	ØUT9[7,8]ZZ	ØUT4[7,8]ZZ
Abdominal, Endoscopic	ØUTC4ZZ	ØUT9[4,F]ZZ	ØUT44ZZ
Abdominal, Open	ØUTCØZZ	ØUT9ØZZ	ØUT4ØZZ

Radical Vulvectomy

Resection by Site	Code also as appropriate Excision of Inguinal Lymph Nodes by Approach	
Vulva	Right	Left
ØUTM[Ø,X]ZZ	07BH[Ø,4]ZZ	07BJ[Ø,4]ZZ

Non-OR procedure combinations

Note: The following table identifies procedure combinations that are considered Non-OR even though one or more procedures of the combination are considered valid DRG OR procedures

Insertion With Removal of Intraluminal Device

Code as appropriate Insertion of Intraluminal Device into Hepatobiliary Duct	Code also as appropriate Removal of Intraluminal Device by Approach and Site			
	Via Natural or Artificial Opening		External	
	Hepatobiliary Duct	Pancreatic Duct	Hepatobiliary Duct	Pancreatic Duct
ØFHB7DZ	ØFPB[7,8]DZ	ØFPD[7,8]DZ	ØFPBXDZ	ØFPDXDZ

Appendix M: Coding Exercises and Answers

Using the ICD-10-PCS tables construct the code that accurately represents the procedure performed.

Medical Surgical Section

Procedure	Code
1. Excision of malignant melanoma from skin of right ear	
2. Laparoscopy with excision of endometrial implant from left ovary	
3. Percutaneous needle core biopsy of right kidney	
4. EGD with gastric biopsy	
5. Open endarterectomy of left common carotid artery	
6. Excision of basal cell carcinoma of lower lip	
7. Open excision of tail of pancreas	
8. Percutaneous biopsy of right gastrocnemius muscle	
9. Sigmoidoscopy with sigmoid polypectomy	
10. Open excision of lesion from right Achilles tendon	
11. Open resection of cecum	
12. Total excision of pituitary gland, open	
13. Explantation of left failed kidney, open	
14. Open left axillary total lymphadenectomy	
15. Laparoscopic-assisted vaginal hysterectomy	
16. Right total mastectomy, open	
17. Open resection of papillary muscle	
18. Total retropubic prostatectomy, open	
19. Laparoscopic cholecystectomy	
20. Endoscopic bilateral total maxillary sinusectomy	
21. Amputation at right elbow level	
22. Right below-knee amputation, proximal tibia/fibula	
23. Fifth ray carpometacarpal joint amputation, left hand	
24. Right leg and hip amputation through ischium	
25. DIP joint amputation of right thumb	
26. Right wrist joint amputation	
27. Trans-metatarsal amputation of foot at left big toe	
28. Mid-shaft amputation, right humerus	
29. Left fourth toe amputation, mid-proximal phalanx	
30. Right above-knee amputation, distal femur	
31. Cryotherapy of wart on left hand	
32. Percutaneous radiofrequency ablation of right vocal cord lesion	
33. Left heart catheterization with laser destruction of arrhythmogenic focus, A-V node	
34. Cautery of nosebleed	
35. Transurethral endoscopic laser ablation of prostate	
36. Percutaneous cautery of oozing varicose vein, left calf	
37. Laparoscopy with destruction of endometriosis, bilateral ovaries	
38. Laser coagulation of right retinal vessel, percutaneous	
39. Thoracoscopic pleurodesis, left side	
40. Percutaneous insertion of Greenfield IVC filter	
41. Forceps total mouth extraction, upper and lower teeth	

Procedure	Code
42. Removal of left thumbnail	
43. Extraction of right intraocular lens without replacement, percutaneous	
44. Laparoscopy with needle aspiration of ova for in vitro fertilization	
45. Nonexcisional debridement of skin ulcer, right foot	
46. Open stripping of abdominal fascia, right side	
47. Hysteroscopy with D&C, diagnostic	
48. Liposuction for medical purposes, left upper arm	
49. Removal of tattered right ear drum fragments with tweezers	
50. Microincisional phlebectomy of spider veins, right lower leg	
51. Routine Foley catheter placement	
52. Incision and drainage of external anal abscess	
53. Percutaneous drainage of ascites	
54. Laparoscopy with left ovarian cystotomy and drainage	
55. Laparotomy and drain placement for liver abscess, right lobe	
56. Right knee arthrotomy with drain placement	
57. Thoracentesis of left pleural effusion	
58. Phlebotomy of left median cubital vein for polycythemia vera	
59. Percutaneous chest tube placement for right pneumothorax	
60. Endoscopic drainage of left ethmoid sinus	
61. External ventricular CSF drainage catheter placement via burr hole	
62. Removal of foreign body, right cornea	
63. Percutaneous mechanical thrombectomy, left brachial artery	
64. Esophagogastroscopy with removal of bezoar from stomach	
65. Foreign body removal, skin of left thumb	
66. Transurethral cystoscopy with removal of bladder stone	
67. Forceps removal of foreign body in right nostril	
68. Laparoscopy with excision of old suture from mesentery	
69. Incision and removal of right lacrimal duct stone	
70. Nonincisional removal of intraluminal foreign body from vagina	
71. Right common carotid endarterectomy, open	
72. Open excision of retained sliver, subcutaneous tissue of left foot	
73. Extracorporeal shockwave lithotripsy (ESWL), bilateral ureters	
74. Endoscopic retrograde cholangiopancreatography (ERCP) with lithotripsy of common bile duct stone	
75. Thoracotomy with crushing of pericardial calcifications	
76. Transurethral cystoscopy with fragmentation of bladder calculus	
77. Hysteroscopy with intraluminal lithotripsy of left fallopian tube calcification	
78. Division of right foot tendon, percutaneous	

Procedure	Code
79. Left heart catheterization with division of bundle of HIS	
80. Open osteotomy of capitate, left hand	
81. EGD with esophagotomy of esophagogastric junction	
82. Sacral rhizotomy for pain control, percutaneous	
83. Laparotomy with exploration and adhesiolysis of right ureter	
84. Incision of scar contracture, right elbow	
85. Frenulotomy for treatment of tongue-tie syndrome	
86. Right shoulder arthroscopy with coracoacromial ligament release	
87. Mitral valvulotomy for release of fused leaflets, open approach	
88. Percutaneous left Achilles tendon release	
89. Laparoscopy with lysis of peritoneal adhesions	
90. Manual rupture of right shoulder joint adhesions under general anesthesia	
91. Open posterior tarsal tunnel release	
92. Laparoscopy with freeing of left ovary and fallopian tube	
93. Liver transplant with donor matched liver	
94. Orthotopic heart transplant using porcine heart	
95. Right lung transplant, open, using organ donor match	
96. Transplant of large intestine, organ donor match	
97. Left kidney/pancreas organ bank transplant	
98. Replantation of avulsed scalp	
99. Reattachment of severed right ear	
100. Reattachment of traumatic left gastrocnemius avulsion, open	
101. Closed replantation of three avulsed teeth, lower jaw	
102. Reattachment of severed left hand	
103. Right open palmaris longus tendon transfer	
104. Endoscopic radial to median nerve transfer	
105. Fasciocutaneous flap closure of left thigh, open	
106. Transfer left index finger to left thumb position, open	
107. Percutaneous fascia transfer to fill defect, right neck	
108. Trigeminal to facial nerve transfer, percutaneous endoscopic	
109. Endoscopic left leg flexor hallucis longus tendon transfer	
110. Right scalp advancement flap to right temple	
111. Bilateral TRAM pedicle flap reconstruction status post mastectomy, muscle only, open	
112. Skin transfer flap closure of complex open wound, left lower back	
113. Open fracture reduction, right tibia	
114. Laparoscopy with gastropexy for malrotation	
115. Left knee arthroscopy with reposition of anterior cruciate ligament	
116. Open transposition of ulnar nerve	
117. Closed reduction with percutaneous internal fixation of right femoral neck fracture	
118. Trans-vaginal intraluminal cervical cerclage	
119. Cervical cerclage using Shirodkar technique	
120. Thoracotomy with banding of left pulmonary artery using extraluminal device	
121. Restriction of thoracic duct with intraluminal stent, percutaneous	

Procedure	Code
122. Craniotomy with clipping of cerebral aneurysm	
123. Nonincisional, transnasal placement of restrictive stent in right lacrimal duct	
124. Catheter-based temporary restriction of blood flow in abdominal aorta for treatment of cerebral ischemia	
125. Percutaneous ligation of esophageal vein	
126. Percutaneous embolization of left internal carotid-cavernous fistula	
127. Laparoscopy with bilateral occlusion of fallopian tubes using Hulka extraluminal clips	
128. Open suture ligation of failed AV graft, left brachial artery	
129. Percutaneous embolization of vascular supply, intracranial meningioma	
130. Percutaneous embolization of right uterine artery, using coils	
131. Open occlusion of left atrial appendage, using extraluminal pressure clips	
132. Percutaneous suture exclusion of left atrial appendage, via femoral artery access	
133. ERCP with balloon dilation of common bile duct	
134. PTCA of two coronary arteries, LAD with stent placement, RCA with no stent	
135. Cystoscopy with intraluminal dilation of bladder neck stricture	
136. Open dilation of old anastomosis, left femoral artery	
137. Dilation of upper esophageal stricture, direct visualization, with Bougie sound	
138. PTA of right brachial artery stenosis	
139. Transnasal dilation and stent placement in right lacrimal duct	
140. Hysteroscopy with balloon dilation of bilateral fallopian tubes	
141. Tracheoscopy with intraluminal dilation of tracheal stenosis	
142. Cystoscopy with dilation of left ureteral stricture, with stent placement	
143. Open gastric bypass with Roux-en-Y limb to jejunum	
144. Right temporal artery to intracranial artery bypass using Gore-Tex graft, open	
145. Tracheostomy formation with tracheostomy tube placement, percutaneous	
146. PICVA (percutaneous in situ coronary venous arterialization) of single coronary artery	
147. Open left femoral-popliteal artery bypass using cadaver vein graft	
148. Shunting of intrathecal cerebrospinal fluid to peritoneal cavity using synthetic shunt	
149. Colostomy formation, open, transverse colon to abdominal wall	
150. Open urinary diversion, left ureter, using ileal conduit to skin	
151. CABG of LAD using pedicled left internal mammary artery, open off-bypass	
152. Open pleuroperitoneal shunt, right pleural cavity, using synthetic device	
153. Percutaneous placement of ventriculoperitoneal shunt for treatment of hydrocephalus	
154. End-of-life replacement of spinal neurostimulator generator, multiple array, in lower abdomen	
155. Percutaneous insertion of spinal neurostimulator lead, lumbar spinal cord	

Procedure	Code
156. Percutaneous replacement of broken pacemaker lead in left atrium	
157. Open placement of dual chamber pacemaker generator in chest wall	
158. Percutaneous placement of venous central line in right internal jugular, with tip in superior vena cava	
159. Open insertion of multiple channel cochlear implant, left ear	
160. Percutaneous placement of Swan-Ganz catheter in pulmonary trunk	
161. Bronchoscopy with insertion of Low Dose, Pd-103 brachytherapy seeds, right lung	
162. Open insertion of interspinous process device into lumbar vertebral joint	
163. Open placement of bone growth stimulator, left femoral shaft	
164. Cystoscopy with placement of brachytherapy seeds in prostate gland	
165. Percutaneous insertion of Greenfield IVC filter	
166. Full-thickness skin graft to right lower arm, autograft (do not code graft harvest for this exercise)	
167. Excision of necrosed left femoral head with bone bank bone graft to fill the defect, open	
168. Penetrating keratoplasty of right cornea with donor matched cornea, percutaneous approach	
169. Excision of abdominal aorta with Gore-Tex graft replacement, open	
170. Total right knee arthroplasty with insertion of total knee prosthesis	
171. Tenonectomy with graft to right ankle using cadaver graft, open	
172. Mitral valve replacement using porcine valve, open	
173. Percutaneous phacoemulsification of right eye cataract with prosthetic lens insertion	
174. Transcatheter replacement of pulmonary valve using of bovine jugular vein valve	
175. Total left hip replacement using ceramic on ceramic prosthesis, without bone cement	
176. Aortic valve annuloplasty using ring, open	
177. Laparoscopic repair of left inguinal hernia with marlex plug	
178. Autograft nerve graft to right median nerve, percutaneous endoscopic (do not code graft harvest for this exercise)	
179. Exchange of liner in femoral component of previous left hip replacement, open approach	
180. Anterior colporrhaphy with polypropylene mesh reinforcement, open approach	
181. Implantation of CorCap cardiac support device, open approach	
182. Abdominal wall herniorrhaphy, open, using synthetic mesh	
183. Tendon graft to strengthen injured left shoulder using autograft, open (do not code graft harvest for this exercise)	
184. Onlay lamellar keratoplasty of left cornea using autograft, external approach	
185. Resurfacing procedure on right femoral head, open approach	
186. Exchange of drainage tube from right hip joint	
187. Tracheostomy tube exchange	
188. Change chest tube for left pneumothorax	
189. Exchange of cerebral ventriculostomy drainage tube	

Procedure	Code
190. Foley urinary catheter exchange	
191. Open removal of lumbar sympathetic neurostimulator lead	
192. Nonincisional removal of Swan-Ganz catheter from right pulmonary artery	
193. Laparotomy with removal of pancreatic drain	
194. Extubation, endotracheal tube	
195. Nonincisional PEG tube removal	
196. Transvaginal removal of brachytherapy seeds	
197. Transvaginal removal of extraluminal cervical cerclage	
198. Incision with removal of K-wire fixation, right first metatarsal	
199. Cystoscopy with retrieval of left ureteral stent	
200. Removal of nasogastric drainage tube for decompression	
201. Removal of external fixator, left radial fracture	
202. Trimming and reanastomosis of stenosed femorofemoral synthetic bypass graft, open	
203. Open revision of right hip replacement, with readjustment of prosthesis	
204. Adjustment of position, pacemaker lead in left ventricle, percutaneous	
205. External repositioning of Foley catheter to bladder	
206. Taking out loose screw and putting larger screw in fracture repair plate, left tibia	
207. Revision of totally implantable VAD port placement in chest wall, causing patient discomfort, open	
208. Thoracotomy with exploration of right pleural cavity	
209. Diagnostic laryngoscopy	
210. Exploratory arthrotomy of left knee	
211. Colposcopy with diagnostic hysteroscopy	
212. Digital rectal exam	
213. Diagnostic arthroscopy of right shoulder	
214. Endoscopy of maxillary sinus	
215. Laparotomy with palpation of liver	
216. Transurethral diagnostic cystoscopy	
217. Colonoscopy, discontinued at sigmoid colon	
218. Percutaneous mapping of basal ganglia	
219. Heart catheterization with cardiac mapping	
220. Intraoperative whole brain mapping via craniotomy	
221. Mapping of left cerebral hemisphere, percutaneous endoscopic	
222. Intraoperative cardiac mapping during open heart surgery	
223. Hysteroscopy with cautery of post-hysterectomy oozing and evacuation of clot	
224. Open exploration and ligation of post-op arterial bleeder, left forearm	
225. Control of post-operative retroperitoneal bleeding via laparotomy	
226. Reopening of thoracotomy site with drainage and control of post-op hemopericardium	
227. Arthroscopy with drainage of hemarthrosis at previous operative site, right knee	
228. Radiocarpal fusion of left hand with internal fixation, open	
229. Posterior approach spinal fusion at L1-L3 level with BAK cage interbody fusion device, open	
230. Intercarpal fusion of right hand with bone bank bone graft, open	

Procedure	Code
231. Sacrococcygeal fusion with bone graft from same operative site, open	
232. Interphalangeal fusion of left great toe, percutaneous pin fixation	
233. Suture repair of left radial nerve laceration	
234. Laparotomy with suture repair of blunt force duodenal laceration	
235. Perineoplasty with repair of old obstetric laceration, open	
236. Suture repair of right biceps tendon (upper arm) laceration, open	
237. Closure of abdominal wall stab wound	
238. Cosmetic face lift, open, no other information available	
239. Bilateral breast augmentation with silicone implants, open	
240. Cosmetic rhinoplasty with septal reduction and tip elevation using local tissue graft, open	
241. Abdominoplasty (tummy tuck), open	
242. Liposuction of bilateral thighs	
243. Creation of penis in female patient using tissue bank donor graft	
244. Creation of vagina in male patient using synthetic material	
245. Laparoscopic vertical (sleeve) gastrectomy	
246. Left uterine artery embolization with intraluminal biosphere injection	

Obstetrics

Procedure	Code
1. Abortion by dilation and evacuation following laminaria insertion	
2. Manually assisted spontaneous abortion	
3. Abortion by abortifacient insertion	
4. Bimanual pregnancy examination	
5. Extraperitoneal C-section, low transverse incision	
6. Fetal spinal tap, percutaneous	
7. Fetal kidney transplant, laparoscopic	
8. Open in utero repair of congenital diaphragmatic hernia	
9. Laparoscopy with total excision of tubal pregnancy	
10. Transvaginal removal of fetal monitoring electrode	

Placement

Procedure	Code
1. Placement of packing material, right ear	
2. Mechanical traction of entire left leg	
3. Removal of splint, right shoulder	
4. Placement of neck brace	
5. Change of vaginal packing	
6. Packing of wound, chest wall	
7. Sterile dressing placement to left groin region	
8. Removal of packing material from pharynx	
9. Placement of intermittent pneumatic compression device, covering entire right arm	
10. Exchange of pressure dressing to left thigh	

Administration

Procedure	Code
1. Peritoneal dialysis via indwelling catheter	
2. Transvaginal artificial insemination	
3. Infusion of total parenteral nutrition via central venous catheter	
4. Esophagogastroscopy with Botox injection into esophageal sphincter	
5. Percutaneous irrigation of knee joint	
6. Systemic infusion of recombinant tissue plasminogen activator (r-tPA) via peripheral venous catheter	
7. Transabdominal in vitro fertilization, implantation of donor ovum	
8. Autologous bone marrow transplant via central venous line	
9. Implantation of anti-microbial envelope with cardiac defibrillator placement, open	
10. Sclerotherapy of brachial plexus lesion, alcohol injection	
11. Percutaneous peripheral vein injection, glucarpidase	
12. Introduction of anti-infective envelope into subcutaneous tissue, open	

Measurement and Monitoring

Procedure	Code
1. Cardiac stress test, single measurement	
2. EGD with biliary flow measurement	
3. Right and left heart cardiac catheterization with bilateral sampling and pressure measurements	
4. Temperature monitoring, rectal	
5. Peripheral venous pulse, external, single measurement	
6. Holter monitoring	
7. Respiratory rate, external, single measurement	
8. Fetal heart rate monitoring, transvaginal	
9. Visual mobility test, single measurement	
10. Left ventricular cardiac output monitoring from pulmonary artery wedge (Swan-Ganz) catheter	
11. Olfactory acuity test, single measurement	

Extracorporeal or Systemic Assistance and Performance

Procedure	Code
1. Intermittent mechanical ventilation, 16 hours	
2. Liver dialysis, single encounter	
3. Cardiac countershock with successful conversion to sinus rhythm	
4. IPPB (intermittent positive pressure breathing) for mobilization of secretions, 22 hours	
5. Renal dialysis, 12 hours	
6. IABP (intra-aortic balloon pump) continuous	
7. Intra-operative cardiac pacing, continuous	
8. Intraoperative ECMO (extracorporeal membrane oxygenation), central	
9. Controlled mechanical ventilation (CMV), 45 hours	
10. Pulsatile compression boot with intermittent inflation	

Extracorporeal or Systemic Therapies

Procedure	Code
1. Donor thrombocytapheresis, single encounter	
2. Bili-lite phototherapy, series treatment	
3. Whole body hypothermia, single treatment	
4. Circulatory phototherapy, single encounter	
5. Shock wave therapy of plantar fascia, single treatment	
6. Antigen-free air conditioning, series treatment	
7. TMS (transcranial magnetic stimulation), series treatment	
8. Therapeutic ultrasound of peripheral vessels, single treatment	
9. Plasmapheresis, series treatment	
10. Extracorporeal electromagnetic stimulation (EMS) for urinary incontinence, single treatment	

Osteopathic

Procedure	Code
1. Isotonic muscle energy treatment of right leg	
2. Low velocity-high amplitude osteopathic treatment of head	
3. Lymphatic pump osteopathic treatment of left axilla	
4. Indirect osteopathic treatment of sacrum	
5. Articulatory osteopathic treatment of cervical region	

Other Procedures

Procedure	Code
1. Near infrared spectroscopy of leg vessels	
2. CT computer assisted sinus surgery	
3. Suture removal, abdominal wall	
4. Isolation after infectious disease exposure	
5. Robotic assisted open prostatectomy	
6. In vitro fertilization	

Chiropractic

Procedure	Code
1. Chiropractic treatment of lumbar region using long lever specific contact	
2. Chiropractic manipulation of abdominal region, indirect visceral	
3. Chiropractic extra-articular treatment of hip region	
4. Chiropractic treatment of sacrum using long and short lever specific contact	
5. Mechanically-assisted chiropractic manipulation of head	

Imaging

Procedure	Code
1. Noncontrast CT of abdomen and pelvis	
2. Intravascular ultrasound, left subclavian artery	
3. Fluoroscopic guidance for insertion of central venous catheter in SVC, low osmolar contrast	
4. Chest x-ray, AP/PA and lateral views	
5. Endoluminal ultrasound of gallbladder and bile ducts	
6. MRI of thyroid gland, contrast unspecified	
7. Esophageal videofluoroscopy study with oral barium contrast	

Procedure	Code
8. Portable x-ray study of right radius/ulna shaft, standard series	
9. Routine fetal ultrasound, second trimester twin gestation	
10. CT scan of bilateral lungs, high osmolar contrast with densitometry	
11. Fluoroscopic guidance for percutaneous transluminal angioplasty (PTA) of left common femoral artery, low osmolar contrast	

Nuclear Medicine

Procedure	Code
1. Tomo scan of right and left heart, unspecified radiopharmaceutical, qualitative gated rest	
2. Technetium pentetate assay of kidneys, ureters, and bladder	
3. Uniplanar scan of spine using technetium oxidronate, with first-pass study	
4. Thallous chloride tomographic scan of bilateral breasts	
5. PET scan of myocardium using rubidium	
6. Gallium citrate scan of head and neck, single plane imaging	
7. Xenon gas nonimaging probe of brain	
8. Upper GI scan, radiopharmaceutical unspecified, for gastric emptying	
9. Carbon 11 PET scan of brain with quantification	
10. Iodinated albumin nuclear medicine assay, blood plasma volume study	

Radiation Therapy

Procedure	Code
1. Plaque radiation of left eye, single port	
2. 8 MeV photon beam radiation to brain	
3. IORT of colon, 3 ports	
4. HDR brachytherapy of prostate using low dose palladium-103, unidirectional source	
5. Electron radiation treatment of right breast, with custom device	
6. Hyperthermia oncology treatment of pelvic region	
7. Contact radiation of tongue	
8. Heavy particle radiation treatment of pancreas, four risk sites	
9. LDR brachytherapy to spinal cord using iodine	
10. Whole body Phosphorus 32 administration with risk to hematopoetic system	

Physical Rehabilitation and Diagnostic Audiology

Procedure	Code
1. Bekesy assessment using audiometer	
2. Individual fitting of left eye prosthesis	
3. Physical therapy for range of motion and mobility, patient right hip, no special equipment	
4. Bedside swallow assessment using assessment kit	
5. Caregiver training in airway clearance techniques	
6. Application of short arm cast in rehabilitation setting	
7. Verbal assessment of patient's pain level	
8. Caregiver training in communication skills using manual communication board	

Procedure	Code
9. Group musculoskeletal balance training exercises, whole body, no special equipment	
10. Individual therapy for auditory processing using tape recorder	

Mental Health

Procedure	Code
1. Cognitive-behavioral psychotherapy, individual	
2. Narcosynthesis	
3. Light therapy	
4. ECT (electroconvulsive therapy), unilateral, multiple seizure	
5. Crisis intervention	
6. Neuropsychological testing	
7. Hypnosis	
8. Developmental testing	
9. Vocational counseling	
10. Family psychotherapy	

Substance Abuse Treatment

Procedure	Code
1. Naltrexone treatment for drug dependency	
2. Substance abuse treatment family counseling	
3. Medication monitoring of patient on methadone maintenance	
4. Individual interpersonal psychotherapy for drug abuse	
5. Patient in for alcohol detoxification treatment	
6. Group motivational counseling	
7. Individual 12-step psychotherapy for substance abuse	
8. Post-test infectious disease counseling for IV drug abuser	
9. Psychodynamic psychotherapy for drug dependent patient	
10. Group cognitive-behavioral counseling for substance abuse	

New Technology

Procedure	Code
1. Infusion of terlipressin via peripheral venous catheter	
2. Transcatheter dilation of left peroneal artery with 2 SAVAL stents	

Answers to Coding Exercises

Medical Surgical Section

	Procedure	Code
1.	Excision of malignant melanoma from skin of right ear	0HB2XZZ
2.	Laparoscopy with excision of endometrial implant from left ovary	0UB14ZZ
3.	Percutaneous needle core biopsy of right kidney	0TB03ZX
4.	EGD with gastric biopsy	0DB68ZX
5.	Open endarterectomy of left common carotid artery	03CJ0ZZ
6.	Excision of basal cell carcinoma of lower lip	0CB1XZZ
7.	Open excision of tail of pancreas	0FBG0ZZ
8.	Percutaneous biopsy of right gastrocnemius muscle	0KBS3ZX
9.	Sigmoidoscopy with sigmoid polypectomy	0DBN8ZZ
10.	Open excision of lesion from right Achilles tendon	0LBN0ZZ
11.	Open resection of cecum	0DTH0ZZ
12.	Total excision of pituitary gland, open	0GT00ZZ
13.	Explantation of left failed kidney, open	0TT10ZZ
14.	Open left axillary total lymphadenectomy	07T60ZZ (RESECTION is coded for cutting out a chain of lymph nodes.)
15.	Laparoscopic-assisted vaginal hysterectomy	0UT9FZZ
16.	Right total mastectomy, open	0HTT0ZZ
17.	Open resection of papillary muscle	02TD0ZZ (The papillary muscle refers to the heart and is found in the *Heart and Great Vessels* body system.)
18.	Total retropubic prostatectomy, open	0VT00ZZ
19.	Laparoscopic cholecystectomy	0FT44ZZ
20.	Endoscopic bilateral total maxillary sinusectomy	09TQ8ZZ, 09TR8ZZ
21.	Amputation at right elbow level	0X6B0ZZ
22.	Right below-knee amputation, proximal tibia/fibula	0Y6H0Z1 (The qualifier *High* here means the portion of the tib/fib closest to the knee.)
23.	Fifth ray carpometacarpal joint amputation, left hand	0X6K0Z8 (A *complete* ray amputation is through the carpometacarpal joint.)
24.	Right leg and hip amputation through ischium	0Y620ZZ (The *Hindquarter* body part includes amputation along any part of the hip bone.)
25.	DIP joint amputation of right thumb	0X6L0Z3 (The qualifier *low* here means through the distal interphalangeal joint.)
26.	Right wrist joint amputation	0X6J0Z0 (Amputation at the wrist joint is actually complete amputation of the hand.)
27.	Trans-metatarsal amputation of foot at left big toe	0Y6N0Z9 (A *partial* amputation is through the shaft of the metatarsal bone.)
28.	Mid-shaft amputation, right humerus	0X680Z2
29.	Left fourth toe amputation, mid-proximal phalanx	0Y6W0Z1 (The qualifier *High* here means anywhere along the proximal phalanx.)
30.	Right above-knee amputation, distal femur	0Y6C0Z3

	Procedure	Code
31.	Cryotherapy of wart on left hand	0H5GXZZ
32.	Percutaneous radiofrequency ablation of right vocal cord lesion	0C5T3ZZ
33.	Left heart catheterization with laser destruction of arrhythmogenic focus, A-V node	02583ZZ
34.	Cautery of nosebleed	093K7ZZ
35.	Transurethral endoscopic laser ablation of prostate	0V508ZZ
36.	Percutaneous cautery of oozing varicose vein, left calf	0Y3J3ZZ
37.	Laparoscopy with destruction of endometriosis, bilateral ovaries	0U524ZZ
38.	Laser coagulation of right retinal vessel, percutaneous	085G3ZZ (The *Retinal Vessel* body-part values are in the *Eye* body system.)
39.	Thoracoscopic pleurodesis, left side	0B5P4ZZ
40.	Percutaneous insertion of Greenfield IVC filter	06H03DZ
41.	Forceps total mouth extraction, upper and lower teeth	0CDWXZ2, 0CDXXZ2
42.	Removal of left thumbnail	0HDQXZZ (No separate body-part value is given for thumbnail, so this is coded to *Fingernail*.)
43.	Extraction of right intraocular lens without replacement, percutaneous	08DJ3ZZ
44.	Laparoscopy with needle aspiration of ova for in vitro fertilization	0UDN4ZZ
45.	Nonexcisional debridement of skin ulcer, right foot	0HDMXZZ
46.	Open stripping of abdominal fascia, right side	0JD80ZZ
47.	Hysteroscopy with D&C, diagnostic	0UDB8ZX
48.	Liposuction for medical purposes, left upper arm	0JDF3ZZ (The *Percutaneous* approach is inherent in the liposuction technique.)
49.	Removal of tattered right ear drum fragments with tweezers	09D77ZZ
50.	Microincisional phlebectomy of spider veins, right lower leg	06DY3ZZ
51.	Routine Foley catheter placement	0T9B70Z
52.	Incision and drainage of external anal abscess	0D9QXZZ
53.	Percutaneous drainage of ascites	0W9G3ZZ (This is drainage of the cavity and not the peritoneal membrane itself.)
54.	Laparoscopy with left ovarian cystotomy and drainage	0U914ZZ
55.	Laparotomy and drain placement for liver abscess, right lobe	0F9100Z
56.	Right knee arthrotomy with drain placement	0S9C00Z
57.	Thoracentesis of left pleural effusion	0W9B3ZZ (This is drainage of the pleural cavity)
58.	Phlebotomy of left median cubital vein for polycythemia vera	059C3ZZ (The median cubital vein is a branch of the basilic vein)
59.	Percutaneous chest tube placement for right pneumothorax	0W9930Z
60.	Endoscopic drainage of left ethmoid sinus	099V4ZZ
61.	External ventricular CSF drainage catheter placement via burr hole	009630Z
62.	Removal of foreign body, right cornea	08C8XZZ

Procedure	Code
63. Percutaneous mechanical thrombectomy, left brachial artery	03C83ZZ
64. Esophagogastroscopy with removal of bezoar from stomach	0DC68ZZ
65. Foreign body removal, skin of left thumb	0HCGXZZ (There is no specific value for thumb skin, so the procedure is coded to *Hand*.)
66. Transurethral cystoscopy with removal of bladder stone	0TCB8ZZ
67. Forceps removal of foreign body in right nostril	09CKXZZ (Nostril is coded to the *Nasal muscosa and soft tissue* body-part value.)
68. Laparoscopy with excision of old suture from mesentery	0DCV4ZZ
69. Incision and removal of right lacrimal duct stone	08CX0ZZ
70. Nonincisional removal of intraluminal foreign body from vagina	0UCG7ZZ (The approach *External* is also a possibility. It is assumed here that since the patient went to the doctor to have the object removed, that it was not in the vaginal orifice.)
71. Right common carotid endarterectomy, open	03CH0ZZ
72. Open excision of retained sliver, subcutaneous tissue of left foot	0JCR0ZZ
73. Extracorporeal shockwave lithotripsy (ESWL), bilateral ureters	0TF6XZZ, 0TF7XZZ (The *Bilateral Ureter* body-part value is not available for the root operation FRAGMENTATION, so the procedures are coded separately.)
74. Endoscopic retrograde cholangiopancreatography (ERCP) with lithotripsy of common bile duct stone	0FF98ZZ (ERCP is performed through the mouth to the biliary system via the duodenum, so the approach value is *Via Natural or Artificial Opening Endoscopic*.)
75. Thoracotomy with crushing of pericardial calcifications	02FN0ZZ
76. Transurethral cystoscopy with fragmentation of bladder calculus	0TFB8ZZ
77. Hysteroscopy with intraluminal lithotripsy of left fallopian tube calcification	0UF68ZZ
78. Division of right foot tendon, percutaneous	0L8V3ZZ
79. Left heart catheterization with division of bundle of HIS	02883ZZ
80. Open osteotomy of capitate, left hand	0P8N0ZZ (The capitate is one of the carpal bones of the hand.)
81. EGD with esophagotomy of esophagogastric junction	0D948ZZ
82. Sacral rhizotomy for pain control, percutaneous	018R3ZZ
83. Laparotomy with exploration and adhesiolysis of right ureter	0TN60ZZ
84. Incision of scar contracture, right elbow	0HNDXZZ (The skin of the elbow region is coded to *Lower Arm*.)
85. Frenulotomy for treatment of tongue-tie syndrome	0CN7XZZ (The frenulum is coded to the body-part value *Tongue*.)
86. Right shoulder arthroscopy with coracoacromial ligament release	0MN14ZZ

Procedure	Code
87. Mitral valvulotomy for release of fused leaflets, open approach	02NG0ZZ
88. Percutaneous left Achilles tendon release	0LNP3ZZ
89. Laparoscopy with lysis of peritoneal adhesions	0DNW4ZZ
90. Manual rupture of right shoulder joint adhesions under general anesthesia	0RNJXZZ
91. Open posterior tarsal tunnel release	01NG0ZZ (The nerve released in the posterior tarsal tunnel is the tibial nerve.)
92. Laparoscopy with freeing of left ovary and fallopian tube	0UN14ZZ, 0UN64ZZ
93. Liver transplant with donor matched liver	0FY00Z0
94. Orthotopic heart transplant using porcine heart	02YA0Z2 (The donor heart comes from an animal [pig], so the qualifier value is *Zooplastic*.)
95. Right lung transplant, open, using organ donor match	0BYK0Z0
96. Transplant of large intestine, organ donor match	0DYE0Z0
97. Left kidney/pancreas organ bank transplant	0FYG0Z0, 0TY10Z0
98. Replantation of avulsed scalp	0HM0XZZ
99. Reattachment of severed right ear	09M0XZZ
100. Reattachment of traumatic left gastrocnemius avulsion, open	0KMT0ZZ
101. Closed replantation of three avulsed teeth, lower jaw	0CMXXZ1
102. Reattachment of severed left hand	0XMK0ZZ
103. Right open palmaris longus tendon transfer	0LX50ZZ
104. Endoscopic radial to median nerve transfer	01X64Z5
105. Fasciocutaneous flap closure of left thigh, open	0JXM0ZC (The qualifier identifies the body layers in addition to fascia included in the procedure.)
106. Transfer left index finger to left thumb position, open	0XXP0ZM
107. Percutaneous fascia transfer to fill defect, right neck	0JX43ZZ
108. Trigeminal to facial nerve transfer, percutaneous endoscopic	00XK4ZM
109. Endoscopic left leg flexor hallucis longus tendon transfer	0LXP4ZZ
110. Right scalp advancement flap to right temple	0HX0XZZ
111. Bilateral TRAM pedicle flap reconstruction status post mastectomy, muscle only, open	0KXK0Z6, 0KXL0Z6 (The transverse rectus abdominus muscle (TRAM) flap is coded for each flap developed.)
112. Skin transfer flap closure of complex open wound, left lower back	0HX6XZZ
113. Open fracture reduction, right tibia	0QSG0ZZ
114. Laparoscopy with gastropexy for malrotation	0DS64ZZ
115. Left knee arthroscopy with reposition of anterior cruciate ligament	0MSP4ZZ
116. Open transposition of ulnar nerve	01S40ZZ
117. Closed reduction with percutaneous internal fixation of right femoral neck fracture	0QS634Z
118. Trans-vaginal intraluminal cervical cerclage	0UVC7DZ
119. Cervical cerclage using Shirodkar technique	0UVC7ZZ
120. Thoracotomy with banding of left pulmonary artery using extraluminal device	02VR0CZ
121. Restriction of thoracic duct with intraluminal stent, percutaneous	07VK3DZ

Procedure	Code
122. Craniotomy with clipping of cerebral aneurysm	03VG0CZ (The clip is placed lengthwise on the outside wall of the widened portion of the vessel.)
123. Nonincisional, transnasal placement of restrictive stent in right lacrimal duct	08VX7DZ
124. Catheter-based temporary restriction of blood flow in abdominal aorta for treatment of cerebral ischemia	04V03DJ
125. Percutaneous ligation of esophageal vein	06L33ZZ
126. Percutaneous embolization of left internal carotid-cavernous fistula	03LL3DZ
127. Laparoscopy with bilateral occlusion of fallopian tubes using Hulka extraluminal clips	0UL74CZ
128. Open suture ligation of failed AV graft, left brachial artery	03L80ZZ
129. Percutaneous embolization of vascular supply, intracranial meningioma	03LG3DZ
130. Percutaneous embolization of right uterine artery, using coils	04LE3DT
131. Open occlusion of left atrial appendage, using extraluminal pressure clips	02L70CK
132. Percutaneous suture exclusion of left atrial appendage, via femoral artery access	02L73ZK
133. ERCP with balloon dilation of common bile duct	0F798ZZ
134. PTCA of two coronary arteries, LAD with stent placement, RCA with no stent	02703DZ, 02703ZZ (A separate procedure is coded for each artery dilated, since the device value differs for each artery.)
135. Cystoscopy with intraluminal dilation of bladder neck stricture	0T7C8ZZ
136. Open dilation of old anastomosis, left femoral artery	047L0ZZ
137. Dilation of upper esophageal stricture, direct visualization, with Bougie sound	0D717ZZ
138. PTA of right brachial artery stenosis	03773ZZ
139. Transnasal dilation and stent placement in right lacrimal duct	087X7DZ
140. Hysteroscopy with balloon dilation of bilateral fallopian tubes	0U778ZZ
141. Tracheoscopy with intraluminal dilation of tracheal stenosis	0B718ZZ
142. Cystoscopy with dilation of left ureteral stricture, with stent placement	0T778DZ
143. Open gastric bypass with Roux-en-Y limb to jejunum	0D160ZA
144. Right temporal artery to intracranial artery bypass using Gore-Tex graft, open	031S0JG
145. Tracheostomy formation with tracheostomy tube placement, percutaneous	0B113F4
146. PICVA (percutaneous in situ coronary venous arterialization) of single coronary artery	02103D4
147. Open left femoral-popliteal artery bypass using cadaver vein graft	041L0KL
148. Shunting of intrathecal cerebrospinal fluid to peritoneal cavity using synthetic shunt	00160J6
149. Colostomy formation, open, transverse colon to abdominal wall	0D1L0Z4
150. Open urinary diversion, left ureter, using ileal conduit to skin	0T170ZC
151. CABG of LAD using pedicled left internal mammary artery, open off-bypass	02100Z9

Procedure	Code
152. Open pleuroperitoneal shunt, right pleural cavity, using synthetic device	0W190JG
153. Percutaneous placement of ventriculoperitoneal shunt for treatment of hydrocephalus	00163J6
154. End-of-life replacement of spinal neurostimulator generator, multiple array, in lower abdomen	0JH80DZ (Taking out of the old generator is coded separately to the root operation Removal)
155. Percutaneous insertion of spinal neurostimulator lead, lumbar spinal cord	00HV3MZ
156. Percutaneous replacement of broken pacemaker lead in left atrium	02H73JZ (Taking out the broken pacemaker lead is coded separately to the root operation Removal.)
157. Open placement of dual chamber pacemaker generator in chest wall	0JH606Z
158. Percutaneous placement of venous central line in right internal jugular, with tip in superior vena cava	02HV33Z
159. Open insertion of multiple channel cochlear implant, left ear	09HE06Z
160. Percutaneous placement of Swan-Ganz catheter in pulmonary trunk	02HP32Z (The Swan-Ganz catheter is coded to the device value Monitoring Device because it monitors pulmonary artery output.)
161. Bronchoscopy with insertion of Low Dose Pd-103 brachytherapy seeds, right lung	0BHK81Z, DB11BBZ
162. Open insertion of interspinous process device into lumbar vertebral joint	0SH00BZ
163. Open placement of bone growth stimulator, left femoral shaft	0QHY0MZ
164. Cystoscopy with placement of brachytherapy seeds in prostate gland	0VH081Z
165. Percutaneous insertion of Greenfield IVC filter	06H03DZ
166. Full-thickness skin graft to right lower arm, autograft (do not code graft harvest for this exercise)	0HRDX73
167. Excision of necrosed left femoral head with bone bank bone graft to fill the defect, open	0QR70KZ
168. Penetrating keratoplasty of right cornea with donor matched cornea, percutaneous approach	08R83KZ
169. Excision of abdominal aorta with Gore-Tex graft replacement, open	04R00JZ
170. Total right knee arthroplasty with insertion of total knee prosthesis	0SRC0JZ
171. Tenonectomy with graft to right ankle using cadaver graft, open	0LRS0KZ
172. Mitral valve replacement using porcine valve, open	02RG08Z
173. Percutaneous phacoemulsification of right eye cataract with prosthetic lens insertion	08RJ3JZ
174. Transcatheter replacement of pulmonary valve using of bovine jugular vein valve	02RH38Z
175. Total left hip replacement using ceramic on ceramic prosthesis, without bone cement	0SRB03A
176. Aortic valve annuloplasty using ring, open	02UF0JZ
177. Laparoscopic repair of left inguinal hernia with marlex plug	0YU64JZ
178. Autograft nerve graft to right median nerve, percutaneous endoscopic (do not code graft harvest for this exercise)	01U547Z
179. Exchange of liner in femoral component of previous left hip replacement, open approach	0SUS09Z (Taking out of the old liner is coded separately to the root operation Removal)

Procedure	Code
180. Anterior colporrhaphy with polypropylene mesh reinforcement, open approach	ØJUCØJZ
181. Implantation of CorCap cardiac support device, open approach	Ø2UAØJZ
182. Abdominal wall herniorrhaphy, open, using synthetic mesh	ØWUFØJZ
183. Tendon graft to strengthen injured left shoulder using autograft, open (do not code graft harvest for this exercise)	ØLU2Ø7Z
184. Onlay lamellar keratoplasty of left cornea using autograft, external approach	Ø8U9X7Z
185. Resurfacing procedure on right femoral head, open approach	ØSURØBZ
186. Exchange of drainage tube from right hip joint	ØS2YXØZ
187. Tracheostomy tube exchange	ØB21XFZ
188. Change chest tube for left pneumothorax	ØW2BXØZ
189. Exchange of cerebral ventriculostomy drainage tube	ØØ2ØXØZ
190. Foley urinary catheter exchange	ØT2BXØZ (This is coded to *Drainage Device* because urine is being drained.)
191. Open removal of lumbar sympathetic neurostimulator lead	Ø1PYØMZ
192. Nonincisional removal of Swan-Ganz catheter from right pulmonary artery	Ø2PYX2Z
193. Laparotomy with removal of pancreatic drain	ØFPGØØZ
194. Extubation, endotracheal tube	ØBP1XDZ
195. Nonincisional PEG tube removal	ØDP6XUZ
196. Transvaginal removal of brachytherapy seeds	ØUPH71Z
197. Transvaginal removal of extraluminal cervical cerclage	ØUPD7CZ
198. Incision with removal of K-wire fixation, right first metatarsal	ØQPNØ4Z
199. Cystoscopy with retrieval of left ureteral stent	ØTP98DZ
200. Removal of nasogastric drainage tube for decompression	ØDP6XØZ
201. Removal of external fixator, left radial fracture	ØPPJX5Z
202. Trimming and reanastomosis of stenosed femorofemoral synthetic bypass graft, open	Ø4WYØJZ
203. Open revision of right hip replacement, with readjustment of prosthesis	ØSW9ØJZ
204. Adjustment of position, pacemaker lead in left ventricle, percutaneous	Ø2WA3MZ
205. External repositioning of Foley catheter to bladder	ØTWBXØZ
206. Taking out loose screw and putting larger screw in fracture repair plate, left tibia	ØQWHØ4Z
207. Revision of totally implantable VAD port placement in chest wall, causing patient discomfort, open	ØJWTØWZ
208. Thoracotomy with exploration of right pleural cavity	ØWJ9ØZZ
209. Diagnostic laryngoscopy	ØCJS8ZZ
210. Exploratory arthrotomy of left knee	ØSJDØZZ
211. Colposcopy with diagnostic hysteroscopy	ØUJD8ZZ
212. Digital rectal exam	ØDJD7ZZ
213. Diagnostic arthroscopy of right shoulder	ØRJJ4ZZ
214. Endoscopy of maxillary sinus	Ø9JY4ZZ
215. Laparotomy with palpation of liver	ØFJØØZZ
216. Transurethral diagnostic cystoscopy	ØTJB8ZZ
217. Colonoscopy, discontinued at sigmoid colon	ØDJD8ZZ
218. Percutaneous mapping of basal ganglia	ØØK83ZZ
219. Heart catheterization with cardiac mapping	Ø2K83ZZ
220. Intraoperative whole brain mapping via craniotomy	ØØKØØZZ

Procedure	Code
221. Mapping of left cerebral hemisphere, percutaneous endoscopic	ØØK74ZZ
222. Intraoperative cardiac mapping during open heart surgery	Ø2K8ØZZ
223. Hysteroscopy with cautery of post-hysterectomy oozing and evacuation of clot	ØW3R8ZZ
224. Open exploration and ligation of post-op arterial bleeder, left forearm	ØX3FØZZ
225. Control of post-operative retroperitoneal bleeding via laparotomy	ØW3HØZZ
226. Reopening of thoracotomy site with drainage and control of post-op hemopericardium	ØW3DØZZ
227. Arthroscopy with drainage of hemarthrosis at previous operative site, right knee	ØY3F4ZZ
228. Radiocarpal fusion of left hand with internal fixation, open	ØRGPØ4Z
229. Posterior approach spinal fusion at L1-L3 level with BAK cage interbody fusion device, open	ØSG1ØAJ
230. Intercarpal fusion of right hand with bone bank bone graft, open	ØRGQØKZ
231. Sacrococcygeal fusion with bone graft from same operative site, open	ØSG5Ø7Z
232. Interphalangeal fusion of left great toe, percutaneous pin fixation	ØSGQ34Z
233. Suture repair of left radial nerve laceration	Ø1Q6ØZZ (The approach value is *Open*, though the surgical exposure may have been created by the wound itself.)
234. Laparotomy with suture repair of blunt force duodenal laceration	ØDQ9ØZZ
235. Perineoplasty with repair of old obstetric laceration, open	ØWQNØZZ
236. Suture repair of right biceps tendon (upper arm) laceration, open	ØLQ3ØZZ
237. Closure of abdominal wall stab wound	ØWQFØZZ
238. Cosmetic face lift, open, no other information available	ØWØ2ØZZ
239. Bilateral breast augmentation with silicone implants, open	ØHVØ9JZ
240. Cosmetic rhinoplasty with septal reduction and tip elevation using local tissue graft, open	Ø9ØKØ7Z
241. Abdominoplasty (tummy tuck), open	ØWØFØZZ
242. Liposuction of bilateral thighs	ØJØL3ZZ, ØJØM3ZZ
243. Creation of penis in female patient using tissue bank donor graft	ØW4NØK1
244. Creation of vagina in male patient using synthetic material	ØW4MØJØ
245. Laparoscopic vertical (sleeve) gastrectomy	ØDB64Z3
246. Left uterine artery embolization with intraluminal biosphere injection	Ø4LF3DU

Obstetrics

Procedure	Code
1. Abortion by dilation and evacuation following laminaria insertion	1ØAØ7ZW
2. Manually assisted spontaneous abortion	1ØEØXZZ (Since the pregnancy was not artificially terminated, this is coded to *Delivery* because it captures the procedure objective. The fact that it was an abortion will be identified in the diagnosis code.)
3. Abortion by abortifacient insertion	1ØAØ7ZX

Procedure	Code
4. Bimanual pregnancy examination	10J07ZZ
5. Extraperitoneal C-section, low transverse incision	10D00Z1
6. Fetal spinal tap, percutaneous	10903ZA
7. Fetal kidney transplant, laparoscopic	10Y04ZS
8. Open in utero repair of congenital diaphragmatic hernia	10Q00ZK (Diaphragm is classified to the *Respiratory* body system in the *Medical and Surgical* section.)
9. Laparoscopy with total excision of tubal pregnancy	10T24ZZ
10. Transvaginal removal of fetal monitoring electrode	10P073Z

Placement

Procedure	Code
1. Placement of packing material, right ear	2Y42X5Z
2. Mechanical traction of entire left leg	2W6MX0Z
3. Removal of splint, right shoulder	2W5AX1Z
4. Placement of neck brace	2W32X3Z
5. Change of vaginal packing	2Y04X5Z
6. Packing of wound, chest wall	2W44X5Z
7. Sterile dressing placement to left groin region	2W27X4Z
8. Removal of packing material from pharynx	2Y50X5Z
9. Placement of intermittent pneumatic compression device, covering entire right arm	2W18X7Z
10. Exchange of pressure dressing to left thigh	2W0PX6Z

Administration

Procedure	Code
1. Peritoneal dialysis via indwelling catheter	3E1M39Z
2. Transvaginal artificial insemination	3E0P7LZ
3. Infusion of total parenteral nutrition via central venous catheter	3E0436Z
4. Esophagogastroscopy with Botox injection into esophageal sphincter	3E0G8GC (Botulinum toxin is a paralyzing agent with temporary effects; it does not sclerose or destroy the nerve.)
5. Percutaneous irrigation of knee joint	3E1U38Z
6. Systemic infusion of recombinant tissue plasminogen activator (r-tPA) via peripheral venous catheter	3E03317
7. Transabdominal in vitro fertilization, implantation of donor ovum	3E0P3Q1
8. Autologous bone marrow transplant via central venous line	30243G0
9. Implantation of anti-microbial envelope with cardiac defibrillator placement, open	3E0102A
10. Sclerotherapy of brachial plexus lesion, alcohol injection	3E0T3TZ
11. Percutaneous peripheral vein injection, glucarpidase	3E033GQ
12. Introduction of anti-infective envelope into subcutaneous tissue, open	3E0102A

Measurement and Monitoring

Procedure	Code
1. Cardiac stress test, single measurement	4A02XM4
2. EGD with biliary flow measurement	4A0C85Z
3. Right and left heart cardiac catheterization with bilateral sampling and pressure measurements	4A023N8

Procedure	Code
4. Temperature monitoring, rectal	4A1Z7KZ
5. Peripheral venous pulse, external, single measurement	4A04XJ1
6. Holter monitoring	4A12X45
7. Respiratory rate, external, single measurement	4A09XCZ
8. Fetal heart rate monitoring, transvaginal	4A1H7CZ
9. Visual mobility test, single measurement	4A07X7Z
10. Left ventricular cardiac output monitoring from pulmonary artery wedge (Swan-Ganz) catheter	4A1239Z
11. Olfactory acuity test, single measurement	4A08X0Z

Extracorporeal or Systemic Assistance and Performance

Procedure	Code
1. Intermittent mechanical ventilation, 16 hours	5A1935Z
2. Liver dialysis, single encounter	5A1C00Z
3. Cardiac countershock with successful conversion to sinus rhythm	5A2204Z
4. IPPB (intermittent positive pressure breathing) for mobilization of secretions, 22 hours	5A09358
5. Renal dialysis, 12 hours	5A1D80Z
6. IABP (intra-aortic balloon pump) continuous	5A02210
7. Intra-operative cardiac pacing, continuous	5A1223Z
8. Intraoperative ECMO (extracorporeal membrane oxygenation), central	5A15A2F
9. Controlled mechanical ventilation (CMV), 45 hours	5A1945Z
10. Pulsatile compression boot with intermittent inflation	5A02115 (This is coded to the function value *Cardiac Output*, because the purpose of such compression devices is to return blood to the heart faster.)

Extracorporeal or Systemic Therapies

Procedure	Code
1. Donor thrombocytapheresis, single encounter	6A550Z2
2. Bili-lite phototherapy, series treatment	6A601ZZ
3. Whole body hypothermia, single treatment	6A4Z0ZZ
4. Circulatory phototherapy, single encounter	6A650ZZ
5. Shock wave therapy of plantar fascia, single treatment	6A930ZZ
6. Antigen-free air conditioning, series treatment	6A0Z1ZZ
7. TMS (transcranial magnetic stimulation), series treatment	6A221ZZ
8. Therapeutic ultrasound of peripheral vessels, single treatment	6A750Z6
9. Plasmapheresis, series treatment	6A551Z3
10. Extracorporeal electromagnetic stimulation (EMS) for urinary incontinence, single treatment	6A210ZZ

Osteopathic

Procedure	Code
1. Isotonic muscle energy treatment of right leg	7W06X8Z
2. Low velocity-high amplitude osteopathic treatment of head	7W00X5Z
3. Lymphatic pump osteopathic treatment of left axilla	7W07X6Z
4. Indirect osteopathic treatment of sacrum	7W04X4Z
5. Articulatory osteopathic treatment of cervical region	7W01X0Z

Other Procedures

Procedure	Code
1. Near infrared spectroscopy of leg vessels	8E023DZ
2. CT computer assisted sinus surgery	8E09XBG (The primary procedure is coded separately.)
3. Suture removal, abdominal wall	8E0WXY8
4. Isolation after infectious disease exposure	8E0ZXY6
5. Robotic assisted open prostatectomy	8E0W0CZ (The primary procedure is coded separately.)
6. In vitro fertilization	8E0ZXY1

Chiropractic

Procedure	Code
1. Chiropractic treatment of lumbar region using long lever specific contact	9WB3XGZ
2. Chiropractic manipulation of abdominal region, indirect visceral	9WB9XCZ
3. Chiropractic extra-articular treatment of hip region	9WB6XDZ
4. Chiropractic treatment of sacrum using long and short lever specific contact	9WB4XJZ
5. Mechanically-assisted chiropractic manipulation of head	9WB0XKZ

Imaging

Procedure	Code
1. Noncontrast CT of abdomen and pelvis	BW21ZZZ
2. Intravascular ultrasound, left subclavian artery	B342ZZ3
3. Fluoroscopic guidance for insertion of central venous catheter in SVC, low osmolar contrast	B5181ZA
4. Chest x-ray, AP/PA and lateral views	BW03ZZZ
5. Endoluminal ultrasound of gallbladder and bile ducts	BF43ZZZ
6. MRI of thyroid gland, contrast unspecified	BG34YZZ
7. Esophageal videofluoroscopy study with oral barium contrast	BD11YZZ
8. Portable x-ray study of right radius/ulna shaft, standard series	BP0JZZZ
9. Routine fetal ultrasound, second trimester twin gestation	BY4DZZZ
10. CT scan of bilateral lungs, high osmolar contrast with densitometry	BB240ZZ
11. Fluoroscopic guidance for percutaneous transluminal angioplasty (PTA) of left common femoral artery, low osmolar contrast	B41G1ZZ

Nuclear Medicine

Procedure	Code
1. Tomo scan of right and left heart, unspecified radiopharmaceutical, qualitative gated rest	C226YZZ
2. Technetium pentetate assay of kidneys, ureters, and bladder	CT631ZZ
3. Uniplanar scan of spine using technetium oxidronate, with first-pass study	CP151ZZ
4. Thallous chloride tomographic scan of bilateral breasts	CH22SZZ
5. PET scan of myocardium using rubidium	C23GQZZ
6. Gallium citrate scan of head and neck, single plane imaging	CW1BLZZ
7. Xenon gas nonimaging probe of brain	C050VZZ
8. Upper GI scan, radiopharmaceutical unspecified, for gastric emptying	CD15YZZ
9. Carbon 11 PET scan of brain with quantification	C030BZZ
10. Iodinated albumin nuclear medicine assay, blood plasma volume study	C763HZZ

Radiation Therapy

Procedure	Code
1. Plaque radiation of left eye, single port	D8Y0FZZ
2. 8 MeV photon beam radiation to brain	D0011ZZ
3. IORT of colon, 3 ports	DDY5CZZ
4. HDR brachytherapy of prostate using low dose palladium-103, unidirectional source	DV10BB1
5. Electron radiation treatment of right breast, with custom device	DM013ZZ
6. Hyperthermia oncology treatment of pelvic region	DWY68ZZ
7. Contact radiation of tongue	D9Y57ZZ
8. Heavy particle radiation treatment of pancreas, four risk sites	DF034ZZ
9. LDR brachytherapy to spinal cord using iodine	D016B9Z
10. Whole body Phosphorus 32 administration with risk to hematopoetic system	DWY5GFZ

Physical Rehabilitation and Diagnostic Audiology

Procedure	Code
1. Bekesy assessment using audiometer	F13Z31Z
2. Individual fitting of left eye prosthesis	F0DZ8UZ
3. Physical therapy for range of motion and mobility, patient right hip, no special equipment	F07L0ZZ
4. Bedside swallow assessment using assessment kit	F00ZHYZ
5. Caregiver training in airway clearance techniques	F0FZ8ZZ
6. Application of short arm cast in rehabilitation setting	F0DZ7EZ (Inhibitory cast is listed in the equipment reference table under E, *Orthosis.*)
7. Verbal assessment of patient's pain level	F02ZFZZ
8. Caregiver training in communication skills using manual communication board	F0FZJMZ (Manual communication board is listed in the equipment reference table under M, *Augmentative/ Alternative Communication.*)

Procedure	Code
9. Group musculoskeletal balance training exercises, whole body, no special equipment	F07M6ZZ (Balance training is included in the motor treatment reference table under *Therapeutic Exercise*.)
10. Individual therapy for auditory processing using tape recorder	F09Z2KZ (Tape recorder is listed in the equipment reference table under *Audiovisual Equipment*.)

Mental Health

Procedure	Code
1. Cognitive-behavioral psychotherapy, individual	GZ58ZZZ
2. Narcosynthesis	GZGZZZZ
3. Light therapy	GZJZZZZ
4. ECT (electroconvulsive therapy), unilateral, multiple seizure	GZB1ZZZ
5. Crisis intervention	GZ2ZZZZ
6. Neuropsychological testing	GZ13ZZZ
7. Hypnosis	GZFZZZZ
8. Developmental testing	GZ10ZZZ
9. Vocational counseling	GZ61ZZZ
10. Family psychotherapy	GZ72ZZZ

Substance Abuse Treatment

Procedure	Code
1. Naltrexone treatment for drug dependency	HZ94ZZZ
2. Substance abuse treatment family counseling	HZ63ZZZ
3. Medication monitoring of patient on methadone maintenance	HZ81ZZZ
4. Individual interpersonal psychotherapy for drug abuse	HZ54ZZZ
5. Patient in for alcohol detoxification treatment	HZ2ZZZZ
6. Group motivational counseling	HZ47ZZZ
7. Individual 12-step psychotherapy for substance abuse	HZ53ZZZ
8. Post-test infectious disease counseling for IV drug abuser	HZ3CZZZ
9. Psychodynamic psychotherapy for drug dependent patient	HZ5CZZZ
10. Group cognitive-behavioral counseling for substance abuse	HZ42ZZZ

New Technology

Procedure	Code
1. Infusion of terlipressin via peripheral venous catheter	XW03367
2. Transcatheter dilation of left peroneal artery with 2 SAVAL stents	X27U395